Practical Pediatric
Otolaryngology

Practical Pediatric Otolaryngology

Editors

Robin T. Cotton, M.D.
Department of Otolaryngology—Head
  and Neck Surgery and Pediatrics
University of Cincinnati
Director, Department of Pediatric
  Otolaryngology
Children's Hospital Medical Center
Cincinnati, Ohio

Charles M. Myer, III, M.D.
Department of Otolaryngology and
  Maxillofacial Surgery
University of Cincinnati
Children's Hospital Medical Center
Cincinnati, Ohio

Associate Editors

David Albert, F.R.C.S.
Consultant Pediatric Otolaryngologist
Great Ormond Street Hospital for
  Children
London, United Kingdom

Peter J. Koltai, M.D.
Section of Pediatric Otolaryngology
Cleveland Clinic Foundation
Cleveland, Ohio

Brian J. Wiatrak, M.D.
Department of Surgery
Division of Otolaryngology—Head and
  Neck Surgery
The University of Alabama at Birmingham
The Children's Hospital of Alabama
Birmingham, Alabama

**John M. Graham, M.A.,
F.R.C.S., D.M.**
Consultant ENT Surgeon
Royal National Throat, Nose and Ear
  Hospital
London University
London, United Kingdom

Scott C. Manning, M.D.
Department of Otolaryngology
University of Washington School of
  Medicine
Children's Hospital and Regional
  Medical Center
Seattle, Washington

**George H. Zalzal, M.D.,
F.A.C.S., F.A.A.P.**
Department of Otolaryngology and
  Pediatrics
George Washington University
Chairman, Department of Otolaryngology
Children's National Medical Center
Washington, DC

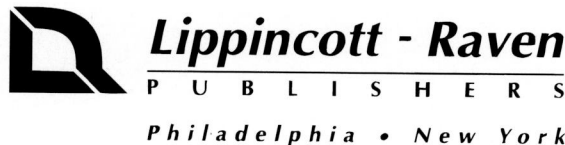

Lippincott - Raven
PUBLISHERS
Philadelphia • New York

Acquisitions Editor: Kathey Alexander
Developmental Editor: Anne M. Sydor
Manufacturing Manager: Dennis Teston
Production Manager: Cassie Moore
Production Editor: Rita Madrigal
Cover Designer: Kevin Kall
Indexer: Susan Lohmeyer
Compositor: Maryland Composition

Printed and bound in China

9 8 7 6 5 4 3 2 1

Library of Congress Cataloging-in-Publication Data
Practical pediatric otolaryngology / editors, Robin T. Cotton, Charles M. Myer III : associate editors, David Albert ... [et al.].
    p.   cm.
Includes bibliographical references and index.
ISBN 0-397-51720-3
1. Pediatric otolaryngology. I. Cotton, Robin T. (Robin Thomas), 1941- . II. Myer, Charles M.
[DNLM: 1. Otorhinolaryngologic Diseases—in infancy & childhood.
2. Otorhinolaryngologic Diseases—diagnosis.
3. Otorhinolaryngologic Diseases—therapy. WV 140 P895 1998]
RF47,C4P73 1998
S18.92′09751—dc21
DNLM/DLC
for Library of Congress   98-17722
                                                                              CIP

To our families,
whose patience, understanding, and selflessness
have allowed us to succeed and prosper
in academic medicine.

Contents

Contributing Authors

David Albert, F.R.C.S.
Consultant Pediatric Otolaryngologist
Great Ormond Street Hospital for Children
Great Ormond Street
London WC1N 3JH
United Kingdom

Thomas M. Andrews, M.D., F.A.C.S., F.A.A.P.
Clinical Assistant Professor
Departments of Otolaryngology and Pediatrics
University of South Florida
801 Sixth St. South, #7535
St. Petersburg, Florida 33701

Denis Ayache, M.D.
Pediatric ENT Department
Hôpital d'Enfante Armand-Trousseau
26 Ave. du Docteur Arnold Netter
Paris 75012
France

C. Martin Bailey, F.R.C.S.
Consultant Otolaryngologist
Department of Pediatric Otolaryngology
Great Ormond Street Hospital For Children
Great Ormond Street
London WC1N 3JH
United Kingdom

Thomas J. Balkany, M.D., F.A.C.S., F.A.A.P.
Hotchkiss Distinguished Professor
Departments of Otolaryngology, Neurological Surgery, and
    Pediatrics
University of Miami
Director, University of Miami Ear Institute
1666 N.W. 10th Avenue, Suite 306
Miami, Florida 33136

Robert G. Berkowitz, F.R.A.C.S.
Director, Department of Otolaryngology
Royal Children's Hospital
Flemington Road
Parkville, Victoria 3053
Australia

David J. Beste, M.D.
Associate Professor of Surgery—Otolaryngology
Department of Surgery
Medical College of Wisconsin
9000 W. Wisconsin Avenue
P.O. Box 1997
Milwaukee, Wisconsin 53213

**Maria A. K. Bitner-Glindzicz, M.B.B.S.,
    Ph.D.**
Lecturer in Clinical Genetics
Department of Clinical and Molecular Genetics
Institute of Child Health
30 Guilford Street
London WC1N 1EH
United Kingdom

C. M. Bower, M.D.
Department of Otolaryngology
University of Arkansas for Medical Sciences
Arkansas Children's Hospital
Little Rock, Arkansas 72205

Linda Brodsky, M.D.
Professor of Otolaryngology and Pediatrics
State University of New York at Buffalo
School of Medicine and Biomedical
    Sciences
Department of Pediatric Otolaryngology
The Children's Hospital of Buffalo
219 Bryant Street
Buffalo, New York 14222-2006

Peter D. Bull, M.B., F.R.C.S.
Consultant Otolaryngologist
Sheffield Children's Hospital
Honorary Clinical Lecturer in
    Otolaryngology
University of Sheffield
Western Bank
Sheffield S10 2TH
United Kingdom

Sukgi S. Choi, M.D.
Associate Professor of Otolaryngology and Pediatrics
Department of Otolaryngology
Children's National Medical Center
George Washington University
111 Michigan Avenue, NW
Washington, D.C. 20010

Mark A. Clymer, M.D.
Facial Plastic and Reconstructive Surgery
Indiana West, PC
4106 South 7th Street
Terre Haute, Indiana 47802

Harvey L. Coates, M.D.
Department of Otolaryngology
Princess Margaret Hospital for Children
208 Hampden Road
Perth, 6008
Australia

Robin T. Cotton, M.D.
Professor of Otolaryngology—Head and Neck Surgery, and
    Professor of Pediatrics
University of Cincinnati
Director, Department of Pediatric Otolaryngology
Children's Hospital Medical Center
3333 Burnet Avenue, OSB 3
Cincinnati, Ohio 45229–3039

Michael J. Cunningham, M.D.
Associate Professor of Otology and Laryngology
Harvard Medical School
Surgeon in Otolaryngology
Massachusetts Eye and Ear Infirmary
243 Charles Street
Boston, Massachusetts 02114–3096

Craig S. Derkay, M.D.
Associate Professor
Department of Otolaryngology and Pediatrics
Eastern Virginia Medical School
825 Fairfax Avenue, Suite 510
Norfolk, Virginia 23507

Rick A. Friedman, M.D., Ph.D.
Assistant Professor
House Ear Clinic, Inc.
2100 West Third Avenue
Los Angeles, California 90057

Éréa-Noël Garabédian, M.D.
Professor of Medicine
Pediatric ENT Department
Hôpital d'Enfante Armand-Trousseau
26 Ave. du Docteur Arnold Netter
Paris 75012
France

Sharon E. Gibson, M.D.
Clinical Assistant Professor
Department of Otolaryngology
Tufts University Medical School
Department of Surgery
Division of Otolaryngology
Brown University Medical School
Director of Pediatric Otolaryngology
Hasbro Children's Hospital
Rhode Island Hospital
Providence, Rhode Island 02905

John M. Graham, M.A., F.R.C.S., D.M.
Consultant ENT Surgeon
Royal National Throat, Nose and Ear Hospital
London University
330 Grays Inn Road
London WCIX 8DA
United Kingdom

Kenneth M. Grundfast, M.D.
Professor
Department of Otolaryngology—Head and Neck
    Surgery
Georgetown University Medical Center
3800 Reservoir Road, NW
Washington D.C. 20007

Gerald B. Healy, M.D.
Professor
Department of Otology and Laryngology
Harvard Medical School
Children's Hospital
300 Longwood Avenue
Boston, Massachusetts 02115

Annelle Hodges, Ph.D.
Department of Otolaryngology (D48)
University of Miami
P.O. Box 016960
Miami, Florida 33101

Lauren D. Holinger, M.D.
Professor of Pediatric Otolaryngology
Department of Otolaryngology—Head and Neck
    Surgery
Northwestern University Medical School
Section of Bronchoesophagology
Children's Memorial Hospital
303 E. Chicago Avenue-Searle 12–569
Chicago, Illlinois 60614

Andrew J. Hotaling, M.D.
Associate Professor
Departments of Otolaryngology—Head and Neck Surgery and
    Pediatrics
Loyola University Medical Center
2160 South First Avenue
Maywood, Illinois 60153–3304

Margaret A. Kenna, M.D.
Associate Professor of Otology and Laryngology
Harvard Medical School
Department of Otolaryngology
Children's Hospital
300 Longwood Avenue
Boston, Massachusetts 02115

Karen Iler Kirk, Ph.D.
Assistant Professor
Department of Otolaryngology—Head and Neck Surgery
Indiana University School of Medicine
702 Barnhill Drive
Indianapolis, Indiana 46032

Evelyn A. Kluka, M.D.
Associate Professor
Department of Otolaryngology
Louisiana State University Medical School
2020 Gravier Street, Suite A
New Orleans, Louisiana 70112

Peter J. Koltai, M.D., F.A.A.P., F.A.C.S.
Professor of Surgery and Pediatrics
Section of Pediatric Otolaryngology
Cleveland Clinic Foundation
9500 Euclid Avenue
Cleveland, Ohio 44195–4939

Ann W. Kummer, Ph.D.
Director, Speech Pathology Department
Field Service Associate Professor
Department of Pediatrics
University of Cincinnati
Children's Hospital Medical Center
3333 Burnet Avenue
Cincinnati, Ohio 45229–3039

Michelle B. Lierl, M.D.
Adjunct Associate Professor of Clinical Pediatrics
Department of Pediatrics
Division of Allergy, Immunology, and Pulmonary Medicine
University of Cincinnati
Children's Hospital Medical Center
3333 Burnet Avenue
Cincinnati, Ohio 45229–3039

Adrian R. Lloyd-Thomas, M.D.
Consultant Anesthetist
Department of Paediatric Anaesthesia
Great Ormond Street Hospital for Children
Great Ormond Street
London WC1N 3JH
United Kingdom

Scott C. Manning, M.D.
Associate Professor and Chief of Pediatric Otolaryngology
Department of Otolaryngology
University of Washington School of Medicine
Children's Hospital and Regional Medical Center
4800 Sand Point Way, N.E., CH-62
Seattle, Washington 98105–0371

Lawrence J. Marentette, M.D., F.A.C.S.
Associate Professor and Director, Cranial Base
    Program
Department of Otolaryngology—Head and Neck
    Surgery
University of Michigan
1500 East Medical Center Drive, Room TC 1904
Ann Arbor, Michigan 48109–0312

Bradley F. Marple
Department of Otolaryngology
University of Texas
Southwestern Medical Center
5223 Harry Hines Blvd.
Dallas, Texas 75235–9035

J. Scott McMurray, M.D.
Assistant Professor
Division of Otolaryngology—Head and Neck
    Surgery
Department of Pediatrics
University of Wisconsin Clinical Science Center
600 Highland Avenue
Madison, Wisconsin 53792–3236

Richard T. Miyamoto, M.D.
Indiana University School of Medicine
Riley Hospital, Suite 0860
702 Barnhill Drive
Indianapolis, Indiana 46032

Claire K. Miller, M.S.
Speech Pathologist
Department of Speech Pathology
University of Cincinnati
Children's Hospital Medical Center
3333 Burnet Avenue, Pavilion 4-22
Cincinnati, Ohio 45229–3039

Charles M. Myer, III, M.D.
Professor
Department of Otolaryngology and Maxillofacial
    Surgery
University of Cincinnati
Children's Hospital Medical Center
3333 Burnet Avenue
Cincinnati, Ohio 45229-3039

Jodi K. Paetsch, M.S.
Aural Rehabilitation Audiologist
Department of Audiology
University of Cincinnati
Children's Hospital Medical Center
3333 Burnet Avenue
Cincinnati, Ohio 45229–3039

Angie J. Pengilly
Speech Therapist
University of Singapore
Singapore

Peter D. Phelps, M.D., F.R.C.S., F.R.C.R., D.M.R.D.
Consultant Radiologist
X-Ray Department
Royal National Throat, Nose, and Ear Hospital
Grays Inn Road
London WC1X 8DA
United Kingdom

William P. Potsic, M.D.
E.M. Newlin Professor of Otorhinolaryngology—Head and Neck Surgery
University of Pennsylvania, and The Children's Hospital of Philadelphia
34th and Civic Center Boulevard
Philadelphia, Pennsylvania 19104

Christopher A.J. Prescott
Professor
Department of Otolaryngology
University of Cape Town
The Red Cross War Memorial Children's Hospital
Klipfontein Road, Rondebosch
Cape Town 7700
South Africa

David W. Proops, B.O.S. (Honorary), M.B.Ch.B., F.R.C.S.
Consultant ENT Surgeon
Department of Otolaryngology—Head and Neck Surgery
University Hospital
Edgbaston
Birmingham B15 2TH
United Kingdom

Vito C. Quatela, M.D., F.A.C.S.
Associate Professor
Facial Plastic and Reconstructive Surgery
University of Rochester
Strong Memorial Hospital
973 East Avenue
Rochester, New York 14607

Gayle P. Riemer, M.A.
Clinical Director
Department of Audiology
University of Cincinnati
Children's Hospital Medical Center
OSB-3, 3333 Burnett Avenue
Cincinnati, Ohio 45229–3039

Richard M. Rosenfeld, M.D., M.P.H.
Associate Professor
Department of Otolaryngology
SUNY Health Science Center at Brooklyn
Long Island College Hospital
Division of Pediatric Otolaryngology
University Hospital of Brooklyn
450 Clarkson Avenue, Box 126
Brooklyn, New York 11203

Michael A. Rothschild, M.D.
Assistant Professor
Departments of Otolaryngology and Pediatrics
Mount Sinai School of Medicine
One Gustave L. Levy Place, Box 1189
New York, New York 10029

Colin D. Rudolph, M.D., Ph.D.
Associate Professor
Department of Pediatrics
University of Cincinnati
Children's Hospital Medical Center
3333 Burnet Avenue
Cincinnati, Ohio 45229–3039

Craig W. Senders
Professor
Department of Otolaryngology—Head and Neck Surgery
University of California, Davis Medical Center
2500 Stockton Boulevard
Sacramento, California 95817

Gail G. Shapiro, M.D.
Clinical Professor
Department of Pediatrics
University of Washington
4540 Sand Point Way NE
Seattle, Washington 98105

Sally R. Shott, M.D.
Associate Professor
Department of Otolaryngology and Maxillofacial Surgery
University of Cincinnati
Children's Hospital Medical Center
3333 Burnet Avenue, OSB 3110
Cincinnati, Ohio 45229–3039

Kevin A. Shumrick, M.D.
Clinical Professor
Department of Otolaryngology
Division of Facial Plastic Surgery and Maxillofacial Trauma
University of Cinncinnati Medical Center
231 Bethesda Avenue, M.L. #528
Cincinnati, Ohio 45267–0528

Susan Snashall, M.D.
Consultant Audiological Physician
Department of Audiological Medicine
St. George's Hospital
Blackshaw Road
London SW17 OQT
United Kingdom

Yoram Stern, M.D.
Department of Otolaryngology
University of Cincinnati
Children's Hospital Medical Center
3333 Burnet Avenue
Cincinnati, Ohio 45229–3039

Jonathan M. Sykes, M.D.
Associate Professor
Department of Otolaryngology—Head and Neck
    Surgery
University of California, Davis Medical Center
2521 Stockton Boulevard, Suite 7200
Sacramento, California 85817

N. Wendell Todd, M.D.
Professor of Otolaryngology and Pediatrics
Department of Otolaryngology
Emory University
1365 Clifton Road
Atlanta, Georgia 30322

Pierre A. Vauthy, M.D.
Director, Pediatric Pulmonary Medicine and
    Critical Care
Department of Pediatrics
Children's Medical Center of Northwest Ohio
2142 North Cove Boulevard
Toledo, Ohio 43606

David L. Walner, M.S., M.D.
Assistant Professor
Department of Otolaryngology/
    Bronchoesophagology
Rush Presbyterian–St. Lukes Medical
    Center
1653 W. Congress Parkway
Chicago, Illinois 60612

Milton Waner, M.D.
Department of Otolaryngology
University of Arkansas for Medical Sciences
Arkansas Children's Hospital
800 Marshall Street
Little Rock, Arkansas 72202

Brian J. Wiatrak, M.D.
Associate Professor of Surgery and Pediatrics
Department of Surgery
Division of Otolaryngology—Head and Neck Surgery
The University of Alabama at Birmingham
The Children's Hospital of Alabama
1600 7th Avenue South, Suite 320
Birmingham, Alabama 35233–1711

J. Paul Willging, M.D.
Associate Professor
Department of Otolaryngology and Maxillofacial Surgery
University of Cincinnati
Children's Hospital Medical Center
3333 Burnet Aenue
Cincinnati, Ohio 45229–3026

George H. Zalzal, M.D., F.A.C.S., F.A.A.P.
Professor of Otolaryngology and Pediatrics
George Washington University
Chairman, Department of Otolaryngology
Children's National Medical Center
111 Michigan Avenue, NW
Washington, D.C. 20010-2970

Preface

Practical Pediatric Otolaryngology is designed to be a user-friendly book that can be pulled off the shelf to answer a clinical problem quickly. The chapters, written primarily by practicing pediatric otolaryngologists, guide the clinician through the process of making a diagnosis and determining appropriate treatment in a reliable and cost-efficient manner. Algorithms allow the reader to understand more closely how the authors approach a particular problem. The Pearls and Perils boxes capture key points that are especially troubling for the practitioner. Case studies presented as the final section of the book illustrate challenging applications of the information provided elsewhere in the text.

Practical Pediatric Otolaryngology is for all clinicians treating children with ear, nose, and throat disorders. It will serve as a valuable resource for those seeking practical advice and sound clinical judgment.

Robin T. Cotton, M.D.
Charles M. Myer, III, M.D.

Acknowledgments

No text of this magnitude can be completed without the cooperation of many individuals. Our section editors were given a great deal of responsibility and performed admirably. Their academic expertise and connections allowed us to assemble a globally diverse group of authors, enabling us to provide readers with a unique text. These individuals worked closely with the authors chosen for individual chapters to produce a book with a relatively uniform appearance and a structured framework.

In any undertaking of this magnitude, capable and efficient secretarial and administrative staff is crucial. Within our own institution, our thanks are given to Marcia Holmes and Jackie Drillien for their coordination of this project with Lippincott–Raven. Judy Ladrigan was indispensable with her expert word processing. Lastly, we would like to thank Kathey Alexander and Anne Sydor from the publisher for their patience, persistence, and knowledge which have allowed this project to be completed. These two individuals have worked hard to produce a quality product while respecting the many commitments and projects that our authors have been working on simultaneously.

Practical Pediatric Otolaryngology

General Considerations

Section Editor
David Albert

1

Special Considerations in the Assessment of the Pediatric Otolaryngology Patient

David J. Beste

HISTORICAL BACKGROUND

All otolaryngologists are trained in routine pediatric otolaryngology. The subspecialty of pediatric otolaryngology is relatively new and is well described as care for "special problems for special children in a special place" (1). Pediatric otolaryngology originates from the desire of pediatricians and other pediatric specialists to have colleagues with an interest and experience in "special children." Children with disabilities such as prematurity, genetic abnormalities, syndromes, cerebral palsy, and pediatric cancers require more intensive and collaborative care than adults. The development of pediatric hospitals and medical centers hastened the need for teams of pediatric specialists in medical, surgical, laboratory, and rehabilitation services.

The development of pediatrics in the late nineteenth century brought an understanding that infants and children were not small adults but were physiologically and emotionally different. Pediatric hospitals, beginning in Europe and spreading to the United States, brought the understanding that the care of infants and children requires special resources. In the last two decades, pediatric specialists in neonatology used the resources to achieve remarkable successes in preventing premature infant mortality. However, as the survival of severely premature infants improved, infants were left with aerodigestive tract complications involving the airway, voice, swallowing, ears, speech, and hearing.

Pediatric otolaryngologists endeavor to study the anatomic, physiologic, and psychological influences on the growth and development of the auditory, communicative, and aerodigestive systems of infants and children.

PATIENT ASSESSMENT

Environment

The examination rooms for the pediatric otolaryngologist should be cheerful and bright, and provide children with stimulation. A neat, clean, and modern decor is better than making the area too childish or decorating it in only primary colors. A variety of simple, quiet toys and reading materials for a spectrum of children should be available in the room. Nontoxic chalk and a chalkboard at an accessible height allow for creative play and can be used for parental education.

Parents will frequently bring grandparents, siblings, or aunts and uncles to the examination. If an otolaryngologist cannot work with these common distractions, a practice devoted to pediatric otolaryngology will become frustrating and that will be demonstrable in patient interactions. But crowded, noisy, and distracting consultations are not the best conditions to convey necessary health-care information. Asking to speak to parents without the other children present can be helpful if there is another adult to care for them in the reception area. However, parents should not be given the idea that office personnel will routinely provide child care for children during the office visits. Optimally, the examination room should be large enough to accommodate both parents, the patient, as well as two other individuals. A soft, large, cushioned bench works better than chairs for providing an adaptable seating area for parents, active children, and their belongings.

Special Considerations

Children are very good at perceiving the emotional state of adults around them, including their parents and the physician. Parents have reason to be apprehensive and anxious concerning their child's health and the examination procedures that will be performed. Parental anxiety is likely to be even higher for patients referred to the pediatric otolaryngologist for possible surgical treatment. An ongoing awareness of the child's and parents' expressed emotional state, as well as nonverbal clues, helps the physician to alter his or her behavior before and during contact with the child (2).

A child's cooperation is best obtained and maintained when the physician presents a kind and friendly manner. The physician's demeanor while taking the pediatric otolaryngologic history and performing the physical examination is expressed both verbally and nonverbally. Each physician possesses a unique deportment, and each learns a variety of techniques to reassure a child and gain a child's confidence. At the beginning of a visit, contacts are made with a child visually, preferably by eye-to-eye contact; verbally, by words of greeting and introduction; and tactilely, during the physical examination. The quality and manner of these contacts impart to the child and parents the attitude and personality of the physician. Gentleness can be conveyed by comfortable eye contact, soft voice volume and inflection, and unhurried soft physical contact(2).

Any parent can attest that sometimes children are irrational and inconsolable, largely depending on the child's temperament and age. In particular, a 2- to 4-year-old child's developmental state allows active cooperation or active uncooperation. These children have a sense of self that is dependent on control of their own body and its functions, commonly expressed in their negativism (3). However, a child's past experiences with physicians and nurses as well as fear of possibly painful procedures unquestionably influence the child's attitude.

If a child is particularly uncooperative for an examination, the physician's response must continually be unconditionally positive and respecting. It can be an extremely frustrating situation when a child, sometimes with the passive consent of the parents, cannot be examined or treated. The physician should understand that the child is responding only out of fear. It should be made clear to the child and the parents that they are still respected, and that the physician understands this behavior is normal and expected. Decisions may then be made as to the use of physical restraint or sedation. The otolaryngologist has the option of bringing the child for a return office visit or to the operating theater for administration of a general anesthetic. A general anesthetic's risks should be carefully weighed based on the chronicity and severity of the clinical situation.

Children with special needs, such as syndromic children, and their parents deserve particular care and attention. They frequently will require more time, which requires an adjustment in the clinic schedule. Special needs children can be as cooperative as normal children and it is best to evaluate their level of function while taking the history. It is frequently advisable to ask for parental suggestions as to the best technique to approach and examine these children.

The process of the office visit includes ending with a summary for the parents of historical and physical findings, pathophysiology, and rationale for treatment (2). This clarification of the visit details, and sometimes negotiating or contracting for further clinical evaluation or treatment, may require patience and repetition. The explanation of treatment rationales for common conditions such as otitis media and sinusitis may be confusing or controversial to even well-educated parents.

Explaining the treatment options and educating the parents are important to make the treatment plan understandable and to improve compliance. Educational materials including videotapes and printed material are important tools for improving parental insight and ultimately compliance.

History

Historical information, particularly information documenting the need for future pediatric surgery, will require appropriate corroborating proof from the primary-care physician's records. As managed care and preauthorization become an everyday reality, the details of previous care which are only available from the pediatrician are necessary. The parents' memory is not considered adequate as sometimes it is inaccurate. It is best to review the records with the parents, reiterating the number and diagnoses of documented visits and associated treatments. Not infrequently, available records are incomplete and the parents' explanation in the pediatric otolaryngologist's note satisfies the review process. Unfortunately, medical care is complex and memories are often inaccurate, so more documentation will undoubtedly be required in the future.

Most physicians are accomplished at obtaining histories of illnesses in adults. It is important that some children, particularly adolescents, be encouraged to participate in this part of the examination. Parents desire to remain spokespersons for their teenagers, treating them as children. The teens themselves may be reluctant to express their feelings and symptoms, but they can be made to feel responsibility for their own care. Most often, if given the opportunity, the teens and parents make the change to this new patient-physician relationship.

Lap Examination

The lap examination of a child maximizes parental participation. The child gets the advantage of close physical contact and the feeling of safety with the parent. In this way, tension is diminished for both the parent and the child and the physician has an opportunity to observe the parent's caretaking behavior (4).

An ear, nose, and throat (ENT) examining chair works well for the routine examination of the pediatric patient. It allows a parent to hold an infant or child for the lap examination (Fig. 1), which is preferable to an examination with the child laying supine on an examination table. Children feel particularly exposed and helpless in the supine position. A parent may hold the child on the lap, with the child's legs between the parent's legs. One arm reaches around the child's thorax and abdomen, holding both the child's hands and arms. The parent's remaining arm and hand extends around the child's head from the frontal to the occipital area. Alternating the hand positions allows visualization of the opposite ear. This technique can allow good exposure to all the necessary areas for examination. It may occasionally be necessary to assist the parent when the child is large or the parent is unable to restrain the child. Children who have been in the office a few times learn that they will only be examined when in the chair, and will be less anxious before the examination and settle down more quickly afterward.

After an examination if there has been a struggle, it is best to let the child "retreat" with the parent to the area of the examination room farthest from the examiner. The examiner should verbally reinforce to the child that the examination is completed. For hearing-impaired children, learning and using the sign for "done" can be helpful. If the examiner retreats to the opposite corner, the child may feel less threatened and may settle down more quickly. Using some type of small positive reinforcement, such as stickers, acknowledges to the child the successful completion of the examination.

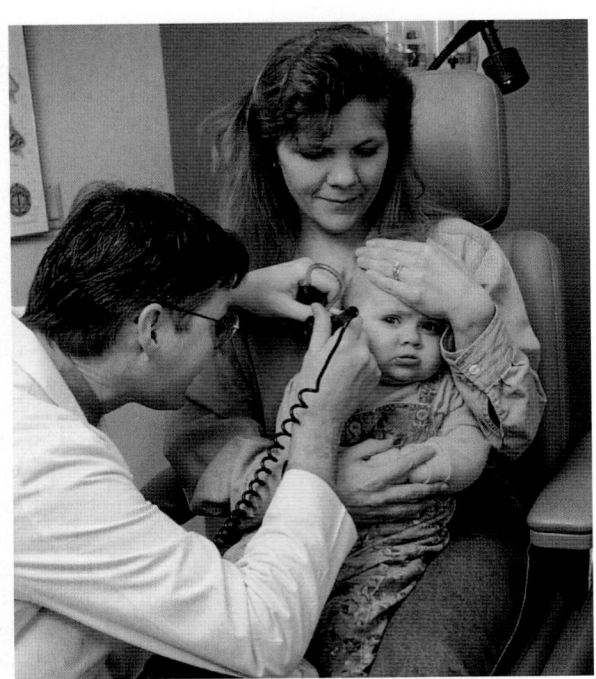

FIGURE 1 Lap examination for a toddler.

Physical Examination

The pediatric otolaryngologist has a particularly difficult physical examination to perform. It is more intrusive for the child than are many other examinations. The head and neck region has the highest concentration of sensory input in a child's body. The physician must be as unobtrusive as possible and still perform an assessment of these sensitive areas.

The least intrusive part of the examination is the visual and audible inspection of the child. Unfortunately, some children, particularly toddlers, will hide from even visual inspection, however, most infants and children will allow observation if they do not understand they are being observed. Respiratory inspection includes evaluation of respiratory rate and effort, retractions, mouth breathing, and audible stridor. Auditory inspection includes evaluating responses to sound, lip reading, and vocal responses. Swallowing activity can be observed when the child is feeding by bottle or given finger foods. Sleep evaluation can include observation for stridor, snoring, retractions, and apnea in sleeping infants. The quiet, simple, and patient inspection of a child during the history taking and physical examination can provide a wealth of information if carefully undertaken.

The pneumotoscopic examination can be particularly problematic because tympanic membrane color, anatomy, and movement are altered in distraught children. Undoubtedly, children's agitation causes inaccuracies in the assessment and contributes to overdiagnosis of otitis media. Ear examinations are the most disquieting part of the examination for small children and infants. Pneumatic otoscopy is a practiced art that requires equipment in proper working condition and a relatively still child. A pneumotoscope with an appropriately sized speculum should be placed in the ear with a good seal. The motion of the posterior superior tympanic membrane is most indicative of middle-ear status. The Paradise specula have soft and pliable tips which are useful in obtaining a seal in an irregularly shaped ear canal.

The nasal examination can be performed simply, particularly if made into a "peekaboo" game with small infants. Taking the otoscope with or without a speculum, the physician can entrance the infant by repetitively getting closer with the speculum during this game (Fig. 2). The happy and smiling examiner can dispel fear and entertain a frequently

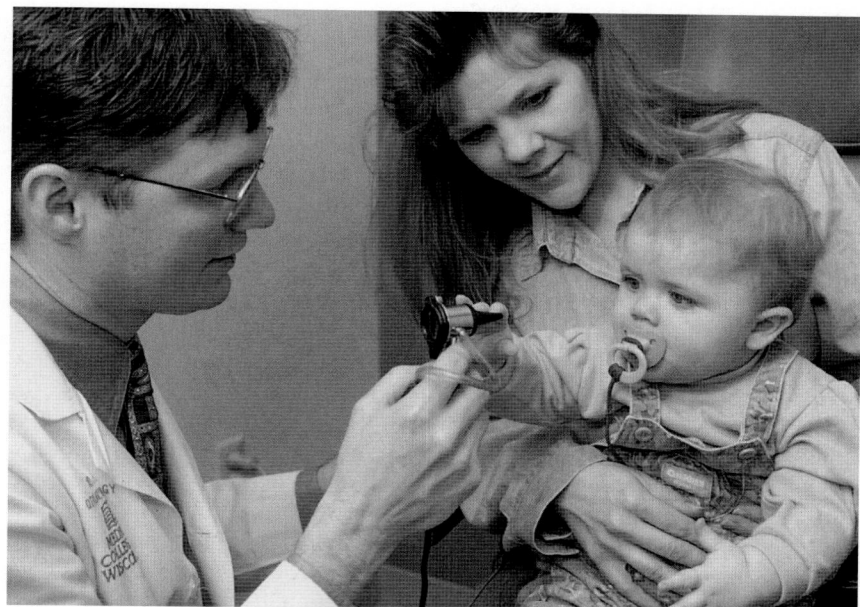

FIGURE 2 Peekaboo game acquaints infants and toddlers with the physician and the otoscope.

laughing infant. The child's nasal tip may then be elevated and the anterior nasal vault examined. Older children will allow the nasal speculum to be used, but only after being acquainted with it. Beginning with a demonstration of the instrument's ability to gently spread the child's fingers, the physician then warns the child about the speculum's ability to tickle the hair (vibrissae) inside of the nose. An inspection of the nares, septum, and inferior and middle turbinates can then be quickly performed with a headlight.

Topical decongestion and anesthesia of the nose for more examination is best accomplished with a 50:50 mixture of 1% phenylephrine hydrochloride (Neo-Synephrine) and 2% lidocaine. This combination provides the expected decongestion and anesthesia and is advantageous in that it does not require the paperwork and risks of having the controlled substance cocaine in the clinic. Parents also require less explanation regarding the use of this mixture than cocaine. In infants the mixture can be applied with a small eyedropper or on cotton wool applicators, and in older children can be applied by spray.

The use of tongue depressors for examination of the oral cavity is another portion of the examination feared by many patients. In cooperative children the fear can be avoided by having the child sit up in the "sniffing position" having the child open the mouth widely, protrude the tongue, and pant "like a puppy." If the child can cooperate, an evaluation of the oropharynx, palatal mobility, tonsils, and frequently the epiglottis can be easily accomplished.

The cervical examination is usually easily accomplished by a quick visual examination and experienced palpation of the neck. When necessary, bimanual examination of the submandibular triangles may be performed safely in children without teeth or those old enough to cooperate.

Developmental Issues

A basic knowledge of childhood development is fundamental, especially because of the role of pediatric otolaryngology in the team evaluating and treating hearing and speech disorders. An understanding of age-related norms is important in the screening evaluation of children during the otolaryngologic examination. A major advantage of taking a pediatric otolaryngology fellowship is the opportunity to gain a more thorough understanding of child development and to integrate this into the pediatric otolaryngologic assessment. The four main areas of development are gross motor, fine motor, cognitive, and speech and language. Speech pathologists are invaluable consultants because they routinely evaluate and treat delays in speech and language development (see Chapter 4). The pediatric specialists of the child development team are particularly useful resources for cases in which autism is suspected. Pediatric audiologists offer significant advantages in the evaluation and treatment of children. First, it is their preference to test and deal with children. Second, they develop an expertise with children. This is particularly useful in determining when a child has a malingering or functional hearing loss. A young child with autism frequently presents to the otolaryngologist or audiologist with attention difficulties that are attributed to hearing difficulties. The otolaryngologist involved in pediatric care can suggest an appropriate referral to the child development team.

Syndromic Evaluations

The pediatric otolaryngologist should have an awareness of syndromes as they impact on the developing infant and child. The otolaryngologic implications of these syndromes, and the impact and risks of common surgical treatments, should be understood prior to medical or surgical treatment. There are some common syndromes involving the head and neck with which the pediatric otolaryngologist should be thoroughly familiar. These include Pierre Robin syndrome, velocardiofacial syndrome, Apert's syndrome, CHARGE association, and Treacher Collins syndrome (see Chapter 41). However, a close cooperation with a medical geneticist is useful and necessary for identification of less common syndromes. It is beneficial for the child and parents to contact or join a local or national support group. The medical geneticist frequently has contacts with these local and national syndrome support groups, and the Internet also offers a commonly used contact and information network.

Procedures in the Clinic

Examinations and procedures for the pediatric otolaryngologic patient can be challenging at best or traumatic at worst for all involved. The use of restraints for an infant or child is often the most safe, humane, and expedient method for the situation. Restraint of the child requires at least one other individual to monitor the child while the physician performs the procedure. There are multiple options for restraint of children. Parental control can be obtained when the parent sits holding the child or lies over the child. This provides the advantage of familiarity of the patient to the individual doing the restraint. Additionally the parent knows the child is safe and unharmed and can discontinue the restraint when he or she desires. It is unfortunate when a parent is unable or unwilling to provide adequate restraint of the child during an office visit (4). In those situations where the child cannot or will not cooperate, the physician may suggest an alternative method of restraint to be used with parental or guardian approval.

The use of the commercially available "papoose" provides a safe and generally accepted instrument for restraint (Fig. 3). It offers a wide variety of options in restraining the head and appendages. The most widely available model has a hard plastic backboard, which may be uncomfortable. After having been restrained with this device, some children become uncontrollable and inconsolable at the mere sight of it in an examination room. A normal twin-size bed sheet offers another alternative. It is a familiar object to infants and children and can be folded to provide a soft restraint with both arms at the patient's side; it is adequate for otologic and head and neck examinations and procedures (Fig. 4). This does require at least one other individual to lie over the child, immobilizing knee flexion and head movement (Fig. 5).

Procedures are best performed without the use of sedation or pharmacologic agents. Flexible nasopharyngoscopy and laryngoscopy without the use of general anesthesia can be easily and routinely performed in most adults; however, in a child it may be a traumatic and invasive experience. Flexible endoscopy can be exceptionally productive in gaining information that is unable to be obtained in any other way, but may be minimally

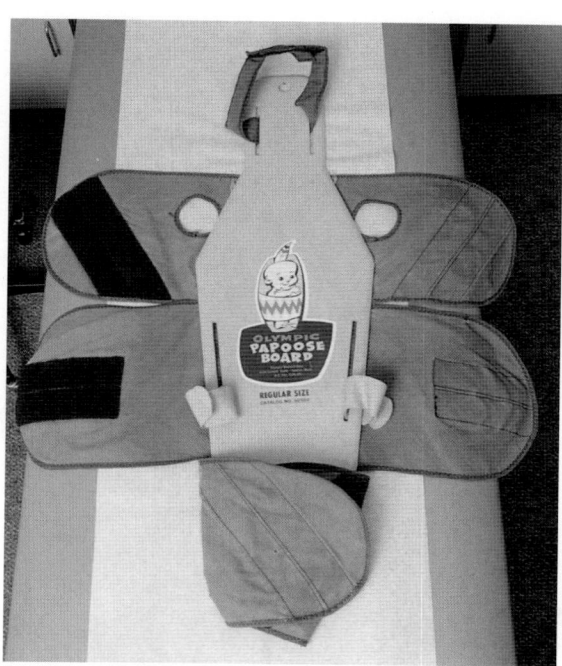

FIGURE 3 Commercially available papoose.

useful if the child is crying or uncooperative. The goals of conscious sedation in these situations are to reduce anxiety, prevent or provide relief from pain, and when appropriate, block memory of disquieting and intrusive procedures. The American Academy of Pediatrics states that conscious sedation should preserve protective reflexes, retain the patient's ability to maintain a patent airway, and permit appropriate responses to physical stimulation and verbal commands (5). The use of conscious sedation in a clinic setting must be accompanied by appropriate precautions such as physiologic monitoring and having equipment available for cardiorespiratory resuscitation.

The use of midazolam has been a boon to these examinations. Midazolam offers advantages over other benzodiazepines: It has a rapid anxiolytic onset and short duration of action. The onset and duration of action are shortest when given intravenously, and progressively increases with nasal and oral administration. Intravenous use frequently causes amnesia, but oral or nasal administration less reliably results in amnesia. Although midazolam is approved for intravenous use, there is an extensive number of references regarding its nasal and oral use in children. Its use has been described for endoscopic, anesthesiologic, dental, radiologic, and emergency room procedures (6–9). The physician using midazolam must be familiar with its use and monitor respiration with pulse oximetry and vital signs until recovery. The drug's muscle relaxant effects last longer than its antianxiety effects so it is important to warn parents to maintain physical contact with their child to avoid injuries. These disinhibited children tend to test their limits while under the influence of midazolam. A child should have parental supervision for a 4 to 6-hour period within a safe environment after receiving the medication.

Video Equipment for Special Procedures

During a special procedure such as flexible laryngoscopy and nasopharyngoscopy, three activities must be simultaneously accomplished. The patient must be controlled and monitored, the equipment must be appropriately manipulated for the patient's comfort and optimal viewing of the area of interest, and the anatomic area of interest must be investigated for a diagnosis. The patient is controlled as appropriate for age by use of the lap examination or by wrapping in a sheet. If mature enough, the patient may sit without assistance. The parents and a clinic nurse are present during these examinations to help

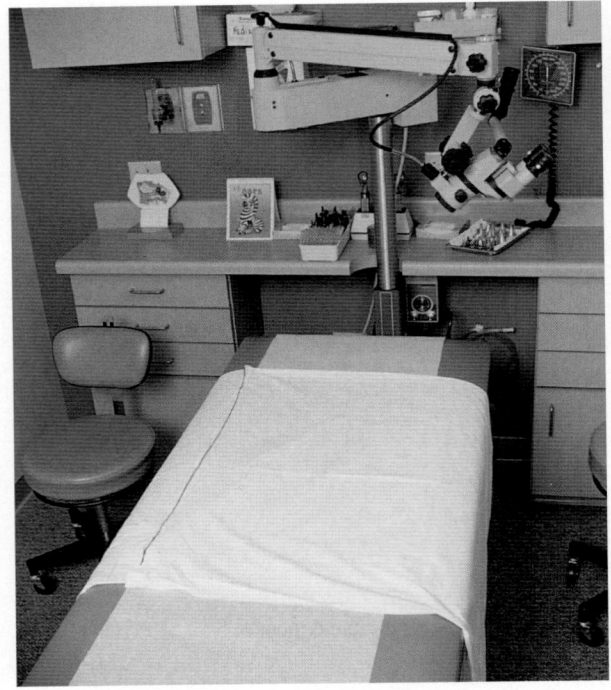

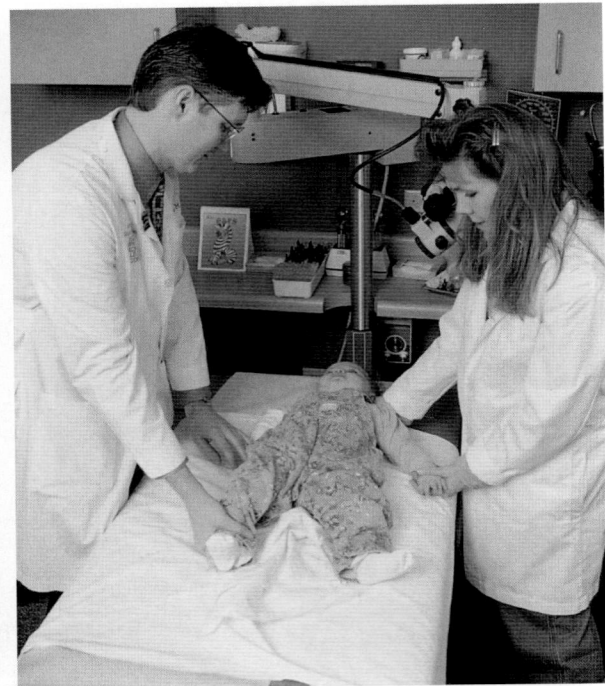

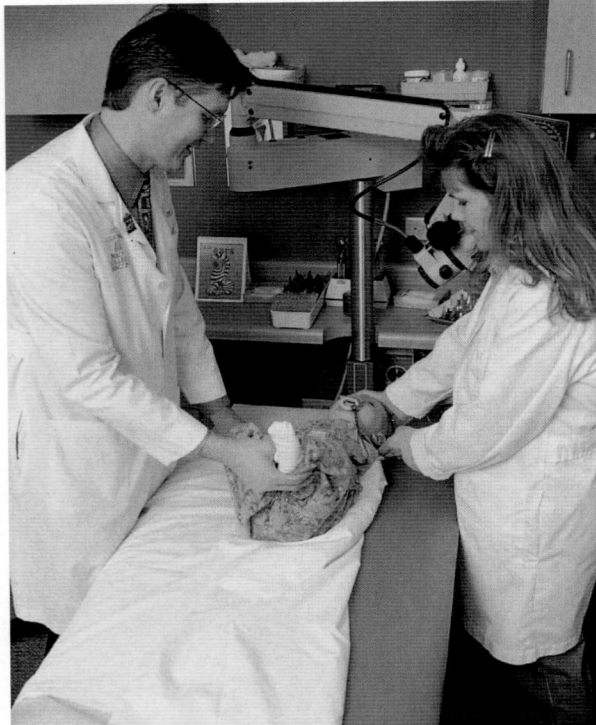

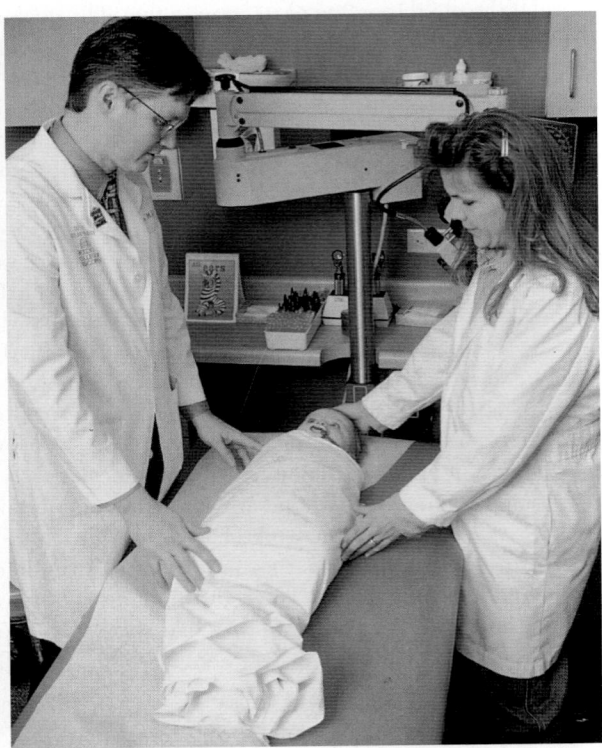

FIGURE 4 Sequence of sheet wrap. **A:** Sheet is positioned horizontally folded two-thirds over itself. **B:** Sheet is brought over right arm and under trunk. **C:** Sheet is brought over left arm and under trunk. **D:** Remaining sheet is wrapped over and around patient.

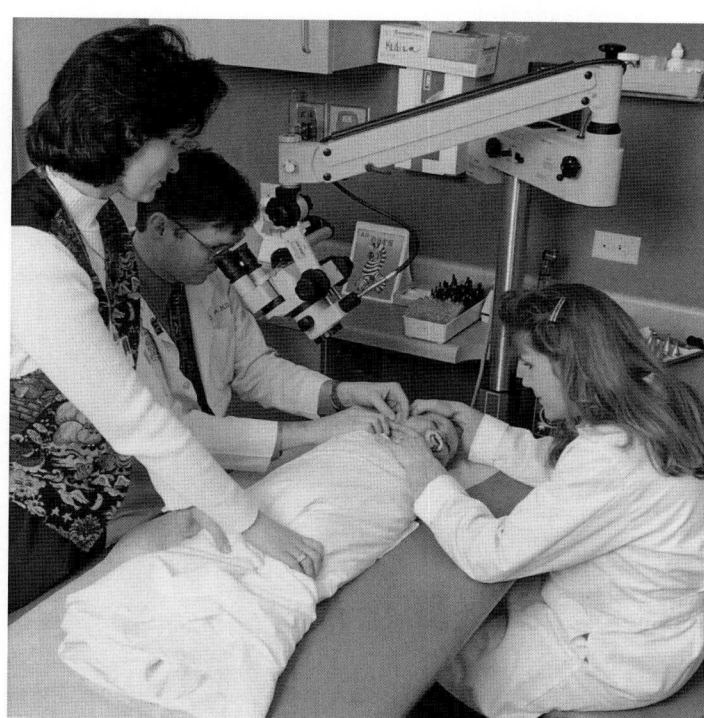

FIGURE 5 Examination under the microscope. The physician has both hands free for microscopic examination while the mother and nurse hold the child.

with control of the child and to monitor the patient's responses. The otolaryngologist is responsible for the remaining activities of endoscope manipulation and diagnosis.

The major advantage of a camera and videotape recorder adapted to the flexible laryngoscope is that it allows the operator to concentrate on manipulation for the patient's comfort, and optimal viewing of the area of interest. The examiner can be confident that the observations have been recorded so the assessment of the area of interest can be analyzed under less stressful and hurried circumstances. The dynamic evaluation of palatal and laryngeal motion need not be repeated as frequently because the videotape can be reviewed multiple times. This ultimately reduces the duration of the examination for uncomfortable patients.

Additionally, the camera allows for more distance between the physician and the child, making the evaluation less intrusive. Allowing an older child to observe the examination on a monitor can provide a distraction for the child and give the child some sense of control. Review of the videotape with the parents and other health professionals after the procedure is greatly appreciated and a wonderful teaching aid.

It is particularly beneficial to have appropriately sized flexible nasopharyngoscopes and laryngoscopes for neonatal, infant, and pediatric evaluations. With adequate decongestion and topical anaesthesia, flexible laryngoscopes with an external diameter less than 3.5 mm consistently fit through the nasal airways of normal neonates and premature infants. All major manufacturers of endoscopic equipment now have video cameras adaptable for pediatric flexible endoscopes. Video equipment prices have made office use reasonable and the image quality is constantly improving. A moderately priced office setup would include a xenon light source, video camera, monitor, and videotape recorder (Fig. 6). A microphone input is invaluable to determining the timing of respiratory and voice dynamics, adding another level of information over images without sound. A video image printer is an extra for still documentation in the patient's medical record. Presenting a photograph of a lesion or anatomic abnormality is also helpful for the parents to understand their child's condition.

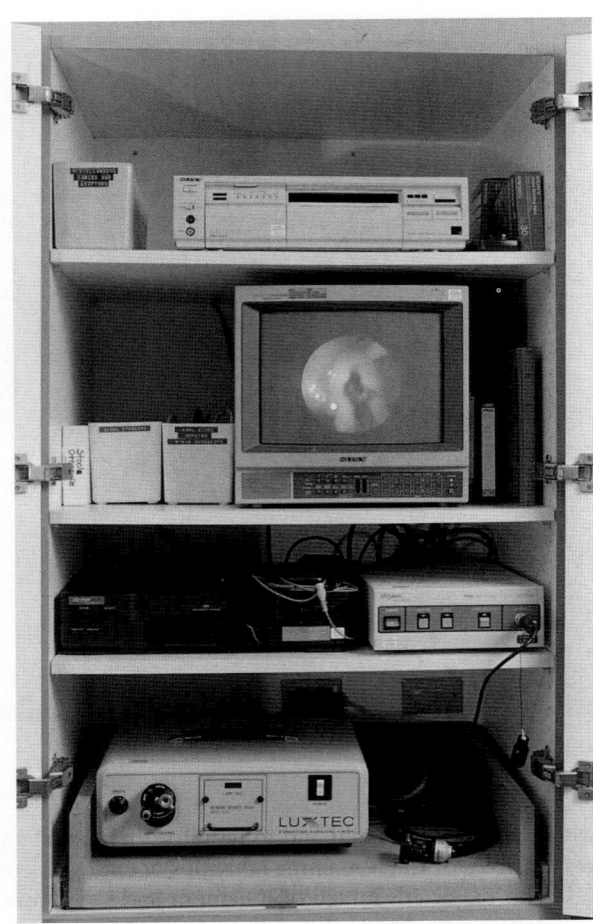

FIGURE 6 Office equipment for the video imaging of upper aerodigestive endoscopy. Top shelf—video image printer; second shelf—monitor; third shelf—VHS video recorder, microphone, and camera; bottom shelf—halogen light source.

Inpatient Consultation

Pediatric otolaryngologists participate in a different culture at a pediatric hospital. There is a dedication to and an enjoyment of children shared by all personnel in the hospital. This sense of purpose and nurturing gives pediatric hospitals a similarity that adult hospitals do not share. Within the pediatric hospital there are subcultures in the neonatal and pediatric intensive care units as well as the oncology unit, emergency room, and operating room. The pediatric otolaryngologist needs to gain experience and confidence to participate in these special environments. Communication with the nurses, support staff, and physicians is more important than in an adult hospital because the personnel take on the role of child advocate and protector. This is understandable when one remembers that the patients cannot protect themselves or communicate effectively. Parents cannot be present at their child's bedside at all times, so the staff acts in the parents' stead to help the new consultant. Verbal or telephone communication with the pediatric medical housestaff, attending physicians, and parents prevents many potential problems.

A successful consultation begins with clearly defined questions determined by the attending service. In most teaching institutions, the task of transmitting a consultation request to the appropriate service is commonly given to the least experienced of the pediatric housestaff. When notified of a consultation, the otolaryngologist consultant must be prepared to help the housestaff by asking those questions that will improve the patient's care. By clearly defining the otolaryngology service's role, the consultant can provide improved service and give clear communication to the parents and attending physicians.

Parents desire the consultant to expediently answer the questions posed by the admitting physician. They are frequently anxious and have unreasonable expectations that the specialist will have the definitive answer about the child's often complex condition. The otolaryngologist consultant should stress the need for physician teamwork and cooperation to diagnose and implement a treatment plan. Personal feelings about past management should be left at the door. It is helpful to begin by giving a brief description of the extent of otolaryngology and an initial explanation of the consultant's expected role in the child's case. It is best to tell the parents the questions asked by the attending physician, immediately setting forth the scope of the consultant's services. At the completion of the consultation, the otolaryngologist should inform the parents that a change in plans previously discussed with their physicians must be cleared with the attending physicians. The parents must understand that the attending physician is ultimately responsible for implementing the consultant's plan. Prompt communication with the attending services after a consultation improves understanding between services and optimizes the child's care.

Special Pediatric Units

The otolaryngologist fills special niches on pediatric hospital units. On the hematology, oncology, and transplant units, the pediatric otolaryngologist commonly participates in the urgent evaluation of the septic patient, and treatment of sinusitis and otitis media. Additionally, control of epistaxis and treatment of other head and neck hemorrhagic disorders are emergent services routinely requested. In the neonatal intensive care unit, airway evaluation and treatment of premature and congenitally malformed neonate infants are commonplace for the pediatric otolaryngology service. The pediatric otolaryngologist augments the services of anesthesiology, pediatric intensivists, and pulmonologists, providing emergency airway access and treatment of airway lesions.

There is a danger that pediatricians may consider otolaryngologists as only niche players, relegating them to roles as "tonsillectomists," ear "tubists," or nosebleed experts. The importance of otolaryngology goes beyond participating as niche players on the pediatric team. The advances in otolaryngology, often developed on the adult otolaryngologic services, can advance and improve pediatric care. It is the pediatric otolaryngologist's role to introduce these services to the pediatricians and children's hospitals, sometimes by performing the services or sometimes by referring to adult otolaryngologist specialists. Otolaryngology has unique perspectives in head and neck anatomy and physiology and has an expanding scope of services, including skull base surgery, placement of vascularized grafts to the head and neck, care of cleft lip and palate, and cochlear implantation. These are just a few recent advances in otolaryngologic care. The mission of any otolaryngologist specializing in pediatrics is to maintain contact with the growing medical and surgical advances in otolaryngology.

⊕ MANAGEMENT OF COMPLICATIONS

There is a wide range of variation in parenting skills and techniques, but the pediatric otolaryngologist should become familiar with signs of abnormal parenting. If suspicious of a deficit in parenting skills, the pediatric otolaryngologist should use the available services of pediatric psychiatry, psychology, and social services. In cases of suspected abuse, the appropriate referral should be made to a child abuse treatment center, sexual abuse treatment center, or the local police. This reporting is required by law in all 50 of the United States. Child abuse may be defined as any injury inflicted on a child. Eighty-two percent of the primary complaints resulting in referral to social services were localized to the head and neck but a large percentage of these cases also had other bodily areas involved (10).

Munchausens syndrome is a disorder in which an individual seeks repeated medical or surgical treatment for factitious illnesses. Munchausens syndrome by proxy (MSP) is a disorder of the parent or caretaker who causes factitious illnesses in a child. A high mortality has been identified in its victims. The presentation of MSP is highly variable and physicians should be cautious of suspicious circumstances or illnesses that do not respond to customary treatments. A pattern of behavior must be documented before the diagnosis of MSP can be made, which means that it is unlikely that the diagnosis can be made in the first visit to the physician (11).

In both abuse and MSP cases, complaints referred to the ear, nose, and throat may present with symptoms of life-threatening apnea, caustic ingestions, and foreign bodies (12). The early consideration of MSP demands the involvement of an experienced team usually made up of pediatricians, psychiatrists, and social services personnel. This team is essential for long-term successful treatment (12).

⚙ REFERENCES

1. Bluestone C. Pediatric otolaryngology: past, present and future. *Arch Otolaryngol Head Neck Surg* 1995;121:505–508.
2. Galazka S. Clinical magic and the art of examining children. *J Fam Pract* 1984;18:229–232.
3. Moss JR. Helping young children cope with the physical examination. *Pediatr Nurs* 1981; 17–20.
4. Smilkstein G. Procedures in family practice: the pediatric lap examination. *J Fam Pract* 1977;4:743–745.
5. American Academy of Pediatrics Committee on Drugs. Guidelines for monitoring pediatric patients during and after sedation for diagnostic and therapeutic procedures. *Pediatrics* 1992;1992:1110–1115.
6. Fuks AB, Kaufman E, Ram D, Hovav S, Shapira. Assessment of two doses of intranasal midazolam for sedation of young pediatric dental patients. *J Pediat Dent* 1994;16:301–305.
7. Yealy D, Ellis J, Hobbs G, Moscati RM. Intranasal midazolam as a sedative for children during laceration repair. *Am J Emerg Med* 1992;10:584–587.
8. Harcke HT, Grissom LE, Meister MA. Sedation in pediatric imaging using intranasal midazolam. *Pediatr Radiol* 1995;25:341–343.
9. Theoux M, West DC, Corddy DH, et al. Efficacy of intranasal midazolam in facilitating suturing of lacerations in preschool children in the emergency department. *Pediatrics* 1993;91:624–627.
10. Willging JP, Bower CM, Cotton RT. Physical abuse of children: a retrospective review and an otolaryngology perspective. *Arch Otolaryngol Head Neck Surg* 1992;118:584–590.
11. Eminson D, Postlewaite RJ. Factitious illness: recognition and management. *Arch Dis Child* 1992;67:1510–1516.
12. Mitchell I, Brummitt J, DeForest J, Fischer G. Apnea and factitious illness (Munchausen syndrome) by proxy. *Pediatrics* 1993;810–814.

D. J. Beste: Department of Surgery—Otolaryngology and Human Communication, Medical College of Wisconsin, Milwaukee, Wisconsin 53201.

• *Practical Pediatric Otolaryngology*
• edited by Robin T. Cotton and Charles M. Myer, III
• Lippincott-Raven Publishers, Philadelphia © 1999

2

Adenotonsillar Disease in Children

Linda Brodsky

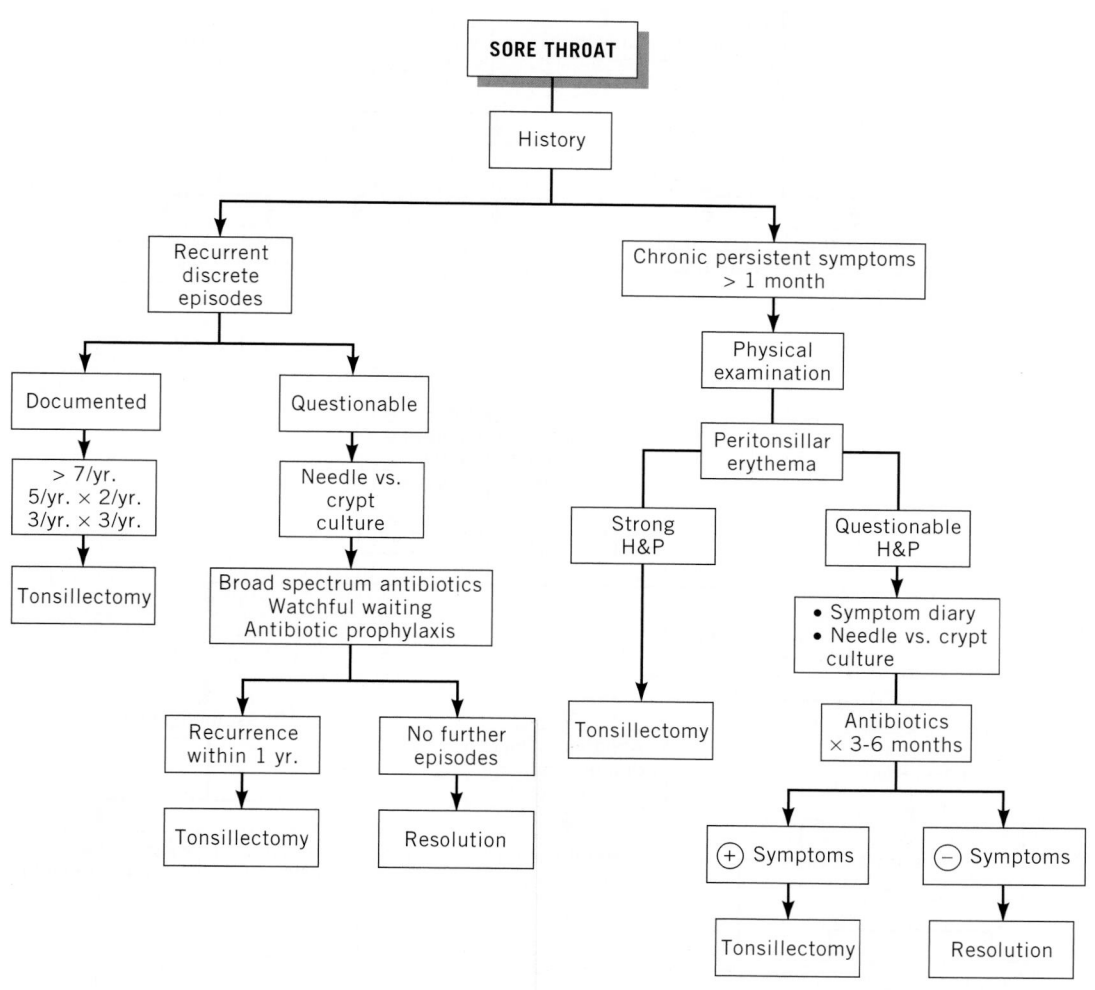

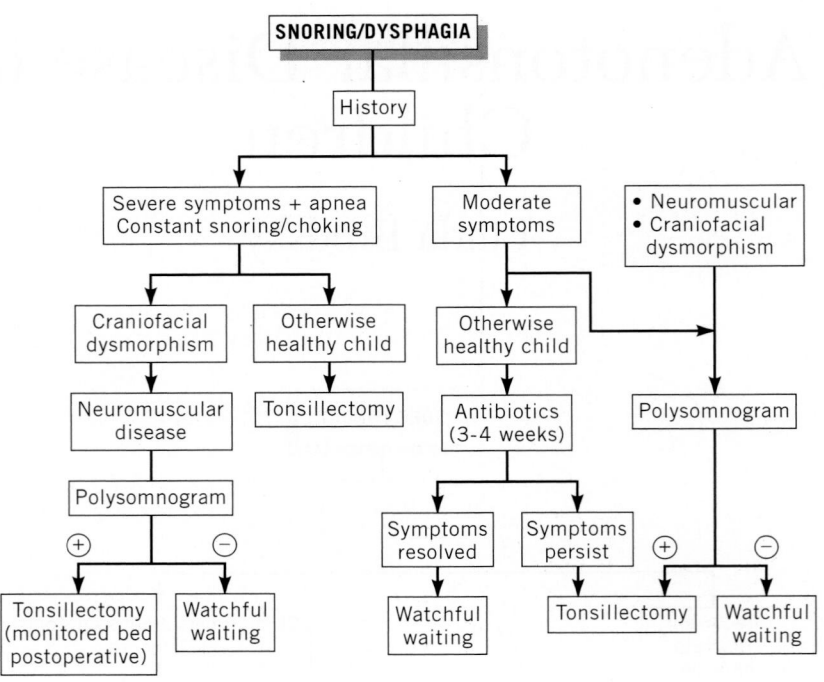

SNORING/DYSPHAGIA

History

- Severe symptoms + apnea / Constant snoring/choking
  - Craniofacial dysmorphism → Neuromuscular disease → Polysomnogram
    - (+) → Tonsillectomy (monitored bed postoperative)
    - (−) → Watchful waiting
  - Otherwise healthy child → Tonsillectomy
- Moderate symptoms
  - Otherwise healthy child → Antibiotics (3-4 weeks)
    - Symptoms resolved → Watchful waiting
    - Symptoms persist → Tonsillectomy
- • Neuromuscular • Craniofacial dysmorphism → Polysomnogram
  - (+) → Tonsillectomy
  - (−) → Watchful waiting

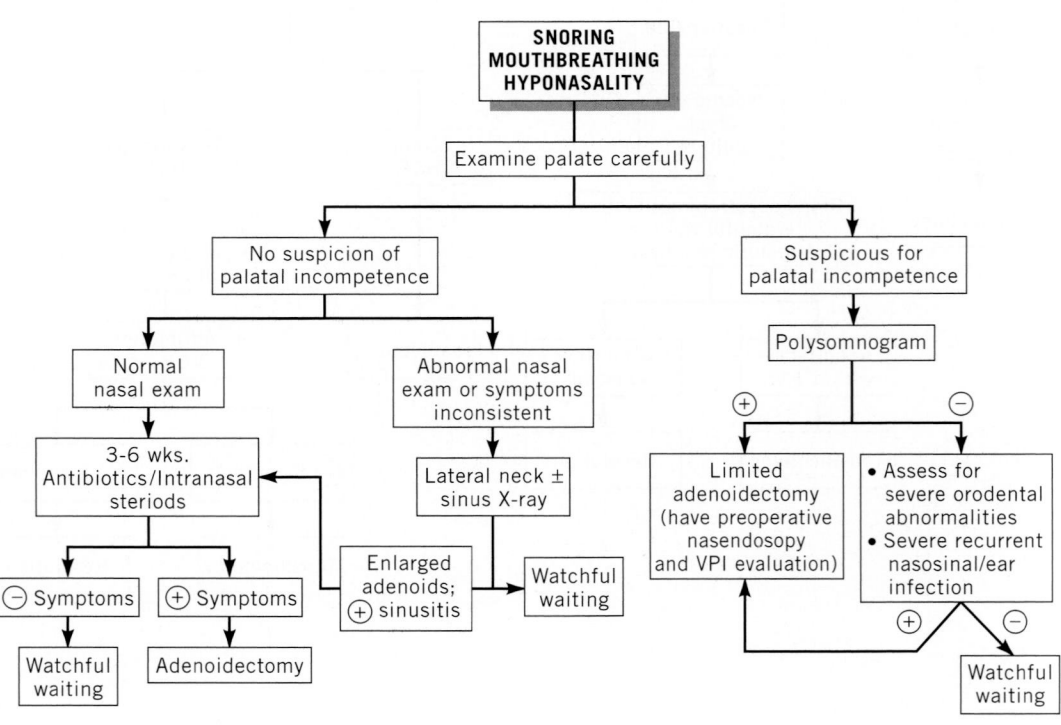

SNORING MOUTHBREATHING HYPONASALITY

Examine palate carefully

- No suspicion of palatal incompetence
  - Normal nasal exam → 3-6 wks. Antibiotics/Intranasal steriods
    - (−) Symptoms → Watchful waiting
    - (+) Symptoms → Adenoidectomy
  - Abnormal nasal exam or symptoms inconsistent → Lateral neck ± sinus X-ray
    - Enlarged adenoids; (+) sinusitis
    - Watchful waiting
- Suspicious for palatal incompetence → Polysomnogram
  - (+) → Limited adenoidectomy (have preoperative nasendosopy and VPI evaluation)
  - (−) → • Assess for severe orodental abnormalities • Severe recurrent nasosinal/ear infection
    - (+) → Limited adenoidectomy
    - (−) → Watchful waiting

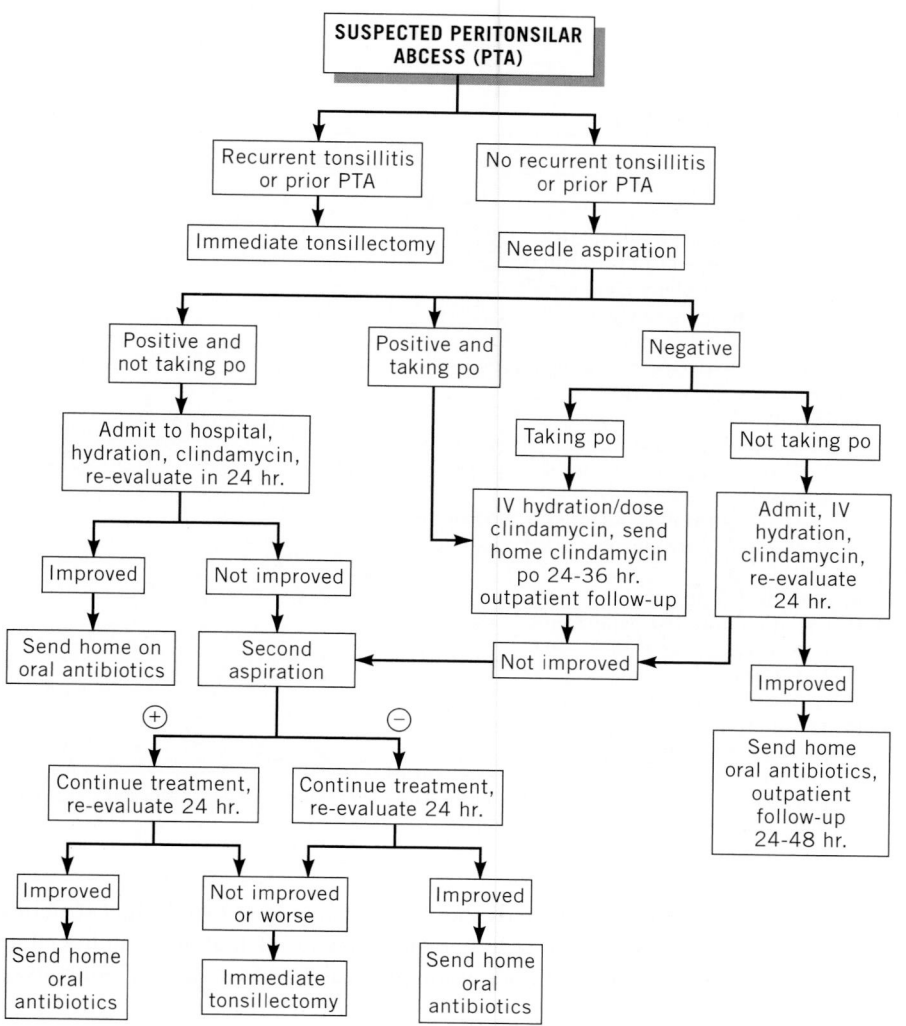

Diseases of the tonsils and adenoids are among the most common problems seen by physicians who care for children. The impact of both infection and obstruction from tonsil and adenoid disease on the child's health may not be localized just to the tonsil or adenoid alone. Major ill effects on the related anatomic structures of the nose and paranasal sinuses, the upper aerodigestive tract, and eustachian tube–middle-ear complex are well established (1,2). Thus, understanding the classification, pathophysiology, evaluation, and treatment of disease processes encountered in the tonsils and adenoids is not only important but also of great practical benefit to the practicing otolaryngologist.

A standardized, well-accepted classification system for diseases of the tonsils and adenoids has been notably absent. Recent attempts to create guidelines for surgical intervention were made more difficult due to the lack of agreement on nomenclature and classification of adenotonsillar disease. Table 1 presents a classification system that is clinically relevant, parallels currently used matrices for surgical indications, and is supported by scientific concepts available in the most recent literature. Important points to remember about clinical classification of adenotonsillar disease are as follows:

1. The most common problems encountered in children are infection and obstructive hypertrophy/hyperplasia[1].

---

[1] *Hypertrophy* refers to an expansion of the lymphoid follicles (B cells) found in large tonsild; *hyperplasia* frefers to an increase in the absolute number of all the cells that are found in the tonsil. The former is used most often in the literature and will be used in this chapter; the latter is preferred by this author because the term *hyperplasia* describes the actual process that is occurring—that of increased cellularity in the whole tonsil, not just the B-cell component (i.e., the lymphoid follicles)(3,4).

TABLE 1: Classification System

I. Infection[a]
   A. Tonsil (palatine)
     1. Acute tonsillitis
     2. Recurrent acute tonsillitis
     3. Chronic (persistent) tonsillitis
   B. Adenoid (nasopharyngeal tonsil)
     1. Acute nasopharyngitis
     2. Recurrent acute nasopharyngitis
     3. Chronic (persistent) nasopharyngitis
II. Obstruction[a]
   A. Tonsil
     1. Acute obstructive tonsillar hypertrophy
     2. Chronic obstructive tonsillar hypertrophy
   B. Adenoid
     1. Acute obstructive adenoid hypertrophy
     2. Chronic obstructive adenoid hypertrophy
III. Miscellaneous
   A. Peritonsillar abscess
   B. Unilateral tonsillar hypertrophy
     1. Neoplastic
     2. Infectious
   C. Lingual tonsillitis/lingual tonsillar hypertrophy
   D. Tonsillolithiasis
   E. Hemorrhagic tonsillitis

[a] Infection and obstruction may occur simultaneously. This then requires a dual classification, e.g., recurrent acute tonsillitis with obstructive tonsillar hypertrophy.

   2. Clinically, the tonsils and adenoids should be evaluated as two distinct structures.
   3. Classification is based on pathophysiologic mechanisms that are manifest in a specific clinical history, pertinent findings on physical examination, and judicious use of laboratory evaluation.

With these principles and the current information available about the clinical-pathologic correlates of adenotonsillar disease in mind, the use of a "decision tree" approach allows the clinician to think efficiently, yet scientifically, about each particular patient's problem. The greater the depth of understanding of these mechanisms and their clinical manifestations, the more readily one will be able to both recognize and treat *not only* the common and rare presentations *but also* the clinical variations inherent in patient care that cannot be readily dictated by guidelines. Each section dealing with a particular clinical problem has a summary of the relevant pathophysiologic correlates and a clinical evaluation and treatment plan. Since the evaluation and treatment of adenotonsillar disease has been so ill-defined in the past, a brief historical overview is presented in order to gain this important perspective.

HISTORICAL BACKGROUND

Preantibiotic Era

The first reference to tonsillectomy was found in the writings of Celsus in the first century C.E., but it was not until the eighteenth and nineteenth centuries that the development of appropriate instrumentation resulted in widespread performance of tonsillectomy (5). Tonsillitis was a greatly feared disease that could result in death from overwhelming infection or airway obstruction. George Washington succumbed to "the quinsy" (peritonsillar abscess) and it is likely that the fictional character Beth in Louisa May Alcott's *Little Women* died from the insidious effects of mitral valve stenosis and cardiac failure resulting from a streptococcal tonsillitis complicated by rheumatic fever.

Thus, in the preantibiotic era, tonsillectomy was the only available method to relieve the patient of enlarged or chronically infected tonsils. Tonsillectomy was performed frequently and often with little scientific basis—many people now alive in their seventh and eighth decades of life will recall entire families of children going to their general practitioner's office for tonsillectomy. Not until the early 1950s, when antimicrobials became widely available, did the pendulum swing away from an automatic "surgical" approach to the tonsils.

The first adenoidectomy was performed in the late nineteenth century by Wilhelm Meyer. Conductive deafness from middle-ear effusion was cured in a woman with this problem by adenoidectomy (6). The apparent inaccessibility of the adenoids made surgery quite difficult until the advent of general anesthesia and in particular, endotracheal intubation. However, soon the adenoids were being removed for "infections" of the ear, high-arch palate, poor appetite, general debility, stupidity, convulsion, night sweats, snoring, enuresis, thick speech, the inability of infants to suck, frequent colds, pyrexia, chronic catarrh of the nose and nasopharynx, epistaxis, anosmia, upset stomach, asthma, hay fever, stammering and croupy cough" (6). Precursors to many of the more modern surgical indications for adenoidectomy can be gleaned from this rather interesting list found in a 1920s otolaryngology textbook.

Modern Times—The Antibiotic Era

With the advent of antimicrobials, the approach to infectious diseases in general, and to infection in the tonsils and adenoids in particular, was altered considerably. The use of antibiotics was credited, at least in part, with a decrease in systemic complications from infection with group A beta-hemolytic streptococcus (GABHS). The rate of tonsillectomy and adenoidectomy for recurrent or chronic infection was greatly decreased; however, several decades later, complications from upper-airway obstruction secondary to adenotonsillar hypertrophy began to emerge.

At approximately the same time, the field of immunobiology exploded with the development of radioimmunoassay techniques. Interest in the tonsils and adenoids as first-line immune organs increased. Pediatric specialization, particularly pediatric infectious disease and pediatric otolaryngology, infused interested clinicians into the research arena. Understanding the pathogenesis of chronic diseases in the tonsils, adenoids, and related structures has led to the successful development of alternative medical and surgical strategies for treatment.

This chapter brings together the scientific principles of pathophysiologic mechanisms, precise clinical evaluation, and some of the most current thinking in regards to the treatment of adenotonsillar disease. Evaluation strategies highlighting the role of a detailed thorough history and physical examination (7), and judicious use of throat cultures and other laboratory and radiologic tests (8,9) are discussed. Nonsurgical treatment modalities such as watchful waiting (10), long-term broad-spectrum antibiotics, prophylactic antibiotics, immune stimulation (11), and replacement of the bacteria important in local homeostasis (12) are also presented. The role of surgery in each situation is highlighted. The specific situations of unilateral tonsillar hyperplasia, peritonsillar abscess, lingual tonsillitis, hemorrhagic tonsillitis, and tonsillolithiasis are discussed separately. Finally, a discussion of the relative merits of the surgical techniques in use today and the range of debate regarding preoperative assessment and postoperative management is presented.

PATIENT ASSESSMENT AND TREATMENT RECOMMENDATIONS

For each clinical classification depicted in Table 1, the proposed pathophysiology, clinical history, physical examination, laboratory assessment, preferred treatment, and complications (with their management) are described.

Tonsil Infection

Acute and Recurrent Acute Tonsillitis

Acute tonsillitis is defined as an infection in the tonsils that is characterized by sore throat, odynophagia, fever, and general malaise. Physical examination usually reveals the tonsils to be enlarged (although this is not always the case), erythematous, exudative, and sometimes accompanied by enlarged, tender, cervical lymph nodes. The illness is usually self-limiting within 10 to 14 days; however, significant morbidity from the illness itself, as well as both local and systemic complications (such as rheumatic fever or acute glomerulonephritis), may result without treatment. The presence of GABHS infection demonstrated on throat culture is not *necessary* to diagnose "acute tonsillitis." Many other potentially pathogenic bacteria, which are not usually present in the cores of normal healthy tonsils, may be present in the crypts of tonsils with infection (13). Furthermore, surface cultures will fail to identify up to 60% of GABHS, which can persist deep in the crypts. Most episodes of acute tonsillitis are diagnosed by a primary-care physician who may be unfamiliar as to the diagnostic criteria. The otolaryngologist can facilitate an accurate evaluation and thereby help both the patient and the referring physician by discussing recurrent sore throats caused by tonsillitis with the above knowledge in hand.

The exact pathogenesis of a single episode of tonsillitis is still unclear. It is likely that obstruction of the crypts of the tonsils (possibly from an antecedent infection) results in multiplication and invasion of small numbers of potentially pathogenic bacteria ordinarily found in the crypts of "normal" tonsils (13). With recurrent episodes of tonsillitis, the type and number of bacterial species found in the tonsils between episodes shift from a flora of commensals to one in which greater numbers and varieties of pathogens are found (14). This situation is similar to that seen with recurrent acute otitis media (AOM) in which subsequent infections require alternative broad-spectrum antibiotics to accommodate these changes (15). Pathologically, tonsils removed because of a history of recurrent infection are more likely to harbor GABHS and have microscopic pathology demonstrating chronic cryptitis, epithelial hyperkeratosis, and microabscesses in the tonsillar parenchyma. Immunologic function is compromised and is characterized by a decrease in the ability to produce local immunoglobulins (16), a decrease in the number of antigen-presenting cells (17), and a shift in the relative numbers of T cells (3). Clinically these patients may at first glance have normal-appearing tonsils; however, the careful examiner will be able to identify subtle physical findings (described later) which have been correlated to these pathologic changes.

Recurrent acute tonsillitis is defined variably (depending on the source) as more than four episodes in one calendar year or seven episodes in 1 year, five episodes per year for 2 years, or three episodes per year for 3 years (18). The stricter indications have received the widest acceptance and are preferred except in situations where concurrent medical disease such as diabetes mellitus, cardiac compromise, seizure disorders, immunodeficiency, or other chronic illnesses are made worse by acute infection. Of note is that many children with a history of recurrent acute tonsillitis are often asymptomatic between infections; their tonsils often return to their normal size and appearance. However, the astute clinician may identify some of the more subtle findings associated with recurrent acute infection, including peritonsillar erythema seen on the anterior tonsillar pillars as they come around to the edge of the soft palate; increased debris in the tonsillar crypts; multiple dilated, surface blood vessels; and a loss of the normal tonsil architecture resulting in fewer crypts and a smooth glistening surface.

The use of a throat culture to establish the diagnosis of "acute tonsillitis" is controversial. The development of the rapid streptococcal screen has too often led the primary-care practitioner to neither diagnose nor treat "tonsillitis" unless GABHS is cultured. This is problematic since infection with other potentially pathogenic bacteria may not only be contributing to the acute illness but also be responsible for the recurrent nature of the disease, even in the absence of cultured GABHS. Furthermore, surface culture swabs are only accurate in identifying 40% to 60% of GABHS; deep crypt or core culture by needle aspiration has been suggested to increase the yield (19). Empiric treatment based on strict diagnostic criteria established with a careful history and precise physical examination may be more appropriate to produce symptomatic relief and perhaps fewer recurrences. In certain instances, culture of the tonsil crypts by direct surface swab or by needle aspiration may yield important information to help establish the presence of interfering or potentially pathogenic bacteria. Culture-directed use of antimicrobials may be more effective in eradicating the infection and forestalling bacterial resistance. However, others have advocated the empiric use of broad-spectrum antibiotics such as amoxicillin–clavulanate potassium (20,21) effective against beta-lactamase–producing microorganisms, or antibiotics (clindamycin) effective against anaerobic microorganisms such as *Bacteroides melaninogenicus* (22). The increasingly troublesome problem of drug resistance compels the physician to prescibe antibiotics thoughtfully. Knowledge of current geographically specific drug susceptibilities must be used and tempered with the severity of the illness and potential untoward effects when there are other medical problems exacerbated by the tonsil infection. Likewise, timely intervention with tonsillectomy can also have a positive benefit on reducing antimicrobial resistance, since pharyngotonsillitis is one of the most common diseases for which antibiotics are given in the United States today.

The use of the antistreptolysin-O (ASO) titer to determine recent GABHS infection is helpful when differentiating infection from colonization with GAGHS or when the diagnosis of recurrent tonsillitis is questionable. Although a single titer is of limited value, elevated titers may help to guide further treatment, particularly in the presence of an impressive physical examination. Alternatively, in questionable situations, evaluation of the child *by the otolaryngologist* during one or more acute episodes over a period of time may be necessary to establish the role of medical or surgical management.

The carrier state for GABHS is not an absolute indication for tonsillectomy. Treatment with rifampin or clindamycin may be effective in eliminating the bacteria. When medical treatment fails, the decision to do a tonsillectomy should be modulated by the child's environment. Is reinfection occurring at school or home? Does the child have a chronic illness made worse by infection? Is someone in the family immunosuppressed? If these factors are present, tonsillectomy should be recommended.

The usual treatment for acute tonsillitis (which must be differentiated from other more common causes of sore throat, such as acute pharyngitis in which the posterior pharyngeal wall and soft palate are diffusely erythematous with little or no involvement of the tonsils and cervical lymph nodes) is antibiotic therapy. Even in the absence of cultured GABHS, clinical improvement in symptoms has been documented. When the patient is "strep negative," the number of previous episodes and assessment of the overall clinical presentation might help to guide the decision to treat. Penicillin is the treatment of choice for patients with few, discrete episodes; however, as the frequency of the episodes increases, the bacteriology changes (20) and antimicrobial therapy should similarly be altered. Before tonsillectomy is contemplated (and in the absence of contributing medical or psychosocial problems), a prolonged course of antibiotics, perhaps directed by deep crypt culture or tonsil core needle aspiration, may be sufficient to break the cycle of infection. Approximately 32% of children with recurrent acute tonsillitis will respond to medical management (with prophylaxis over 6 months or a prolonged course—30 days of broad-spectrum antibiotics) and avoid tonsillectomy (Brodsky et al. unpublished data, 1995–1996). The precise role of prophylaxis has yet to be established; however, even in severely affected children, watchful waiting may result in a 20% improvement rate during 1 year's observation (10). The long-term outcomes of alternative therapies to tonsillectomy are essentially unknown. Recent advances in replacing the absent normal oral flora (12) and immune stimulation (13) have been successfully used in Europe, but have not yet been adopted in the United States as treatment modalities for tonsillar disease.

Recommendations for tonsillectomy are *guided* by the number of episodes. However, severity (as measured by number of days lost from school or work or need for hospitalization), patient age, and the presence of extenuating factors such as diabetes mellitus, cystic fibrosis, significant heart or kidney disease, neurologic disease exacerbated by acute febrile illnesses (such as seizures), and the presence of immunocompromise in patient or family members are additional factors that need to be considered and strengthen the case for tonsillectomy. The patient's and parents' attitudes toward the illness should also be solicited, as one family unit may suffer little from recurrent infection, while another may be overwhelmed by the situation.

Special Situations in Acute Tonsillitis

Acute Infectious Mononucleosis   The differential diagnosis of acute tonsillitis may include acute infectious mononucleosis (IM), caused by the Epstein-Barr virus (EBV), a highly lymphotropic virus. Acute IM is a very common infection and usually presents in early childhood as an uncomplicated viral infection with sore throat and lymphadenopathy. Not surprisingly, most cases of acute IM go undiagnosed. Most children have persistently elevated levels of IgG anti–viral capsid antigen (anti-VCA) (denoting past infection) by age 5 years. When infection occurs in the adolescent or young adult, it is usually much more severe and can have significant complications. The virus itself is a polyclonal B-cell activator and causes diffuse swelling of the lymphoid tissue of Waldeyer's ring, neck, axilla, and groin. Severe odynophagia may result in dehydration; rapid and severe enlargement of the tonsils and adenoids may result in acute airway obstruction; concomitant peritonsillar abscesses have also been described.

The history almost always includes a relatively rapid onset of symptoms that usually have been treated (unsucessfully) with antibiotics. The general appearance of the patient is quite poor, with overwhelming lethargy and malaise. Muffled voice and difficulty handling one's secretion may also be present. On physical examination a white, cheesy exudate covers most of the tonsil. Lymphadenopathy in the neck, axilla, and groin is usually impressive but may be absent in early phases of the disease. An enlarged liver or spleen, especially if tender, should alert the clinician to an increased severity of the illness. Laboratory evaluation should include a throat culture for coexisting bacterial infection, a complete blood cell count with differential to identify atypical lymphocytes, and a serologic test to establish EBV as the etiology of the disease. The monospot test is unreliable in the early phase of the disease or in children less than 5 years old. IgM anti-VCA levels above 1:10 and IgG anti-VCA levels above 1:320 are good evidence of acute or recent infection. Convalescent sera showing elevated IgG anti-VCA levels are diagnostic. When liver or spleen involvement is suspected, liver function test results need to be monitored.

Treatment includes hydration, relief from airway obstruction (systemic steroids, placement of a nasopharyngeal tube), and treatment of a bacterial infection when present. The routine use of steroids in IM is controversial, as some believe it may result in overwhelming infection; however, rapid relief of obstruction and improvement in the general well-being of the patient is the usual response. If antibiotics are prescribed, neither ampicillin nor erythromycin should be used, owing to the tendency for a diffuse maculopapular rash to develop with the former (Fig. 1) and liver enzyme changes with a secondary hepatitis to occur with the latter.

Systemic Complications—Rheumatic Fever and Acute Glomerulonephritis   Rheumatic fever is a systemic, multisystem disease that is characterized by arthritis, fever, carditis, choreiform movement, emotional lability, and less frequently, subcutaneous nodules and a characteristic rash (erythema marginatum). Infection with GABHS from invasive infection in the skin or throat is the etiology. The most serious morbidities come from rheumatic heart disease, with the possibility of recurrent attacks, once established. Recurrence is prevented by *lifelong* antimicrobial prophylaxis with penicillin.

Acute post-streptococcal glomerulonephritis is a self-limited disease that results from a previous skin or pharyngeal infection from a nephritogenic strain of GABHS. Clinical manifestations can range from mild to critical and include an abrupt onset with dark-col-

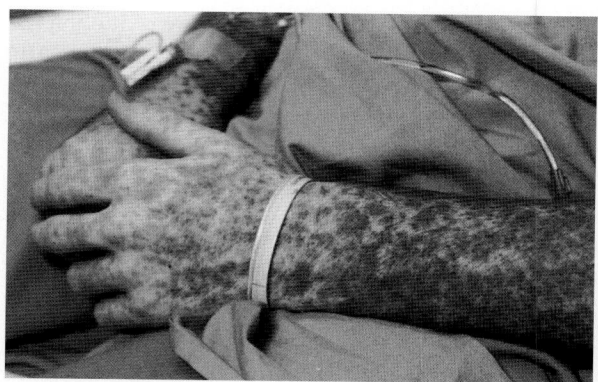

FIGURE 1 Severe maculopapular rash in a teenager with acute infectious mononucleosis.

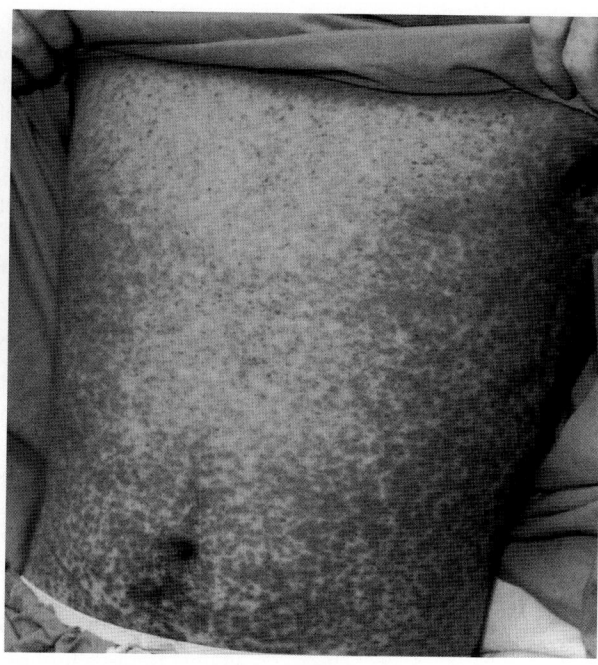

ored urine, facial edema, and decreased urination. Malaise, low-grade fever, flank or abdominal pain, and irritability are common. Progression to acute renal failure, congestive heart failure, and electrolyte imbalance may occur and requires supportive therapy for 10 to 20 days. Complete resolution is the rule if recognized and treated promptly.

Chronic or Persistent Tonsillitis

Although most patients present with a history of discrete, recurrent episodes of tonsillitis as described in the previous section, a smaller number of patients present with a persistent sore throat secondary to chronic, persistent tonsillar infection. Pathologic correlates have been established for this entity (23,24) and include histopathologic evidence of chronic cryptitis, epithelial hyperkeratosis, and microabscesses in the tonsillar parenchyma.

The clinical presentation of chronic (persistent) tonsillitis has not been studied in depth. The duration and severity of sore throat are often difficult to establish. Symptom diaries may be helpful in questionable cases. In general, sore throat or pain with swallowing, lasting longer than 4 weeks, may be consistent with persistent tonsillitis. Symptoms should be present for at least half the day (thus excluding morning sore throats, which are commonly seen in patients with nocturnal nasal obstruction who live in dry environments) and are usually present for perhaps 10 of 14 days. Associated symptoms include halitosis, tonsillolithiasis, chronic fatigue, and chronic or recurrent cervical lymph node pain and tenderness.

The physical examination can be very helpful in these patients, although the findings are often subtle. The tonsils may have dilated surface vessels and loss of crypt architecture, resulting in smooth surface and fewer crypts. Tonsillar or peritonsillar erythema is frequently present. Palpation of the tonsil, although somewhat uncomfortable for the patient, may express exudates from debris in the tonsil crypts, highly suggestive of chronic tonsillitis. The size of the tonsils does not seem to correlate with the symptoms; thus, small tonsils may be found as commonly as large ones. Tender, sometimes enlarged cervical nodes are usually present, and may be the only manifestation in some patients.

Supportive laboratory information is likewise difficult to obtain. Surface cultures may miss 40% to 60% of the bacteria found in the cores of tonsils. Culture of needle aspiration core material although difficult to obtain in younger children, may yield more accurate information. However, sufficient evidence exists as to the nature of the microbial flora present in chronic disease for the clinician to proceed with empiric therapy. Administration of broad-spectrum antibiotics effective against beta-lactamase–producing microorganisms or antibiotics effective against *B. melaninogenicus* for 10 to 20 days can be justified. Some have advocated 90 days of therapy with penicillin, to treat for potential actinomycosis infection (25).

Establishing a recent infection with EBV by serology is also important; sore throat after acute IM may persist for 3 to 6 months. If the sore throat is present for longer, and antimicrobial therapy is ineffective in relieving symptoms, tonsillectomy is considered.

PEARLS AND PERILS

1. Acute airway obstruction from tonsillitis is a medical and sometimes surgical emergency. High-acuity nursing, airway precautions, and the judicious use of antibiotics and steroids are important management points.
2. When in doubt about the stability of the airway, secure it with a nasopharyngeal tube (trumpet in older patients, an appropriately cut endotracheal tube in younger ones).
3. Chronic obstructive tonsillar hypertrophy often has an underlying bacterial etiology. A therapeutic trial with a broad-spectrum antibiotic that is effective against beta-lactamase–producing microorganisms, given for 20 to 30 days, may prove to be effective in reducing the size of the tonsils enough to relieve the obstruction (for more than 1 year) in 15% to 20% of children.
4. A history of throat infection is very often absent in the presence of large obstructing tonsils, and in the absence of obstructing symptoms even very severe enlargement of the tonsils may not necessarily be problematic for the child.
5. In children with craniofacial dysmorphism or neuromuscular weakness, smaller tonsils (and adenoids) may still play a significant role in upper-airway obstruction.
6. Clinical evaluation with symptoms and signs highly supportive of obstruction do not warrant evaluation with polysmnography. However, when the history and physical examination findings are disparate (rendering the diagnosis unclear) *or* when there is a potentially medically complicating problem, polysomnography will be required not only for diagnosis, but also for safe perioperative management.

Adenoid Infection

Historically the adenoids have been considered as part of the lymphoid tissue of Waldeyer's ring and were removed automatically along with the tonsils. Recognition of the anatomic considerations (relationship to nose and paranasal sinuses anteriorly and eustachian tube laterally) that are unique to the adenoids has led to a more precise consideration of the indications for adenoidectomy. The adenoids are almost always considered for removal based not only on the presence of disease in the adenoids themselves but also on the presence of disease in the related structures of the middle-ear–eustachian tube–mastoid complex and the nose and paranasal sinuses. Recurrent viral or bacterial infection, environmental and food allergies, as well as extraesophageal reflux are all described as contributing to chronic inflammation in the upper aerodigestive tract and nasopharynx resulting in chronic nasopharyngitis or adenoiditis.

Recurrent or Chronic Adenoid Infection

Recurrent or chronic infection in the adenoids *without obstructive hypertrophy* may manifest as recurrent AOM, persistent middle-ear effusion, or recurrent or chronic rhinosinusitis.

Clinical presentation usually (but not necessarily) includes chronic or recurrent nasal discharge. The character of the discharge can be quite variable and not necessarily green or yellow. However, clear nasal discharge, especially when associated with a history of itchy eyes or nose and multiple episodes of sneezing, should prompt evaluation for concomitant allergic rhinitis. If sinusitis is also present, it is usual that chronic cough, especially nocturnal, may be present in more than 80% of children (26). Chronic nasal congestion with snorting or sniffing is often described and in younger children may interfere with eating. "My child always has a cold" or "keeps a cold all winter long" is a frequent observation by parents. The history may also reveal that every episode of otitis is preceded by an upper respiratory tract infection or that the child has frequent bouts of "sinusitis."

Positive findings on the physical examination may be quite difficult to establish. Direct visualization of the adenoids in children is difficult due to less than optimal cooperation in younger children in whom the disease is most prevalent. Therefore, indirect findings must be sought to provide relevant, albeit, less precise, clinical information. A postnasal drip and nasal discharge can suggest infection in the nasopharynx, nose or paranasal sinuses. When in doubt, especially in older children, in whom adenoids are less likely to cause problems, direct nasopharyngoscopy by either flexible or rigid endoscopes is very useful. In children undergoing adenoidectomy for recurrent (and perhaps persistent) otitis media, nasopharyngeal swab may offer information to guide antibiotic therapy for treatment [otitis media with effusion (OME)] or prophylaxis (recurrent AOM) (26,27).

If the adenoids are recommended for removal because of recurrent AOM, documentation of a recent episode of AOM is necessary. A well-documented history of three or more episodes in 6 months or four or more episodes in 12 months is also necessary. (Many children have fever and ear pain treated with antibiotics after a telephone conversation with the primary-care physician. In these cases, the diagnosis may not be firm enough for the otolaryngologist to recommend surgery on either the adenoids or the ears.)

Prophylactic antibiotic therapy for recurrent AOM has failed when one or more episodes of AOM occur during 3 months of prophylaxis. Amoxicillin is the preferred antibiotic for prophylaxis by this author, because of the rare but potentially serious blood dyscrasias seen with the use of sulfonamides, which also require monitoring of the white blood cell count. Prophylaxis is most effective in children in whom the middle-ear effusion from the acute episode has cleared. However, one recent report advocates the use of prophylaxis for up to 6 months in the presence of middle-ear effusion (27). Although its effectiveness in preventing recurrent AOM may have been demonstrated, the effects of prolonged middle-ear effusion on hearing and the general healthy ear structures were unfortunately underplayed. For recurrent AOM, placement of tympanostomy tubes, as a reasonable alternative to prophylaxis, is a decision made on a case-by-case basis in consultation with the family, primary-care physician, and otolaryngologist together. The age of the child, prior treatment, time of year, and other extenuating factors are all considered. The role of adenoidectomy in this situation to prevent otitis media must also be individualized. The presence of a strong clinical picture implicating the adenoids may make the decision easier for the clinician and family. Other compelling factors to be considered include the presence of congenital deafness, otitis-triggered febrile seizures, speech and language delay, craniofacial anomalies (including cleft palate), and neurodevelopmental disorders with impaired cognition.

The benefits from adenoidectomy for persistent middle-ear effusion have been studied in depth (28,29,30). The size of the adenoids does not seem to be relevant to outcome in these children. The bacteriology in these cases has been shown to shift from the normal nasopharyngeal flora with predominance of *Streptococcus viridans* and *Neisseria* species, to potentially pathogenic bacteria, particularly *Hemophilus influenzae* and *Branhamella catarrhalis* (31). Furthermore, a change in the structure of the overlying mucosa from one that is approximately one-third each pseudostratified ciliated columnar epithelium, specialized squamous epithelium, and transitional epithelium to one that is overwhelmingly a specialized squamous epithelium is noted. A shift in the regulatory T-cell population has also been observed (32).

In children with symptoms associated with adenoid disease (frequent nasal obstruction or recurrent or chronic nasal discharge), particularly in children ages 4 to 8 years, adenoidectomy, *regardless of the preoperative size of the adenoids*, is beneficial in reducing the need for another set of typanostomy tubes in up to 50% of children. Thus, in a child with severe ear disease, especially those undergoing placement of a second set of tubes, or when clinical examination supports the presence of repeated or chronic adenoid infection, adenoidectomy should be recommended simultaneously.

Adenoidectomy for the treatment of sinusitis has been suggested but well-designed clinical studies are lacking. In a review of 625 children undergoing adenoidectomy, of those with documented (n = 52) or strongly suspected (n = 273) sinusitis (by symptoms and x-ray findings), adenoidectomy was effective in eliminating the sinusitis symptoms in 55% to 70% of those children followed for an average of 2 years (33). Often prophylaxis will be effective in controlling the symptoms of sinusitis (34); however, the duration of therapy is usually prolonged and well-established guidelines have yet to be presented. It is not unusual for children with sinusitis to require prophylaxis during several seasons, especially if there are developmental delays present in the immune system.

Complications from recurrent or chronic adenoid infection are relatively rare, but in younger children can include chronic upper-airway obstruction with failure to thrive.

Tonsil Obstruction

Acute Obstructive Tonsillar Hypertrophy

Acute upper-airway obstruction from tonsil enlargement almost always results from an acute infection. Acute tonsillitis alone, especially in young children, peritonsillar abscess (unilateral or rarely bilateral), and acute IM (described in detail earlier) are the most common underlying etiologies. Rarely lymphoma or atypical mycobacterial infection of the tonsil will present as an airway obstruction; however, prior symptoms of change in the voice or nocturnal breathing patterns may be elicited. An acute onset of a severe sore throat with difficulty swallowing associated with loud, often irregular breathing while awake and snoring while asleep should alert the clinician to the possibility of impending upper-airway obstruction. Often the family will dismiss the presence of "snoring," even when accompanied by "pauses" (apneas), because snoring is culturally acceptable and not always associated with the concept that the child might be dangerously ill. Acute onset of drooling is another important sign of upper aerodigestive obstruction.

The physical examination is most notable in that the child will sit upright, in a head-forward position, and will not be able to control his or her secretions. The voice is quite muffled, and audible, stertorous breathing is present. Careful examination of the oral cavity and oropharynx may be done; significant trismus with a soft-palate bulge is suspicious for peritonsillar abscess.

Treatment of the airway must be instituted often before confirmatory laboratory testing can be accomplished. Unless there is serious concern about epiglottitis (which is very unusual today and rarely presents with a concomitant tonsillitis), a lateral neck airway film does not add any information that cannot be gleaned from the physical examination. Treatment decisions are based on the severity of the airway distress. Children who become very irritable, disoriented, combative, or lethargic may be experiencing impending airway obstruction. The patient should be admitted to the hospital and placed in a monitored bed where both adequate nursing and medical surveillance are available. Antibiotics for acute infection and steroids in patients with acute IM are started. A nasopharyngeal tube should be available for placement. If peritonsillar abscess is the cause, and the patient is cooperative, bedside needle aspiration by an experienced senior clinician may be attempted; however, if any doubt as to the stability of the airway exists, airway securement in the operating room is preferred. Awake intubation over a bronchoscope in the most severely affected patients should be considered; preparation for tracheotomy may be needed as well.

Sudden relief of both acute (and chronic) upper-airway obstruction may result in the development of acute postobstructive pulmonary edema. The clinical presentation can be somewhat confusing—despite adequate ventilation, the oxygen saturation remains low, lung compliance is decreased, and in some patients pink, frothy sputum will be suctioned from the endotracheal tube. The pathogenesis of this situation is based on the sudden changes in intrathoracic pressures, which then lead to extravasation of fluid from the pulmonary vasculature into the alveoli. Prompt recognition can be lifesaving. Positive end-expiratory pressure is administered and intravenous diuretics are given. An intraoperative chest x-ray film may be obtained. If the pulmonary edema is severe enough to cause significant congestive heart failure, use of morphine and digitalis may be necessary. Admission to an intensive care unit with resolution over 48 to 72 hours is the usual course of events when prompt recognition and treatment occur.

Chronic Obstructive Tonsillar Hypertrophy

The pathophysiology of tonsillar hypertrophy has received much attention during the last 10 to 15 years. Once regarded as a normal physiologic response, tonsillar enlargement results from a complex set of circumstances that in any one child, may result in pathologically enlarged tonsils.

Upper-airway obstruction occurs when the airway resistance increases secondary to a decrease in the area of the airway. Both the oropharyngeal muscles and the tonsils collapse into the airway. Children with poor neuromuscular control or constricted airways from craniofacial dysmorphic or anatomic altertions are at greater risk for collapse and obstruction, even with lesser degrees of adenotonsillar hypertrophy. In children with clinically enlarged tonsils, with and without clinical symptoms of airway obstruction, the size of the oropharynx in the lateral dimension was found to be narrower in children with obstruction (35). Enlarged tonsils are more often infected with *H. influenzae* (4) and have altered bacterial homeostasis, with fewer commensal bacteria found in the tonsillar crypts, and of those potentially pathogenic bacteria that do infect the tonsil, the bacterial concentration is greater (3,16,36,37,38). Immunologic alterations have been described and include a decreased ability to respond to antigenic stimulation, alterations in the location and number of antigen-presenting cells, and changes in the regulatory T cells and B-cell function (3,4,16).

Vigilance in the pursuit of both the obvious and the more discrete clinical manifestations of disease is important. Unless a history of sleep disturbances can be elicited, the problem often goes undiagnosed. Snoring is the most common complaint. Usually it is described as loud, often with snorting, choking, and pauses lasting for 10 to 30 or 40 seconds. Parents will describe the child as "snoring like a truck driver" or "snoring louder than his or her father." Restless sleep, with the child often found in unusual or bizarre positions, is a sensitive indicator (39). A child who sleeps in the sniff position or with the neck hyperextended is not uncommonly described. Associated symptoms to be sought include morning headaches, secondary enuresis (resumed bedwetting in a child who was previously dry), daytime hypersomnolence with napping and lethargy, and changes in behavior patterns—especially a deterioration in school performance and general well-being. Dysphagia with choking episodes can be present. Meats, in particular, seem to be avoided by children with symptomatic obstructive tonsillar hypertrophy. Growth disturbances, which can be demonstrated on the child's growth chart, may be seen. Failure to thrive can be attributed to decreased oral intake as well as increased caloric expenditures associated with the increased work of breathing. In the most severe cases a child can present with congestive heart failure from cor pulmonale. Some children present with awake obstructive apnea. Stertorous, snorty breathing that is readily heard by those nearby is the usual clinical presentation. A *history of throat infection is very often absent and is not necessary for the tonsils to be pathologically enlarged. Similarly, in the absence of obstructive symptoms, even very severe enlargement of the tonsils may not necessarily be a problem for the child's upper aerodigestive tract.*

The physical examination should include assessment of the general well-being of the child. Height and weight plotted on an up-to-date growth curve can be quite revealing and previous records should be sought from the primary-care physician. Obstruction can occur with lesser degrees of tonsillar enlargement in children with neuromuscular weakness or craniofacial anomalies, especially those associated with midface hypoplasia such as Down syndrome or Crouzon's syndrome or mandibular hypoplasia such as seen in children with Treacher Collins syndrome. Thus, attention to underlying medical problems and particularly to craniofacial dysmorphism is mandatory.

Examination of the oral cavity and oropharynx can be challenging. Tongue extrusion and gagging can make the tonsils seem larger than they actually are. Thus, the child should be instructed to open the mouth gently with the tongue resting gently on the floor of the mouth. Visual inspection alone, without depressing the tongue, will often reveal the size and shape of the tonsils. When a long soft palate, prominent tongue, or a small oropharynx makes visualization difficult, two tongue depressors are gently placed on the midportion of the tongue, anterior to the circumvallate papillae, to depress the tongue without gagging the child (Fig. 2). Tonsil size is measured on a scale of 0 to +4 (11) (Fig. 3), based on the percent obstruction of the oropharynx in the lateral dimension. When the inferior pole of the tonsil is not visible with this maneuver, sometimes further tongue depression is needed to assess the inferior pole (Fig. 4). Asymmetric enlargement comparing the upper pole and lower pole can result in hypopharyngeal obstruction. This area is the narrowest part of the pharynx with the greatest chance for obstruction, particularly when the child is asleep and muscle tone is reduced.

Objective measures of the physiologic effects of obstructing tonsils (and adenoids) are difficult to obtain. The sleep polysomnogram, which is a multichannel recording of the patient's sleep, is expensive and often not available in many settings. Furthermore, accepted definitions for abnormal findings in children are not standardized, and the ef-

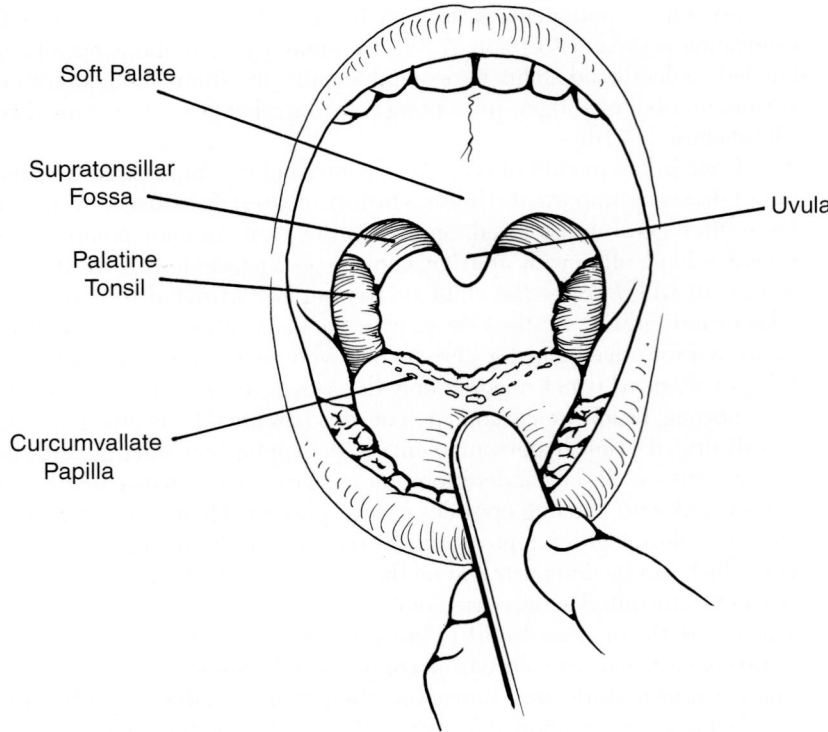

FIGURE 2 The tonsils are examined with the tongue lying on the floor of the mouth and two tongue depressors gently pressing down anterior to the circumvallate papillae. This prevents gagging, which is associated with medialization of the tonsils and a false impression of obstructing tonsils. (From ref. 7, with permission.)

Soft Palate

Supratonsillar Fossa

Palatine Tonsil

Curcumvallate Papilla

Uvula

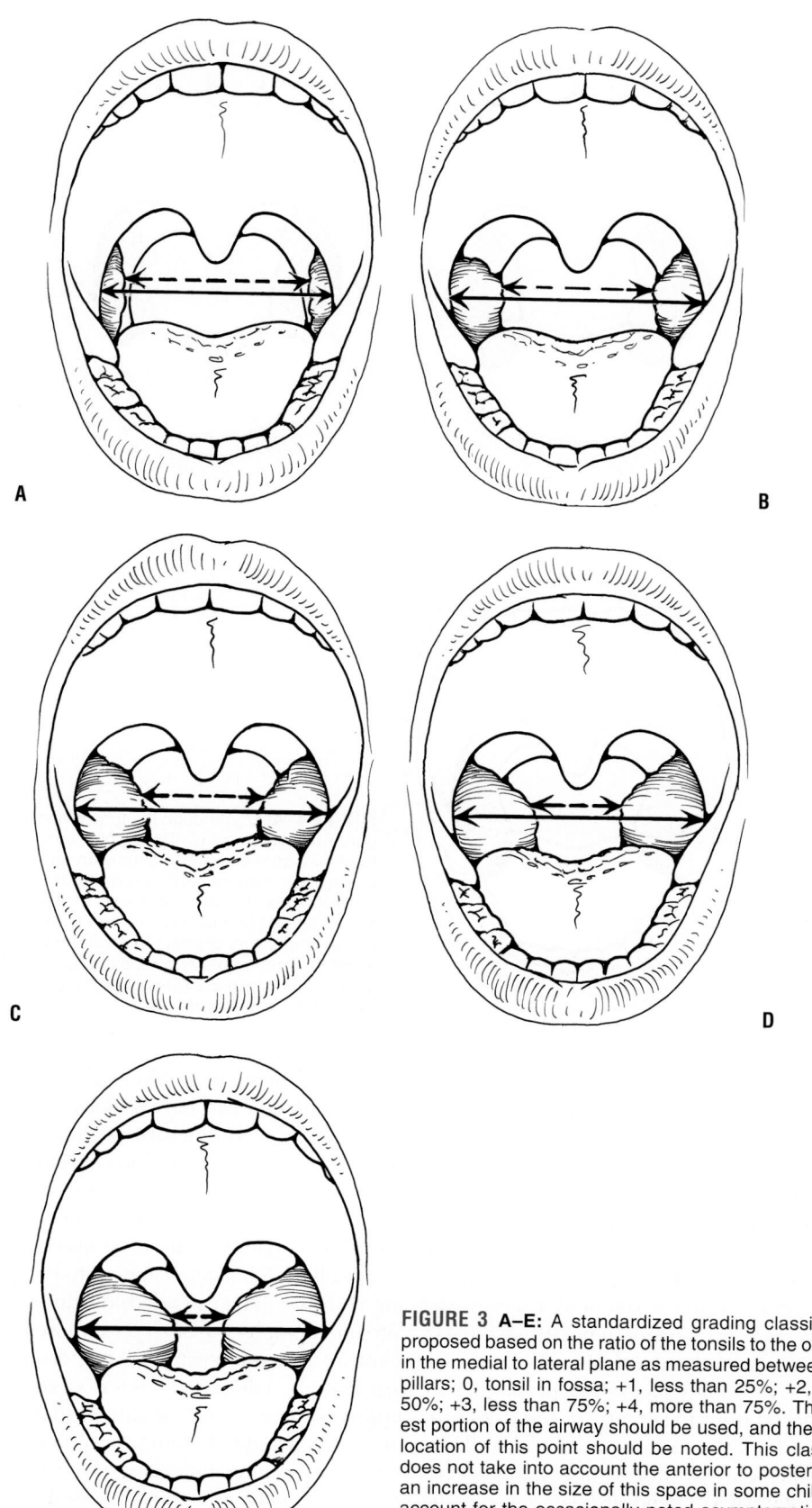

FIGURE 3 A–E: A standardized grading classification is proposed based on the ratio of the tonsils to the oropharynx in the medial to lateral plane as measured between anterior pillars; 0, tonsil in fossa; +1, less than 25%; +2, less than 50%; +3, less than 75%; +4, more than 75%. The narrowest portion of the airway should be used, and the anatomic location of this point should be noted. This classification does not take into account the anterior to posterior space; an increase in the size of this space in some children may account for the occasionally noted asymptomatic massive tonsillar hypertrophy. (From ref. 7, with permission.)

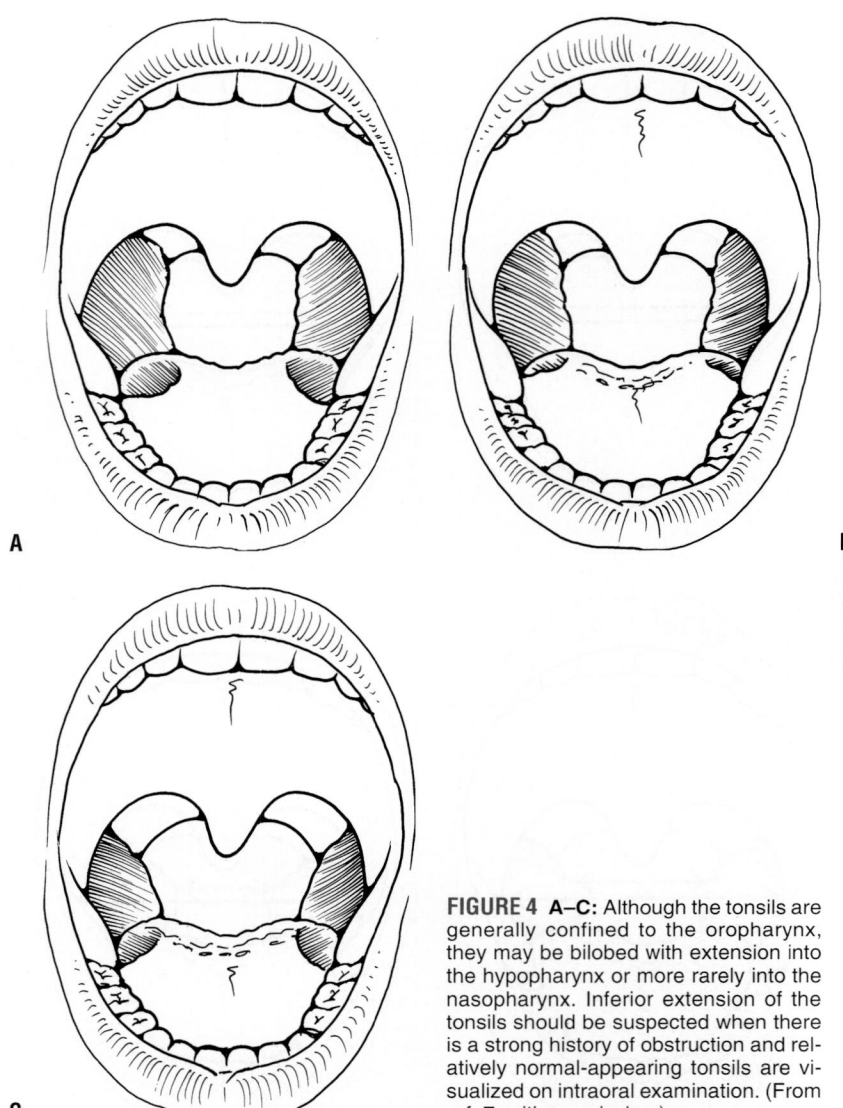

FIGURE 4 A–C: Although the tonsils are generally confined to the oropharynx, they may be bilobed with extension into the hypopharynx or more rarely into the nasopharynx. Inferior extension of the tonsils should be suspected when there is a strong history of obstruction and relatively normal-appearing tonsils are visualized on intraoral examination. (From ref. 7, with permission.)

fects of lesser degrees of obstruction on the growth and well-being of children are unknown. There is evidence that partial obstructive hypoventilation can have serious sequelae. Alternative methods such as audiotape and videotape recording of the child's sleep can be misleading and are often inaccurate. The reliance on oximetry alone fails to address the issue of apneas and hypopneas without oxygen desaturation. Sleep sonography has been found to correlate with polysomnography (40); however, it has not yet enjoyed widespread use. Thus, it is advocated that clinical examination is the most useful and should be as detailed as possible. The most sensitive clinical indicators appear to be snoring, pauses, gasping, frequent arousals, sleeping with the neck extended, daytime sleepiness, and chronic mouth breathing (39,41). Polysomnography is reserved for those children in whom the diagnosis is in doubt (the clinical signs and symptoms are disparate), the possibility of a severe problem is so great that physiologic parameters must be established prior to surgery, or the risk of the surgery is so great for that patient that the diagnosis of obstruction must be as well documented as possible before proceeding with tonsillectomy with or without adenoidectomy. Cardiac examination using electrocardiography (ECG), echocardiography and chest x-ray films may be required to establish the presence or absence of early right-sided heart strain.

Recent studies demonstrated that approximately 30% of tonsils will reduce in size significantly enough to relieve the child of obstructive symptoms if treated with broad-spectrum antibiotics for 3 to 6 weeks (Brodsky et al., unpublished data, 1995–1996). Relapse rates are about 50% within 6 to 9 months and tend to correlate with patient age—younger patients are more likely to have a relapse presumably due to their smaller airway size. However, since most children do not respond to this therapy, tonsillectomy (with or without adenoidectomy—see next section) should be offered to the patient and family.

PEARLS AND PERILS

1. Diagnosis is made difficult unless clear-cut clinical criteria are recognized and followed—the use of throat cultures alone may be insufficient to establish a diagnosis of acute or recurrent tonsillitis.
2. When the diagnosis of recurrent acute *tonsillitis* is questionable, offer to examine the child during a "typical" acute episode so as to rule out lingual tonsillitis, pharyngitis, or sinusitis as the true underlying etiology.
3. Chronic (persistent) tonsillitis presents with different symptoms and physical findings. The symptoms may include halitosis, fatigue, frequent sore throat, and enlarged and tender neck nodes. Physical examination may reveal increased debris in the crypts, peritonsillar erythema, loss of crypt architecture, and tender cervical lymph nodes. Symptom diaries may be helpful in establishing the presence and severity of the disease.
4. The carrier state of group A beta-hemolytic streptococcus may not be an absolute indication for tonsillectomy (see text).
5. Recurrent episodes of tonsillitis should be treated with broad-spectrum antibiotics, which may eradicate alternate pathogens or interfering bacteria. Amoxicillin-clavulanate and clindamycin can be used.
6. In children for whom the surgical indications are "borderline" in nature, or for the family who is cautious about the concept of surgery, watchful waiting or chronic antibiotic prophylaxis, or both, are reasonable alternatives and may be considered for 6 to 12 months.

Adenoid Obstruction

Acute Obstructive Adenoid Hypertrophy

Acute nasal airway obstruction is almost always associated with an infection in the nose, paranasal sinuses, and nasopharynx (i.e., adenoids). Younger children in particular, whose airways are smaller, may present with an acute viral or bacterial infection that is so severe that nasal obstruction results in impaired respiration. In infants up to about the age of 6 months, who rely primarily on nasal breathing, nasal obstruction can be life-threatening. Older children may develop acute nocturnal respiratory disturbances with snoring, restless sleep, and apneas, as described earlier. The inability to eat and breathe simultaneously is a common complaint in both acute and chronic obstruction. The child may also experience a sore throat from mouth breathing or postnasal secretions coating the pharynx.

Owing to the close anatomic relationships of the related structures of the nose, paranasal sinuses, and nasopharynx, it is often impossible to localize exactly the initial site of infection leading to obstruction. However, since the microbiology of these three problems—acute rhinitis, acute sinusitis, and acute nasopharyngitis—is similar, *when acute nasal airway obstruction is present*, empiric treatment with broad-spectrum antibiotics and both topical and systemic decongestants should be started. Infants and children less than 1 year old sometimes need hospitalization for monitoring, hydration, vigorous local nasal care, and systemic antibiotics.

Chronic Obstructive Adenoid Hyperplasia

The pathophysiology of chronic obstructive adenoid hyperplasia has received much attention in the recent literature (42,43). Like the tonsils, enlargement of the adenoids is still regarded as a normal physiologic response by some clinicians; however, when a normal response causes an abnormal physiologic state (i.e., obligate mouth breathing, obstructive snoring, and voice changes), then the "normal" response is exaggerated and potentially harmful to the patient.

Positioned in the nasopharynx, an anatomic space that can be thought of as a rigid box on three sides that serves as a conduit for air and rhinonasal secretions, the adenoids are particularly important in the pathophysiology of nasal obstruction. Direct intraoperative measurements of both the adenoids and the nasopharynx in obstructed and nonobstructed otherwise healthy children reveal that increased adenoid size (and not the nasopharyngeal size) is responsible for the obstruction.

Alterations in the microbiology are found with enlarged adenoids—normal homeostasis is disrupted with a decrease in the concentrations of commensals and an increase in the frequency of isolation of potential pathogens (43). Furthermore, as the adenoids become larger, and the microbiology shifts, the surface mucosa transforms from a mixed mucosa of about one-third each pseudostratified ciliated columnar, specialized squamous (for antigen presentation), and mixed to primarily specialized squamous epithelia. This results in mucociliary stasis and further contributes to pathologic enlargement of the adenoids.

Obstructive adenoid hypertrophy (OAH) is most readily diagnosed by history and physical examination. The triad of obligate (or near constant) mouth breathing, snoring, and hyponasal voice is seen. Concomitant symptoms often include persistent rhinorrhea, postnasal drip, and chronic cough, but are quite nonspecific and can also be seen with allergic rhinitis and chronic sinusitis, both of which may be present and contributing to the obstruction and to the ongoing antigenic challenge that is resulting in the adenoid enlargement. Snoring occurs in more than 85% of children with obstructing adenoids (33), and is much less frequent in children undergoing adenoidectomy for other reasons. Associated symptoms of obstructive sleep apnea, as described earlier for the tonsils, may be present from obstructing adenoids alone and should be sought during the discussions with the family.

The physical examination is challenged by the need to identify the exact location(s) of the nasal obstruction and the relative contribution of the adenoids. Observation of the child during the discussions of history with the parents may help to establish the mouth breathing as obligate or not. The child may have the classic "adenoid facies" (open-mouthed posture, flat midface, dull appearance, and dark discoloration under the eyes); however, this appearance may be seen in children with chronic nasal obstruction from other causes. Oro-facial-dental abnormalities with alterations in the maxillary-mandibular relationship may be apparent.

Alterations in the nasality of speech may be very apparent in normal conversation, oftentimes making the child's speech difficult to understand. Comparison of directed utterances of phrases that emphasize nasal emissions such as "Mickey Mouse" or "milkman" with those that do not such as "baseball" may be performed. Others suggest using nasal pinching during speech to listen for changes in nasalance as a method for determining nasality. A decrease in nasal resonance (hyponasality) is most often associated with obstructing adenoids and to a much lesser degree with severe obstructive allergic rhinitis.

Anterior rhinoscopy can be readily accomplished by using the otoscope head with a large ear speculum, or in older children, the nasal speculum attachment. Children are familiar with this equipment, it is already in hand, and it provides both illumination and magnification. Thus, the anterior nasal mucosa, septum, and nasal secretions are assessed. With isolated OAH, one often sees normal nasal mucosa, a normal septum, and rarely scant secretions sitting on the floor of the nose. When the nasal mucosa is inflamed from either allergic or infectious causes, a nasal smear may help direct therapy to alleviate the effects of underlying allergies or sinusitis, which can interfere with the assessment of the precise role the adenoids are playing in the nasal obstruction. Nasal mucus from the area of the middle turbinate is swabbed with a nasopharyngeal swab, and is examined microscopically (Wrights, stain). The presence of eosinophils suggests allergies; bacteria and polymorphonuclear neutrophil leukocytes (PMNs) suggest infection. Based on the nasal smear, a therapeutic trial of antibiotics, topical nasal or systemic steroids, antihistamines, or a combination of these agents, may be utilized to determine their effects on the nasal obstruction. Often enough relief of symptoms will occur to avoid surgery on the adenoids.

When the clinical picture remains unclear, the use of either indirect mirror or direct flexible fiberoptic nasopharyngoscopy will be necessary to view the adenoids. The role of lateral neck radiographs is somewhat controversial. In children who exhibit the typical signs and symptoms of OAH, an x-ray study is not necessary to confirm what is clinically apparent. Some authors correlated the adenoid-nasopharyngeal ratio or the air column width to adenoid size; however, their use of a two-dimensional radiograph to assess a complex, three-dimensional space, the disregard of the relationship of the adenoids to the posterior choanae, and finally, the presence of mucus that may be overlying moderately sized adenoids (and thus causing a functional obstruction not well demonstrated on x-ray films) make this a less than optimal examination. Other factors that contribute to the lack of usefulness of these x-ray films include inconsistent patient positioning, variations in technique, and lack of cooperation from the child, who may be crying or unable to close the mouth during the examination (both resulting in relatively different palatal positions, which will have an effect on measurements). The use of the lateral neck film may be helpful and should be limited to the assessment of *possible* OAH, particularly in the presence of nasal mucosal disease or in children in whom the history and physical examination findings are disparate and the child is uncooperative for direct nasopharyngeal examination as described earlier.

Assessment of palatal integrity is mandatory during the assessment of the adenoids. Palatal abnormalities may either mimic or be masked by the hyponasality of OAH. A submucous cleft palate can be readily identified by the presence of a bifid uvula, notched hard palate, and midline diastasis of the musculature (Fig. 5). A history of nasal regurgi-

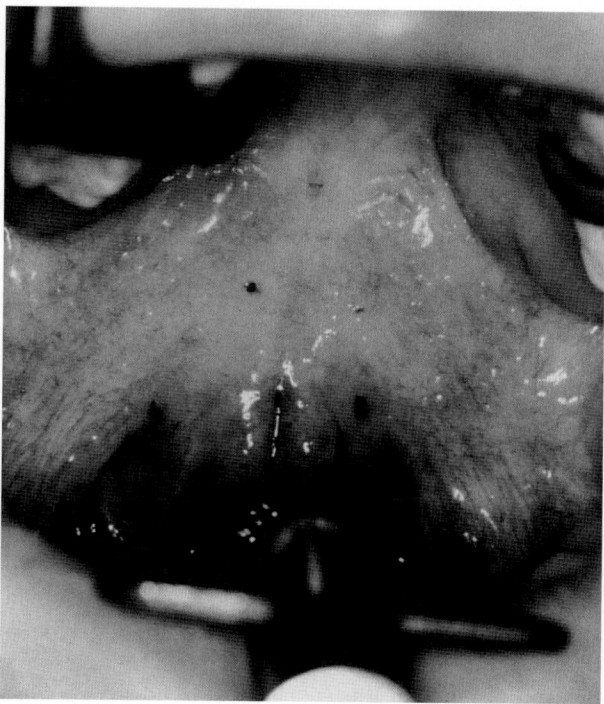

FIGURE 5 Submucous cleft palate seen intraoperatively before pharyngeal flap surgery. Note the bifid uvula, zona pelucida, and hard-palate notch.

tation of liquids, a family history of velopharyngeal insufficiency (VPI) or clefting, or any suspicion of hypernasal or mixed nasal speech should prompt direct visualization of the nasal surface of the palate to assess for occult submucous cleft palate. Similarly, when an adenoidectomy is undertaken in a very young child, particularly if there is any craniofacial dysmorphism, the possibility of postoperative VPI should be discussed before surgery.

Before an adenoidectomy is performed a trial of broad-spectrum antibiotics for 3 to 6 weeks may be helpful. The simultaneous use of topical nasal steroids also has been promoted by some (44). If the symptoms do not resolve, adenoidectomy is indicated for obstruction associated with awake or asleep airway obstruction, hyponasality interfering with speech, and mouth breathing that has secondary symptomatology of oro-dental-facial abnormalities (best confirmed by a dentist), dry mouth or lips, and chronic sore throats. The complications of failure to thrive, congestive heart failure from right-sided heart strain, and postobstructive pulmonary edema such as described earlier can all occur with OAH. Persistent VPI after adenoidectomy (more than 2 months after surgery) most often responds to a course of speech therapy. On rare occasions severe cases require corrective surgery.

PEARLS AND PERILS

1. The triad of hyponasality, snoring, and mouth breathing almost always indicates enlarged, obstructing adenoids.
2. Lateral neck films may be very misleading if patient cooperation or positioning is poor, or if choanal adenoids or mucostasis are causing the obstruction.
3. Normal nasal mucosa and nasal septum on physical examination and the presence of hyponasal speech and mouth breathing are the typical physical findings when adenoids alone are responsible for the obstruction.
4. The otoscope head is a handy, useful tool to examine a child's nasal cavity.
5. The adenoids are always evaluated separately from the tonsils.

Special Situations in the Tonsils—Peritonsillar Abscess, Unilateral Tonsillar Enlargement, Tonsillolithiasis, Hemorrhagic Tonsillitis, and Lingual Tonsillitis

Peritonsillar Abscess

Until recently, the pathophysiology of peritonsillar abscess has been described as arising from direct extension of an acute tonsillitis into the peritonsillar space. Recent study revealed that peritonsillar abscess is most likely from an infection of a minor salivary gland that sits on the superior pole of the tonsil (most often) (45), but can be found in the middle or inferior pole as well (personal observation). Clinical experience supports this as yet to be widely accepted proposal—the bacteriology is almost always *Staphylococcus aureus* or mixed oral anaerobes (often found in salivary gland infections), the clinical presentation is not always heralded by recurrent sore throats or even evidence of tonsillitis in the ipsilateral or contralateral tonsil, and the recurrence rate is low (less than 10%) and parallels the low recurrence rates for bacterial sialadenitis.

Sore throat, muffled voice, and trismus are the clinical hallmarks of peritonsillar abscess. Often an episode of tonsillitis will have occurred within the past several weeks. An inability to swallow, drooling, fever, and odynophagia are seen. Peritonsillar abscess is seen more frequently in older children and teenagers.

Severe trismus, with an inability to open the mouth more than 2.0cm, challenges the clinician in the physical examination as well as treatment. Intraoral examination usually reveals a soft-plate bulge just superior and lateral to the superior pole of the tonsil. Usually this collection of pus pushes the tonsil inferiorly and medially. Often, but not always, there will be uvular deviation; however, absence of this sign may mislead the clinician and should not be relied on. When the abscess is lateral or inferior to the tonsil, the palatal bulge and tonsil displacement might not be as prominent as the trismus, which is usually worse. Interestingly, the tonsils themselves can be normal in appearance; tender cervical nodes complete the picture. When in doubt about the diagnosis, the clinician should obtain a complete blood cell count with differential. Unusual vascular malformations or parapharyngeal tumors can also present with a clinical picture similar to a peritonsillar abscess and confuse an inexperienced practitioner.

The treatment of choice in the acute phase will depend on the previous history. All patients receive clindamycin for coverage of *S. aureus* and oral anaerobes. If it is a first abscess, without an antecedent history of recurrent or persistent tonsillitis, the patient undergoes needle aspiration, hydration, and treatment with antibiotics, and the abscess will almost always resolve (46). Interval tonsillectomy is not needed as the recurrence rate is very low. In the case of recurrent abscess or a history of recurrent or persistent tonsillitis, immediate bilateral tonsillectomy is performed—a 6.1% recurrence rate in the contralateral side has been noted if both tonsils are not removed (47). The postoperative recovery of immediate tonsillectomy is similar to that of elective tonsillectomy, and the dissection is easier at the time of infection rather than after 6 weeks when fibrosis of the peritonsillar tissues occurs. In a young child who will not cooperate for needle aspiration and in whom antibiotics are not effective within 24 to 48 hours, an immediate tonsillectomy is performed (48).

Two complications of particular concern are acute airway obstruction, particularly during induction of anesthesia if the abscess is large, and spontaneous drainage with aspiration of pus. Both can be avoided with careful technique and experienced clinicians performing the needle aspiration and administering the anesthetic. It is most important that the surgeon and anesthesiologist work closely during airway securement.

Unilateral Tonsillar Enlargement

The pathophysiology of a unilaterally "enlarged" tonsil is most often due to the asymmetric anatomic position of two equally sized tonsils. However, infrequently, a child will present with true unilateral tonsil hypertrophy, the etiology of which must be established. Unusual infections, such as atypical mycobacteria infection, fungal infection, and actinomycosis, are most common. Neoplastic processes, particularly lymphoma, are also to be considered.

The clinical presentation is often insidious—change in voice or new-onset progressive snoring is common. A neck mass may be noticed and physical examination will reveal a unilaterally enlarged tonsil. Often the appearance of the substance of the tonsil will differ from that on the contralateral side.

Diagnostic excisional biopsy must be performed. If extension beyond the tonsil is suspected, appropriate imaging studies such as computed tomography of the neck (with contrast enhancement) or magnetic resonance imaging might be indicated. Preoperative consultation with the pathologist will ensure proper processing of the tonsil specimen. Pathologic examination for caseating granulomas or actinomycosis is also done. Cultures should be sent for routine anaerobic and aerobic bacterial, fungal, and mycobacterial studies. Preoperative consultation with an oncologist (if a high index of suspicion for malignancy exists) is prudent, and particularly helpful if a bone marrow biopsy might be required and could be painlessly performed while the child is under general anesthesia. Treatment, of course, depends on the underlying etiology and is almost always multidisciplinary in nature.

Tonsillolithiasis

Tonsillar concretions are formed from debris (food, dead bacteria, immune cells, and crypt epithelial cells) that collect in the tonsillar crypts. Tonsilloliths may present as malodorous breath or on occasion, as the expectoration of cheesy, foul-tasting lumps. Often, the patient will be able to express these from the tonsil crypts.

Cautery with topical silver nitrate has been recommended in adults. Its usefulness in children is questionable as usually the tonsillolithiasis is diffusely present. Use of a water pick is similarly limited; antibiotics are usually ineffective. The treatment of choice is tonsillectomy, which is almost always successful in correcting the problem.

Hemorrhagic Tonsillitis

An infrequent presentation of both acute and chronic tonsillitis is hemorrhage from the tonsils. Usually, dilated surface vessels, seen in chronic tonsillitis, account for the bleeding; however, diffuse parenchymal bleeding has also been noted (Fig. 6) (49). Rarely a previously unrecognized coagulopathy will present in this fashion; IM may also be the underlying etiology.

Treatment is directed toward local control of the bleeding. If unsuccessful, immediate tonsillectomy is warranted.

Lingual Tonsillitis

The lingual tonsils sit at the base of the tonsil and continue down into the vallecula. They are often forgotten in the differential diagnosis of acute and chronic sore throats and upper-airway obstruction.

Indirect mirror or direct flexible fiberoptic laryngoscopy is required to visualize the lingual tonsils. Erythema and enlargement may indicate an infection, which should be treated similarly to chronic infection or obstruction in the tonsils and adenoids.

When there is no response to medical therapy, then surgical removal is recommended. Suspension microlaryngoscopy with CO_2 laser excision is recommended by some and hot knife cautery excision, by others (50).

SURGICAL CONSIDERATIONS

Tonsillectomy and Adenoidectomy

Indications

Tonsillectomy with or without adenoidectomy is the most commonly performed major, pediatric surgical procedure in the United States today. Indications for surgical intervention are continually undergoing revision. Furthermore, no consensus exists as to

FIGURE 6 Hemorrhagic tonsillitis from dilated surface blood vessels. (From ref. 7, with permission.)

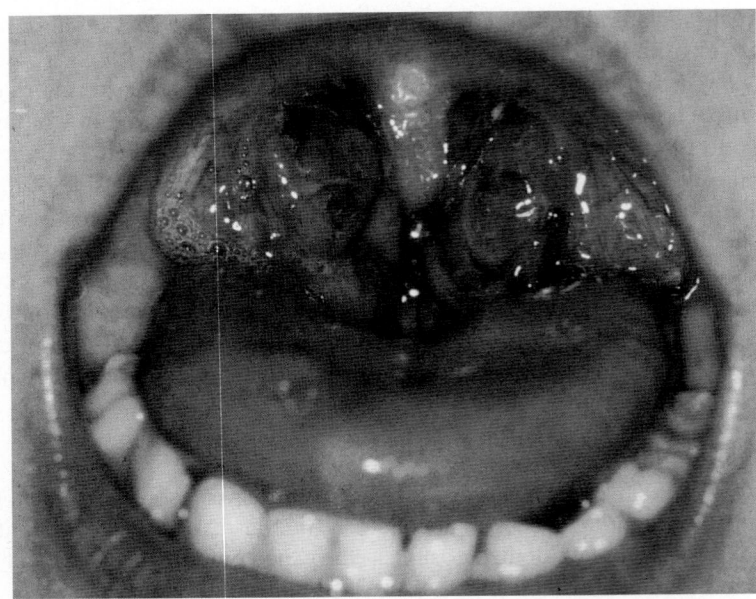

TABLE 2: Current Indications for Tonsillectomy with or without Adenoidectomy

	Tonsils	Adenoids
Infection		
1. Recurrent tonsillitis[a] (≥ 7/yr, 5/yr × 2 yr, 3/yr × 3 yr)	+	−
2. Persistent, chronic tonsillitis	+	−
3. Recurrent otitis media unresponsive to medical or previous placement of tubes	−	+
4. Chronic/recurrent nasopharyngitis	−	+
5. Chronic/recurrent sinusitis	−	+
Obstruction		
1. Hypertrophy with obstruction unresponsive to medical treatment (acute and chronic) with or without obstructive apnea, severe dysphagia, and failure to thrive		
a. If adenoids enlarged only	−	+
b. If tonsils enlarged only	+	−
c. If tonsils and adenoids enlarged	+	+
2. Nasal obstruction with speech abnormalities, orodental abnormalities	−	+
Miscellaneous		
1. Recurrent peritonsillar abscess or peritonsillar abscess with previous history of recurrent/persistent tonsillitis	+	−
2. Unilateral tonsillar hypertrophy	+	−
3. Hemorrhagic tonsillitis	+	−
4. Chronic tonsillolithiasis	+	−

[a] Indications may be less strict when concomitant medical conditions are made worse by infections.

either the appropriate preoperative evaluation or the appropriate medical management that should precede tonsillectomy with or without adenoidectomy for every child. Thus, developing guidelines is difficult and should be an ongoing process. A summary of the current indications for tonsillectomy and adenoidectomy is listed in Table 2.

Preoperative Evaluation

Careful preparation of the family and child is the key to a smooth, successful recovery. Often tonsillectomy with or without adenoidectomy is the first surgical procedure a child undergoes. A detailed description of the day's events with particular attention to the postoperative recovery (which is made difficult by vomiting, sore throat, and bleeding) should be discussed. Family history regarding bleeding, reactions to anesthesia (to assess for the potential of malignant hyperthermia), and other contributing medical problems should be elucidated. The cost-effectiveness of an evaluation for the presence of coagulopathies is still debated; however, the evaluation should be undertaken if there is a family history of bleeding disorder, if there is easy bruisability or bleeding in the child, or for a child less than 6 years old who has never had surgery without complication. When indicated, a partial thromboplastin time and bleeding time are sufficient screening parameters. The hematocrit is determined in all patients in case a preoperative baseline value is required to assess the severity of a postoperative hemorrhage.

Children with Down syndrome may require a flexion-extension cervical spine x-ray film in order to evaluate for C1-2 dislocation, which could compromise the spinal cord. However, this examination has limitations in younger children in whom the structures of interest are not yet ossified. Thus, another approach to the child with Down syndrome is to perform all such surgeries with the neck flexed instead of extended.

Surgical Technique

Techniques vary widely for tonsillectomy and less so for adenoidectomy. Careful dissection of the tonsil in the subcapsular plane can be performed with a cold knife technique, hot knife, and laser, hemostasis, can be obtained with suction electrocautery, bipolar cautery, suture, topical astringents, and vasoconstrictors.

Adenoids are generally removed transorally with indirect mirror visualization of the nasopharynx and adenoid tissue. In this way, complete removal, particularly at the posterior choanae, can be achieved and a low rate of revision adenoidectomy can prevail. Hemostasis is by pressure/packing or by suction coagulation.

Recent preliminary data (51) show that the technique of microbipolar dissection tonsillectomy, described in 1993 (52), results in a significantly reduced bleed rate and a faster rate of recovery with earlier resumption of normal diet and activity. Thus, it is the preferred technique of this author. At the end of the procedure, suctioning of the stomach to remove any gastric contents may be done.

Postoperative Care

By far the greatest controversy in tonsillectomy with or without adenoidectomy exists over discharge criteria and timing. In properly selected individuals, early discharge from the same-day surgery unit can be facilitated by judicious use of intraoperative pain medications, anti emetics, and fluid replacement and supplementation. Some surgeons give intravenous antibiotics and steroids as well as topical or injectable anesthetics, sometimes combined with vasoconstrictors. However, the reported increased postoperative bleeding rate seen after administration of injectable vasoconstrictors makes their use questionable. Requirements to drink or urinate post operatively before discharge are not necessary. However, an experienced examiner should visualize the pharynx for palatal swelling and fresh bleeding. Usually antibiotics are started orally for 10 days after oral feeding is established.

Children who should be considered for overnight observation are those who may be at higher risk for complications from the procedure in the immediate postoperative period. These children (and families)

1. Are less than 3 years old.
2. Experience poor oral intake or vomiting or are at additional risk of bleeding.
3. Have complex cardiac disease, seizures, cerebral palsy, neuromuscular disorders, craniofacial anomalies, or severe asthma.
4. Live more than 1 hour from the hospital (or less in inclement weather).
5. Have limited resources and there is a question of the ability to provide adequate early postoperative care.
6. Experience excessive parental or child anxiety about early discharge.

MANAGEMENT OF COMPLICATIONS

The most common immediate complications after tonsillectomy with or without adenoidectomy are bleeding, protracted vomiting, and severe pain leading to decreased oral intake and dehydration. Appropriate parent education will result in prompt recognition and treatment.

Late complications (after the first 3 to 5 days) are uncommon and include delayed tonsillar hemorrhage, nasopharyngeal/choanal stenosis after adenoidectomy, pharyngeal stenosis after tonsillectomy, otitis media with effusion, and velopharyngeal insufficiency (as discussed earlier).

SUMMARY

Effective evaluation and treatment of diseases of the tonsils and adenoids is quite challenging. The clinician who endeavors to understand the changing concepts in disease pathogenesis, medical management options, indications for surgery, surgical technique and intraoperative care, and postoperative management will be better positioned to give the most up-to-date care to the children she or he treats.

❉ REFERENCES

1. van Cauwenberge PB, Bellussi L, Maw AR, Paradise JL, Solow B. The adenoid as a key factor in upper airway infections. *Int J Pediatr Otorhinolaryngol* 1995;32 (Suppl):S71–S80.
2. Deutsch ES, Isaacson GC. Tonsils and adenoids: an update. *Pediatrics* 1995;161:17–21.
3. Brodsky L, Moore L, Stanievich J. The immunology of tonsils in children: the effect of bacterial load on the presence of B and T-cell subsets. *Laryngoscope* 1988;98:93–98.
4. Brodsky L, Moore L, Stanievich J. The role of *Haemophilus influenzae* in the pathogenesis of tonsillar hypertrophy in children. *Laryngoscope* 1988;98,10:1055–1060.
5. Curtin J. The history of tonsil and adenoid surgery. *Tonsils Adenoids* 1987;20:415–419.
6. Ruben RJ, Weg N. Contraindications to adenoidectomy. *Bull NY Acad Med* 1975;51:817–827.
7. Brodsky L. Modern assessment of tonsils and adenoids. *Pediatr Clin North Am* 1989;36:1551–1569.
8. DeDio RM, Tom LW, McGowan KL, Wetmore RF, Handler SD, Potsic WP. Microbiology of the tonsils and adenoids in a pediatric population. *Arch Otolaryngol Head Neck Surg* 1988;114:763–765.
9. Gaffney RJ, Freeman DJ, Walsh MA, Cafferkey MT. Differences in tonsil core bacteriology in adults and children: a prospective study of 262 patients. *Respir Med* 1991;85:383–388.
10. Freeland AP, Curley JWA. The consequences of delay in tonsil surgery. *Otolaryngol Clin North Am* 1987;20:405–408.
11. Careddu P, Biolchini S, Alfano S, Zavatinni G. Pidotimod in the prophylaxis of recurrent acute tonsillitis in childhood. In:Galioto GB, ed. *Tonsils: a clinically oriented update*. Basel:Karger, 1991.
12. Roos K, Holm SE, Grahn E, Lind L. Interfering alpha-streptococci as a protection against recurrent streptococcal pharyngotonsillitis. *Adv Otorhinolaryngol* 1992;47:142–145.
13. Mitchelmore IJ, Reilly PG, Hay AJ, Tabaqchali S. Tonsil surface and core cultures in recurrent tonsillitis: prevalence and anaerobes and beta-lactamase producing organisms. *Eur J Clin Microbiol Infect Dis* 1994;13:542–548.
14. Brook I, Yocum P, Foote PA Jr. Changes in the core tonsillar bacteriology of recurrent tonsillitis: 1977–1993. *Clin Infect Dis* 1995;21:171–176.
15. Faden H, Bernstein J, Stanievich J, Brodsky L, Ogra P. Effect of prior antibiotic treatment on middle ear disease in children. *Ann Otol Rhinol Laryngol* 1992;101:87–91.
16. Koch J, Brodsky L. Qualitative and quantitative immunoglobulin production by specific bacteria in chronic tonsillar disease. *Laryngoscope* 1995;105:42–48.
17. Brodsky L, Frankel S, Gorfein J, Rossman J, Noble B. The dendritic cell in normal and diseased tonsils in children. *Acta Otolaryngol Suppl (Stockh)* 1995;523:98–100.
18. Paradise J, Bluestone C, Bachman R, et al. Efficacy of tonsillectomy for recurrent throat infection in severely affected children. *N Engl J Med* 1984;310:674–683.
19. Shamim A, Alghamdi S, Kameswaran M, Shenoy AK, Thomas R, Okafor BC. Is fine needle aspiration of the tonsil superior to a surface swab for isolating its core flora in recurrent tonsillitis? *Ann Saudi Med* 1996;16:50–52.
20. Brook I. Treatment of patients with acute recurrent tonsillitis due to group a beta haemolytic streptococci:a prospective randomized study comparing penicillin and amoxicillin/clavulanate potassium. *J Antimicrob Chemother* 1989;24:227–233.
21. Brook I, Leyva F. The treatment of the carrier state of group A beta-hemolytic streptococci with clindamycin. *Chemo* 1981;27:360–367.
22. Jensen JH, Larsen SB. Treatment of recurrent acute tonsillitis with clindamycin. An alternative to tonsillectomy? *Clin Otolaryngol* 1991;16:498–500.
23. Lotter A, Allen G. Recent observations on the bacteriology of tonsillitis. *Ear Nose Throat J* 1975;54:23–26.
24. Bieluch V, Martin E, Chasin W, Tally F. Recurrent tonsillitis: histologic and bacteriologic evaluation. *Ann Otol Rhinol Laryngol* 1989;98:332–335.
25. Pransky S, Feldman S, Kearns D, Seid A, Billman G. Actinomycosis in obstructive tonsillar hypertrophy and recurrent tonsillitis. *Arch Otolaryngol* 1991;117:883–885.
26. Lusk R, Lazar R, Muntz H. The diagnosis and treatment of recurrent and chronic sinusitis in children. *Pediatr Clin North Am* 1989;36:1411–1421.
27. Faden H, Waz MJ, Bernstein JM, Brodsky L, Stanievich J, Ogra PL. Nasopharyngeal flora in the first three years of life in normal and otitis-prone children. *Ann Otol Rhinol Laryngol* 1991;100:612–615.

28. Gates G, Avery C, Prhoda TJ, Cooper JC. Effectiveness of adenoidectomy and tympanostomy tubes in the treatment of chronic otitis media with effusion. *N Engl J Med* 1987;317: 1444–1451.

29. Avery C, Gates G, Prhoda TJ. Effect of adenoidectomy upon children with chronic otitis media with effusion. *Laryngoscope* 1988;98:58–63.

30. Berman S, Roark R, Luckey D. Theoretical cost effectiveness of management options for children with persisting middle ear effusions. *Pediatrics* 1994;93:353–363.

31. Faden H, Stanievich J, Brodsky L, Betstein J, Ogra P. Changes in nasopharyngeal flora during otitis media of childhood. *Pediatr Infect Dis* 1990;9:623–626.

32. Brodsky L, Koch R. Bacteriology and immunology of normal and diseased adenoids in children. *Arch Otolaryngol Head Neck Surg* 1993;119:821–829.

33. Behar P, Pizzuto M, Poje C, Duffy L, Behar J, Brodsky L. The role of adnoidectomy in the treatment of pediatric sinusitis. *Arch Otolaryngol* 1998 (*in press*).

34. Gandhi A, Brodsky L, Ballow M. Benefits of antibiotic prophylaxis in children with chronic sinusitis:assessment of outcome predictors. *Allergy Proc* 1993;14:37–43.

35. Brodsky L, Adler E, Stanievich JF. Naso- and oropharyngeal dimensions in children with obstructive sleep apnea. *Int J Pediatr Otorhinolaryngol* 1989;17:1–11.

36. Toner J, Stewart T, Campbell J, Hunter J. Tonsil flora in the very young tonsillectomy patient. *Clin Otolaryngol* 1986;11:171–174.

37. Brodsky L, Nagy M, Volk M, Moore L, Stanievich J. The relationship of tonsil bacterial concentration to surface and core cultures in chronic tonsillar disease in children. *Int J Pediatr Otorhinolaryngol* 1991;21:33–39.

38. Koch R, Brodsky L. Effect of specific bacteria on lymphocyte proliferation in diseased and nondiseased tonsils. *Laryngoscope* 1993;103:1020–1026.

39. Goldstein NA, Sculerati N, Walsleben JA, Bhatia N, Friedman DM, Rapoport DM. Clinical diagnosis of pediatric obstructive sleep apnea validated by polysomnography. *Otolaryngol Head Neck Surg* 1994;111:611–617.

40. Potsic W. Comparison of polysomnography and sonography for assessing regularity of respiration during sleep in adenotonsillar hypertrophy. *Laryngoscope* 1987;97:1430–1437.

41. Potsic WP. Assessment and treatemnt of adenotonsillar hypertrophy in children. *Am J Otolaryngol* 1992;13:429–464.

42. Brodsky L, Koch J. Anatomic correlates of normal and diseased adenoids in children. *Laryngoscope* 1992;102:1268–1274.

43. Brodsky L, Koch RJ. The bacteriology and immunology of normal and diseased adenoids in children. *Arch Otorhinolaryngol* 1993;119:821–829.

44. Demain JG, Goetz DW. Pediatric adenoidal hypertrophy and nasal airway obstruction: reduction with aqueous nasal beclomethasone. *Pediatrics* 1995;95:355–364.

45. Passy V. Pathogenesis of peritonsillar abscess. *Laryngoscope* 1994;104:185–190.

46. Weinberg E, Brodsky L, Stanievich J, Volk M. Needle aspiration of peritonsillar abscess in children. *Arch Otorhinolaryngol* 1993;119:169–172.

47. Sorensen JA, Godballe C, Andersen NH, Jorgensen K. Peritonsillar abscess: risk of disease in the remaining tonsil after unilateral tonsillectomy a chaud. *J Laryngol Otol* 1991;105:442–444.

48. Brodsky L, Sobie S, Korwin D, Stanievich J. Peritonsillar abscess in children: a prospective study. *Laryngoscope* 1988;98:780–783.

49. Brodsky L, Levy S, Stanievich J. Hemorrhagic tonsillitis. *Laryngoscope* 1989;99:15–18.

50. Brodsky L. Lingual tonsillectomy. In:Bailey BJ, ed. *Atlas of head and neck surgery—otolaryngology*. Philadelphia:Lippincott-Raven, 1996:814–815.

51. Brodsky L, Pizzuto M, Gendler J, Duffy L. Microbipolar dissection vs. cold knife/suction cautery tonsillectomy in children: preliminary results of a prospective study. *Acta Otolaryngol Suppl (Stockh)* 1996;523:256–258.

52. Andrea M. Microsurgical bipolar cautery tonsillectomy. *Laryngoscope* 1993;103:1177–1178.

L. Brodsky: Department of Otolaryngology and Pediatrics, School of Medicine and Biomedical Sciences, State University of New York at Buffalo, Buffalo, New York; and Department of Pediatric Otolaryngology, Children's Hospital of Buffalo, Buffalo, New York 14222.

- *Practical Pediatric Otolaryngology*
- edited by Robin T. Cotton and Charles M. Myer III
- Lippincott-Raven Publishers, Philadelphia © 1999

3

Central and Obstructive Apnea

Michael A. Rothschild

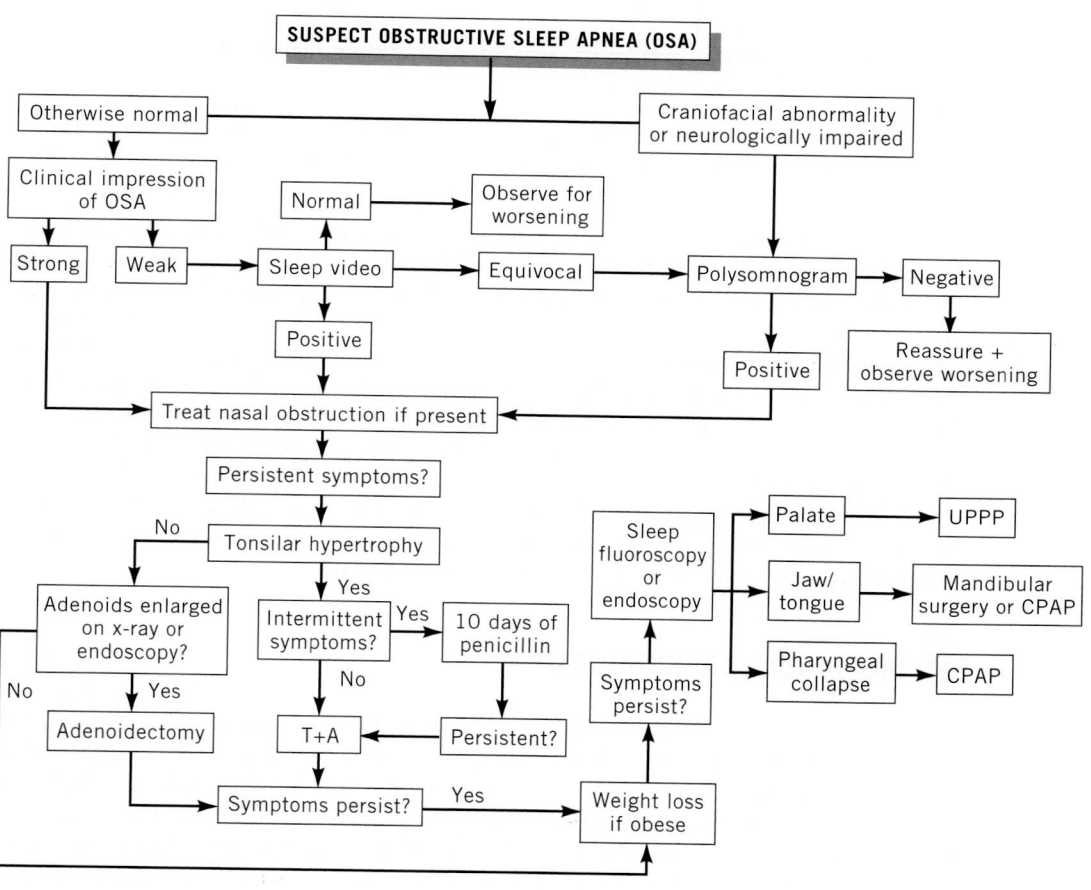

continued on next page

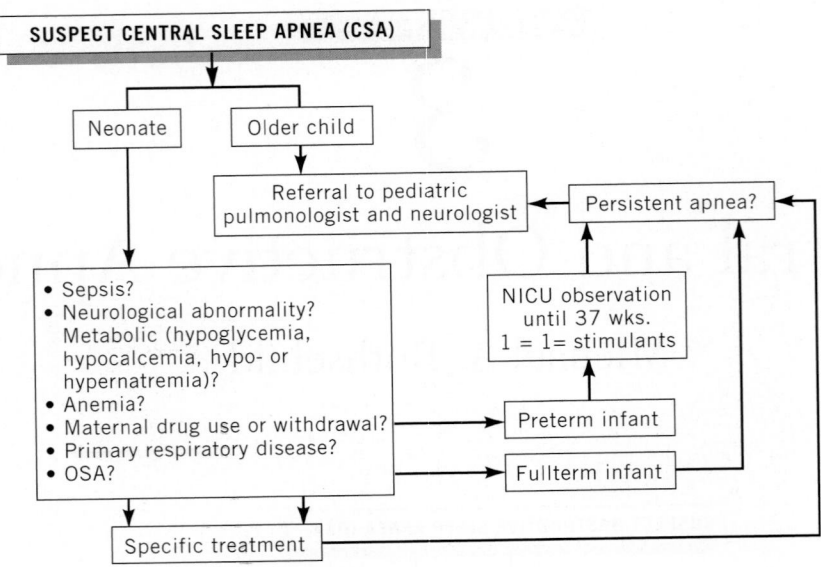

"Damn that boy; he's gone to sleep again. Joe! Joe!" (Sundry taps on the head with a stick, and the fat boy, with some difficulty, roused from his lethargy.)—Charles Dickens, *The Pickwick Papers*, 1837

This chapter encompasses two very different conditions, with the common thread of life-threatening apnea. Obstructive apnea is likely to be more familiar to the reader, given the prevalence of its most common etiology (adenotonsillar hypertrophy). The practicing otolaryngologist may spend considerable time managing this entity. Central apnea, on the other hand, is typically a disease of very young infants, and is rarely in the clinical province of the head and neck surgeon. Nevertheless, the two may coexist, and familiarity with the entire spectrum of respiratory disturbances is important for those who undertake to care for such children. While apnea may occur during waking hours, this is unusual and beyond the scope of a chapter oriented toward routine clinical practice. Therefore, the remainder of the discussion focuses on sleep disordered breathing—alterations in respiration arising due to the central nervous system depression or the reduction of pharyngeal tone that accompany the sleep state.

HISTORICAL BACKGROUND

As the quote from Dickens suggests, sleep disorders have been long recognized, but were not systematically studied before the middle of this century (1). During the 1950s and 1960s, the condition today known as obstructive sleep apnea (OSA) was explored. Adenotonsillar hypertrophy and obesity were determined to be predisposing factors, and the sequelae of hypoventilation, daytime somnolence, cardiac arrhythmia, and right-sided heart failure were also described. Later work centered on palatine redundancy and pharyngeal collapse, as the interplay of the various levels of nocturnal airway obstruction was noted (2). Finally, the understanding of central apnea (CA) provided further detail in the study of sleep architecture, especially in very young infants.

Sleep apnea, a subset of the broader category of sleep disordered breathing, has been well characterized by accurate and reproducible data from polysomnography (PSG) laboratories. Criteria for classifying adult patients with sleep apnea arose from sleep laboratory results over the past three decades, and more recently, pediatric standards have been published as well (3). Sleep disturbance in children has been cited as a contributing factor to a variety of behavioral disorders. These are more commonly a cause for concern than the relatively rare end-stage cardiac disease of long-standing, untreated OSA. Research into apnea in newborns has been driven by the need to identify possible etiologies for the sudden infant death syndrome (SIDS), although any connection between apnea and SIDS is at this point unclear.

PATIENT ASSESSMENT: OBSTRUCTIVE SLEEP APNEA

Sleep apnea may result from obstruction at a number of sites in the upper airway (i.e., between the nares and the larynx). OSA is caused by either fixed anatomic obstruction (such as adenotonsillar hypertrophy) or collapse of an otherwise patent pharynx. The upper airway has a tendency to collapse in the presence of negative pressure associated with inspiration and airflow. This is balanced by the muscular tone of the palate, pharynx, and tongue. Assuming that the patient has no dyspnea when awake, OSA is caused by the inability of the airway to remain patient with the loss of muscle tone during sleep, due to either severe narrowing, abnormally weak resting tone, or a combination of both (Fig. 1). Gravity may also contribute to obstruction by causing soft tissue prolapse during supine sleep in susceptible children.

Restricted airflow due to anatomic structures may cause apnea despite partial airway patency. Reduction in cross-sectional area results in an increase in the speed of the airstream, as the patient attempts to maintain a constant tidal volume. Intraluminal air pressure is inversely proportional to the rate of flow (Bernoulli's principle), so the negative pressure of inspiration is accentuated. When this pressure reaches the point that the pharyngeal musculature can no longer maintain patency (the critical closing pressure), collapse and obstructive apnea occur. At this point, the inspiratory efforts increase, resulting in further collapse of the airway and continued obstruction. This cycle is broken by partial arousal, an increase in pharyngeal tone, and repositioning of the airway or the entire body. In this manner, airflow is restored. This corresponds to the intermittent gasping and unrest often reported by the parents of children with OSA.

History

Typically, the signs of pediatric OSA are first noted by the parents. They may be concerned about the child's snoring, although often the apneic events themselves are apparent and a source of great anxiety. Parents may report keeping a vigil at bedside, intervening with frequent repositioning or partial arousal. Needless to say, this is problematic for both the parents and the child.

Features of OSA include daytime somnolence, behavioral problems (such as inattentiveness, hyperactivity, or irritability), and persistent enuresis. Mouth breathing is a general sign of nasal obstruction, and may be associated with OSA. Patients with nasal obstruction have a number of typical findings, including "adenoid facies" (open-mouthed stance), pectus excavatum, and rhinorrhea. In addition, the voice may have a hyponasal quality, arising from a lack of nasal resonance.

When interviewing the parents, it is important to identify signs that differentiate significant sleep disordered breathing (including both apneas and hypopneas) from snoring. After careful questioning, they may report neck extension, brief awakenings, exacerbation of obstruction when supine, and frequent positional changes. The untrained eye may not detect subtle or hidden findings such as paradoxical chest wall motion or intercostal and supraclavicular retractions. However, the characteristic gasping after partial arousal is generally noticed.

It is also important—as with any condition—to determine the duration of the signs that are suggesting OSA. Young children may have a marked lymphoid reaction during acute upper respiratory tract infections, with transient adenotonsillar hypertrophy. In many patients therefore, nocturnal dyspnea may resolve spontaneously or following antibiotic therapy. Adenotonsillectomy is still indicated if these episodes are frequently recurrent and troubling in and of themselves, even if there is improvement between infections. In addition, lymphoid tissue may rapidly hypertrophy, owing to neoplasm or other lymphoproliferative disorders. Such acute OSA may be fatal if not rapidly managed (4).

Certainly, at the initial evaluation of any OSA patient, congenital craniofacial anomalies should be specifically noted. Although such patients have typically been diagnosed in early infancy, subtle nonsyndromic abnormalities may be first noted when sleep apnea

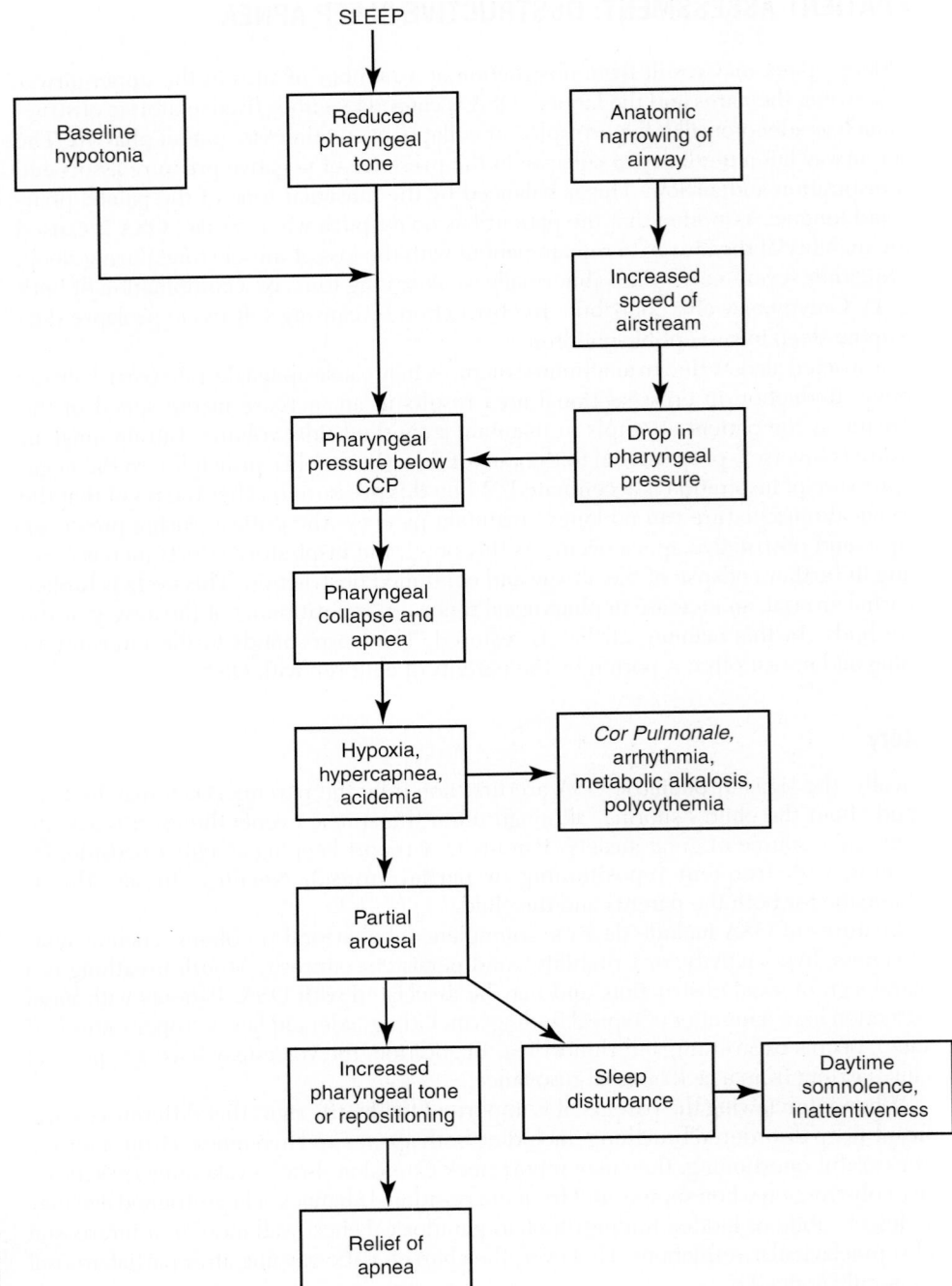

FIGURE 1 The physiology of obstructive sleep apnea and its complications. CCP, critical closing pressure.

develops. These patients fall into two groups, those characterized by hypoplasia of the lower face with obstruction at the level of the tongue base, and those noted to have relative midface hypoplasia (with nasal obstruction or nasopharyngeal narrowing) (5).

The former group is typified by the Pierre Robin sequence (PRS), the etiology of which is likely some type of intrauterine interference with mandibular growth, resulting in posterosuperior tongue displacement (glossoptosis) and potential clefting of the palate (Fig. 2). While the airway obstruction is generally not severe enough to cause asphyxia while awake, during sleep the relaxation of the pharyngeal and tongue base musculature may be enough to cause intermittent apnea and arousal. Therefore, these patients often

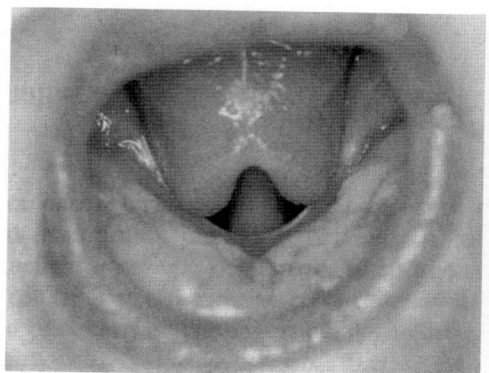

A

FIGURE 2 A, B: A child with Pierre Robin sequence, demonstrating the typical recessed mandible and posterior displacement of the tongue (glossoptosis). (From ref. 27, with permission.)

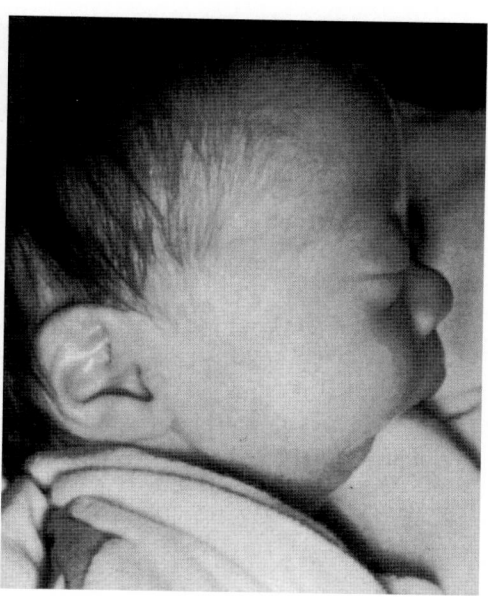

B

present with symptoms of OSA in early infancy, which tends to improve with mandibular growth and increasing muscular tone. PRS may be isolated or associated with other anomalies (which tends to worsen the clinical course) 6. A variety of other conditions are grouped with PRS in the context of mandibular hypoplasia and airway obstruction. These include branchial arch abnormalities such as the Treacher Collins and Goldenhar's syndromes, as well as Nager's, Hallermann-Streiff, and Brachmann-de Lange syndromes.

Patients with midfacial hypoplasia have a different clinical course. Nasal obstruction alone can be a cause of significant dyspnea in the first 2 months of life (the period of obligate nasal respiration). This is the case in children with choanal atresia, who require immediate correction in the perinatal period. However, patients with midfacial hypoplasia generally do not have complete nasal obstruction. Therefore, they will present with OSA later in childhood as general somatic growth outdistances the hypoplastic maxilla. The nocturnal difficulties may be maximized during the peak in relative volume of adenoid tissue (between ages 1 and 3), adding to the obstruction of the narrow nasal vault. Craniosynostosis patients fall into this category (Crouzon's, Apert's and Pfeiffer's syndromes) (7). Patients with Down syndrome also have a high incidence of OSA (8), which may be related to nasopharyngeal narrowing as well as macroglossia, hypotonia, and obesity.

Another setting for OSA is reduced pharyngeal resting tone, in which the tongue, palate, and pharyngeal musculature is weak and compliant even during waking hours. This is occasionally seen in neonates with hypotonia, and tends to improve with growth and development. In addition, this type of OSA may be acquired, and is often seen in neurologically devastated children. Such OSA is particularly pronounced in the supine position, due to posterior prolapse of the tongue or epiglottis.

One more unusual cause of OSA is seen in the child who has undergone surgery to compensate for velopharyngeal insufficiency (VPI). In VPI, there is inadequate closure of the soft palate against the posterior pharyngeal wall, resulting in hypernasal speech (excessive nasal resonance) or nasal reflux, or both. VPI may be primary, occur after adenoidectomy, or persist after repair of a cleft palate. Several surgical approaches to this problem have been described, the most common of which is the pharyngeal flap. In this procedure, a myomucosal flap is rotated up from the posterior pharyngeal wall and anchored to the palate, with the intent of partially obstructing the nasopharynx and improving the VPI. OSA and VPI represent opposite ends of the spectrum of nasopharyngeal obstruction, and if the flap is too bulky, OSA may result.

Physical Examination

There are two typical and contrasting body types associated with pediatric obstructive sleep apnea. The child with isolated adenotonsillar hypertrophy is often thin. This is thought to be caused by the increased work of breathing at night, or (rarely) from actual dysphagia related to pharyngeal obstruction. Nasal obstruction in young children may limit feeding as well, since respiration cannot continue during swallowing. This is most obvious in the continuous swallowing of bottle feeding, but occurs in older patients as well. Adenotonsillectomy has the greatest likelihood of success in these cases.

Obese children may have OSA related to abundant pharyngeal soft tissue. These patients are more likely to have multiple contributing factors including tonsillar hypertrophy, pharyngeal collapse, tongue prolapse, as well as restriction of diaphragmatic and chest wall excursion. Nevertheless, adenotonsillectomy may still be effective, by reducing oropharyngeal level obstruction, which increases airflow, countering the tendency of the airway to collapse at other levels.

Once OSA is suspected, the upper aerodigestive tract should be evaluated from the nares to the larynx. Nasal obstruction from reactive mucosal congestion or from structural anomaly (e.g. deviated septum) may be the sole cause of sleep disturbance, as mentioned earlier. By increasing nasal airflow, the lower portions of the pharynx may be "stented" open, compensating for collapse at other sites. This is the physiology behind a device sold as a cure for snoring, in which the nasal valve (a cartilaginous passage in the external nose) is dilated by an adhesive strip bonded to a metal spring. Certainly, in the absence of true nasal valve collapse, the patient is better served by identifying the underlying cause of nasal obstruction and treating it primarily.

The oropharynx should be examined for tonsillar hypertrophy. The typical "snorer's throat" may be noted, with a reduced anteroposterior diameter and long, floppy soft palate. The high arched palate or recessed upper lip seen in maxillary hypoplasia may result in daytime nasal obstruction as well as OSA. Adenoid hypertrophy generally exists along with tonsillar hypertrophy, and does not need independent documentation. However, if the tonsils are small or absent, and the voice is hyponasal, flexible endoscopy is indicated to examine the nasal cavity and nasopharynx for adenoid hypertrophy or other obstruction. Lateral neck films are frequently used to document adenoid hypertrophy, but endoscopy is more accurate and will demonstrate other pathology not seen on radiographs (such as pharyngeal collapse or tongue base obstruction). If the endoscopist is skilled, and the child is properly prepared, then nasal endoscopy will be well-tolerated. On the other hand, if the tonsils are enlarged and tonsillectomy is planned, it is not necessary to subject the child to the stress of endoscopy or the radiation and expense of lateral neck films, as the adenoids may be directly examined under general anesthesia.

The mandible should be assessed, as should the tongue. Obstruction at this level may be very difficult to treat, and may cause persistent symptoms after adenotonsillectomy. The clinician should make note of a reduced diameter in the hypopharynx, a large or posteriorly prolapsing tongue, and any degree of retrognathia or micrognathia. Obesity should be specifically noted, as this lessens the likelihood of success in treating OSA surgically. The obese child's health is at risk even in the absence of sleep apnea, and efforts toward weight loss should be initiated and maintained even after OSA has resolved.

The relationship of growth hormone (GH) and OSA is still unclear, but GH levels seem to be reduced in patients with sleep apnea, returning to normal after restoration of adequate nocturnal respiration. Furthermore, patients with acromegaly are known to be at risk for OSA, presumably because of abundant soft tissue in the tongue base, hypopharynx, and supraglottic larynx. These patients may also demonstrate muscle weakness that can contribute to pharyngeal collapse, as well as CA. Although apnea is rarely the presenting symptom of acromegaly, it should be specifically investigated in this disease. Fortunately, such apnea related to overproduction of GH generally resolves with successful treatment of the primary endocrine disorder, and surgery of the upper aerodigestive tract is rarely necessary.

Investigation

Sleep apnea is formally graded using PSG data. The sleep laboratory report includes the frequency of apneic events, as well as the physiologic effect (usually measured as the number and severity of desaturations, arrhythmias, and arousals). Hypopneas are also of interest, as a reduction in airflow can result in sleep disturbance without complete cessation of respiration. The respiratory disturbance index (RDI) is the number of apneas or hypopneas per hour, while the sleep disturbance index is the number of arousals per hour. The duration of each apnea is measured and used to determine whether or not it is a significant "apneic event". However, the duration itself is less important than the outcome (arousal and hypoxia) in determining the ultimate effect on mental status, right-sided heart function, and cardiac rhythm. CA is also detected, although arousal is less likely and desaturation less common when compared to obstructive events. In addition, PSG data include end tidal carbon dioxide concentration (which approximates arterial levels), electrooculogram (eye movements), submental and extremity electromyograms, and electroencephalogram to better characterize sleep architecture.

PSG is an expensive and somewhat invasive procedure, and is therefore not routinely performed on all children suspected of having OSA. Patients with complex head and neck anomalies or neurologic disease are typically referred for PSG. This is because such children often require multiple or complementary interventions, and an objective record of the nature of OSA is useful in long-term management. On the other hand, otherwise normal children with large tonsils and a clinical history strongly consistent with OSA may undergo tonsillectomy and adenoidectomy without PSG. Surgical results in these children are generally excellent, although there is some controversy in the literature regarding the correlation of the history with PSG evidence of OSA.

Frequently, the clinical history is equivocal, and the tonsils are only moderately enlarged. In this case, a sleep videotape is very helpful. The parents are instructed to capture the typical nocturnal dyspnea that prompted them to seek medical help. No effort is made to capture the entire night's sleep, but rather a representative sample. The assumption here is that if the OSA is clinically significant, the parents should be able to demonstrate it with a well-chosen 5- to 10- minute segment. Instructions are also given to capture the torso as well as the head in the frame, and to remove (or at least pull up) enough clothing to reveal intercostal retractions and paradoxical respiratory motion (i.e., abdominal retraction during chest wall expansion). Of course, the sound track should be recorded as well.

Audiotapes may be used successfully as well, if the parents do not have access to videotape equipment. However, the added information provided by video is useful, especially in differentiating the silence of apnea from the silence of transient abatement of snoring due to repositioning and improved airflow. If there is still a question as to the presence of apnea after observing a videotape or listening to an audiotape, the patient may be referred for PSG. While there is a good deal of clinical experience using tape studies in making the diagnosis of OSA, formal validation of this method is only now emerging in the literature.

Many health insurance corporations require objective documentation of sleep disturbance before authorizing adenotonsillectomy, or before allowing an overnight stay following the procedure. For this reason, home sleep studies have become popular as a method of providing evidence of sleep apnea. These studies are less comprehensive than full PSG, but can provide information regarding airflow, respiratory effort, and in some cases, oxygen saturation. They are less invasive and less expensive than PSG, and take place in the more familiar home environment. Unfortunately, they may be unreliable, owing to technical problems maintaining the electrodes on sleeping children outside of a supervised laboratory. Furthermore, some of these devices are prone to excessive artifact that may make the data difficult to interpret. While this type of investigation may prove necessary in some managed-care situations, audiotape or videotape studies are generally accepted as well. The availability of such services should not be interpreted to mean that a diagnosis of sleep disordered breathing on clinical grounds is impossible.

In addition to apnea, other significant respiratory disturbances may occur during sleep. As mentioned earlier, *hypopnea* refers to a diminution of airflow without cessation of respiration. The upper-airway resistance syndrome (UARS) implies an increase in intrathoracic negative pressure in the absence of significant apnea or hypopnea (9). These conditions may cause symptoms similar to OSA (e.g., daytime somnolence). For this reason, the results of any investigation must be interpreted by a clinician caring for the individual patient. Even in the absence of true apnea, sleep disordered breathing may be associated with significant sleep disturbance and daytime symptoms, and will respond to appropriate treatment.

If the cause of OSA remains unclear after a thorough physical examination, airway fluoroscopy may be helpful. In this study, a lateral cineradiograph of the upper airway is performed and recorded on videotape. Ideally, this should be done during normal sleep, since the use of sedatives may result in pharyngeal hypotonia that does not represent the patient's baseline. Children with daytime symptoms suggesting OSA (mouth breathing, hyponasal speech, dyspnea during feeding) may demonstrate collapse of the airway on fluoroscopy while awake. This study is helpful in pinpointing the level of obstruction, and tailoring therapy appropriately (10).

It is also important to reassure parents whose children have been thoroughly evaluated and found not to have significant nocturnal respiratory disturbance. Simple snoring is caused by vibratory motion in the soft palate associated with partial airway obstruction, but should not be associated with hypoxia, arousal, daytime symptoms, or cardiac complications. Parents should understand the nature of the problem, and possible solutions. Surgical therapy for snoring is typically limited to patients for whom marital harmony is threatened, and therefore rarely used in children. Snoring related to adenotonsillar hypertrophy alone should resolve with growth, and therefore adenotonsillectomy is not typically justified. However, weight loss in obese children or treatment of nasal obstruction can improve airflow and reduce palatine vibration.

👥 TREATMENT RECOMMENDATIONS: OBSTRUCTIVE SLEEP APNEA

Treatment of OSA is, of course, individualized. The most common etiology in children is adenotonsillar hypertrophy, and the vast majority of these patients are cured by tonsillectomy and adenoidectomy. Even without apparently massive tonsils, this surgery is often successful as tonsillar enlargement can be hidden from direct inspection by the palatoglossal fold ("iceberg tonsils"). Furthermore, tonsils may prolapse during sleep, causing greater impingement on the airway than is apparent on physical examination. Even a small increase in pharyngeal cross-sectional area may be enough to prevent development of the critical closing pressure. In all cases of tonsillectomy, consent is also obtained for adenoidectomy since it is expected that these two organs hypertrophy together. If the adenoid pad is then found to be small and nonobstructing, adenoidectomy is not performed so as to avoid the remote risk of complications such as VPI or nasopharyngeal stenosis.

As mentioned earlier, only if the tonsils are extremely small is it necessary to preoperatively evaluate the adenoids for hypertrophy. If a patient is scheduled for adenoidectomy and there is any question as to the contribution of the tonsils to airway obstruction, consent is also obtained for possible tonsillectomy. With the patient under general anesthesia, and the mouth gag in position, it is possible to directly examine the tonsils more thoroughly than in the office setting. Should the tonsils seem to have a large component hidden from view, they should be removed as well. In discussing these possibilities with parents, it is useful to describe tonsils and adenoids as different parts of the same organ (Waldeyer's ring of lymphoid tissue). In this case, the need for combined treatment is more easily understood, as is the contribution of both tonsils and adenoids to obstruction of the airway.

The technique of adenotonsillectomy is varied among surgeons, and unlikely to affect the ultimate success of the operation. It is important to initially palpate the tonsils to exclude the presence of large ectatic vessels at risk for injury. In addition, the palate should be examined to determine if an occult submucous cleft is present. This may be suggested by the presence of a bifid uvula with palpation, revealing a muscular diastasis in the soft palate or a notch in the posterior edge of the hard palate.

The author's preferred method of excision is electrocautery dissection of the tonsils in a subcapsular plane while holding firm, medially directed traction. Hemostasis is by judicious cauterization of bleeding points with a suction cautery, and no attempt is made to completely coagulate the entire bed. Punctuate arterial bleeding is controlled by hemostat and cautery. A dental mirror is used for hemostasis in the superior pole, which is both a common site of bleeding and difficult to visualize directly (Fig. 3). Adenoidectomy is then performed with curettes under visual control using a dental mirror (Fig. 4), with subsequent suction cautery hemostasis. If submucous cleft is present, the surgeon should perform a "superior-half" adenoidectomy (Fig. 5), in which the obstructed choanae are unblocked while leaving a cushion of tissue at the level of contact between the palate and the pharynx. This lessens the risk of postoperative VPI.

Patients undergoing adenotonsillectomy receive intraoperative dexamethasone (1 mg per kilogram, with a maximum dose of 12 mg) to reduce postoperative pain and dysphagia (11). In addition, ampicillin is given (40 mg per kilogram intravenously) followed by oral amoxicillin (20 mg per kilogram per day in three doses), substituting clindamycin in the case of penicillin allergy (15 mg per kilogram per day in three doses). This is continued for 5 days to reduce the foul taste and odor of necrotic debris in the pharynx (12).

Postoperative pain management is primarily by acetaminophen. The first dose is given as a rectal suppository (20 to 30 mg per kilogram) prior to emergence from anesthesia, providing analgesia during the postoperative period without relying on oral medication. Narcotics act as respiratory depressants, and are therefore avoided in children with OSA. In any case, narcotics are rarely needed in this setting, since the typical patient with OSA has tonsils that are easily dissected from their beds in a clean subcapsular plane. This is in contrast to patients undergoing tonsillectomy for recurrent pharyngitis with a scarred peritonsillar space from repeated infection.

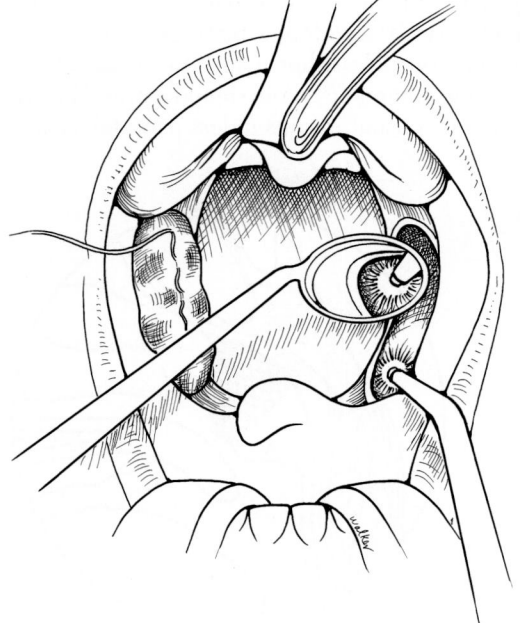

FIGURE 3 The dental mirror is used to allow precise hemostasis in the superior tonsillar pole with the suction cautery.

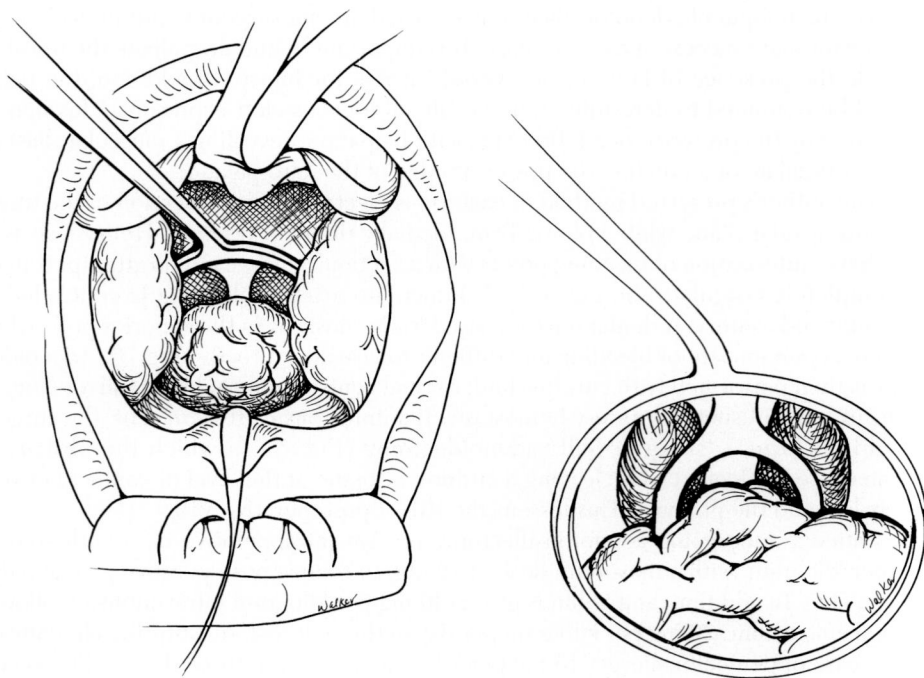

FIGURE 4 **A, B:** The dental mirror is used to visualize the adenoids, which allows for more precise and thorough removal of tissue with an adenoid curette.

A

B

Aspirin is not used for 2 weeks before or after surgery, and other nonsteroidal anti-inflammatory agents (NSAIDs) that may interfere with coagulation are also avoided in the perioperative period. Although this point is somewhat controversial, the few studies that have been done tend to support this last recommendation (13). Certainly, given the lack of a major analgesic advantage of NSAIDs and the apparent increase in both intra-operative blood loss and late hemorrhage, few clinicians use these drugs in tonsillectomy patients.

Diet is unrestricted except for the prohibition of sharp-edged foods (e.g., pretzels or chips) for the first 2 postoperative weeks. Providing palatable foods helps to maintain oral intake, and strict liquid diets do not reduce the risk of delayed hemorrhage. The parents are informed preoperatively that the delayed postoperative hemorrhage rate is 2% to 4% and that the most common time for bleeding is 5 to 10 days following surgery (during eschar separation). They are instructed not to fly or make other major travel plans for 2 weeks after surgery, and to immediately go to the emergency room should any oral bleeding be noted. This approach enhances informed consent, results in less parental anxiety

FIGURE 5 If submucous cleft is suspected, a "superior-half" adenoidectomy is performed, removing just enough tissue to unblock the choanae while leaving tissue at the level of contact between the soft palate and the pharynx.

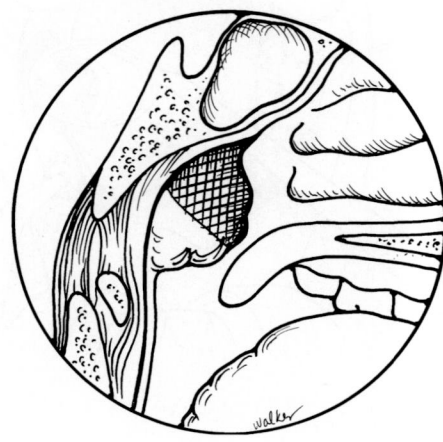

should bleeding occur, and provides for quicker evaluation by the surgeon. All such patients should be evaluated rapidly, as a small amount of bleeding may herald major hemorrhage a short time later.

Obstruction of the nasal vault may be chronic and tenacious despite aggressive medical and surgical therapy, especially when arising from inhalant allergies or recurrent sinusitis. Nevertheless, specific treatment should be pursued. A deviated septum, although common, is rarely a significant cause of nasal obstruction in children. Turbinate hypertrophy unresponsive to medical management may be addressed by resection or cautery. The former risks crusting and postoperative hemorrhage (lessened by the submucosal approach) while the latter risks recurrent nasal obstruction, especially if unipolar electrodes are used. Surgical technique in the treatment of nasal obstruction is fairly complex, and since this is rarely a major factor in pediatric OSA, it will not be discussed here in greater detail.

A less common cause of OSA in children is palatine-level obstruction. A long, floppy soft palate may prolapse against the posterior pharyngeal wall during sleep, resulting in snoring or apnea. Redundant mucosa in the region of the oropharynx may have the same results. Uvulopalatopharyngoplasty (UPPP) has been primarily applied to adult patients. This operation is very effective in selected individuals, and involves removing the tonsils and the posterior edge of the soft palate (including the uvula). The resultant mucosal defect is then closed with absorbable sutures. This procedure risks the development of VPI, and it is uncommonly performed on young children.

Children who have OSA following pharyngeal flap surgery may be helped by thinning the obstructing tissue band enough to relieve the nasopharyngeal obstruction, enlarging the lateral ports. Hopefully, enough of the flap will be retained so as to prevent recurrence of VPI. Of course, OSA is potentially fatal, while VPI is not. Therefore, if thinning of the flap is inadequate, the flap must be removed entirely.

Surgery on the lower jaw is reserved for patients in whom the more conservative measures, as already outlined, have failed, and in whom the apparent site of obstruction is at the level of the tongue base. Cephalometric radiographs will reveal the precise degree of micrognathia or retrognathia, and its contribution to airway obstruction. Most such procedures involve osteotomies of the mandible with advancement. Similarly, the hyoid bone may be suspended anteriorly from the mandible for patients with OSA related to tongue base or hypopharyngeal-level collapse. There is limited experience with these procedures for OSA, and they are generally not done in young children in whom significant future mandibular growth is anticipated.

A variety of devices and procedures have been developed for infants in whom airway obstruction results from congenital micrognathia or glossoptosis (as with the PRS). These strategies include using an apparatus to pull the mandible or tongue anteriorly, supports to fix a sleeping infant in pronation, nasopharyngeal airway stents, and tongue-lip adhesion to distract the tongue forward. All of these approaches rely on the assumptions that OSA in these children results solely from posterior prolapse of the tongue, and that it tends to resolve with growth and development. While the latter assumption is generally true, the former has not been borne out by direct endoscopic observations, which suggest that obstruction may also arise from lateral pharyngeal collapse (14). In any event, most of these devices are technically impractical. Furthermore, they all imply a degree of airway obstruction beyond that appropriate for conservative management (slow feeding, prone positioning, and observation for spontaneous improvement). Such severe obstruction is best treated with a temporary tracheotomy, which will more reliably relieve both OSA and difficulties with feeding related to airway obstruction.

While OSA related to mandibular hypoplasia tends to improve with growth, children with maxillary hypoplasia often suffer worsening OSA with age. Nasal- and nasopharyngeal-level obstruction is frequently seen in patients with isolated midface hypoplasia and those with craniosynostoses. Partial nasal obstruction in the perinatal period is treated with topical humidification (saline drops), judicious suctioning, and occasionally nasal steroids. Although some clinicians will use nasopharyngeal stents as a temporizing measure, the same caveat applies as in patients with micrognathia—severe obstruction is better treated with a temporary tracheotomy (15). These patients may eventually require craniofacial surgery. Midface advancement (e.g., by Le Fort III osteotomy) has been advocated but is technically difficult and not uniformly successful. Soft-palate split has also been recommended in selected cases to enlarge the nasopharyngeal airway.

Continuous positive airway pressure (CPAP) is administered by a snugly fitting nasal mask that is strapped over the face during sleep. When positive pressure is maintained, the collapsing airway is stented open. The advantages of CPAP include the avoidance of surgery and the ability to treat transient OSA with short-term therapy. In addition, some conditions (such as diffuse pharyngeal collapse or obesity) do not have simple surgical solutions short of tracheotomy. Apart from OSA that is the result of a prolapsing supraglottic obstruction (as in acquired laryngomalacia), CPAP effectively treats a wide variety of conditions. The disadvantages are discomfort and the difficulties small children have in tolerating the apparatus. Certainly, if a specific structure can be addressed surgically in a patient who is an acceptable operative risk (e.g., adenotonsillectomy), it is preferable to avoid prolonged dependence on a CPAP machine. However, in selected patients, CPAP may avoid tracheotomy and effectively relieve OSA. A more costly form of airway support is available: bi-level positive airway pressure (BIPAP). This is better-tolerated at high pressure levels since the device can be set to provide lower pressure during exhalation.

As mentioned earlier, patients with devastating neurologic injury may demonstrate pharyngeal hypotonia and airway collapse during sleep. An ethical question in this situation is how aggressive one should be in treating OSA, since in the absence of cardiac complications (arrhythmia or cor pulmonale), there may be no benefit in pursuing specific therapy. Management would most likely involve either CPAP or tracheotomy, both of which place an additional burden on the caregivers. Occasionally, such a patient will suffer from isolated epiglottic prolapse and will benefit from laryngoplasty (16).

PEARLS AND PERILS

1. Polysomnography provides a great deal of useful information, but is not necessary in the evaluation of all cases of suspected obstructive sleep apnea (OSA). It is most useful in complex patients with multifactorial OSA who may require serial interventions and objective interval evaluation.
2. Hypopnea and the upper-airway resistance syndrome can result in symptoms of OSA in the absence of complete apnea, and are treated in a similar fashion.
3. Sleep videotape is a readily available, noninvasive, and helpful diagnostic tool in cases where the parent history is equivocal. Care must be taken to frame the child's head and torso and to record the sound at high volume. Enough of the child's torso should be exposed to demonstrate chest wall motion, intercostal retractions, and paradoxical respiratory patterns.
4. Children undergoing adenotonsillectomy for OSA should generally be observed overnight in a monitored setting. Surgical edema, retained anesthetic agents, reduced respiratory drive, and postobstructive pulmonary edema may all contribute to respiratory distress on the first postoperative night.
5. Preoperative discussion with parents before adenotonsillectomy should include
   The possibility of persistent OSA (especially if the child is obese).
   The incidence of postoperative hemorrhage and instructions on what to do if this occurs.
   The anticipated change in voice as nasal obstruction is relieved, and resonance is increased.
   The possibility of adenoidal regrowth.
   Instructions on diet (no sharp-edged foods for 2 weeks, but otherwise unrestricted).
   Instructions on pain control (acetaminophen, no nonsteroidal antiinflammatory drugs, avoid narcotics).

Apnea monitors may be used for CA (see below), but have not been widely used in patients with OSA. This is because OSA is more likely to have a definable and treatable primary cause, while CA is more likely to be treated expectantly, waiting for maturation of the respiratory control mechanism. Furthermore, apnea monitors which work by detecting chest wall motion and not oxygen saturation may not differentiate respiratory efforts against obstruction from normal chest excursion until development of late sequelae (e.g., bradycardia or agonal respiration).

Finally, remember that obesity can contribute to OSA, and should be addressed in treating any such patient. This does not necessarily mean deferring other treatment indefinitely. Adenotonsillectomy, CPAP, or UPPP is frequently helpful even in the presence of obesity, and certainly should not be withheld pending weight loss. Obesity has many contributing factors—dietary, genetic, psychological, and cultural—and may persist despite the clinician's best efforts.

ⓘ MANAGEMENT OF COMPLICATIONS: OBSTRUCTIVE SLEEP APNEA

Complications of OSA can be categorized as neurologic, cardiovascular, hematologic, and metabolic. Behavioral problems such as inattentiveness and somnolence are the result of sleep disturbance, and tend to improve with the restoration of normal sleep architecture. Potentially irreversible neurologic injury and developmental delay may be caused by repeated hypoxia in severe OSA. Many syndromic children have been considered mentally retarded as a feature of their underlying dysmorphism, when aggressive treatment of OSA may have markedly improved their cognitive abilities.

Pulmonary vascular resistance is increased by chronic hypoxia or hypercapnia, and may lead to acquired right-sided heart failure or cardiomegaly (cor pulmonale). This is thought to be due to increased vascular tone in the pulmonary arterial vessels. In addition, apnea is associated with cardiac arrhythmia in both infants and older patients. Bradycardia is a common associated finding in neonates, and may progress to asystole if the apnea is not relieved. This and other bradyarrhythmias (such as conduction blocks) are linked to vagal reflexes. Hypoxia can cause ventricular ectopy as well as bradycardia by stimulating peripheral chemoreceptors.

Chronically hypoxic patients develop polycythemia due to increased erythropoiesis, which can also elevate pulmonary artery pressures (by sludging in the microvasculature). Similarly, hypoxic episodes may cause patients with sickle cell disease to suffer a crisis with small-vessel obstruction. Chronic carbon dioxide retention causes an increased tolerance to hypercapnia in the brainstem respiratory center. The primary stimulus to breathe may thus become the compensatory hypoxic respiratory drive, and these patients can become apneic following relief of OSA or if given supplemental oxygen. This is similar to the situation found in adults with chronic obstructive pulmonary disease.

Finally, young infants with the chronic respiratory acidosis of OSA will develop a compensatory metabolic alkalosis. This can lead to reduced tissue oxygen delivery despite the presence of adequate oxygen saturation. If the same patients have nasal airway obstruction, they will experience difficulty with feeding. Thus, impaired peripheral metabolism and malnutrition can lead to both failure to thrive and interference with cognitive development. All of these complications are best treated by managing the underlying OSA, although chronic systemic changes may be slow to resolve.

Complications of Treatment

The treatment of OSA may result in complications as well. The most feared early complication of adenotonsillectomy is hemorrhage. While the occasional cooperative adolescent or adult may allow control with silver nitrate cautery in the examining chair, young children should be returned to the operating room. This provides for thorough examination and better hemostasis, which is especially important in a patient with a small blood volume and lesser margin of safety. Odynophagia is also seen universally after tonsillectomy, and occasionally requires admission for intravenous hydration.

The first night after adenotonsillectomy for OSA is associated with a small but significant risk of increased respiratory distress (17), potentially due to a number of factors. Surgical edema may not reach its peak in the palate and pharynx until several hours after surgery. Residual anesthetic agent may take 12 hours or more to be completely eliminated, resulting in reduced pharyngeal muscular tone and respiratory drive. The reduction in carbon dioxide retention and an increase in blood oxygen saturation after successful surgery may result in CA, owing to the patient's increased tolerance for hypercapnia and reliance on hypoxic respiratory drive. Finally, there is the possibility of pulmonary edema following the relief of long-standing partial airway obstruction (18). For these reasons, patients undergoing adenotonsillectomy for significant OSA should be in a monitored setting on the first postoperative night (the pediatric intensive care unit, the recovery room, or a dedicated observation unit).

There is some controversy in the literature regarding this recommendation, and there is a growing experience with outpatient surgery of all types as a response to financial pressures. If the patient has severe enough OSA to warrant surgery, it is the author's opinion that at this point the costs of overnight observation are generally outweighed by the benefits of ensuring adequate resolution of airway obstruction. However, every patient should be evaluated individually, and some patients may be appropriate for discharge after shorter periods of observation (e.g., healthy patients over age 3 with isolated adenotonsillar hypertrophy).

Late complications of both UPPP and adenotonsillectomy include VPI and nasopharyngeal stenosis. VPI is more common, and may be associated with an unsuspected submucous cleft of the soft palate or other form of palatine dysfunction. Removal of the adenoids can unmask occult VPI that was compensated for by nasopharyngeal lymphoid tissue. This is often transient, and improves as the patient becomes better able to form an appropriate palatopharyngeal seal during phonation. Even in the absence of true VPI, parents will notice a change in the child's voice as nasal obstruction is relieved and resonance is increased. Because of this, all parents are told preoperatively to expect a change away from the familiar hyponasal quality (an anticipated outcome and not a complication).

Nasopharyngeal stenosis is a very serious complication that may occur after aggressive adenoidectomy resulting in a near-circumferential open wound in the pharynx that heals by contracture. The patient may be left with a pinhole opening to the nasopharynx, or complete obstruction. Local tissue flap reconstruction, often requiring multiple stages, is required to correct this problem (19).

Adenoid regrowth after surgery occurs on occasion. In tonsillectomy, the excised tissue is encapsulated, and is dissected cleanly from the tonsillar bed. The adenoids, however, are a carpet of submucosal lymphoid tissue in the nasopharynx, and are usually "shaved" with a curette or other cutting instrument (although some recommend the use of cautery only so as to avoid the complication of VPI). Despite the method used, there is a chance for regrowth of obstructing tissue since it is impossible to remove all lymphoid material from the nasopharynx (and inadvisable to try to do so). It is important to discuss this with the parents preoperatively, and to also mention the expected eventual regression of adenoid tissue should this occur.

Nasal CPAP may quickly overcome OSA, but its very success harbors a potential complication. Sleep-deprived patients who are able to eventually sleep may enter a state known as *rebound*, in which the rapid eye movement phase (REM sleep) is accentuated, and respiratory drive may be reduced, resulting in central sleep apnea (CSA). Furthermore, relief of hypoxia and hypercapnia may also result in CSA due to chronic changes in the central respiratory control mechanism as described earlier. For this reason, CPAP is typically initiated in a sleep laboratory so that the first night's sleep is under monitored conditions.

⚉ PATIENT ASSESSMENT: CENTRAL APNEA

CA (or periodic breathing) is the cessation of respiratory efforts, and is primarily a disease of early infancy. Premature infants are especially prone to such apnea, and for this reason the PSG duration criteria for an apneic event are 10 seconds in adults, 15 seconds in infants, and 20 seconds in preterm newborns. These patients are thought to have apnea related to an immaturity of central control mechanisms (20), which fail to respond normally to rising carbon dioxide levels by increasing respiratory efforts. This is accentuated during sleep as the ventilatory drive is further depressed. In addition, respiratory muscle activity may be discoordinated in neonates, resulting in glottic closure and tongue prolapse during inspiration, adding an obstructive component to CA.

Apnea usually presents within the first week of life, and may delay discharge from the newborn nursery. However, significant apnea with bradycardia or hypoxia is rare in full-term neonates and typically abates by 37 weeks' gestational age in premature infants. It is important to realize that respiratory depressants may make former premature infants at risk for new, life-threatening apnea. Because of this, overnight monitoring is recommended after general anesthesia for these children up to 60 weeks after conception (21), and some centers follow this protocol for all infants under 5 months of age.

Persistent apnea warrants a search for an underlying cause, especially in full-term infants. Just as with sepsis, very young infants do not localize physical findings well and systemic conditions may present as apnea. Possible etiologies to be considered include infections (particularly with the respiratory syncytial virus), metabolic disorders including hypoglycemia and hypocalcemia, maternal drug use and withdrawal, subclinical seizure activity, increased intracranial pressure, or other occult neurologic disease. The Arnold-Chiari syndrome involves caudal displacement of the brainstem or nuclear dysgenesis. This can result in both bilateral vocal cord paralysis and CA, causing hypoxia even following tracheotomy for airway obstruction. Reflux of gastric contents may irritate vagal afferents resulting in "reflex apnea." This may also result in aspiration and laryngospasm (which adds an obstructive component). Finally, the child should be closely observed during apnea to rule out the possibility that the apnea is primarily obstructive. The clinician should look for respiratory efforts and increased airflow with manual jaw opening. On rare occasion, if no treatable cause is found, an infant may be discharged home with an apnea monitor. PSG is occasionally used in infants, but the standards for normal sleep architecture in these patients have only recently emerged (22). In this case, pH probe monitoring is also included to detect gastroesophageal reflux.

In some cases, apneic events are not detected until after discharge of the newborn from the hospital. Parents may bring an apparently well child to the emergency department, terrified after having found the infant limp or cyanotic. A history is frequently given of a rapid response to stimulation, and cardiopulmonary resuscitation may have even been initiated. The term for this condition is an *apparent life-threatening event* (ALTE). It is not known whether such patients would have become cases of SIDS had the parents not intervened; certainly few caregivers would simply observe such a child for spontaneous improvement. It may be that the infant is frequently cycling through unnoticed episodes of apnea without ill effect. In any case, ALTE should be evaluated as already described for apnea of infancy, to rule out any treatable etiology and to initiate monitoring if appropriate.

CA may be associated with a few other conditions that rarely afflict children. Hyperventilation results in hypocapnia and occasionally CSA. In this case, the patient's response to carbon dioxide is normal, but the blood carbon dioxide level is low and apnea results when sleep further depresses respiration. This is generally seen in adults at high altitudes, and is uncommon in children. In contrast, congenital central alveolar hypoventilation (CCAH) is a primary failure of respiratory drive, while the Cheyne-Stokes breathing pattern implies cyclical apnea usually related to congestive heart failure or central nervous system disease. In these conditions, the patient has an abnormally reduced response to rising carbon dioxide levels.

CCAH is also known as Ondine's curse—named for the mythologic nymph who cursed her unfaithful human lover by requiring conscious effort for him to breathe. In this disease, there is a primary failure of the autonomic mechanism that controls breathing. Some cases are associated with Hirschprung's disease (23), implying a common autonomic neural dysgenesis. Rarely, Ondine's curse may be first noted in adult men. When arising later in life, apnea may actually be the secondary result of an acquired insult to the central nervous system (such as multiple sclerosis or a space-occupying lesion). CCAH typically presents with sleep hypopnea, as the tendency toward disordered breathing is diminished during waking hours. In addition, these children display hypotonia, cor pulmonale, other signs of autonomic dysfunction (such as syncope), and a measurably impaired respiratory response to hypercapnia. Mortality is high unless treatment is initiated promptly.

⏩ TREATMENT RECOMMENDATIONS: CENTRAL APNEA

Apnea of infancy or prematurity is generally self-limited and improves with maturation of the central nervous system. Individual events resolve with tactile stimulation, or spontaneously if observation is continued. Nevertheless, if CSA is severe, these patients are at risk for the complications described previously (such as failure to thrive, psychomotor retardation, and cor pulmonale). A more controversial point is whether or not to institute home cardiorespiratory monitoring for infants with lesser degrees of apnea, in hopes of avoiding SIDS.

SIDS is perhaps one of the most terrifying specters of parenthood. Despite considerable attention and research, the underlying cause of SIDS remains elusive (24). Unlike OSA (with its characteristic findings and its typically indolent course), SIDS—as the name implies—is sudden and by definition unpredictable. One large study failed to reveal a correlation between SIDS and apnea in the 29 of 10,000 monitored infants (25), and there is little data to demonstrate any connection between apnea and sudden death.

Because of the lack of supporting data, most academic neonatology centers recognize that home monitoring of otherwise healthy infants with apnea is unlikely to be beneficial. Furthermore, it may add to familial stress through false alarms and interference with the normal bonding process. Nevertheless, such monitoring is often instituted by clinicians. In the individual case, there may be considerable pressure from the parents to provide a monitor, as well as the physician's strong instinct to err on the side of safety given the general state of ignorance regarding the etiology of SIDS. This pressure is even stronger in a family that has already lost one child in this manner, despite the lack of evidence for the utility of monitoring. Such parents may take turns standing watch all night over a sleeping infant. Many clinicians believe that the "security" of short-term monitoring is appropriate even though this has not been shown to prevent SIDS in siblings of victims.

If an apnea monitor is to be used, caregivers must be fully instructed in the application of the device, and understand when false alarms are occurring. Furthermore, they must develop some degree of clinical acumen, and be able to assess the child's respiratory patterns, skin pallor or cyanosis, and degree of respiratory discomfort. The monitor is not a panacea, and is no substitute for a thorough medical evaluation and continued vigilance for new signs and symptoms by the physician. The American Academy of Pediatrics's "supine sleep" campaign has probably contributed more to reducing SIDS mortality than has home monitoring, although the physiologic reason for its success is still unclear (26). It is important to remember that the reverse of this recommendation holds true for some infants, including those with gastroesophageal reflux or OSA related to retrognathia or glossoptosis, who should be positioned prone for sleep.

Respiratory stimulants are occasionally used in patients with CSA, although generally not by otolaryngologists. Medications such as doxapram and the methylxanthines (caffeine and theophylline) may be used for CSA expected to be transient, and are generally not continued beyond 2 months after full term. Side effects of agitation and irritability limit their long-term use. Additionally, there is some experience using CPAP in neonates with apnea, although generally not outside of a hospital nursery. This may be beneficial in infants with both mild central and obstructive apnea that is expected to be transient.

CA or hypoventilation that does not resolve and requires chronic treatment (such as in Ondine's curse) is usually managed by assisted ventilation. There are four strategies for this approach: positive-pressure ventilation through tracheotomy, noninvasive respiratory support (BIPAP), negative-pressure ventilation, and respiratory pacing. Tracheotomy has the advantage of providing access for pulmonary toilet, which is useful in children with other neurologic disorders who are at risk for aspiration. BIPAP provides variable ventilatory support in inspiration and expiration, and is useful when partial ventilation is required. Negative-pressure ventilation (using the cuirass apparatus) assists with respiration by causing expansion of the chest wall and entrainment of air. Diaphragmatic or phrenic nerve stimulation by an implantable pacemaker is a more recent option, and is effective in children with CCAH syndrome.

PEARLS AND PERILS

1. Premature infants are prone to apneas of longer than 20 seconds, and continue to be at risk until approximately 37 weeks after conception.
2. Former premature infants are at increased risk for postoperative apnea following general anesthesia, and should be monitored overnight when younger than 60 weeks after conception. Some centers extend this precaution to term infants undergoing surgery before the age of 5 months.
3. Central apnea in a full-term neonate should not be considered idiopathic "apnea of infancy" until all other causes are ruled out. This includes sepsis, seizure activity and other neurologic disorders, metabolic disorders, obstructive apnea, and maternal substance abuse.
4. Central apnea is most concerning when cyanosis and bradycardia accompany the episodes. These infants are more likely to benefit from specific treatment or monitoring.
5. There is no consensus on the etiology of sudden infant death syndrome (SIDS), but simple apnea without cyanosis or bradycardia is unlikely to be causative. Home cardiorespiratory monitoring has not been shown to reduce the rate of SIDS, but it is still used for selected infants with significant apnea.

⬤ MANAGEMENT OF COMPLICATIONS: CENTRAL SLEEP APNEA

CSA can have many of the same systemic complications as OSA, including psychomotor retardation, arrhythmia, and failure to thrive. These sequelae are most common if the CSA is chronic and untreated. Despite intensive investigation, the link between CA and SIDS remains unproved, and only children with severe episodes involving cyanosis and bradycardia are presumed to be at increased risk for sudden death.

⬤ REFERENCES

1. Aserinsky E, Kleitman N. Regular occurring periods of eye motility and concomitant phenomena during sleep. *Science* 1953;118:273.
2. Koopmann C, Moran W. Sleep apnea—an historical perspective. *Otolaryngol Clin North Am* 1990;23:571–575.

3. Marcus CL, Omlin KJ, Basinki DJ et al. Normal polysomnographic values for children and adolescents. *Am Rev Respir Dis* 1992;146:1235–1239.

4. Hague K, Catalano P, Rothschild M, Strauchen JA, Fyfe B. Posttransplant lymphoproliferative disease presenting as sudden respiratory arrest in a 3 year old child. *Ann Otol Rhinol Laryngol* 1997;106(3):244–247.

5. Rothschild MA. Craniofacial abnormalities and upper airway obstruction. *Curr Opin Otolaryngol Head Neck Surg* 1995;3:396–401.

6. Tomaski S, Zalzal G, Saal H. Airway obstruction in the Pierre Robin sequence. *Laryngoscope* 1995;105:111–114.

7. Kakitsuba N, Sadaoka T, Motoyama S, et al. Sleep apnea and sleep-related breathing disorders in patients with craniofacial synostosis. *Acta Otolaryngol Suppl (Stockh)* 1994;517:6–10.

8. Jacobs In, Gray RF, Todd NW. Upper airway obstruction in children with Down syndrome. *Arch Otolaryngol Head Neck Surg* 1996;122:945–950.

9. Newman JP, Clerk AA, Moore M, Utley DS, Terris DJ. Recognition and surgical management of the upper airway resistance syndrome. *Laryngoscope* 1996;106:1089–1093.

10. Gibson SE, Myer CM III, Strife JL, O'Connor DM. Sleep fluoroscopy for localization of upper airway obstruction in children. *Ann Otol Rhinol Laryngol* 1996;105:678–683.

11. April MM, Callan ND, Nowak DM, Hausdorff MA. The effect of intravenous dexamethasone in pediatric adenotonsillectomy. *Arch Otolaryngol Head Neck Surg* 1996;122:117–120.

12. Telian SA, Handler SD, Fleisher GR, Baranak CC, Wetmore RF, Potsic WP. The effect of antibiotic therapy on recovery after tonsillectomy in children. A controlled study. *Arch Otolaryngol Head Neck Surg* 1986;112:610–615.

13. Gunter JB, Varughese AM, Harrington JF, et al. Recovery and complications after tonsillectomy in children:a comparison of ketorolac and morphine. *Anesth Analg* 1995;81:1136–1141.

14. Sher AE, Shprintzen RJ, Thorpy MJ. Endoscopic observations of obstructive sleep apnea in children with anomalous upper airway: predictive and therapeutic value. *Int J Pediatr Otorhinolaryngol* 1986;11:135–146.

15. Sirotnak J, Brodsky L, Pizzuto M. Airway obstruction in the Crouzon syndrome: case report and review of the literature. *Int J Pediatr Otorhinolaryngol* 1995;31:235–246.

16. Woo P. Acquired laryngomalacia: epiglottis prolapse as a cause of airway obstruction [see comments]. *Ann Otol Rhinol Laryngol* 1992;101:314–320.

17. Rothschild MA, Catalano P, Biller HF. Ambulatory pediatric tonsillectomy and the identification of high-risk subgroups. *Otolaryngol Head Neck Surg* 1994;110:203–210.

18. Guffin TN, Har el G, Sanders A, Lucente FE, Nash M. Acute Postobstructive pulmonary edema. *Otolaryngol Head Neck Surg* 1995;112:235–237.

19. Cotton RT. Nasopharyngeal stenosis. *Arch Otolaryngol* 1985;111:146–148.

20. Henderson Smart DJ, Pettigrew AG, Campbell DJ. Clinical apnea and brain-stem neural function in preterm infants. *N Engl J Med* 1983;308:353–357.

21. Kurth CD, Spitzer AR, Broennle AM, Downes JJ. Postoperative apnea in preterm infants. *Anesthesiology* 1987;66:483–488.

22. Kahn A, Dan B, Groswasser J, Franco P, Sottiaux M. Normal sleep architecture in infants and children. *J Clin Neurophysiol* 1996;13:184–197.

23. el Halaby E, Coran AG. Hirschsprung's disease associated with Ondine's curse: report of three cases and review of the literature. *J Pediatr Surg* 1994;29:530–535.

24. Bergman A. Wrong turns in sudden infant death syndrome research. *Pediatrics* 1997;99:119–121.

25. Southall DP, Richards JM, Rhoden KJ, et al. Prolonged apnea and cardiac arrhythmias in infants discharged from neonatal intensive care units: failure to predict an increased risk for sudden infant death syndrome. *Pediatrics* 1982;70:844–851.

26. Positioning and SIDS: American Academy of Pediatrics Task Force on Infant Positioning and SIDS. *Pediatrics* 1992;89:1120–1126.

27. Andrews TM. Airway obstruction in craniofacial anomalies. In: Myer CM III, Cotton RT, Shott SR, eds. *The pediatric airway*. Philadelphia: JB Lippincott Co., 1995;247–261.

M. A. Rothschild: Departments of Otolaryngology and Pediatrics, Mount Sinai School of Medicine, Mount Sinai Medical Center, New York, New York 10029.

• *Practical Pediatric Otolaryngology*
• edited by Robin T. Cotton and Charles M. Myer, III
• Lippincott-Raven Publishers, Philadelphia © 1999

4

Assessment of Speech and Language Disorders in Children

Ann W. Kummer

Verbal communication depends on the development of normal speech and language skills. These skills affect the way an individual is able to function in society, and impact most activities of daily living. Unfortunately, an estimated 6-million children under the age of 18 have a speech or language disorder, as estimated by the National Institutes of Health (1). Boys make up about two-thirds of this population. Many children identified as late or slow talkers at the age of 2 continue to have language problems at the age of 4 (2). At this time, the risk of developing learning problems is very high, and the communication disorder can have a negative impact on the child's social interactions and relationships. Since a communication disorder can have a significantly adverse effect on the developing child, the development of communication skills should be closely monitored, particularly in the preschool years.

Pediatricians and parents often consult with an otolaryngologist when a young child demonstrates communication difficulties. The first assumption may be that the poor speech or lack of adequate speech is due to faulty hearing. Another assumption may be that the speech difficulty is due to an abnormality of the oral cavity or vocal tract. Although the otolaryngologist may feel comfortable assessing anatomic or physiologic abnormalities, the physician may have more difficulty in determining the nature of the communication disorder, the actual cause in many cases, and the appropriate method of treatment.

The purpose of this chapter is to give an overview of normal speech and language development, and to discuss common speech and language disorders in children. This chapter is also meant to be used by the physician as a guide to the assessment of communication disorders in patients who present in the office. This information should help the otolaryngologist to adequately address the concerns of parents, and to know when to initiate a referral to a speech-language pathologist for further evaluation and treatment.

DEFINITIONS

Speech

Speech, or *articulation*, can be defined as the physical production of individual sounds. Speech requires the rapid movement of the oral articulators, such as the lips, tongue, jaw, and velum. This movement for articulation must be made in coordination with respiration and phonation in order to form individual speech sounds. These sounds are then combined and produced in sequence to form spoken words. The term *phonology* is sometimes used in association with articulation. *Phonology* refers to the rules that govern the combination of sounds into syllables and words.

Language

While speech is a physical component of verbal communication, language is the cognitive component. *Language* can be defined as the meaning or the message conveyed back and forth between individuals. Verbal language requires the use of words, phrases, and sentences to convey information to the listener. Language also can take other forms or modalities, such as reading and writing, signs, and even facial expressions and gestures.

HOW SPEECH IS PRODUCED

With every instrument that is capable of producing sound, there are usually three key components: (a) a vibrating mechanism that can be set in motion to produce sound, (b) a stimulating mechanism that can set the vibration in motion, and (c) a resonating mechanism to reinforce or amplify the sound. In human speech, the vocal folds are the vibrating bodies, the force of breath pressure is the stimulating force, and the cavities of the vocal tract provide the mechanism for resonating the sound energy. The acoustic product is then altered for different speech sounds by varying the size and shape of the oral cavity through the placement and movement of the articulators.

Respiration and Phonation

Respiration not only is important for life support, but also is important for speech. The air pressure from the lungs is what provides the motivating force for phonation and the energy for speech. During quiet breathing, the inspiratory and expiratory phases are fairly equal in duration. During speech, however, there is a quick period of inspiration prior to the initiation of an utterance. Air pressure, through expiration, is then maintained under the vocal folds during the entire utterance. The expiratory phase may be short or relatively long, depending on the length of the produced utterance. The inspiratory and expiratory phases are controlled by the speaker during speech production.

Phonation is the sound that is produced when the vocal folds begin to vibrate. This sound, or voice, is used for the production of all vowel sounds. It is used for only about half of the consonant sounds, however, as discussed below.

Resonance

Resonance refers to the sound quality that occurs as the sound energy from the vocal folds resonates, or vibrates, as it travels through the cavities of the vocal tract. The size and shape of the pharyngeal cavity, oral cavity, and nasal cavity all affect the overall acoustic product of the voice. The function of the velopharyngeal valve controls the amount of sound energy that enters the oral cavity and nasal cavity for each produced sound. Too much sound energy in the nasal cavity during speech results in *hypernasality*, whereas too little nasal resonance results in *hyponasality*. An abnormal blockage of sound energy anywhere in the vocal tract will cause *cul-de-sac resonance*. (Resonance disorders are discussed in Chapter 50.)

Articulation

Individual speech sounds, in contrast to letters, are often referred to as *phonemes*. For example, /ch/ is two letters, but only one speech sound or phoneme. Phonetic symbols, rather than the letters, are usually used in speech pathology, but the English letters are used in this chapter. Phonemes are classified as either vowels or consonants. This classification is based on the amount of obstruction in the oral cavity during production.

Vowels are produced with a relatively open oral cavity. The sound energy from the vocal folds and the air pressure from the lungs pass through the oral cavity with very little obstruction. The acoustic product is the result of the shape of the oral cavity, as defined by the position of the tongue and the lips. Vowels tend to be classified by tongue height (high, mid, or low), tongue position (front, central or back), and lip rounding (present or absent).

Consonants are produced by partial or complete obstruction of the oral cavity during production. Consonants are classified by the place of articulation, manner of articulation, and voicing. Table 1 shows the classification of consonants based on these parameters.

The *place of articulation* is the point in the vocal tract where the greatest constriction is found. There are seven points of constriction along the vocal tract from the lips to the glottis. Therefore, for classification of phonemes by place of articulation, there are bilabial sounds (p, b, m, w), labiodental sounds (f, v), dental sounds (voiceless th and voiced th), alveolar sounds (t, d, s, z, n, l), palatal sounds (sh, zh, ch, j, r, y), velar sounds (k, g, ng), and the glottal sound (h).

The *manner of production* refers to the way in which the sound is produced and the amount of blockage of the airstream. *Plosives* (p, b, t, d, k, g), sometimes referred to as *stop-plosives* or even *stops*, are sounds that are produced with total blockage somewhere along the vocal tract, followed by a sudden release of the air pressure and sound. *Fricatives* (f, v, th, s, z, sh, zh, and h) are sounds that are produced with the articulators close enough together to cause a friction sound when the airstream is forced through the narrow passage. *Affricates* (ch and j) are produced by combining a plosive and a fricative and producing both at the same time. For example, /ch/ is produced by combining /t/ plus /sh/. The /j/ sound is produced by combining /d/ plus /zh/. Some fricatives and affricates are also called *sibilants* (s, z, sh, zh, ch, j) since they are characterized by their high-frequency energy. When sibilant sounds are produced, the sound and air are forced between the tongue and alveolar ridge and also between the closed teeth. *Nasals* (m, n, ng) are produced with complete closure somewhere in the oral cavity and the velum down. As a result, sound energy resonates in the oral cavity and the nasal cavity, and much of the air pressure and sound are released in the nasal cavity. *Liquids* (l, r) are produced with many variations, depending on the position in the word and the phonemic context. Finally, *glides* (w and y), which are also called *semivowels*, are produced with gliding movement and minimal constriction of the oral cavity.

Voicing refers to the vibration of the vocal folds during the sound production. Although all vowels and most consonants are *voiced* during production, some consonants are actually *voiceless*. The consonants that are classified as plosives, fricatives, and affricates occur in voiced/voiceless cognate pairs. Although they are produced at the same place of articulation and with the same manner, one is voiceless and the other is voiced (p/b, t/d, k/g, f/v, s/z, sh/zh, th as in "thin"/th as in "then," and ch/j). Voiced phonemes are

TABLE 1: Classification of English Phonemes according to Place of Articulation, Manner of Articulation, and Voicing

Manner of Articulation	Voicing	Place of Articulation						
		Bilabial	Labiodental	Dental	Alveolar	Palatal	Velar	Glottal
Plosives	Voiceless	p	—	—	t	—	k	—
	Voiced	b	—	—	d	—	g	—
Fricatives	Voiceless	—	f	th (thin)	s	sh	—	h
	Voiced	—	v	th (then)	z	zh	—	—
Affricates	Voiceless	—	—	—	—	ch	—	—
	Voiced	—	—	—	—	j	—	—
Nasals	Voiced	m	—	—	n	—	ng	—
Liquids	Voiced	—	—	—	l	r	—	—
Glides	Voiced	w	—	—	—	y	—	—

typically produced with less intraoral breath pressure than their voiceless cognates, owing to the blockage of the vocal folds at the level of the glottis.

PEARLS AND PERILS

1. At 2 months:
   Watches the speaker's face.
   Cries are differentiated by needs.
   Coos with vowel sounds.
2. At 4 to 6 months:
   Localizes to sound.
   Coos with intonation.
   Vocalizes to others.
3. At 6 to 9 months:
   Responds to name.
   Recognizes names of family members.
   Responds to simple commands accompanied by a gesture.
   Uses gesture for communication (pointing, reaching, waving for hi or bye).
   Imitates actions (as in peek-a-boo).
   Babbles using early developmental consonants (i.e., b, m, w, d, n, g).
4. At 10 to 12 months:
   Begins to point to some body parts following a command.
   Follows simple, one-part commands (i.e., Get your shoe).
   Gives objects to others upon verbal request.
   Jargons with different sound combinations.
   May begin to use first words.
5. At 12 to 18 months:
   Can identify many objects and pictures following a verbal command.
   Follows commands easily.
   Listens more to the meaning of conversations.
   Uses several single words.
   Communicates with a combination of words and gestures.
6. At 18 to 24 months:
   Understands concepts (adjectives, pronouns, plurals).
   Follows compound and complex commands.
   Uses two-to three-word combinations.
   Tries to tell about experiences.
   Begins to use more speech sounds such as fricatives (f, s, sh).
7. At 2 to 3 years:
   Shows interest in explanations for "why" and "how" questions.
   Uses phrases and short sentences for communication.
   Begins to use more complex morphologic and syntactic forms.
8. At 3 to 4 years:
   Uses long and structurally complex sentences.
   Tells stories and relates experiences from the past.
   Errors in syntax include regularization of irregular forms.
   Speech is intelligible to all listeners, although minor articulation errors are noted.

In connected speech, articulation is influenced by the stress of individual phonemes and the intonation of the utterance. *Stress* is related to increased muscular effort and subglottic pressure during the production of a syllable. Stressed syllables are produced with greater articulatory precision and are longer in duration than unstressed syllables.

In addition, they tend to be higher in pitch and intensity. *Intonation* refers to the frequent changes in pitch throughout an utterance, as controlled by the rate of vibration of the vocal folds and the tension of the muscles of the larynx. Although there are changes in pitch throughout connected speech, there tends to be a drop in pitch at the end of each statement and an increase in pitch at the end of a question. Both stress and intonation are used for emphasis and also to help to convey meaning.

As can be noted above, speech is a very complicated act that requires the coordination of respiration, phonation, and the manner and placement of articulation. Movement must be done quickly and accurately, and with appropriate stress and intonation. Speech also must be produced in conjunction with cognition and language function for communication. Any errors or breakdown in this coordinated process can be symptomatic of a communication disorder.

NORMAL DEVELOPMENT

In assessing articulation and language disorders in children, it is important to have a clear understanding of what is normal at each developmental stage. Of course, children do not begin speaking with perfect articulation and structurally complex sentences. The development of these skills occurs gradually over a period of 6 or more years. During the course of speech and language learning, normal "developmental errors" are noted and these errors should not be mistaken for an abnormality or disorder.

Both articulation and language skills begin to develop at birth. Although these skills develop concurrently, each component is discussed separately for the sake of clarity.

Speech (Articulation)

Articulation development actually begins with the birth cry. With early cries, the infant must coordinate respiration, phonation, and oral movement in order to produce sound.

Vocal play and purposeful sound making begin around 2 months when the infant begins to coo. *Cooing* consists of sighs and various vowel sounds that are produced as a form of vocal play. This is an important stage of articulation development since the child begins to learn to manipulate the oral mechanism to produce sounds in a purposeful manner. In addition, the child learns to associate tactile-kinesthetic sensations with an acoustic result, thus developing an important oral-auditory feedback loop. Cooing becomes more intonated by the ages of 4 to 6 months as the child learns to produce contrasts in pitch, amplitude, and resonance. *If the infant is not cooing by 4 months, the physician should monitor this infant's development very closely.*

At around 6 months, sound production changes with the onset of babbling. *Babbling* is characterized by the production of consonant sounds in a repetitive manner (i.e., "ma ma ma," "ba ba ba," etc.). During the babbling stage, the child learns to produce many of the "early developmental phonemes" or speech consonants, including the bilabial sounds (p, b, m, w), lingual-alveolar sounds (t, d, n), and velar sounds (k, g). As with cooing, babbling is an important stage of normal development since it provides the child with an opportunity to practice sound production for speech, and also helps to develop an auditory feedback loop that allows the child to learn to produce certain sounds purposefully. *If the child is not babbling by 8 or 9 months, this may indicate a potential problem.*

Jargon is the next stage and usually begins between the ages of 9 and 10 months. With jargon, the child uses these early developmental sounds in a variety of combinations rather than in a repetitive manner. In addition, various intonational patterns are used. It may seem as if the child is actually speaking, but using a foreign language. In fact, many parents will report that their child is talking in sentences but just cannot be understood. Of course, jargon is merely sound practice and not actually meaningful speech.

During the first year of life, most of the early developmental sounds need to be well established since they lay the ground work for the development of sounds in the next stage. *If the child is not producing a variety of these sounds by the age of 12 months, this may indicate reason for concern.*

The next stage of articulation development involves the acquisition of some of the "fricative" sounds (such as f, s, z, sh). Not only are these sounds more difficult to produce than the early developmental sounds, they also require the assistance of teeth. Most of the fricative sounds should develop between 12 months and 2 years.

Once fricatives are acquired, the child should begin to produce the affricate phonemes (ch and j). The child must have acquired both the plosive and fricative sounds individually before these phonemes can be combined to produce the affricate sounds.

By age 3, the child should have acquired the use of most speech sounds. As a result, the speech should be intelligible most of the time, although some sounds may be incorrectly produced. If the child's speech is difficult to understand at this point, a referral for a speech pathology evaluation is indicated.

The last sounds to be developed are usually /l/, /r/, /th/, and /v/. Many children have difficulty with one or more of these speech sounds up to the age of 6. *By the age of 6, the child should have essentially "perfect" speech with no errors in articulation. If articulation errors persist after this age, a referral for professional help is indicated.*

Language

At birth, the infant is aware of sounds in the environment, and startles or cries in response to loud or sudden noises. Expressive language also begins to develop at birth and begins with early cries. Although early cries are reflexive and are stimulated by physical or environmental conditions, the infant soon learns that these cries bring about a caregiver's response. As a result, the infant begins to use crying and various vocalizations to bring about this response. Most parents are able to discriminate their infant's cries of hunger versus the cries of pain, or cries of needing attention.

By 2 months, the infant begins to attend to a speaker's face and responds to the speech by maintaining eye contact. The infant coos and produces sounds spontaneously.

Around 4 months, the infant localizes to sound. He or she also begins to vocalize directly to others with cooing, and learns to imitate and to take turns in a communicative situation. In the first 6 months, the infant is taking in all that he or she hears in the environment and may be beginning to understand that speech has meaning. However, the infant does not demonstrate much understanding at this point.

PEARLS AND PERILS

1. History of cleft palate or submucous cleft
2. Craniofacial anomalies
3. Significant dental malocclusion or macroglossia
4. Hearing loss or chronic middle-ear effusion
5. Sensory or perceptual difficulties
6. Laryngeal or vocal fold pathology
7. History of traumatic brain injury
8. Neuromotor disease or dysfunction
9. History of prematurity or traumatic birth history
10. History of significant feeding or swallowing difficulties
11. History of developmental delay
12. Psychosis or autism
13. Environmental deprivation for a variety of reasons, including long-term hospitalization

---

Between 6 to 9 months, the child begins to show that he or she is associating meaning to the sound combinations heard in speech. The child looks up in response to his or her name and seems to recognize the names of family members. The child responds to simple commands that are accompanied by a gesture. He or she also begins to communicate with gestures, such as pointing, reaching, and waving for hi or bye. The child starts to imitate others in play, such as peekaboo, and also imitates vocalizations with babbling.

By 10 to 12 months, the child should be able to point to some body parts when they are named. The child demonstrates understanding by giving objects to others upon request and responding to many simple, one-part commands. He or she babbles and jargons to others and occasionally uses single words in addition to the gestures for communication. Following the first birthday, the child's receptive language seems to increase greatly. Of course comprehension ability precedes production so the child is able to understand far more than he or she is able to say or produce.

First words begin to emerge anywhere between the ages of 9 and 18 months. Most children use one or two words by the first birthday. Of interest is the fact that many first words sound much like babbling using the early developmental phonemes (i.e., mama, dada, bye-bye). They become true words when these sound combinations are used in an appropriate and meaningful way.

Between 12 and 18 months, the child shows a great increase in understanding of language. He or she identifies many common objects and pictures following a verbal request and follows commands more easily. The child seems to listen to the meaning of conversation. He or she begins to use more single words and communicates with a combination of words and gestures.

Between 18 and 24 months, the child begins to understand more complex language. He or she shows an understanding of some concepts (such as adjectives, possessive pronouns, and plural forms) and can follow many compound and complex commands. At this stage, the child also begins to combine words together for short utterances. Most children begin combining two, three, and even four words together around the same time. *The child should be at least combining two words together for short utterances by the age of 2.*

Between the ages of 2 and 3, the child's receptive language abilities progress to the point where he or she is understanding long and complex sentences, and even shows an interest in explanations of "why" and "how." The child seems to understand most forms of syntax and follows everyday conversation easily. From this point on, receptive language continues to develop, but primarily in the area of vocabulary. Expressively, the child begins using phrases and short sentences for communication, and begins to use more complex syntactic and morphologic forms.

By the age of 3, the child should be communicating with long and structurally complex sentences. The child is able to tell stories and relate experiences that happened in his or her past. The child will continue to make errors of syntax, particularly regularizing irregular forms, as in "I talk gooder than you." Speech should be clear enough to be understood most of the time. At this point, the child begins to develop pragmatic skills for some of the social rules of conversation.

Speech and language development is very individual and minor variations occur in the rate and sequence of development. However, the physician should be knowledgeable of what is expected during the stages of development, and proactive in screening for communication difficulties. *Whenever there is a suspicion that the child is not developing speech or language skills normally, the child should be referred to a speech-language pathologist for a professional evaluation.*

SPEECH DISORDERS

Articulation Disorder

An articulation disorder is characterized by difficulty producing speech sounds in comparison to the ability of age-matched peers. This difficulty is usually with consonants, although in severe disorders, even vowel distortions are noted. As a result of this difficulty, speech may be unpleasant or distracting to the listener. In more severe disorders, the speech may be hard to understand or even unintelligible. Poor speech intelligibility is a primary characteristic of an articulation disorder.

PEARLS AND PERILS

1. Have the child repeat the following sentences while noting articulation errors:

p	Popeye plays putt putt.
b	Buy baby a bib.
m	My mommy makes lemonade.
w	Wade in the water.
y	You have a yellow yo-yo.
h	He has a big horse.
t	Take teddy to town.
d	Do it for Daddy.
n	Nancy is not here.
k	I like cookies and cream.
g	Go get the wagon.
ng	Put the ring on her finger.
f	I have five fingers.
v	Drive a van.
l	I like lollipops.
s	I see the sun in the sky.
z	Zip up your zipper.
sh	She went shopping.
ch	I eat cherries and cheese.
j	John told a joke to Jim.
r	Randy has a red fire truck.
th	Thank you for the toothbrush.
blends	splash, sprinkle, street

When a child has difficulty with articulation, he or she may compensate by trying to produce sounds in an easier way. As a result, speech may be characterized by speech sound omissions, sound substitutions, or distortions. In addition, slurring and overall oral inactivity may be noted.

Omissions occur when the child has so much difficulty with the motor requirements for speech that he or she leaves out sounds in words, most commonly middle and final sounds. In many cases, the child will have difficulty combining consonants in blends (i.e., pl, st, dr, etc.). Examples of typical patterns of sound omissions are as follows:

I ri the bu to coo. (I ride the bus to school.)
Daey bo a cu. (Daddy broke a cup.)
My ca a do ah paying ousi. (My cat and dog are playing outside.)

In more severe cases, the child may omit all consonants, and only produce vowel sounds with a grunt (glottal stop) in place of the consonants. Of course, this causes speech to be essentially unintelligible.

Substitutions are noted when an incorrect sound is substituted for the correct one. Most commonly, the child will substitute a sound that is easier to produce and developed early, for a sound that is harder to produce and therefore developed later. Some common examples of sound substitutions are as follows:

t/k	I eat tate and tooties.
d/g	I'm a dood dirl.
p/f	I have pive pingers.

t/s   I tee the tun in the ty.
w/l   I wike wowwe pops.
w/r   The wabbit is wunning.

When substitution errors are noted, they usually occur on many different sounds. In fact, the child may use only the early developmental sounds, such as plosives and nasals, as substitutions for the later developing consonants. In a more severe case, the child may only use one or two consonants as a substitution for all other speech sounds.

Distortions occur when the child is attempting to produce the sound correctly, but the articulatory placement is incorrect, resulting in an altered sound. A common distortion occurs with the production of the /r/ sound. Many children have difficulty with the motor requirements of this sound. As a result, the tongue may not be high enough or retracted enough for the appropriate placement, thus causing distortion. Other common distortions are *lisps*, which occur on sibilant or "teeth sounds" (s, z, sh, ch, j). An anterior or *frontal lisp* occurs when the tongue is articulating against or between the incisors. This distortion sounds almost like a /th/ sound that is not as sharp or "sibilant" as the correct sound should be. A *lateral lisp* occurs when the tongue tip or dorsum articulates against the alveolar ridge or palate, stopping the anterior movement of the airstream. As a result, the airstream is redirected laterally, causing a slurpy, slushy type of sound. At times, saliva can be seen bubbling at the sides of the mouth during speech.

Some patients demonstrate oral-motor dysfunction that causes distortion of all speech sounds, particularly in connected speech. A *dysarthria* is a type of articulation disorder that is the result of neurologic dysfunction associated with cerebral palsy or acquired neurologic damage. Dysarthria is characterized by poor movement of all of the articulators, causing slow, slurred, and inarticulate speech. Respiration, phonation, and resonance also may be affected. As a result, dysarthric speech is usually hypernasal, and utterances can be short and choppy due to poor respiratory support.

An *apraxia of speech*, also known as *verbal apraxia*, is another motor speech disorder. In this case, the patient has difficulty with motor planning and sequencing of movements. Although the child may be able to move the oral structures normally for feeding and other nonspeech activities, he or she demonstrates difficulty coordinating movements required for speech. As a result, the speech is characterized by many inconsistent substitutions, many sound omissions, sound and syllable reversals, and even obvious struggle behaviors during speech production. Speech is best when producing single sounds or words, but breaks down when the child is combining the sounds and words to produce the longer utterances of connected speech.

The causes of articulation disorders include structural anomalies, such as a history of cleft palate or velopharyngeal insufficiency (VPI). If the VPI causes a significant leak of air pressure into the nasal cavity during speech, there may be inadequate air pressure in the oral cavity for the normal production of sounds.

Dental abnormalities, particularly anterior crossbite or class III malocclusion, often can affect speech sound production. For normal speech production, the maxillary arch should overlap the mandibular arch. If the anterior maxillary teeth are retrusive relative to the mandible or are inside the mandibular arch, this can interfere with the movement of the tongue during speech, causing faulty articulation.

Hearing loss, especially a sensorineural loss, can affect speech sound perception and learning, thus affecting articulation production. Even chronic otitis media has been shown to affect speech development.

As mentioned previously, oral-motor dysfunction is also a common cause of articulation disorders, particularly apraxia of speech and dysarthria. Oral-motor dysfunction can be noted as a result of neurologic damage, but also is noted in patients with no other apparent neurologic problems.

Contrary to popular belief, *ankyloglossia*, commonly known as *tongue-tie*, usually does not interfere with speech production. Whether the lingual frenulum has an anterior attachment on the tongue tip or is unusually short, the tongue tip is usually unrestricted enough for adequate elevation and protrusion for speech. The tongue only needs to elevate slightly to the alveolar ridge for the /l/ sound, and must protrude only to the back of the maxillary incisors for the /th/ sound. If ankyloglossia is noted in a patient with an articulation disorder, it is usually just coincidental. Most speech-language pathologists agree that a frenulectomy is not indicated for speech purposes in almost all patients with ankyloglossia.

Phonology Disorder

A *phonology disorder* is much like an articulation disorder in that the patient demonstrates speech sound substitutions, omissions, and distortions, making the speech difficult to understand. The cause, however, is not related to structural or functional difficulties, but due to a faulty "rule" that the child is using in producing speech patterns. For example, the child may always produce the /t/ sound as a substitution for sibilant sounds (s, z, sh, ch, j). Therefore, treatment would focus not on the individual sounds but instead on correcting the rule for all of the affected sounds.

Fluency Disorder

A *fluency disorder*, commonly known as *stuttering*, is also a type of speech disorder. Stuttering occurs when the child demonstrates an abnormal amount of repetitions, hesitations, prolongations, or blocks in the normal flow or rhythm of speech. These disruptions often are accompanied by facial tension, forceful eye blinks, or secondary movements such as foot stomping.

The cause of stuttering is still not fully understood. What is known is that stuttering seems to be a learned behavior that is developed by children who may have a predisposition for the problem. Articulation and language problems also are noted frequently in these patients.

In assessing the child's speech fluency, it is important to note that all normal speakers have dysfluencies in speech. These dysfluencies tend to be mild and usually are not even noticed by the listeners. Dysfluencies in normal speakers will increase in situations where the speaker is nervous, anxious, upset, or even tired.

Normal dysfluencies are particularly common in young children between the ages of 2 and 6. During this time, the child is just learning to articulate sounds and to put words together appropriately for sentences. Therefore, speech production is somewhat challenging. In addition, young children tend to be very excitable, which further increases the likelihood of dysfluencies. Many children go through a period of months with enough dysfluencies that their speech could be described as "stuttering." In most cases, the speech improves without intervention by the time the child enters school.

When parents express concerns about stuttering, it is very important to reassure them that in the preschool years, this is usually normal. It is very important that they ignore the dysfluencies when they occur by not pointing them out to the child, correcting the speech, or telling the child to slow down. They should try to give the child their full attention during speech and make the speaking situations as easy and non-threatening as possible. In many cases, counseling by a speech-language pathologist will help the parents to understand what to do and why in dealing with these speech problems at home.

In some cases, the dysfluencies persist longer than 6 to 8 months, or become severe enough that the child expresses concern about his or her speech. The child may even avoid speaking situations for fear that he or she may stutter. Tension with speech may be visible and there may also be some secondary characteristics such as eye blinks, foot stomping, or head jerks. When the symptoms become this severe, this would be considered true stuttering. In this case, direct intervention by a speech-language pathologist is indicated.

LANGUAGE DISORDERS

Language assessment can be difficult and challenging for a variety of reasons. With children, it is important to consider the child's chronologic and mental age, and compare his or her skills with what is expected for that developmental level. Therefore, knowledge of normal language development is very important. Another consideration is the child's cultural and linguistic background. For example, it is widely understood that black Americans often use a dialect that has its roots in Africa. This dialect has rules of syntax that are often different from standard English (3). In assessing language skills, it is important to be able to distinguish language disorders from dialectical differences. Finally, language assessment can be difficult in view of the extremely complex nature of language. It is important to evaluate all aspects of language in order to completely rule out a language disorder or language delay.

It should be noted that a *language disorder* is characterized by deviant language skills or problems that are not seen during the course of normal development. A *language delay* is characterized by a normal, although unusually slow, progression of language development.

In evaluating a child's language skills, it is important to consider both receptive and expressive language. In addition, there are three basic components of both receptive and expressive language that all children must develop. These components are the content, the form, and the use.

Receptive language, also referred to as *comprehension*, is the child's ability to understand the language of others. This is demonstrated by his or her responses to questions or requests, and the ability to follow directions. Children with a receptive language disorder may demonstrate difficulty understanding the speech of others. They may be unable to follow commands as their same-aged peers and they may have difficulty answering questions appropriately. Some children with receptive language disorders demonstrate an *echolalia*. For example, the child is asked, "How old are you?" and responds with "Old are you." With echolalia, the child may echo all or part of a question or command that he or she does not understand, while responding appropriately when he or she does understand. Since children need to be able to understand language meaning and form before they are able to generate language, children with receptive language disorders also demonstrate expressive language problems.

Expressive language refers to the child's ability to create language in order to convey a message. Children with expressive language disorders may have limited vocabulary skills or use words inappropriately. They may have difficulty formulating sentence structures. As a result, they may use short, "telegraphic" phrases and sentences, or faulty sentence structures.

The *content* of language, called *semantics*, is the meaning of the words, phrases, and sentences that are used for communication. Comprehension and expression of the meaning of a word are always dependent on the child's ability to conceptualize perceptual and functional characteristics of a word, and categorize these features. For example, the word "chair" has perceptual features of a seat for one person and it usually has four legs. The functional feature is that it is something that one can sit in. These perceptual and functional features help the child to categorize objects that can be called "chair" from those that are similar, such as "table" and "sofa."

Children with semantic problems have difficulty categorizing words based on these perceptual and functional features and they have difficulty associating words with meaning. They may also have difficulty retrieving from long-term memory those words that they know and want to use. As a result of these problems, these children often have limited vocabulary skills, demonstrate word-finding difficulties, or may frequently use words inappropriately. In comparison to their peers, their utterances contain proportionally more concrete words, such as nouns and verbs, and fewer abstract words, such as adjectives, adverbs, prepositions, articles, and conjunctions. Children with semantic problems have particular difficulty with abstract language, such as understanding concepts, figurative language, and words with multiple meanings.

The *form* of language involves syntax and morphology. *Morphology* refers to the rules that govern the structure of words. Children with morphology problems have difficulty understanding and using the rules of words for appropriate verb tense, plurals, possessives, prefixes and suffixes, and comparatives. *Syntax* refers to the structure of the sentences. Children with syntax problems may have difficulty with word order and the use of words that have little meaning, but form the "glue" for the sentence. As a result, they may use improper sentence structures or omit the smaller words, such as prepositions, articles, and conjunctions. This may cause the sentences to be somewhat "telegraphic" in nature. They may also use improper forms of words, such as the "to be" verbs (is, am, are) or forms of "do" (do, did, does). Examples of problems with syntax and morphology include the following:

That a ball.
Him go school.
What he is doing?
Mommy Daddy go shopping.
How he break that?
Him are running.

In the course of normal development, children will learn the rules of syntax and morphology long before they learn the exceptions to the rules. As a result, they may make frequent errors in syntax and morphology as they apply the rule inappropriately. Examples are as follows:

I got stang by a bee.
I hurted my toe.
I have two feets.

Since in this case the child has learned a rule and is applying the rule in a novel situation, these errors actually represent very good language learning. Errors of regularizing irregular noun and verb forms should *not* be considered characteristics of a language disorder in the preschool and early school years.

Finally, the *use* of language is referred to as *pragmatics*. Pragmatics involves the rules of conversation and the communicative intent of the spoken language. Children with pragmatic disorders may not understand certain rules of conversation, such as the following:

You begin a conversation with a greeting.
All of your utterances must relate to the topic at hand.
You need to let the listener know if you decide to change the topic.
You reference all pronouns before using them.
You base your conversation on what the listener knows.
Your conversation and responses should be appropriate for the situation.
You end a conversation in a certain way, usually by saying "good-bye."

Children who have difficulty with pragmatics may have clear speech and normal sentence structures. However, they may not reference the topic or even pronouns in their conversations. Their comments are often socially inappropriate or off the topic. It may be difficult to understand the message that they are trying to convey because they just do not make any sense. The child may also have difficulty understanding sentences with inferred meanings. For example, the sentence "Could you please pass the salt?" is actually a command and does not require an affirmative answer. Expressions or idioms, such as "Two heads are better than one" may be interpreted literally, with no understanding of the deeper meaning.

Causes of language disorders include hearing loss, mental retardation, environmental deprivation, or neurologic damage or dysfunction. The term *aphasia* refers to an acquired language disorder resulting from neurologic damage.

PREREQUISITES FOR NORMAL COMMUNICATION DEVELOPMENT

Although most children are able to develop communication skills normally, there are certain prerequisites for this development. These prerequisites include the physical ability to produce sounds and language, and the ability to perceive speech and language. In addition, there are several prerequisites for the ability to learn speech and language skills.

The *physical prerequisites* include an intact central nervous system which includes head and neck control, normal control over respiration and phonation, and normal oral-motor skills. In addition, intact oral and pharyngeal cavities, and normal laryngeal structures are important. Finally, the auditory system must be adequate for normal speech perception.

Learning prerequisites include intelligence, which is an important prerequisite for all kinds of learning, including learning of communication skills. If the child is developmentally delayed, communication abilities would be expected to be commensurate with developmental age, not chronologic age.

Environmental stimulation is another important prerequisite for speech and language learning. Just as in learning a foreign language, the more the child is exposed to language, the faster he or she will develop it. If the child's exposure to the speech and language of others is limited, then language learning will be delayed.

Motivation is another factor in the learning process. Many children under the age of 2 are able to communicate adequately through the use of gestures, or by having an older sibling do the talking for them. As long as this system is sufficient to meet the communication needs of the child, the child will not learn to communicate by talking. Around the age of 3, when the child wants to tell about experiences, this system is no longer effective and the child will often develop speech and language skills rapidly at this time.

Sensory perception is important for speech and language learning. Although hearing is obvious, the importance of visual perception cannot be understated. As noted already, children learn the meaning of words by associating what they perceive (usually visually) with the word. Without vision, common words that are coded and categorized based on visual perception (i.e., boy, big, red, sky, etc.) would be very hard to learn and understand.

PEARLS AND PERILS

1. Review the medical and developmental history. Look for factors that could cause or contribute to a communication disorder, or would place the child at risk for communication difficulties.
2. Do a complete oral examination to rule out structural defects, specifically submucous cleft palate, macroglossia, and significant dental malocclusion.
3. If voice or resonance problems are suspected, do an endoscopic evaluation of velopharyngeal function and vocal fold function.
4. Examine the patient for dysmorphic features or evidence of a syndrome.
5. Evaluate for chronic middle-ear effusion and do a hearing test to rule out hearing loss.
6. Refer the patient directly to a speech-language pathologist or to a program where these services are offered (i.e., school for the deaf, developmental evaluation center, etc.). Be sure to send information regarding specific concerns, and include all pertinent information obtained from the history review and examination.

SCREENING FOR COMMUNICATION DISORDERS

It is important to routinely screen all preschool children for speech and language problems, particularly those who are between the ages of 2 and 5. Screening for communication difficulties can be done directly through formal assessment, indirectly through informal observation, or merely by interviewing the parents.

Formal screening for communication disorders can be somewhat time-consuming and the examiner still can miss subtle deficits, particularly in the area of language. However, a formal assessment can be of value in allowing the physician to sample the child's communicative abilities using a structured format. Formal tests include the Fluharty Preschool Speech and Language Screening Test (4), which can be used to screen children from ages 2 to 6 years in the areas of articulation, vocabulary, and receptive and expressive language. The Denver Developmental Screening Test (5) can be used with children from birth to 6 years to test various aspects of development, including speech and language. The Receptive-Expressive Emergent Language Scale (REEL) (6) and the Clinical Linguistic and Auditory Milesone Scale (CLAMS) (7,8) are both used to screen children from birth to 3 years through observation and parent report.

An informal assessment also can be done and can usually yield enough information to make a decision regarding the need for referral. Speech and language can be screened informally by means of the following:

- Asking the child to point to certain objects or follow certain commands.
- Listening to the child's spontaneous speech while he or she is talking to a parent or playing.
- Eliciting communication by saying such things as the following:
  - What do you want to be when you grow up? Why?
  - What does a (fireman) do?
  - Tell me how you make a peanut butter and jelly sandwich.
  - Explain the game of baseball to me.
- Having the child repeat words or sentences, such as those listed in the articulation screening test. (Even in repeating, the child will use his or her own form of articulation, and will usually revert to his or her own form of syntax and morphology.)

Finally, the physician can screen for communication problems merely by interviewing the parents regarding their observations and concerns. The physician might ask the parents questions such as the following:

Do you have any concerns regarding your child's communication abilities?
Do you understand your child's speech most or all of the time?
How well do strangers understand your child's speech?
When your child is talking, how many words does he or she put together at a time?
Does your child leave out words in the sentence?
Is your child communicating as well as other children the same age?
Have your child's communication skills improved in the last 3 months?

Parents are usually very good observers of their own children, and can often effectively compare their child's communication skills with those of siblings or peers. A study by Glascoe (9) showed that skillful observation of the child combined with identification of parental concern is sensitive to most speech and language problems. At the same time, this screening method is more cost-effective and less time-consuming. A simple rule of thumb is that if the parents are worried about their child's speech and language development, a referral for evaluation is usually appropriate.

Once screening is completed, the child's communication skills should be compared to what is expected at the child's developmental level. If the child seems delayed in development, or demonstrates any of the problems noted on the "Indications for Referral" list, the physician should evaluate for any medical problems that could cause or contribute to the communication disorder. Once this is done, then a referral should be made to a speech-language pathologist for complete assessment and intervention.

---

1. At 12 months:

    The child was a quiet infant who seldom cooed or babbled.

    The child is very quiet or has limited vocalizations.

    The child does not vocalize with consonant sounds (such as b, m, d, and n).

    The child shows evidence of significant feeding problems.

    Development of motor milestones appears significantly delayed.

2. At 18 months:

    The child uses mostly vowel sounds and gestures for communication.

    The child does not use any meaningful single words.

    The child cannot follow simple commands.

    The child cannot point to body parts or common objects following a verbal request.

3. At 2 years:

    The child does not combine words for short utterances (i.e., Get doggie. Go bye-bye.).

    The child cannot follow two unrelated commands (i.e., Go get your shoes and give them to Daddy.).

4. At 3 years:

    The child does not communicate with complete sentences.

    Sentences are short, "telegraphic," or incomplete.

    The child echoes parts of questions or commands rather than responding appropriately.

    The speech is usually hard to understand.

    There are many omissions of consonants in speech.

5. At 4 years or older:

    Sentence structures are noticeably defective and short.

    The child frequently uses words inappropriately.

    The child has difficulty expressing ideas or conveying what happened in an event.

    The speech is somewhat difficult to understand, especially by strangers.

6. At 6 years:

    The child has difficulty producing any speech sounds.

7. At any age:

    The vocabulary size is limited in comparison to peers of his or her age.

    The child is embarrassed or self-conscious about his or her speech.

    An abnormal number of dysfluencies are noted and have persisted over many months.

    Dysfluencies are accompanied by facial tension and secondary behaviors.

    The voice is abnormal in pitch, quality, or resonance.

REFERRAL FOR TREATMENT

If a communication disorder is suspected or the child does not have prerequisite skills for normal communication, then a referral should be made to a qualified speech-language pathologist for evaluation and treatment. Speech-language pathologists are found in hospitals, private practice, health-care agencies, home health, and school settings.

The prerequisites of speech and language development can be evaluated even in infancy. At that age, the speech-language pathologist may opt to enroll the child in formal treatment if problems are noted, or work with the parents through home programs. Formal therapy is usually started around the age of 2 or 3 if problems are noted. Even if therapy is not recommended at that time, the speech-language pathologist can provide parents with developmentally appropriate activities for use in stimulating speech and language development in the home.

TIMETABLE FOR INTERVENTION

Early intervention is very important for children with communication disorders and can ultimately affect the long-term prognosis for normal communication skills. Intervention is best started during the preschool years. At this time, the brain is particularly receptive to speech and language learning (which is why normal children are able to learn a foreign or second language much faster than their parents). Since this is a critical period of normal speech and language learning, intervention for communication disorders should be done at this time to take advantage of this receptivity to speech and language learning.

Early intervention is also important owing to the factor of habit strength. Since speech and language skills are used every day, patterns of communication become strongly habituated early in development. If those patterns are faulty, they may be harder to change as the child becomes older due to the habit strength factor.

Finally, early intervention is important because a communication disorder can affect a child's social and emotional development, and seriously impair the child's ability to learn in school. An investment in early intervention can pay off in the future in regards to treatment and educational costs.

⊛ REFERENCES

1. Office of Scientific and Health Reports. Developmental speech and language disorders: hope through research. Bethesda, MD: National Institute of Neurological and Communicative Disorders and Stroke; 1988;88–2757.
2. National Deafness and Other Communication Disorders Advisory Board. Research in human communication. Bethesda, MD: National Institute on Deafness and Other Communication Disorders; 1991;92–3317.
3. Emerick LL, Haynes WO. *Diagnosis and evaluation in speech pathology*, 3rd ed. Englewood Cliffs: Prentice-Hall, 1986.
4. Fluharty NB. *Fluharty preschool speech and language screening test*. Boston: Teaching Resources Corporation, 1978.
5. Frankenberg WK, Cobbs JB. Denver developmental screening test. *J Pediatr*, 1967;71: 181–191.
6. Bzoch KR, League R. *Receptive-expressive emergent language scale*. Gainesville, FL: Computer Management Resources, 1991.
7. Capute AJ, Accardo PJ. Linguistic and auditory milestones during the first two years of life. *Clin Pediatr* 1978;17:847–853.
8. Capute AJ, Shapiro BK, Palmer FB. Marking the milestones of language development. *Contemp Pediatr* 1987;4:24–41.
9. Glascoe FP. Can clinical judgement detect children with speech-language problems? *Pediatrics* 1991;87:317–322.

A. W. Kummer: Speech Pathology Department, Children's Hospital Medical Center, Cincinnati, Ohio 45229–3039.

- *Practical Pediatric Otolaryngology*
- edited by Robin T. Cotton and Charles M. Myer, III
- Lippincott-Raven Publishers, Philadelphia © 1999

5

Pediatric Voice Disorders

Angie J. Pengilly

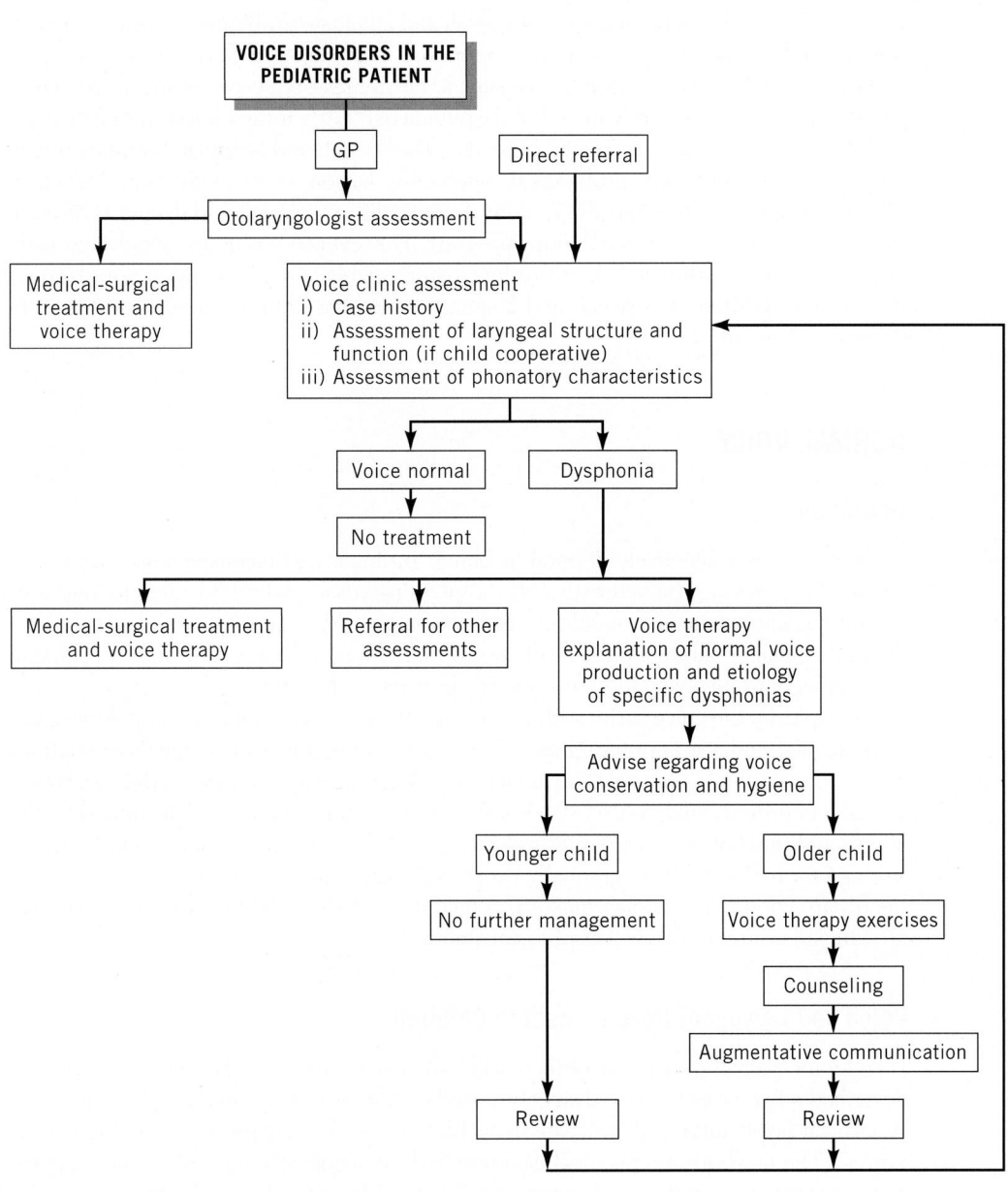

This chapter describes and discusses different aspects of voice in children. It includes the assessment, diagnosis, management, and treatment of the pediatric voice, highlighting the value of a team approach, including the child's parents or caregivers and teachers.

Humans are social beings and communication is an important characteristic, be it through spoken or written words. Language may also be expressed using nonverbal forms (e.g., signs) (1). The voice plays many roles in the verbal communication process. It helps the audibility of speech and distinguishes different consonant sounds (e.g., the voiceless sound "s" and the voiced sound "z"); (2) signals prosodic features (e.g., pitch, stress, rhythm, and pause variations and shades of feeling and emotion) (3); and identifies features such as age, gender, education and intelligence, and socioeconomic and regional roots (3).

Dysphonia (the abnormal voice) in school-aged children is relatively common and estimates of incidence range from 6% to 40% (4,5). Dysphonia alone or in combination with other developmental or acquired speech and language problems can render speech unintelligible, generating a social and emotional handicap. Furthermore, listener perceptions of personality and appearance such as cleanliness, honesty, kindness, and pleasantness have been negatively linked to dysphonia (6). Early intervention therefore is essential for optimum developmental outcome. The speech and language therapist is well equipped to prevent voice problems through close liaison with caregivers and teachers (4), ensure appropriate referrals (7), contribute to the assessment and diagnosis of voice problems, and oversee a voice therapy program. However, referrals are not always made (4). Furthermore, although voice disorders feature highly in recommended prioritization systems for children (4), speech and language therapists are often under confident in their management (8).

NORMAL VOICE

Definition

Normal voice is subjectively defined as being "ordinary and inconspicuous" (3) and as having the following characteristics (4): (a) pleasing voice quality; (b) suitable loudness; (c) appropriately balanced nasal and oral resonance; (d) a speaking fundamental frequency (modal or habitual pitch level) appropriate for age, gender, and size; (e) suitable voice inflections involving loudness and pitch; and (f) adequate rate.

In children the voice varies with the degree of cognitive, emotional, and physical development. Loudness is predominantly influenced by motor control. Quality variations result from vocal fold physical growth factors, changes in shape and size of the vocal tract, and fine neuromuscular control (9). Vocal fundamental frequency is determined by the length and mass of the vocal folds and tension (10). Infants have short vocal folds, resulting in a high pitch that gradually drops with laryngeal growth until puberty. Voice breaks are common in adolescence (3). Voice use is influenced by social and cognitive growth and awareness as well as physical abilities (9).

Voice and Laryngeal Development in Children

Developmentally the structure of the vocal fold changes with age. Hirano and Bless (11) described a five-layer vocal fold structure in the adult larynx: epithelium of the mucosa; superficial layer, intermediate layer deep layer of the lamina propria; and the vocalis muscle. The newborn has no vocal ligament and the whole structure of the lamina propria is nearly uniform. Layer structure development is only achieved by the end of adolescence. There is evidence that the immaturity of children's vocal folds may increase susceptibility to microtrauma and nodule formation (12).

Hirano and Bless (11) described the mechanism of phonation:

As the subglottal pressure increases against the closed glottis, the bilateral vocal folds are blown apart and the glottis opens. The vocal folds keep moving laterally until the subglottal pressure drops to a specific level. At the maximum opening, the upper part of the vocal fold edge (the so-called "upper lip") keeps moving laterally while the lower part of the edge (the so-called "lower lip") is moving medially. At a certain point in time, the upper lip also begins moving medially. Initially, the medial movement of the vocal folds results primarily from the recoiling force. As the vocal folds approach each other, narrowing the glottis, a negative pressure caused by the Bernoulli effect is built up in the glottis. This negative pressure sucks the vocal folds into close contact. The contact usually takes place first at the lower lip of the edge of the vocal folds.

The contact area of the vocal fold increases until the subglottic pressure becomes high enough to blow apart the vocal folds. This aeromechanical action is repeated and results in phonation.

The voice serves important communicative functions; for example, an infant's cry may indicate discomfort or hunger (3). Abnormality of the cry is an important signal to caregivers and physicians. It can indicate abnormal pathology that may be potentially life-threatening (e.g., neurologic disorders, tumors, and endocrine disease) and must not be overlooked (13). Baken (14) concluded that most laryngeal disorders do not influence mean significantly. However, in some pathologies (e.g., unilateral vocal fold paralysis), the variability and range of fundamental frequency are affected adversely.

Differences in infant and child larynges in contrast to the adult larynx have been carefully described (3, 15). The larynx is initially high in the vocal tract (at the level of C3–4), dropping to level C6–7 at 15 years (15). Subepithelial tissue is more vascular and less dense in young children and therefore more liable to posttraumatic or inflammatory edema (12). The size of the vocal folds increases with age and general body growth from 6 to 8 mm in the newborn to up to 8 to 16 mm in the adult (15). Of interest, there is little difference in male and female pitch and frequency until puberty (16). There is a marked drop in pitch at puberty in boys related to as increase in male hormone levels (17). The thyroid angle in the boys narrows from 110 degrees to 90 degrees (15). Titze (17) described how vocal fold thickening occurs due to an increase in the bulk of the thyroarytenoid muscle and results in "chest or modal voice." As the folds thicken and become more rectangular, muscle patterns controlling vocal fold vibration need to change. Difficulty controlling this may result in frequent changes of register (between that of the child and adult voice) during development, which continues until about the age of 20 years.

VOICE DISORDERS

Definitions

Aphonia is voice without a determinable laryngeal tone. The voice is whispered or breathy. *Dysphonia* is voice judged by the listener to be abnormal with regard to quality, loudness, pitch, flexibility, or their combinations (16). Perceptual rating of voice is a very difficult task. Judgments of voice quality are influenced by many variables such as characteristics of the speaker, listener judgment (training and experience included), designation of standards, phonetic content of sample read or spoken, and loudness, pitch, and rate (18).

Perceptual and Acoustic Characteristics

Perceptual

A child is described as having a voice problem if the voice is distracting or unpleasant to listeners and is abnormal enough to interfere with communication (4). Difficulties may occur with one or more of the following subjective characteristics.

Voice Quality

Disturbances are often caused by laryngeal dysfunction, that is, in sound production at or near the vocal fold level (8). Andrews (18) described four main quality disturbances:

1. Breathiness—excess air leak during phonation due to the incomplete adduction of the vocal folds during the closed phase of the vocal fold vibratory cycle. The amount of breathiness relates to the degree of vocal fold closure.
2. Harshness—aperiodicity of the vibration. There is an unpleasant "edge" to the voice, hard onsets, and overadduction of the folds. The vocal tract exhibits increased tension, effort, and constriction.
3. Hoarseness—air leakage and noise (aperiodicity of vibratory pattern) in the signal. In severe cases there are usually aphonic periods or voice breaks. Wilson (4) defined hoarseness as a mixture of breathiness and harshness.
4. Vocal fry/creak—described as similar to a creaking door. The vibratory pattern is relaxed and produced at a very low pitch. It is sometimes used at the end of sentences, especially when the child is tired.

Loudness

A child may talk too loudly, attracting attention to herself or himself, or too softly to be heard (4). Everyday conversational speech may exhibit levels between 77 and 82 decibels (18). A hearing test is mandatory for children with loudness problems.

Pitch

Pitch is the subjective perception of frequency. Abnormalities include inappropriately high or low speaking fundamental frequency, narrow pitch range, and excessive pitch breaks (4). Diplophonia is a double voice characterized by two distinct pitches heard simultaneously (9).

Rate and Prosody

Speech may be too fast or slow, and with inappropriate stress and intonation (4).

Other Features

Children may complain of vocal fatigue after long periods of talking, becoming hoarse by the end of the day. They may be unable to complete sentences as the air supply runs out, resulting in breathy voice. Phonation range may be reduced, interfering with singing. Strain or struggle may be evidenced as a result of excessive amounts of tension and fatigue due to vocal effort. The voice may have tremor (9).

Resonance Problems

Nasal resonance may be regarded as a parameter of voice quality (4, 15), although the focus of this chapter is on the phonatory characteristics. Inadequate velopharyngeal closure often results in hypernasal resonance primarily carried on vowels, abnormal nasal emission (air escape) on consonant sounds, and sometimes compensatory phonatory and consonant errors. Papsin (19) commented that hypernasality can occur following adenoidectomy, though it usually resolves without treatment within a few months. In children with cleft palate or suspected submucous cleft, adenoidectomy must be judiciously performed, if at all, to diminish the chance of acquired postoperative hypernasality.

Acoustic

Colton and Casper (9) described how the study of sound can provide important information about movements of the vocal folds and how many acoustic signs are possibly associated with any pathology. There is, however, often a lack of one-to-one mapping between specific acoustic parameters and perceptual categories (15). Instrumental analysis can be performed to show the fundamental frequency curve of the speaking voice (Fig. 1).

Differing fundamental frequencies are associated with differing phonation types. In

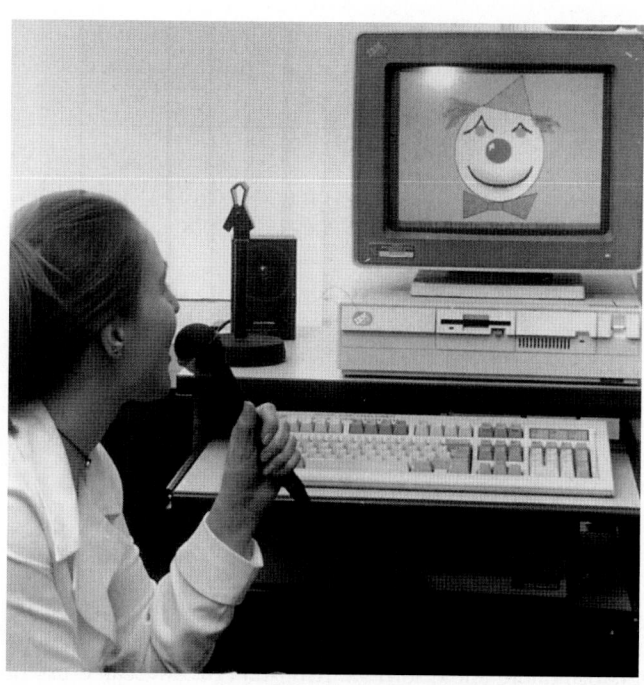

FIGURE 1 Speech viewer.

modal voice the average range is 94 to 287 Hz (20); in falsetto phonation, pitch is high (the average for a man being 275 to 634 Hz); in creak, pitch is low (the mean fundamental frequency being 34.6Hz and the average range for male speakers 24 to 52 Hz).

Interpretation of acoustic data is limited by the lack of normative data available for children [see (4,14)]. Furthermore, patients with a phonatory problem can have normal acoustic features. The differences between normal and pathologic voices can be so small that they are not shown in acoustic signs (9). Measures cited frequently include fundamental frequency, which corresponds to perceived vocal pitch; amplitude; spectral noise; maximum phonation time; and the S/Z ratio.

Fundamental Frequency

To measure frequency, clinical measures are taken of mean fundamental frequency; frequency variability, which is presumed associated with monopitch; phonation range; and pitch perturbation or jitter (the vocal fold irregularity of vibration). Vocal cord pathology can result in dysphonia by causing increased aperiodicity of the vocal folds (9). Boone and McFarlane (10) also suggested measuring habitual (modal) pitch. Normative data for children (girls and boys independently) are available for different ages (4, 14).

Amplitude

The overall or average sound pressure level (SPL) refers to an utterance's average level (a sustained vowel or spontaneous sentence). Measured in decibels, it gives an indication of vocal fold vibration strength. Dynamic range is the range of vocal intensities someone can produce. Perturbation (shimmer) is the variation in amplitude of vocal fold tone from one cycle to the subsequent cycle. Poor neural control or growths on the vocal folds may affect this (9).

Spectral Noise

Colton and Casper (9) described how this is aperiodic, random energy in the voice occurring in particular frequency bands or throughout the whole frequency range. Noise levels are normally low; abnormal voices exhibit increased levels. The level of noise is measured directly using the harmonics to noise ratio. Ratios greater than one (expected for normal speakers) indicate that harmonic energy is greater than noise energy. Spectral noise levels can also be measured indirectly using a spectrogram. Elevated noise levels are associated with an abnormal frequency or the creation of extra unwanted sound sources at the vocal fold level.

Maximum Phonation Time

This is the maximum time a child can sustain voice on one breath (18), for example, while saying "ah" (4). Short times reflect an inefficiency of the phonatory or respiratory system (9).

S/Z Ratio

The maximum durations of s and z are also used as a measure of efficiency of phonation and respiration. The duration of the voiceless s infers duration of the exhalation phase. The duration of voiced z indicates how long the vocal fold vibratory pattern can be sustained. If it is significantly shorter, it indicates the presence of lesions that increase mass or poor laryngeal control (18).

CLASSIFICATION

Many classification systems for voice disorders exist (Table 1). There is an ongoing debate about the terminology for nonorganic disorders. Aronson (16) advocated use of the term *psychogenic voice disorders* to refer to all voice disorders without organic laryngeal pathology. However, Morrison and Rammage (15) advocated a classification of musculoskeletal voice disorders separating "psychogenic" and "functional" disorders. They proposed that *functional* describes voice disorders attributed primarily to incorrect vocal technique, for example, poor coordination of respiratory, resonatory, articulatory, and phonatory gestures, excessive or reduced laryngeal valving, improper control of loudness and pitch dynamics, or extraordinary voice-use demands. Some are associated with secondary pathologies, for example, nodules. The term *psychogenic* is used to refer to voice disorders characterized by muscle misuse that clearly have a primary psychoemotional etiology. They identify six patterns of muscle-misuse voice disorders, classified by glottic and supraglottic shapes and postures seen on endoscopy.

The overlap between organic and function or psychogenic etiologies is well documented in the literature. Generally, voice disorders are viewed on a continuum between organic and functional etiologies. Their interaction renders it difficult at times to distinguish between them (4).

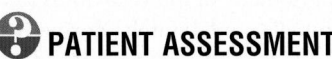 PATIENT ASSESSMENT

Indications

Investigation is advocated for an abnormal cry (13) and dysphonia of 2 to 3 weeks, duration (4). Children may be referred to laryngologists, to speech-language pathologists, or to a multidisciplinary team. Ideally assessment should be carried out in a specialized pediatric voice clinic specifically equipped to examine and quantify the degree of vocal disability (21). In such a clinic, both otolaryngologists and speech and language therapists can contribute to assessment and diagnosis. The assessment of dysphonia must always include visualization of the vocal tract to exclude potentially sinister pathology (i.e., glottic web, recurrent respiratory papilloma) (19).

Referrals for older children are often initiated by unfamiliar adults. Teachers may first notice the dysphonia and encourage parents to seek expert advice. Boone and McFarlane (10) suggested the use of a voice screening program in public schools by speech pathologists for the early identification of dysphonic children.

TABLE 1 A Classification of Children's Voice Disorders and Their Associated Voice Characteristics after Wilson 1987

Classification	Perceptual and/or Acoustic Characteristics	Reference
1. Organic Voice Disorder		
Subglottic stenosis—congenital and acquired	Hoarseness	50
	Harshness, whisper	Clary et al (unpublished)
	Low or high pitch	Clary et al (unpublished)
	Reduced loudness	49
	Inadequate pitch range	50
Laryngeal web	Hoarseness	Holinger, Johnston and Schiller 1954 in ref. 4
	Weak or absent cry	
Vocal cord sulcus	High pitch	Moore 1971 in ref. 4
	Hoarse, breathy voice	Greison 1984 in ref. 4
Underdeveloped vocal cords	Breathy voice	West and Ansberry in ref. 4
Vocal fold palsy	Abnormal cry	16
	Breathiness and weakness	3
	Hoarseness, monotone and soft voice	4
Papillomata	Hoarseness and aphonia	de Weese and Saunders 1982 in ref. 4
Laryngeal trauma	Hoarseness, breathiness and aponia	Holinger and Schild 1972 in ref. 4
Structural deviations in velopharyngeal area, oral cavity and nose	Hypernasality, hyponasality and nasal emission of sounds	4
	Hoarseness	McDonald and Baker 1951 in ref. 4
Neurologic problems	Cerebral palsy is associated with a variety of voice problems depending on the type of cerebral palsy (e.g., interruption of voicing and reverse phonation)	Mysak 1971 in ref. 4
Mental retardation	Hoarse, husky hypo- or hypernasality monotone, rate and volume disorders.	Schlanger and Gottsleben 1957 in ref. 4
Hearing loss	Vary with type and degree (e.g., in severe hearing loss: breathiness, harshness, hyper/hyponasality, monotonous pitch, loudness problems, slow rate)	4
2. Organic Changes From Voice Abuse		
Nodules, polyps and keratosis	Hoarseness	4
Ventricular band phonation	Hoarseness	4
	Low pitch .	4
	Restricted pitch range	4
	Vocal fry	4
Nonspecific laryngitis	Hoarseness	4
3. Functional Voice Disorder		
Disturbed mutation	Maintains high pitched prepubertal voice	4
Psychological	Conversation aphonia or dysphonia	4
	Hoarseness, harshness, and breathiness	
Elective mutism	Selective nonvocalization	4
Imitation of others	Any symptom	4
4. Voice Disorders Due to Contributing Factors		
Allergy, upper respiratory conditions	Difficult to determine exact nature of their influence	4
Premenstrual tension	Hoarseness	4

Case History

Case history is mandatory to explore causes of voice disorder and contributing factors [e.g., see (4)]. In the process of taking a case history, the clinician can also establish a relationship with the parents and child (9). Language tailored to the child's and parent's or caretaker's level is used to gain information on voice history and medical details, for example, episodes of intubation, psychological factors, and previous therapy (4,10,16). The child's parent or caretaker provides information about the child in his or her natural environments. Information from the teacher, friends, and family is also useful.

The interview may be conducted by the speech-language pathologist alone (15) or with members of a multidisciplinary team. The multidisciplinary team should always include an otolaryngologist and speech-language pathologist and may also include other professionals such as a psychiatrist, social worker, audiologist, physiotherapist, and medical electronics engineer (3). The concept of the joint multidisciplinary voice clinic in pediatrics is emerging.

Medical Examination

Ear-nose-throat (ENT) assessment of laryngeal structure, and when possible function, is essential for children with voice disorders, to determine the nature of the dysphonia and to exclude possible malignancy or papillomas. Flexible nasendoscopy is one technique developed for this purpose and indirect laryngoscopy is a conventional method of assessment.

Successful reports of video nasendoscopy in children as young as 3 years (22) and even 2 years (23) have been described in the literature. Lotz et al (23) cited an 87% success rate for nasendoscopies in children between ages 3 and 6. Sometimes the opportunity is taken to examine palatal function at the same time. Clinical style and experience of working with children are very important. Sufficient time needs to be allowed for each child to settle into the examination. The child should be given an explanation about what will happen in language at an appropriate developmental level. Nasendoscopy usually involves the use of a topical anesthetic either sprayed or placed on cotton wool in one nostril. The spray is demonstrated in the air and then on the child's hand before it is put in the nostril (small amounts first). Some surgeons use an anesthetic packing that is left for approximately 5 to 10 minutes. In contrast, some do not use any local anesthetic. When flexible nasendoscopy is used at the author's institution, many children become distressed during the examination, often after the instillation of topical anesthetic.

The child is shown the equipment and the procedure is explained using true statements. For example, "You will feel something in your nose, but it won't hurt" (23). The child signals if he or she is uncomfortable as the scope is passed, and adjustments are made accordingly. Encouragement and rewards (e.g., bravery certificate for having cooperated) are an integral part of the technique.

Use of rigid endoscopes and stroboscopy has recently been advocated for children over 5 years old (24). This approach provides larger, clearer visual images of the child's larynx and enables a view of mucosal waves on stroboscopy. Hirano and Bless (11) described items to be assessed, such as symmetry of movements, amplitude, and mucosal wave as well as their interpretations. Trained observers use stroboscopy in combination with other assessment techniques to obtain quantitative and qualitative data on vocal function and dysfunction. They recommend a protocol of saying /i/ at normal pitch and loudness for at least 2 seconds, then gradually increasing loudness, and elevating and lowering the pitch. Vocal attack is checked by having the patient produce a syllable chain of /i/ repetitions at a rapid rate, if possible. Sustained vowels can only be used as the endoscope intrudes orally, preventing consonant or speech production. Several authors reported the successful use of a brief examination with the 70-degree rigid endoscope, with stroboscopy, without local anesthesia (12, 24) (Fig. 2).

Video recording is advocated as this allows repeated visualization of what may only

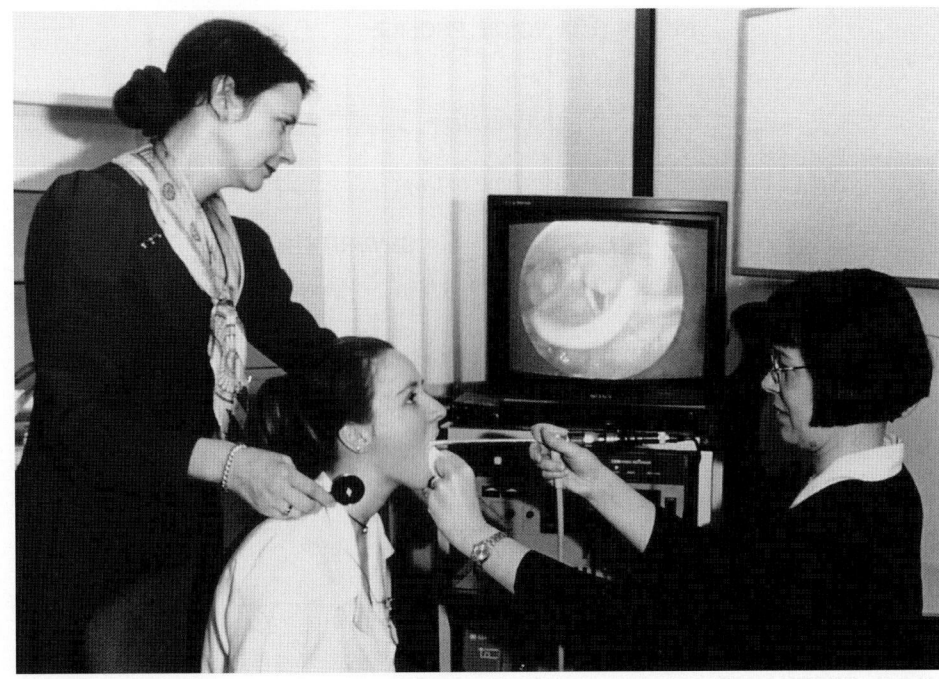

FIGURE 2 Rigid stroboscopy. (From ref. 21, with permission.)

be a brief examination, facilitating interpretation. It also permits permanent recordings of vocal fold patterns for comparison with subsequent evaluations. With the video recorder equipment it is possible to detect deviations in vocal tract physiology and anatomy (10).

If rigid endoscopy and flexible endoscopy fail, a microlaryngoscopy under general anesthesia may be necessary. Successful voice clinic outcomes are preferable and are related to adequate preparation and clinician skill and style. The pediatric environment is considered crucial to successful examination in children.

Other assessments may include radiologic and ultrasound examinations (i.e., for documentation of unilateral vocal cord paralysis), x-ray films for diagnosing laryngeal lesions and velopharyngeal function, and computed tomography of the larynx.

Phonatory Examination

This takes the form perceptual assessment, acoustic assessment, and other assessment.

Perceptual Assessment

Several subjective assessments have been reported for the description of voice, for example, the Vocal Profile Analysis Protocol (20) and the Buffalo III Voice Profile (4). The subjective rating of voice is considered to be extremely difficult. Furthermore, it is generally accepted that no instrumental technique can substitute for the trained "ear" (3) (Fig. 3).

Acoustic Assessment

Instruments now available use signal acquisition and processing techniques and computer software [e.g., Kay Elemetrics Computerized Speech Laboratory (CSLTM) Model 4300B] to provide analyses such as intensity, pitch, and spectral displays. The Multi-Dimensional Voice Program (MDVP) performs measurements of many specific acoustic parameters including jitter, shimmer, and noise to harmonic ratio.

"Perceptual-acoustic evaluation provides the critical information link between physiological voice function and a listener's perception of the resultant acoustic speech signal" (15). For research purposes, taped voice samples may be analyzed in university voice

BUFFALO III VOICE PROFILE

Name _____ Birth Date _____ Age _____ Sex _____

Rater _____ Date _____ Time of Day _____ Place _____

SEVERITY RATING

	Normal	Mild	Moderate	Severe	Very Severe
1. **LARYNGEAL TONE** Breathy Harsh Hoarse	1	2	3	4	5
2. **PITCH** Too High Too Low	1	2	3	4	5
3. **LOUDNESS** Too Loud Too Soft	1	2	3	4	5
4. **NASAL RESONANCE** Hypernasal Hyponasal	1	2	3	4	5
5. **ORAL RESONANCE** Throatiness	1	2	3	4	5
6. **BREATH SUPPLY** Amount	1	2	3	4	5
7. **MUSCLES** Hypertense Hypotense	1	2	3	4	5
8. **VOICE ABUSE** Amount and Degree	1	2	3	4	5
9. **RATE** Too Fast Too Slow	1	2	3	4	5
10. **SPEECH ANXIETY** Amount and degree	1	2	3	4	5
11. **SPEECH INTELLIGIBILITY**	1 100%	2 75%	3 50%	4 25%	5 0%
12. **OVERALL VOICE RATING**	1	2	3	4	5

COMMENTS:

Adequate Aspects   Aspects for Improvement

1. _____   1. _____

2. _____   2. _____

3. _____   3. _____

FIGURE 3 Buffalo III voice profile. (From ref. 4, with permission.)

laboratories, or with specialist equipment. Acoustic recordings (analog or digital) need to be of high quality and it is recommended that recordings are made in a soundproof room, with a unidirectional microphone with good feedback suppression, a wide frequency range, and a low distortion factor (15).

A minimal protocol for acoustic analysis, if the child is cooperative, is "three trials of two different sustained vowels, one open and low, the other high and closed, and repetition or oral reading of a standard sentence which samples several different vowels and voiced segments, such as: `I will be ready to go soon'" (15). The parameters usually assessed are fundamental frequency, amplitude of vocal fold vibrations, aperiodicity of vibration, coordination, and timing measures (18). Results need to be interpreted in the context of normal values for phonatory function in childhood (4,14).

Fundamental frequency can also be measured using an oscilloscope and amplitude by a sound level meter. A phonetogram is clinically helpful as it shows a display of physiologic ranges for intensity and fundamental frequency and for interactions of these parameters (15).

Careful interpretation of digital acoustic measures has been advocated. Several variables such as recording equipment and environment need to be taken into account. Hillman et al (25) suggested that limitations are not well enough understood by practicing clinicians. With a disordered voice signal, it is not possible to ascertain whether accurate measures are being obtained in all patients.

Other Assessment

Electrolaryngography or electroglottography records changes in electrical impedance across the larynx to measure vocal cord contact during phonation. As well as giving acoustic information, frequency of vocal fold vibration can be calculated and displayed against time (Fx) and other parameters (26). The waveform shape (Lx) corresponds to vocal fold vibration patterns. Waveforms corresponding to normal, breathy, harsh, vocal fry, and burp voice qualities have been described (27).

The myoelastic-aerodynamic theory of phonation indicates that aerodynamics are important in evaluating voice functions (18). The quantity of air and its pressure can be measured using phonatory flow rates and volumes, and intraoral pressure and resistance measures (15). Such equipment is expensive and usually laboratory based. Also there are few normative data available for children (5).

In conclusion, clinicians rely on gathering many kinds of information from many sources to reach a diagnosis. Although instrumental measures are useful when they confirm what a clinician hears in a voice, the process of analysis and synthesis of diagnostic information is dependent on clinical knowledge and expertise rather than technological ability and knowledge. Experienced clinicians will appreciate that they must interpret data from computer-based systems carefully. They need to understand the rationale for their use, and be aware of their drawbacks (18).

TREATMENT RECOMMENDATIONS

Medical and Surgical Treatment

Structural abnormalities of the vocal folds may require medical or surgical treatment such as use of the carbon dioxide laser for children with papillomas and endoscopic or open surgery for subglottic stenosis (15).

In many patients, however, initial treatment will be voice therapy and perhaps a nonspecific medical treatment such as corticosteroids for laryngeal inflammation (28). When voice therapy and medical management have been undertaken and fail, phonosurgery may be indicated (24). The general view is that phonosurgery should be avoided before the age of 10 years (12) because the integrity of the vibrating margin of the folds is put at risk by surgery (18). Experienced clinicians, however, advise operative treatment earlier for benign vocal fold lesions in motivated children (12).

Family Counselling

Most children with dysphonia exhibit vocal hyperfunction, using excessive force and effort during speech, and most voice therapy programs (4,29) place emphasis on identifying such vocal abuse and misuse, outlining specific steps for reducing their occurrence (10) (Fig. 4).

Explanations regarding normal voice production and the etiology of their specific dysphonia can be given to even young children. The level and degree of instruction will depend on the age of the child (4), but the instruction aims to increase the understanding of therapy procedures, thereby motivating the child and the family in therapy.

Advice on voice conservation (such as avoidance of vocal abuses) and hygiene (avoidance of laryngeal irritants such as very dry atmospheres and spicy foods) is given to all patients with hyperkinetic dysphonia (3).

Patient motivation and cooperation are needed for improvement to occur. Success is rewarded rather than failure highlighted (4). The whole family, teacher, and class may need to be included in the therapeutic process. When there is prolonged voice abuse that appears to have a psychological basis, it is advisable to refer the child to a clinical psychologist.

Voice rest is a principle sometimes advocated, particularly following surgery. For children, compliance is not easy; in some patients a reduction in voice use may be sufficient, together with the encouragement of gentle voice use.

Voice Therapy—General Principles

Treatment in preschool children is mainly conservative, aimed at improving vocal hygiene and modifying vocal abuse (10). School-aged children are generally able to understand the principles of voice production and use, and are usually keen to try out a variety of phonatory behaviors in voice therapy (30).

Voice therapy techniques may include any or all of a number of therapeutic approaches. For example, techniques such as listening training, relaxation techniques, breathing exercises, posture modification, and development of prosody (3,4) are advocated. Trial and error methods of searching for the most efficient voice using facilitating approaches include techniques such as chewing, inhalation phonation, yawn-sigh, and elimination of hard glottal attack (10). Visual biofeedback has been reported as particularly useful for dysphonic patients, using instrumentation such as Visi Pitch and laryngography (31).

There are now voice therapy programs specifically for children (4,30). Several factors are particularly pertinent (29). First, children tend to lack any awareness of the problem. Therapy needs to develop their awareness of communication and characteristics of their own behavior to enhance motivation for change. Second, it is important to gear the language used to children's developmental levels and to teach "voice characteristic" concepts to children during the early stages of the therapy program, such as what "hoarseness" is. The family and other significant adults, for example, teachers, are very important in the child's therapy program. The family's awareness and collaboration are vital. Last, therapy for children differs from adult therapy, because children are developing and changing as therapy progresses. Treatment needs to be designed to suit their developmental stage. Most of all, therapy tasks need to be relevant to the child, in language that is meaningful to the child, and tied to specific concrete events and situations (Fig. 5).

Therapeutic Techniques for Specific Dysphonias

Vocal Nodules

The most common lesion found in children with dysphonia is the vocal nodule (4). Voice abuse and misuse have been described as causing the majority of functional voice problems, which can lead eventually to tissue changes of the vocal folds with nodule for-

FIGURE 4 Poor voice use. (From ref. 30, with permission.)

Name _____   Date _____

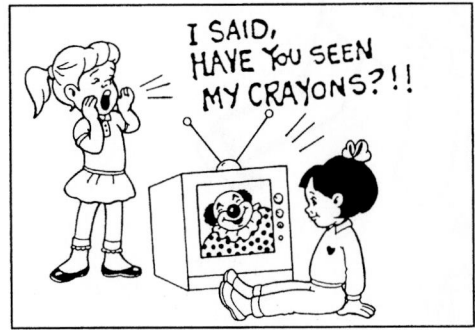

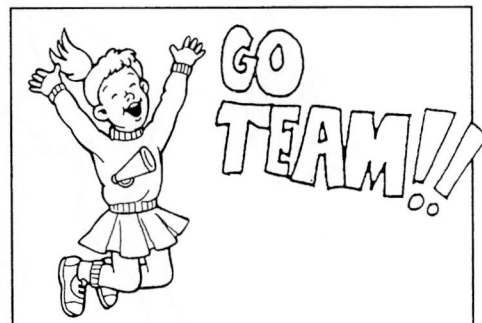

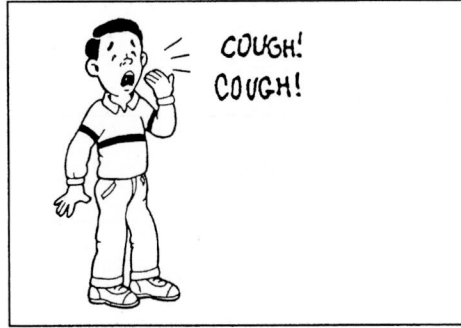

Draw a picture of a person using poor voice habits.

Circle the things you think might be bad for your voice.

1. Shouting in the lunchroom.
2. Raising your shoulders when you breathe in.
3. Singing along loudly with tapes.
4. Drinking 8 glasses of water a day.
5. Wearing socks with holes in the heels.
6. Talking on the phone for 3 hours.
7. Chewing gum.
8. Clearing your throat each time you speak.
9. Laughing loudly and harshly.
10. Touching your toes 10 times.
11. Making a noise like a locomotive.
12. Forgetting to brush your teeth.

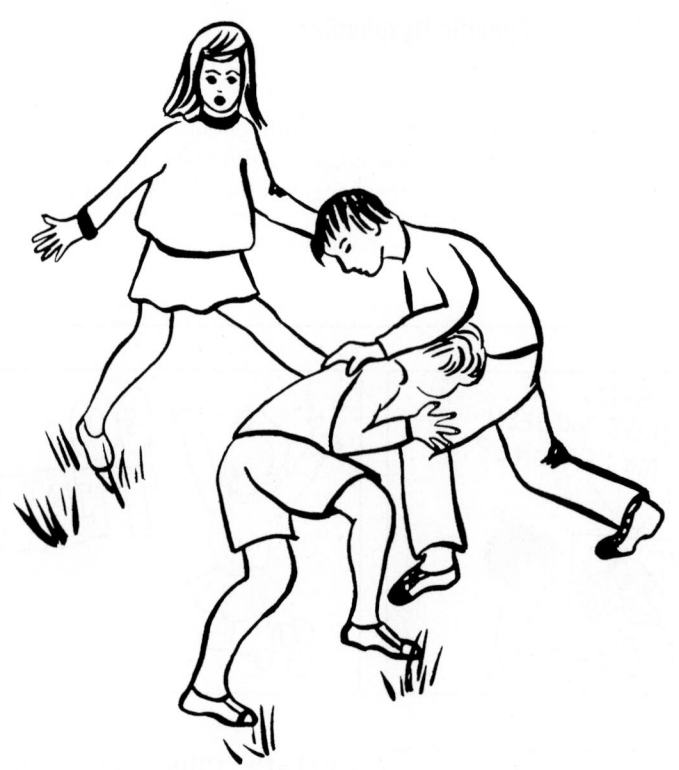

VOICE THERAPY CHART

Purpose: _____ Eliminating voice abuse _____

Name _____ Jill _____ Date ____ Nov. 4–8 ____ Week # _____ 1 _____

PLACE EVENT		Wrestling					Soccer					Swimming				
DAY		1	2	3	4	5	1	2	3	4	5	1	2	3	4	5
N U M B E R S (MINUTES)	30															
	25											22				
	20	20														
	15						18						11			
	10		10											10		
	5			5				9	4						5	
	0				0	0				0	0					0

FIGURE 5 Voice therapy chart. (From ref. 4, with permission.)

mation (10). Examples of misuse include increased strain or tension reflected in hard glottal attack, and inappropriate pitch level. Vocal abusive behaviors tend to be harsher than misuse and more likely to traumatize the vocal fold mucosa (9). (e.g., excessive coughing, screaming, prolonged loudness). Different authors have stressed psychosomatic aspects affecting voice aggression, immaturity, and inability to cope with situations that are stressful (32). Poor vocal hygiene can contribute to the dysphonia (3); for example, older children and adolescents may smoke cigarettes, drink alcohol, and work in dusty places. Of note, "loud" or large families are conducive to poor voice habits.

Vocal nodules are more common in boys than girls, with presentation peaking between the ages of 5 and 10 years (32). There is ongoing controversy as to whether the lesions disappear spontaneously at puberty (33). Vocal nodules are usually described as benign swellings at the junction of the anterior and middle thirds of the vocal folds (34). In the early stages they are soft and pliable, later becoming larger and fibrotic (10). The presenting symptom is hoarseness, with occasional coughing and frequent throat clearing. The hoarseness is exacerbated with increased voice use during the day and with deterioration of the condition. If the nodules are large, habitual pitch may be lowered considerably. However, nodule size is not directly related to the degree of dysphonia (34). There is some evidence that vocal fold immaturity in children increases their susceptibility to vocal nodules (12).

Controversy surrounds the role of the speech-language pathologist working with this condition. To date there has been no conclusive study identifying the best treatment regime. The literature consists only of a few studies: The efficacy of therapy has been questioned (32,35); however there is also a report of successful therapy (7). Ford et al (36) found that 10 of 20 patients with vocal nodules who did not respond to therapy had microwebs. These may be coincidental or representative of another expression of the response to trauma factors known to produce vocal nodules, but the voice team should ensure no vocal web is present. Ruscello et al (6) found listeners' perceptions of dysphonic children to be negative, providing strong support for early therapy. Delay until after puberty may be detrimental to peer relationships, self-esteem, and social development.

Allen et al (33) suggest that unsuccessful therapy may be related to the therapy itself. Generalist speech-language pathologists, with no opportunity to keep up-to-date, may be inadequately trained to treat this population. This is particularly so given that children with vocal nodules from only a very small percentage of typical caseloads. This provides support for the increasing role of specialist pediatric voice therapists working with this unique population.

Furthermore, in looking at outcomes, there are flaws. Vocal improvement is generally rated using subjective terminology. None of the studies cited results of acoustic analysis to support their findings. The need for objective measures to quantify subjective ratings of voice has been identified in the literature (25).

Current treatment tends to be conservative rather than involve early surgery (12,32), which is arguably not necessary in children and possibly harmful (34). Any injury to the vocal fold margin can cause lasting vocal disability and the nodules would be likely to recur promptly if the etiologic factors were not successfully identified and eliminated. More recently, however, Benjamin and Croxon (37) reported success with surgical removal of nodules and questioned the value of voice therapy even by experienced clinicians. Also Hirschberg et al (38) cited a retrospective study of 179 children comparing results of vocal hygiene, voice therapy, surgery, and no treatment for vocal nodules and polyps. Eighty-nine percent showed improvement by surgery at 1 month after the operation, 40% showed some improvement following voice therapy, and only 6% of patients showed improvement practicing vocal hygiene after about 7 months. Surgery was recommended for patients distressed due to hoarseness who required immediate improvement. If voice improvement was not urgent, voice therapy was recommended. If patients were not motivated, vocal hygiene was recommended—results not being expected anyway due to noncompliance.

Despite the lack of scientific evidence, in the author's opinion, voice therapy should always be considered as a first-line approach. Surgical procedures alone are unlikely to have long-lasting effects unless coincidental with advantageous spontaneous changes in laryngeal structure and function (possibly associated with puberty) or changes in other predisposing and precipitating factors such as patterns of voice abuse and misuse or emotional state. In children for whom voice therapy alone has not been sufficient, surgery may be indicated. If the child and family are unmotivated to participate in therapy, regular reviews rather than a surgical approach are advocated to reinforce advice on voice conservation and hygiene, to assess for changes in attitude toward therapy (particularly if the dysphonia increases or if vocal demands on the child increase), and to assess possible effects of puberty.

This review highlights the need for a systematic study to assess the effects of puberty on the dysphonic voice, due to vocal nodules, and to compare that outcomes of voice therapy and surgical intervention for vocal nodules, using specialist voice therapists to rate children's voices before and after therapy and comparing them with normal controls. Acoustic analysis should be used to quantify the perceptual findings.

Vocal Fold Palsy

Vocal fold palsy may be congenital or acquired, unilateral or bilateral (3). Aronson (16) described how vagus nerve lesions may be intramedullary, extramedullary, or extracranial. Some or all of the branches of the vagus may be affected, with resulting paralysis (immobility) or paresis (weakness) of laryngeal muscles and aphonia or dysphonia. The location of the lesion along the nerve pathway, and whether one or both nerves are involved, will determine the degree of dysphonia. Usually there is abductor palsy with unilateral vocal cord palsy due to, for example, birth trauma, idiopathic factors, chemotherapy, or trauma (19). There is a reasonably good prognosis for recovery in infants and children (39).

Most authors described mixed findings for voice function: abnormal cry (16), breathiness and weakness (3,4), hoarseness, monotone and soft voice (4), short maximum phonation time and loss of mucosal waves (3), changes of pitch and problems with fine control (4), and lack of ability to produce the lowest notes of the vocal range (3). Clinically a normal cry can often be reported, further clouding the diagnosis of this lesion (19). There have been few scientific studies to substantiate reports. Hoarseness has been more commonly associated with unilateral palsy whereas normal voices may occur with bilateral involvement (39). When both cords are in a median position, the voice is good (4). Most authors advocate voice therapy for unilateral or bilateral vocal fold palsy (3,4,10,16).

Therapy techniques include effort closure, elimination of excess muscular tension, a trial and error search for the optimum pitch and loudness involving the least physical effort, and counselling for emotional problems arising from the voice disorder (16).

Alternative surgical approaches are advocated for patients who do not make progress with therapy (3). Arytenoidectomy may be indicated for bilateral involvement (3). However, airway improvement may be at the expense of voice (40), although from clinical experience this is not always the case. As arytenoidectomy is nonreversible, it should not normally be considered until the age of 10 years (28). Medialization laryngoplasty-thyroplasty may be required for unilateral vocal fold palsy (3). Because it is reversible, it may be suitable at an earlier age, although the worldwide experience of pediatric thyroplasty is still quite small (28). The indications for phonosurgery in pediatric populations are only now being developed (19).

In extreme cases of bilateral vocal fold palsy patients may need to learn to use an electrolarynx. When the vocal folds are paralyzed in an abducted position, phonation is not possible (10).

Long-Term Tracheostomy

The presence of a tracheostomy for more than 1 month may be associated with developmental problems, as tracheostomized babies are often sicker than nontracheostomized babies and may have additional developmental delays and problems that can delay or interfere with their acquisition of speech (19).

The presence of a tracheostomy tube may also interfere with vocalization, making it difficult or even impossible. For voicing there needs to be some air leak around the cannula and through the larynx. Lack of phonation causes an inability to babble and develop expressive language. Bleile (41) described how the long-term status of language at the age of approximately 5 years has been documented and was commensurate with nonverbal intelligence.

A considerable number of tracheostomized children appear delayed when compared to children of their own age. The children may also have language delays when they enter school and further research is advocated. Virtually all have extensive speech and language therapy intervention for their communication difficulties. Most investigators recommend intervention as essential to achieving a good outcome. Intervention involves assessment of phonation and choice of therapy among the options available (40).

Therapy Options to Facilitate Expressive Communication   A child who can achieve phonation spontaneously (with or without finger occlusion or by using chin dipping to cover the tracheostomy tube) is a candidate for a one-way speaking valve (e.g., Rusche, Passy-Muir, De Santi). With one-way *speaking valves*, enhancements of communicative development have been reported (42), with improvements such as clearer and easier vocalization; normalized vocal quality, pitch, intensity, and intonation; increased vocalizations and babbling; and increased appetite. The choice of valve appears related to the preference of the surgeon, speech and language therapist, and parent or child. All require medical consultation and referral. Therapy involves desensitization of the child to the valve and reinforcement of all vocalizations (42). Papsin (19) advised that these speaking valves on occasion can become jammed closed with an accumulation of debris and secretions. Children must be able to remove the valve consistently on their own before it can be used without adult supervision. Caution must be exercised with younger children and those with other muscular weakness or incoordination. Some older children may benefit from use of a fenestrated tube (42) in conjunction with a speaking valve.

The *electrolarynx* generates a vibratory sound source. When held against the child's neck, the electrolarynx transmits the sound into the vocal tract for speech production (42). It is a short-term option useful for aphonic children who had developed expressive speech and language before tracheostomy. Electrolarynxes are expensive. Another therapeutic use is for children who have never babbled. The child needs to be able to hold it and to have good oral-motor movements. Therapy procedures include desensitizing the child to the device (noise and vibration) by letting him or her feel it on the arm or leg, and oral imitation activities (42).

Silverman and McGowan (42) reported how air trapped in the cheeks can be modified by the articulators to produce "buccal speech." Although reportedly insufficient for intelligible speech, it has been described as useful for aphonic children, for example, getting attention and making simple requests, even if using imprecise words. Procedures are often discovered by the children in nonvocal oral-motor play, and speech-language pathologists can encourage it by positively reinforcing its use. Esophageal speech may be particularly difficult for children, especially young children.

Therapy Options Facilitating Nonoral Communication   Aphonic children who have reached a cognitive developmental level of at least 9 months and who have sufficient motor skills benefit from an introduction of *sign language* (in America Signed English and American Sign Language) to communicate (42). In the United Kingdom the popular system is Makaton.

Picture communication boards or computer systems are useful for children with motor problems that preclude the use of electrolarynxes or the development of sign language. Children must show the cognitive ability to associate meanings with symbols (42).

Subglottic Stenosis

This disorder involves narrowing of the subglottis, and the glottis may also be involved. It may be congenital or acquired; the latter is associated with a "scarred contracted laryngeal opening" (43). Children may present with hoarse voice, limited exercise tolerance, stridor, "croup," and a history of failed extubation (44).

Although normal growth allows a small number of children to be decannulated (45), widening of the stenosis can be surgically achieved using endoscopic resection or laryngotracheal reconstruction (LTR) with rib grafting to augment the airway, permitting decannulation.

Results of voice studies following LTR suggest that the majority of children have abnormal voices. Percentages vary from 21% (46) to 93% (47). There have been numerous variables across studies, for example, subject selection criteria, uses of various types of stents and for varying durations, vocal rehabilitation factors, and voice assessment methodologies.

Quality has been described as harsh, whisper (48), rough with elements of breathiness (49), and hoarse (50). Pitch has been found to be high or low (48), in the region of 100 to 130 Hz, as compared to other similarly aged control children (49). Volume is reduced (49), pitch range is inadequate, maximum phonation time is shortened (50), speed of vocal fold vibration is random (49), and inhalation phonation with some associated articulatory problems and decreased speech intelligibility have been reported (50).

Videolaryngoscopic findings include anterior commissure blunting, supraglottic vibration during phonation and abnormal vocal fold mobility (48), poor or incomplete movement of one or both arytenoids (51), arytenoid fixation (50), and vocal cords at different levels resulting in vertical asymmetry during vibration (51). Surgical techniques are continuously evolving, with the aim of improving voice outcome (51).

Very few studies have reported voice assessment findings prior to LTR. Many children are tracheostomized and aphonic before surgery and are unfortunately often too young to be cooperative for voice assessments. Studies that exist, such as that by Zalzal et al (47), have methodologic flaws such as small subject numbers, lack of control data, mixed pathology prior to LTR, varying numbers and types of surgical procedures previously undertaken, and omission of objective measures.

A voice assessment is recommended after LTR. Voice therapy aims to eliminate supraglottal phonation using inhalation phonation techniques as described by Boone and McFarlane (10). Traditional voice therapy techniques may then strengthen the voice. Occasionally, when glottal voice is not possible due to pathology, supraglottal phonation needs to be encouraged as a substitute voice.

Ventilated Children

One speaking valve—the Passy-Muir—fits in line into a ventilator (18) and enables the ventilator-dependent child who has an air leak around the tracheostomy tube to speak.

Another option for ventilated patients who require a cuffed tracheostomy tube is the use of a speaking tracheostomy tube (18) (Figs. 6 and 7). Gas travels through an extra air line exiting via a slit just superior to the cuff, and then continues up through the glottis and vocal tract. Occluding the port of a Y-piece at the proximal end directs air to allow phonation.

Puberphonia

During puberty there is usually a change in the speaking fundamental frequency of the voice due to laryngeal growth (voice mutation). In boys the pitch lowers by about an octave and in girls, by about three to four semitones (4). In most boys complete mutation of the voice takes place within 3 to 6 months (16). Disturbed mutation is usually psychogenic in origin. It may be organic or functional or a combination of the two (e.g., psychological involvement, juvenile personality, and sexual conflicts (4).

On laryngoscopy excessive tension may be noted, particularly in the posterior carti-

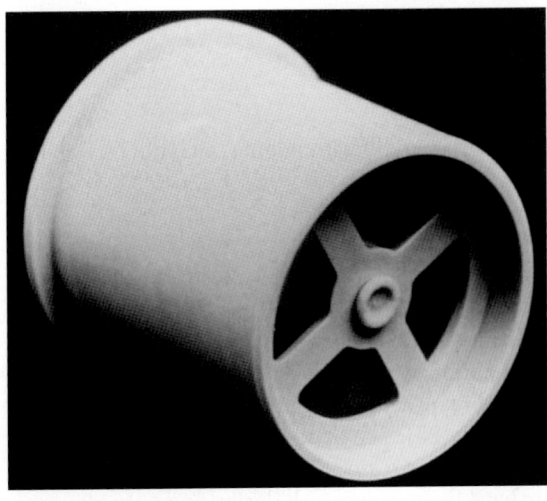

FIGURE 6 Passy-Muir speaking valve. (By kind permission of Passy-Muir Inc.)

laginous area. There may be restriction of vocal fold vibration (to the anterior membranous portion) and the larynx may be elevated (18).

Speech therapy is the appropriate treatment using either voice therapy techniques or visual biofeedback (18). The Speech Viewer is particularly helpful. Counseling is frequently an integral part of therapy.

Laryngeal Webs

Wilson (4) described how these consist of thin connective tissue and range in size. They are associated with weak, hoarse, or absent cry. Usually pitch raises in proportion to the shortening of the free margins of the vocal folds. Treatment is usually surgical and if required, voice therapy after web removal (4).

Ventricular Band Phonation

Boone and McFarlane (10) described how production of this phonation type involves vibration of approximating ventricular folds, which, being large in mass, usually results in a low-pitched voice, limited pitch variability, and monotonous speech. They further suggested that the voice, which is usually hoarse, may be a successful compensatory method of phonating when severe pathology (e.g., severe papilloma) precludes true vocal fold vibration. Sometimes, in diplophonia, both true and false cords vibrate simultaneously. It may also be caused by vocal abuse, psychological stress, or surgery or can present congenitally in the presence or absence of true vocal cords (4). When there is no

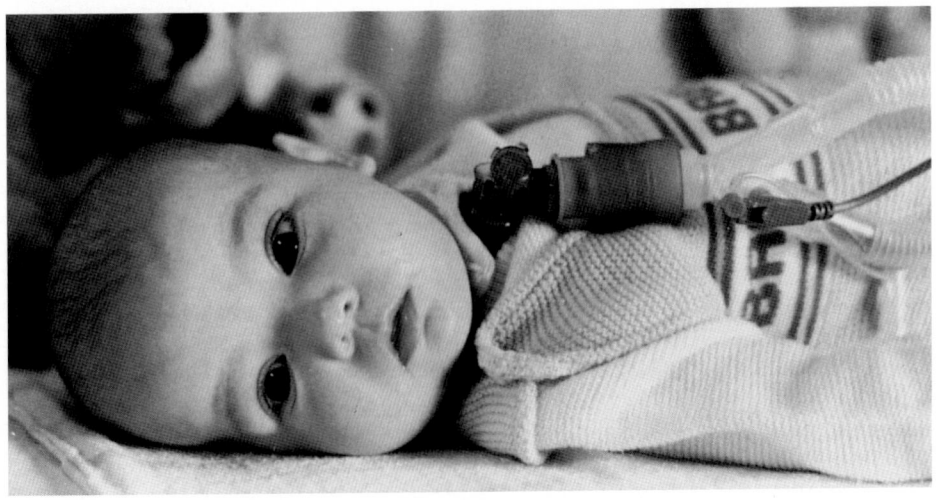

FIGURE 7 Ventilated baby using a Passy-Muir speaking valve. (By kind permission of Passy-Muir Inc.)

persisting pathology of the true cords, voice therapy to restore glottal phonation is usually successful (10).

Vocal Cord Edema

The superficial layer of the lamina propria can fill with edema in conditions such as vocal abuse or laryngitis (3).

Efficacy of Voice Therapy

Do children benefit from voice therapy? Benjamin and Croxon (37) suggested that children find it hard to cooperate even with specialist clinicians, possibly generating further problems of conflict between family members. Speech and language therapists and pathologists generally believe that intervention with voice-disordered patients can be very successful. Their views are based on perceptual judgments, patient reports, and results of post-treatment laryngeal examinations (25). The need for objective investigations to evaluate the effects of voice therapy has been stressed (25). There are very few studies reported in the literature, and many have flaws in research design and outcome measures. The reports are essentially descriptive, none employing a valid experimental design to assess effects (25).

⚙ REFERENCES

1. Morley ME. *The development and disorders of speech in childhood*. Edinburgh: Churchill Livingstone, 1972.
2. Borden GJ, Harris KS. *Speech science primer*, 2nd ed. Baltimore: Williams & Wilkins, 1984.
3. Greene MCL, Mathieson L. *The voice and its disorders*. London: Whurr, 1989.
4. Wilson DK. *Voice problems of children*, 3rd ed. Baltimore: Williams & Wilkins, 1987.
5. Zajac DJ, Farkas Z, Dindzans LJ, Stool SE. Aerodynamic and laryngographic assessment of pediatric vocal function. *Pediatr Pulmonol* 1993;15:44–51.
6. Ruscello DM, Lass NJ, Podbesek J. Listeners' perceptions of normal and voice-disordered children. *Folia Phoniatr* 1988;40:290–296.
7. Deal RE, McClain B, Sudderth JF. Identification, evaluation, therapy, and follow-up for children with vocal nodules in a public school setting. *J Speech Hear Disord* 1976;41:390–397.
8. Shearer WM. Diagnosis and treatment of voice disorders in school children. *J Speech Hear Disord* 1972;37:215–221.
9. Colton RH, Casper JK. *Understanding voice problems*. Baltimore: Williams & Wilkins, 1990.
10. Boone DR, McFarlane SC. *The voice and voice therapy*, 4th ed. Englewood Cliffs, NJ: Prentice-Hall, 1988.
11. Hirano M, Bless DM. *Videostroboscopic examination of the larynx*. San Diego: Whurr, 1993.
12. Schalen L, Rydell R. Dysphonia in children: not necessarily due to voice abuse. *Voice* 1995; 4:44–45.
13. Cohen SR, Thompson JW, Geller KA, Birns JW. Voice change in the pediatric patient. *Ann Otol Rhinol Laryngol* 1983;92:437–443.
14. Baken RJ. *Clinical measures of speech and voice*. London: Taylor and Francis Ltd, 1987.
15. Morrison M, Rammage L. *The management of voice disorders*. London: Chapman and Hall Medical, 1994.
16. Aronson AE. *Clinical voice disorders*, 3rd ed. New York: Thieme, 1990.
17. Titze I. Voice research. Critical periods of vocal change: puberty. *NATS J* 1993;(Jan/Feb).
18. Andrews ML. *Manual of voice treatment*. San Diego: Singular Publishing Group, 1995.
19. Papsin BC. Personal communication, 1996.
20. Laver J. *The gift of speech*. Edinburgh: Edinburgh University Press, 1991.
21. Papsin BC, Pengilly AJ, Leighton SEJ. The developing role of a paediatric voice clinic: a review of our experience. *J Laryngol Otol* 1996;110:1022–1026.
22. D'Antonio LA, Chiat D, Lotz W, Netsell R. Pediatric videonasendoscopy for speech and voice evaluation. *Otolaryngol Head Neck Surg* 1986;94:578–583.
23. Lotz WK, D'Antonio LL, Chait DH, Netsell RW. Successful nasoendoscopic and aerodynamic examinations of children with speech/voice disorders. *Int J Pediatr Otorhinolaryngol* 1993;26:165–172.

24. Cornut G, Troillet-Cornut A. Childhood dysphonia: clinical and therapeutic considerations. *Voice* 1995;4:70–76.

25. Hillman RE, DeLassus Gress C, Hargrave J, Walsh M, Bunting G. The efficacy of speech-language pathology intervention: voice disorders. *Semin Speech Lang* 1990; 11: 297–310.

26. Abberton E, Fourcin A. Electrolaryngography. In: Code C, Ball M, eds. *Experimental clinical phonetics*. Croom Helm, 1984:62–78.

27. MacCurtain F, Fourcin AJ. Applications of the electroglottograph wave form display. In: Lawrence V, ed. *Transcripts of the tenth symposium: care of the professional voice*. Part I. New York: The Voice Foundation, 1982:51–57.

28. Albert D. Personal communication, 1996.

29. Andrews ML. *Voice therapy for children*. London: Longman, 1986.

30. Flynn PT, Andrews ML. *Using your voice wisely and well*. Tucson: Communication Skill Builders, 1990.

31. Hirson A, Fawcus R. Visual feedback in the management of dysphonia. In: Fawcus M, ed. *Voice disorders and their management*, 2nd ed. London: Chapman and Hall, 1991.

32. Toohill RJ. The psychosomatic aspects of children with vocal nodules. *Arch Otolaryngol* 1975; 101:591–595.

33. Allen MS, Pettit JM, Sherblom JC. Management of vocal nodules: a regional survey of otolaryngologists and speech-language pathologists. *J Speech Hear Res* 1991;34:229–235.

34. Von Leden H. Vocal nodules in children. *Ear Nose Throat J* 1985;64:29–41.

35. Kay NJ. Vocal nodules in children—aetiology and management. *J Laryngol Otol* 1982;96: 731–736.

36. Ford CN, Bless DM, Campos G, Leddy M. Anterior commissure microwebs associated with vocal nodules: detection, prevalence, and significance. *Laryngoscope* 1994;104:1369–1375.

37. Benjamin B, Croxen G. Vocal nodules in children. *Ann Otol Rhinol Laryngol* 1987;96: 530–533.

38. Hirschberg J, Dejonckere PH, Hirano M, Mori K, Schultz-Couton H-J, Vrticka K. Symposium voice disorders in children. *Int J Pediatr Otorhinolaryngol* 1995;32[Suppl]:S109–S125.

39. Gentile RD, Miller RH, Woodson GE. Vocal cord paralysis in children 1 year of age and younger. *Ann Otol Rhinol Laryngol* 1986;95:622–625.

40. Tucker HM. Vocal cord paralysis in small children: principles in management. *Ann Otolaryngol Rhinol Laryngol* 1986;95:618–621.

41. Bleile KM. Children with long term tracheostomies. In: Bleile KM, ed. *The care of children with long-term tracheostomies*. San Diego: Singular Publishing Group, 1993.

42. Silverman McGowan J, Bleile KM, Fus L, Baranas E. Communication disorders. In: Bleile KM, ed. *The care of children with long-term tracheostomies*. San Diego: Singular Publishing Group, 1993.

43. Evans JNG. Stenosis of the larynx. In: Evans JNG, ed. *Scott-Brown's otolaryngology*, 5th ed. Paediatric otolaryngology. London: Butterworth, 1987:495–502.

44. Morrisey MSC, Bailey CM. Diagnosis and management of subglottic stenosis after neonatal ventilation. *Arch Dis Child* 1990;65:1103–1108.

45. Bailey CM. Surgical management of acquired subglottic stenosis. *J Laryngol Otol Suppl* 1988; 17:45–48.

46. Smith RJH, Catlin FI. Laryngotracheal stenosis: a 5-year review. *Head Neck* 1991;13: 140–144.

47. Zalzal GH, Loomis SR, Derkay MD, Murray SL, Thomsen J. Voice quality of decannulated children following laryngeal reconstruction. *Laryngoscope* 1991;101:425–429.

48. Clary RA, Pengilly A, Bailey M, et al. Analysis of voice outcomes in paediatric patients following surgery for laryngotracheal stenosis *Arch Otolaryngol Head Neck Surg* 1996;122: 1189–1194.

49. Sell D, MacCurtain F. Speech and language development in children with acquired subglottic stenosis. *J Laryngol Otol Suppl* 1988;17:35–38.

50. Smith ME, Marsh JH, Cotton RT, Myer CM. Voice problems after pediatric laryngotracheal reconstruction: videolaryngoscopic, acoustic and perceptual assessment. *Int J Pediatr Otorhinolaryngol* 1993;25: 173–181.

51. Smith ME, Mortelliti AJ, Cotton RT, Myer CM. Phonation and swallowing considerations in pediatric laryngotracheal reconstruction. *Ann Otolaryngol Rhinol Laryngol* 1992;101: 731–738.

A.J. Pengilly: Department of Speech Therapy, The University of Singapore, Singapore.

• *Practical Pediatric Otolaryngology*
• edited by Robin T. Cotton and Charles M. Myer, III
• Lippincott-Raven Publishers, Philadelphia © 1999

6

Sialorrhea

C. Martin Bailey

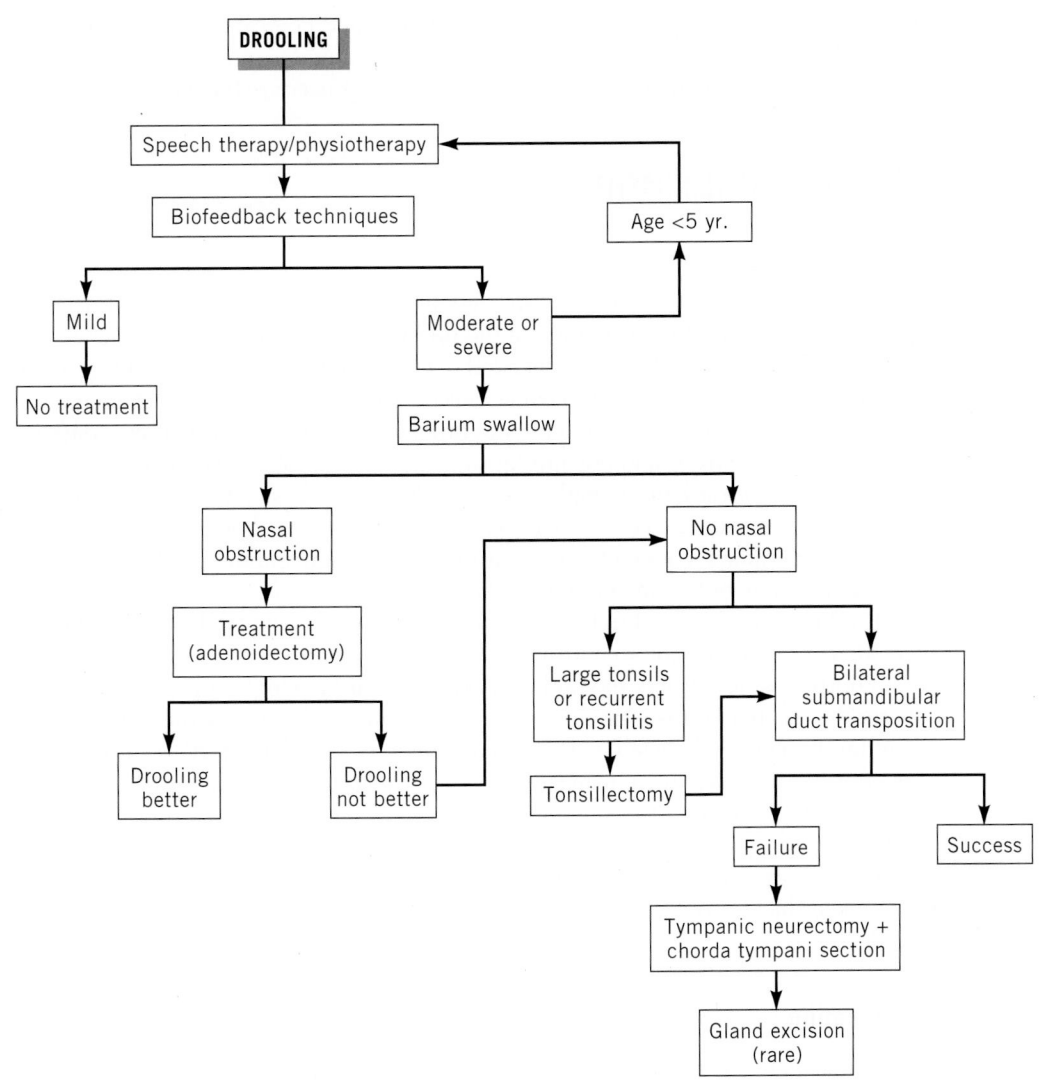

HISTORICAL BACKGROUND

Sialorrhea, or drooling, is a common problem among neurologically impaired children and reflects a failure of coordination of the muscles of the tongue, palate, and face that act in the first stage of swallowing. There is excessive pooling of saliva in the anterior part of the mouth, and consequent overspill. Children with cerebral palsy comprise the largest group afflicted by this problem, and it often isolates them from society more than any of their other handicaps.

Dissatisfaction with the results of physiotherapy, medical treatment, and even radiotherapy prompted an evaluation of surgical options. Interest in the surgical treatment of drooling developed from the description in 1967 of a technique by Wilkie (1), which consisted of bilateral submandibular gland excision and rerouting of the parotid ducts into the tonsillar fossae. Since then, a number of other procedures that aim to reduce saliva production, redirect salivary flow, or do both have been described. In 1968 Enfors and Lundberg (2) and in 1969 Laage-Hellman (3) described transposition of the submandibular ducts into the tonsillar fossae. In 1970 Goode and Smith (4) reported the results of bilateral chorda tympani section and bilateral tympanic neurectomy, so dividing the parasympathetic secretomotor fibers to the submandibular and parotid glands respectively. In 1978 Glass et al (5) and in 1979 Dundas and Peterson (6) reported the outcome of bilateral submandibular gland excision with bilateral parotid duct ligation, claiming less morbidity than that associated with the Wilkie procedure but with equal success.

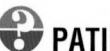 **PATIENT ASSESSMENT**

History

Objective methods of measuring drooling are difficult to perform and may not necessarily correlate well with the magnitude of the problem to patients, parents, teachers, and nursing staff (7). A careful history is needed to establish the severity of dribbling, noting the number of bibs or tops that become soaked with saliva and require changing each day. Factors that aggravate the tendency to drool are determined, such as concentration on a task in hand, stress, and posture (in some children dribbling becomes very severe when they lean forward, for example, over schoolwork on a desk). An assessment is made of the degree of voluntary control that can be exerted over the drooling, and a judgment is formed regarding the patient's awareness of the problem and the psychosocial effects that it has on him, or her and on the family and school friends.

It is important to establish the severity of neurodevelopmental delay, and in particular the degree of oromotor control and swallowing ability, as this influences the outcome of treatment. Parents should be asked how well the child can eat and drink: the poorer the ability to initiate the first stage of swallowing, the poorer the result of treatment for drooling is likely to be. At this point, enquiry should be made regarding previous efforts with conservative management, in particular, speech therapy/physiotherapy and biofeedback techniques aimed at improving jaw elevation, lip closure, and tongue control.

If there is a history of recurrent tonsillitis, tonsillectomy will be needed prior to submandibular duct transposition in order to prevent the risk of retrograde submandibular sialadenitis.

Examination

On examination, any factors causing nasal obstruction must be assessed: nasal obstruction tends to cause mouth-breathing, and this predisposes to dribbling, but it must be remembered that a mouth-open facies is usual in the child with cerebral palsy. Particular attention must be paid to head control (lolling with neck flexion increases drooling), tongue control, and swallowing ability. A crude but useful assessment of tongue control can be derived from the patient's ability to protrude the tongue on request. Excoriation of the skin around the mouth may result from severe drooling. The size of the tonsils can be important: If they are very large, relocation of the submandibular ducts behind the anterior faucial pillars will be difficult and preliminary tonsillectomy will be necessary.

Investigations

Further investigations are seldom needed. However, if there is clinical evidence of any disorder of the second or third stage of swallowing, a barium swallow study should be performed to exclude the possibility of chronic aspiration, spastic esophageal disease, or esophageal stricture (8).

PEARLS AND PERILS

1. Ensure relief of any nasal obstruction, to minimize mouth-open facies.
2. Beware the severely handicapped child with head lolling in flexion (you cannot defeat gravity!).
3. Do not consider surgery until the age of 5 to 6 years. Drooling has a natural tendency to improve as children grow older, and this happens more slowly in the neurologically damaged child (9).
4. Each child should have at least 6 months of oral training to improve oral-motor skills before surgery.

 TREATMENT RECOMMENDATIONS

Author's Preferred Method: Bilateral Submandibular Duct Transposition

Following the original descriptions of submandibular duct transposition (2,3), the technique has been widely adopted by others (8,10–13). Each submandibular duct is dissected out and rerouted through a submucosal tunnel to open posteriorly in the tonsillar fossa.

Tonsillectomy is not routinely necessary, but should be undertaken prior to submandibular duct transposition in patients who have recurrent tonsillitis, as otherwise there is a risk of retrograde submandibular sialadenitis. Tonsillectomy *after* duct transposition may be difficult without damaging the ducts! Preliminary tonsillectomy should also be done if the tonsils are very large, making relocation of the ducts behind the anterior faucial pillars difficult. The author's preference is to perform the tonsillectomy, if indicated, 3 months before duct transposition, although others are prepared to combine the two procedures (9).

The operation is carried out with the patient positioned as for a tonsillectomy, with general anesthesia maintained via a nasotracheal tube taken out of the operative field through the head drape. A side mouth gag or dental prop is inserted, and a small pharyngeal pack is used to prevent the accumulation of blood in the pharynx. The surgeon works from the head of the patient: a headlight can be helpful when working posteriorly at the fauces, but most of the procedure is best performed using an overhead operating light.

A malleable retractor is used to retract the tip of the tongue and flatten the floor of the mouth, which is infiltrated around the sublingual papillae with about 2 mL of adrenaline (epinephrine) 1:200,000. An elliptical incision 2.5 cm long and 1 cm wide is then made around the sublingual papillae, and the "island" of mucosa thus created is carefully elevated. This large island is divided in the midline between the papillae to leave a smaller mucosal island around the opening of each submandibular duct (Fig. 1): Each island is tagged laterally (to avoid the duct) with a 4-0 black silk suture.

With gentle traction on the suture, the submandibular duct is identified and separated from the sublingual salivary gland by sharp dissection. The duct is then dissected out until the lingual nerve is visualized, or the deep part of the gland is reached, thus mobilizing a length of 2 to 3 cm (Fig. 2). The use of "peanut" swabs wrung out in a solution of adrenaline (epinephrine) 1:1,000 is a valuable aid to dissection and hemostasis during this delicate part of the procedure.

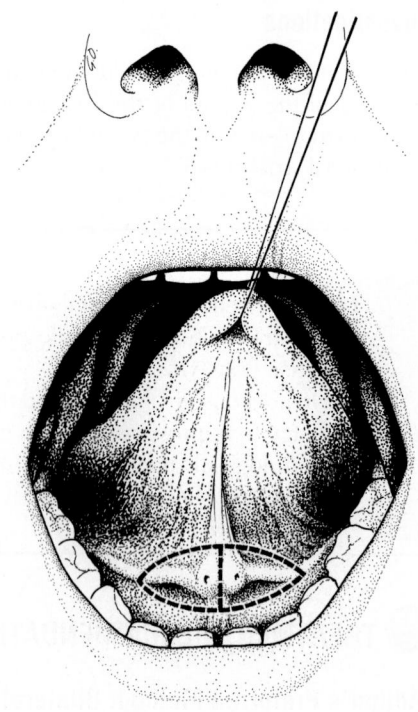

FIGURE 1 Elliptical incision around sublingual papillae. (From ref. 13, with permission.)

A pair of fine, slightly curved artery forceps is then used to create a submucosal tunnel from the lateral end of the incision, at the deepest point of the dissection alongside the duct, to the tonsillar fossa just behind the base of the anterior faucial pillar. A firm "push" on the forceps is required to penetrate the palatoglossus and enter the tonsillar fossa. During this maneuver the tongue is retracted with a 1–0 black silk suture placed through its lateral border as far posteriorly as possible (Fig. 3). A heavy silk suture is grasped with the artery forceps in the tonsillar fossa and pulled back through the tunnel: It is then tied to the "tagging" suture on the mucosal island and used to pull the duct

FIGURE 2 Dissection of the submandibular duct. (From ref. 13, with permission.)

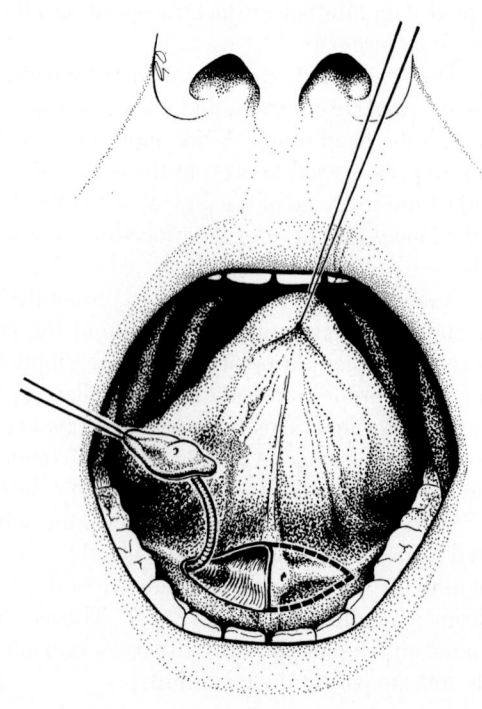

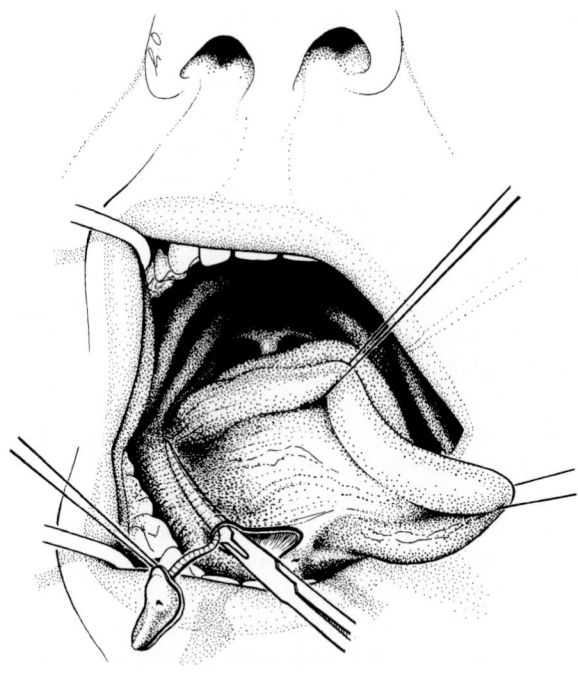

FIGURE 3 Creation of the submucosal tunnel. (From ref. 13, with permission.)

through the tunnel, taking care to avoid kinking or twisting. A single 4-0 polyglactin 910 (Vicryl) suture is employed to secure the mucosal island to the edge of the faucial incision within the tonsillar fossa (Fig. 4). The same method is used on the other side, and the sublingual incision is left unsutured.

Postoperatively there is some swelling of the floor of the mouth for 24 to 48 hours, and sometimes swelling of the submandibular glands as well, but there is seldom any difficulty in encouraging an adequate intake of oral fluids. Patients generally remain in the hospital for 3 nights following surgery, until they are eating and drinking well. An initial outpatient evaluation of the success of the operation is made after 4 weeks, but the child is assessed again 3 months and 1 year postoperatively.

FIGURE 4 The duct is passed through the tunnel. (From ref. 13, with permission.)

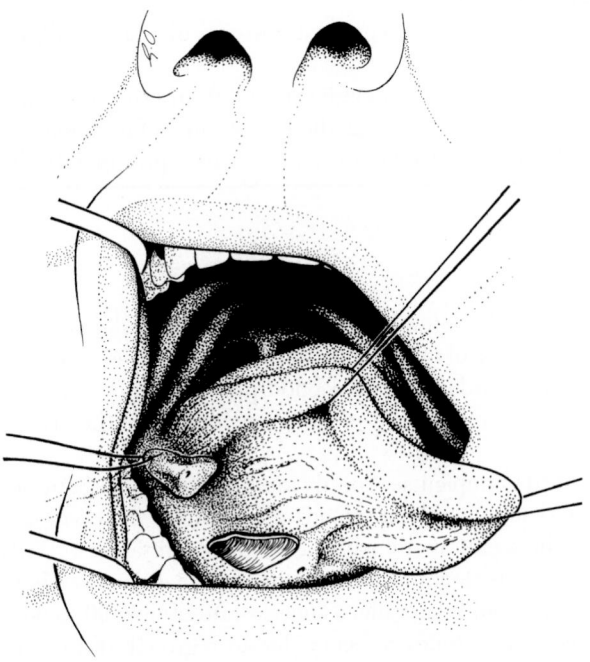

The technique has a high rate of success (80% to 100% in the series cited above), and minimal morbidity with few complications (infection, ranula formation). Furthermore, no external incisions are required as the dissection is intraoral. The initial improvement seems to be well maintained in the long term (14,15), despite the experience reported by some (16). Indirect evidence by radioisotope scanning indicates continued function of the submandibular glands at near-normal secretion rates following the procedure (10,17). The operation is logically directed at the glands responsible for 70% of total resting salivary secretion (18). Furthermore, in patients who drool, the problem is not one of excessive production of saliva but of the inability to swallow it satisfactorily. Redirecting the flow of saliva so that it is more easily swallowed thus corrects the fundamental defect while maintaining normal function; the sense of taste and the quantity of saliva produced are not affected. In particular, the risk of xerostomia is avoided.

Crysdale modified his technique in 1988 to include intraoral excision of the sublingual glands (9). This is done primarily to eliminate the risk of postoperative ranula formation, although it also reduces saliva production by 5%. However, it does substantially add to the procedure and increases the risk of damage to the lingual nerves. The incidence of postoperative ranula formation is relatively low (less than 10%), and most of the cysts either resolve spontaneously or require no more than simple marsupialization (see below), and so the author's preference is to leave the sublingual glands *in situ*.

The operation of bilateral submandibular duct transposition is technically straightforward, has a high rate of success with a low morbidity, and entails no external scars. It is the procedure of choice for the drooling patient in whom speech therapy or physiotherapy has proved unhelpful. However, it is important that the expectations of all concerned are realistic: substantial improvement can be expected, but it is rare to totally eliminate drooling. In particular, preoperative neurologic status is more predictive of surgical outcome than severity of sialorrhea, with the more severely handicapped children deriving less benefit (15).

PEARLS AND PERILS

1. Preliminary tonsillectomy is unnecessary unless there is a history of recurrent tonsillitis or the tonsils are very large.
2. Prophylactic antibiotic cover is essential to prevent postoperative submandibular sialadenitis.
3. The sublingual incision in the floor of the mouth is best left unsutured in order to minimize postoperative swelling and reduce the risk of ranula formation.
4. The result of surgery should not be judged until at least 4 weeks postoperatively.

Other Methods

Denervation procedures have a place for those few patients in whom submandibular duct transposition fails to achieve adequate control of drooling. In this circumstance, bilateral tympanic neurectomy with unilateral chorda tympani section probably represents the best compromise, in order to preserve some sense of taste and minimize the risk of xerostomia.

Tympanic neurectomy and chorda tympani section divide the parasympathetic secretomotor fibers to the parotid and submandibular glands respectively, via a tympanotomy approach to the middle ear. The secretomotor pathway to the minor salivary glands is unaffected, as it follows a different route, together with that for lacrimation (19). However, even when both nerves are sectioned bilaterally, a success rate of only 50 to 80% can be expected (4,12,20), and late failure tends to occur due to regrowth of preganglionic fibers along the multiple anatomic communications that are known to exist between the parasympathetic fibers of the glossopharyngeal nerve and the nervus intermedius (19).

Initial failure to control dribbling has been attributed to incomplete sectioning of all branches of the tympanic plexus on the promontory (12), but although there is sensory branching of Jacobson's nerve on the promontory, the parasympathetic neurons are said to course through the middle ear without branching (21). Initial failure is more likely to be due to the patient's inability to swallow well enough to clear even a reduced amount of saliva from the mouth. If both nerves are sectioned bilaterally, loss of taste to the anterior two-thirds of the tongue is inevitable, and xerostomia is said to be a risk. Complications are rare, but the procedure is contraindicated in any patient with a unilateral sensorineural hearing loss because of the remote risk of surgically damaging the only-hearing ear. Furthermore, it would seem wise to separate the operation on each ear by 3 to 6 months rather than risk complications developing simultaneously on both sides.

Parotid duct ligation is another second-line technique that can be useful if residual drooling is mainly watery (9). Combining this with *bilateral submandibular gland excision* (essentially a modification of the Wilkie procedure) is an approach supported by some authors (16), but one that the current author regards as a last resort. It leaves two external scars, and can cause xerostomia: indeed, it could be said that patients who require such radical surgery to control their drooling are probably unsuitable candidates for surgery.

⊕ MANAGEMENT OF COMPLICATIONS

Submandibular swelling is common immediately after duct transposition, and usually subsides spontaneously, presumably as edema of the ducts resolves and saliva again flows freely. Occasionally it can be persistent, if Wharton's duct has been kinked or become stenosed, but even so is likely to settle without treatment, owing to atrophy of the gland. Exceptionally it may be necessary to excise a gland that remains swollen and uncomfortable.

Submandibular sialadenitis should not occur in the immediate postoperative period if appropriate antibiotic cover has been used. If it should develop later, then conventional treatment with antibiotics and sialogogues is called for. Rarely, recurrent sialadenitis may require gland excision.

Ranula formation occurs in about 10% of patients treated by submandibular duct transposition alone (14,22). A simple ranula is an intraoral epithelial-lined cyst arising from partial obstruction of the distal end of a sublingual gland duct, whereas a plunging ranula is an extravasation pseudocyst with just a connective tissue lining that develops following disruption of the duct. A plunging ranula may extend from the floor of the mouth down into the fascial planes of the neck and achieve considerable size (23). The sublingual glands each have about 15 ducts, half of which open directly into the submandibular duct and the remainder separately on the sublingual papilla. All these ducts therefore are divided during the operation of submandibular duct transposition, but presumably reestablish drainage as the mucosal incision in the floor of the mouth heals. If adequate drainage does not become reestablished, and the gland does not atrophy, then sublingual salivary secretions will become trapped submucosally and a ranula is likely to develop: this is possibly more likely to happen if the mucosal incision is sutured instead of being left to heal by secondary intention. However, most simple ranulas are small, many burst and resolve spontaneously, and those that do not are easily treated by intraoral marsupialization. The rare plunging ranulas are more difficult to manage, and demand excision of the sublingual salivary glands that are their secretory source if recurrence is to be prevented; but they are so uncommon that routine excision of the sublingual glands as part of every submandibular duct transposition operation seems difficult to justify.

✴ REFERENCES

1. Wilkie TF. *Can J Surg* 1967;10:60–67.
2. Enfors B, Lundberg A. *Sv Lakartidningen* 1968;65:4416–4417.
3. Laage-Hellman JE. *Nord Med* 1969;82:1522.
4. Goode RL, Smith RA. *Laryngoscope* 1970;80:1078–1089.
5. Glass LW, Nobel GL, Vecchione TR. *Plast Reconst Surg* 1978;62:523–526.
6. Dundas DF, Peterson RA. *Plast Reconst Surg* 1979;64:47–51.
7. Ekedahl C, Hallen O. *Acta Otolaryngol* 1973;75:464–469.
8. Cotton RT, Richardson MA. *Otolaryngol Head Neck Surg* 1981;89:535–541.
9. Crysdale WS, Gaffney RJ. In: Bluestone CD, Stool SE, Kenna MA, eds. *Pediatric otolaryngology*. Philadelphia: WB Saunders, 1996;974–983.
10. Ekedahl C. *Acta Otolaryngol* 1974;77:215–220.
11. Guerin RL. *Arch Otolaryngol* 1979;105:535–537.
12. Crysdale WS. *Laryngoscope* 1980;90:775–783.
13. Bailey CM, Wadsworth PV. *J Laryngol Otol* 1985;99:1111–1117.
14. Burton MJ, Leighton SEJ, Lund WS. *J Laryngol Otol* 1991;105:101–103.
15. Mankarious LA, Bottrill ID, Huchzermeyer PM, Bailey CM. *Otolaryngol Head Neck Surg* 1998 (*in press*).
16. Shott SR, Myer CM, Cotton RT. *Otolaryngol Head Neck Surg* 1989;101:47–50.
17. Hotaling AJ, Madgy DN, Kuhns LR, Filipek L, Belenky WM. *Arch Otolaryngol* 1992;118:1331–1333.
18. Scheyer L, Levine L. *J Appl Physiol* 1955;7:508–512.
19. Parisier SC, Blitzer A, Binder WJ, Friedman WF, Marovitz WF. In: Silverstein H, Norrell H, eds. *Neurological survey of the ear*. Birmingham, AL: Aesculapius Publishing, 1977;4–18.
20. Michel RG, Johnson KA, Patterson CN. *Arch Otolaryngol* 1977;103:94–97.
21. Parisier SC, Blitzer A, Binder WJ, Friedman WF, Marovitz WF. *Otolaryngology* 1978;86:308–321.
22. Crysdale WS, Mendelsohn JD, Conley S. *Laryngoscope* 1988;98:296–298.
23. Balakrishnan A, Ford GR, Bailey CM. *J Laryngol Otol* 1991;105:667–669.

C.M. Bailey: Great Ormond Street Hospital for Children, London, WC1N 3JH, United Kingdom.

- *Practical Pediatric Otolaryngology*
- edited by Robin T. Cotton and Charles M. Myer, III
- Lippincott-Raven Publishers, Philadelphia © 1999

7

Clinical Genetics in Pediatric Otolaryngology

Maria A. K. Bitner-Glindzicz

When healthy parents have a child with a facial malformation or hearing loss, the questions that they tend to ask are "Why has this happened?," "What can be done?," and "Will it happen again?," and if the overall clinical picture is complex, they will ask about diagnosis and prognosis. The clinical geneticist has a part to play in trying to answer some of these questions, particularly those concerning recurrence risk and diagnosis of rare inherited syndromes. This chapter outlines why a knowledge of clinical genetics might be useful to the practicing physician, and uses mainly the genetics of hearing loss to illustrate how advances in clinical molecular genetics may make a valuable contribution to the information given to parents.

HEARING LOSS

Approximately 1 in 1,000 of the United States population is born deaf or develops a profound hearing loss in early childhood (1–3). The proportion of cases due to environmental factors is decreasing, probably owing to two factors; improving neonatal intensive care and rubella immunization programs (4). What is evident from population-based studies is that at least *half* of all cases of profound hearing loss are attributable to genetic causes (3,4) and this proportion appears to be increasing, possibly owing to an increase in marriages among the deaf.

Given this observation, it is likely that genetic causes of hearing loss are not rare but rather are unrecognized, being difficult to distinguish from those cases with an environmental etiology. Sometimes hearing loss may be due to new mutation in the affected individual (proband) or due to nonexpression of a dominant gene in one of the parents (nonpenetrance), in which case both parents hear normally. However, it is possible that a degree of underdiagnosis still exists in clinical practice, particularly when there is a single individual affected with hearing impairment in a family.

It may be possible to identify children whose hearing loss is genetic in origin and in some cases, to pick out patients who have a genetically determined hearing loss, by careful history taking and clinical examination followed by special investigations. Despite this approach, it still may not be possible in a single individual to be sure whether the cause of the hearing loss is indeed genetic and therefore counseling must be based on empirical data only. In clinical genetic practice, deafness can be usefully divided into nonsyndromic (in which there are no extraauditory features) and syndromic (where deafness is one of a constellation of clinical features), of which there are over 400 entries in the London Dysmorphology Database (5). Physical examination and investigation aim particularly to select patients with syndromic forms of hearing loss, which account for 30% of all genetically determined hearing loss. Clinically, it is important to try to identify those cases with an obvious genetic cause, whether syndromic or nonsyndromic, in order to make a diagnosis, which may have important prognostic implications for the patient and for their relatives. Scientifically, identification is also important as it enables the study of individuals and families with the same condition in whom a genetic change has resulted in hearing loss. This may provide information about the function of the identified gene at the molecular level in the normal hearing process, of which little is known at the present time.

PEARLS AND PERILS: Syndrome Diagnosis

1. Prognosis—syndromic diagnoses of Alport's syndrome, Marshall Stickler syndrome, and branchio-oto-renal (BOR) syndrome may have prognostic implications for the patient (e.g., renal insufficiency in Alport's syndrome, renal malformation in BOR, and retinal detachment in Stickler's syndrome).
2. Recurrence risk to parents.
3. Offspring risk to child.
4. Prenatal diagnosis for serious, syndromic conditions.
5. Research implications—information about normal ear development, the normal auditory transduction process, and the etiology of deafness.

Given that there is an even chance of a particular patient having a genetically determined hearing loss, what is there in the patient's history and physical examination that might lead the otorhinolaryngologist to consider a genetic cause?

When taking the history for the first time, the physician needs to consider the possibility of a genetic etiology and determine whether there are any other clinical features that will help to make a diagnosis. Perhaps the most important part of the history is the family history (See "Pearls and Perils."). It should not be assumed that there is no family

---

PEARLS AND PERILS: Family History and Examination

1. Is there a family history?
2. Are there any associated clinical features in the family?
   a. Major, i.e., renal failure, visual loss, developmental delay
   b. Minor, i.e., facial asymmetry, ear pits, repaired cleft palate (or high-arched palate) (See next "Pearls and Perils.")
3. Do not assume there is no family history just because the parents appear to be normally hearing. Parents' hearing should be evaluated by audiograms.
4. Ask about the hearing status of the parents, their siblings and parents, as well as the siblings of the affected child.
5. Ask specifically about consanguinity because it will not necessarily be volunteered.
6. Minor associated features will be missed unless the patient is examined with these in mind.
7. Examine the parents and unaffected siblings for minor features.

---

history simply because the parents of the patient appear to hear normally. Parents should be asked specifically whether they themselves have a hearing loss. A parent with a mild unilateral hearing loss may not associate this with the child's severe bilateral hearing loss. Variable expression of dominant genes in particular may give rise to this phenomenon. Furthermore, it is well documented that the effect of dominant genes may be reduced in penetrance and so the effects of the gene may appear to skip a generation altogether, parents who have normal hearing may themselves have parents with early-onset hearing loss, a fact that may not come to light unless specifically sought. In the case of X-linked

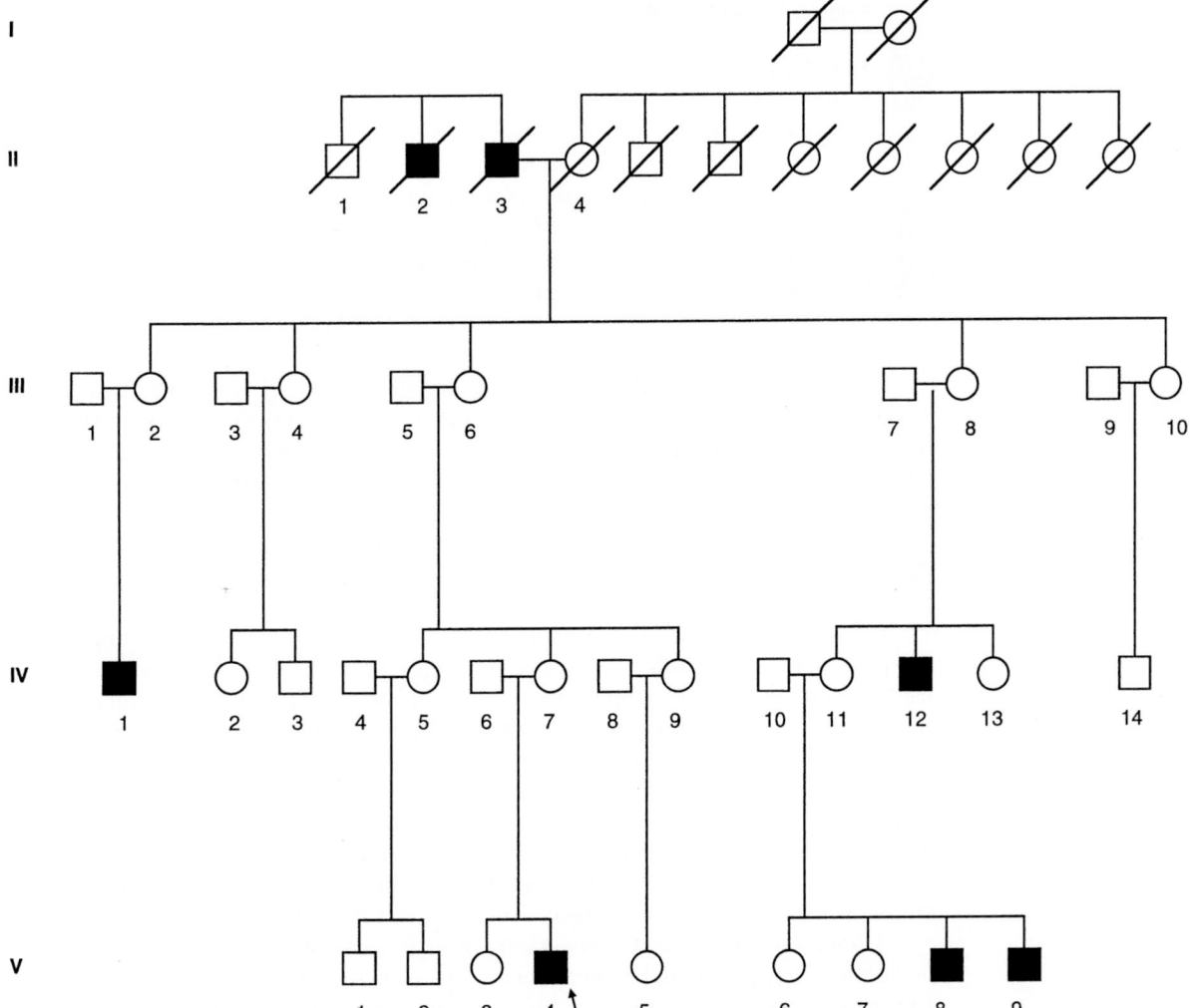

FIGURE 1 Only an extended family history from the parents of an individual V$_4$ reveals a clear pattern of X-linked hearing loss.

hearing loss, both parents may have normal hearing and a relevant family history may only come to light upon further questioning (Fig. 1). Finally, if after thorough discussion and construction of the family tree, no other relative with hearing loss is identified, a specific enquiry should be made as to whether the parents are related. If two such hearing parents have a child with a congenital or early-onset hearing loss, it is likely that this is autosomal recessive in origin, and there is a significant recurrence risk. The parents may welcome referral to a geneticist for further discussions.

In addition to the family history, the pregnancy and birth history and the rubella status of the mother should be ascertained when seeking a cause for a child's hearing loss. Attention should be paid to the developmental history of the child; isolated motor delay may be the first sign of vestibular dysfunction and global developmental delay may prompt the search for a syndrome diagnosis with the help of a geneticist. Emerging visual problems may be indicated by history and through developmental screening procedures.

Physical examination of the child may occasionally lead to a syndrome diagnosis. However, the rarity of many syndromes and their clinical variability, combined with the nonspecificity of some associated clinical features, can make syndromic diagnosis difficult. In addition, a diagnosis that is difficult to make in the early years may be more obvious as the child grows older. Despite these problems, one should examine all children with hearing loss carefully and certain features should be particularly borne in mind as they may be easily overlooked.

PEARLS AND PERILS: Physical Examination

1. External ears. Check the size, shape, and position. Are there any pits or tags?
2. Eyes. Check the spacing, color, and eyebrows. Are there any lacrimal problems?
3. Neck. Are there cysts or fistulas? Does the neck appear short?
4. Pigmentation. Check limbs and trunk as well as enquiring specifically.
5. Hands and feet. Are the fingers and joints normal?
6. At a first glance does the child appear dysmorphic?
7. Does he or she look like the parents?
8. Is there any facial asymmetry?

Indeed one may have to specifically ask oneself, is the child dysmorphic in any way? Are the external ears normal in shape and position? Are the eyes normally spaced and do they slant up or down? Are the irides and sclerae normal? Is the nose unusual or prominent? Is the overall appearance coarse at all? Is the face symmetric? Is the neck normal or short? Are there any cysts, fistulas, or swellings? In trying to decide whether or not the child looks like the parents, it may be helpful to ask the parents to bring photographs of themselves as children. Many facial features are very subtle and can be overlooked unless specifically sought.

Preauricular ear pits, for example, although common in the general population, when found in a child with hearing loss may suggest that the child has branchio-oto-renal (BOR) syndrome and supporting features may be seen in other family members. A small branchial cyst indicates a similar diagnosis but can be easily hidden by clothing or by an unwilling child who looks otherwise normal and nondysmorphic. Unusual pigmentation, heterochromia of the iris, or unusually blue irides, for example, may not be noted and are not diagnostic in themselves but may lead the clinician to look for other features of Waardenburg's syndrome (WS) in the child or the parents. The palate should always be examined, as it may, with other features, prompt a syndrome diagnosis, for example, Marshall Stickler syndrome if associated with characteristic facial dysmorphism.

A brief look for unusual pigmentation or birthmarks over the limbs and trunk may be helpful (e.g., pigmented or depigmented patches seen in WS, or lentigines seen in LEOPARD syndrome—*l*entigines, *e*lectrocardiographic defects, *o*cular hypertelorism, *p*ulmonary stenosis, *a*bnormal genitalia, *r*etardation of growth, and *d*eafness). Inspection

---

PEARLS AND PERILS: Investigations

1. Audiologic testing of first-degree relatives (at least pure-tone audiometry).
2. Baseline ophthalmologic examination (may lead to a syndromic diagnosis, e.g., lenticonus and macular flecks seen in Alport's syndrome, retinitis pigmentosa seen in Usher's syndrome, high myopia seen in Marshall Stickler syndrome; a baseline assessment may be useful if the child develops visual problems later in childhood).
3. Serology for congenital infection (e.g., TORCH screen—*t*oxoplasmosis, *r*ubella, *c*ytomegalovirus, and *h*erpes).
4. Urinalysis (simple dipstick test or urine microscopy may lead to a diagnosis of Alport's syndrome).
5. Electrocardiogram (to exclude a prolonged QT interval seen in Jervell and Lange-Nielsen syndrome; although this condition is rare, the investigation is cheap and should be performed in all children with congenital hearing loss).
6. Chromosome analysis if the patient is dysmorphic or has multiple malformations.
7. Computed tomography scan of the inner ear if the child has a profound or progressive hearing loss.

---

2. Hypoplasia of the facial bones—zygomatic, malar, and mandibular hypoplasia. Micrognathia may occasionally be of such a severe degree that it gives rise to respiratory obstruction.
3. Downward slanting of the palpebral fissures with lower-eyelid colobomata and a paucity of eyelashes medial to the coloboma.
4. Cleft palate, which occurs in about 35% [reviewed in (7)]. Gorlin et al. (7) mentioned the incidence of pharyngeal incompetence secondary to agenesis of the soft palate, submucous cleft palate, and immobile soft palate.

This common autosomal dominant condition is likely to present to the pediatric otorhinolaryngolist. The parents of all children with Treacher Collins syndrome should be referred to a geneticist for counseling. It is important to determine whether, in the absence of a family history, the child's parents are minimally affected or even nonpenetrant gene carriers, or whether the condition in the child represents a new mutation. Deciding whether or not other family members are gene carriers can be extremely difficult in some cases as the expressivity of the gene is variable (8). Since the gene has now been identified (9), it is theoretically possible to see whether a mutation in the *Treacle* gene of the affected child was inherited from a parent or has arisen *de novo* (as is the case in 60% of patients). In families where the recurrence risk is high, prenatal diagnosis, combining mutation detection and detailed ultrasound scanning, may be used to assess the degree of severity of the condition in an affected child.

In summary, the child with Treacher Collins syndrome may present to the otorhinolaryngologist for a number of reasons. Genetic referral is important for the following reasons:

1. If there is a family history, parents need to be aware of the recurrence risk, the range of severity of the condition, and the availability and limitations of prenatal diagnosis.
2. When there is no obvious family history, it is important to determine whether or not one parent has minor features and is a gene carrier, or whether recurrence risk in a future pregnancy is low. Radiology of the skull of the parents may be of help—the occipitomental view of the zygomatic complex may be helpful (8) and mutation detection may be possible.
3. Rarely, children have facial features reminiscent of Treacher Collins syndrome but additional features that point to other diagnoses with different recurrence risks. For example, children with Nager's syndrome or Miller syndrome have preaxial (i.e., radial x-ray abnormalities) and postaxial (i.e., ulnar) limb abnormalities in addition to facial features.

Branchio-oto-renal Syndrome

The combination of ear pits, branchial fistulase, clefts or cysts, and hearing loss was described by many authors in the nineteenth century but it was not until 1975 that Melnick et al (10) highlighted concomitant renal anomalies. Penetrance of the mutant gene in this condition is high but once again *expressivity* is variable (i.e., the majority of those who carry the mutant gene show *some* feature but the range of severity is wide).

The clinical features include the following:

1. Malformation of the external ears (cup or lop ears, microtia) and ear pits (shallow blind depressions the size of a pinhead situated anterior to attachment of the helix, or in the attachment of the helix itself).
2. Branchial fistulas, clefts, sinuses, or cartilaginous nodules that may present to the otorhinolaryngologist. Patients occasionally give a history of a relative who has had "fish parts" removed from the neck.
3. Hearing loss that is highly variable and may occur in 85% to 90%. The loss may be conductive, sensorineural, or mixed and may be associated with morphologic abnormalities of the temporal bone and sometimes of the ossicles (11).

4. Renal malformations that vary in severity from agenesis to milder asymptomatic findings such as hydronephrosis, crossed renal ectopia, diverticula, and caliceal cysts.

A number of rarer associations found in BOR syndrome are reviewed elsewhere (11).

The gene was localized to chromosome 8q12–22 by linkage analysis and the observation of a cytogenetic aberration in a patient with BOR and trichorhinophalangeal syndrome. Genetic and physical mapping of the region led to the identification of the mutant gene, which is the human homologue of a gene first described in *Drosophila* flies called *eyes absent* (12). Studies in the mouse showed that this gene is expressed in the developing otic vesicle, the cochlear and vestibular neuroepithelium, and the condensing mesenchyme of the middle ear. In addition, it is expressed in the developing kidney but not demonstrated in the developing collecting duct system or in the branchial arches. A variety of mutations in the coding sequence of the gene have been demonstrated and all are predicted to disrupt the gene product. It is postulated that the disease arises due to reduced gene dosage. Mutation detection in families should become available in the near future.

Waardenburg's Syndrome

WS is one of the auditory pigmentary disorders. It is inherited as an autosomal dominant condition with a frequency of about 2 to 3 per 100,000 (1). Clinical and genetic studies have shown that WS may be usefully classified into different subtypes. Of these, types I and II are the most common and are distinguished clinically by facial appearance and have been found to be caused by mutations in different genes.

WS refers to the combination of hearing loss with white forelock, heterochromia irides (different-colored eyes), and skin pigmentary changes (Fig. 3). The facial feature that distinguishes between type I and II WS is dystopia canthorum (lateral displacement of the medial canthi of the eyes), which is usually apparent on inspection and breeds true within families (i.e., either all or none of the family members show the feature). Dystopia may be seen in association with synophrys (bushy, fused eyebrows) and a high, broad nasal root. Diagnostic criteria for WS have been compiled by the Waardenburg Consortium and the reader is referred to other texts for full clinical descriptions (7,13).

Of most interest to the otorhinolaryngologist is the hearing impairment observed in this condition. The loss is sensorineural, congenital, and either unilateral or bilateral. It

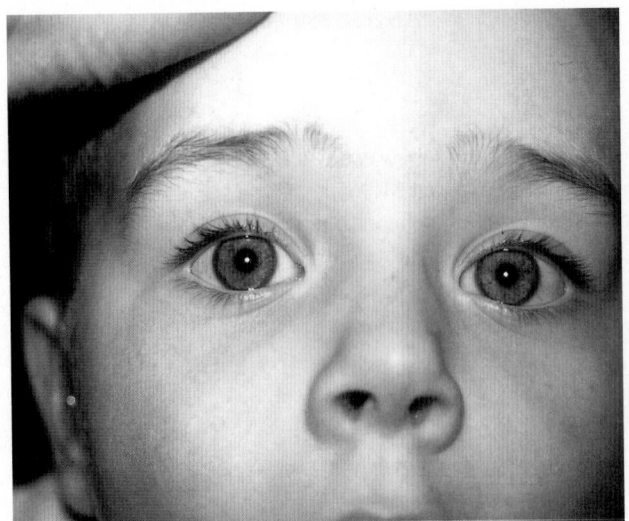
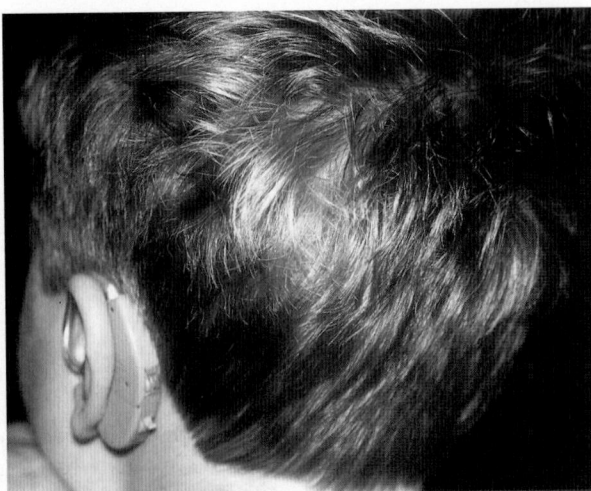

A   B

FIGURE 3 Child with Waardenburg's syndrome. **A:** Note the subtle heterochromia of the irides. There is no dystopia canthorum, making this likely to be type II Waardenburg's syndrome. **B:** Note the gray patch of hair in the same child.

is usually nonprogressive but not always so. The hearing loss tends to be more common in families with type II WS (7,14), with the incidence being 70% to 80% in type II compared with 20% to 50% in type I. Most importantly, it may vary in severity between affected family members, ranging from profound to no loss at all. This is obviously an important point to highlight in genetic counselling—a presenting child may have a minor hearing loss but parents should be counseled that subsequent children may need to have careful assessment of auditory function during childhood.

Abnormalities of vestibular function have been less well studied than those of the auditory system. In a single large family with type I WS investigated by Marcus (15), there was a high incidence of vestibular hypofunction that was not always found in association with hearing loss.

Genetic linkage studies showed that the mutant gene in families with type I WS maps to chromosome 2q35 and mutations have been found in the *PAX3* gene, a transcription factor expressed in the early embryo (13). The gene in about 20% of type II WS families maps to chromosome 3p and mutations have been found in the transcription factor *MITF*. The remaining families with type II WS show no linkage to the known loci and the genes are unmapped at the present time.

Alport Syndrome

Alport syndrome describes the association of nephritis and progressive sensorineural hearing loss. There may be characteristic eye signs and in some families there is an association with the presence of leiomyomatosis of the esophagus, trachea, and vulva. There is genetic heterogeneity and the condition is usually transmitted in an X-linked dominant manner although cases of autosomal recessive and rarely autosomal dominant transmission exist.

In the X-linked form of the disease, female patients are less severely affected than male patients. In boys, the renal disease is characterized by hematuria in early childhood, which is initially microscopic but may become macroscopic during intercurrent infection. This is later associated with a deterioration in renal function during adolescence, progressing to renal failure and death by 20 to 40 years. In females patients the condition is milder, with microscopic hematuria apparent by 20 years. In some families this may be the only renal symptoms in female members, whereas in others there is progression to renal failure in a similar manner to their affected male relatives. Confirmation of diagnosis usually requires a renal biopsy, with the specimen showing variable thinning and thickening and splitting of the glomerular basement membrane at electron microscopy.

The hearing loss is progressive and variable, occurring at a later age in female patients. In boys the hearing is normal in early childhood, with a hearing loss starting during the second decade and progressing during adolescence. High frequencies tend to be more affected although in early-onset forms, progression may eventually involve the lower tones also. Again the picture in female patients is also variable, with hearing loss being milder and of later onset or even undetectable in some. Subclinical hearing loss may become apparent only on pure-tone audiometry, and research has shown that some female carriers of X-linked Alport syndrome may have a mid-frequency notch on Audioscan testing (16).

Specific eye signs may be helpful in making a diagnosis of Alport syndrome. Anterior lenticonus and macular flecks may be seen and there may be progression to myopia in patients with early-disease. Rarely the anterior lenticonus progresses to anterior capsule cataract followed by rupture of the anterior lens capsule. Ophthalmologic examination of female patients, at risk of being carriers may be helpful in assigning carrier status, but unfortunately normal findings on examination do not completely rule out the possibility of being a carrier.

Genetic counseling is important for families in whom the diagnosis is made. The variable but potentially serious nature of the condition needs to be outlined as although the lifespan of female patients is usually normal, 50% to 75% of affected male patients required renal replacement therapy by 20 to 40 years, compared with 10% to 35% of female patients (17).

Considerable progress has been made in the elucidation of the defect underlying Alport syndrome. The X-linked form is caused by mutation of the gene *COL4A5*, which encodes the alpha-5 subunit of collagen. IV. A wide variety of mutations in the gene have been reported but mutation detection is only available in about 40% of cases, partly because of the very large size of the gene. However, carrier detection and prenatal diagnosis may still be available by linkage (i.e., tracking the inheritance of the mutation-bearing chromosome through the family) when the pattern of inheritance is clearly X-linked and the diagnosis firm. Alport's syndrome in which leiomyomatosis occurs is due to deletion of both *COL4A5* and *CO4A6* genes, which lie adjacent to each other on the long arm of the X chromosome.

Furthermore, rarer cases of recessive Alport's syndrome (approximately 10% of cases of Alport syndrome), in which male and female patients are affected with equal severity, may be caused by mutations in the genes *COL4A3* and *COL4A4* on chromosome 2 (18).

Pendred's Syndrome

Pendred originally described the combination of goiter and congenital sensorineural hearing loss in 1896 (19), and many cases have been reported since then. Fraser's study (20) comprises the largest number of cases described to date and outlines the autosomal recessive mode of inheritance, natural history, and variability of the condition. Furthermore, the prevalence of this condition among deaf adults of 7.5 per 100,000, observed by Fraser in the British population, suggests that it is a common cause of congenital hearing loss.

The goiter classically appears in late childhood or sometimes in adolescence, and according to Fraser (20) most goiters are euthyroid. However, in the study by Johnsen et al. (21), as many as 50% of the goiters were found to be hypothyroid. The goiter is described as initially diffuse but may later become nodular, and those that are subject to surgery tend to recur.

The most common pattern of hearing loss is that of bilateral moderate to severe loss, worse in the high frequencies. The onset is usually prelingual but later onset has also been reported. Recent data suggest that there may be abnormalities of vestibular function, either bilateral vestibular failure or unilateral vestibular hypofunction, in a major proportion of patients, with normal vestibular function in the remainder (22). Mondini's malformation of the cochlea has been observed using computed tomography scanning. Dilated endolymphatic ducts and widened vestibular canals have also been demonstrated using magnetic resonance imaging.

The thyroid defect in Pendred's syndrome is one of organification of iodine, which is revealed by the perchlorate discharge test. Under normal circumstances, radioactive iodine given by injection is organified. When this process is defective, perchlorate provokes a rapid discharge of unorganified iodine from the gland. Thus, radioactivity measured over the gland falls dramatically after administration of perchlorate as the unbound iodine is excreted. In normal individuals the radioactive iodine is bound and organified so that when perchlorate is given, there is little discharge of iodine and radioactivity measured over the gland remains high. Discharge of 10% or less is taken to be normal. Pendred's syndrome is not the only cause of a positive result on the perchlorate discharge test; autoimmune thyroiditis is another cause. For this reason, it is useful to measure thyroid autoantibodies, especially when the overall clinical picture is not characteristic of Pendred's syndrome.

The molecular defect underlying this condition is not yet known and it is likely to be caused by mutation in a single gene. Two groups recently mapped the gene to chromosome 7q (23,26) and the gene responsible has recently been identified (25).

Goldenhar Syndrome

Various terms (hemifacial microsomia, first and second branchial arch syndrome, oculoauriculovertebral dysplasia) have been used to describe this condition. The main features include facial asymmetry, malformed external ears, and an epibulbar dermoid (in which cases the term *Goldenhar syndrome* is usually applied). Other facial features may include microtia, stenosed or atretic auditory canals, ossicular malformations, preauricular skin tags, micrognathia, and macrostomia. Diagnosis of this condition should also prompt a search for vertebral, cardiac, and renal anomalies that may also be associated, hence the term *oculoauriculovertebral dysplasia*. The majority of such cases are sporadic in nature, and so recurrence risks are low, but occasional dominant families with remarkable intrafamilial variability and incomplete penetrance have been described. Therefore, both parents should be examined carefully and asked about the family history of associated features.

The etiology of this interesting condition is unknown at present.

CHARGE Association

This acronym stands for *c*oloboma, congenital *h*eart disease, choanal *a*tresia, *r*etardation, *g*enital anomalies, and *e*ar (deafness). The choanal atresia in these children means that they present frequently to the pediatric otorhinolaryngologist in the neonatal period requiring surgery. In addition to the features just listed, children may also present with cleft lip and palate, tracheoesophageal fistula, and oral frenulae. Many have abnormal pinnae and a high proportion have a hearing loss. This is often mixed, the middle-ear component being secondary to choanal atresia, cleft palate, or ossicular malformations. The sensorineural component may range from mild to severe or even profound.

In addition to the features just mentioned, renal malformations are common and should always be sought. There is a significant mortality associated with this condition due to the combination of upper-airway and cardiac problems.

In most patients the condition is sporadic but occasional dominant families and siblings have been reported. A recurrence risk of 6% is usually quoted.

CONCLUSIONS

Despite recent progress in the elucidation of the molecular basis of some craniofacial malformation and deafness syndromes, a great deal remains unknown. Although carrier detection based on mutation screening in families can now be offered for conditions such as Treacher Collins syndrome, WS, and BOR syndrome, little information can be given regarding the prediction of disease severity. This is particularly disappointing to those wishing to have children, as many fear passing on genes that will cause serious malformation or profound sensory impairment such as deafness. Prenatal diagnosis, although theoretically possible, cannot be based on mutation detection alone. Hopefully, future research will enable the elucidation of factors that influence disease severity caused by a particular mutation and will possibly allow the moderation of gene expression by environmental factors.

SUMMARY

When presented with a deaf child or one with a malformation, it is worth thinking about the possibility of a genetic etiology. One needs to ask direct questions when taking a family history, and to ask specifically about features known to be associated with syndromes, in family members as well as the proband (i.e., renal failure, visual problems, etc.). When examining the child, it is useful to look particularly for the minor features associated with common syndromes. Finally, one should consider referral to a clinical geneticist on the grounds that there may be important implications for the parents, and for other family members.

✸ REFERENCES

1. Fraser G. *The causes of profound deafness in childhood*. Baltimore: The Johns Hopkins University Press, 1976.
2. Newton VE. Aetiology of bliateral sensorineural hearing loss in young children. *J Laryngol Otol Suppl* 1985;10: 1–57.
3. Morton NE. Genetic epidemiology of hearing impairment. In: Ruben RJ, van der Water TR, Steel KP, eds. *Genetics of hearing impairment*. Ann N Y Acad Sci 1991;630:16–31.
4. Marazita M, Ploughman L, Rawlings B, Remington E, Amos K, Nance W. Genetic epidemiological studies of earlyonset deafness in the U.S. school age population. *Am J Med Gene*. 1993;46:486–491.
5. Winter R, Baraitser M. *London dysmorphology database*. Oxford: Oxford University Press, 1996.
6. Phelps PD, Poswillo D, Lloyd GAS. The ear deformities in mandibulofacial dysostosis. *Clin Otorthinolaryngol* 1981;6:15–28.
7. Gorlin RJ, Toriello HV, Cohen MM. *Hereditary hearing loss and its syndromes*. Oxford: Oxford University Press, 1995:62–65.
8. Dixon MJ, Marres HAM, Edwards SJ, Dixon J, Cremers CWRJ. Treacher Collins syndrome: correlation between clinical and genetic linkage studies. *Clin Dysmorphol* 1994;3:96–103.
9. Treacher Collins Collaborative Group. Positional cloning of a gene involved in the pathogenesis of Treacher Collins syndrome. *Nat Genet*. 1996;12:130–136.
10. Melnick M, Bixler D, Silk K, Yune H, Nance WE. Autosomal dominant branchio-oto-renal dysplasia. *Birth Defects* 1975;II:121–128.
11. Chen A, Francis M, Ni L, et al. Phenotypic manifestations of branchio-oto-renal syndrome. *Am J Med Gene* 1995;58:365–370.
12. Abdelhak S, Kalatzis V, Heilig R, et al. A human homologue of the drosophila eyes absent gene underlies branchio-oto-renal (BOR) syndrome and identifies a novel gene family. *Nat Genet*. 1997;15:157–164.
13. Read AP, Newton VE. Waardenburg syndrome. In: Martini A, Read A, Stephens D, eds. *Genetics and hearing impairment*. London: Whurr Publishers, 1996:157–165.
14. Liu XZ, Newton VE, Read AP. Waardenburg syndrome type II: phenotypic findings and diagnostic criteria. *Am J Med Gene*. 1995;55:95–100.
15. Marcus RE. Vestibular function and additional findings in Waardenburg's syndrome. *Acta Otolaryngol Suppl* 1968;229:1–30.
16. Sirimanna KS, France E, Stephens SDG. Alport's syndrome: can the carriers be identified by audiometry? *Clin Otolaryngol* 1995;20:158–163.
17. Flinter FA. Molecular genetics of Alport's syndrome. *Q J Med* 1993;86:289–292.
18. Mochizuki T, Lemmink HH, Maryama M, et al. Identification of mutations in the $\alpha 3$(IV) and $\alpha 4$(IV) collagen genes in autosomal recessive Alport syndrome. *Nat Genet*. 1994;8:77–82.
19. Pendred V. Deaf mutism and goitre. *Lancet* 1896;2:532.
20. Fraser GR. Association of congenital deafness with goitre (Pendred's syndrome). *Ann Hum Genet*. 1965;28:201–248.
21. Johnsen T, Larsen C, Friis J, HougaardJensen FH. Pendred's syndrome: acoustic, vestibular and radiological findings in 17 unrelated patients. *J Laryngol Otol* 1987;101:1187–1192.
22. Luxon L. Neuro-otological findings in Pendred's syndrome. *European workgroup on genetics of hearing impairment*. Milan; Italy, 1996.
23. Coyle B, Coffey R, Armour JA, et al. Pendred syndrome (goitre and sensorineural hearing loss). *Nat Genet* 1996;12:421–423.
24. Sheffield VC, Kraiem Z, Beck JC, et al. Pendred syndrome maps to chromosome 7q21–34 and is caused by an intrinsic defect in thyroid iodine organification. Nat Genet 1996;12:424–426.
25. Everett LA, Glaser B, Beck JC, et al. Pendred syndrome is caused by mutations in a putative sulphate transporter gene (POS). *Nat Genet* 1997;17:411–422.

• *Practical Pediatric Otolaryngology*
• edited by Robin T. Cotton and Charles M. Myer, III
• Lippincott-Raven Publishers, Philadelphia © 1999

M.A.K. Bitner-Glindzicz: Department of Clinical and Molecular Genetics, Institute of Child Health, London WC1N 1EH, United Kingdom.

8

Chronic Cough

Lauren D. Holinger

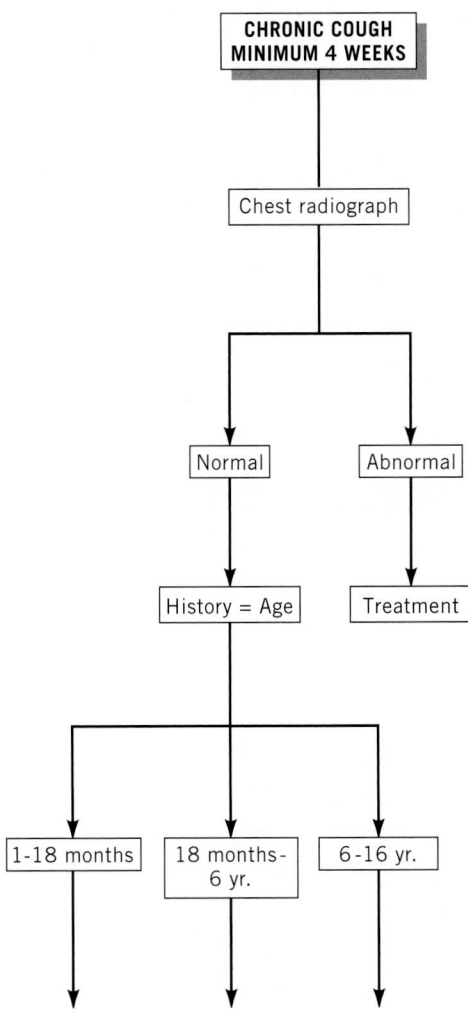

continued on next page

continued

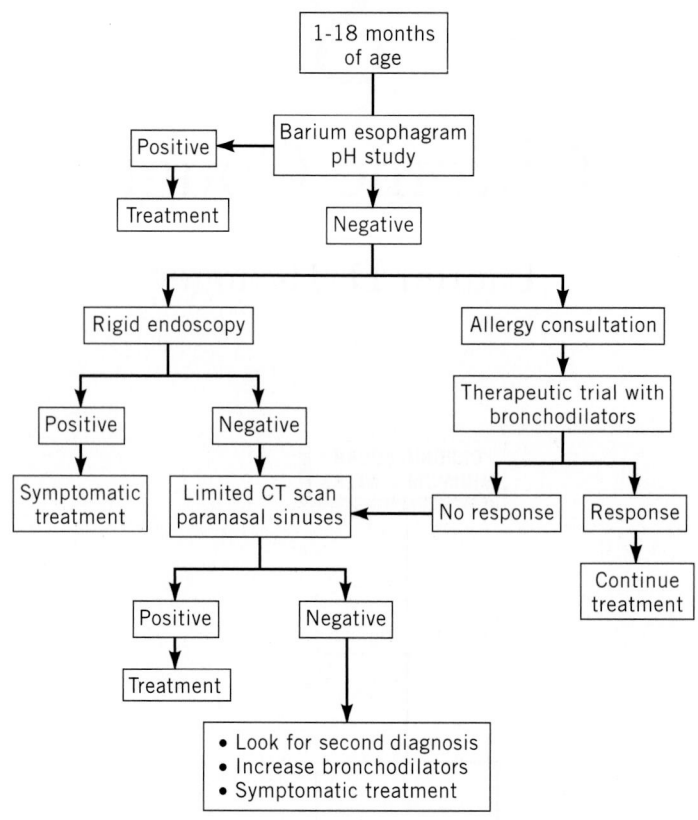

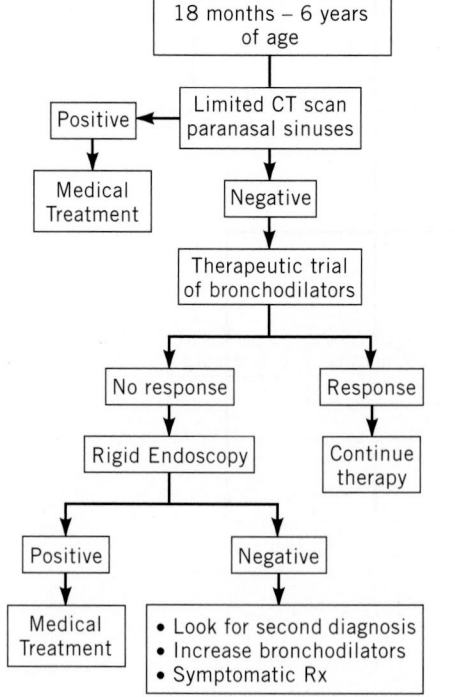

continued on next page

118

continued

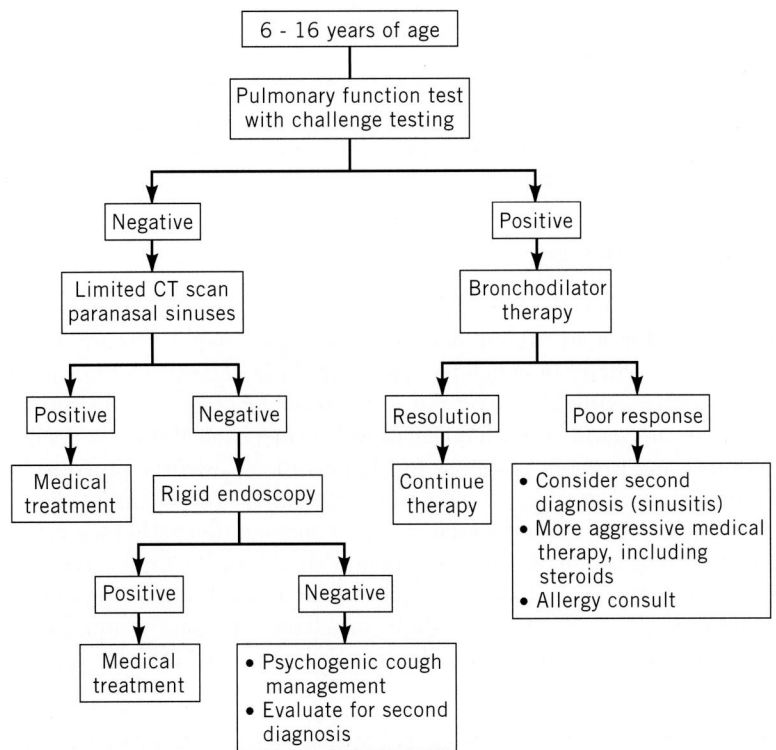

OVERVIEW

A single normal cough is a sudden, violent expiratory expulsion of air after deep inspiration and closure of the laryngeal sphincter. Cough is an important defense mechanism that maintains health by removal of (a) abnormal secretions, exudate, or inflammatory products; (b) foreign bodies; and (c) all irritating sensations from the respiratory tract. It can be an important factor in the spread of infection, a symptom of an underlying disease, or a distressing problem itself, causing complications and great concern to the patient and family, in addition to many sleepless nights. If persistent, it may lead to irritation of the larynx and tracheobronchial tree, vomiting, failure to thrive, exhaustion, or more serious complications, such as fracture of ribs, pneumothorax, pneumomediastinum, and rupture of rectus abdominis muscles.

Cough is one of several means by which the lungs are protected and cleared. Other mechanisms include (a) the gag reflex; (b) mucociliary clearance, which was described in detail by Hilding (1); (c) phagocytosis by alveolar macrophages, which can provide important information regarding the etiology of the cough; and (d) lymphatic drainage.

Cough is the reason for 6.7% of all pediatric office visits (2), and chronic cough is a common reason for referral to the pediatric bronchoscopist. There is a broad range of causes of chronic cough in children and bronchoscopy plays an important role in the evaluation. In this chapter, the differential diagnosis of chronic cough is explored. The diagnostic approach to this problem is presented and therapeutic options are discussed.

"The cough is the watchdog of the lungs," observed Chevalier Jackson more than 70 years ago (3). He pointed out that the function of cough is to protect the lungs from a "dangerous intruder" or an "internal enemy." Although cough has important functions in both health and disease, two considerations are of paramount importance. First, the cough itself may be detrimental to the well-being of the infant or child, even leading to serious complications (4). Second, as Clerf (5) pointed out, chronic persistent cough is a symptom of an underlying disorder and cannot be well managed on the basis of only a presumptive or inferential diagnosis. The proper management therefore does not involve symptomatic or nonspecific therapy, but is initially directed at identifying the underlying disorder. Correct treatment is possible only after a precise diagnosis has been established. Symptomatic treatment is rarely necessary to prevent the complications of cough or to ease a child's distress.

The Cough Reflex Arc

The afferent limb is the first of the three phases of the cough reflex arc. Stimulation of a cough receptor or an afferent neuron initiates the cough reflex arc (Fig. 1). The sensory nerve fibers (irritant or cough receptors) are located between the ciliated pseudostratified columnar epithelial cells of the airway from the pharynx to the terminal bronchioles. Receptors are sensitive to chemical as well as mechanical stimuli, responding to chemical fumes and irritants as well as touch, intrinsic or extrinsic pressure from masses, inflammation, foreign objects, and particulate matter. They adapt readily.

Cough receptors are found in greater concentration within the larynx, at the carina, and at the bifurcation of large and medium-sized bronchi. Other receptors are located in the nose and paranasal sinuses (afferent: trigeminal nerve), pharynx (afferent: glossopharyngeal nerve), external auditory canal and tympanic membrane, pleura, stomach (afferent: vagus nerve), pericardium and diaphragm (afferent: phrenic nerve), and

FIGURE 1 Anatomy of the cough reflex arc. The afferent limb includes the receptors and afferents. The cough center is the coordinating locus of the cough. The afferent limb carries impulses to the muscles that affect the cough. (From ref. 6, with permission.)

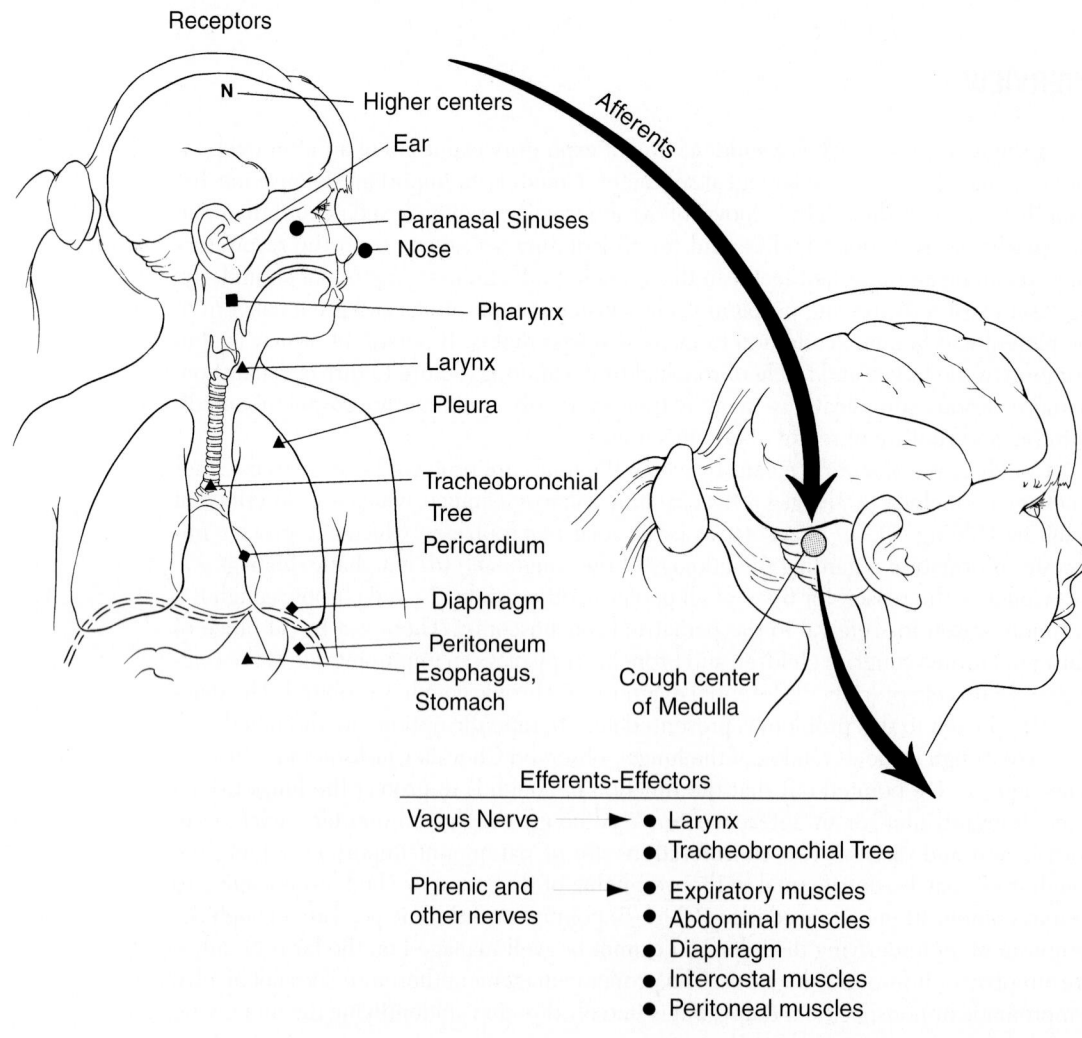

esophagus (6). Impulses are transmitted primarily by the vagus nerve to the "cough center" of the brain, located diffusely in the medulla.

The cough center in the medulla is the central coordinating locus of the cough (4). This area of the brainstem integrates impulses and coordinates the complicated expiratory muscle activity that constitutes an effective cough.

The efferent limb of the cough reflex arc emanates from the cough center. Efferent impulses travel to the musculature of the larynx and tracheobronchial tree (efferent: vagus nerve), intercostal muscles, diaphragm, abdominal wall, and pelvic floor (efferent: phrenic nerve and third cervical to second sacral spinal motor nerves).

PATIENT ASSESSMENT

Multifarious conditions in the upper half of the body can produce cough. Virtually any disorder that stimulates a cough receptor or the afferent neurons of the cough reflex arc (see Fig. 1) can produce a cough. A comprehensive list of the conditions that can cause cough (in infants and children with a normal-appearing chest radiogram) is provided (Table 1).

TABLE 1: Etiology of Chronic Cough in Children

Asthma	Cough-variant asthma
Infectious	Chronic sinusitis; chronic Waldeyer's ring infection; pertussis, parapertussis, adenovirus infection, tuberculosis, chronic bronchitis, parasitic infections
Congenital	
Airway narrowing	Aberrant innominate artery, vascular rings (double aortic arch, etc.); foregut anomalies; bronchogenic cyst, esophageal duplication; subglottic stenosis, tracheomalacia; tracheal and bronchial stenosis; web
Aspiration	Gastroesophageal reflux, esophageal incoordination, tracheoesophageal fistula, cleft larynx; neurologic: vocal fold paralysis, pharyngeal incoordination, achalasia; cricopharyngeal achalasia
Other	Tracheobronchial tree abnormalities; cystic fibrosis; primary ciliary dyskinesia; congenital heart disease; bronchopulmonary dysplasia
Psychogenic	Psychogenic cough
Traumatic	Foreign body: airway, nasal, external auditory canal
Environmental	Cigarette smoking: active, passive; low humidity; allergies (without bronchospasm); industrial pollutants
Otologic	Cerumen, foreign body, infection, neoplasm, hair in the external auditory canal
Neoplastic	Subglottic hemangioma; recurrent respiratory papillomatosis; bronchial adenoma; mediastinal, causing tracheobronchial compression
Medications	Angiotensin-converting enzyme inhibitors; inhalational agents; neuromuscular blocking agents
Other	Cardiovascular: rheumatic fever, congestive

TABLE 2: Diagnostic Protocol for Evaluation of Chronic Cough in Children

History
  Age
  Character, duration of symptoms
  Immunizations
Physical examination
  Nose, pharynx, larynx, sinuses, neck, chest, ears
Radiologic examination
  Posteroanterior and lateral
  Airway films
  Paranasal sinus CT scan
  Barium esophagram/UGI
Nuclear medicine
  Reflux scan
24-hr pH probe
Pulmonary function studies
  Spirometry or flow-volume curves (before and after
    bronchodilators: bronchoprovocation, methacholine
    challenge testing)
Laboratory studies
  Sputum culture and Gram's stain, CBC with differential
  Nasal smear for cytology, nasal epithelial biopsy for
    ciliary motility and ultrastructure, nasal swab for
  pertussis; fluorescent antibody titers
  Fungal titers, viral titers
  Quantitative immunoglobins
  Alpha-1-antitrypsin
  HIV: ELISA, Western blot
Skin tests
  Sweat chloride, allergy testing
  PPD test
Consultations
  Allergy, pulmonary, infectious disease, cardiology,
    gastroenterology
Endoscopy
  Indications—depend on
    Severity of symptoms
    Duration of symptoms (> 6–8wk)
    History or PE suggestive of foreign body aspiration,
      obstructive lesion
    Failure to diagnose by other means
  Studies
    Cultures: bacterial, viral, acid-fast bacteria, fungal,
      chlamydia
    Cytology: eosinophils, macrophages (fat, hemosiderin
      stains)
    Stains: Gram, Giemsa
    Biopsies: H & E, electron microscopy for ciliary
      ultrastructure (if no motility seen with light
      microscopy)

CT, computed tomography; UGI, upper gastrointestinal; CBC, complete blood cell count; HIV, human immunodeficiency virus; ELISA, enzyme-linked immunosorbent assay; PPD, purified protein derivative; PE, physical examination; H & E, hematoxylin and eosin.

Clinical Evaluation

Infants and children with chronic cough for more than 4 weeks are evaluated by the following diagnostic protocol: (a) history, (b) physical examination, and (c) chest radiograph (if not done recently). When clinically indicated and possible (age precludes some studies), some of the studies outlined in Table 2 are selected. Consultation is freely sought from the pediatric allergy, pulmonology, infectious disease, gastroenterology, and cardiology services.

The evaluation of each patient is individualized based on the initial history, the age of the patient, and the studies completed prior to the initial visit.

History

Several factors in the history may help determine the cause of the chronic cough. The age of the patient at the onset of the cough is probably of greatest importance (6):

Birth to 18 Months: Cough-variant asthma, aberrant innominate artery, and gastroesophageal reflux are the three most common causes of chronic cough. Primary tracheomalacia, subglottic stenosis, and sinusitis, as well as other congenital conditions such as cystic fibrosis and bronchogenic cyst, also need to be considered.

Eighteen months to 6 Years: Sinusitis is the most frequent diagnosis; cough-variant asthma is the second. Subglottic stenosis and gastroesophageal reflux are less frequent considerations.

Six to 16 Years: Cough-variant asthma, psychogenic cough, and sinusitis are the most common cause of chronic cough.

In *infants*, passive smoke exposure may cause a chronic cough, but more often is merely an exacerbating factor. Aspiration causing chronic cough in infants is likely to be related to congenital anomalies such as tracheoesophageal fistula or cleft larynx. Chlamydia, rubella, cytomegalovirus, and respiratory syncytial virus may cause chronic cough in infants, as can cystic fibrosis or other suppurative lung diseases and cough-variant asthma.

In the *school-aged child*, bronchial foreign body, cystic fibrosis or other suppurative lung disease, passive exposure to tobacco or smoke, or postnasal drip may be implicated. Common factors include cough-variant asthma, active or passive smoking, *Mycoplasma pneumoniae* infection, psychogenic cough, or postnasal drip.

At *any age*, causes of chronic cough include cough-variant asthma; viral, mycoplasma, or pertussis infection; or therapy with angiotensin-converting enzyme inhibitors such as captopril.

The nature of the cough is a second important characteristic. A loose productive cough suggests suppurative lung disease, while a dry, brassy cough occurs when tracheal irritation is present. Hawking or throat clearing suggests that sinusitis, gastroesophageal reflux, or allergic rhinitis is causing postnasal drip. A paroxysmal cough is often noted in pertussis, pertussis syndrome, or cystic fibrosis. A bizarre, loud cough that disappears at night is usually due to psychogenic (habit) cough.

Sputum production may offer other diagnostic clues. Clear sputum may be seen with asthma; purulent sputum is noted with cystic fibrosis, primary ciliary dyskinesia, immune deficiencies, and localized bronchiectasis. Bloody sputum may occur with cystic fibrosis, foreign body aspiration, bronchiectasis, hemosiderosis, or pulmonary embolism.

A diurnal pattern of chronic cough may be of significance. Nocturnal cough shortly after retiring suggests gastroesophageal reflux or postnasal drip (from allergies or sinusitis). Nocturnal cough in the early morning hours may be due to asthma. Morning cough is typical of suppurative lung disease such as cystic fibrosis. A cough that disappears at night after daytime prominence suggests a psychogenic etiology. Finally, a cough during feeding is likely to be due to aspiration.

Many patients referred for evaluation of chronic cough have had previous trials of medication. Partial response to therapy suggests a diagnosis. If antibiotics have helped, suppurative lung disease or sinusitis is likely. If bronchodilators are useful, then asthma is a probable diagnosis. A response to corticosteroids is not very helpful since asthma and airway inflammation of almost any cause will respond. Absence of a response to corticosteroids suggests either an anatomic problem or psychogenic cough. Improvement after treatment with antihistamines is noted when allergies and postnasal drip cause a chronic cough.

Inspiratory stridor is due to pathology and airway narrowing in the larynx or cervical trachea. Coughing with expiratory wheezing suggests asthma or bronchial narrowing from an intrabronchial foreign body. Seasonal variation suggests asthma. Cold air may exacerbate asthma as may various airborne allergens. Infections are a more prominent cause of chronic cough in the winter. Concomitant allergy or eczema suggests that asthma may be present. Growth failure is rare, but suggests significant disease such as cystic fibrosis or severe asthma. Exposure to others with infection or chronic cough should be determined. Day-care and school exposures should not be neglected in the initial history taking.

Physical Examination

The patient's general health and nutrition are noted. If they are impaired, significant disease such as cystic fibrosis, severe asthma, or immune deficiency may be present. Allergic rhinitis, conjunctivitis, or hypertrophy of pharyngeal lymphoid follicles is seen with asthma or allergic disease.

The ears are examined as cough may occur with stimulation of the external auditory canal or tympanic membrane. When chronic cough is associated with otitis media and sinusitis, asthma or primary ciliary dyskinesia may also be present. Nasal polyps suggest cystic fibrosis or asthma.

Occasionally, a patient with chronic cough may have an increase in anteroposterior diameter of the thorax. This may be due to cystic fibrosis or severe asthma. Careful auscultation of the chest may reveal adventitial sounds in patients with a chronic cough. Diffuse wheezing suggests asthma, while localized wheezing suggests bronchial obstruction such as with a foreign body, bronchomalacia, or a tumor. Crackles are found when pneumonia or pulmonary fibrosis is present.

Laboratory Investigations

Diagnostic testing is directed by data from the history and physical examination and consideration of the most likely causes of chronic cough in the child's age group. Infection and cough-variant asthma are the most common causes of chronic cough and are considered early in the workup. Primary ciliary dyskinesia and alpha-1-antitrypsin deficiency are rare; they are specifically tested for when there is only a reasonable clinical likelihood that one of these conditions is present and the more common entities have been ruled out.

Irwin et al (7) developed the anatomic approach to the diagnosis of chronic cough in 1981. Since their approach was based on data from adults, it cannot be used for children. However, the philosophy of investigating common causes first using a stepwise approach is logically and medically sound. Table 2 lists diagnostic studies that may be useful in the diagnosis of chronic cough in children.

Following the initial history taking, physical examination, and review of the chest radiograph and all other available data, an individualized plan is developed for each patient. The least traumatic, safest, and most cost-effective studies or investigations are planned to identify the most likely diagnosis as promptly as possible (see Table 2).

While many patients are referred specifically for endoscopic examination, not all undergo bronchoscopy. The diagnosis is occasionally apparent after the preliminary evaluation, and when a child responds to specific therapy, there is no need for bronchoscopy. The following studies are particularly effective in each age group for establishing a precise diagnosis (6):

Birth to 18 months: endoscopy; barium esophagram, radionuclide reflux scan; therapeutic trial of bronchodilators

Eighteen months to 6 years: paranasal sinus computed tomography (CT); therapeutic trial of bronchodilators; endoscopy

Six to 16 years: pulmonary function studies (with methacholine challenge testing); endoscopy; paranasal sinus CT

Endoscopy may include bronchoalveolar lavage (BAL). The findings by BAL may be considered to confirm the diagnosis of aspiration since it is the most effective means of obtaining alveolar macrophages to stain for lipid—indirect evidence of aspiration. Vocal fold mobility is also evaluated prior to induction of general anesthesia in patients who may be aspirating.

PEARLS AND PERILS

1. Cause of cough varies with age. Some diagnoses are considerably more common in certain age groups.
2. Obtaining posteroanterior and lateral chest radiographs is the first step in evaluating the patient.
3. Patient evaluation is individualized on the basis of the following:
   a. The results of studies previously completed
   b. What is most cost-effective
   c. What is least invasive
   d. What is most likely to establish the correct diagnosis

 TREATMENT RECOMMENDATIONS

Treatment is carried out appropriately after the underlying cause of the cough has been determined. Symptomatic treatment of cough is rarely necessary and rarely effective. Treatment of individual conditions is as follows.

Cough-variant asthma is the most common cause of chronic cough (Table 3). Thirty-two percent of children in one study suffered from this disorder (6) The cough is typically a dry hacking cough that may be more irritating at night. It can occur at any age. Bronchoscopy may reveal normal findings, may show laryngotracheal inflammation secondary to the mechanical trauma of coughing, or may reveal a second disorder (such as subglottic stenosis). The workup is remarkable in that there is generally a paucity of other findings when cough-variant asthma occurs alone. When the child is old enough to cooperate, pulmonary function studies with methacholine challenge confirm the diagnosis. A therapeutic trial of bronchodilators is useful for diagnostic purposes in children too young to undergo pulmonary function testing.

Interestingly, cough-variant asthma is the most common incorrect diagnosis at the time of referral to a specialist (6). Bronchodilator therapy has been tried in most of these children. A few of these patients are noncompliant or undertreated. A short course of steroids may be necessary to control bronchospasm when the child has an infection (such as a viral respiratory tract infection or sinusitis).

Cough-variant asthma can have any of five complicating characteristics: (a) The cough continues because of undertreatment; (b) the cough continues because of noncompliance with recommended medication; (c) the cough is frequently associated with sinusitis, which exacerbates the problem; (d) sinusitis is often misdiagnosed as cough-variant asthma; and (e) 43% of patients with cough-variant asthma have a second condition as well, most commonly sinusitis, subglottic stenosis, or gastroesophageal reflux (6). It is in this most challenging group (termed *mixed*) that thorough evaluation, particularly sinus CT and endoscopy, is necessary if the reason for failed therapy of cough-variant asthma is to be determined. Treatment of one of the two causes of cough in this mixed group typically results in an improvement of symptoms. However, when the cough does not completely resolve, one must consider the possibility of a coexisting condition that also causes cough.

TABLE 3: Etiology of Chronic Cough[a]

Diagnosis	No. of Patients	%
Cough-variant asthma	23	32
Sinusitis	17	23
Gastroesophageal reflux	11	15
Aberrant innominate artery	9	12
Psychogenic cough	7	10
Unknown	6	8
Subglottic stenosis	5	7
Tracheomalacia	3	4
Cystic fibrosis	1	1
Viral bronchitis	1	1
Bronchogenic cyst	1	1
Bronchial foreign body	1	1
Subtotal	85	110
Mixed		
Cough-variant asthma		
+Subglottic stenosis	3	4
+Sinusitis	3	4
+Gastroesophageal reflux	2	2
+Aberrant innominate artery	1	1
+Psychogenic cough	1	1
Gastroesophageal reflux		
+Cystic fibrosis	1	1
+Aberrant innominate artery	1	1
Bronchial foreign body		
+Subglottic stenosis	1	1
Subtotal	13	18
Total	72	100

[a]Etiology of chronic cough in 72 infants and children with normal chest radiographs (6). Thirteen patients had more than one diagnosis and are termed *mixed*. These account for the 18% apparent excess diagnoses.

Sinusitis is the second most frequent diagnosis. These patients may be incorrectly or incompletely diagnosed as having cough-variant asthma, having failed bronchodilator therapy prior to evaluation. Limited CT of the paranasal sinuses is standard for diagnosing and following these patients (8).

All children can be managed successfully by oral medication, although maintenance antibiotics are sometimes necessary to prevent a recurrence of symptoms (6). Operative intervention is not required. Some children require continuous oral antibiotic therapy for 4 or even 6 weeks before the cough subsides. Children who have an inhalant allergy contributing to rhinorrhea, cough, and recurrent sinusitis need to have this treated appropriately.

Gastroesophageal reflux is a particularly important consideration in the birth to 18-month age group (6). It may be associated with failure to thrive, apnea, pneumonia, exacerbation of asthma (9), and dysphagia. Evaluation includes barium swallow studies that may also reveal tracheoesophageal fistula, vascular ring, or aspiration. Radionuclide reflux scan and 24-hour pH probe are more sensitive should the esophagram results be negative. Esophagoscopy (with biopsy) also can be useful in diagnosing reflux esophagitis. Surgery is reserved for rare, severe gastroesophageal reflux that fails to respond to medical management.

Psychogenic cough is typically a dry hacking cough occurring in the adolescent. Onset usually occurs with a viral respiratory tract infection during the school year. The cough is present only during the waking hours and is unaccompanied by systemic signs. Before making this diagnosis, the physician should perform an evaluation to exclude other common causes of chronic cough. Tracheitis observed at bronchoscopy with psychogenic cough is probably secondary to the cough rather than a cause of cough.

Children do not continue to lose large amounts of time from school after their evaluation and bronchoscopy, although symptoms may have been so severe that an entire year of school has to be repeated. Psychiatric consultation may be obtained but ongoing psychotherapy for the child and family is rarely indicated.

Aberrant innominate artery is diagnosed in about 10% of patients; all are younger than 18 months (6). Resolution of symptoms occurs over several months. Worsening of the cough is common during respiratory infections. The diagnosis is suggested by lateral airway films that show compression of the anterior trachea just below the thoracic inlet. Bronchoscopy is necessary for confirmation.

Subglottic stenosis is typically found with a second diagnosis as well: tracheomalacia, cough-variant asthma, or bronchial foreign body. Endoscopy is diagnostic and resolution of cough occurs without surgical intervention.

Pertussis causes a dramatic cough in infants and children, and is suspected and diagnosed frequently prior to referral for bronchoscopy. It is a self-limited disease that rarely continues for more than 8 weeks, although it used to be known as "100-day cough."

The otorespiratory reflex is mediated by Arnold's nerve, the auricular branch of the tenth cranial nerve (10), and is a rare cause of chronic cough. Careful examination of the ears, with removal of cerumen and any hairs in contact with the tympanic membrane or the opposite wall of the external auditory canal, is carried out during initial physical examination.

Drug-induced cough or bronchospasm can be produced by three groups of drugs: angiotensin-converting enzyme inhibitors, inhalational agents, and neuromuscular blocking agents (11). Captopril and enalapril, common angiotensin-converting enzyme inhibitors, produce a cough that is dry and persistent and has a female predominance. Symptoms develop within days to months of beginning therapy and resolve within 1 to 2 weeks after stopping the medication. Bronchial hyperreactivity is the likely mechanism for cough. Treatment is avoidance of the offending drugs.

Inhalational agents include aerosolized medications delivered by metered-dose inhalers. The inert propellants and dispersants of albuterol, metaproterenol, and beclomethasone have been identified as offenders. Sulfite sensitivity may produce a cough in susceptible patients who are taking isoproterenol (Isuprel), isoetharine (Bronkosol), or racemic epinephrine. The mechanism is thought to be the nonspecific irritant effect of the inhaled particle.

Neuromuscular blocking agents can produce bronchospasm. This group includes *d*-tubocurarine, alcuronium, atracurium, vecuronium, and pancuronium (11).

PEARLS AND PERILS

1. Two or more diagnoses need to be considered when the diagnosis is not readily apparent.
2. When there is no response to therapy:
   a. The condition is being undertreated,
   b. The family or patient is noncompliant,
   c. The diagnosis is incorrect, or
   d. The therapy is incorrect.
3. Oral antibiotic therapy for sinusitis may take as long as 6 weeks for the patient to respond.
4. Initial aggressive therapy may be necessary to control cough-variant asthma. Often a brief course of steroids is necessary.

While the cause of cough may remain undetermined despite exhaustive diagnostic evaluation, most patients will eventually experience spontaneous resolution of symptoms, often weeks to months following failure of therapeutic trials of bronchodilators or antibiotics.

Once the etiology of the cough has been determined, specific therapy is initiated with the exception of those patients for whom expectant management is deemed more appropriate, for example, patients with an aberrant innominate artery. More than 80% will have complete resolution of the cough (12). A few will continue to cough but show subjective improvement. More than one-fourth will require ongoing medication, particularly those with cough-variant asthma.

MANAGEMENT OF COMPLICATIONS

Persistent cough may lead to irritation of the larynx and tracheobronchial tree, vomiting, failure to thrive, exhaustion, or more acute complications such as fracture of ribs, pneumothorax, pneumomediastinum, and rupture of the rectus abdominis muscles. It is therefore necessary to promptly identify the underlying cause or causes of the cough and treat the condition or conditions specifically.

REFERENCES

1. Hilding AC. Experimental studies on some little understood aspects of the physiology of the respiratory tract and their clinical importance. *Trans Am Acad Ophthalmol Otolaryngol* 1961;65:475–495.
2. McLemore T, Delozier T. Summary: national ambulatory medical care survey. *Advance data from vital and health statistics*, no. 88, 1985. Hyattsville, MD: Public Health Service; 1987; (PHS) 87–1250.
3. Jackson C. Postulates on cough reflex in some of its medical and surgical phases. *Ther Gaz* 1920;44:609.
4. Irwin RS, Rosen MJ, Braman SS. Cough: a comprehensive review. *Arch Intern Med* 1977; 137:1186–1191.
5. Clerf LH. Cough as a symptom. *Med Clin North Am* 1947;31:1393–1399.
6. Holinger LD, Sanders AD. Chronic cough in infants and children: an update. *Laryngoscope* 1991;101:596–605.
7. Irwin RS, Corrao UM, Pretter MR. Chronic persistent cough in the adult: the spectrum and frequency of causes and successful outcome of specific therapy. *Am Rev Respir Dis* 1981;123: 413–417.
8. McAllister W, Lusk R. Comparison of plain radiographs and coronal CT scan in infants and children. *AJR* 1989;153:1259–1264.
9. Irwin RS, French CL, Curley FJ, Zawacki JK, Bennett FM. Chronic cough due to gastroesophageal reflux. Clinical diagnostic and pathogenic aspects. *Chest* 1993;104:1511–1517.
10. Todisco T. The oto-respiratory reflex. *Respiration* 1982;43:354–358.
11. Meeker DP, Wiedman HP. Drug-induced bronchospasm. *Clin Chest Med* 1990;11:163–175.
12. Irwin RS, Demers RR. Management of the patient with cough. *Compr Ther* 1979;5:43–49.

L.D. Holinger: Department of Otolaryngology—Head and Neck Surgery, Northwestern University Medical School, and Section of Bronchoesophagology, Children's Memorial Hospital, Chicago, Illinois 60614.

- *Practical Pediatric Otolaryngology*
- edited by Robin T. Cotton and Charles M. Myer, III
- Lippincott–Raven Publishers, Philadelphia © 1999

9

Immunodeficiency Disorders

Michelle B. Lierl

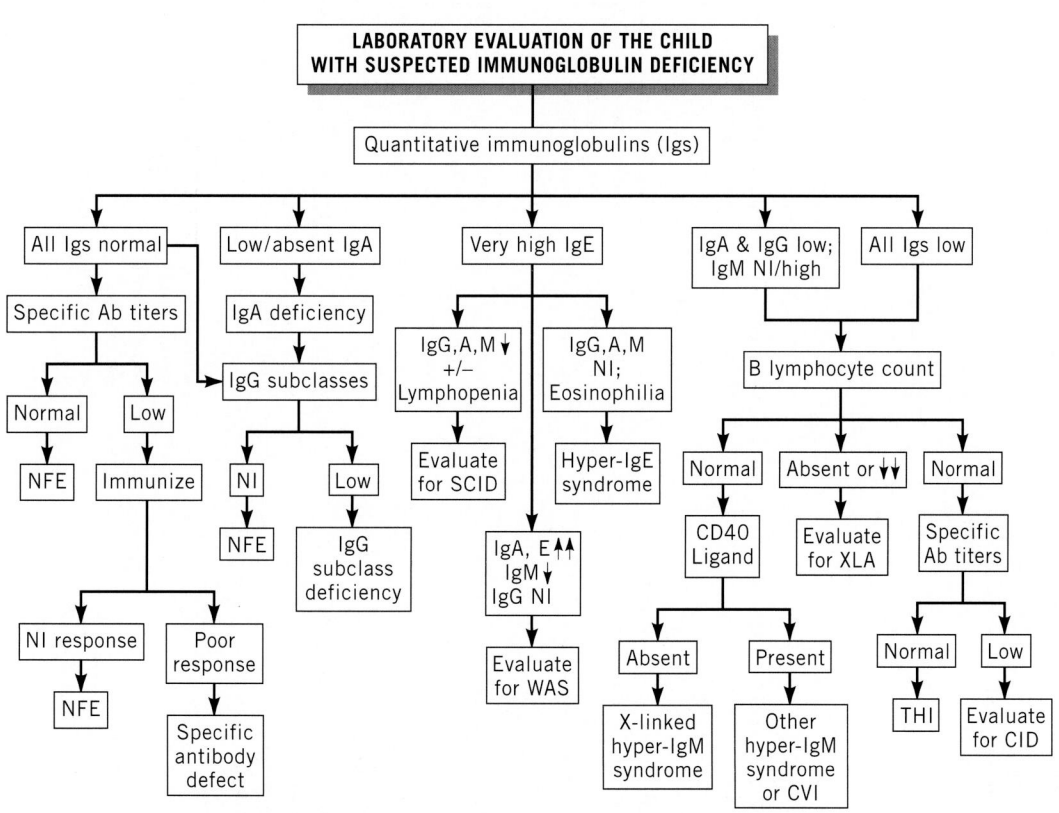

Igs, immunoglobulins; Ab, antibodies; NFE, no further evaluation; NI, normal; SCID, severe combined immunodeficiency; WAS, Wiskott-Aldrich syndrome; CVI, common variable immunodeficiency; XLA, X-linked agammaglobulinemia; THI, transient hypogammaglobulinemia of infancy; CID, combined immunodeficiency.

OVERVIEW

The immune system is a complex array of different types of effector cells and cell products that interact to protect the body from infectious agents and malignancies. Many different types of immunodeficiency syndromes, resulting from defects in one or more elements of the immune system, have been described. This discussion is limited to those immune deficiency syndromes that are likely to present with recurrent upper respiratory tract infections.

Table 1 summarizes the clinical characteristics of the syndromes discussed in this chapter.

TABLE 1: Characteristics of Immunodeficiency Diseases That Can Present with Recurrent Upper Respiratory Tract Infections

Disease	Inheritance	Immunologic Abnormalities	Age at Onset of Symptoms	Sites of Infection	Infecting Organisms	Physical Examination[b]	Associated Findings
IgA deficiency	Autosomal recessive; unknown; (can also be acquired, secondary to infection or drug therapy)	IgA low or absent; IgG and IgM normal	Variable; usually first year of life	Otitis media, sinusitis, bronchitis, pneumonia, gastrointestinal	Usual pediatric pathogens[a]; Giardia lamblia	Signs of allergy (some patients); signs of collagen vascular disease	Allergic rhinoconjunctivitis, asthma, eczema, urticaria; autoimmune diseases; anti-IgA antibody; malignancy
IgG subclass deficiency	Unknown	One or more IgG subclasses low or absent; total IgG normal	After 6 mo	Otitis media, sinusitis, bronchitis, pneumonia	Usual pediatric pathogens[a]	Normal except for intercurrent infection	None
Specific antibody defect	Unknown	Normal immunoglobulin levels; no rise in antibody titer after infection or immunization	After 6 mo	Otitis media, sinusitis, pneumonia, pneumococcal sepsis	Usual pediatric pathogens[a]; Streptococcus pneumoniae prominent	Sometimes, persistent lymphadenopathy	None
Transient hypogammaglobulinemia of infancy	Unknown	Low IgG, IgA, IgM but normal B-cell numbers and rise in antibody titers after immunization	After 6 mo	Otitis media, sinusitis, bronchitis, pneumonia; oral candidiasis	Usual pediatric pathogens[a]; Candida albicans	Normal except for intercurrent infection	None
X-linked agammaglobulinemia	X-linked recessive	Very low to absent immunoglobulins; no mature B cells	After 6 mo	Otitis media, sinusitis, bronchitis, pneumonia, sepsis; meningitis; osteomyelitis; septic arthritis; cellulitis; gastroenteritis; CNS	Usual pediatric pathogens[a]; Pseudomonas sp.; enteroviruses (poliovirus, echovirus, coxsackievirus)	Hypoplastic tonsils, adenoids, and lymph nodes	Neutropenia; chronic echovirus dermatomyositis-encephalitis

	Inheritance	Immunologic abnormalities	Age of onset	Site of infection	Common pathogens	Physical findings	Complications
Common variable immunodeficiency	Autosomal recessive; autosomal dominant; unknown	Low IgG; IgA and IgM low to absent; low specific antibody titers; variable T-cell abnormalities	Usually after puberty; occasionally in childhood	Sinusitis, otitis media, bronchitis, pneumonia; GI	*Hemophilus influenzae*, *S. pneumoniae*, staphylococci; *Mycoplasma pneumoniae*; herpes simplex herpes zoster; *G. lamblia*, fungi, mycobacteria, *Pneumocystis carinii*	Malnutrition; signs of autoimmune diseases	Autoimmune diseases; malignancies
Hyper-IgM syndrome	X-linked or autosomal recessive (can also be secondary to congenital rubella)	IgM normal to very high; IgG IgA and IgE low	After 6 mo	Otitis media, sinusitis, pneumonia; GI; cutaneous or soft tissue	Usual pediatric pathogens[a]; *P. carinii*; *G. lamblia*; *Cryptosporidium*	Enlarged tonsils, adenoids, lymph nodes, spleen, and liver; oral ulcers	Neutropenia (persistent or cyclic); autoantibody production (thrombocytopenia, hemolytic anemia, hypothyroidism, arthritis); warts; malignancies
Wiskott-Aldrich syndrome	X-linked recessive	Inability to form antibody to polysaccharide antigens; low IgM, very high IgA and IgE, normal or high IgG; various T-cell defects	Before 6 mo	Otitis media, sinusitis, pneumonia; stomatitis; cutaneous	Usual pediatric pathogens[a]; viral (cytomegalovirus, varicella, herpes simplex); *P. carinii*	Eczema, petechiae; hepatosplenomegaly; cervical adenopathy; herpetic skin lesions and/or conjunctivitis	Hematologic: thrombocytopenia with small platelets, eosinophilia, anemia, lymphopenia; severe adverse reactions to immunizations; hemorrhage: GI, pulmonary, CNS; arthritis; malignancies

continued

TABLE 1: *(Continued)*

Disease	Inheritance	Immunologic Abnormalities	Age at Onset of Symptoms	Sites of Infection	Infecting Organisms	Physical Examination[b]	Associated Findings
Ataxia-telangiectasia syndrome	Autosomal recessive	Variable immunoglobulin abnormalities: deficiency of IgA, IgG, and/or IgM; IgG subclass deficiency; poor specific antibody responses; variable T-cell defects	Variable; infancy to 5 yr	Sinusitis, bronchitis, pneumonia	Usual pediatric pathogens[a]; viral	Neurologic: cerebellar ataxia, slurred speech, choreoathetoid movements, drooling, strabismus, mask-like facies, muscle atrophy, diminished reflexes; telangiectasia: bulbar conjunctivae, facial, extremities	Excessive chromosomal breakage; granulocytopenia, lymphopenia, eosinophilia; cerebral atrophy; cardiac aanomalies; Malignancy
Immunodeficiency—centromeric instability facial anomaly syndrome	Autosomal recessive	Low to absent immunoglobulin levels; normal B-cell number; T cells low or normal; natural killer cells impaired	First year of life	Sinusitis, otitis media, pneumonia	Usual pediatric pathogens[a]; viral	Facial anomalies (see text)	Chromosomes 1 and 16 structural abnormalities; failure to thrive; malabsorption; mental retardation
Hyper-IgE syndrome	? Autosomal dominant with variable penetrance	Extremely elevated IgE; poor specific antibody responses; deficiency of memory T cells; decreased or absent lymphoproliferative responses to antigen	Variable; usually first year of life	Cutaneous and pulmonary abscesses; sinusitis, otitis media, orbital/periorbital cellulitis	*S. aureus*; usual pediatric pathogens[a]; fungi (*C. albicans, Aspergillus* sp, *Trichophyton* sp.; gram-negative bacteria	Coarse facial features in most patients; eczematous skin lesions; furunculosis	Eosinophilia (peripheral blood and sputum); intermittent granulocyte chemotactic defects in some patients; osteopenia

Neutrophil defects	Various	Various defects in oxidative burst, chemotaxis, phagocytosis	Early infancy	Cutaneous abscesses and cellulitis; stomatitis; periodontitis; recurrent sinusitis, otitis, pneumonia; suppurative adenitis; osteomyelitis; GI fistulas	*S. aureus; Pseudomonas, Serratia,* other enterobacteria, *Aspergillus, Candida*	Variable with different defects; lymphadenopathy, hepatosplenomegaly, cutaneous scarring	Impaired wound healing; delayed separation of the umbilical cord (esp. in leukocyte adhesion defects); various anomalies associated with specific syndromes
Pediatric AIDS	(Perinatal or parenteral transmission)	Depletion of CD4+ T cells; hypergammaglobulinemia with poor specific antibody production	Variable; infancy through the first few years of life	Otitis media, sinusitis, pneumonia; oral/esophageal candidiasis; GI	Usual pediatric pathogens[a]; *P. carinii,* other protozoa; fungal; viral; mycobacterial (*M. tuberculosis, M. avium-intracellulare*)	Failure to thrive; lymphadenopathy, hepatosplenomegaly, parotitis; oropharyngeal candidiasis, chronic herpes stomatitis	Lymphoid interstitial pneumonitis; encephalopathy; endocrinopathies; anemia, neutropenia, thrombocytopenia; malignancy; cardiomyopathy; nephropathy

[a]The usual pediatric bacterial respiratory pathogens include *Branhamella catarrhalis, Streptococcus pneumoniae, Hemophilus influenzae,* group A streptococcus, and *Staphylococcus aureus.*

[b]Physical examination findings listed in this table are those found in *addition* to the signs of chronic sinopulmonary infections that are typical of all these disorders.

CNS, central nervous system; GI, gastrointestinal.

Primary Immunodeficiencies

Primary immunodeficiencies are those caused by developmental abnormalities. The most common of these, and the most likely to present with recurrent respiratory tract infections, are the *antibody deficiency syndromes.*

Selective IgA deficiency is the most common antibody deficiency syndrome, affecting about 1 in 500 to 700 people of the general population. In this condition, all the immunoglobulins are present in normal concentration except for IgA, which is absent or significantly below the lower limit of normal. Secretory IgA levels are usually low also. T-cell function and specific antibody responses of IgG and IgM are normal. The deficiency appears to be due to a defect in the final maturation stages of the B cell, since normal numbers of IgA-bearing B lymphocytes are found in IgA-deficient patients.

Most individuals with selective IgA deficiency, especially those with a "partial" deficiency (i.e., the IgA level is more than 2 standard deviations below the normal range, but above 5mg per deciliter), are completely asymptomatic. However, IgA-deficient individuals have a higher incidence than the general population of diseases in three categories: recurrent infections (respiratory, gastrointestinal), allergic diseases, and autoimmune diseases. The infectious and allergic diseases can be attributed to the loss of the mucosal barrier function of IgA. Increased mucosal penetration of microbes leads to recurrent infections; increased penetration of allergens induces IgE-mediated allergic responses. The etiology of the increased incidence of collagen vascular diseases in these patients is less well understood, but might also relate to increased systemic exposure to various antigens with subsequent development of cross-reactive autoantibodies.

In patients who have a combination of IgA deficiency and an IgG subclass deficiency (see below), recurrent infection is a more prominent presentation and less likely to resolve with increasing age (1,2).

Circulating antibodies to IgA are present in 30% to 40% of patients who have complete absence of IgA. These patients can have severe anaphylactic reactions if they receive IgA-containing blood products.

IgG subclass deficiencies are also common in the population. In this condition, the total serum IgG level is normal, but one or more of the four IgG subclasses is absent or the level is significantly low (3). As in selective IgA deficiency, not all affected individuals are symptomatic. Those who are symptomatic present with recurrent bacterial respiratory infections (sinusitis, otitis media, bronchitis, and pneumonia).

The natural history of children with IgG subclass deficiencies and recurrent infection is variable. Most affected individuals present during early childhood, and the recurrent infections tend to become less problematic with increasing age. The subjects in most studies of IgG subclass deficiencies and recurrent infections are children, although affected adults have also been reported (4). Only a few studies have retested IgG subclass levels over the course of several years. The data from these studies show that the deficiency may or may not resolve over time (5).

Because of the finding of IgG subclass deficiencies in asymptomatic individuals, many immunologists question the clinical relevance of an IgG subclass deficiency as an isolated abnormality (6,7). The ability to form appropriate antibody responses to specific infectious agents is considered a better reflection of the patient's immune competence.

Defects in specific antibody formation have been observed in patients with and those without IgG subclass deficiency. In these patients, little or no antibody is produced after infection or immunization. Some patients are able to respond to certain kinds of antigen, but not to others (8). In particular, a poor response to polysaccharide antigens has been observed in patients presenting with recurrent respiratory tract infections (9,10). This finding probably has clinical relevance, since most of the common respiratory bacterial pathogens have polysaccharide capsules. The antibody response to polysaccharide antigens is predominantly an IgG2 subclass response; in some patients, a defective response to polysaccharide antigens is associated with an IgG2 subclass deficiency. The IgG1 and

IgG3 subclasses are chiefly responsible for responses to protein antigens such as tetanus and diphtheria toxoids, and viral antigens (3).

Transient hypogammaglobulinemia of infancy represents a maturational delay in the infant's production of immunoglobulins. The normal newborn has very low levels of endogenous antibody production, but is protected by maternal IgG that crosses the placenta during the third trimester of pregnancy. The maternal IgG is gradually catabolized, resulting in a physiologic nadir in antibody levels at the ages of 3 to 6 months. In the normal infant, endogenous antibody production in response to antigenic stimulation results in a subsequent rise of total IgM and IgG antibody levels. Infants with transient hypogammaglobulinemia fail to produce endogenous antibody at the normal time, so that their levels of IgG, IgA, and sometimes IgM "bottom out" at the ages of 3 to 6 months and remain quite low for several months. In most cases, antibody production begins to increase by the age of 1 year and antibody levels usually reach normal the ages of by 2 to 3 years (although in some infants, normal levels are not achieved until 4 to 5 years). IgA levels tend to rise the most slowly, and some patients have persistent IgA deficiency (11). Even while the antibody levels are low, a good specific antibody response to immunizations can usually be demonstrated (12).

Infants with transient hypogammaglobulinemia can be asymptomatic or can present with recurrent respiratory tract infections including otitis media, sinusitis, pneumonia, and pharyngitis. Serious systemic infections are not characteristic of this condition. The usual age at which recurrent infections begin is around 6 months. Infants born prematurely may present at an earlier age with very low levels of IgG, since they have missed part or all of the third trimester of pregnancy during which maternal IgG transfer occurs.

X-linked agammaglobulinemia (XLA) (Bruton's disease) is a congenital condition characterized by a complete or nearly complete absence of circulating B cells and plasma cells. IgA and IgM are absent, and IgG levels are absent or very low. The disease is inherited as an X-linked recessive disorder. These boys usually present after the age of 6 months with recurrent bacterial infections (13) (Fig. 1). Surprisingly, despite the profound antibody deficiency, as many as 21% of children with XLA do not manifest unusual problems until as late as 3 to 5 years (14). In addition to upper and lower respiratory tract infections, episodes of septicemia, meningitis, osteomyelitis, and septic arthritis are common. Cell-mediated immunity is normal in these patients, and most viral infections are handled normally. However, vaccine-associated poliomyelitis is a significant risk following immunization with a live polio vaccine. These patients are also prone to develop chronic echovirus or coxsackievirus infection with slowly progressive meningoencephalitis and a dermatomyositis-like syndrome.

In addition to the antibody deficiency syndromes, various types of *combined im-*

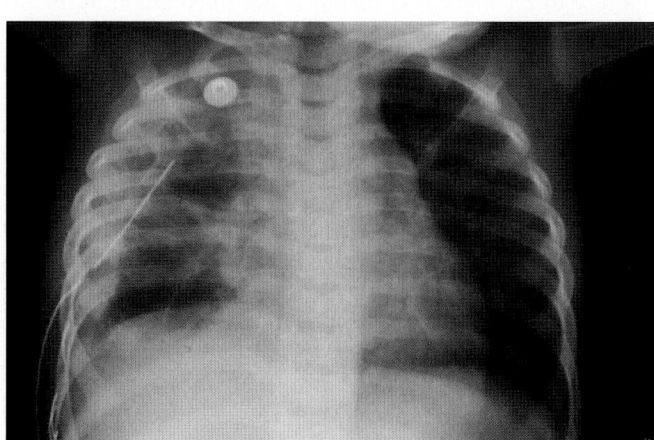

FIGURE 1 This 1½-year-old boy had a history of several episodes of otitis media and pharyngitis, but was otherwise well until he presented with acute onset of fever, cough, and dyspnea. Chest x-ray films showed pneumonia and empyema; culture of the pleural effusion grew *Streptococcus pneumoniae*. He was treated with antibiotics and chest tube drainage and recovered uneventfully. Seven months later he again developed an acute febrile illness with generalized malaise, and blood cultures grew *Pseudomonas aeruginosa*. Immunologic evaluation was performed at this time, and revealed absence of IgG, IgM, and IgA. Lymphocyte enumeration revealed absence of mature B cells, with normal numbers and subtypes of T cells. He was diagnosed with X-linked agammaglobulinemia and begun on immunoglobulin replacement therapy. He remained free of infection for the ensuing 2 years.

munodeficiencies can present with recurrent respiratory tract infections. In combined immunodeficiencies, there are defects in both the B and T lymphocyte–mediated immune responses. Most patients with combined immunodeficiencies show clinical signs of T-lymphocyte dysfunction, such as opportunistic infections with fungi, viruses, and protozoa; but they also have a high incidence of sinusitis, otitis media, and bronchopneumonia.

The *severe combined immunodeficiency syndromes* usually present early in infancy with severe chronic lung disease, chronic diarrhea, failure to thrive and debilitation, and chronic oral thrush. While upper respiratory tract infections are often a part of the clinical picture, it is usually obvious that these children have a serious immunologic problem. They are unlikely to present, undiagnosed, to the otolaryngologist.

Common variable immunodeficiency (CVI) is a clinical syndrome in which a previously well child or adult develops recurrent bacterial infections and hypogammaglobulinemia (15). Because of the marked variability in clinical presentation and laboratory abnormalities it is presumed that several different defects can lead to this syndrome. Most patients have normal numbers of mature B lymphocytes, but the B cells are unable to mature to plasma cells and produce specific antibody. Various defects in T-lymphocyte subsets and function have been observed in patients with CVI, and it is suspected that abnormalities in the interactions between the T and B lymphocytes result in the inability to produce normal antibody responses (16).

The clinical presentation of CVI is similar to that of XLA except for the age of onset. Symptoms most often develop during the second or third decade of life, although CVI is occasionally diagnosed in young children. Recurrent bacterial respiratory tract infections are the most prominent manifestation, and progression to bronchiectasis is not unusual in untreated patients. Recurrent attacks of herpes simplex and herpes zoster are also seen in many patients with CVI. Gastrointestinal symptoms, due to parasitic or bacterial infections, are a frequent problem. Adult patients are also afflicted with an increased incidence of autoimmune diseases and malignancies.

Hyper-IgM syndrome is a rare condition in which the levels of IgA, IgG, and IgE are low but the serum IgM level is normal or high. It is usually inherited as an X-linked recessive trait, although a few cases of autosomal recessive and autosomal dominant inheritance have been reported. The underlying defect is an abnormality in a T-lymphocyte membrane protein known as the *CD40 ligand*, which binds to a receptor called CD40 on B lymphocytes and other antigen-presenting cells. Without the CD40 ligand on the T cells, the patient's B cells are unable to produce memory B lymphocytes and are unable to switch from producing IgM to producing other types of immunoglobulin (17). The result is a profound defect in the ability to produce antibody in response to infection.

The clinical presentation is that of recurrent upper respiratory tract infections and pneumonia, usually beginning after the age of 6 months (18). In addition to the usual bacterial pathogens, pneumonia due to *Pneumocystis carinii* is not uncommon in infants with hyper-IgM syndrome (Fig. 2). Infections of the skin and soft tissues, particularly peritonsillar or paratracheal soft tissue infections, can be a serious problem (19,20). In children who are not diagnosed at an early age, the chronic antigenic stimulation of the B-lymphocyte system can lead to massive hypertrophy of the lymphoid tissue. The presenting complaint is sometimes upper-airway obstruction due to enlarged tonsils and adenoids. In these children, the serum IgM levels are often extremely high, whereas earlier in infancy the IgM levels may be normal. Some of the IgM antibodies can function as autoantibodies, resulting in hemolytic anemia, thrombocytopenia, arthritis, and other autoimmune disorders. Gastrointestinal disease and malabsorption, sometimes due to parasitic infections, are also frequent problems. Neutropenia develops in about half of the patients with hyper-IgM syndrome, and manifests as persistent or recurrent problems with stomatitis and oral ulcers.

Wiskott-Aldrich syndrome is characterized by eczema, thrombocytopenia with small

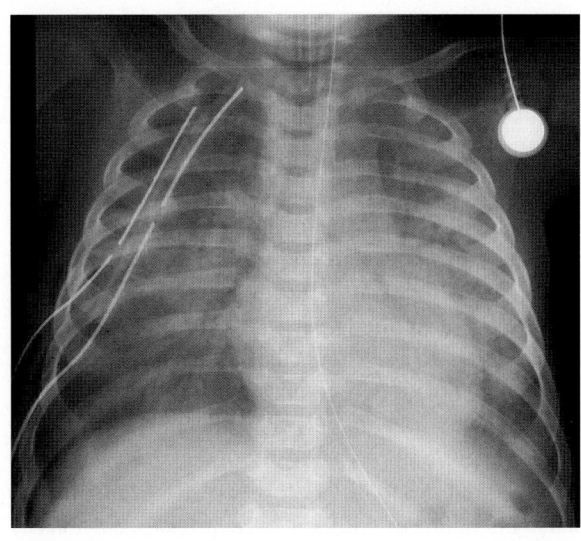

FIGURE 2 This 7½-month-old boy presented with a 2-month history of pneumonia. Chest x-ray films revealed diffuse interstitial disease. A lung biopsy specimen was positive for *Pneumocystis carinii.* Levels of IgG and IgA were very low, but IgM levels were in the normal range. The numbers of mature B and T cells were normal. The CD40 ligand was found to be defective. He was diagnosed with hyper-IgM syndrome and was treated with immunoglobulin replacement and trimethoprim-sulfa prophylaxis for *Pneumocystis* infection.

platelets, and recurrent infections. The mode of inheritance is X-linked recessive. The immunologic defect is complex, with abnormal T-lymphocyte function and poor responses to polysaccharide antigens. Typically, measurements of serum antibody concentrations reveal a normal level of IgG, high levels of IgA and IgE, and a low level of IgM.

Affected boys present clinically in infancy, often with petechiae or an episode of bleeding. With the development of eczema, petechiae are seen in the excoriations. Chronic otitis media with draining ears is typically the first infectious problem, often accompanied by bouts of bronchitis and pneumonia. Pneumococcal sepsis and meningitis can be complicating developments. During episodes of infection, the thrombocytopenia becomes more severe and may result in serious hemorrhage into the lungs, gastrointestinal tract, or brain. In addition to infections with encapsulated bacteria, patients with Wiskott-Aldrich syndrome are susceptible to viral infections, especially herpetic stomatitis, cytomegalovirus, and varicella, and to *P. carinii* pneumonia (21).

Ataxia-telangiectasia syndrome is a complex one characterized by sinopulmonary infections, progressive ataxia, and telangiectasia. The immune defect is variable, usually consisting of a combination of depressed T-lymphocyte function, IgA deficiency, and deficiencies in one or more of the IgG subclasses (22). The underlying defect is unknown. The mode of inheritance appears to be autosomal recessive.

Clinically, the first manifestation of the syndrome is usually the ataxia, which begins sometime between infancy and the age of 5 years (23). It begins as a cerebellar ataxia and progresses to a state of generalized muscle weakness and atrophy with choreoathetoid movements and cranial nerve dysfunction. Some patients are mentally retarded. The development of telangiectasia on the bulbar conjunctivae occurs between the ages of 1 and 6 years. Many patients eventually develop telangiectases on the nose, ears, antecubital and popliteal areas, hands, and feet.

The recurrent respiratory tract infections begin during childhood, and often progress to bronchiectasis. As the neuromuscular disease progresses, recurrent aspiration probably plays a role in the development of chronic pulmonary disease. Both bacterial and viral pathogens are involved.

Patients with ataxia-telangiectasia syndrome are also susceptible to a variety of malignancies.

Immunodeficiency–centromeric instability–facial anomaly (ICF) syndrome is a recently described disorder that can present to the otolaryngologist because of severe recurrent respiratory tract infections and facial anomalies. The facial anomalies consist of macroglossia, epicanthal folds, hypertelorism, and a flat nasal bridge. Serum immunoglobulin levels are low to absent, despite a normal number of B cells. T-cell numbers and natural killer cell activity may be low. Chromosomal anomalies are identifiable in peripheral blood lymphocytes (24).

Hyper-IgE syndrome is a primary immunodeficiency of unknown etiology, characterized by recurrent staphylococcal abscesses and extremely elevated levels of serum IgE. Despite the clinical resemblance to chronic granulomatous disease, no consistent defect of neutrophil function has been identified in hyper-IgE syndrome. Eosinophilia of the blood and sputum is common; abnormalities in cell-mediated immunity are demonstrable in more than half the patients. Although the serum levels of IgG, IgA, and IgM are normal in most patients, defective IgG antibody recall responses have been reported. Several cases of familial occurrence have been reported; the apparent mode of inheritance is autosomal dominant with incomplete penetrance.

The clinical manifestations usually begin early in infancy. While furunculosis and cutaneous abscesses are the most frequent manifestations, sinusitis, otitis media, and lung abscesses are also common. There is a marked propensity to form persistent pneumatoceles following episodes of pulmonary infection. In addition to *Staphylococcus aureus* and the usual pediatric bacterial pathogens, fungal infections of the sinuses and pneumatoceles are common (25) (Fig. 3). Many patients have a chronic pruritic dermatitis, but there are usually no respiratory symptoms suggestive of allergy despite the markedly elevated IgE levels. Other associated findings include pronounced osteopenia, and coarse facial features in most patients.

Defects in neutrophil number or function have various clinical presentations that often include the upper respiratory tract. Several forms of neutropenia or chemotactic disorders present with chronic periodontitis or oral stomatitis, or both. In chronic granulomatous disease, recurrent cutaneous abscesses are the most prominent feature, but recurrent sinusitis, otitis media, and pneumonia are also frequent complications.

Secondary Immunodeficiencies

Secondary immunodeficiencies occur when a previously normal immune system is damaged by malnutrition, metabolic disease, protein wasting, drugs, surgery, or infection. Many of these patients will present with recurrent respiratory tract infections, in addition to signs and symptoms of their underlying disease process. The only secondary immunodeficiency that is addressed in detail in this chapter is the immunodeficiency secondary to human immunodeficiency virus (HIV) infection.

Pediatric acquired immunodeficiency syndrome (AIDS), caused by infection with HIV type (HIV-1), is rapidly increasing in incidence worldwide. Acquisition of HIV-1 in children is now mainly through perinatal transmission, although some older children were infected through contaminated blood products.

The time course of the HIV infection is variable. Usually no definite symptoms are noted in perinatally infected infants, despite widespread viral dissemination to the lymphoid tissue, central nervous system (CNS), and internal organs. Antiviral immune responses develop within the first several weeks, and the amount of circulating free virus decreases. The asymptomatic period that follows the infection varies in duration from a few months to several years; during this time the virus continues to infect and destroy CD4+ (helper) T lymphocytes. When the CD4+ T-cell population is significantly depleted, the patient becomes symptomatic with recurrent infections (26).

In the early stages of pediatric AIDS, recurrent upper respiratory tract infections such as sinusitis and otitis media are common. These children might be distinguished from the usual pediatric patients by the presence of persistent oral candidiasis or paroti-

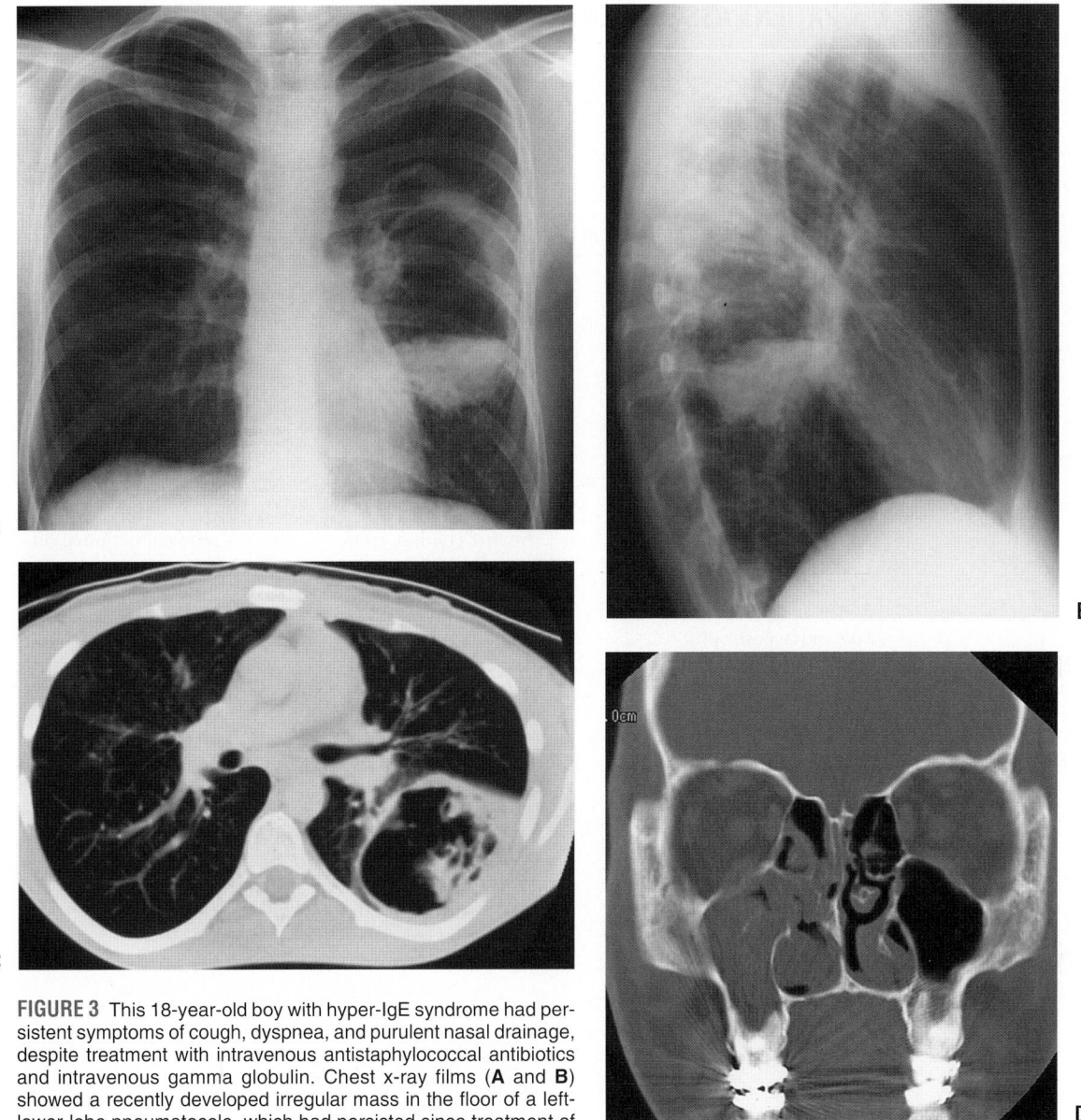

FIGURE 3 This 18-year-old boy with hyper-IgE syndrome had persistent symptoms of cough, dyspnea, and purulent nasal drainage, despite treatment with intravenous antistaphylococcal antibiotics and intravenous gamma globulin. Chest x-ray films (**A** and **B**) showed a recently developed irregular mass in the floor of a left-lower-lobe pneumatocele, which had persisted since treatment of a staphylococcal lung abscess 1 year previously. Computed tomography (CT) of the pneumatocele (**C**) revealed a fungating mass typical of an aspergilloma; cultures of the resected mass confirmed the diagnosis of aspergilloma. CT of the sinuses (**D**) showed extensive disease of the right maxillary and ethmoidal sinuses, with significant bone loss. Cultures of the sinuses also grew *Aspergillus fumigatus*. Surgical drainage and antifungal therapy resulted in marked clinical improvement, and he remained stable on chronic antifungal and antistaphylococcal therapy.

tis, or both (27). Diffuse lymphadenopathy and hepatosplenomegaly are less often present during the earlier stages of pediatric AIDS. As the disease progresses, the patient not only continues to manifest recurrent respiratory tract infections but also begins to present with more serious infections, as well as various systemic signs of illness such as failure to thrive, chronic diarrhea, chronic lung disease, and involvement of various organ systems such as the CNS, heart, kidneys, and liver.

🜂 PATIENT ASSESSMENT

The differential diagnosis of the patient with suspected immunodeficiency because of recurrent respiratory tract infections is shown in Table 2.

TABLE 2: Differential Diagnosis of the Child with Recurrent Respiratory Tract Infections

Diagnosis	Characteristics	Diagnostic Procedures
Allergic rhinitis	Itchy nose and eyes; sneezing; pale nasal mucosal edema; clear nasal secretions	Typical history and physical findings; good response to antihistamines and/or intranasal cromolyn or steroid therapy; positive skin tests to relevant aeroallergens
Recurrent viral URIs due to high exposure levels (day-care center syndrome)	Healthy appearing, thriving child; normal lymphoid tissue; exposure to several other children	Typical history and physical examination
Adenoid hypertrophy	Chronic mouth breathing; snoring and/or sleep apnea; nasal obstruction by physical examination	Flexible rhinoscopy or x-rays of the lateral airway
Immunodeficiency	Recurrent bacterial infections; +/– family history; +/– findings on physical examination (see Table 1)	Immunologic laboratory testing (see Fig. 1)
Cystic fibrosis	Thick nasal secretions; chronic sinusitis with nasal polyposis; recurrent bronchitis +/– pneumonia; clubbing of digits; pseudomonas or staphylococcus in sputum culture; +/– malabsorption and failure to thrive	Sweat chloride and/or genetic testing
Aspirin triad	Steroid-dependent asthma; chronic rhinosinusitis and nasal polyposis; exacerbations of respiratory disease after ingestion of NSAIDs	Aspirin challenge
Immotile cilia syndrome	Chronic sinusitis, otitis media, bronchitis; recurrent pneumonia; 50% have situs inversus; male infertility; positive family history	Mucus clearance studies; cilia biopsy for electron microscopic examination

URIs, upper respiratory tract infections; NSAIDs, nonsteroidal antiinflammatory drugs.

History

A thorough history is essential in the evaluation of the child with recurrent infection. The following points should be carefully addressed.

Does the Child Really Have Recurrent Bacterial Infections?

Most children who present to an immunodeficiency clinic with the chief complaint of recurrent "sinus infections" turn out to have either allergic rhinitis or frequent viral upper respiratory tract infections due to high exposure levels.

Allergic rhinitis can usually be distinguished by a careful history. The rhinorrhea with allergic rhinitis is typically clear and thin, rather than thick and purulent as it would be with sinusitis. The nose, eyes, and throat are usually itchy; the parents will report that the child frequently rubs the eyes and nose and makes peculiar sounds in the throat in an attempt to scratch the itch. Fits of sneezing are common. In many patients, there is a clear history of exacerbations of symptoms with exposure to allergens such as pets, house dust, grass, and molds. In some cases of perennial allergic rhinitis, however, when the patient has chronic year-round symptoms due to constant exposure to indoor allergens, the picture is less clear-cut. The symptoms of itching and sneezing are often less prominent in these patients; their complaints are more of daily nasal congestion and rhinorrhea. Episodes of sinusitis and otitis media are frequent complications of allergic rhinitis, owing to obstruction of the eustachian tubes and sinus ostia by the edema and inspissated mucus.

Frequent viral respiratory tract infections are especially common in very young children attending day-care centers, or in children starting school for the first time after spending their preschool years at home. While this situation represents a normal stage in the acquisition of immunity to the common community viral pathogens, it can create considerable stress for parents. A subset of children have a tendency to develop marked febrile responses to minor viral infections. Thus, while every child in the class has the same cold, these children will develop a fever. Day-care center policy will then dictate that the parent take time off from work and take the child home, and the child will not be allowed to return until the fever is gone for 24 hours. Not only does this worry the parent ("Why does my child get so much sicker than all the other children?"), but also it can result in a considerable number of missed workdays. The parent often responds to this situation by pressuring the child's physician to "do something" to help the child get better faster, which translates into a diagnosis of otitis media or sinusitis and a prescription for an antibiotic. After several such episodes, the child has a history of recurrent bacterial respiratory tract infections and is referred for otolaryngologic intervention or immunologic evaluation. While this scenario is common, it can be difficult to sort out in retrospect from the child who truly has recurrent bacterial infections. Distinguishing features include the epidemiologic history (i.e., the infections occur when the child has been exposed to children with viral illnesses) and the nature of the rhinorrhea, which is usually clear early in the course of the viral upper respiratory tract infection, only becoming purulent during the last few days.

Age of Onset

The age of onset of the infections helps categorize the likely causes. For example, children who begin to experience illness within the first weeks of life probably have a severe combined immunodeficiency, a neutrophil defect, or Wiskott-Aldrich syndrome. Infants who are initially well and then begin to manifest recurrent respiratory tract infections after about the age of 6 months are likely to have an antibody defect. Children whose symptoms begin later in childhood or in adolescence may have CVI.

Type of Infection

The type of infection is important. As mentioned already, frequent viral respiratory tract infections, sometimes complicated by otitis media, are common in normal infants and young children. Recurrent bacterial or fungal infections are more significant. In antibody deficiency syndromes, combined immunodeficiencies, and pediatric AIDS, the most common infecting organisms are the usual pediatric pathogens: *Moraxella catarrhalis, Streptococcus pneumoniae, Hemophilus influenzae,* group A streptococcus, and occasionally *S. aureus.* In neutrophil defects such as chronic granulomatous disease and in hyper-IgE syndrome, *S. aureus* or fungi (*Candida, Aspergillus species*) are often cultured from the sinuses. Fungal infections are also suggestive of AIDS, or other combined immunodeficiencies. A history of *P. carinii* pneumonia is suggestive of hyper-IgM syndrome, pediatric AIDS, or a combined immunodeficiency with significant T-lymphocyte dysfunction.

Sites of Infection

The sites of infection are important. Children presenting with recurrent episodes of otitis media and sinusitis, and no history of more serious infections, may have a selective antibody deficiency or could be in the early stages of pediatric AIDS. A prominent history of recurrent bronchitis and pneumonia and a history of frequent or chronic diarrhea are more typical of CVI or AIDS, although some patients with selective IgA deficiency also present with these symptoms. Patients with a history of pneumonia, sepsis, meningitis, or other serious infections are more likely to have XLA, advanced stages of AIDS, Wiskott-Aldrich syndrome, or another form of combined immunodeficiency. Patients with a history of recurrent cutaneous and pulmonary abscesses should be evaluated for chronic granulomatous disease or other neutrophil defects, and for hyper-IgE syndrome. A history of poliomyelitis following immunization with the live attenuated polio vaccine is typical of XLA or severe combined immunodeficiency syndromes.

Pattern of Infectious Episodes

The pattern of infectious episodes should be carefully elucidated. The typical pattern in a child with an immunodeficiency is that their infections respond (though sometimes more slowly than normal) to antibiotic treatment, only to recur within 1 to 2 weeks after discontinuing antibiotics. Infections tend to occur year-round, although somewhat less frequently in the summer months. Children whose recurrent upper respiratory tract infections are due to chronically obstructed eustachian tubes or sinus ostia will present with this same pattern of recurrence. The occurrence of infections most often during the warmer months of the year is strongly suggestive of allergic rhinitis as the underlying cause. Children with recurrent viral infections due to high exposure levels, on the other hand, usually have significantly more infections during the winter and spring respiratory viral seasons, and are relatively well throughout the summer and early fall months.

Family History

The family history is important, and in suspected cases of immunodeficiency it is worthwhile to solicit information from grandparents and other members of the extended family. Since many of the immunodeficiency syndromes have a recessive mode of inheritance, it is often necessary to look beyond the immediate family for a history of children who experienced recurrent infections or died in infancy or childhood. In families with selective IgA deficiency, there can be a history of individuals with collagen vascular disorders, allergic diseases, or recurrent infections. Patients with CVI sometimes have family members with other antibody deficiency syndromes such as selective IgA deficiency or IgG subclass deficiency. When boys are suspected to have one of the X-linked recessive disorders (XLA, chronic granulomatous disease, or Wiskott-Aldrich syndrome), look to the maternal uncles for a history of similar problems. A careful parental history should also be taken, looking for risk factors for AIDS (history of transfusions of blood products, illicit intravenous drug use, sexual promiscuity, or bisexuality).

Medication History

The medication history can also be helpful. Long-term treatment with phenytoin can cause IgA deficiency. The use of immunosuppressive agents can result in secondary immunodeficiency.

Physical Examination

The purposes of the physical examination of the child with recurrent respiratory tract infection are threefold: to identify any current site(s) of infection, to look for complications of chronic infection, and to note associated abnormalities that may be clues to the presence of an underlying immunodeficiency or other cause for the patient's symptoms.

Signs of Acute Infection

Nose   In acute sinusitis, the nasal mucosa is usually edematous and erythematous. Copious purulent nasal secretions and postnasal drainage are common. These findings do not distinguish bacterial sinusitis from a viral upper respiratory tract infection, particularly during the second week when the secretions caused by a viral infection become purulent in appearance. When maxillary sinusitis is present, rhinoscopy can sometimes demonstrate secretions draining from the maxillary ostia. If no secretions are seen in the nose in the upright position, the patient should be asked to bend forward with the head hanging down for several seconds. Due to disruption of the ciliated epithelial lining of the sinuses, secretions often puddle in the maxillary sinuses in the upright position and drain only when the ostia are positioned "downhill." Similarly, copious postnasal drainage may occur when the patient is lying supine. Erythematous streaks and folliculitis are often present on the posterior part of the pharynx, due to the drainage of purulent secretions.

Examination of the face in the patient with acute sinusitis usually reveals intraorbital puffiness or discoloration, but this is a nonspecific finding associated with nasal mucosal edema of any cause. Erythema is sometimes present over the infected sinus. Tenderness to light pressure over an infected sinus can be a useful marker of sinus inflammation, but is difficult to assess in young children. Transillumination of the sinuses is not an accurate means of assessment for sinusitis.

Other signs of acute sinusitis include fever, cough, halitosis, decreased appetite, and sometimes vomiting of purulent mucoid material. When frontal sinusitis is present, careful neurologic examination is indicated, to rule out intracranial extension of the infection. Erosion of the infection through the posterior plate of the frontal bone can result in development of an epidural, subdural, or brain abscess, or meningitis. Cavernous sinus thrombosis is another potential complication of acute or chronic sinusitis. The findings of photophobia, loss of vision, meningismus, hyperreflexia, clonus, seizures, focal weakness, or a change in mental status should prompt immediate imaging of the brain. Extension of maxillary sinusitis into the orbit should also be considered. Periorbital erythema, proptosis, or loss of extraocular muscle function indicates the presence of an orbital extension of the infection.

Ears   Examination of the ears in patients with acute otitis media reveals hyperemia and dullness of the tympanic membrane, with varying degrees of outward bulging and loss of the usual landmarks. A purulent effusion is sometimes visible behind the tympanic membrane. Spontaneous perforation can result in drainage of pus into the external auditory canal. If the tympanic membrane is intact, pneumatic otoscopy shows decreased mobility.

Extension of the infection into the mastoid sinus results in erythema, swelling, and tenderness over the mastoid; the pinna is sometimes displaced forward. Intracranial extension of infection in the form of abscess, meningitis, or lateral sinus thrombosis is also possible, especially in the immunodeficient child. Facial nerve paralysis, due to erosion of the infection into the facial canal in the middle ear, is a rare complication of acute otitis media.

Mouth and Throat   The tonsils should be inspected carefully, looking for evidence of purulent infection or asymmetry suggestive of a tonsillar abscess. A bulge in the posterior part of the pharynx can also indicate an abscess. Oropharyngeal candidiasis or periodontitis might also be noted in patients with immunodeficiency conditions.

Lungs   A careful pulmonary examination should always be performed in children with recurrent upper respiratory tract infection, looking for signs of lower respiratory tract disease. The findings of diffuse rhonchi and productive cough are suggestive of bronchitis. The presence of tachypnea, nasal flaring, or rales on auscultation indicates pneumonia. Areas of decreased air exchange can be associated with consolidated pneumonia, pulmonary abscess, or empyema. Splinting of the chest on deep inspiration, due to pleuritic chest pain, is seen with pneumonia or pleural effusion.

Skin   The skin should be examined carefully for areas of cellulitis or abscess. Careful inspection of the anus will identify an anal abscess or rectoanal fisula, and an abdominal examination can identify hepatomegaly, splenomegaly, or intraabdominal abscess.

Signs of Chronic Infection

Signs of chronic infection are useful in distinguishing the child with a significant problem from those with benign recurrent viral upper respiratory tract infections.

The general health and nutritional status of the child can appear normal in the presence of selective antibody deficiency syndromes, whereas failure to thrive and debilitation are seen with the more serious immunodeficiencies.

Scarring and thickening of the tympanic membranes indicate recurrent episodes of otitis media; perforations and chronic purulent drainage are not uncommon in children with immunodeficiencies.

Children with chronic sinusitis often have excoriations and impetiginous lesions of the nostrils and philtrum due to the chronic purulent drainage. Posterior pharyngeal follicular erythema due to postnasal drainage is also common. Nasal polyposis can develop even in very young children with chronic sinusitis; this finding should always prompt an evaluation for cystic fibrosis, but can also be seen in children with antibody deficiency syndromes. In patients with long-standing nasal obstruction, the typical facial deformity caused by chronic mouth breathing develops.

Recurrent episodes of bronchopneumonia result in the development of bronchiectasis in many patients with immunodeficiencies. This manifests on physical examination as a congested cough; coarse crackles and rhonchi are heard on auscultation. Clubbing of the digits often develops. Radiographic studies are necessary to confirm the diagnosis of bronchiectasis (Fig. 4).

Associated Abnormalities

Associated abnormalities can be a clue to the presence of some of the antibody deficiency syndromes (see Table 1). Facial dysmorphisms should be noted. The skin should be examined carefully for eczematous or autoimmune rashes, telangiectasia, petechiae, or scars from previous abscesses. Examination of the joints for signs of arthritis is also important. A thorough neurologic examination can reveal early signs of ataxia or chronic encephalitis.

Laboratory Evaluation

The laboratory evaluation of the child with suspected immunologic defects should be guided by the clinical presentation; a full battery of immunologic testing need not be ordered on every child.

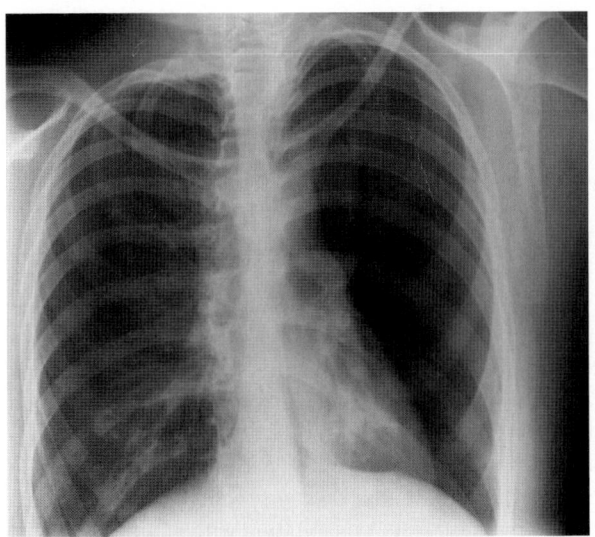
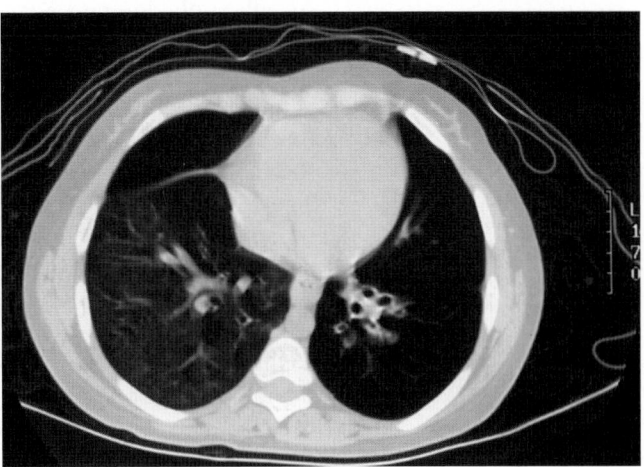

FIGURE 4 Chest x-ray film (**A**) and computed tomography scan (**B**) showing bronchiectasis of both lower lobes.

Blood Cell Counts

The complete blood cell count (CBC) and differential provides much useful information and can sometimes point toward a specific diagnosis.

The finding of anemia can be associated with the autoimmune conditions accompanying certain immunodeficiency syndromes (see Table 1).

Thrombocytopenia can occur secondary to autoimmune phenomena, but when the platelet size is small, Wiskott-Aldrich syndrome should be suspected.

Neutropenia can also be secondary to autoimmune disease or can be a primary abnormality leading to recurrent infection. In patients with cyclic neutropenia, repeated CBCs must be performed every other day for several weeks, to demonstrate the regular cyclic fluctuations in neutrophil counts. Markedly elevated neutrophil counts are seen in patients with leukocyte adhesion molecule defects, and also during acute infections.

Since most lymphocytes are T lymphocytes, the finding of lymphopenia is suggestive of a combined immunodeficiency with T-cell involvement.

Significant eosinophilia can be seen in patients with hyper-IgE syndrome, Wiskott-Aldrich syndrome, and other combined immunodeficiencies.

Measurement of Immunoglobulins

Quantitative measurement of immunoglobulins should be undertaken in patients in whom an antibody defect is suspected. The characteristic patterns of immunoglobulin defects in the various disorders are shown in Table 1. It is important to remember that the normal levels of each immunoglobulin increase with age. For example, an IgG level of 300mg per deciliter, which would be considered significantly low in a 10-year-old, is well within the normal range for a 6-month-old. Use a laboratory that reports age-specific normal ranges for immunoglobulin levels. The finding of very high levels of all classes of immunoglobulins is characteristic of pediatric AIDS, as well as a much rarer congenital immunodeficiency known as Nezelof's syndrome.

Measurement of IgG Subclasses

IgG subclasses can be measured in patients who have a clinical picture suggestive of an antibody defect, but have normal total immunoglobulin levels. Again, age-specific normal ranges should be taken into account in interpreting these results.

Measurement of Antibody Titers

Specific antibody titers are useful measures of appropriate *in vivo* immune responses. A single postvaccination titer can be measured for tetanus, diphtheria, or *H. in-*

fluenzae type b in children who have received their primary immunizations with these vaccines. If the vaccine has not yet been administered, or if initial antibody levels are low, specific antibody responses can be measured before and 3 to 4 weeks after immunization. A fourfold rise in titer is generally considered to represent an adequate antibody response. The response to polysaccharide antigens is usually assessed by measurements of antipneumococcal titers, taken before and 3 to 4 weeks after administration of the pneumococcal vaccine. (Although *H. influenzae* type b is also an encapsulated organism, the vaccine in current use has the polysaccharide antigen conjugated to a protein toxoid antigen, resulting in a vigorous antibody response even in children who are unable to respond to polysaccharide antigens alone.) A good response to polysaccharide antigens is not seen in normal children until around the age of 2 years.

The tests mentioned above (CBC and differential, measurements of immunoglobulin levels and subclasses and of specific antibody levels) are widely available through commercial laboratories. These tests can be ordered by the otolaryngologist, with consideration of the presentation and differential diagnosis of the patient. Careful selection of a laboratory with excellent quality control and pediatric age-specific normal ranges is essential. If abnormalities are detected by these tests, consultation with an immunologist can provide recommendations for further evaluation and treatment.

Neoantigen Testing

Some patients have already been given intravenous immunoglobulin replacement prior to being evaluated for specific antibody responses. In these patients the usual specific antibody titers cannot be used, since the exogenous IgG contains significant titers against the common human pathogens and vaccines. Measurement of antibody responses to neoantigens (i.e., antigens to which humans are not usually exposed) is useful in this instance. Bacteriophage ϕX174 is an example of a neoantigen used in this way. The ϕX174 testing is performed by a research laboratory, and extensive data are available regarding primary and secondary IgG and IgM responses to this antigen (28). While the assay is not available through commercial laboratories, immunologists in some referral centers are able to arrange for this testing.

Lymphocyte Cell Marker Studies

Lymphocyte cell marker studies utilize antibodies against known molecules on the cell surfaces of lymphocytes to identify and count the lymphocyte subsets.

In patients in whom the immunoglobulin levels are very low or absent, B-cell enumeration is necessary to distinguish XLA from other forms of hypogammaglobulinemia. The CD19 or CD20 marker identifies B lymphocytes.

In patients in whom a combined immunodeficiency is suspected, T lymphocytes and natural killer cells should also be enumerated. The CD3 marker detects all mature T cells. Helper (CD4+) and suppressor/cytotoxic (CD8+) T cells are also measured. Normally, the helper:suppressor ratio is about 2:1. In conditions characterized by T-cell deficiency, the total number of T lymphocytes can be low, or the helper-suppressor ratio can be abnormal. In HIV infection, the CD4+ cell counts are monitored periodically. When they start to drop, this heralds the onset of clinical AIDS.

Natural killer cells are identified by the CD16 and CD56 markers.

Lymphocyte Stimulation Tests

Lymphocyte stimulation testing is performed by exposing lymphocytes *in vitro* to either antigens, such as tetanus or candida, or mitogens (substances derived from plants that cause lymphocytes to become activated and proliferate). The lymphocytes are then cultured with radiolabeled thymidine, and their proliferation can be measured by the uptake of the labeled thymidine into their nuclei. Stimulants specific for B cells and for T cells, as well as those requiring the normal interaction of T and B cells, can be utilized.

Studies of lymphocyte cell surface markers and mitogen or antigen stimulation responses should be undertaken in consultation with an immunologist. These assays must be performed in a specialized immunology laboratory to obtain reliable results.

Genetic Studies

Specific genetic studies can be performed to confirm the diagnosis of some of the more severe immunodeficiency diseases, if initial testing yields results consistent with these diagnoses. For example, mutation analysis of the *Btk* gene (which codes for Bruton tyrosine kinase) reveals abnormalities of this gene in most patients with XLA. Absence of the CD40 ligand on activated CD4+ T cells confirms the diagnosis of X-linked hyper-IgM syndrome. These tests are available through research laboratories, and can be arranged for by the immunology consultant.

Neutrophil Studies

Neutrophil studies should be performed in patients who present with a significant component of cutaneous or pulmonary abscesses. Measurement of oxidative burst activity, either by the nitroblue tetrazolium (NBT) assay or by chemiluminescence, is the test for chronic granulomatous disease. Assays for random chemokinesis and directional chemotaxis, phagocytosis, and staphylococcal killing are useful for assessing other functional aspects of the neutrophils. Leukocyte adhesion molecules should also be assayed. Unfortunately, extensive neutrophil studies are not widely available, and neutrophils do not survive mailing well. To obtain reliable results from neutrophil studies, it is necessary to send the *patient* to the site of a laboratory capable of performing the above-mentioned assays.

Complement Assays

Complement assays are generally not useful in patients presenting with recurrent upper respiratory tract infections. Complement defects are rare, and more often present with autoimmune diseases than with recurrent infections. In the occasional patient with recurrent severe pyogenic infections in whom none of the more common immunologic defects can be identified, assays of the complement system could be considered. The measurement of components C3 and C4, or the CH_{50}, are sufficient to screen for defects in the early part of the complement pathway, and are available through most commercial laboratories. Deficiencies in the late components, C5 through C9, have been associated in rare instances with recurrent neisserial infections. Assays for these late complement components are not as widely available and the immunology consultant should be asked for recommendations regarding a reliable laboratory.

PEARLS AND PERILS

1. Keep in mind the differential diagnosis of recurrent upper respiratory tract infections.
2. In evaluating a patient with suspected immunodeficiency, consider the time course, sites of infection, and type of pathogens, to guide the laboratory evaluation.
3. If minor abnormalities are detected on immunologic tests obtained during an acute infection, repeat the tests a few weeks later when the patient is well. Often, mildly depressed cell counts or immunoglobulin levels are part of the response to acute infection rather than reflecting an underlying abnormality.
4. For all patients with severe or unusual immunodeficiency syndromes, consult a pediatric immunologist for help with comprehensive immunologic evaluation and long-term management.

🌀 TREATMENT RECOMMENDATIONS

The management of patients with immunodeficiency syndromes is determined by the severity of the immunologic defect.

Minor Immunoglobulin Deficiencies

·Minor immunoglobulin deficiencies such as IgA deficiency, IgG subclass deficiencies, partial defects in specific antibody response, and transient hypogammaglobulinemia of infancy should be managed conservatively, if possible.

1. Decreasing exposure to infectious agents (e.g., careful handwashing by the patient and caretakers, avoidance of exposure to large groups of children) helps somewhat to decrease the incidence of infection.
2. Prophylactic antibiotics [once-daily amoxicillin or sulfisoxazole (Gantrisin)] have been used, often with good results, to decrease the recurrence rates of sinusitis and otitis media. It is important to remember that when a patient does develop an infection while taking a prophylactic antibiotic, the infecting organism is relatively resistant to that antibiotic. An antibiotic with a broader spectrum of activity should be used to treat the infection. With the recent development of increasing resistance of microbial pathogens to antibiotics, it might become necessary to rethink the practice of long-term use of prophylactic antibiotics.
3. Measures that promote drainage of the sinuses and middle-ear cavities are effective in decreasing infections. Conservative measures include the use of saline or hypertonic saline lavages to promote sinus drainage. The early use of decongestants during viral infections can also help to keep the sinus ostia, and possibly the eustachian tubes, patent. In cases where polypoid tissue is developing secondary to repeated infections, the use of intranasal steroid sprays can cause regression of the obstructing tissue.

Some children with minor immunodeficiencies, especially IgA deficiency, have associated allergic rhinitis. Control of the edema and secretions caused by the allergic rhinitis helps to maintain patency of the eustachian tubes and sinus ostia. Institution of environmental control measures to decrease allergen exposure, and the regular use of topical cromolyn, intranasal steroid sprays, or oral antihistamine-decongestant combinations are effective for most patients. Patients who fail to respond to these measures should receive allergen immunotherapy.

In many cases surgical intervention is necessary for children with immunodeficiencies and recurrent otitis media or sinusitis. Placement of ventilating tubes can be very effective in controlling the problem of recurrent otitis media in these children. In some cases functional endoscopic sinus surgery is needed to reestablish sinus drainage pathways (Fig. 5). Following the surgery, a prolonged course of intranasal steroids is advisable to prevent recurrence of the obstruction.

Careful and consistent application of the above-mentioned measures is often sufficient to control these conditions. As mentioned already, many children with the minor antibody deficiency syndromes show clinical improvement as they grow older. In some, however, the clinical course is more severe and persists into adulthood. With IgA deficiency, no further specific therapy is available. Repeated sinus surgical procedures may be necessary. To prevent the development of bronchiectasis and chronic pulmonary disease, aggressive antibiotic therapy and chest physiotherapy should be instituted at the onset of each respiratory infection.

For the IgG deficiency syndromes, specific replacement therapy is available in the form of intravenous immunoglobulin (IVIG) preparations. These preparations contain IgG concentrated from hundreds of blood donors, and thus have a good representation of specific antibody to most pathogens. All the IgG subclasses are present in IVIG. Traces of IgA are also present, and this can pose a problem for patients with IgA deficiency and anti-IgA antibodies (see below). The blood donor screening process and ster-

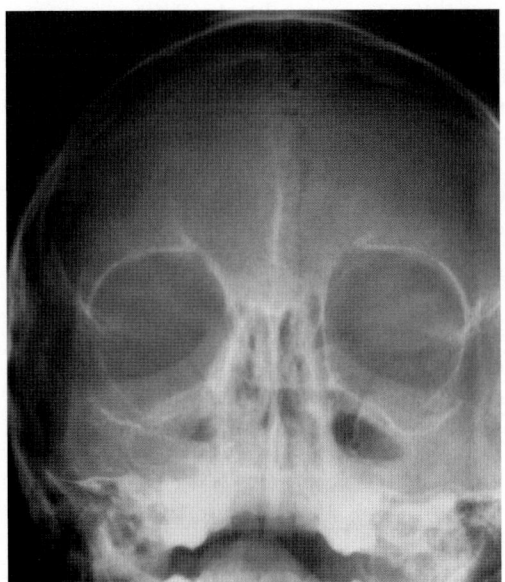
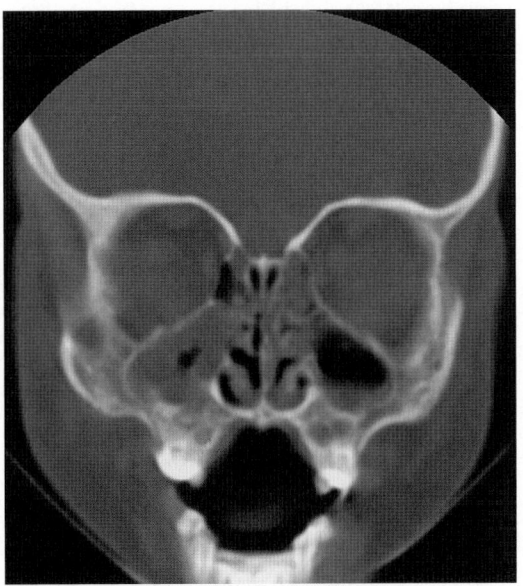

A   B

FIGURE 5 This 4-year-old boy presented with chronic sinusitis and asthma. Immunologic studies were normal except for a low level of the IgG2 subclass, and absence of specific antibody response to pneumococcal vaccine. He also had significant allergies. Despite prolonged treatment with antibiotics and intranasal steroids as well as intensive asthma therapy, his symptoms persisted. These sinus x-ray films (**A**) and computed tomography scan (**B**) were obtained during the sixth week of treatment with amoxicillin–clavulanate potassium (Augmentin). There was diffuse disease involving the ethmoidal and maxillary sinuses and obstruction of the osteomeatal complex. Functional endoscopic sinus surgery was performed. The patient improved but subsequently had repeated relapses of the sinus disease, until age 5 when he was begun on intravenous immunoglobulin therapy. The chronic sinusitis resolved, and further treatment now focuses on control of the allergic rhinitis and asthma.

ilization techniques used in the preparation of IVIG appear to be very effective in preventing viral contamination of the product; there has never been a reported case of transmission of HIV or hepatitis B via IVIG. (There was a problem with hepatitis C transmission through Gammagard, in 1994; this has now been resolved and Gammagard is back on the market.)

Since the serum half-life of IgG is about 25 days, IVIG is usually given every 4 weeks. The usual dose for IgG subclass deficiency is 200 to 400mg per kilogram. The dose for specific antibody defects is usually at least 400mg per kilogram, in order to give sufficient specific antibody. During a significant acute infection, exogenous antibody against the pathogen can be consumed. Thus, if a patient develops pneumonia, sepsis, or another serious infection, an extra dose of IVIG should be given along with antibiotic therapy.

Treatment of patients with the minor antibody deficiency syndromes with IVIG should be given for several-month blocks of time, with periodic reassessment of the need for continued therapy. Generally, the young child with recurrent respiratory tract infections should be treated through the fall, winter, and spring. If the response to treatment is good and the child is clinically well, the IVIG can be discontinued through the summer months. If infections recur, replacement therapy should be restarted and continued for another year. If the child remains well through the summer, IgG subclasses or antibody titers can be retested 4 to 5 months after administration of the last dose of IVIG, when most of the exogenous antibody will be gone. If results have normalized, the child can remain off of IVIG. If the results are still abnormal, but the child is clinically well, a decision can be made whether to resume the replacement therapy or to wait and see how the child does during the next winter. In some cases, even though the antibody defect persists, the patient is eventually able to discontinue IVIG replacement therapy.

Patients who have both IgG subclass deficiency and IgA deficiency, and who require IVIG treatment, should be tested for anti-IgA antibody. If anti-IgA antibody is found,

IVIG should be given only with extreme caution. Gammagard is the IVIG preparation with the lowest IgA content, and should be used for patients with anti-IgA antibodies. While many such patients tolerate Gammagard infusions without reactions, the treatments should always be given in a facility where anaphylaxis can be treated (these patients are not candidates for home infusions). The infusion should be started at a slow rate and gradually increased as tolerated. Epinephrine and diphenhydramine hydrochloride (Benadryl) should be available at the bedside. For patients who have complete absence of IgA but do not have anti-IgA antibody, it is still advisable to use Gammagard for IgG replacement, as the subsequent development of anti-IgA antibody might be less likely with less IgA exposure.

Treatment with IVIG is rarely necessary for patients with transient hypogammaglobulinemia of infancy. Careful infection avoidance measures, with or without prophylactic antibiotic therapy, usually suffice to keep these children relatively healthy. The immunoglobulin levels should be monitored every 6 months until they normalize, to confirm the diagnosis.

Conditions with Major Defects in Immunoglobulin Production

Conditions with major defects in immunoglobulin production, such as XLA, CVI, hyper-IgM syndrome, AIDS, severe defects in specific antibody formation, and the combined immunodeficiencies, require more aggressive therapy. These patients should always be managed in conjunction with an immunologist.

IVIG therapy is always indicated for these conditions, and should be given throughout life. The usual dose is 400mg per kilogram every 4 weeks, with extra doses given during acute infections. Some patients require higher doses to remain free of infection, and some patients do better when the IVIG is given every 3 weeks.

Antibiotic prophylaxis to prevent. *P. carinii* pneumonia, usually trimethoprim-sulfamethoxazole, is necessary for patients with a component of T-cell dysfunction (e.g., AIDS, combined immunodeficiencies, hyper-IgM syndrome). Some patients with CVI and XLA do better when kept on a daily dose of amoxicillin or sulfisoxazole. Aggressive antibiotic therapy should be begun early in the course of any acute infection.

Preventative measures, as just outlined, are also essential in these more severely affected patients. Surgical interventions in the form of ventilating tubes or sinus drainage procedures are often required. During surgery for refractory sinusitis or otitis media, cultures for aerobic and anaerobic bacteria, fungi, and mycobacteria should be obtained to help guide antimicrobial therapy.

Immunizations are ineffective in patients with severe antibody defects. However, routine childhood immunizations are recommended for children with AIDS, with the exception that inactivated poliovirus vaccine should be used in place of the usual live oral vaccine. Live viral vaccines, especially poliovirus, are contraindicated in patients with XLA and in any patient with T-cell dysfunction. Patients with T-cell defects who are exposed to chickenpox should be given either acyclovir prophylaxis or a dose of varicella-zoster immune globulin unless they are receiving IVIG, which contains protective titers against varicella.

A discussion of the antiviral and immune modulator treatment for AIDS is beyond the scope of this chapter. A good update on this topic is included in the reference list (29).

Some of the combined immunodeficiencies have a poor prognosis, even with good supportive care as outlined. Bone marrow transplantation is a treatment option for severely affected patients with certain conditions such as Wiskott-Aldrich syndrome.

Neutrophil Defects and Hyper-IgE Syndrome

Treatment of patients with neutrophil defects or hyper-IgE syndrome includes good skin care. Cuts and abrasions should be cleansed thoroughly with antibacterial soap and covered with clean dressings. Daily prophylactic treatment with antistaphylococcal antibiotics (e.g., trimethoprim-sulfamethoxazole, dicloxacillin) helps to decrease the incidence of abscess. When abscesses do develop, surgical incision and drainage are usually necessary; deep-seated or extensive abscesses should be treated with intravenous antibiotics. Surgical drainage of the sinuses and middle ears is also often indicated. If fungal infection of the sinuses, lungs, or other internal organs develops, surgical drainage is essential. Treatment of acute bacterial or fungal infections should be guided wherever possible by culture results. It is generally recommended that patients who have been treated for a fungal infection continue to receive prophylactic antifungal treatment indefinitely thereafter.

Patients with hyper-IgE syndrome sometimes have defective specific antibody responses (30). These patients can benefit from IVIG therapy.

Interferon gamma, given subcutaneously on a three times per week schedule, has been shown to be effective in decreasing the incidence of serious infections in some patients with chronic granulomatous disease (31). Granulocyte colony-stimulating factor is effective for treatment of conditions associated with significant neutropenia.

PEARLS AND PERILS

1. Good supportive and preventative care is essential for all immunodeficient patients, and may be sufficient for many patients with minor immunodeficiencies.
2. Intravenous gamma globulin replacement, when used judiciously and in appropriate doses, can be a highly effective treatment modality for many patients with antibody deficiency syndromes.
3. Be aggressive with antibiotic therapy, preventatively and early in the course of each infection.
4. Whenever possible, obtain cultures to guide antibiotic and antifungal therapy.

CONCLUSIONS

Immunodeficiency diseases are not uncommon in the population of pediatric patients referred to an otolaryngologist because of recurrent otitis media or sinusitis, or both. Familiarity with these diseases, their clinical presentations, and laboratory findings can facilitate an early diagnosis, thus allowing institution of appropriate management of the underlying problem and minimizing complications.

REFERENCES

1. Björkander J, Bake B, Oxelius VA, Hanson LA. Impaired lung function in patients with IgA deficiency and low levels of IgG2 or IgG3. *N Engl J Med* 1985;313:720–724.
2. Ugazio AG, Out TA, Plebani A, et al. Recurrent infections in children with "selective" IgA deficiency: association with IgG2 and IgG4 deficiency. *Birth Defects* 1983;19:169–171.
3. Schur PH. IgG subclasses—a review. *Ann Allergy* 1987;58:89–99.
4. Björkander J, Bengtsson U, Oxelius VA, Hanson LA. Symptoms in patients with lowered levels of IgG subclasses, with or without IgA deficiency, and effects of immunoglobulin prophylaxis. *Monogr Allergy* 1986;20:157–163.
5. Shakelford PG, Granoff DM, Polmar SH, et al. Subnormal serum concentrations of IgG2 in children with frequent infections associated with varied patterns of immunologic dysfunction. *J Pediatr* 1990;116:529–538.
6. Nahm MH, Macke K, Kwon OH, Madassery JV, Sherman LA, Scott MG. Immunologic and clinical status of blood donors with subnormal levels of IgG2. *J Allergy Clin Immunol* 1990;85:769–777.
7. Shackelford PG. IgG subclasses: importance in pediatric practice. *Pediatr Rev* 1993;14:291–296.

8. Umetsu DT, Ambrosino DM, Quinti I, Siber GR, Geha RS. Recurrent sinopulmonary infection and impaired antibody response to bacterial capsular polysaccharide antigen in children with selective IgG-subclass deficiency. *N Engl J Med* 1985;313:1247–1251.

9. Ambrosino DM, Umetsu DT, Siber GR, et al. Selective defect in the antibody response to *Haemophilus influenzae* type b in children with recurrent infections and normal serum IgG subclass levels. *J Allergy Clin Immunol* 1988;81:1175–1179.

10. Zora JA, Silk HJ, Tinkelman DG. Evaluation of postimmunization pneumococcal titers in children with recurrent infections and normal levels of immunoglobulin. *Ann Allergy* 1993; 70:283–287.

11. McGeady SJ. Transient hypogammaglobulineamia of infancy: need to reconsider name and definition. *J Pediatr* 1987;110:47–50.

12. Tiller TL, Buckley RH. Transient hypogammaglobulinemia of infancy: review of the literature, clinical and immunologic features of 11 new cases, and long-term follow-up. *J Pediatr* 1978;92:347–353.

13. Lederman HM, Winkelstein JA. X-linked agammaglobulinemia: an analysis of 96 patients. *Medicine* 1985;64:145–156.

14. Harmaszewski RA, Webster ADB. Primary hypogammaglobulinaemia: a survey of clinical manifestations and complications. *Q J Med* 1993;86:31–42.

15. Strober W, Eisenstein E, Jaffe JS, Cunningham-Rundles C. New insights into common variable immunodeficiency. *Ann Intern Med* 1993;118:720–730.

16. Jaffe JS, Eisenstein E, Sneller MC, Strober W. T-cell abnormalities in common variable immunodeficiency. *Pediatr Res* 1993; 33[Suppl]: S24–S28.

17. Conley ME, Larche M, Bonagura VR, et al. Hyper IgM syndrome associated with defective CD40-mediated B cell activation. *J Clin Invest* 1994;94:1404–1409.

18. Nortarangelo LD, Duse M, Ugazio AG. Immunodeficiency with hyper-IgM. *Immunodef Rev* 1992;3:101–122.

19. Barkin RM, Bonis SL, Elghammer RM, Todd JK. Ludwig angina in children. *J Pediatr* 1975; 87:563–565.

20. Kyong CU, Virella G, Fudenberg HH, Darby CP. X-linked immunodeficiency with increased IgM: clinical, ethnic, and immunologic heterogeneity. *Pediatr Res* 1978;12:1024–1026.

21. Hong R. Disorders of the T-cell system. In: Stiehm ER, ed. *Immunologic disorders in infants & children*. Philadelphia: WB Saunders, 1996;363–368.

22. Fiorilli M, Businco L, Pandolfi F, Paganelli R, Russo G, Aluti F. Heterogeneity of immunological abnormalities in ataxia-telangiectasia. *J Clin Immunol* 1983;3:135–141.

23. Boder E, Sedgwick RP. Ataxia-telangiectasia: a familial syndrome of progressive cerebellar ataxia, oculocutaneous telangiectasia, and frequent pulmonary infection. *Univ S Calif Med Bull* 1957;9:15–27.

24. Smeets DF, Moog U, Weemaes CM, et al. ICF syndrome: a new case and review of the literature. *Hum Genet* 1994;94:240–246.

25. Buckley RH. Disorders of the IgE system. In: Stiehm ER, ed. *Immunologic disorders in infants & children*. Philadelphia: WB Saunders, 1996;413–420.

26. Pantaleo G, Graziosi C, Fauci A. The immunopathogenesis of human immunodeficiency virus infection. *N Engl J Med* 1993;328:327–335.

27. European Collaborative Study. Children born to women with HIV-1 infection: natural history and risk of transmission. *Lancet* 1991;337:253–260.

28. Pyun KH, Ochs HD, Wedgwood RF, Yang X, Heller SR, Reimer CB. Human antibody responses to bacteriophage φX174: sequential induction of IgM and IgG subclass antibody. *Clin Immunol Immunopathol* 1989;51 252–263.

29. Tudor-Williams G, Pizzo PA. Pediatric human immunodeficiency virus infection. In: Stiehm ER, ed. *Immunologic disorders in infants & children*. Philadelphia: WB Saunders, 1996; 510–552.

30. Sheerin KA, Buckley RH. Antibody responses to protein, polysaccharide, and φX 174 antigens in the hyperimmunoglobulinemia E (hyper IgE) syndrome. *J Allergy Clin Immunol* 1991;87:803–811.

31. International Chronic Granulomatous Disease Cooperative Study Group. A controlled trial of interferon gamma to prevent infection in chronic granulomatous disease. *N Engl J Med* 1991; 324: 509–516.

• *Practical Pediatric Otolaryngology*
• edited by Robin T. Cotton and Charles M. Myer, III
• Lippincott-Raven Publishers, Philadelphia © 1999

M.B. Lierl: Department of Pediatrics, Division of Allergy, Immunology and Pulmonary Medicine, University of Cincinnati, Children's Hospital Medical Center, Cincinnati, Ohio 45229–3039.

Anesthesia

Adrian R. Lloyd-Thomas

Pediatric otolaryngology presents anesthesiologists with some of the greatest anesthetic challenges, and success requires a close understanding and cooperation between the anesthesiologist and the surgeon. In this chapter, general considerations are given in the first four sections while specific anesthetic techniques for various aspects of ear-nose-throat (ENT) surgery are presented in the last five sections.

GENERAL PREOPERATIVE PREPARATION

Much routine ENT surgery is performed as an elective outpatient procedure. Careful screening is essential to ensure that children with multisystem problems are identified, and that the child is optimally prepared before surgery.

Investigations

For the majority of operations in fit healthy children, investigations are not required. However, preexisting disease (e.g., pulmonary disorders, muscle disorders, renal disorders with or without hypertension) or a family history of inherited disease (e.g., glycogen storage disorders) should prompt appropriate laboratory and radiologic investigations as indicated by the child's physical status. Anomalies associated with cardiac defects (e.g., CHARGE association), or children with known cardiac defects, should be investigated by echocardiography and electrocardiography. Patients undergoing operations where the anticipated blood loss may exceed 10mL per kilogram require hemoglobin estimation and blood crossmatching. Hemoglobinopathies should be investigated where clinically indicated (e.g., racial group, family history, clinical history).

Starvation

Hitherto periods of preanesthetic starvation have been too long (1). Recommended guidelines are indicated in Table 1. There should be no oral intake for 2 hours before the anticipated start of anesthesia.

Cutaneous Anesthesia

Intravenous induction of anesthesia may be preferred from infancy. Application of (EMLA) cream (eutectic mixture of the local anesthetics lidocaine and prilocaine hydrochloride) to the skin above a suitable vein at the time of the last drink (2 hours preoperatively) will ensure effective topical anesthesia and allow virtually pain-free intravenous induction. If time is short, topical amethocaine gel (4%) is effective within 30 to 45 minutes; moreover, the local vasodilation caused by this preparation may facili-

TABLE 1: Recommended Starvation Period before Elective Surgical Operations

Food	Time to Stop Preoperatively (hr)
Food including cow's milk and formula milk	6
Breast milk	4
Clear fluids	2

(From ref. 1, with permission.)

tate cannulation. Local allergic reactions (usually mild redness) may be seen in 5% to 10% of patients using this preparation. Local angioneurotic edema may occur, which will make venous cannulation almost impossible.

Psychological Preparation

A clear explanation with information (books, photographs, videos, etc.) can do much to allay a child's anxiety before surgery. Many units advocate prior visiting by parents and children, though distance from the hospital may make this impractical. Hospital facilities should be child friendly with a clear demarcation between adult and pediatric units. Infants who cannot participate in this type of preparation may need preanesthesia sedation, but because this will delay recovery, it should be decided on an individual basis.

Preanesthesia Sedation

Preanesthesia sedation (Table 2) may be dangerous if there is airway compromise. In patients suitable for sedation, the oral route is probably the most satisfactory. While preanesthesia sedation is currently avoided in outpatient surgery, it is valuable in inpatient surgery, especially for major procedures that may require techniques of induced hypotension. A relaxed and calm child presenting for anesthesia induction without the catecholamine drive of anxiety will facilitate the production of good surgical conditions.

Prophylaxis Against Emesis

Careful anesthesia, gentle patient handling, and avoidance of gaseous gastric distention can do much to reduce postanesthesia nausea and vomiting. If intravenous induction is used, propofol is associated with a lower incidence of nausea and vomiting. Avoidance of opioids, the most common cause of anesthesia-induced nausea and vomiting, will help to minimize emesis but at the potential risk of poor pain control. The advent of 5-hydrox-

TABLE 2: Suggestions for Preanesthesia Medication for Neonates, Infants, and Children[a]

Weight	First Choice		Second Choice	
< 5 kg	Atropine only	20 µg/kg	Atropine only	20 µg/kg
5–10 kg	Triclofos	30–75 mg/kg	Midazolam syrup	0.5 mg/kg
(Atropine may be required also)	**Max. dose:**	1 g	**Max. dose:**	15 mg
10–20 kg	Midazolam syrup	0.5 mg/kg	Temazepam (tablets)	0.5–1.0 mg/kg
	Max. dose:	15 mg		
			Max. dose:	20 mg
> 20 kg	Temazepam (tablets)	0.5–1.0 mg/kg	—	
	Max. dose:	20 mg	—	

[a]Sedation should be avoided in patients with any form of upper-airway obstruction.

ytryptamine (5-HT$_3$) receptor antagonists has revolutionized the control of opioid-induced nausea and vomiting. Administration of between 100 to 200 μg of ondansetron per kilogram before opioid injection will reduce postoperative nausea and vomiting significantly (2). Intraoperative fluid administration may help by delaying requests for oral intake in the postoperative period. Furthermore the first, intake of oral fluid should be when the child requests a drink, not earlier as a result of parental encouragement, which may precipitate nausea and vomiting. Many advocate the use of ice lollies as a first fluid intake following ENT surgery.

PEARLS AND PERILS: Anesthesia-Induced Nausea and Vomiting

Pearls
1. Careful anesthesia
2. Gentle patient handling
3. Prophylactic antiemetics
4. Intravenous fluid bolus intraoperatively
Perils
5. Oral fluids encouraged too early postoperatively
6. Vigorous mask ventilation with gastric distention
7. Opioids without antiemetic

Induction

Inhalational

An inhalational induction of anesthesia requires a calm, gentle, and reassuring approach to the infant. Parental presence at the time of induction can be very helpful, as can the use of flavored masks to offset the unpleasant odor of inhalational anesthetics. The two volatile anesthetic agents, halothane and sevoflurane, are useful as induction agents in children. Halothane is a familiar drug, with a smooth onset of action and a low incidence of airway irritation. Sevoflurane has the advantage of low solubility with consequent rapid onset of action. Moreover, its low pungency makes it acceptable to the child in high concentrations. This allows delivery of an 8% concentration from the outset, with consequent rapidity of effect. Against its use is the high cost, though many use it as an induction agent, switching to a less expensive alternative for the maintenance of anesthesia.

Intravenous

Thiopentone (3 to 5 mg per kilogram) remains the gold-standard intravenous induction agent for children. Propofol (3 to 5 mg per kilogram) may be associated with a reduction in nausea and vomiting and a clear-headed recovery, and permits easy introduction of the laryngeal mask airway (LMA). This may make it advantageous in ambulatory procedures. Its main disadvantage is pain on injection, which may be partially offset by mixing it with lignocaine (1 mg of lignocaine with 10 mg of propofol). Propofol is not licensed in the United Kingdom for induction of anesthesia in children less than 3 years old.

Maintenance of Anesthesia

Minor procedures can be accomplished by using spontaneous respiration with nitrous oxide in oxygen and a volatile agent of choice. More complex surgery, or when the airway will be shared, usually requires tracheal intubation. A wide range of children's tracheal tubes are available. It is well recognized that the cricoid cartilage is the narrowest part of the airway in the prepubescent child. Uncuffed tracheal tubes, which pass with ease (not forced), should be used, and there should be a leak of gas around the tube at an inflation pressure of 20 cm H$_2$O.

TABLE 3: Contraindications to Suxamethonium[a]

Clinical Problem	Condition Causing
Hyperkalemia after suxamethonium administration	Burns
	Tetanus
	Paraplegia
	Muscular dystrophy
Respiratory and jaw muscle rigidity	Dystrophia myotonica
Malignant hyperpyrexia	—

[a]Suxamethonium may be hazardous in these conditions. Patients with undiagnosed muscular dystrophy may experience hyperkalemia following suxamethonium administration. A history of recent-onset clumsiness or weakness should prompt further investigation.

Neuromuscular Blocking Agents

Concern has been expressed widely over the use of suxamethonium in pediatric anesthetic practice. There are still indications for the use of suxamethonium for anesthesia for otolaryngologic procedures and it should be used also for emergency anesthesia in patients with a full stomach. Careful preoperative assessment is mandatory to exclude those conditions in which suxamethonium administration may be hazardous (Table 3). The advent of short-acting, rapid-onset competitive neuromuscular blockers means that suxamethonium can be avoided except in specific circumstances. The expected duration of action of the various neuromuscular blocking drugs available is shown in Table 4. The cardiovascular stability and low incidence of histamine release seen with the newer agents represent an advance.

Monitoring

At all times basic patient monitoring should be applied (Table 5). This is especially important during airway surgery when patient access is restricted. Invasive monitoring should be employed during induced hypotension and major surgery.

SPECIAL CONSIDERATIONS FOR NEONATAL AND INFANT ANESTHESIA

The physiologic immaturity of the neonate and infant results in significant differences from the adult or older child, which require consideration when planning anesthesia. For an in-depth treatise on neonatal anesthesia the reader is referred to the book by Hatch et al (3). This section briefly considers important differences.

The combination of narrow airways (high resistance), a compliant chest wall (low resting functional residual capacity), a high closing volume (ventilation-perfusion mismatch), and a need for high alveolar minute ventilation places the neonate and infant at

TABLE 4: Common Competitive Neuromuscular Blocking Drugs, Their Dose,
                and Duration of Action

Drug	Dose (mg/kg)	Duration of Action (min)
Atracurium	0.5	20–25
Cisatracurium	0.1–0.4	20–50
d-Tubocurarine	0.5	30–40
Mivacurium	0.1	5
	0.2	10–12
Rocuronium	0.6	20–30
Vecuronium	0.1	15–20

TABLE 5: Basic Monitoring Suggested for Every Patient undergoing anesthesia[a]

Pulse oximetry (SpO_2)
Electrocardiography
Noninvasive blood pressure
Inspired/expired gas and vapor analysis
Ventilator alarms
Temperature (especially neonates and infants)
Neuromuscular monitor if using relaxants

[a]Further monitoring may be required, as determined by clinical conditions.

a respiratory disadvantage. Continuous positive airway pressure (CPAP) will help to reduce the effects of a further reduction in functional residual capacity associated with anesthesia. In most cases, with the exception of diagnostic airway assessment, tracheal intubation and mechanical ventilation are essential. Vagotonic reflexes and the vagotonic action of anesthetic agents tend to cause cardiac slowing. In the neonate, in which only 30% of the heart mass is contractile tissue, cardiac output is rate dependent. Moreover, tissue oxygen demand associated with rapid growth requires a cardiac output of two times that of an adult on a weight for weight basis. Adequate atropinization is essential in this group of patients, to prevent bradyarrhythmias.

The pulmonary vascular tree is reactive and the pulmonary circulation may develop hypertension or switch to a transitional state in the setting of hypoxia, acidosis, or hypercapnia. Careful attention to adequacy of ventilation with the maintenance of normoxia and normocapnia will avoid this pitfall. The complexities of anesthesia in patients with associated congenital cardiac anomalies are beyond the scope of this text and the reader is referred to *Pediatric Cardiac Anesthesia* (4).

Renal blood flow, glomerular filtration rate, and the ability to concentrate urine are reduced until the age of 2 years. Both dehydration and sodium and water loads are poorly handled by the immature kidney; furthermore, insensible losses are high in this age group. This requires careful attention to fluid balance (Table 6) (5) There is a higher percentage of extracellular fluid per kilogram in neonates, which results in a higher distribution volume for drugs such as neuromuscular blockers.

It should be remembered that immaturity of the neuromuscular junction means that neonates are sensitive to competitive neuromuscular blocking drugs and relatively resistant to depolarizing blocking drugs. Atracurium remains the neuromuscular blocking drug of choice in this group of patients.

The high surface area to weight ratio, and the immaturity of the shivering and mechanisms sweating with a dependence on oxidative brown fat metabolism to generate heat, mean that the neonate will lose heat readily and the heat generation process will result in an increase in oxygen demand. Careful attention to the preservation of heat loss is essential (Table 7).

TABLE 6: Fluid Requirements for Neonates: Increasing Fluid administration with Increasing Age

	Day 1 (mL/kg/d)	*Rising daily to:*	*Day 5* (mL/kg/d)
Full-term	20–40		120
Premature	60–80		160

TABLE 7: Techniques to Minimize Convective, Conductive, and Radiant Heat Losses

Warm operating room.
Minimize drafts.
Adequate patient dressing (bonnet, clothes).
Adequate coverings (blankets, surgical drapes).
Place foil around limbs.
Hot-air mattress.
Heat and moisture exchanger in anesthesia circuit.
Warmed fluids/volume replacement.

PAIN MANAGEMENT

Neurophysiology

Any injury will result in the activation of peripheral nociceptors, which feed information to the dorsal horn of the spinal column via alpha delta fibers and C fibers. But this is not the only mechanism contributing to a child's perception of pain following surgery. Local release of leukotrienes and prostaglandins will result in the development of primary hyperalgesia around the wound. Repetitive C fiber activity results in dorsal horn prostaglandin release, causing secondary hyperalgesia to develop. Treating this entails the use of a multimodal approach (Table 8).

PEARLS AND PERILS

Pearls
1. Use multimodal approach.
2. Use a preemptive approach to treat before pain is excessive.
3. Give adequate and regular doses.
Perils
4. Don't rely on one agent for analgesia.
5. Failure to give prophylactic antiemetics with opioid analgesia.

Acetaminophen

This highly useful analgesic is very acceptable to children. Fifteen to 20 mg per kilogram is required for analgesia via the oral route, from which absorption is very reliable. Rectal absorption of suppositories is more variable, with doses of 20 mg per kilogram reported to not give even antipyretic plasma levels. A larger dose of 20 to 30 mg per kilogram should be given via this route to achieve satisfactory analgesia; absorption may be delayed so a longer dosing interval is appropriate (8 hours) (6).

TABLE 8: Site and Mode of Action for Analgesic Medications

Analgesic	*Mechanism*
Acetaminophen	Central antiprostaglandin activity
NSAIDs	Reduce prostaglandin release in periphery and dorsal horn
Opioids	Peripheral, dorsal horn, and central opioid receptors
Alpha agonists	Locus ceruleus and bulbospinal pathways and dorsal horn alpha-2-receptor activation

NSAIDs, nonsteroidal antiinflammatory drugs.

TABLE 9: Dosage Recommendations for Commonly Used Nonopioid Analgesics in Children

	Dose (mg/kg)	Dose Interval (hr)
Acetaminophen (max daily dose 90 mg/kg)		
Oral		
Antipyretic	10	6
Analgesic	15–20	6
Rectal		
Antipyretic	15	8
Analgesic	20–30	8
NB: jaundiced neonates max. 5mg/kg		
Ibuprofen		
Oral	5 mg/kg	6
Diclofenac		
Oral	1 mg/kg	8–12
Rectal	1 mg/kg (from 1yr)	8–12
Ketorolac		
Intravenous	0.2–0.5 mg/kg (from 1yr)	6 (max. 8 doses)

Nonsteroidal Antiinflammatory Drugs

In practice there are three useful nonsteroidal antinflammatory drugs (NSAIDs) for children (Table 9). During anesthesia, diclofenac is especially valuable as it can be given by suppository. Ketorolac has been compared with morphine in ENT surgery and found to be as effective, with the added advantage of not having unwanted opioid side effects. NSAIDs should be avoided in children with significant renal impairment. Much discussion occurs on whether they should be used in patients with reversible airway disease. Asthma is increasingly common in urban-dwelling children, with many receiving beta-sympathomimetic therapy at some stage in their life. NSAIDs are such effective analgesics for ENT surgery that it is a pity to exclude a large proportion of patients from their benefits. A satisfactory practical approach is to avoid NSAIDs if a child is on very active asthma treatment (regular inhalation of beta-agonists, cromoglycate, inhaled/oral steroids). If however they are on minimal therapy, NSAIDs may be employed, but parents should be alerted to the possibility of worsening asthma symptoms, upon which they should stop therapy immediately and seek medical advice. Do NSAIDs increase the likelihood of bleeding following ENT surgery, particularly adenotonsillectomy? To date there are no good randomized controlled studies which show that bleeding or the likelihood of a return to surgery is increased by the use of NSAIDs. Their antiplatelet activity should be kept in mind, and in any child for whom there is concern about the bleeding status, NSAID use needs to be carefully considered before therapy is commenced.

Opioids

Opioids remain the mainstay of perioperative analgesia. By their action binding with opioid receptors (mainly mu receptors) analgesia is provided peripherally, in the dorsal horn, and centrally. The duration of action depends on the drug chosen and excretion is dominantly through liver metabolism. By contrast, the newest opioid, remifentanil, is cleared by tissue esterases, resulting in a very predictable and short half-life. As yet there is little experience with this drug in ENT practice. Immature neonatal metabolic pathways mean that there is an unpredictable half-life for these drugs in neonates. They should be used with caution, as neonates are also more sensitive to the depressant effects of these agents. Codeine phosphate (1 mg per kilogram per 8 hours) is a useful supplement to minor analgesics in cases where there is a wish to avoid major opioids.

Opioids have been avoided in traditional ambulatory anesthesia because of the high incidence of nausea and vomiting. The advent of 5-HT$_3$ receptor antagonists given prophylactically, which reduces considerably the likelihood of nausea and vomiting, now allows the use of opioids in this group of patients. Nonopioid analgesics such as buprenorphine and tramadol have ceiling analgesia and patients experience almost as much nausea and vomiting, suggesting that these drugs have few advantages in reducing these side effects.

The choice of intraoperative analgesic should be guided by the experience of the anesthesiologist and the requirements of the individual patient. Postoperative analgesia using opioids will involve the use of morphine for the majority of pediatric patients. If planning to give postoperative morphine analgesia, the author prefers to use it as the intraperative analgesic (100 to 200 µg per kilogram).

With the modern infusion pumps, postoperative analgesia with morphine can be controlled by the patient or a nurse. Opioid analgesia should be given according to clear, locally agreed-upon protocols that include a clear policy for patient observation (pain score, sedation score, respiratory rate, SpO$_2$ monitoring, and volume infused). Suggested programming for patient- and nurse-controlled analgesia is given in Table 10.

Alpha-2-agonists

The realization that noradrenaline (released in the dorsal horn following activation of bulbospinal pathways) was a transmitter involved in suppression of nociception led to the proposal that alpha-2-agonists could be analgesic. At present, clonidine is the most tried of these drugs. It is an effective premedicant (anxiolysis, analgesia, sedation, and dry mouth): moreover, used intraoperatively and postoperatively it affords analgesia (with opioid sparing) yet is devoid of the unwanted opioid side effects. A single dose of 2 to 4 mg per kilogram (maximum 150 µg as premedication 1.0 to 1.5 µg before anesthesia) or an incremental intravenous injection of 1 to 2 µg per kilogram during anesthesia will provide smooth cardiovascular conditions and reduce the requirement for opioids. This is especially valuable in anesthesia for major surgery, where moderate induced hypotension is planned.

Local Anesthesia

Field blocks using lignocaine or bupivacaine, with or without a vasoconstrictor, are a valuable adjunct to general anesthesia in pediatric otolaryngology. Specific nerve blocks can also be employed (e.g., inferior alveolar nerve block for lip surgery, mandibular nerve block for operations on the face).

The maximum single dose of lignocaine should be 4 mg per kilogram without a vasoconstrictor and 6 mg per kilogram with a vasoconstrictor. The maximum dose of epinephrine should be 5 µg per kilogram. The maximum dose of bupivacaine should be 1.5 to 2.0 mg per kilogram.

TABLE 10: Recommended PCA/NCA Pump Programming Based on the Use of Morphine sulfate[a]

Initial Programming	Loading Dose (µg/kg)	Background Infusion (µg/kg/hr)	Bolus Dose (µg/kg)	Lockout (min)
PCA				
< 50kg	50–100	4	10–20	5–15
> 50kg	50–100	0	1–2mg	5–15
NCA	50–100	0–20	10–20	20–60
NCA in intensive care areas	50–100	0–20	10–20	5–10

PCA, patient-controlled analgesia; NCA, nurse-controlled analgesia.

[a]Infusions should be made up as 1 mg per kilogram of body weight of morphine diluted to 50 mL with glucose 5% in those weighing less than 50 kg. In those weighing more than 50 kg, a standard solution of 50 mg in 50 mL of glucose 5% should be employed.

TABLE 11: Clinical Symptoms and Signs in Patients with Chronic Upper-airway Obstruction

Obstructed respiratory movement during sleep
Daytime drowsiness
Snoring
Substernal retraction
Cyanosis
Apnea
Difficulty in swallowing
Failure to thrive
Apparent mental dullness
Rarely right-sided heart failure

ROUTINE EAR-NOSE-THROAT SURGERY

Routine ENT surgery (placement of middle-ear ventilation tubes, adenoidectomy, and tonsillectomy) is common in children. Standard preoperative assessment (see above) should be undertaken but there are specific abnormalities in children presenting for this type of operation that require consideration.

Preoperative Assessment

Chronic Airway Obstruction

It is increasingly recognized that adenotonsillar enlargement can give rise to significant upper-airway obstruction, with periodic apneic episodes or obstructive respiratory movements during sleep. There will often be a characteristic history (Table 11). Rarely this progresses to pulmonary hypertension and right-sided heart failure (cor pulmonale) due to long-standing hypoventilation with hypoxia and hypercapnia. As well as careful clinical assessment, these patients require investigations (Table 12). Identification of this disorder often results in infants presenting for surgery. Adenotonsillectomy techniques differ, and with them the expected blood loss. If blood loss is likely to be more than 5% to 10% of the circulating blood volume, a full blood cell count is essential, as is group and blood crossmatching. In the patients with cor pulmonale, relief of upper-airway obstruction (soft rubber nasal airway) and diuretic therapy are vital before proceeding to surgery. Optimization may take a considerable period.

Coagulopathy

Taking a careful history, including family history, will uncover significant problems for which further investigation may be required. A drug history is vital. Although the use of antiplatelet drugs prior to surgery, for example, NSAIDs, has not been associated with an increased risk of hemorrhage, caution should be exercised, with careful postoperative observation.

TABLE 12: Suggested preanesthesia Investigations in Patients with Long-standing Upper-airway Obstruction

Full blood cell count with group, save and crossmatch
ECG (look for excess right-axis deviation)
If indicated, Echo
Assess right ventricular hypertrophy
Assess pulmonary artery pressure
If Echo data incomplete, cardiac catheterization

ECG, electrocardiography; echo, echocardiography.

TABLE 13: Baseline Preanesthesia Investigations in Patients with Cystic Fibrosis

Full blood cell count
Liver function tests
Coagulation if liver involved
Pulmonary function tests
Chest x-ray films

Cystic Fibrosis

Patients with cystic fibrosis may present for nasal polypectomy. This multisystem disorder gives rise to anesthetic problems, due to chronic obstructive pulmonary disease and cirrhosis. Progressive pulmonary disease will lead to pulmonary hypertension and cor pulmonale. Suggestions for preoperative investigations are given in Table 13. Certain characteristics will make these patients particularly prone to perianesthetic problems (Table 14). Careful preoperative preparation of these patients is vital with adequate physiotherapy, antibiotics, and hydration.

Anesthetic Management

Premedication

Sedation is avoided in ambulatory anesthesia. Atropine premedication is not necessary for routine procedures in older children, but should be used in infants and in patients with chronic airway obstruction. The latter should never be given sedation before anesthesia.

Induction

The method of induction should be chosen, with attention to the individual circumstances of the child. Inhalation induction may be considered superior in the younger patient with airway obstruction.

Airway Maintenance

During induction use of CPAP, by partial occlusion of the open tail of the Jackson-Rees modification of Ayre's T piece, will assist in keeping the airway open. An LMA will facilitate airway control in the operating room during minor surgery such as the insertion of ventilation tubes. Anesthesia must be sufficiently deep before introduction of the LMA or laryngospasm will occur. Once a satisfactory unobstructed airway has been achieved, episodes of desaturation during minor ENT surgery have been shown to be significantly less when using the LMA, compared with a face mask and Guedel airway.

Indeed there are many who would advocate a flexible LMA for adenotonsillectomy when using an anesthetic with spontaneous respiration. Once in position, the LMA is well tolerated at light levels of anesthesia. Moreover, it can be left *in situ* during recovery until removed by the patient. This technique requires experience and is not suited for infants having adenotonsillectomy for chronic airway obstruction, because in them the mask encroaches on the surgical field. Moreover, in these patients insertion of the Boyle-Davis gag may result in obstruction of the LMA.

TABLE 14: Pulmonary Function in Cystic Fibrosis Likely to be Associated with Poor Anesthesia Outcome

Vital capacity of less than 50% predicted
Partial carbon dioxide pressure of > 50 mm Hg
FEV_1/FVC ratio of $< 65\%$
No pulmonary reserve on maximum expiratory flow volume curve

FEV_1, forced expiratory volume in 1 second; FVC, forced vital capacity.

TABLE 15: Clinical signs of hemorrhage in a Child following Tonsillectomy or Adenoidectomy

Fresh blood in mouth or frequent swallowing
Nausea and vomiting of fresh or altered blood
Tachycardia
Restlessness
Pale skin
Sweating
Cold peripheries with poor capillary refill (> 1 sec)
Hypotension (very late sign)[a]

[a]Hypotension is very late sign in children and implies a very significant loss of blood (> 20% of circulating volume). Tonsillectomy bleeding should be detected long before this stage is reached.

Tracheal intubation with an RAE preformed tracheal tube is the more common technique. A small leak should be present on inflation to 20 cm H_2O. Neuromuscular blockade with mechanical ventilation using nitrous oxide and oxygen and a supplement of a volatile agent is probably now the technique of choice. This allows the use of intravenous opioids (the author's choice being fentanyl 3 μg per kilogram for adenoidectomy and 5 μg per kilogram for adenotonsillectomy); as a result of good analgesia, recovery is smoother and more peaceful. Acetaminophen and NSAIDs are given by the rectal route during anesthesia. The anesthesiologist should be careful to check the airway after insertion of the Boyle-Davis gag, to ensure that partial obstruction has not occurred.

At the end of surgery, if spontaneous respiration using a tracheal tube has been chosen, the patient should be extubated deep, after inspection of the pharynx and suction if required. If an LMA has been used, the child may be sent to recovery with the mask in place until he or she removes it. If paralysis with mechanical ventilation has been chosen, careful inspection of the pharynx with suction should be performed, after which residual neuromuscular blockade should be reversed (neostigmine 50 μg per kilogram, atropine 25 μ per kilogram), and the child extubated while either awake or in deep anesthesia. Using mivacurium as a relaxant will avoid the need for reversal of the neuromuscular blockade thereby potentially reducing anticholinesterase-induced postoperative nausea and vomiting. Coughing and straining (increasing venous pressure) should be avoided.

Posttonsillectomy Hemorrhage

Careful postoperative observation is mandatory and signs of hemorrhage should be sought (Table 15). Return to the operating room should be delayed until active resuscitation (plasma expander with or without blood) has been commenced and until there is improvement in clinical state. Induction is hazardous and the operating room should be well prepared (Table 16). Induction should be either by inhalation (head-down, lateral position) or by intravenous rapid sequence, using preoxygenation and

TABLE 16: Operating Room Preparation for Bleeding Tonsils[a]

Experienced assistants
Two laryngoscopes (open + ready)
Two large wall suckers at the head of the table
Forceps
A selection of tracheal tubes with stilettes
Tilting operating table

[a]Anesthesia is hazardous in patients with bleeding following adenotonsillectomy and the operating room must be well prepared and staffed. Anesthesia should not commence until basic resuscitation has taken place, with restoration of the circulating blood volume.

cricoid pressure. The anesthesiologist should choose the technique with which he or she is comfortable. Induction may unmask undertreated hypovolemia and the anesthesiologist should be prepared for immediate volume expansion. The stomach should be emptied with a wide-bore tube as far as is possible, with large blood clots being hard to remove, and the child should be extubated in a lateral head-down position at the end.

NASAL SURGERY

Special considerations for nasal surgery are protection of the airway (tracheal intubation and pharyngeal pack) and minimization of blood loss by topical vasoconstriction. Vasoconstriction can best be achieved using topical cocaine (2% to 4% solution, 20 to 40 mg per milliliter), which may also be employed in an outpatient setting for procedures under local anesthesia. Cocaine blocks the intraneuronal uptake of catecholamines, by which mechanism it sensitizes the myocardium to exogenous epinephrine, inducing arrhythmias during halothane anesthesia. Cocaine 3 mg per kilogram is the upper dose limit, but 1.5 mg per kilogram is the preferred dose during halothane anesthesia. A dose of 1.5 mg per kilogram to the nasal mucosa results in peak plasma levels between 15 and 60 minutes after administration, thereafter gradually decreasing over the next 4 to 6 hours. Toxicity is manifested by agitation and should be treated with benzodiazepines (rectal diazepam 0.2 to 0.4 mg per kilogram).

Choanal Atresia

This is considered in the section on airway surgery.

Nasal Polypectomy

Older children (especially those with cystic fibrosis) may present for nasal polypectomy. The principles of anesthesia management (see above) for cystic fibrosis should be followed. The airway must be protected by use of a reliable oropharyngeal pack. For boys with juvenile nasopharyngeal angiofibromas, massive hemorrhage may occur during surgical excision despite preoperative estrogen therapy or selected embolization of feeding vessels. The anesthesiologist should prepare the patient in such a way that large blood loss can readily be managed (Table 17).

ANESTHESIA FOR MAJOR EAR-NOSE-THROAT SURGERY

The principles of anesthesia for major ENT surgery are similar although the operations performed may be diverse. Any surgery involving the operating microscope will be facilitated by careful attention to minimizing perioperative blood loss (Table 18).

TABLE 17: Anesthetic Preparation for Patients in Whom Major Blood Loss is Anticipated

Large-bore cannulae
Invasive arterial and central venous pressure measurement
Warming blanket
Warmed fluids
Urinary catheter
Temperature monitoring

TABLE 18: Minimizing Perioperative Blood Loss*a*

Psychological preparation
Effective premedication for calm, unstressed induction
Smooth induction of anesthesia
Narcotics and alpha-2-agonists to minimize hypertension during laryngoscopy and intubation
Careful patient positioning
   Reverse Trendelenburg
   Avoid excessive neck rotation
Local anesthetic block with vasoconstriction
Moderate induced hypotension by volatile agents and beta-blockade
(mean arterial pressure, 60 mm Hg)
Controlled ventilation to normocapnia using a slow respiratory rate

*a*Minimizing intraoperative blood loss during delicate surgery requires a multifactorial approach with contributions from both anesthesiologist and surgeon.

Induced Hypotension

Moderate induced hypotension is helpful in providing good operating conditions. However, it is not the only factor. Good topical anesthesia, vasoconstriction, and careful surgical technique are more important. The alpha-2-agonist clonidine, given as premedication, produces a calm and sedated child and will help to obtund hypertension on intubation when given in a dose of 2 to 4 µg per kilogram. Furthermore, by reducing central nervous system sympathetic outflow, it facilitates the induction of mild hypotension by volatile agents. Remifentanil may be a useful opioid in this setting as its breakdown by tissue esterases gives a pharmacokinetic profile in which the half-life is independent of both the dose given and the duration of the infusion. This allows the use of high doses during surgery. A steady slow heart rate is helpful in achieving good surgical conditions. Labetolol (maximum total dose 1mg per kilogram in incremental injections will keep the heart rate and blood pressure controlled. As with all beta-blockers, it should be used with caution in patients with asthma.

Local anesthetic block with vasoconstrictors is helpful. The maximum suggested dose for epinephrine during halothane anesthesia is 1 µg per kilogram but rises to 3 to 5 µg per kilogram during isoflurane or enflurane anesthesia, respectively. An infusion of remifentanil may be used to abolish patient response to surgery (loading dose 1–2 mcg/kg, then infusion of 0.5–10 mcg/kg/min).

Middle-Ear Reconstruction

It is well recognized that nitrous oxide can cause a rise in middle-ear pressures, which may affect adversely the outcome of reconstructive surgery through graft displacement. Such elevations are not seen with oxygen/air/volatile agent anesthesia. Nitrous oxide should be avoided for this type of surgery or at the very least its use should be stopped 45 to 60 minutes before the end of the operation.

AIRWAY ASSESSMENT AND BRONCHOSCOPY

Diagnostic Airway Assessment

Airway abnormalities present challenging problems to both anesthesiologist and surgeon. Clinical expertise and familiarity with a wide range of equipment is essential for the safe management of these children.

Patient Assessment

Airway obstruction can occur at any level in the respiratory tree. Careful patient assessment is essential so that anesthesia can be appropriately handled. Stridor, hoarseness, recurrent croup, cyanotic attacks, wheezing, tachypnea, persistent cough, hemoptysis, and dyspnea are all symptoms of potential airway problems. Examination may reveal severe abnormalities (e.g., cystic hygroma, Pierre-Robin syndrome), while careful observation may give an indication of the severity of the obstruction. Characteristics such as distress, use of accessory muscles, intercostal recession, sternal depression, and tracheal tug will give an indication of the severity of the obstruction. Initial examination should include assessment of the airway in different positions, as relief of airway obstruction may be seen with particular postures. The nature of the stridor may be helpful in indicating the likely level of obstruction (Table 19). Investigations that may help include chest x-ray films, Cincinnati radiographs, head and neck computed tomography scans, and pulmonary function tests including sleep studies, although none of these are relevant for life-threatening respiratory obstruction when immediate intervention is indicated.

Techniques of Airway Management

Airway problems in children are often dynamic, and it is helpful to preserve spontaneous respiration to make a full assessment. This requires good topical anesthesia with or without general anesthesia.

Premedication

Preanesthesia sedatives are precluded in this group of patients except in very specific circumstances (see below). Atropine administration is an important part of preanesthesia preparation. Twenty micrograms per kilogram is given by intramuscular injection 30 minutes preoperatively (maximum 0.5 mg) or 20 μ per kilogram, by intravenous injection at induction. Atropine is required to counteract the vagotonic action of volatile anesthetics and any vagotonic reflexes from airway instrumentation, and most importantly to dry the mucous membranes, thus allowing good topical anesthesia and facilitating the examination. It is preferable to give atropine by intramuscular injection so that the mucous membranes are dry by the time the topical anesthetic is applied. Oral administration is unsatisfactory, as receptor occupancy is low using this route, with consequent poor action (7).

Topical Anesthesia

Although laryngoscopy and bronchoscopy may be performed in the older child using topical anesthesia and sedation, in practice almost all children require general anesthesia as well. Effective topical anesthesia contributes to the success and safety of any airway examination.

If an awake examination is attempted in a child, a full technique of topical anesthesia is required. This will only apply to the occasional case as most children will need general anesthesia as well. The nasal passages can be anesthetized using 1% to 4% cocaine (1.5 to 30 mg per kilogram maximum). This also has the advantage of inducing vasoconstriction. Thereafter, lignocaine spray (4% to 10%) is used to anesthetize the posterior regions of the tongue and pharynx (glossopharyngeal nerve), while a cotton-wool ball moistened with lignocaine (4%) is held in the lateral part of the pharynx (piriform fossa), inducing a block of the internal laryngeal branch of the superior laryngeal nerve. If the larynx cannot be visualized, puncture of the cricoid membrane with a 25-gauge needle, and injection of 1mL of lignocaine will anesthetize the trachea. The total dose

TABLE 19: The Site of an Acute Respiratory Obstruction as Suggested by the Clinical Nature of the Stridor

Stridor	Level of Lesion
Inspiratory	At or above larynx
Hoarseness	Vocal cords involved
Biphasic	At or below larynx
Expiratory	Below larynx

TABLE 20: Examples of Conditions Associated with Airway Abnormalities[a]

Craniofacial dysmorphologies
   Pierre Robin syndrome
   Treacher Collins syndrome
   Goldenhar's syndrome
   Hallerman-Streiff syndrome
   Möbius, syndrome
   Cornelia de Lange syndrome
Glycogen storage diseases
Cystic hygroma

[a]Careful preanesthesia assessment is vital, combined with operating room preparation with a wide range of airway equipment including a fiberoptic bronchoscope.

of lignocaine should not exceed 5 mg per kilogram. Topical anesthesia to this extent will allow awake nasotracheal intubation in those with hard-to-visualize or nonvisualized larynges.

For the more usual case under general anesthesia, topical lignocaine (4% to 10%) by spray is adequate (3 to 5 mg per kilogram maximum). In small infants (weighing less than 5 kg), dilute lignocaine (1% or 4%) is drawn into a syringe and sprayed around the larynx and down the trachea.

Techniques for Tracheal Intubation

The techniques and refinements of intubation for specific conditions and procedures are considered in separate sections but the following text concentrates on individual techniques that may be applied in several areas.

Awake Intubation   This may be appropriate for the older patient with a nonvisualized larynx (Table 20), although its place in infancy and childhood is limited. Mild sedation (fentanyl 1 to 2 μ per kilogram or midazolam 0.1 to 0.2 mg per kilogram, which can be reversed by naloxone and flumazanil, respectively) is given and topical anesthesia is applied to the airway as described earlier. With an optimal extended position, blind nasotracheal intubation can be performed by passing a well-curved tracheal tube through the nose toward the larynx, listening for maximal breath sounds. To ensure that the tube remains curved, pack it in an appropriate position in ice for 20 to 30 minutes before use. On hearing the breath sounds, the physician passes through the larynx. On occasion it may be assisted by a stilette with an anteriorly angulated bend at the tip. Fiberoptic intubation has reduced the place of blind nasal intubation and is discussed below.

Intubation under Anesthesia   In patients with airway problems, inhalational anesthesia with preservation of spontaneous respiration is the optimal method of induction. The use of 100% oxygen will afford a margin of safety should further airway obstruction occur during induction. Halothane remains the volatile agent of choice, permitting a smooth induction without laryngeal irritation, yet through its higher solubility, keeping the patient anesthetized even during brief periods of airway obstruction. The newer volatile agents have such low solubility that recovery is excessively quick.

The use of CPAP will help to keep the airway patent and prevent tracheal collapse. During induction, intravenous access if not already present, should be established. In the straight-forward patient whose airway is easy to maintain under deep inhalational anesthesia, nasotracheal intubation can be facilitated using suxamethonium (1.0 to 1.5 mg per kilogram), after which topical anesthesia should be applied before passage of the tracheal tube.

Intubation should be as atraumatic as possible, with the anesthesiologist carefully guiding the tip of the bevel in such a manner that it does not catch in the right ventricle of the larynx. Thereafter, spontaneous respiration resumes and the child can be positioned for microlaryngoscopy. Anesthesia is maintained using oxygen and halothane with spontaneous respiration. When the surgeon has made an initial examination of the larynx, and when all the instruments are available for bronchoscopy, the nasotracheal tube is withdrawn from the larynx into the posterior region of the pharynx. This allows an unimpeded view of the larynx, while anesthesia is maintained by insufflation of oxygen and halothane, which is inhaled from the pool in the pharynx. The surgeon must ensure that the airway is unimpeded during this phase of the examination.

Bronchoscopy   Anesthesia is maintained by nasopharyngeal insufflation of oxygen and halothane during the changeover from laryngoscopy to bronchoscopy. In pediatric otolaryngology the Stortz ventilating bronchoscope is preferred. Oxygen and halothane can be administered via the side arm, allowing preservation of spontaneous respiration and maintenance of anesthesia. The optical telescope (Hopkins rod) occupies a significant proportion of the internal lumen on the smaller bronchoscopes and presents a marked increase in airflow resistance, retarding passive expiration with the potential development of pulmonary hyperinflation and hypoventilation. Intermittent removal of the telescope, with occlusion of the orifice by a thumb, will permit brief periods of unobstructed ventilation. Alternatively many surgeons now prefer to pass the rod alone, often through the suspension laryngoscope, with anesthesia being maintained by nasopharyngeal insufflation of oxygen and halothane. This technique will only permit a diagnostic assessment, especially in smaller patients in whom the rod also causes significant airway obstruction. At the end of the bronchoscopy, halothane should be turned off, oxygen insufflated, and the bronchoscope withdrawn to sit above the glottic aperture, thereby allowing an assessment of vocal cord function and dynamic laryngeal status.

An alternative technique of general anesthesia, which reduces operating room pollution, is to give propofol by infusion. Anesthesia may be commenced by inhalation or the intravenous route. After application of topical anesthesia, propofol is infused at a rate of 12 to 15mg per kilogram per minute while oxygen is insufflated into the pharynx. The infusion should be stopped when the surgeon commences an examination of vocal cord movement.

Jet Injector Bronchoscope   Sanders injector bronchoscopes are available for pediatric patients and many advocate their use with muscle relaxation because of the potential for superior ventilation. However, they may be hazardous in inexperienced hands. In the child there is often a minimal leak around the bronchoscope, meaning that the infant may be exposed to very high inflation pressures. Furthermore, the use of muscle relaxants will complicate the diagnosis of lesions, such as tracheomalacia, that will not be fully revealed unless there is negative intrathoracic pressure, seen during spontaneous respiration. The author strongly advocates the use of spontaneous respiration used with the Stortz ventilating bronchoscope or the telescope alone.

Postbronchoscopy Stridor   Careful attention to technique will ensure that this occurs rarely, but examinations requiring multiple insertions of the bronchoscope may cause mucosal edema and postoperative stridor. Therapeutic measures are shown in Table 21.

TABLE 21: Therapeutic Measures for Postbronchoscopy Stridor[a]

Nil by mouth—give intravenous fluids
Humidified supplemental oxygen
Nebulized racemic epinephrine (2.25% 1 in 6 dilution)
Electrocardiographic monitoring mandatory
Dexamethasone (0.25 µg/kg stat, 0.1 mg/kg 8 hourly)

[a]Stridor may become manifest in the postanesthesia care unit (PACU), following instrumentation of the upper airway. Dexamethasone may be given in the operating room if stridor is thought likely to occur. Other measures should be instituted if required in the PACU.

Specific Airway Problems

Using the principles just outlined, one can perform a safe diagnostic examination for the wide range of airway abnormalities that may be seen in children. However, special attention is needed in certain specific conditions.

Foreign Body Removal

Administering anesthesia for foreign body removal should follow the principles outlined earlier. Some children will present with acute severe upper-airway obstruction. They should be transferred immediately to the operating room where awake laryngoscopy with, if necessary, insertion of a bronchoscope, may allow removal of the laryngeal/tracheal foreign body.

The more usual clinical presentation of a foreign body is of an object in the distal tracheobronchial tree and there is time for preoperative preparation including atropine premedication. If the foreign body is causing significant obstruction of a main bronchus, induction of anesthesia will be slow because of impaired ventilation. When the anesthesia is sufficiently deep (assessed by the tone of the abdominal muscles, which should be very slack), topical anesthesia should be applied. Spontaneous respiration should be preserved so that the foreign body is not blown more distally by positive-pressure ventilation. Adequate depth of anesthesia is vital throughout the whole examination, as often the size of the foreign body exceeds the internal diameter of the bronchoscope so that once it is held by the forceps the whole assembly is removed as a single movement. If there is a cough at this stage, the foreign body may be lost from the forceps or it may impact in the main airway. If the anesthesiologist is in doubt about the depth of the anesthesia, suxamethonium 0.25 to 0.5 mg per kilogram may be given for optimal relaxation during removal of the bronchoscope. A mask should be applied as soon as the instrument is removed, to maintain or deepen anesthesia in preparation for further examination. Vegetable matter often breaks up and may have to be removed in many parts. Repeated passage of the bronchoscope may predispose mucosal edema and stridor, which should be managed as described (see Table 21).

Laser Surgery

The carbon dioxide laser is widely used to treat, for example, laryngeal papillomas and supraglottic cysts and to perform laser aryepiglottoplasty. The main problem for the anesthesiologist is the potential for ignition of plastic tracheal tubes, all of which can burn. Nitrous oxide also supports combustion, even though the gas mixtures will not absorb a laser beam and therefore cannot be heated. Standard laser precautions should be applied: protecting the patient's eyes and face, and requiring staff to wear goggles. If the child has a tracheostomy, the tracheal tube should be changed for a nonfenestrated silver tube. For children without a tracheostomy, a variety of metal tubes exist and these can be employed with spontaneous respiration. The tube may be withdrawn into the pharynx to treat areas obscured by its presence. The author has found this technique easy to employ, though others argue for paralysis with jet ventilation via the laryngoscope (8) or Venturi jet small-diameter tube ventilation. During any jet ventilation technique the surgeon must ensure that the airway is free of obstruction; otherwise, the patient is exposed to hazardously high airway pressures. Although as a rule preoperative sedatives should be avoided with upper-airway obstruction, many children, for example, with papillomas, have multiple operating room procedures. Used with care, tranquilizers or mild sedative may help to allay fears of the examination in these children who present repeatedly.

The Difficult Intubation

The principles outlined in the previous discussion are employed in the patient with a difficult airway. In essence, patients with difficult airways fall into two groups: firstly, those in whom the larynx may be visualized but obstruction prevents the passage of a normal tracheal tube; and secondly, those in whom visualization of the larynx is impossible. For both types intubation may be difficult and the operating room team should be primed for urgent tracheostomy if this becomes necessary.

The Visualized Larynx

Gentle induction of anesthesia as outlined earlier should permit intubation under deep inhalational anesthesia. Throughout, CPAP will help to prevent airway collapse. Preservation of respiration will provide a pointer to the laryngeal inlet, especially in the presence of obstructive lesions that distort laryngeal anatomy (e.g., cysts, epiglottitis). Physical airway narrowing will only permit the passage of a small tracheal tube. A wide range of tubes of different sizes should be available, especially those of small internal diameter but a long length. Introducers may be helpful. Patients with severe airway narrowing may develop postextubation stridor due to further narrowing caused by intubation-induced mucosal edema. If on initial laryngoscopy the anesthesiologist is clear that subglottic narrowing is present, intubation should be avoided and the examination should proceed, with anesthesia maintained by insufflation of halothane in oxygen via the nasopharynx. Careful diagnostic examination without intubation will help to avoid unnecessary morbidity.

Epiglottitis Immunization with the *Hemophilus influenzae* type b vaccine has markedly decreased the incidence of this condition in early childhood. Management of the patient with suspected epiglottis involves rapid transfer to the operating room, inhalation induction as described above, and after the diagnosis is made, securing the airway with a nasotracheal tube. Bubbles moving in and out with respiration will afford the best clue as to the position of the larynx. More commonly, acute laryngotracheobronchitis is seen, which if severe and unresponsive to steroids demands nasotracheal intubation and intensive care management.

The Nonvisualized Larynx

Lesions likely to cause a nonvisualization of the larynx are listed in Table 20. Involvement of the temporomandibular joints in Still's disease may present as an inability to open the mouth.

The Laryngeal Mask Airway For surgical operations in which intubation is not required, it is often possible to introduce an LMA and achieve good airway control despite being unable to see the larynx. Furthermore, the LMA may act as a guide through which a fiberoptic bronchoscope can be introduced (see below). In the occasional, severely affected patient with high upper-airway obstruction, an LMA can bypass the obstruction, providing a satisfactory airway and permitting anesthesia with spontaneous respiration during the performance of a tracheostomy.

The ability of the patient to tolerate the LMA at very light levels of anesthesia means that it can also be used in the assessment of vocal cord function. Often the technique of withdrawing the bronchoscope into the supraglottis results in a very short period of vocal cord examination because the patient will not tolerate the rigid instrument in the mouth. By using the laryngeal mask, with a fiberoptic bronchoscope passed down through a swivel connector, it is possible to ensure that the patient remains adequately oxygenated yet give the otolaryngologist a lengthy view of the vocal cords, allowing a proper assessment of function.

Fiberoptic Intubation The fiberoptic bronchoscope has revolutionized the approach to the nonvisualized larynx. Intubation may be attempted while the patient is awake, using topical anesthesia as described earlier, or under general anesthesia. With a nasopharyngeal airway in place (this may be the tube to be passed into the trachea), the fiberoptic bronchoscope can be passed down to the pharynx ready for identification of the glottic apertere. A variety of fiberoptic bronchoscopes are now available (Table 22). The lack of

TABLE 22: Presently Available Fiberoptic Intubating Bronchoscopes[a]

External Diameter	Tube Size
2.7 mm	3–4
3.2 mm	4.5–6.0
5.8 mm	6.5 and above

[a]When the bronchoscop passed down a tracheal tube, a very significant proportion of the airway will be lost, leading to high resistance to breathing. If positive-pressure ventilation is used, the high resistance to expiration may lead to gas trapping and the risk of barotrauma.

suction capability on the smallest bronchoscopes is a disadvantage and prior advancement of the nasotracheal tube into the pharynx will help to prevent lens soiling on passage through the nose. Thereafter, the bronchoscope can be guided into the trachea and down to the carina, and the tracheal tube advanced over the bronchoscope into position. A rotating, twisting action is often required to introduce the tube through the larynx. After the position of the tracheal tube is checked, the bronchoscope should be quickly withdrawn because it occupies a large proportion of the internal tube diameter and therefore presents a significant obstruction to respiration.

Variations on this technique have been described. Using a 4.5-mm tube through the nose and guided by the fiberscope to impact in the glottis, a bougie guide can be passed into the trachea. The 4.5-mm tube is then removed and the smaller tube can be passed through the larynx into the final tracheal position. This technique allows the use of a larger fiberscope while placing small nasotracheal tubes in an infant. A further modification is the use of an adult fiberscope to introduce a cardiac catheter wire into the trachea. The cardiac catheter itself is then passed over the wire and the tracheal tube introduced into the trachea over the wire and catheter combination.

Retrograde Translaryngeal Catheters   This technique, well described in texts of anesthesia, is mentioned for the sake of completeness. The author has never employed it and many consider it to be contraindicated in infants.

Tracheostomy   There are occasions when tracheostomy is required, both electively and in an emergency. However, in the latter circumstances every reasonable effort should be made to gain control of the airway. Lifesaving hurried tracheostomy in the cyanosed child is very rarely required. It is far better to gain some control of the airway (even with a cricothyroid cannula), oxygenate the patient, and then perform a controlled tracheostomy. Tracheostomy may be performed under local anesthesia but again this is rarely required.

If the patient is intubated, then anesthesia with controlled ventilation is preferred. If a tracheostomy is being done with just mask anesthesia, then oxygen and halothane with spontaneous ventilation is preferred. Local anesthetic wound infiltration will help to obtund the response to surgery. The patient must be positioned with the head extended and well fixed. One hundred percent oxygen should be given in the 5 minutes before exchange of the oral or nasotracheal tube for the tracheostomy tube. It is vital that the anesthesiologist check the sterile connectors for the chosen tracheostomy tube, to ensure compatibility with the anesthesia circuit. When the trachea is divided, the existing tracheal tube is withdrawn to just above the split and the tracheostomy tube is inserted. Should this fail, the existing tube can be readvanced until a further attempt is made. Once a tracheostomy tube is secure, the head must be returned to the normal position, upon which the anesthesiologist should ensure there is bilateral, even air entry and that ventilation is easy. Single-lung ventilation or unusually high inflation pressures imply that the tracheostomy tube is too long, and this should be adjusted immediately before the patient is awakened or returned to the ward.

AIRWAY SURGERY

Choanal Atresia

This neonatal emergency (see discussion on neonatal anesthetic requirements) requires stabilization with an oral airway through which inhalational anesthesia is introduced. Neuromuscular blockade is followed by orotracheal intubation using an RAE preformed tube. Hand ventilation is advised during positioning of the Dingman (cleft-palate type) gag, thereby ensuring that the tube is unobstructed. Intravenous fluids should be given and continued into the postoperative period. Blood loss may be substantial if significant drilling is required. Preoperative hemoglobin estimation is mandatory and blood transfusion may be required very occasionally. Anesthesia is terminated when the nasal stents are adequately positioned. Spontaneous respiration should resume and the baby is extubated and allowed to breathe through the stents.

Aryepiglottoplasty

Division of the aryepiglottic folds is undertaken for severe laryngomalacia with failure to thrive. The basic principles of airway surgery should be followed. If this is to be done with a laser, insufflation of oxygen and halothane into the nasopharynx with spontaneous ventilation is adequate. Division using instruments is best managed with an RAE tracheal tube held out of the surgical field using the suspension laryngoscope. Hand ventilation is advised throughout the operation to ensure that the tracheal tube is not obstructed by the laryngoscope.

Cricoid Split and Laryngeal Reconstruction

Patients with subglottic stenosis can have this condition relieved by cricoid split or laryngeal reconstruction.

Cricoid Split

Those patients considered for cricoid split will have failed extubation and will present in the operating room intubated from the intensive care unit. A chest x-ray study should be done to check the tube position before the patient goes to the operating room, as a careful estimation of the tube length is required. During anesthesia, which follows the same principles as for tracheostomy (see above), the existing nasotracheal tube will be replaced by one that is the correct size for the age of the child or occasionally one size larger. This will be used to hold the cricoid split apart. After a period of ventilation with 100% oxygen, the existing nasotracheal tube is withdrawn and the new tube is introduced. The surgeon can assist the passage of the new tube to the required position. The length of the new nasotracheal tube must be correct at this time, as once the neck is closed it is very difficult to reintubate the trachea nasally, because the tip of the bevel will tend to impact in the cricoid split, thereby creating a false passage. If this occurs, a fiberscope placed under direct vision may help to guide the nasal tube past the split in the cricoid. Anesthesia using opioids and muscle relaxants is employed for this procedure and this provides adequate conditions for the journey back to the intensive care unit. Depending on the patient's medical state, mechanical ventilation or restoration of spontaneous breathing with CPAP may be used while the nasotracheal tube remains *in situ* for 10 days on the intensive care unit.

Laryngeal Reconstruction

Anterior laryngeal reconstruction may be performed as a single-stage procedure (no tracheostomy, prolonged nasotracheal intubation in the intensive care unit) or as a two-stage procedure (tracheostomy, placement of a Silastic stent, and delayed closure of the tracheostomy). Anterior and posterior reconstructions usually require the presence of a tracheostomy. Full monitoring (including invasive measurement of pressures) is mandatory for this surgery. Access to the patient is very limited during the operation and reliable monitoring and venous access is mandatory.

Single-Stage Reconstruction   Nasotracheal intubation is required and the principles of anesthesia for cricoid split are employed. Costal cartilage is harvested and the wound is then flooded with saline solution. A sustained Valsalva maneuver is employed to ensure that the pleura has not been breached during harvesting, after which the chest wound is closed around a catheter laid adjacent to the intercostal nerves. This catheter is used to give bolus-dose local anesthetics to provide analgesia. The patient is then intubated as described for a cricoid split, after which the graft is placed and the wound closed. Again tube positioning is critical.

Two-stage Reconstruction   Anesthesia is induced via the tracheostomy or intravenously. The technique of using an opioid with muscle relaxation, mechanical ventilation with nitrous oxygen, and a volatile agent is preferred. The tracheostomy is reintubated using a snug-fitting RAE tube, cut to size, or a cuffed flexometallic tube carefully positioned. If the latter is chosen, it has the advantage of protecting the airway, but it must be securely fixed or inadvertent migration with surgical movement may occur, resulting in selective bronchial placement.

The reconstruction follows similar principles to the single-stage procedure but a Silastic stent is placed in the subglottis instead of a nasotracheal tube. At the end of surgery the standard tracheostomy tube is replaced, anesthesia is reversed, and the patient awakened and returned to the intensive care unit, spontaneously breathing with humidified oxygen. Intravenous fluids are continued until feeding is resumed. The stent may cause glottic incompetence and resultant difficulties in swallowing leading to aspiration.

Endoscopic Repair of Cleft Larynx

Anesthesia for repair of a cleft larynx requires use of a tracheal tube (either reinforced or RAE) that held forward by the suspension laryngoscope, allowing the surgeon free access to the posterior region of the larynx. The technique of anesthesia should involve neuromuscular blockade, mechanical or hand ventilation using nitrous oxide and oxygen with a volatile agent supplement, opioids, and if necessary, topical anesthesia. Toward the end of the repair, which is conducted using the suspension laryngoscope and microscope, anesthesia should be lightened so that there is a rapid return of protective laryngeal reflexes at the end of surgery.

SUMMARY

There is no area of surgery more challenging to the anesthesiologist than pediatric otolaryngology. Careful patient assessment, with anesthesia directed to patient safety, while allowing the surgeon optimal access to operate, will result in the best possible outcome for the patient.

⊕ REFERENCES

1. Phillips S, deBorn AK, Hatch DJ. Preoperative fasting for paediatric anaesthesia. *Br J Anaesth* 1994;73:529–536.
2. Morton NS, Camu F, Dorman T, et al. Ondansetron reduces nausea and vomiting after paediatric adeno-tonsillectomy. *Paediatri Anaesth* 1997;7:37–45.
3. Hatch DJ, Sumner ES, Hellmann J. *The surgical neonate: anesthesia and intensive care*. London: Edward Arnold, 1995.

4. Lake C. *Paediatric cardiac anesthesia*. Norwalk, CT: Appleton & Lange, 1995.
5. Bennett EJ, Bowyer DE. Fluid and electrolyte balance. In: Sumner E, Hatch D, eds. *Textbook of paediatric anaesthetic practice*. London: Balliere Tindall, 1985.
6. Southhall, DP, ed. *Prevention and control of pain in children: a manual for healthcare professionals. Report of the Working Party of the Royal College of Paediatrics and Child Health*. London: BMJ Publications, 1997.
7. Gervais HW, El Gindi M, Radermacher PR, et al. Plasma concentration following oral and intramuscular atropine in children and their clinical effects. *Paediatr Anaesth* 1997;7:13–18.
8. Kauffman JA, Little FB, Weeks DB. Proximal large bore jet ventilation for laryngeal laser surgery. *Arch Otolaryngol Head Neck Surg* 1987;113:314.

A.R. Lloyd-Thomas: Department of Paediatric Anaesthesia, Great Ormond Street Hospital for Children, London WC1N 3JH, United Kingdom.

• *Practical Pediatric Otolaryngology*
• edited by Robin T. Cotton
  and Charles M. Myer, III
• Lippincott-Raven Publishers,
  Philadelphia © 1999

Outcomes Research for the Practicing Physician

Richard M. Rosenfeld

Yogi Bera must have been thinking about outcomes research when he noted, "You can observe a lot just by watching," because outcomes researchers learn a lot just by asking. More specifically, they ask patients whether or not they feel and function better after a certain intervention. What a novel and haughty concept—asking patients how they feel rather than judging treatment by objective end points such as radiographs, laboratory tests, or survival curves!

Outcomes research applies new methods for obtaining, rating, and validating the subjective experience of patients and their objective health status (1). In contrast to randomized trials that measure *efficacy* under ideal conditions, outcomes studies measure *effectiveness* in real-life clinical scenarios. Outcomes studies emphasize quality of life in diverse individuals, whereas randomized trials emphasize objective results in patients meeting strict inclusion criteria. Nonetheless, an outcomes study can benefit by including some objective end points, and a randomized trial can benefit by including quality of life measures. The two approaches are mutually beneficial, not mutually exclusive.

The ultimate goal of outcomes research is to help patients, payers, and physicians make rational choices in medical care based on the *effect of such choices on patient's lives* (2). Few practicing physicians would contest this statement, yet even fewer truly understand what is really meant by outcomes research. This chapter provides a selective and nontechnical tour of outcomes research, tailored to the needs of practicing physicians with limited backgrounds in epidemiology and statistics. Guidelines are also offered on how to use quality of life surveys and patient satisfaction questionnaires to enhance clinical practice.

WHAT IS OUTCOMES RESEARCH?

Outcomes research deals with all identified changes in health status and quality of life arising as a consequence of how a health problem is handled. *Health status* is the degree to which a person is able to function physically, emotionally, and socially, with or without aid from the health-care system. In contrast, *quality of life* is the degree to which persons *perceive* themselves as able to function. Both health status and quality of life extend far beyond the usual disease-specific treatment end points used to determine success or failure in clinical trials. A clinical trial may be interested in the hearing improvement achieved with insertion of tympanostomy tubes for otitis media, but an outcomes study would measure the actual and perceived benefits of improved hearing on the child's physical, emotional, and social function.

The definition of outcomes research remains nebulous, because the answer depends on exactly who is asking the question: patient, payer, or physician. The outcomes "movement" is as much political as scientific, based on the premise that health-care outcomes have not received sufficient attention and that physicians know too little about what produces desired health effects. Different approaches to the methods and madness of outcomes research are illustrated below. Readers should realize that concepts continue to evolve, and new approaches are likely to exist by the time this chapter is published.

A Technology of Patient Experience

Paul Ellwood noted in 1988 that our inability to measure and understand health-care outcomes resulted in uninformed patients, skeptical payers, frustrated physicians, and besieged health-care executives (2). In response, he proposed a technology for collaborative action called "outcomes management":

> Outcomes management is a technology of patient experience designed to help patients, payers, and providers make rational medical care–related choices based on better insight into the effect of these choices on the patient's life. Outcomes management consists of a common patient-understood language of health outcomes; a national data base containing information and analysis on clinical, financial, and health outcomes that estimates as best as we can the relation between medical interventions and health outcomes, as well as the relation between health outcomes and money; and an opportunity for each decision-maker to have access to the analyses that are relevant to the choices they must make.

To achieve these goals, Ellwood proposed (a) systematic measurement of the functioning and "well-being of patients," along with disease-specific clinical outcomes, at appropriate time intervals; (b) pooling of clinical and outcome data on a massive scale; (c) analysis and dissemination of results from the segment of the database most appropriate to the concerns of each decision maker; and (d) greater reliance on practice guidelines by physicians when selecting appropriate interventions.

Health-care Stakeholders

The number of individuals and organizations involved in outcomes research has grown rapidly over the past decade. Greater insight into the outcomes movement can be obtained by understanding what each of the stakeholders hopes to gain from the process (3).

Public and private payers seeking to reduce health-care costs may use effectiveness results to ration health care or to establish national guidelines. Reimbursement and purchasing decisions could eventually be linked to quality assessment reflecting desirable or undesirable health outcomes. For hospitals and other health-care organizations, effectiveness results would establish local treatment guidelines, identify opportunities for improvement, and be used for marketing purposes. Patients, the public, and individual providers could use effectiveness data to make informed treatment decisions, particularly when the preferred treatment for an individual patient is not obvious and the patient or caregiver is willing to participate in the decision-making process.

Medical Treatment Effectiveness Program

Since 1989, the Agency for Health Care Policy and Research (AHCPR) has funded special projects known as Patient Outcomes Research Teams (PORTs) (4). These large and complex 5-year undertakings, with average annual budgets of 1 million dollars, represent the leading edge of outcomes research methodology. Emphasis is placed on outcomes that patients understand and care about, such as quality of life, functional capacity, symptom relief, and cost (in contrast to physiologic measures and parameters that focus more on organs than their owners). Questions of cost-effectiveness and appropriateness are additional basic themes in this research.

Each of the PORTs follows a standard research model, which consists of (a) systematic literature review (*metaanalysis*); (b) analysis of variations in practice patterns and patient outcomes (*primary data*), (c) analysis of cost and claims data (*secondary data*), (d) *decision analysis* to define the optimal path to the desired outcome, and (e) strategies for effective *dissemination and assimilation* of research findings. Despite the grandiose goals of the PORTs, the methodology remains embryonic and has not yet been applied to clinical problems confronting the practicing pediatric otolaryngologist.

American Academy of Otolaryngology–Head and Neck Surgery Foundation Outcomes Research Grant

When the American Academy of Otolaryngology–Head and Neck Surgery Foundation (AAO-HNS) introduced its Outcomes Research Small Project Grant in 1996, the purpose was to foster research that would improve the effectiveness and appropriateness of medical practice. Projects supported under the program would develop and disseminate scientific information on the effects of otolaryngology services and procedures on patients' survival, health status, functional capacity, and quality of life. Three main categories of outcomes research were identified: patient-based studies, record-based studies, and process assessment (Table 1).

An ideal patient-based outcomes study would incorporate the principles outlined earlier for the AHCPR PORTs. No effort of this magnitude is yet underway in pediatric otolaryngology (as of July 1996), but smaller efforts are ongoing to develop and validate measures of comorbidity, disease severity, and disease-specific quality of life. Records-based outcomes studies have been more popular because they are easier, faster, and less expensive to design and conduct. Process assessment includes anything that happens between two evaluation points that might affect health. Although not directly related to patient care, the editorial review process is included in this definition (see Table 1) to acknowledge the importance of peer-reviewed publications as a foundation for *evidence-based medicine*.

Outcomes and the Practicing Physician

The foregoing discussion suggests there are two separate, but related, agendas in the outcomes movement. *Outcomes management* by payers and hospitals tries to cut costs by controlling physician and patient access to health-care resources. *Outcomes research* by physicians tries to identify management options that result in the highest overall and disease-specific quality of life for patients. Lest they fall victim to the control paradigm of outcomes management, practicing physicians must participate in—or at least understand the fundamental principles of—outcomes research. The remainder of this chapter aims to facilitate this goal.

TABLE 1: Overview of Outcomes Research

Patient-based outcomes research
Creation and validation of health-related quality of life measures
Creation and validation of disease-specific clinical severity scales
Observational studies of treatment effectiveness
Record-based outcomes research
Analysis of administrative and financial databases
Regional variations in practice patterns and outcomes
Metaanalysis, decision analysis, or cost-effectiveness studies
Analysis of national data sets or population-based surveys
Process assessment
Continuous quality improvement
Patient satisfaction with health-care services
Development of clinical practice guidelines
Editorial peer review process

UNDERSTANDING OUTCOMES RESEARCH

Outcomes studies involve hypothesis-driven research that relies on fundamental principles of epidemiology and statistics for validity. Realizing that for most readers these two disciplines are nothing more than bad memories from medical school, this section highlights the essentials necessary to understand outcomes research.

Crash Course in Epidemiology

Over the past 50 years, the definition of epidemiology has broadened from concern with communicable disease epidemics to encompass all phenomena related to health in populations. Epidemiology brings method to the madness of planning and conducting research studies, including outcomes research.

Epidemiologists are obsessed with avoiding bias and proving causality. *Bias* refers to any trend in the collection, analysis, or interpretation of data that leads to conclusions systematically different from the truth (5). *Causality* is the ability to relate causes to the effects they produce. The fruit of these obsessions is the randomized controlled trial (RCT), which since the Second World War has epitomized successful application of the scientific method to clinical medicine. From an evolutionary perspective, outcomes research is a giant step backward from the RCT because of increased bias and reduced ability to demonstrate causality. Comparing these two types of research (Table 2) is a useful exercise in basic epidemiology.

RCTs and outcomes studies are based on two diametrically opposed philosophies: realism versus empiricism (6). Medical realists believe they can know what actually occurs when someone gets sick or well. Through deterministic reasoning (e.g., RCTs) they seek out mechanisms of illness and therapy, including etiology, pathophysiology, and the mechanisms of action. In contrast, medical empiricists should seek only to observe and demonstrate relationships, not cause and effect. Probabilistic reasoning (e.g., an outcomes study) is used to predict future results based on past experience, whatever the cause. The probabilist (outcomes researcher) plays the odds whereas the determinist (RCT researcher) imagines the underlying process.

The virtues of RCTs are stated in the name itself: control groups and randomization. The presence or absence of a *control group* has a profound influence on data interpretation. An uncontrolled study—no matter how elegant—is purely descriptive (7). Nonetheless, authors of case series or cohort studies often delight in unjustified musings

TABLE 2: Comparison of Randomized Controlled Trials and Outcomes Studies

Characteristic	Randomized Controlled Trial	Outcomes Study
Philosophy	Realism	Empiricism
Goal	Establish cause and effect	Demonstrate relationships
Level of investigator control	Experimental	Observational
Treatment allocation	Random assignment	Routine clinical care
Study design	Parallel groups	Longitudinal cohort
Patient selection criteria	Restrictive	Broad
Typical setting	Hospital or university based	Community based
End point definitions	Objective health status	Subjective quality of life
End point assessment	Blinded	Unblinded
Time frame	Short or intermediate	Long
Statistical analysis	Paired or independent groups	Multivariate regression
Potential for bias	Low	Very high

TABLE 3: Explanations for Favorable Outcomes in Treatment Studies

Explanation	Definition	Solution
Bias	Systematic variation of measurements from their true values; may be intentional or unintentional	Accurate, protocol-driven data collection
Chance	Random variation without apparent relation to other measurements or variables; e.g., getting lucky	Control or comparison group
Natural history	Course of a disease from onset to resolution; may include relapse, remission, and spontaneous recovery	Control or comparison group
Placebo effect	Beneficial effect caused by the expectation that the regimen will have an effect; e.g., power of suggestion	Control or comparison group with placebo
Halo effect	Beneficial effect caused by the manner, attention, and caring of a provider during a medical encounter	Control or comparison group treated similarly
Confounding	Distortion of an effect by other prognostic factors or variables for which adjustments have not been made	Randomization or multivariate analysis
Allocation (susceptibility) bias	Beneficial effect caused by allocating subjects with less severe disease or better prognosis to treatment	Randomization or comorbidity analysis group
Ascertainment (detection) bias	Favoring the treatment group during outcome analysis; e.g., rounding up for treated subjects, down for controls	Blinded outcome assessment
Transfer bias	Inequalities in accounting for all initial patients; e.g., omitting postoperative deaths from survival rates	Intention-to-treat analysis

on efficacy, effectiveness, association, and causality. Without a control or comparison group, it is often impossible to distinguish natural history from treatment effects (Table 3). In the words of Voltaire, "The art of medicine consists in amusing the patient while nature cures the disease."

The placebo and halo effects (see Table 3) may account for on average 70% of good to excellent outcomes in uncontrolled studies (8). The potential for these effects is proportional to the novelty or impressiveness of the treatment given and the setting in which it is administered. Coincidentally, surgical subspecialists often administer novel treatments in impressive settings. Further, patients with chronic disease typically have fluctuating symptoms and seek medical care (and enroll in research studies) when symptoms are at their worst. Thus, the next change is likely to be an improvement (independent of therapy), a phenomenon called *regression to the mean*.

Studies with control or comparisons groups may be performed with or without randomization. In an RCT the investigator randomly assigns patients to treatment or control groups. An RCT is an *experimental* study because conditions are controlled by the investigator for the express purpose of increasing medical knowledge, not for providing clinical care. In contrast, an outcomes study is a form of *observational* research. Treatment decisions occur as part of routine clinical care, without intervention from the investigator other than to record, classify, and analyze. This lack of control predisposes observational studies to numerous hidden biases, only some of which are overcome by using a control group (see Table 3).

A major source of bias in outcomes studies are the individual judgments and other selective decisions that influence clinical management in the absence of randomized assignment (9). Randomization balances baseline prognostic factors—known and unknown—among groups, including severity of illness and the presence of comorbid conditions (e.g., asthma in a sinusitis trial). Because these factors also influence a clinician's decision to offer treatment, nonrandomized studies are prone to *allocation (susceptibility) bias* (see Table 3) and false-positive results (10). A typical example occurs when the survival of surgically treated cancer patients is compared with that of nonsurgical controls (e.g., radiation or chemotherapy). Without randomization, the surgical group will generally have a more favorable prognosis—independent of therapy—because the customary criteria for operability (special anatomic conditions and no major comorbidity) also predispose to favorable results.

RCTs prevent two other biases that plague observational research: detection bias and transfer bias (see Table 3). *Detection bias* occurs when unequal methods of surveillance and identification are applied to treatment and control patients, because observers are affected by their knowledge and prior expectations concerning therapy. Experimental studies can prevent this by double blinding patients and physicians to treatment status, but comparable measures would be unethical in observational research. *Transfer bias* arises from inequalities in accounting for all patients initially entered in the study. For example, if we limit our analysis to only those patients who survived surgery or who were highly compliant with medication use, our success rates would be falsely elevated. RCTs avoid this by analyzing according to intention to treat, rather than completion of treatment. Although not impossible, intention-to-treat analysis can be difficult in observational studies.

If RCTs lie at the top of the epidemiologic food chain, why bother at all with observational studies such as outcomes research? Because as they shed bias and don the gown of causality, RCTs became increasingly divorced from the realities of everyday medical practice. In other words, the price of scientific purity is low relevance to real world situations. Results of RCTs are limited by constraints of selective admission criteria, rigorous therapeutic protocols with measures to ensure compliance, and narrowly defined outcome measures. The treatment end points in RCTs are chosen for their objectivity, and are not necessarily important to patients (or physicians). RCTs are expensive and not always ethical, particularly for surgical therapies. Finally, randomized trials can become outdated quickly and often do not address issues of effectiveness and dissemination.

The outcomes movement has been fueled, in part, by the aforementioned inadequacies of using RCTs to guide medical therapy. Nonetheless, observational (outcomes) treatment comparisons may contain all the biases randomized trials are intended to prevent or reduce. The prognosis and choice of treatment can be affected by baseline comorbidity, the pattern of symptoms, the severity of symptoms, and the pattern of disease progression. When these crucial clinical factors, called *covariates*, are suitably identified and classified, they can be used for adjustments that remove or reduce bias when observational data are used for therapeutic comparisons. Unfortunately, appropriate covariates have not been adequately defined for most diseases. A major part of outcomes research, therefore, is to identify and classify these disease-specific covariates.

Crash Course in Statistics

"Every sensible person promptly associates the term 'statistics' with the thought: 'This is a bunch of lies'," observed August Bier, surgeon and philosopher. If you agree, you might as well skip this section. Regrettably, you will remain half in the dark when it comes to understanding outcomes research, because epidemiology is to statistics as leadership is to management: The epidemiologist (leader) makes sure that the right data are analyzed, but the statistician (manager) makes sure that the data are analyzed right. Great data analyzed poorly are worth as much as poor data analyzed greatly.

Accepting *uncertainty* is the key to understanding outcomes data. Uncertainty is present in all data, because of the inherent variability in biologic systems and in our ability to assess them in a reproducible fashion. Nearly 2,000 years ago Pliny the Elder reported with certainty, "The only certainty is that nothing is certain." For example, if you measure disease-specific quality of life in 20 children with stable disease on 5 days, how likely would it be to get the same mean result each time? Very unlikely, because of random and unpredictable fluctuations in response. Similarly, if you measured quality of life in five groups of 20 children, how likely would it be to get the same results in each group? Again unlikely, because of variations between individuals. We would get a range of similar results, but rarely the exact same result on repetitive trials.

Uncertainty must be dealt with when interpreting data, unless the results are meant to apply only to the particular group of patients in which the observations were initially made. Statisticians consider all clinical measurements to be *estimates* of some "true" value that can never be known, because some degree of unavoidable error is always present. Measurements made on a finite sample of observations are called *point estimates* because the values obtained in other samples are unlikely to be exactly the same. In medicine, however, we seek to pass from observations to generalizations, from point estimates to estimates about other populations. When this process occurs with calculated degrees of uncertainty, we call it *inference*.

Here is a brief example of clinical inference. After treating five patients with vitamin C for intractable vertigo, you remark to a colleague that four had excellent improvement in health status. She asks, "How confident are you of your results?" "Quite confident," you reply, "There were five patients, four improved, and that's 80%." "Maybe I wasn't clear," she interjects, "How confident are you that 80% of vertiginous patients *in general*, whether in your practice or mine, will respond favorably to vitamin C?" "In other words," she continues, "can you *infer* anything about the real effect of vitamin C on vertigo from only five patients?" Hesitatingly you retort, "Maybe I'll have to see a few more patients to be sure."

The real issue, of course, is that a sample of only five patients offers low *precision*. How likely is it that the same results would be found if five new patients were studied? Actually, we can state with 95% confidence that four out of five successes in a single trial is consistent with a range of results from 28% to 99% in future trials. This 95% *confidence interval* may be calculated manually or with a statistical program (11–13), and tells us the *range of results consistent with the observed data*. Thus, if this trial were repeated we could obtain a success rate as low as 28%, not very encouraging compared with the original point estimate of 80%. A broad 95% confidence interval indicates a large amount of uncertainty, whereas a narrow interval indicates much greater precision. All main results in an outcomes study should be accompanied by a 95% confidence interval to aid interpretation.

The uncertainty plot thickens when comparing *two or more groups*, because errors in inference are inevitable. If we conclude the groups are different, they may actually be equivalent (type I statistical error or false positive). If we conclude they are the same, we may have missed a true difference (type II statistical error or false negative). All *statistical tests* (*t* tests, chi-square, etc.) are simply a means of estimating the likelihood of a type I error. The *values* produced by such tests indicate the likelihood that the purported association or relationship under study is really a false-positive finding. For example, if we find an association between passive smoking and otitis media at p = 0.03, there is only a 3% chance that this represents a fortuitous (false-positive) finding.

Outcomes studies use *multivariate analysis* to determine the independent effect of multiple predictor variables on an outcome. Predictors may be disease-specific (tumor stage, treatment administered, etc.) or general (age, sex, socioeconomic status, comorbidity, etc.). Examples of multivariate analysis include logistic and proportional hazards (Cox) regression. Each produces a statistical model that predicts outcomes based on combinations of individual variables. The adequacy of the model as a whole is determined by R^2 (1.0 indicates perfect fit) and its associated *p* value. Each predictor variable has an associated coefficient and *p* value, which reflect the magnitude and significance of any effect on outcome adjusted for all the other variables in the model. Proportional hazards (Cox) regression is widely used in patient-based outcomes studies to determine prognostic factors and to compare treatment regimens after adjustment for imbalances (covariates) between the treatment groups (14).

Outcomes studies are prone to *data dredging* and *post hoc* hypotheses, because of the large number of variables often involved. When a large number of statistical tests are performed, some will be significant by chance alone, because each test has a 5% chance of error. This "multiple *p* value problem" is compounded by extensive subgroup comparisons, but can be avoided by using multivariate analysis. Even with multivariate analysis, however, problems can still arise when hypotheses are formulated *post hoc*—after even the briefest glance at the data—thereby invalidating the probability basis for statistical testing. This is similar to the Texas sharpshooter who shoots an arrow at a barn wall, then runs and draws a bull's-eye around it. Whereas his friends may later applaud his incredible accuracy, his *post hoc* cleverness invalidates its significance.

A statistical test is valid only when the *study sample* (Table 4) is random and representative. Unfortunately, these assumptions are frequently violated or overlooked. A random sample is necessary because most statistical tests are based on probability theory—playing the odds. The odds apply only if the deck is not stacked and the dice are not rigged; that is, all members of the *target population* have an equal chance of being sampled for study. Investigators, however, typically have access to only a small subset of the target population because of geographic or temporal constraints. When they choose an even smaller subset of this *accessible population* to study, the method of choosing (sampling method) affects our ability to make inferences about the original target population.

Of the sampling methods listed in Table 5, only a random sample is theoretically suitable for statistical analysis. Because outcomes research is observational, random samples are rarely feasible. Nonetheless, a *consecutive sample* or *systematic sample* offers a relatively good approximation, and provides data of sufficient quality for most statistical tests. The worst sampling method occurs when subjects are chosen based on convenience or subjective judgments about eligibility. Applying statistical tests to the resulting convenience (grab) sample is the equivalent of asking a professional card counter to help you win a blackjack game when the deck is stacked and cards are missing—all bets are off because probability theory will not apply.

Separating the Good, the Bad, and the Ugly

A good outcomes study is *valid* not only for the subjects studied, but also for similar subjects outside the study. *Internal validity* exists when the study results are credible for the

---

TABLE 4: Glossary of Statistical Terms Related to Sampling and Validity

Term	Definition
Target population	Entire collection of items, subjects, patients, observations, etc., about which we want to make inferences; defined by the selection criteria (inclusion and exclusion criteria) for the study
Accessible population	Subset of the target population that is accessible for study, generally because of geographic or temporal considerations
Study sample	Subset of the accessible population that is chosen for study
Sampling method	Process of choosing a sample from a larger population; the method may be random or nonrandom, representative or nonrepresentative
Selection bias	Error caused by systematic differences between a study sample and target population; examples include studies on volunteers, and those conducted in clinics or tertiary-care settings
Internal study validity	Degree to which conclusions drawn from a study are valid for the study sample; results from proper study design, unbiased measurements, and sound statistical analysis
External study validity (generalizability)	Degree to which conclusions drawn from a study are valid for a target population (beyond the subjects in the study); results from representative sampling and appropriate selection criteria

TABLE 5: Methods for Sampling a Population

Method	How It Is Performed	Comments
Brute force sample	Includes all units of study (charts, patients, laboratory animals, or journal articles) accessible to the researchers	Time-consuming, and unsophisticated; bias prone because missing units are seldom randomly distributed
Convenience (grab) sample	Units are selected on the basis of accessibility, convenience, or subjective judgments about eligibility	Assume this method when none is specified; study results cannot be generalized because of selection bias
Systematic sample	Units are selected using some simple, systematic rule, such as first letter of last name, date of birth, or day of week	Less biased than a convenience sample, but problems may still occur because of unequal selection probabilities
Consecutive sample	Every unit is included over a specified time interval, or until a specified number is reached	Excellent method when intake period is long enough to adequately represent seasonal and other temporal factors
Random sample	Units are assigned numbers, then selected at random until a desired sample size is attained	Best method because all units have a known (and equal) probability of selection; rarely feasible for outcomes studies

specific sample of subjects studied. The preceding sections describe several features of internal validity, including 95% confidence intervals to measure precision, p values to control for chance (random error), and multivariate analysis to adjust for the effects of multiple predictor variables. More importantly, bias should be minimized by protocol-driven data collection using valid and reliable outcome measures. *External validity* exists when the study results are credible for subjects outside the study. Consecutive or systematic samples that are representative of the target population ensure this goal is achieved.

A good outcomes study uses outcome measures that are valid and reliable. For example, the following steps are necessary to construct a quality of life measure: (a) select the items, (b) choose response options, (c) determine reproducibility, (d) determine validity, and (e) determine responsiveness (15). These issues are discussed later in greater detail, but for now let it suffice to say that good outcomes measures rarely arise by divine providence. At a bare minimum the measure should make sense (face validity), should be approved by expert clinicians (content validity), should be reproducible (test-retest validity), and should measure what it is supposed to measure (construct validity). Finally, if the survey is used to measure clinical change, it must be capable of detecting differences when they occur (responsiveness to longitudinal change).

A bad or ugly outcomes study ignores the laws of statistical and epidemiologic gravity (if you missed these laws, reread the two preceding sections). These studies lack control or comparison groups, are conducted without a specific protocol, and often rely on biased data that were not collected in a systematic fashion (e.g., chart review or administrative databases). Patients are selected using judgmental or convenience samples. Outcome measures are limited to simple surveys or questionnaires of unknown validity and reliability. Follow-up is sporadic and incomplete, with low response rates. Comparative statements are made without statistical tests for association or correlation to control for random error. Conclusions tend to reflect the *a priori* biases of the investigators, and are not supported by the data.

Although most readers are comfortable with patient-based outcomes studies, interpreting a records-based or process-based article can be extremely frustrating. Fortunately, several interpretive guides have been published. Readers who are not easily intimidated are invited to peruse the series of "how to" articles written by the Evidence-Based Medicine Working Group on using a metaanalyses (overviews) (16), decision analyses (17), clinical practice guidelines (18), and reports of small-area variations in the outcomes of health services (19).

PEARLS AND PERILS

1. Most outcomes studies use observational data collected during routine patient care, not specifically for research. Consequently, they are prone to biases that randomization avoids including allocation bias, detection bias, transfer bias, and sampling bias.
2. Outcomes studies without a control or comparison group provide descriptive data only; no statements can be made about effectiveness, regardless of how encouraging the results appear.
3. The same laws of statistical gravity apply to outcomes research that apply to all other medical data: random error, uncertainty, and sampling problems. Check for 95% confidence intervals, p values, and representative sampling schemes.
4. Patient-based outcomes studies are nothing more than cohort studies with a quality of life twist. Adjustments must be made for baseline covariates, comorbidity, unequal periods of follow-up, and patients who drop out or are lost to follow-up.
5. Records-based outcomes studies are limited by the quality and completeness of the source material, which was originally collected for administrative (not clinical) reasons. Important clinical covariates may not be recorded, creating biased and misleading results.
6. Outcomes studies of process are always dynamic. Resulting recommendations and guidelines are subject to constant revision as new studies are published.

OUTCOMES RESEARCH AND PEDIATRIC OTOLARYNGOLOGY

This section presents an overview of outcomes research efforts in pediatric otolaryngology. No attempt is made to provide a systematic review of all published studies. Rather, examples are selected to illustrate the virtues, limitations, and embryonic nature of outcomes efforts to date (July 1996). For consistency with the AAO-HNS grant application guidelines, the section is divided into patient-based studies, record-based studies, and studies of process assessment.

Patient-Based Outcomes Research

No large-scale patient-based outcomes research projects have been published in pediatric otolaryngology, nor has the AHCPR funded any PORTs in this area. The AAO-HNS has placed a high priority on effectiveness research, with plans for large-scale studies of otitis media and pediatric sinusitis. A pilot study of outcomes in pediatric rhinosinusitis has been reported (20), the results of which are summarized below.

A cohort study of 41 consecutive children with chronic or recurrent sinusitis, without obstructive adenoid hyperplasia, concluded that a stepped treatment protocol improved the quality of life for children and caregivers (20). The protocol steps were (a) additional antibiotics, (b) adenoidectomy, and (c) functional endoscopic sinus surgery (FESS). Outcome was assessed with a sinusitis response survey, which gave equal weight to caregiver expectations (not met, met, or exceeded), quality of life issues (physician visits, restricted activity days, need for antibiotics, etc.), and response of the three most troublesome symptoms to the final intervention (worse, same, better, or cured). The three major symptoms were elicited by asking "If I could wave a magic wand over your child's head and instantly cure three symptoms of sinusitis, which three would you want them to be?"

Two months after *entering* each step, caregiver expectations were met or exceeded for 32% of children treated with antibiotics, 70% children treated with adenoidectomy, and 89% of children treated with FESS. Based on the number of children *staying* at each step, 83% of children reported improvement or cure of all major symptoms at 12 months and 85% of caregivers felt their expectations had been met or exceeded. The final survey scores showed no significant differences among groups. Because this was not an RCT with concurrent treatment arms, this lack of difference did not indicate equivalence between antibiotics, adenoidectomy, and FESS. Rather, it showed that comparable outcomes could be achieved with any of these measures in a stepped management protocol. The data further suggest that additional antibiotics and adenoidectomy should be considered before FESS, even when clinical symptoms of obstructing adenoids are absent.

Let us now scrutinize this study further. Without an untreated comparison group, we cannot rule out chance, natural history, placebo effect, or halo effect as explanations for the favorable outcomes (see Table 3). Therefore, we *can* say that the stepped protocol is effective after 12 months, but we *cannot* say with certainty exactly what components of the protocol (e.g., surgery, physician attention, perceived efficacy of FESS, passage of time) caused this outcome. Allocation bias and detection bias may also be operating (see Table 3), although transfer bias is eliminated by the 100% follow-up rate. Problems also exist with the survey itself, which has unknown validity and reliability. Finally, the small sample induces low precision and may limit generalizability. Despite these limitations, the study does help caregivers and providers gain some perspective on what to expect from a stepped treatment protocol in routine clinical care.

An interesting mix of outcomes research and basic science is demonstrated in a study by Lee and Rosenfeld (21). The authors hypothesized that the adenoid may serve as a reservoir for bacterial pathogens that cause sinonasal symptoms. A quality of life questionnaire was given to 84 caregivers of children undergoing adenoidectomy, with seven-point questions to assess the frequency and severity of sinonasal infectious symptoms, ear infection symptoms, and nasal obstructive symptoms over the preceding 6 months. Responses for the "how often" (frequency) questions and "how much" (severity) questions were multiplied to produce a symptom impact score from 1 to 49 for each symptom domain. Good validity was demonstrated. Multivariate analysis showed that 48% of the variability in pathogenic bacteria levels within the adenoid core was explained by the sinonasal symptom impact score. Adenoid size (weight) did not correlate with pathogen levels, similar to what has been observed for otitis media.

An active area of patient-based outcomes research in pediatric otolaryngology concerns efforts to develop disease-specific quality of life measures for otitis media, sinusitis, and adenotonsillar disease. A pilot study of 61 children with chronic otitis media compared health-care visits, use of antibiotics, and parental perceptions of hearing and speech problems for the 12 months prior to ventilation tube surgery to the 12 months after surgery (22). Significant decreases were found in total health-care visits, ear-related health-care visits, antibiotic use, and the prevalence of hearing loss. This was an exploratory study, however, that did not produce an outcomes measure for widespread clinical use. Reliable and valid quality of life measures are under development by the American Academy of Pediatrics, the AAO-HNS, as well as independent outcomes researchers.

Record-Based Outcomes Research

A productive area of record-based outcomes research in pediatric otolaryngology has been metaanalysis of RCTs for acute otitis media (AOM) and otitis media with effusion (OME). Metaanalysis is a form of literature review in which the results of studies are *systematically* assembled, appraised, and combined using a predefined protocol to reduce bias and subjectivity. The emphasis is often on numbers over narrative, in order to increase statistical power and to improve estimates of effect size—an index of how much difference exists between two groups. A traditional literature review emphasizes narrative, with strengths and weaknesses of individual studies discussed selectively and informally by one or more experts. Varying degrees of credibility result, because of potential bias in selecting source articles. The differences between narrative reviews and metaanalyses are summarized in Table 6.

Metaanalysis has helped define what to expect from medical treatment of otitis media, based on the more than 200 clinical trials already published (23). A consistent finding has been the relatively modest impact of antibiotics on clinical control (Table 7). Expectations must reflect the need to treat about seven children on average to improve one, above and beyond what would occur from natural history alone. Further, natural history (spontaneous resolution) is a formidable opponent: About 80% of AOM resolves with placebo "treatment," and recurrent AOM decreases by 1.5 to 3.0 annual episodes with placebo "prophylaxis." Note that the questions addressed in the first column of Table 7 are more meaningful and complex than the usual way of summarizing RCTs by statistical significance alone.

Studies of cost-effectiveness and decision analysis often begin where metaanalysis ends. The "bottom-line" efficacy estimates derived in the metaanalysis are combined under various clinical scenarios to determine which offers the highest probability of a successful outcome. For example, Berman et al. (24) determined the most cost-effective treatment for persistent OME to be corticosteroid plus an antibiotic 6 weeks after diagnosis of AOM. The average reader is unlikely to contest this conclusion after trying to decipher the 11 dense numeric tables in the article. Unfortunately, the 16 efficacy estimates in the decision tree are biased and imprecise and make several unproven assumptions for intervention combinations with no published data. The 11 tables, therefore, suffer from the garbage-in garbage-out phenomenon, to which many well-intentioned cost-effectiveness studies succumb. Further, the study occurs in a clinical vacuum, with no discussion of steroid risks, such as behavioral changes, immune suppression, flare-ups of AOM, and disseminated varicella infection.

TABLE 6: Comparison of Narrative (Traditional) Reviews and Metaanalyses

	Narrative Review	Metaanalysis
Research design	Free form	A priori protocol
Literature search	Convenience sample	Systematic sample
Focus	Broad; summarizes a large body of information	Narrow; tests one or two specific hypotheses
Emphasis	Narrative	Numbers
Validity	Variable; high potential for bias in article selection	Good, provided articles are of adequate quality and combinability
Bottom line	Broad recommendations, often based on personal opinion	Estimates of effect size, based on statistical pooling of data
Utility	Provides quick overview of a subject area	Provides summary estimates for decision analysis, cost-effectiveness studies, and practice guidelines

TABLE 7: Implications of Metaanalysis for the Treatment of Otitis Media

Question	Antibiotic Therapy of OME	Steroid Therapy of OME	Antibiotic Therapy of AOM	Prophylaxis of Recurrent AOM
1. Is the result statistically significant?	Yes; confirmed by 3 independent meta analyses	No; low statistical power	Yes; publication bias is unlikely	Yes; publication bias is unlikely
2. What occurs in control group? (natural history)	15%–30% resolution of OME in all affected ears	15%–30% resolution of OME in all affected ears	70%–90% resolution of AOM symptoms, excluding effusion	1.5–3.0 decrease in annual AOM episodes
3. What are the benefits of therapy?	14% increase in short-term control	20%–30% *potential* increase in short-term control	14% increase in clinical control after 7–14	Prevention of 1.5 AOM episodes per year of prophylaxis
4. What data are available on subgroups?	No apparent differences in comparative drug efficacy	Steroid-antibiotic is most likely better than steroid alone	No differences in comparative efficacy in 9 subgroup analyses	Trend toward higher efficacy with sulfisoxazole vs other drugs
5. To whom do the results best apply?	Children not recently treated with antibiotics	Children not recently treated with antibiotics	Children receiving initial empiric therapy for simple AOM	Children with 3 AOM episodes in 6 mo, 4 in 12 mo, or 5 total
6. What are the clinical implications?	Must treat about 7 children to improve 1; therapy is optional	Casual use of steroids is not justified; may benefit selected children	Must treat about 7 children to improve 1; risk of mastoiditis if untreated	Must treat 1 child for 9 mo to prevent 1 episode; risk of accelerated bacterial resistance

AOM, acute otitis media; OME, otitis media with effusion.

A widespread clinical practice that has its roots in records-based outcomes research is the mandatory second opinion for tonsillectomy required by many insurance carriers. After Wennberg et al. (25) reported in 1969 that Vermont hospital service areas had a 13-fold difference in tonsillectomy rates, the State Medical Society and local physicians adopted a second opinion procedure. Four years later, the average rate for all areas had declined 46% and most of the prior small-area variations were eliminated. Small-area variations in tonsillectomy rates are not confined to the United States; similar trends occur in England and Norway (26). Differences among physicians in either their diagnostic style or their belief in efficacy of tonsillectomy are believed responsible for the observed variance. The largest small-area variations generally occur for elective procedures with controversial indications, providing inspiration to writers of record-based outcomes studies.

Process Assessment

A notable example of process assessment is the clinical practice guideline on OME released by the AHCPR in 1994 (27). Clinical guideline development is a major emphasis of recent health policy efforts, driven by economic pressures and a desire to achieve a baseline level of practice in clinical settings. Guideline development is an explicit process, based on highly organized and critical review of the literature, extraction of raw data from primary research sources, and data review by a multidisciplinary panel of experts. Of the 3,600 OME articles identified for initial study, 1,200 were selected for comprehensive review, and 250 were considered appropriate for evidence gathering. The final guideline required several years of sustained effort to produce, cost approximately one million dollars, and was scrutinized by nearly 100 expert peer reviewers before publication.

The target population for the OME guideline is a child age 1 through 3 years who is otherwise healthy except for OME, and has no craniofacial, neurologic, or sensory deficits. Pneumatic otoscopy was endorsed as the preferred method for detecting OME, and a hearing evaluation was recommended when bilateral effusions persist for 3 months. Antibiotics were considered *optional* therapy, because of the minimal impact on resolution seen in metaanalysis (see Table 7). Antihistamine and decongestant preparations were found ineffective, and oral steroids were not recommended based on limited scientific evidence and panel majority opinion. Insertion of tympanostomy tubes was *recommended* for bilateral OME lasting at least 4 months with an associated hearing loss (20-decibel hearing threshold level or worse in the better hearing ear), but were *optional* at 3 months. Adenoidectomy was a clinical option for children age 4 years or older, but tonsillectomy was not recommended at any age for control of OME.

Although the OME guideline is imperfect, it is the most systematic, readable, and clinically relevant overview of the OME literature available. Criticisms raised reflect more the inherent uncertainty of the primary data, not the integrity of the guidelines process. Guidelines are an imperfect way of coping with imperfect data. Readers may debate whether a cutoff of 20 decibels is appropriate for "normal" hearing, whether oral steroids may or may not benefit selected children, and whether children younger than 4 years derive any benefit from adenoidectomy for OME. What is not debatable, however, is the lack of definitive research to support one opinion over the other. The strength of guideline development lies as much in its ability to identify holes in our knowledge base, as in its ability to define rational—and irrational—treatment paradigms.

A delightful example of process assessment run amuck is the attempt by Kleinman et al. (28) to assess the appropriateness of tympanostomy tube insertion. After studying a utilization review database for three private insurers, the authors concluded that with "generous clinical assumptions," surgical recommendations were appropriate for 41% of children, equivocal for 32%, and inappropriate for 27%. Not surprisingly, the sensational results received widespread attention in the lay press despite numerous methodologic flaws in study design. Unfortunately these flaws readily escaped the casual reader who was bombarded with terminology such as "expert panel," "two-round modified Delphi method," and "smart-logic branching algorithms" as an assurance of validity.

Scrutiny of the proprietary criteria cited by Kleinman et al to judge appropriateness showed them to be inconsistent and biased. For example, a child with OME for 120 days and untested hearing is an "equivocal" surgical candidate, but becomes "appropriate" after an audiogram is performed, regardless of whether the results are normal or abnormal. What is being assessed here is the presence or absence of an audiogram, not the appropriateness of surgery. Further, a child with hearing loss is an "equivocal" surgical candidate when OME lasts 91 to 120 days, but paradoxically becomes "inappropriate" when the effusion lasts longer. Surgery was also "inappropriate" when no antibiotics were prescribed beyond those for AOM, in spite of the AHCPR conclusion that antibiotics are a clinical option, not a mandate (or even a recommendation) before surgery. Finally, tube insertion was never judged appropriate for *recurrent* AOM—even after breakthrough infections while on antibiotics—despite several RCTs showing efficacy that matched or exceeded the efficacy of antimicrobial prophylaxis.

The most serious problems with this appropriateness study, however, is that the authors did not compare the utilization review process with a gold standard, and hence the sensitivity and specificity are unknown. Some tape-recorded conversations were reviewed for validity, but the reviewer was the lead author of the article, a prior paid consultant for the insurance firm, and someone who is obviously biased against surgery by the negative editorial tone of the article. A meaningful gold standard would incorporate information from physician- or patient-initiated appeals, second opinions by impartial physicians (who actually examined the child), and direct interviews of caregivers and their children. Not only was this information not sought, it was never even determined if the proposed surgeries were performed.

This article study (28) was elaborated on to illustrate what happens when outcomes research is initiated by insurance companies seeking to cut costs, rather than by concerned physicians seeking to increase effectiveness. What can the critical reader conclude from the Kleinman article? That when data are collected with a utilization review process of unknown sensitivity and specificity, and judged for appropriateness against biased and inconsistent criteria, a lot of surgical recommendations appear inappropriate or equivocal. So much for "appropriateness" research.

Simple studies of process assessment can be performed easily during routine clinical care. For example, Rosenfeld and Sandhu (29) determined the prevalence of injury counseling opportunities in children referred to a pediatric otolaryngologist by surveying caregivers as part of office registration. A random sample of 300 surveys stratified by age showed that the hottest water temperature was unknown by 72% of caregivers, smokers were present in 25% of households, bicycle helmets were not used by 22% of children, car seats or seat belts were not used by 11% of children, and 10% of homes did not have working smoke alarms. Although 98% of caregivers had a regular pediatrician, 91% of families still offered one or more counseling opportunities. This suggests substantial opportunities for surgical specialists to reinforce the prevention foundation laid by primary-care physicians.

USING QUALITY-OF-LIFE MEASURES TO ENHANCE CLINICAL PRACTICE

Physicians can participate in the outcomes movement by using quality-of-life measures in their everyday practice. As noted previously, quality of life reflects the patient's subjective perception of health status. When quality of life improves after physician contact, all stakeholders in the health-care process are more likely to view the situation favorably. In the absence of physician-generated effectiveness data, process-based studies (like the Kleinman fiasco just described) will be the only source of outcomes "data" to judge the medical profession.

Outcomes research is more interested in health-related quality of life (HRQL) than in overall, or general, quality of life. HRQL excludes other widely valued aspects of life that are not typically considered as "health," including income, freedom, and quality of the environment. Although these aspects are important, they are rarely affected by health interventions. In contrast, a HRQL survey focuses on the physical, social, and emotional impact of disease on the individual. Most surveys are self-administered questionnaires, composed of *items* or questions grouped into *domains* that reflect a particular focus of attention. The focus of an HRQL instrument may be generic or disease specific. Generic measures are of particular interest to policy makers; disease-specific measures are of particular interest to patients and clinicians.

This section shows clinicians how to develop, validate, and use a disease-specific HRQL survey in their routine practice. For the remainder of this section, the term *quality-of-life survey* is used for simplicity instead of *disease-specific HRQL survey*. Even if you never design your own survey, you will benefit from a little insight into what makes a good survey good and a bad survey bad. Although the approach is purposefully simplistic, curious readers will find more in-depth information in the numerous articles (15,30) and books (31,32) published on survey development.

Crash Course in Survey Design

A quality-of-life survey is judged by its purpose, reliability, validity, and responsiveness (Table 8). When the purpose of the survey is to evaluate change over time (e.g., effectiveness), the instrument is called an *evaluative* measure. Surveys may also be designed to predict prognosis or to discriminate among individuals with different levels of disease (15). Because effectiveness research is of great interest to physicians, the focus in this section is on evaluative measures.

TABLE 8: Comparison of Discriminative, Predictive, and Evaluative Surveys

	Discriminative Survey	Predictive Survey	Evaluative Survey
Purpose	Discriminates among individuals along a continuum of illness	Predicts outcome or prognosis	Evaluates within-person change over time in effectiveness studies
Content	Emphasizes aspects of the domain that are stable over time	Emphasizes items that correlate well with a gold standard measure	Emphasizes aspects of the domain that respond to clinically significant change
Reliability	Requires good internal consistency and test-retest reproducibility	Requires good internal consistency and test-retest reproducibility	Requires good test-retest reproducibility; internal consistency less important
Validity	Degree to which the survey measures what it is supposed to measure	Degree to which survey results correlate with a gold standard measure	Degree to which the survey measures what it is supposed to measure
Responsiveness	Not applicable	Not applicable	Ability of the survey to detect a clinical difference when one is present

To understand why a survey must be tested before it is used, consider a simple "effectiveness" question asked 1 year after endoscopic sinus surgery: "Knowing what you now know, would you still have had the surgery and would you recommend it to a friend or relative?" When 85% of telephone contacts respond "yes," the investigators report resounding success. But how certain are we that these subjects would respond the same if asked 2 weeks later (test-retest reliability) or if asked by an impartial observer (interobserver reliability)? Further, does the question truly measure effectiveness (validity), or might it reflect natural history, placebo effect, or simply catching the subject on a good day (chance). A "yes" answer might also be caused by the inherent tendency of most people to respond positively (acquiescence bias), by satisfaction with the surgeon independent of the procedure (halo bias), or by the tone in which the question was stated (framing bias). Finally, we do not know what degree of clinical change—if any—is implied by a "yes" answer (responsiveness).

Reliability refers to the stability or reproducibility of a survey result. Recall from our crash course on statistics that all measurements possess some degree of unavoidable random error. Survey results are no exception. We are more likely to discount random error when a self-administered survey shows similar results at two time points for a subject with stable disease (test-retest reliability), or when an oral survey is administered twice by the same interviewer (interobserver reliability) or by different interviewers (intraobserver reliability). A survey must have a *test-retest coefficient of at least 0.70* before it can be recommended for clinical use (a coefficient of 1.00 indicates perfect reliability). This usually requires testing at least 80 subjects to achieve a precision of ± 0.05 (95% confidence interval).

Another form of reliability often mentioned for surveys is *internal consistency*. When measuring a trait, behavior, or symptom, we usually want the scale to be homogeneous—all of the items should be tapping different aspects of the same attribute. If we are measuring the emotional impact of chronic sinusitis on a child, then each item should relate to emotional impact (e.g., irritability, frustration, embarrassment). Therefore, the items should be moderately correlated with each other, as well as the total score for the emotional impact domain omitting that item. Items with Pearson correlation scores less than 0.20 should be discarded or rewritten. A frequently encountered measure of internal consistency is Cronbach's alpha, which should be between 0.70 and 0.90 (higher values suggest redundancy).

Validity refers to how well the survey is measuring what we think (or hope) it is. Validation is actually a process of hypothesis testing, in which we seek correlations between survey items or results and external measures of similar properties (e.g., a gold standard test or a previously validated survey). For example, we are most likely to believe results of a pain question on a sinusitis survey if the response correlates with radiographic disease or with a pain subscale on a general quality of life measure like the SF-36. Similarly, a question on hearing loss should correlate with audiogram results. Correlation coefficients (r) need not be large, but should be about 0.20 to 0.50. Although statisticians have described a veritable grab bag of validity subtypes (construct validity, criterion validity, etc.), the distinctions are subsidiary to the basic principles already noted.

Responsiveness is the ability of a survey to detect change in a patient's condition. An evaluative measure is typically administered before *and* after some intervention of interest, and the difference in scores is noted. The larger this *change score*, the larger the degree of clinical change, regardless of whether the intervention was watchful waiting, an educational program, or medical or surgical treatment.

An astute reader may wonder, "Why bother with change scores? Why not simply ask people how much they have changed?" Although this is a time-honored approach, people simply do not remember how they were at the beginning. People tend to systematically overestimate their initial symptoms, creating exaggerated effectiveness results. Additional bias occurs because retrospective estimates of initial state are highly correlated with the present state, not the true initial state. Consequently, change should not be assessed directly, but indirectly with change scores.

Creating a Simple Survey for Pediatric Use

Surveys developed for adults will rarely—if ever—be useful for children. Assessing a child's quality of life poses immediate problems that are not present with adult measures (33). Developmental change makes it difficult to apply any single measure to all age groups, particularly in the preschool years when change is rapid. Further, parents and professionals often differ substantially in their definition and perception of child well-being. Moreover, children's self-reports of functional status and those of parents do not always correlate. Children in grades 6 to 8 have been able to complete self-administered surveys with assistance, but younger children must be assessed through the response of their caregivers.

Disease-specific HRQL outcome surveys are essentially nonexistent for common disorders such as otitis media, sinusitis, adenotonsillitis, and obstructive sleep apnea syndrome. Clinicians involved in the care of such children are ideally positioned to create new instruments. Innovation is easy when the existing terrain is barren. Enthusiasm, however, must be tempered by the principles of survey design enumerated in the preceding section. An evaluative survey not only must look good and make sense, but also must have a known amount of reliability, validity, and responsiveness. The remainder of this section illustrates this process by showing how to develop a disease-specific HRQL survey for otitis media.

The first step in creating a disease-specific outcomes survey is to define the domains and items (questions) of interest. For example, the Otitis Media Impact Survey (OM-6) in Figure 1 consists of six items representing the domains of physical suffering, hearing loss, speech impairment, emotional distress, activity limitations, and caregiver concerns. Each domain has only a single item, although multiple related items could also have been used. Item content is determined by caregiver interviews, consensus among health providers (physicians, audiologists, etc.), and expert review. Ideally the items are unambiguous, ask only a single question, and are comprehensible to the target population (see Table 4). The target population for the OM-6 is children age 6 months or older with

OTITIS MEDIA IMPACT SURVEY

Instructions: Please help us understand the impact of ear infections or fluid on your child's quality of life by checking one box [x] for each question below. Thank you.

PHYSICAL SUFFERING: Ear pain, ear discomfort, ear discharge, ruptured ear drum, high fever, or poor balance. How much of a problem for your child during the past 4 weeks?

[ ] Not present/no problem   [ ] Hardly a problem at all   [ ] Quite a bit of a problem
                                [ ] Somewhat of a problem   [ ] Very much a problem
                                [ ] Moderate problem   [ ] Extreme problem

HEARING LOSS: Difficulty hearing, questions must be repeated, frequently says "what," or television is excessively loud. How much of a problem for your child during the past 4 weeks?

[ ] Not present/no problem   [ ] Hardly a problem at all   [ ] Quite a bit of a problem
                                [ ] Somewhat of a problem   [ ] Very much a problem
                                [ ] Moderate problem   [ ] Extreme problem

SPEECH IMPAIRMENT: Delayed speech, poor pronunciation, difficult to understand, or unable to repeat words clearly. How much of a problem for your child during the past 4 weeks?

[ ] Not present/no problem   [ ] Hardly a problem at all   [ ] Quite a bit of a problem
     (or not applicable)   [ ] Somewhat of a problem   [ ] Very much a problem
                                [ ] Moderate problem   [ ] Extreme problem

EMOTIONAL DISTRESS: Irritable, frustrated, sad, restless, or poor appetite. How much of a problem for your child during the past 4 weeks as a result of ear infections or fluid?

[ ] Not present/no problem   [ ] Hardly a problem at all   [ ] Quite a bit of a problem
                                [ ] Somewhat of a problem   [ ] Very much a problem
                                [ ] Moderate problem   [ ] Extreme problem

ACTIVITY LIMITATIONS: Playing, sleeping, doing things with friends/family, attending school or day care. How limited have your child's activities been during the past 4 weeks because of ear infections or fluid?

[ ] Not limited at all   [ ] Hardly limited at all   [ ] Moderately limited
                                [ ] Very slightly limited   [ ] Very limited
                                [ ] Slightly limited   [ ] Severely limited

CAREGIVER CONCERNS: How often have you, as a caregiver, been worried, concerned, or inconvenienced because of your child's ear infections or fluid over the past 4 weeks?

[ ] None of the time   [ ] Hardly any time at all   [ ] A good part of the time
                                [ ] A small part of the time   [ ] Most of the time
                                [ ] Some of the time   [ ] All of the time

OVERALL, HOW WOULD YOU RATE YOUR CHILD'S QUALITY OF LIFE AS A RESULT OF EAR INFECTIONS OR FLUID?
(Circle one number)

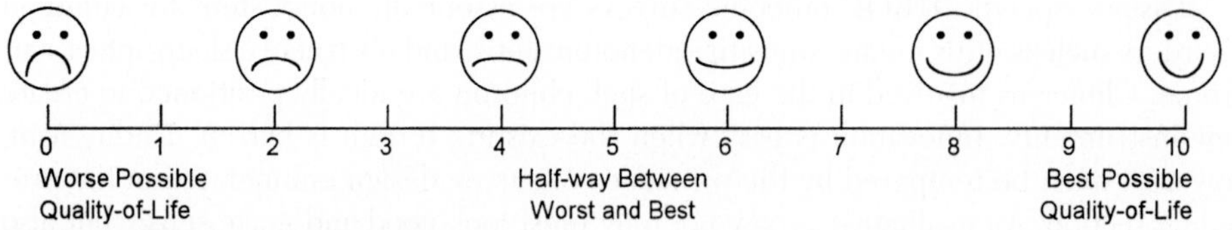

0 1 2 3 4 5 6 7 8 9 10
Worse Possible   Half-way Between   Best Possible
Quality-of-Life   Worst and Best   Quality-of-Life

FIGURE 1 Example of a disease-specific quality-of-life measure for evaluating longitudinal change in outcomes studies of treatment effectiveness.

chronic OME (3 months or longer) or recurrent AOM (3 or more episodes in the past 12 months).

Having defined the items, the next step is to specify the measurement scale for the response. A response scale with seven categories is an efficient way to measure change (34). With a seven-point scale, a change score of 0.5 indicates minimal clinical change, 1.0 suggests moderate change, and 1.5 is consistent with large change. When fewer than five levels are used, reliability and efficiency decrease dramatically. Examples of seven-point Likert scales are shown in the OM-6 (see Fig. 1). Likert scales permit a discrete number of continuous responses that are framed on an agree-disagree continuum. At the bottom of the figure is a global ear-related quality of life question, which is scored using a ten-point visual analog scale (35). Although this survey includes only a global disease-specific question, some investigators recommend that all instruments contain two global ratings: one for overall quality of life and one for health-related issues (36).

The pilot version of the survey should be tested on a small group of representative patients. If it takes too long to complete, or appears too confusing, it must be rewritten. For each question the frequency of the individual responses should be tallied. Responses chosen less than 20% of the time, or more than 80% of the time, must be reassessed. Similarly, if certain questions routinely get a minimal response level, they should be replaced. A final aspect of the pilot test is to check for internal consistency as described earlier.

When the final version of the survey is ready for testing, thought must be given as to what other data will be collected concurrently for validation. For example, a quality of life survey for sinusitis should show some moderate correlation with results of intranasal examination and staging by computed tomography. An otitis media survey should correlated with middle-ear status, otoscopy results, and prior disease burden (antibiotic use and physician visits). The specifics will vary according to the survey purpose, but the basic principle is to show that the survey behaves the way it should, correlating items and domains with appropriate external measures. Another approach is to administer a previously validated general quality of life measure, and to compare survey findings with appropriate subscale values on the general measure. During the validation process a subset of patients with stable disease should complete a second survey *within 2 to 14 days* to determine test-retest reliability.

As an example of survey validation, a presentation of the preliminary results on 186 patients who received the OM-6, 80 of whom were retested for reliability, follows (37). Adequate test-retest reliability was obtained both for the survey score ($r = 0.87$) and the quality-of-life rating ($r = 0.85$). Internal consistency was shown for the related domains of speech impairment versus hearing loss ($r = 0.37$, $p < 0.001$) and activity limitations versus physical suffering ($r = 0.48$, $p < 0.001$). Validity was shown by significant correlations ($p = 0.002$) between middle-ear status (by algorithm) with both the survey score and the caregiver estimate of hearing loss. Significant correlations ($p < 0.001$) were also observed between survey score and quality-of-life rating ($r = 0.64$), doctor's visits past month and physical symptoms ($r = 0.47$), and antibiotics past months and caregiver concerns ($r = 0.26$).

The final aspect of testing an evaluative survey—and perhaps the most important—is to demonstrate responsiveness to change. An easy method to assess responsiveness is to have both the patient and physician independently estimate the perceived degree of clinical change on a seven-point scale, using positive values for improvement and negative values for deterioration. The survey change score (difference between preintervention and postintervention results) is then tested for correlation with the perceived change levels. An alternative way is to calculate the *standardized response mean* (SRM) by dividing the mean change score by its standard deviation (38). Values less than 0.2 denote insensitive instruments, and values more than 0.8 indicate large sensitivity. For the OM-6 the change score showed good correlation with the degree of reported change ($r = 0.66$, $p < 0.001$) and the SRM after tympanostomy tube insertion was 1.7. These preliminary results suggest good responsiveness to longitudinal change.

There is no right or wrong way to design an evaluative survey. The principles and practices outlined should help guide the motivated reader. Using outcomes measures in your practice not only will help demonstrate the effectiveness of the care you provide, but also will give greater insight into the way common disorders impact your patients' lives. The more that patients perceive physician interest in their quality of life, the more enthusiastic they will be about completing outcomes surveys in the office setting.

PEARLS AND PERILS

1. Keep it simple. A beautifully crafted, reliable, valid, and responsive survey is of little use if it is too cumbersome for seamless integration into routine clinical care.
2. Choose questions that fully reflect the diverse physical, emotional, and social impact of the disorder on children and their caregivers. Focus on items likely to change with treatment.
3. Use a seven-point response scale to measure change; scales with fewer than five options or more than ten options are not recommended.
4. A survey needs more than good looks and common sense; it must be tested for reliability and validity. Determining test-retest reliability is particularly important.
5. Retrospective patient estimates of change are prone to numerous biases; measure change by the difference in survey scores before and after the intervention of interest.
6. Survey findings are subject to the same uncertainty as all medical data; 95% confidence intervals are required to show the range of results consistent with the data

---

CONCLUSIONS

This chapter provided an overview of outcomes research, its virtues and limitations, and its potential impact on practicing physicians. Several points deserve reemphasis. Outcomes research is nothing new; it simply places a quality of life twist on old-fashioned cohort studies. As an observational endeavor, however, outcomes studies are subject to all of the biases and distortions that randomized studies so beautifully prevent. Records-based studies and studies of process assessment face the added problem of garbage-in, garbage-out. Because these studies rely on data collected for routine patient care or for administrative purposes, important clinical information related to decision making, prognosis, or outcome is often absent.

Outcomes research and randomized trials are synergistic. There is a need for both the realism of experimental studies and the empiricism of personal experience. Outcomes studies are simply a means for systematically recording and interpreting personal experience. As noted by the United States physician Alvan Barach, we must "remember to cure the patient as well as the disease." Randomized trials focus on disease, but outcomes studies emphasize patients and their subjective perceptions of health status. As Tanenbaum (6) so astutely noted, outcomes research is not "… a new foundation for clinical medicine; it is raw material for the artful practitioner."

By systematically recording their own clinical experience, practicing physicians can participate proactively in the outcomes movement. Satisfaction surveys and quality of life measures can be easily incorporated into most routine clinical encounters. Given the existing void of physician-collected outcomes data, almost any effort is likely to produce new and useful data. As health-care providers we cannot afford to delegate responsibility for monitoring effectiveness to insurers and governmental agencies, whose overriding objectives are to manage cost—not to improve patient care.

REFERENCES

1. Picirillo JR. Outcomes research and otolaryngology. *Otolaryngol Head Neck Surg* 1994;111: 764–769.
2. Ellwood PM. Outcomes management: a technology of patient experience. *N Engl J Med* 1988; 318:1549–1556.

3. Guadagnoli E, McNeil BJ. Outcomes research: hope for the future or the latest rage? *Inquiry* 1994;31:14–24.

4. Maklan CW, Greene R, Cummings MA. Methodological challenges and innovations in patient outcomes research. *Med Care* 1994; 32[Suppl]: JS13–JS21.

5. Last JM, ed. *A dictionary of epidemiology*, 3rd ed. New York: Oxford University Press, 1995.

6. Tanenbaum SJ. Knowing and acting in medical practice: the epistemological politics of outcomes research. *J Health Polit Policy Law* 1994;19:27–44.

7. Moses LE. The series of consecutive cases as a device for assessing outcome of intervention. *N Engl J Med* 1984;311:705–710.

8. Turner JA, Deyo RA, Loeser JD, Von Korff M, Fordyce WE. The importance of placebo effects in pain treatment and research. *JAMA* 1994;271:1609–1614.

9. Feinstein AR. Fraud, distortion, delusion, and consensus: the problems of human and natural deception in epidemiologic science. *Am J Med* 1988;84:475–478.

10. Feinstein AR. Epidemiologic analyses of causation: the unlearned scientific lessons of randomized trials. *J Clin Epidemiol* 1989;42:481–489.

11. Gardner MJ, Altman DG. Confidence intervals rather than p values: estimation rather than hypothesis testing. *BMJ* 1980;292:746–750.

12. Gustafson TL. *TRUE EPISTAT reference manual*. Richardson, TX: Epistat Services, 1994.

13. Mehta C, Patel N. *StatXact: statistical software for exact nonparametric inference*. Cambridge, MA: Cytel Software Corporation, 1991.

14. Katz MH, Hauck WW. Proportional hazards (Cox) regression. *J Gen Intern Med* 1993;8: 702–711.

15. Jaeschke R, Guyatt GH. How to develop and validate a new quality of life instrument. In: Spilker B, ed. *Quality of life assessments in clinical trials*. New York: Raven Press, 1990: 47–57.

16. Oxman AD, Cook DJ, Guyatt GH. Users' guides to the medical literature VI. How to use an overview. *JAMA* 1994;272:1367–1371.

17. Richard WS, Detsky AS. Users' guides to the medical literature VII. How to use a clinical decision analysis. *JAMA* 1995;273:1292–1295, 1610–1613.

18. Hayward RSA, Wilson MC, Tunis SR, et al. Users' guides to the medical literature VIII. How to use clinical practice guidelines. *JAMA* 1995;274:570–574, 1630–1632.

19. Naylor D, Guyatt GH. Users' guides to the medical literature X. How to use an article reporting variations in the outcomes of health services. *JAMA* 1996;275:554–558.

20. Rosenfeld RM. Pilot study of outcomes in pediatric rhinosinusitis. *Arch Otolaryngol Head Neck Surg* 1995;221:729–736.

21. Lee D, Rosenfeld RM. Adenoid bacteriology and sinonasal symptoms in children. *Otolaryngol Head Neck Surg* 1997;116:301–307.

22. Facione N. Quality of life issues in chronic otitis media with effusion: parameters for future study. *Int J Pediatr Otolaryngol* 1991;22:167–179.

23. Rosenfeld RM. What to expect from medical treatment of otitis media. *Pediatr Infect Dis J* 1995;14:731–738.

24. Berman S, Roark R, Luckey D. Theoretical cost effectiveness of management options for children with persisting middle ear effusions. *Pediatrics* 1994;93:353–363.

25. Wennberg JE, Blowers L, Parker R, Gittelsohn AM. Changes in tonsillectomy rates associated with feedback and review. *Pediatrics* 1977;59:821–826.

26. McPherson K, Wennberg JE, Hovind OB, Clifford P. Small-area variations in the use of common surgical procedures: an international comparison of New England, England, and Norway. *N Engl J Med* 1982;307:1310–1314.

27. Stool SE, Berg AO, Berman S, et al. Otitis media with effusion in young children. Clinical practice guideline, no. 12. Rockville, MD: Agency for Health Care Policy and Research, Public Health Service, US Dept. of Health and Human Services; July 1994;94–0622.

28. Kleinman LC, Kosecoff J, Dubois RW, Brook RH. The medical appropriateness of tympanostomy tubes proposed for children younger than 16 years in the United States. *JAMA* 1994; 271:1250–1255.

29. Rosenfeld RM, Sandhu S. Injury prevention counseling opportunities in pediatric otolaryngology. *Arch Otolaryngol Head Neck Surg* 1996;122:609–611.

30. Kessler RC, Mroczek DK. Measuring the effects of medical interventions. *Med Care* 1995; 33[Suppl]: AS109–AS119.

31. Streiner DL, Norman GR. *Health measurement scales: a practical guide to their development and use*, 2nd ed. Oxford: Oxford Medical Publications, 1995.

32. Fink A. *The survey handbook*. Thousand Oaks, CA: SAGE Publications, 1995.
33. Rosenbaum P, Cadman D, Kirpalani H. Pediatrics: assessing quality of life. In: Spilker B, ed. *Quality of life in clinical trials*. New York: Raven Press, 1990;205–215.
34. Juniper EF, Guyatt GH, Willan A, Griffith LE. Determining a minimal important change in a disease-specific quality of life questionnaire. *J Clin Epidemiol* 1994;47:81–87.
35. Hadorn DC, Uebersax J. Large-scale health outcomes evaluation: how should quality of life be measured? Part I—calibration of a brief questionnaire and a search for preference subgroups. *J Clin Epidemiol* 1995;48:5:607–618.
36. Gill TM, Feinstein AR. A critical appraisal of the quality of quality-of-life measurements. *JAMA* 1994;272:619–626.
37. Rosenfeld RM, Goldsmith AJ, Tetlus L, Belzano A. Quality of life for children with otitis media. *Arch Otolaryngol Head Neck Surg* 1997;123:1049–1054.
38. Gliklich RE, Hilinski JM. Longitudinal sensitivity of generic and specific health measures in chronic sinusitis. *Qual Life Res* 1995;4:27–32.

R.M. Rosenfeld: Department of Otolaryngology, SUNY Health Science Center at Brooklyn; Division of Pediatric Otolaryngology, University Hospital of Brooklyn; and Department of Otolaryngology, Long Island College Hospital, Brooklyn, New York 11201.

• *Practical Pediatric Otolaryngology*
• edited by Robin T. Cotton
  and Charles M. Myer, III
• Lippincott-Raven Publishers,
  Philadelphia © 1999

12

Hearing Assessment in Infants and Children

N. Wendell Todd

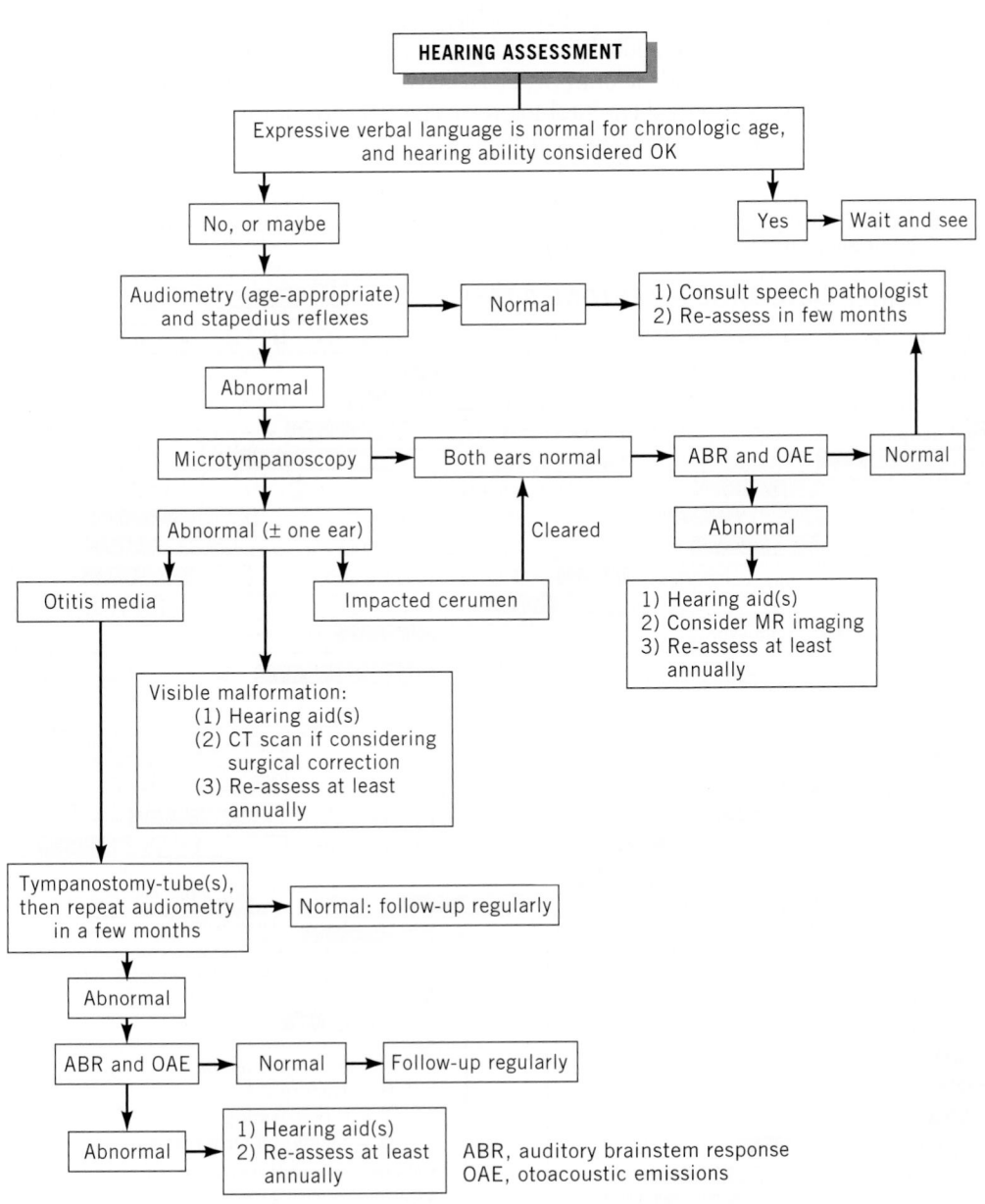

ABR, auditory brainstem response
OAE, otoacoustic emissions

Hearing is assessed to determine if the auditory apparatus functions sufficiently for the child to develop aural–verbal language. The assessment of the efferent limb of aural–verbal communication, i.e., expressive verbal language, is necessary (1,2). That a child has normal (or better, for age) expressive verbal language is itself the best evidence that the child has adequate audition (Fig. 1).

Some practitioners think that the assessment of hearing in infants and small children is impossible. That is incorrect. Nevertheless, the assessment of hearing in infants and small children is difficult and challenging and requires repeated testing—sometimes with quite sophisticated equipment and concomitant professional personnel. The use of a battery of observations and tests, with cross-checking, is necessary.

An aspect of Murphy's law applies here: tests that truly measure auditory communicative input are either of poor sensitivity and specificity (e.g., behavioral observational audiometry), or too sophisticated to use with a child until age 5 years or so (e.g., tests of central auditory processing).

With increasing experience that cochlear implantation can facilitate aural–verbal communication in profoundly hearing impaired patients, the distinction between "sensory" (i.e., cochlear) and "neural" (i.e., VIII nerve and central nervous system) hearing loss is no longer of just theoretical interest. The tools for distingushing cochlear from neural hearing loss are clinically available.

FIGURE 1 Language developmental milestones, illustrated by the Early Language Milestone Scale-2, by Coplan. (From ref. 3, with permission.)

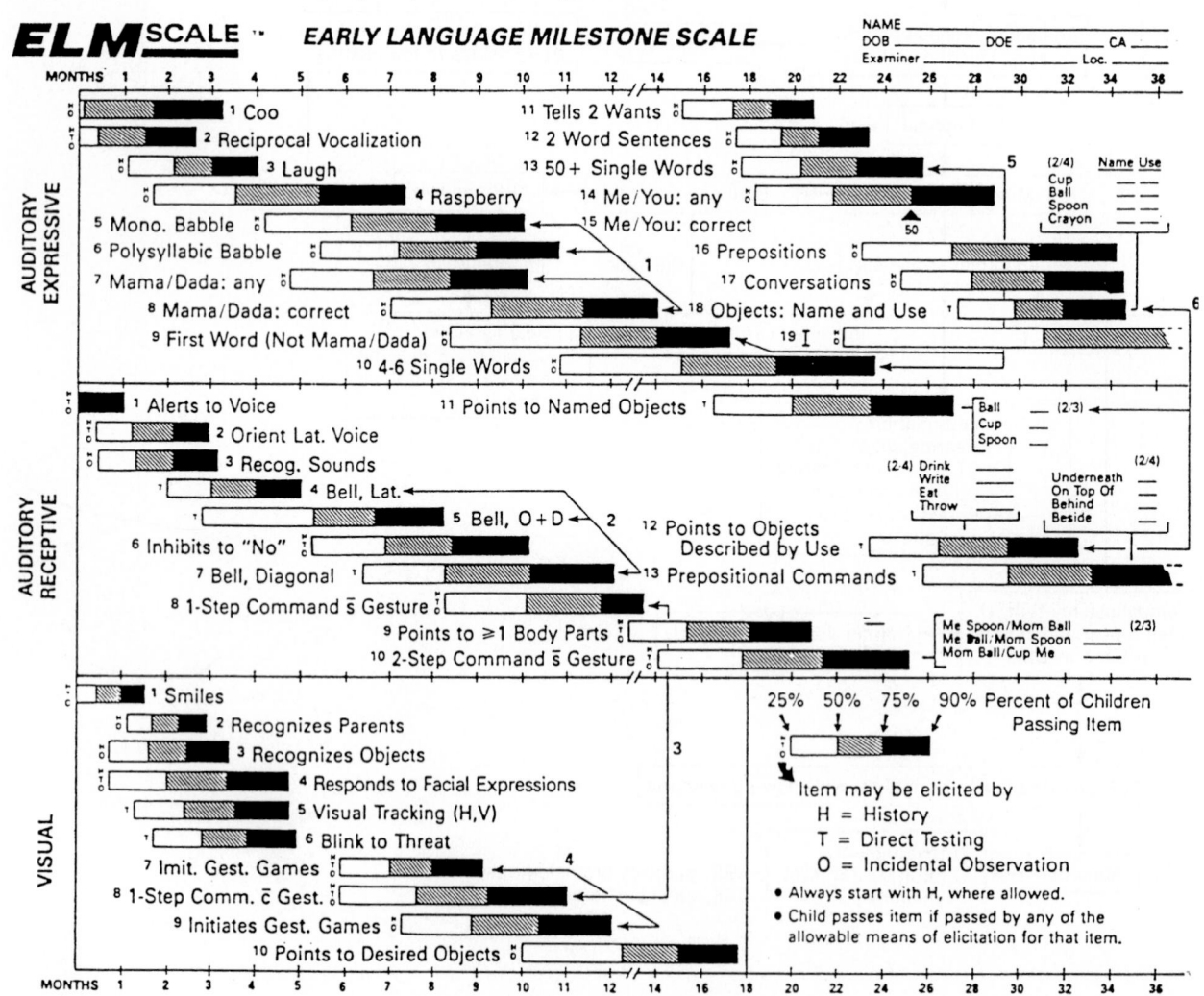

BEHAVIORAL OBSERVATION AUDIOMETRY

Although it is often plagued by high numbers of false-negative and false-positive responses (4,5), behavioral observation audiometry has been demonstrated by astute clinicians to be useful in term gestation babies. Preterm babies are more difficult to assess behaviorally.

The technique appears deceptively simple to the casual spectator. To the unsuspecting baby, a sound is presented sufficiently loud to provoke arousal (generalized body movement), a startle reflex (a jump), or the so-called auropalpebral reflex (i.e., eye blinking by the awake baby, or eyelid tightening by the asleep baby). The stimulus must be auditory only. Low-frequency sounds (those lower than about middle C on a piano, or a distant railroad train) can often be felt, i.e., are tactile stimuli rather than being heard. Visual cues are omitted. For a response to be valid, it must be time related to the stimulus. Stimuli typically used are speech, narrow-band noise, warble tones, or noisemakers. The term threshold is not applicable for behavioral observational auditometry, rather the term *minimal response level* (i.e., the least level of sound stimulus for noting a response) is appropriate (Table 1).

Behavioral observation audiometry offers negligible ear-specific information, rather it offers an estimate of the auditory function of the baby's better hearing ear and also demonstrates that the nervous and skeletal systems work sufficiently well to exhibit a response.

After about age 6 months, children tend to lose interest in repeatedly responding to such sounds—unless something repeatedly tweaks their interest (Table 2).

REINFORCEMENT AUDIOMETRY

In a sound-treated room, the child is positioned between two loudspeakers. The usual stimuli are speech and narrow bands of noise are centered on the octaves of clinical testing (0.25, 0.5, 1, 2, and 4 kHz). Warble tones likewise are centered. Stimuli are presented in alternating ascending and descending intensities, changing the center frequency of the stimulus. If the child's head turns toward the loudspeaker that provided the stimulus, a positive response is noted. To maintain the child's interest in the task of responding to the sound stimuli, an animated mechanical toy is activated (e.g., a dancing

TABLE 1: Expected Sound Intensity Necessary for Unconditioned Responses by Normal Infants

Age (mos)	Noisemaker (dBSPL)	Warbled Pure Tones (dBHL)	Speech (dBHL)	Normal Response	Startle to Speech (dBHL)
1.5–4	55	70	47	Eye widening, shift, or blink; quieting	65
4–7	45	51	21	Head turn toward sound	65
9–13	30	38	8	Direct localization to side and below	65
21–24	25	26	3	Direct localization above and below ear level	65

[a]Both false-negative and false-positive results limit the usefulness of behavioral audiometry in infants. Note that the intensity of the noisemakers is presented in dB sound pressure level. In the so-called speech frequencies (0.5, 1, and 2 kHz), 10 dBSPL is approximately zero dBHL.

(Adapted from ref. 6, with permission.)

TABLE 2: Subjective Response Audiometry: Applicability, Requirements, Responses, and Reliability[a]

Item	Behavioral Observation Audiometry	Reinforcement Audiometry	Play Audiometry	Regular (Adult) Audiometry
Age	<6 months	6–24 months	2–4 years	≥ 5 years
Equipment, environment	Quiet room or sound booth	Sound booth	Sound booth	Sound booth
Stimulus	Rattles, horns; narrow band or warble tones; speech	Speech, warble tones	Speech, pure tones	Speech, pure tones
Delivery	Sound field	Sound field	Headphones	Headphones
Response	"Scare the baby" e.g., eyes blink	Head turnings, reinforced by activating an animated toy	Conditioned tasks, e.g., place a block into a can	Raise hand
Limits of normal (dBHL)	30	20	15	15
Reliability	Poor to fair	Good	Good to excellent	Excellent

[a]Applicable ages are only approximations. The developmental age of the patient should be considered when choosing a test. Note that a larger sound booth is required for reinforcement audiometry than is needed for testing in which the stimulus can be delivered by headphone.

monkey near the speaker that elicited the response (Fig. 2). Another response reinforcement strategy is to provide candy or another tangible prize each time the child makes a specified response to an auditory test stimulus. This technique, termed *tangible reinforced operant conditioning audiometry* is useful for hard-to-test patients of all ages. With such reinforcements, children typically will cooperate enough to allow the determination of minimal response level for several frequencies. Although responses additional to head turning were accepted when visual reinforcement audiometry was initially

FIGURE 2 Setup for visual reinforcement audiometry.

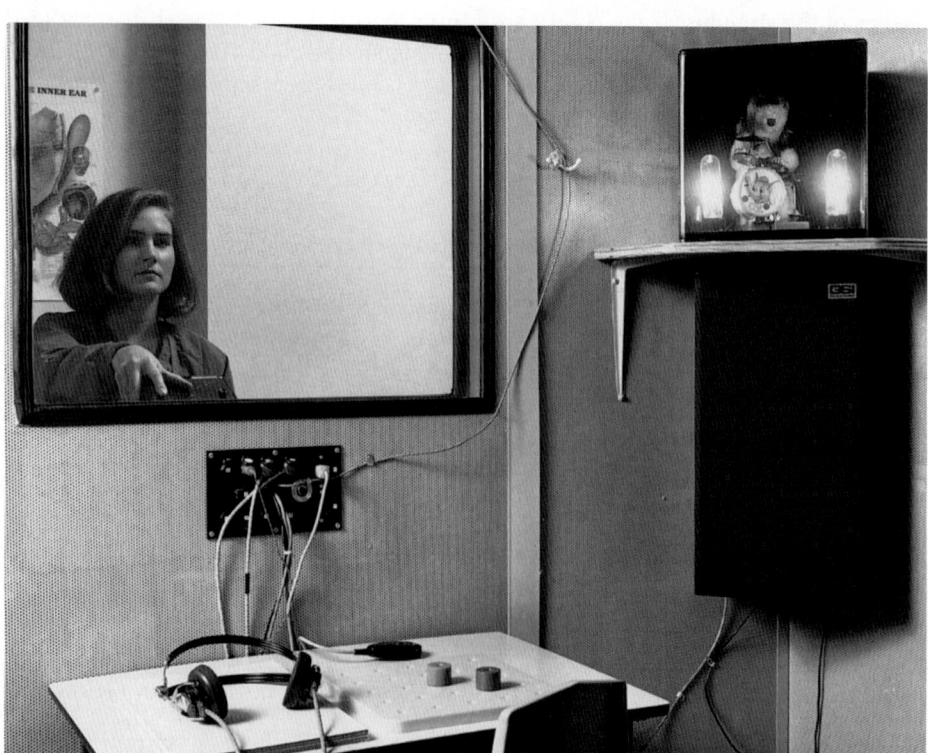

described in 1969, present opinion suggests that the head-turning response is associated with more reliable results.

Reinforcement audiometry, like behavioral response audiometry, has additional limitations. Usually, only scant ear-specific information is obtainable (unless the patient can tolerate insert tubephones). The better ear's thresholds are approximated—the worse ear could have profound hearing loss. Calibration of the sound booth and equipment is problematic. The American National Standards Institute (ANSI) 1996 standard for audiometers gives specific values for warble tones and narrow bands of noise in a sound field (7). The maximum output of the speakers is typically about 80 dBHL (hearing level) and the highest frequency deliverable about 4 kHz.

PEARLS AND PERILS

1. Why calibrate test equipment?
   Calibration is performed to optimize confidence that the measurement is truthful. Equipment must be electroacoustically calibrated to reference standards (provided by ANSI and the International Electrotechnical Commission). Calibration at regular intervals is mandated by a number of professional and regulatory groups (e.g., the American Speech and Hearing Association, the Occupational Safety and Health Act). A daily biologic listening check is good practice. For example, is there background noise (e.g., hum, static) in the headphone? Are the pure tones clear in quality? (Table 3).

2. What is the cross-check principle?
   The cross-check principle involves checking a synthesis of a patient's data for meaningful interpretation. Does the information "add up"? Does the information make sense? For example, −8 to +6 dB is the acceptable range for the speech reception threshold (SRT) to jibe with the average of thresholds for pure tones of 0.5, 1, and 2 kHz (Table 4). Another example: there is an inconsistency if a patient can converse with you at typical conversational loudness, but has bilateral voluntary pure tone thresholds of 60 dBHL from 0.5 through 4 kHz (Table 5). In normal infants, the threshold for wave V elicited by clicks, whose energy is centered in the 2- to 4-kHz range, is generally equivalent to the thresholds found on behavioural audiometry to narrow band noise and warbled tones centered at 2 and 4 kHz.

3. What is a decibel and dBSPL, dBHL, dBnHL, dBSL, and dB(A)?
   The decibel, one-tenth of a bel (Alexander Graham Bell's unit for the intensity of sound), is the unit of measure of the intensity of sound. Commonly abbreviated as dB, it is based on the logarithm of a ratio between an output sound and a reference. There is a good historic reason for using a logarithmic scale: loudness (the subjective perception of sound) is nearly linearly related to the logarithm of the ratio of the output intensity divided by the intensity of the reference. The decibel scale is thus relative to an arbitrary reference intensity. For dBSPL (i.e., sound pressure level), the reference intensity is 20 μPa, which is the same as 0.0002 μbar and 0.0002 dyne/cm².

   Mathematically,

   $$\text{dbSPL} = (10) \log_{10}\left(\frac{\text{output intensity}}{\text{intensity reference}}\right)^2 = (20) \log_{10}\left(\frac{\text{output intensity}}{\text{reference intensity}}\right)$$

   So, if the output intensity equals the reference intensity, then the parenthetical expression is 1; as the log of 1 is zero, the output would be 0 dBSPL. Note the requirement to know the intensity of the reference standard.

   dBHL (dB hearing level) is dBSPL adjusted to audiometric 0 at each frequency (Fig. 3). That is, a fudge factor is introduced to dBSPL to get dBHL. A 1,000 Hz pure tone with an intensity of 17 dBSPL is the same as 10 dBHL.

Some auditory stimuli, e.g., clicks, do not have accepted reference standards of intensity. "dBnHL" is the intensity that each laboratory should establish (and monitor), with 0 dBnHL being the click intensity for normal persons to identify 50% of stimuli.

dBSL (dB sensation level) is determined for each individual patient and is referenced to that patient's voluntary threshold for the particular stimulus (e.g., pure tone or speech). The words for determining speech discrimination scores are often presented at 40 dBSL, that is, 40 dB more intense than the patient's SRT.

dB(A) is not a measurement of patient hearing. Rather, it is a measure of the intensity of noise (e.g., in a work environment). The measure is weighted so that some frequencies are at different dBSPL than are other frequencies. These fudge factors differ from the fudge factors for defining audiometric zero (dBHL) (see Fig. 3).

4. What is a threshold?

Unlike the picturesque vision of the bride carried across the "threshold" of the doorway into her new home, the psychophysical definition of "threshold" is vexing. The auditory threshold is the dividing line from no sensation to the onset of sensation. In determining voluntary thresholds in pediatric audiometry, the *method of limits* is typically used: the testee indicates either a "Yes, I heard it" or a "No, I didn't hear anything" response; stimuli are presented in ascending and descending intensities, in an alternating fashion, to focus on the threshold.

A commonly utilized threshold is the (SRT), which is the intensity at which the testee responds correctly to 50% (or a few percentage points more) of the spondee words presented. The SRT is *not* "the softest level at which spondee words can be accurately identified." Patients, even children, must understand something of the concept of threshold (i.e., they must understand that guessing is necessary for the testing to be accurately done) in order for "threshold" to be reasonably measured. Patients who respond only when certain of hearing/understanding the spondee give falsely elevated thresholds.

5. "Because he talks so loudly, I think his hearing is poor."

Perhaps this mother's concern correctly depicts the son's elevated bone-conducted thresholds in his better hearing ear. Remember that one's own vocalizations travel to the cochleae by both air and bone conduction. So, if the better hearing ear's cochlear thresholds are elevated, the boy has to speak comparatively loudly to hear himself. The more common finding clinically, however, is that such a patient's bone-conducted thresholds are satisfactory—and that the patient talks loudly for other reasons (often behavioral).

In a quiet environment, if the examiner asks the child in a soft voice, near a whisper, to count serially, the loud-talking youngster with bilateral conductive hearing loss will often speak softly after one or two dozen numbers.

A soft-spoken but hard-of-hearing patient is commonly encountered. Such a patient is likely to have bilateral conductive hearing loss, which is often amenable to surgical correction.

6. What is recruitment?

Recruitment (abnormal loudness growth) is a peculiar situation in which an ear has reduced dynamic range, that is, the range (in dB) from the threshold of sound detection to the threshold of intolerable loudness is narrowed. Behaviorally, the patient complains of sounds being too loud. Normal dynamic range for speech is from 0 dBHL (by definition) to about 90 dBHL. Recruitment is a sign of pathology in the cochlea. At stapedius reflex testing, recruitment is suspected when the reflex is elicited at less than 70 dBSL. During auditory evoked potential testing, recruitment is indicated by a steep latency–intensity plot (see Fig. 5).

De-recruitment may be considered the antithesis of recruitment. It is a sign of retrocochlear pathology (e.g., cerebellopontine angle neoplasm).

7. What is masking? When is it needed?

Masking is sound, different from the test stimulus, presented to the non-test ear. Masking is administered to ensure that the test ear is truly the ear being tested. Masking should be done when (a) the audiometric configuration of a patient's two ears differ greatly (e.g., when the signal intensity is 40 dB or more than the bone conduction threshold in the non-test ear), or (b) when the bone conduction thresholds are being checked in an ear that seems to have a conductive loss (i.e., an air–bone gap) of 10 dB or more.

TABLE 3: Sources of Variance in Audiometric Testing[a]

Factor	Source of Variance
Room	Noise levels Reverberation Calibration

Equipment	Voltage stability
	Calibration
	   Frequency
	   Intensity
	   Reference standard
	   Rise–fall times
	Distortion of stimulus
	Intermittent faults

Sound delivery mode (see Table 6)	Sound field Headphone Insert phone Bone oscillator
Test technique	Instructions Ascending, descending, hybrid Stimulus duration Interstimulus duration Manual, semiautomatic Response-indicating method

Tester	Attention
	Response criteria
	Motivation
	Personality
	   Interpretation
	   Expectancy bias

Testee	Motivation Comprehension of instructions Judgement criteria Detection variance Learning effect Circadian effect Attention, comfort (e.g., wet diaper), fatigue Temporary threshold shift, e.g. the "tone decay" (abnormal adaptation) of retrocochlear lesions True fluctuating hearing impairment

[a]In such testing, the cooperative patient is expected to respond voluntarily to the auditory stimulus. (Adapted from ref. 22, with permission.)

TABLE 4: Summary Features of Patients With Various Types of Hearing Problems

| Parameter | Type of Hearing Loss | | | |
	Conductive	Sensory	Neural	Factitious
observation	soft-spoken, visually attentive	loud-spoken, visually attentive	loud-spoken, visually attentive	variable
tuning fork tests	AC<BC	AC>BC[a]	AC>BC	variable
voluntary audiometry	boneconducted stimuli elicit responses at lower intensities than do air-conducted stimuli	high intensity stimuli uncomfortable	discrimination ability rolls-over at high intensities	inconsistencies common
tympanometry	abnormal	normal	normal	normal
stapedius reflex	absent	present (at low sensation level)	present (at high SL), but decays	normal
otoacoustic emissions	absent	abnormal	normal	normal
auditory brainstem response	delayed wave I	abnormal (short latencies)	abnormal (long latencies), or absent	normal
management	surgery	hearing aid(s); if profound and bilateral, maybe cochlear implant	therapy in cued speech, and speech-reading	psychiatric

[a]AC>BC indicates that air-conducted stimuli elicit better responses than do bone-conducted stimuli.

Observing the patient's communicative ability practically allows assessing the better-hearing ear's receptive capability. Similarly, in the absence of contralateral masking, sound field observational audiometry tests the better-hearing ear. Lip-reading necessitates visual attentiveness to the speaker's face. Patients with years of severe sensory loss often have monotonal speech that lacks musicality and sibilants (i.e. they have "deaf speech"). A patient's results of the auditory tests must be consistent. Do the findings "add up"? Do they correlate? In locating the facial nerve during surgery, reliance on one single landmark (e.g. the cochleariform process) can be dangerous, as the presumptive landmark may, in fact, not be the landmark. Otherwise stated, the cross-check principle is endorsed.

TABLE 5: Degrees of Hearing Impairment for Children, as Related to Hearing Threshold Level (i.e., dBHL) in the Better Hearing Ear

Degree of Loss	Average Threshold (0.5, 1, 2 kHz, in dBHL)	What Can Be Heard Without Amplification	Probable Needs
None: normal range	≤15	All speech sounds	None
Borderline	16–25	May miss unvoiced consonants (e.g., s, x, z)	Preferential seating; surgery, assitive listening device, or hearing aid(s) may help
Mild	26–40	Misses 25–50% of classroom discussions	Preferential seating; must have improved hearing by surgery and/or hearing aids
Moderate	41–65	Misses most speech sounds at normal conversational level	All of the above, plus consider special classroom situation
Severe	66–95	Hears no sound of normal conversation	All of the above, plus special classroom situation
Profound	≥96	Hears essentially no sounds	Manual (sign) communication or successful cochlear implant with aggressive habilitation

[a]Note that children with one normal hearing ear, or at least a permanent mild loss in the other ear, have difficulty localizing sounds, as well as difficulty understanding speech in a noisy or reverberant environment. In contrast to mild hearing loss in children, adults with previously established aural communication skills can perform adequately at the same thresholds. As an example, the audiometric standard for a U.S airline transport pilot is to have unaided pure tone thresholds (at 0.5, 1, 2, and 3 kHz) for the better (and worse) ears of at least 35 (35), 30 (50), 30 (50), and 40 (60) dbHL, respectively (26).

(Adapted from ref. 6, with permission.)

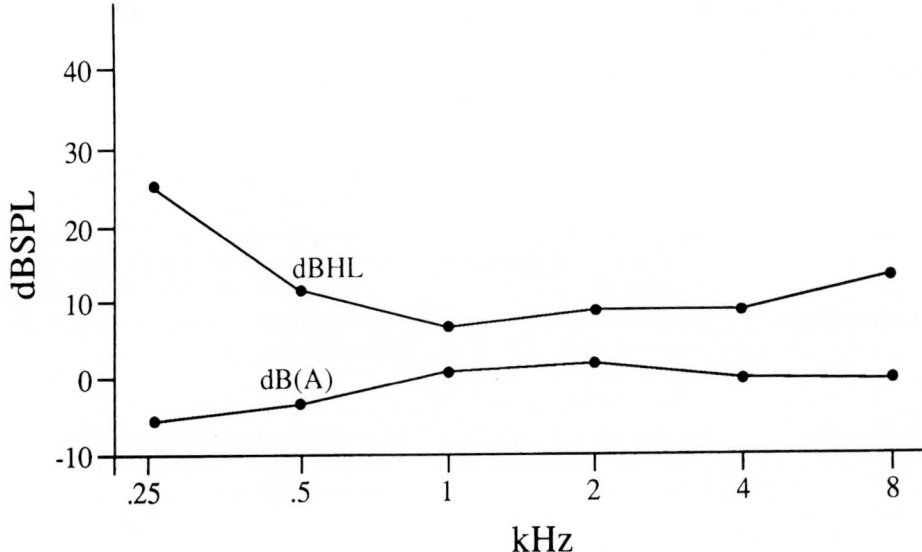

FIGURE 3 Fletcher–Munson plot showing the intensity (in dBSPL) of a pure tone at which normal persons respond to 50% of the stimuli presented. This line depicts zero dB hearing level (dBHL). Also plotted is the dB(A) zero dB line. The A-scale weighting, which correlates fairly well with people's sense of loudness, is used to evaluate noise environments. In 1974 the U.S. Environmental Protection Agency recommended limiting the 24-hour equivalent A-weighted sound pressure level to 70 dB. The assumption was that such noise, over a period of 40 years, would worsen the 4-kHz threshold by less than 5 dB in 96% of the population.

PLAY AUDIOMETRY

Applicable for children from about 2 to 4 years of age, play audiometry affords a reliable audiogram that may be ear specific. Testing requires an experienced clinician. Sound stimuli may be presented by loudspeaker, headphone, or bone oscillator, as the child will tolerate. Positive responses are conditioned motor activities (e.g., dropping blocks in a bucket, pointing to a picture, or identifying a toy). The testor must guard against false responses.

Play audiometry can be challenging to the examiner, who must concentrate on the patient's behavior while simultaneously operating the audiometer. In preparation for testing, an initial time of semistructured play with the child is necessary to minimize fear and maximize cooperation. The challenge is to prepare the child to respond to an auditory stimulus by a playful action, rather than playing randomly. Furthermore, the child must understand the concept that it is appropriate to respond to even very soft sounds. The examiner needs to be creative in picking play audiometry tasks appropriate to the child's development, ability, and interests.

CONVENTIONAL (I.E., ADULT-TYPE) AUDIOMETRY

The standard audiologic battery includes (a) both air-conducted and bone-conducted pure tone thresholds for each ear, (b) the speech reception threshold for each ear, and (c) speech discrimination scores. Acoustic stimuli may be delivered by headphone, insert ear canal phone, or bone oscillator. The non-test ear should be masked whenever there is a possibility that the stimulus is heard in the non-test ear, i.e., when the auditory stimulus is intense enough to be carried through the skull and to stimulate the non-test ear.

For speech reception threshold and speech discrimination score determinations, most clinicians working with children prefer the flexibility of the "monitored live voice" stimulus modality. The words presented for determining speech reception threshold are standardized selected spondees—two-syllable words with approximately equal emphasis placed on each syllable (e.g., airplane, cookbook, mushroom, pancake, hot dog). For speech discrimination testing, a standard list of single-syllable phonetically balanced words (e.g., love, jar, kite, moon) are presented, and the percentage correctly repeated by the testee is reported;

TABLE 6: Comparison of Modes of Sound Delivery During Audiologic Testing: Advantages and Disadvantages

Delivery Technique	Advantages	Disadvantages
Sound field	Does not touch patient	Tests better hearing ear; calibration variable with objects in field; exact positioning in field is crucial maximum output about 80 dBHL
Headphone	Ear-specific information; can mask contralateral ear; traditional	Assume nominal ear canal volume; force of the phone may collapse canal; assumes nil leakage beneath the phone
Insert tubephone	Ear-specific information; prevent canal collapse; latencies 0.8–0.9 msec less than with headphone	May be painful;tube may be obstructed by cerumen
Bone oscillator	The only clinical way to measure bone-conducted thresholds	Nominal distortion values are more lenient than for headphones and insert tubephones

a score of 90% or more is generally considered normal. Such "discrim" testing has problems. Some words may be unfamiliar and thus more difficult to identify. The binary scoring scheme (the response is either right or wrong) itself offers no information as to patterns of phoneme confusion. Moreover, the testing environment cannot determine real-life ability to understand speech. If a patient does not allow testing with a long list of words (e.g., 50), the likelihood of measurement error increases. For example, on a 25-word list, if the score is 92% correct, the expected variation (95% confidence interval) is from 72% to 100%; that is, the range of measurement error decreases as the number of elements increases.

Advantages and disadvantages of the various methods of delivering sound stimuli are summarized in Table 6. Some persons dislike some of the delivery techniques. Firm stabilization of the bone oscillator placement is often problematic. Some persons consider the output of a well-functioning bone oscillator output to be monotonal, distorted, or artificial.

Conventional audiometry cannot always be applied to those age 5 years and older. Patient age for accomplishing this testing is quite variable, depending on maturity, intelligence, trust, developmental age, and presence or absence of handicap or learning disability.

ACOUSTIC IMMITTANCE TESTING

The ear absorbs sound, unlike a microphone that converts acoustical energy into an electrical form, but does not absorb. Acoustic immittance testing indirectly measures the amount of sound that is being absorbed, by directly measuring the intensity of a tone remaining in the external ear canal. Maximum sound absorption occurs when the pressure differential across the tympanic membrane is zero. Therefore, middle ear pressure can be measured by this technique, known as tympanometry (Fig. 4). Acoustic immitance testing is helpful in determining whether a patient does or does not have middle ear effusion.

Contraction of the stapedius muscle changes the acoustic immittance of the middle ear. (Recall that the stapedius muscle, innervated by the VIIth cranial nerve, attaches via its tendon to the stapes.) Acoustic (also known as stapedius) reflexes, measurable clinically since the early 1970s, can infer the healthy functioning of the auditory afferent limb to the brainstem, and the efferent limb through the facial nerve and the middle ear. A sufficiently intense sound will elicit contraction of the stapedius muscle bilaterally and consensually in the normal person, increasing the stiffness of the middle ear and decreasing sound absorption. As for other measurements, ANSI standards exist for acoustic immittance testing (8).

For hearing assessment, the presently available clinical measure of the stapedius reflex is the threshold—the stimulus intensity at which a change in middle ear stiffness/compliance occurs to 50% of stimuli. The range for stapedius reflex thresholds in normal persons is 70 to 100 dBHL, the median being 85 dBHL for pure tone stim-

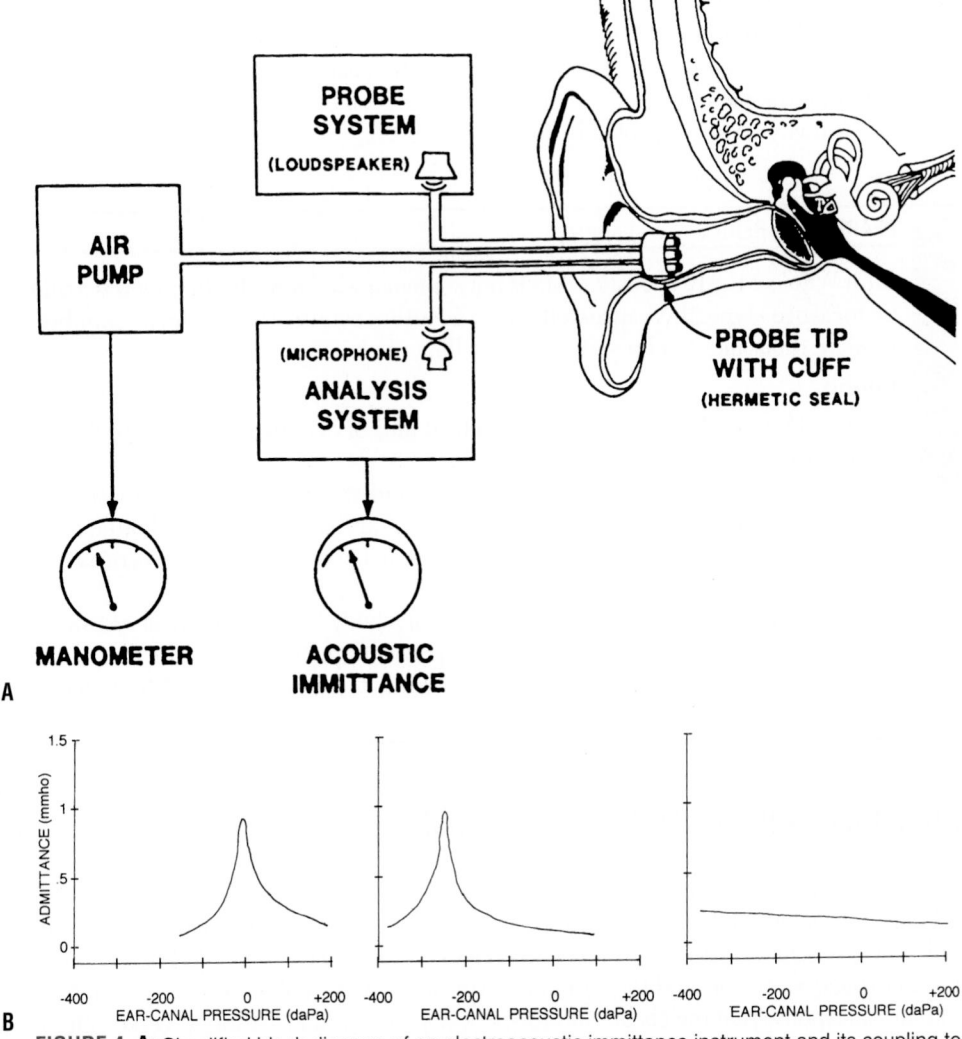

FIGURE 4 A: Simplified block diagram of an electroacoustic immittance instrument and its coupling to the human ear. The instrument is coupled to the ear by means of a probe tip that is hermetically sealed in the ear canal by means of a soft rubber cuff. The probe tip contains openings connected to the three basic subsystems of the instrument. One opening is directed from an air pump system used to introduce air pressure changes in the ear canal during tympanometry. Another probe tip opening connects the loudspeaker of a probe system to the ear canal for the introduction of probe tones and/or reflex-activating signals. The probe tip also connects the microphone of an analysis system to the ear canal to monitor sound pressure levels. The probe and analysis systems indirectly estimate the acoustic immittance of the ear by monitoring sound pressure levels in the ear canal (at the probe tip). The acoustic immittance at the tympanic membrane is proportional to the sound pressure level of the probe tone developed in the ear canal. (From ref. 9, with permission.) **B:** The three general types of tympanograms. On the left is that of a normal ear, with the tympanometric peak pressure within 50 daPa of atmospheric pressure. In the center is a tympanogram showing the peak pressure at −250 daPa, which may simplistically be interpreted as subnormal amounts of air getting through the eustachian tube into the middle ear. On the right is a flat tympanogram (showing no peak); as the acoustic admittance is low, the plot is consistent with middle ear effusion. If the acoustic admittance were quite high, the right plot would be consistent with an open tympanic membrane. Each illustrative tympanogram was obtained with a 226-Hz probe tone; as test conditions were nominal (20°C, at standard sea level atmospheric pressure), compensation was not necessary. Currently available acoustic immittance instruments measure acoustic admittance, not impedance. The unit for acoustic immittance is the acoustic mmho. At nominal conditions with a probe tone of 226 Hz, 1 mL of air has an admittance of 1 acoustic mmho.

uli of 0.5, 1, 2, and 4 kHz. The reflex is normally elicited at a lower intensity when broadband noise is the stimulus; this is the basis for the ill-named sensitivity prediction with the acoustic reflex (SPAR) test. The test is ill-named because it does not predict sensitivity, rather, if the patient's data are in the normal region of the bivariate plot, then additional sensitivity testing is probably not required (10).

PEARLS AND PERILS

mho Who is Mo? In acoustics, Mo is not someone you know. Rather, *mho* is a unit of measure, typically expressed as its one-thousandth (milli-) form (mmho). fr. *milli*, thousand + *mho*, (backward spelling of *ohm*).

mmho

1. One-thousandth of a mho is the practical unit of conductance equal to the reciprocal of the ohm.
2. In acoustics, at nominal conditions (20°C and standard sea level atmospheric pressure) with a 226-Hz probe tone, 1 mL of air has an acoustic admittance of 1 acoustic mmho and an acoustic impedance magnitude of 1,000 acoustic Ω; the SI unit is m³/Pa·s.
3. In electricity, the SI unit of conductance of a body with an electrical resistance of 1 Ω, allowing 1 A of current to flow per volt applied; an electrical mho is a synonym for a siemens (Sir William *Siemens*, German-born British engineer, 1823–1883).

AUDITORY EVOKED POTENTIAL RESPONSE

Known in the vernacular as *brain wave hearing test*, auditory evoked potential studies became widely used clinically with the availability of systems that electronically amplify and average tiny stimulus-induced voltages (about 5 μV) embedded in the background voltages. A short auditory stimulus, typically a click of about 0.1 msec duration, initiates a response that travels the auditory neural pathways and are identifiable with superficial (i.e., scalp) electrodes. To be identifiable from background electrical activity, highly synchronous firing must occur. The most effective stimuli for evaluating specific frequencies are tone pips. The acoustic energy of clicks is in the 2- to 4-kHz range.

Of the four general regions of auditory evoked voltages, the brainstem auditory evoked response is used clinically in children (Table 7 and Fig. 5) (11). The initial response region, that of electrocochleography, requires electrode placement near (and the nearer the better)

TABLE 7: Auditory Evoked Voltages: Comparison of the Various Types

Type	Electrode Placement	Latency Epoch	Effect of Anesthesia[a]	Portion of System Tested	Repeatability[b]
Electrocochleography	Promontory	<2 msec	None	Peripheral (external ear canal through cochlear nerve)	Excellent
Brainstem response	Surface	<10 msec	None	Brainstem	Good
Middle responses, i.e., "thalamus"	Surface	10–100	Marked	Most	Fair
Long latency, i.e., "cortical"	Surface	100–600	Marked	Entire	Poor

[a]If the anesthetic, or the technique of its delivery to the patient, alters the pressure differential across the tympanic membrane from zero, then a conductive hearing impairment may be introduced; such conductive hearing impairment confounds testing.

[b]Repeatability of waveforms is a hallmark of valid evoked potentials. Of the four types of auditory evoked potentials, only the brainstem auditory evoked potential studies are commonly used cliniclaly in children.

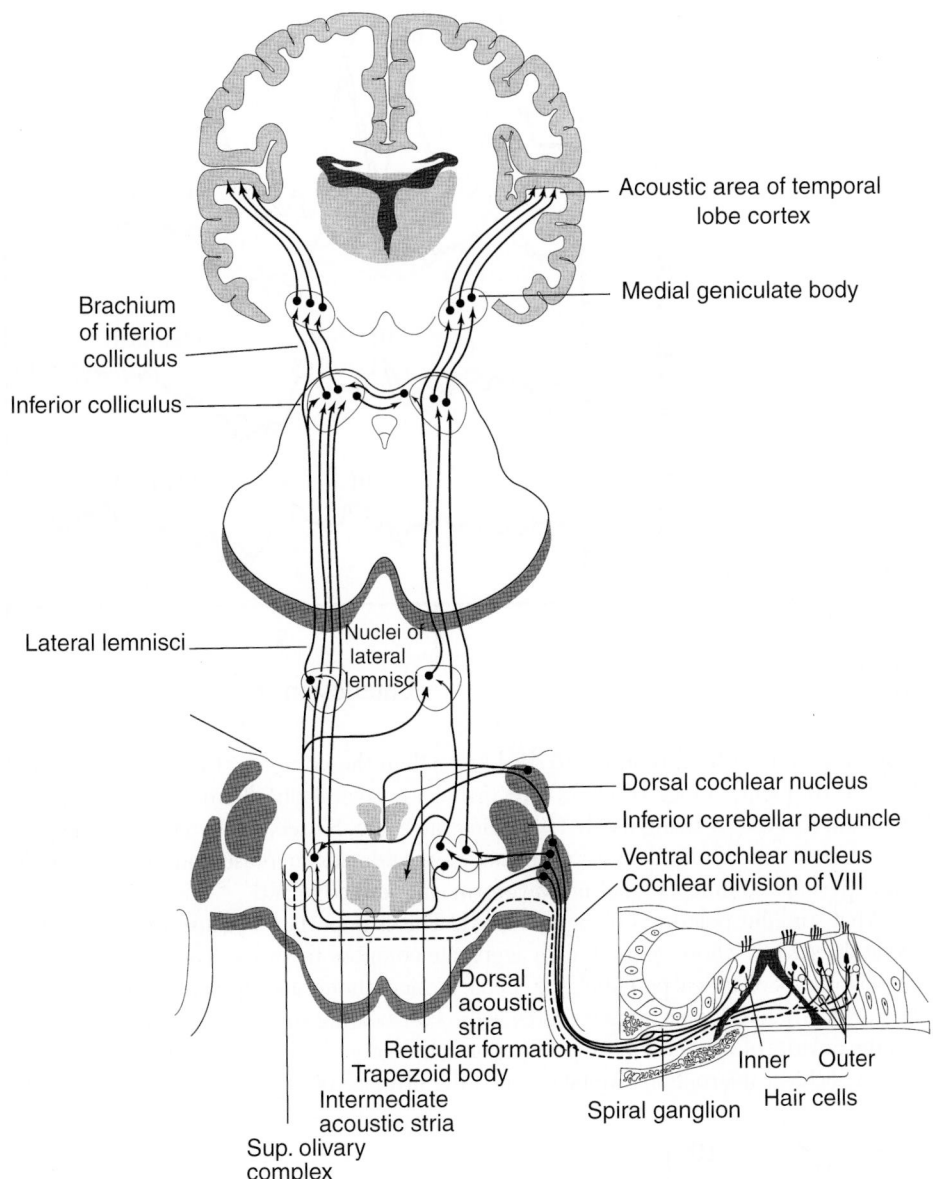

Acoustic area of temporal lobe cortex

Medial geniculate body

Brachium of inferior colliculus

Inferior colliculus

Lateral lemnisci

Nuclei of lateral lemnisci

Dorsal cochlear nucleus

Inferior cerebellar peduncle

Ventral cochlear nucleus
Cochlear division of VIII

Dorsal acoustic stria

Reticular formation

Trapezoid body

Intermediate acoustic stria

Sup. olivary complex

Spiral ganglion

Inner   Outer

Hair cells

FIGURE 5 Schematic of ear and neural projections. (From ref. 11, with permission.) Although the voltage generator sites for the brainstem auditory evoked response are not exactly known, their approximate locations can be remembered by the mnemonic ECOLI: wave I is largely generated by *E*ighth nerve action potentials; wave II in the *C*ochlear nuclei; wave III in the superior *O*livary complex; IV in the *L*ateral lemniscus; and wave V in the *I*nferior colliculus.

The neural connections to hair cells are complex. Some understanding of the additional complexity is needed to interpret tests clinically that distinguish sensory (i.e., hair cell lesions) from neural hearing loss. As shown, the neurons having their cell bodies in the spiral ganglion (located in Rosenthal's canal of the bony modiolus) are afferent (i.e., centripetal). There are two types of such afferent neurons. About 90% to 95% are large bipolar type I auditory neurons: they connect the inner hair cells to the cochlear nuclei, are myelinated, and have large cell bodies. The remaining afferent neurons are type II, characterized as small, unmyelinated, and connecting the outer hair cells to cochlear nuclei. Not shown in the illustration are the olivocochl fibers, which are efferent (i.e., centrifugal) to outer hair cells; their fibers traverse the ganglion (24).

the generator, i.e., a needle electrode on the bony covering of the cochlea. This requires a general anesthetic. The placement of an electrode on the lateral aspect of the tympanic membrane can be difficult, even in a sedated child. The generators of brainstem auditory evoked voltages are infratentorial and are not influenced by narcosis or general anesthesia. Patient age, however, does influence wave latencies until about age 24 months (Figs. 6 and 7).

Many (a thousand or more) clicks are utilized so that the evoked electroencephalographic (EEG) pattern can be recognized from noise (EEG and measurement artifact). The auditory evoked response is buried in background noise whose magnitude is 10 to 30 times that of the signal (12). The interrelationship of noise and signal can be expressed as:

$$\text{signal-to-noise ratio} = \left(\frac{\text{signal amplitude}}{\text{noise amplitude}}\right)\sqrt{\text{number of samples}}$$

The recording of brainstem auditory evoked EEG waveforms is objective, and test–retest repeatability is excellent intra-lab. Intrasubject latencies for waves I, III, and V are generally no longer than 0.3 msec, and probably never exceed 0.5 msec (13). Gen-

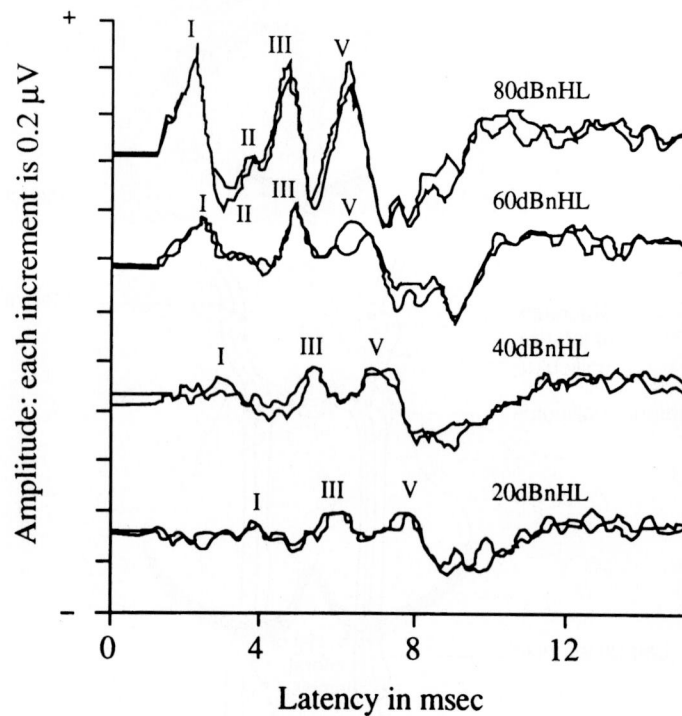

FIGURE 6 Auditory evoked brainstem response of a normal subject. Filter settings of 100 and 3,000 Hz. Rarefaction click stimuli at a rate of 21.1/sec. At each stimulus intensity, 2,048 responses were averaged. Note how the amplitude of wave V decreases and the absolute latency of wave V increases, as stimulus intensity is decreased.

erally, wave V threshold is about 15 dB higher than the voluntary thresholds for 2 to 4 kHz, the frequency range of clicks. Nevertheless, several pitfalls must be recognized. What stimulus rate is being used? High click rates, e.g. 80/sec, allow rapid data acquisition but stress the auditory system in that wave latencies increase and amplitudes decrease, perhaps so much so that no waveform can be recognized.

What stimulus polarity is being delivered? This is important because wave I is generated at three sites, whose generators in aggregate compose the wave. The hair cells generate two forms of electrical potential, the cochlear microphonic and the summating potential. The cochlear microphonic, whose source is the hair-bearing surface of the cell, is in phase with the polarity of the auditory stimulus, that is, a condensation (compression) sound wave elicits a cochlear microphonic voltage that is the inverse voltage of a rarefaction wave. By

FIGURE 7 This latency–intensity plot (mean, ± 2 SD) of wave V is for normal patients age 2 years and older, for a clinic that uses filter settings of 100 and 3,000 Hz, average of 2,048 responses at each stimulus intensity, and insert tubephone-delivered clicks at 21.1/sec. The normal plot is between the two lines that are defined by the round dots. (Note that 0.9 msec has been added to the time of stimulus delivery, to adjust for using a tubephone rather than a headphone to deliver the click stimuli.) As Gorga et al. (25) emphasize, wave V latency is typically about 1 msec longer in term newborns than it is in normal persons age 2 years and older. The triangles depict findings of an ear with cochlear-type hearing loss.

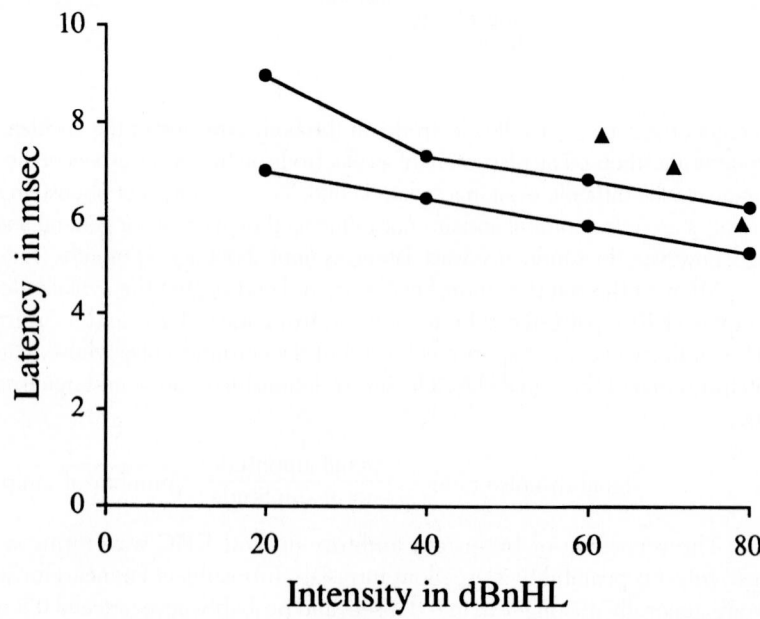

contrast, the summating potential, whose source is the depolarization of the hair cell itself, is not affected by polarity of the auditory stimulus. The eighth nerve action potential, also termed the whole nerve or compound action potential, is the aggregated discharge of many auditory neurons. (Each inner hair cell relates to about 20 to 30 neurons.) If a patient's wave I is completely generated by the cochlear microphonic potential, that wave I's polarity flops upside down with alternating stimulus polarity and would be averaged to zero. By contrast, that patient's wave I is identifiable in a run of compression clicks and identifiable (although inverted) in a run of rarefaction clicks. Hence a patient with auditory neuropathy studied only with alternating polarity clicks could be labeled as having sensorineural hearing loss, when in fact the lesion is neural. A hearing aid benefits the patient with sensory (i.e., cochlear) loss but not neural loss; patients suffering an auditory neuropathy are probably best served by cued speech or manual methods of communication.

What filter setting is used? The one commonly used is 100 to 3,000 Hz. Changing the lower limit of the bandwidth from 100 to 50 Hz makes noise increase, but the wave V amplitude also increases, while wave V latency also increases (12). How is the waveform presented? Note that electroencephalographers conventionally plot negative voltages upward on the page, whereas auditory testors plot positive voltages upward. Is the patient normothermic? The hypothermia of physiologic sleep, nearly 1°C, is associated with 0.2 msec prolongation of wave V latency (14).

OTOACOUSTIC EMISSIONS

The cochlea generates sounds recordable in the external ear canal, as discovered by Kemp (15). The elucidation of the mechanism of generation of these sounds by Brownell (16) has resulted in the clinical acceptance of otoacoustic emissions measurements. Persons with an intact peripheral auditory system, but with an isolated neural hearing loss, have intact otoacoustic emissions (17,18).

Some background information may facilitate an understanding of otoacoustic emissions. The inner hair cells are the receptors of auditory stimuli, and they relay the signal through the spiral ganglion cells into the afferent portion of the eighth nerve. The outer hair cells are motile, the motility being related cycle by cycle to the acoustic stimulus. With low-level auditory stimulation, outer hair cells augment (presumably via the tectorial membrane) the stimulation of the inner hair cells. In response to high levels of auditory stimulation, the olivocochlear fibers convey the message to the outer hair cells to stiffen, with resultant dampening of the stimulation of the inner hair cells. At high levels of auditory stimulation, the outer hair cells dampen (presumably via the tectorial membrane) the stimulation of the inner hair cells. The augmentation and dampening effect of the outer hair cells is exponentially, not linearly, related to the intensity of auditory input. Succinctly, the inner hair cells are sensory and the outer hair cells are accessory motor in function.

The motility of outer hair cells produces sounds that are transmissible through the intact, functioning middle ear, identifiable in the external ear canal (with amplification, so that they can be sorted from background noise). The measurement of otoacoustic emissions is objective evidence of functioning outer hair cells. Nonfunctioning outer hair cells produce a sensory (i.e., cochlear) hearing loss of about 40 to 50 dBHL. Patients with this problem can have auditory brainstem evoked responses. Sensory hearing loss worse than about 40 to 50 dBHL is associated with the additional loss of inner hair cell function.

TABLE 8: Comparison of the Types of Otoacoustic Emissions

Name	Stimulus	Response
Spontaneous	None	Normal, most in 1–3-kHz range
Transient evoked	Click	Kemp's "echo"
Stimulus frequency evoked	One continuous pure tone	In stimulus frequency
Distortion product evoked[a]	Two continuous pure tones	Frequency specific

[a]In children, the distortion product type of evoked emissions is the most applicable.

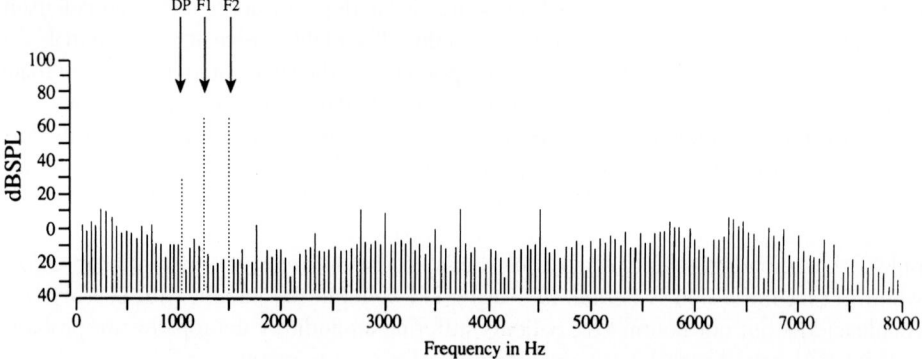

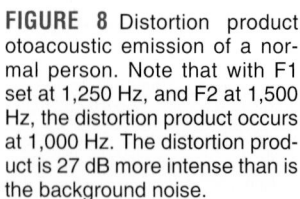

FIGURE 8 Distortion product otoacoustic emission of a normal person. Note that with F1 set at 1,250 Hz, and F2 at 1,500 Hz, the distortion product occurs at 1,000 Hz. The distortion product is 27 dB more intense than is the background noise.

Of the four types of otoacoustic emissions, two are presently recognized as clinically useful: the transient evoked type and the distortion product type of emission (Table 8). Transient evoked otoacoustic emissions are extracted from the stimulus sound on the basis of time delay, so responses can be detected up to about 5 kHz. These emissions permit testing of the olivocochlear complex. Normally, contralateral noise stimulation activates the olivocochlear complex (bilaterally), and suppresses the transient emission more than 1 dB in the test ear (19).

Distortion product otoacoustic emissions allow testing of frequencies of 0.5 through 8 kHz, depending on what stimulation frequencies (F1 and F2) are chosen. By convention, F1 is lower than F2. That is, if two tones of F1 and F2 are presented to the ear, then a third tone (the distortion product) is produced by outer hair cells. The distortion product response is a pure tone whose frequency can often be expressed by the formula: $FDP = (2F1) - (F2)$. The magnitude of the distortion product is dependent on F1 and F2, as well as on the intensity of F1 and F2—termed L1 and L2, for level of intensity of F1 and F2, respectively. A ratio of F2 to F1 of 1.22 is often chosen (Fig. 8).

Emissions are mature in babies of only 32 weeks of gestation (4), about 2 years earlier than brainstem auditory evoked response maturation. In neonates, distortion product emissions can be detected, on the average, in about two-thirds of the acquisition time of transient emissions (20). Spontaneous otoacoustic emissions come from the majority of normal ears.

CENTRAL AUDITORY PROCESSING

Central auditory processing problems may be considered analogous to central blindness, of which cortical blindness is the glaring example. There is no argument that some patients seem to suffer with problems of central auditory processing. However, when confronted with a patient with a central auditory processing problem, most physicians express dismay. Not the least of the dismay is the muddied distinction of this problem from dyslexia, retardation, behavior issues, auditory deprivation effect, and attention deficit disorder.

Additional aspects contribute to the dismay. What diagnostic tests identify the problem? The answer is "many"—but test meaningfulness is suspect. As Cherry (21) has noted, "There are no reported longitudinal studies that follow large groups of children (pass vs. fail) over time to validate test results." Another dismaying question is: What can be done to help the patient with a problem of central auditory processing? At least one answer is optimizing the signal-to-noise ratio (23). Normal persons, of course, also process auditory stimuli better when the signal-to-noise ratio is increased.

ACKNOWLEDGMENTS

Among those who read all or part of the manuscript and offered advice were Jolie C. Fainberg, MA, Lara E. Johnson, MEd, and Richard T. Jackson, PhD. This work was supported by the Lions of Georgia.

✦ REFERENCES

1. Matkin ND. Early recognition and referral of hearing-impaired children. *Pediatr Rev* 1984;6:151–156.
2. Ruben RJ. Language screening as a factor in the management of the pediatric otolaryngic patient. *Arch Otolaryngol Head Neck Surg* 1991;117:1021–1025.
3. Coplan J. *The early language milestone scale*, 2nd ed (ELM-2). Austin, TX: PRO-ED, 1993.
4. Bonfils P, Francois M, Avan P, Londero A, Trotoux T, Narcy P. Spontaneous and evoked otoacoustic emissions in preterm neonates. *Laryngoscope* 1992;102:182–186.
5. Hirsch A. Behavioral tests: applications and limitations in comparison with brainstem response audiometry. *Acta Otolaryngol* 1991;Suppl 482:118–125.
6. Northern JL, Downs, MP. *Hearing in children*, 3rd ed. Baltimore: Williams & Wilkins, 1984.
7. American National Standards Institute, c/o Acoustical Society of America. American National Standard Specification for Audiometers. S3.6–1996, 1996, New York, N.Y.
8. American National Standards Institute, c/o Acoustical Society of America. American National Standard Specifications for Instruments to Measure Aural Acoustic Impedance and Admittance (Aural Acoustic Immittance). S3.39–1987(R1996), 1987, New York, N.Y.
9. Katz J, ed. *Handbook of clinical audiology*, 4th ed. Baltimore: Williams & Wilkins, 1994.
10. Wilson RH, Margolis RH. Acoustic reflex measurements. In: Rintelman WF, ed. *Hearing assessment*. Austin, TX: PRO-ED, 1990:247–319.
11. Netter FH. In: Silverstein H, Wolfson RJ, Rosenberg S, eds. *Clinical symposia* Summit, NJ: Ciba-Geigy 1992;44.
12. Hall III JW. *Handbook of auditory evoked responses*. Needham Heights, MA: Allyn and Bacon, 1992.
13. Oyler RF, Lauter JL, Matkin ND. Intrasubject variability in the absolute latency of the auditory brainstem response. *J Am Acad Audiol* 1991;2:206–213.
14. Litscher G. Continuous brainstem auditory evoked potential monitoring during nocturnal sleep. *Int J Neurosci* 1995;82:135–142.
15. Kemp DT. Stimulated acoustic emissions from within the human auditory system. *J Acoust Soc Am* 1978;64:1386–1391.
16. Brownell WE. Outer hair cell electromotility and otoacoustic emissions. *Ear Hear* 1990;11:82–92.
17. Monroe JAB, Krauth L, Arenberg IK, Prenger E, Philpott P. Normal evoked otoacoustic emissions with a profound hearing loss due to a juvenile pilocytic astocytoma. *Am J Otology* 1996;17:639–642.
18. Starr A, Picton TW, Sininger Y, Hood LJ, Berlin CI. Auditory neuropathy. *Brain* 1996;119:741–753.
19. Berlin CI, Hood LJ, Cecola RP, Jackson DF, Szabo P. Does type I afferent neuron dysfunction reveal itself through lack of efferent suppression? *Hear Res* 1993;65:40–50.
20. Brass D, Kemp DT. Quantitative assessment of methods for the detection of otoacoustic emissions. *Ear Hear* 1994;15:378–389.
21. Cherry R. In: Katz J, Stecker N, Henderson D, eds. *Central auditory processing: a transdisciplinary view*. St. Louis: Mosby-Year Book 1992;129–139.
22. Hannley M. *Basic principles of auditory assessment*. San Diego: College-Hill, 1986.
23. Crandell CC, Samaldino JJ, Flexer C. *Sound-field FM amplification: theory and practical applications*. San Diego: Singular, 1995.
24. Brown MC. Anatomical and physiological studies of type I and type II ganglion neurons. In: Merchan MA, Juiz JM, Godfrey DA, Mugnaini E, eds. *Mammalian cochlear nuclei: organization and function*. New York: Plenum, 1993;43–54.
25. Gorga MP, Kaminski JR, Beauchaine KL, Jesteadt W, Neely ST. Auditory bainstem reponses from children three months to three years of age: normal patterns of response II. *J Speech Hear Res* 1989;32: 281–288.
26. Federal Aviation Administration. *Medical Standards*. September 16, 1996.

RECOMMENDED READINGS

Berlin CI, ed. *Hair cells and hearing aids*. San Diego: Singular, 1996.
Gerber SE, ed. *The handbook of pediatric audiology*. Washington: Gallaudet, 1996.

N.W. Todd: Departments of Otolaryngology and Pediatrics, Emory University School of Medicine, Atlanta, Georgia 30322.

• *Practical Pediatric Otolaryngology*
• edited by Robin T. Cotton and Charles M. Myer, III
• Lippincott–Raven Publishers, Philadelphia © 1999

13

Congenital and Acquired Hearing Loss: Etiology and Management

N. Wendell Todd

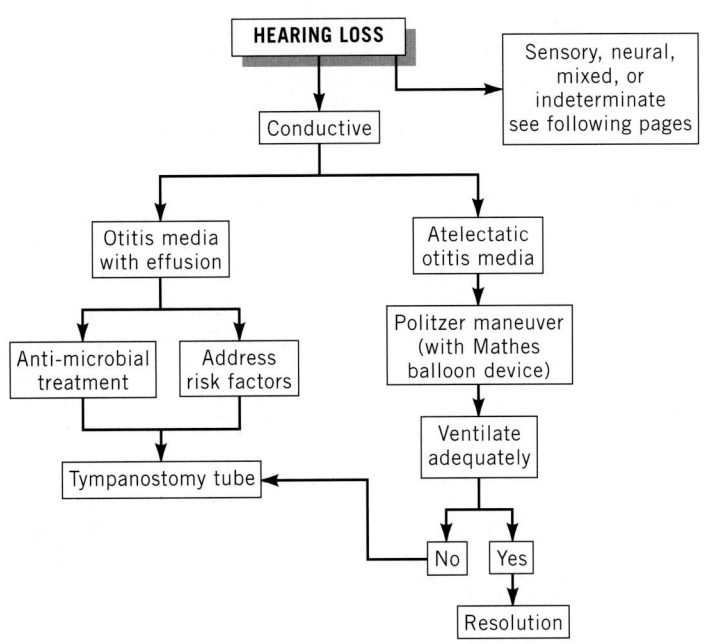

continued on next page

continued

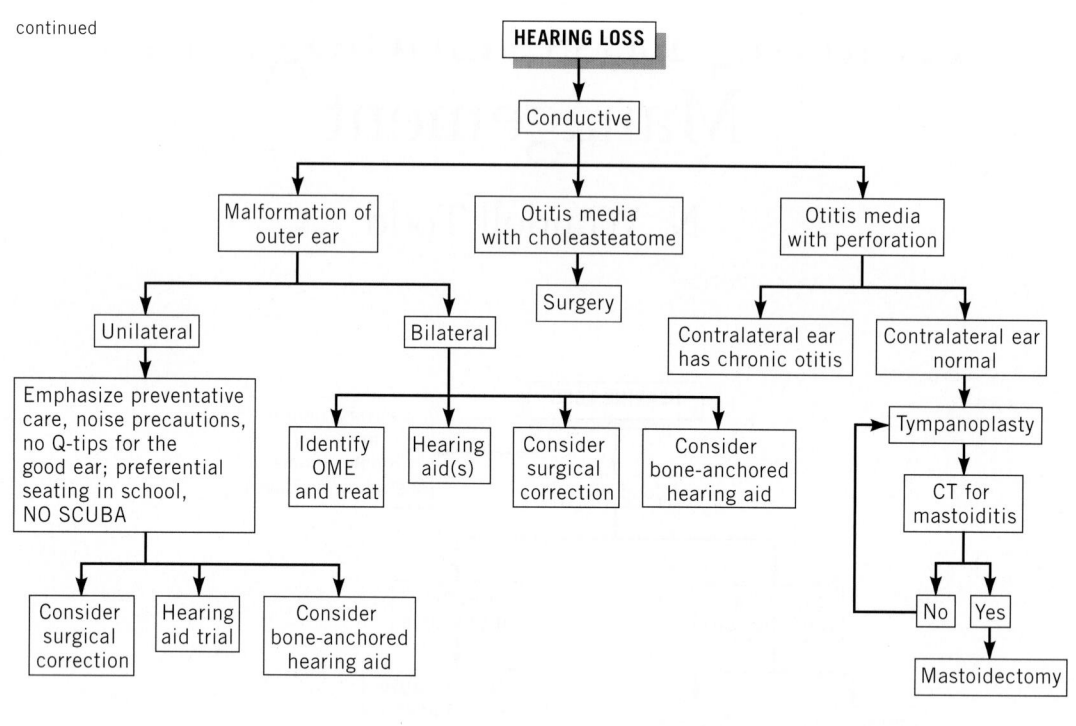

HEARING LOSS

Conductive

- Malformation of outer ear
  - Unilateral
    - Emphasize preventative care, noise precautions, no Q-tips for the good ear; preferential seating in school, NO SCUBA
      - Consider surgical correction
      - Hearing aid trial
      - Consider bone-anchored hearing aid
  - Bilateral
    - Identify OME and treat
    - Hearing aid(s)
    - Consider surgical correction
    - Consider bone-anchored hearing aid
- Otitis media with choleasteatome
  - Surgery
- Otitis media with perforation
  - Contralateral ear has chronic otitis
  - Contralateral ear normal
    - Tympanoplasty
      - CT for mastoiditis
        - No
        - Yes
          - Mastoidectomy

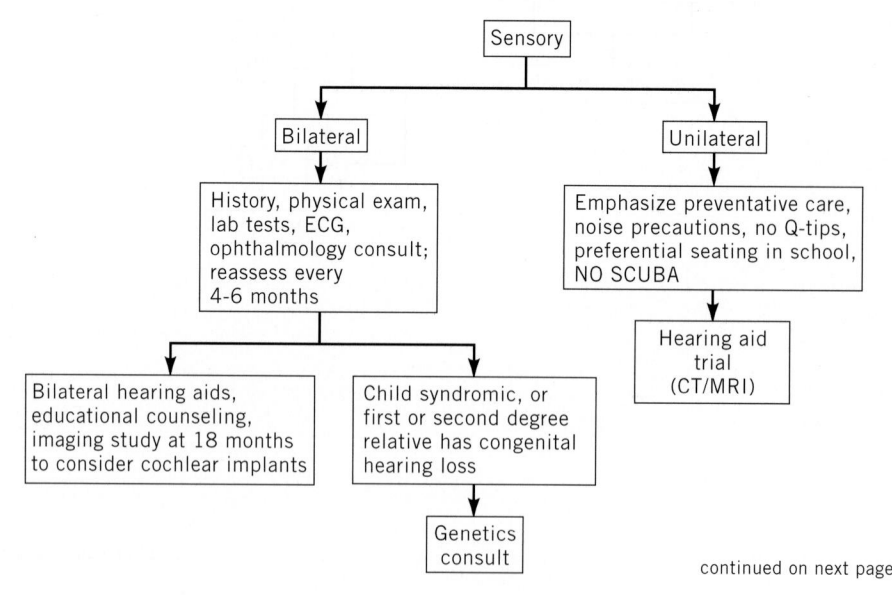

Sensory

- Bilateral
  - History, physical exam, lab tests, ECG, ophthalmology consult; reassess every 4-6 months
    - Bilateral hearing aids, educational counseling, imaging study at 18 months to consider cochlear implants
    - Child syndromic, or first or second degree relative has congenital hearing loss
      - Genetics consult
- Unilateral
  - Emphasize preventative care, noise precautions, no Q-tips, preferential seating in school, NO SCUBA
    - Hearing aid trial (CT/MRI)

continued on next page

continued

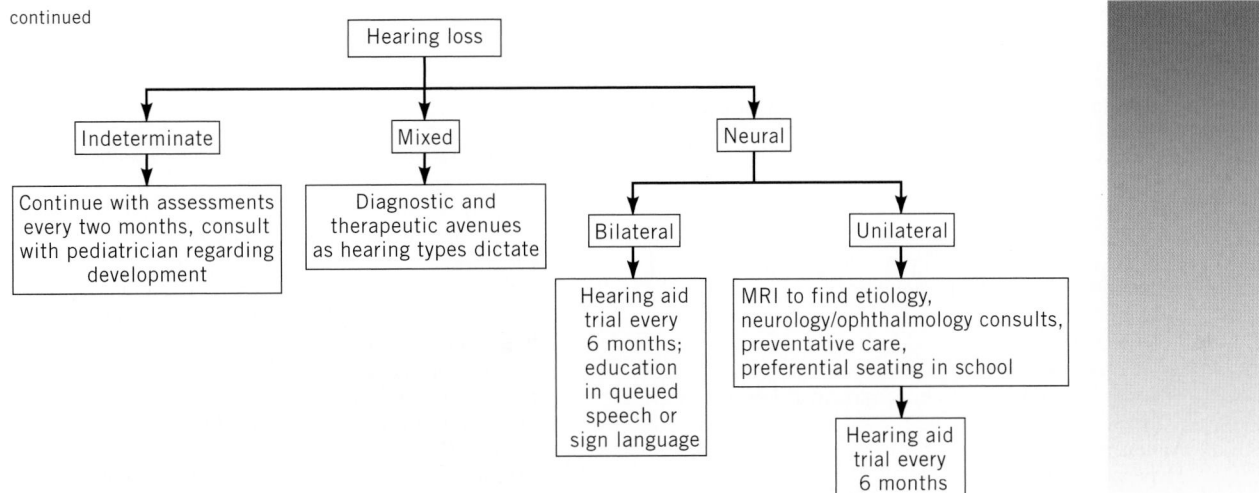

The physician must concomitantly address two avenues of concern about the child with hearing loss. The first is diagnostic, sometimes regarded as esoteric and academic, and not important. Is the hearing loss genetic or acquired? Was the hearing loss present at birth or during early infancy, or later? Is the child otherwise normal-appearing? Are there associated features (syndromic)? Is the hearing loss conductive or sensorineural (Table 1)? The practical value of the first avenue is to understand the cause of lost hearing, how to improve hearing, and how to counsel the parents about the risks for hearing loss in family members.

The second avenue of concern is that of therapy, or management: What can be done about it? Sign language, pharmacotherapeutics, amplification, or surgery? Practicality is the reason that the diagnostic and therapeutic avenues should be addressed concomitantly. Rarely do patients solely seek the diagnosis, rather, a patient seeks relief of the problem. The diagnostic avenue leads and connects to the therapeutic avenue.

Testing a child's hearing is difficult, with the paradox that the rigorous tests assess the peripheral auditory system and the less rigorous tests assess auditory–verbal communication. Test–retest variability is a problem in behavioral audiometry. Moreover, the child's hearing may change during the following months or years. Hence, longitudinal assessment and care are mandatory. The patient seems best served by repeated examinations in conjunction with confirming and analyzing historical data, by the same team of otolaryngologist and audiologist. The hearing-impaired pediatric patient (especially appropriate is the archaic definition of patient: one who suffers, endures, or is victimized) is optimally attended in a milieu of trust and gentleness. Parents, families, audiologists and physicians grieve for the child with the hearing loss in stages similar to those of adjusting to the reality of other losses (e.g. death): denial, guilt, depression, anger, and anxiety. Trust and empathy are the foundations for nurturing a sense of control and coping.

Otitis media and congenital aural atresia are addressed in Chapters 14, 16, and 20.

🧩 PATIENT ASSESSMENT

A history, for both the child and the family, is the most valuable item for establishing an etiology. Gestational age? Birth weight? Normal weight for gestational age? Remember that the frequency of congenital malformations is increased in children small for gestational age. Low Apgar scores are associated with impaired hearing. Ask about motor development and confirm by your own observations. Balance problem? A 4-year-old who performs ballet (or bicycling or skate-boarding) well does not have disequilibrium. Ask about vision and syncope. Ask the family if they really think the child is hearing impaired, and if the hearing aid(s) is of benefit. Tinnitus? Aural fullness? Ask how the child is doing in school. How is the child's vision when illumination is poor? Can the child see

TABLE 1: Guide to the Etiologic Classification of Sensorineural Hearing Loss

Congenital (aplasia or dysgenesis of at least part of cochlea)
  Genetic (i.e., defective zygote)
    Hearing loss alone
      Cochlear dsyplasias
        Bony: identifiable by computed tomography;
        includes large vestibular aqueduct,
        Mondini type, etc.
        Membranous
    Hearing loss with other abnormalities (syndromes)
      Waardenburg's: white forelock; variably colored
        irises
      Albinism
      Hyperpigmentation
      Onychondystrophy
      Pendred's: abnormal thyroid
      Jervell Lange-Nielsen: long QT interval
      Usher's: progressive retinitis pigmentosa
      Chromosome abnormality, e.g., XO, monosomy 18q and
       18p
      CHARGE association[a]
      Mitochondrial disorders
  Nongenetic (i.e., acquired intrauterine)
    Hearing loss alone
      Ototoxic poisoning: aminoglycosides, quinine
    Hearing loss maybe with other abnormalities
      Infections
      Rubella
        Cytomegalic inclusion virus
        Bacterial
        Toxoplasmosis
        Syphilis[b]
      Poisons: thalidomide
      Metabolic disorders: hypothyroidism (cretinism)[b]
      Kernicterus (usually Rh incompatibility)
      Radiation in first trimester
      Prematurity
      Birth trauma, anoxia

Delayed (degenerative changes in at least part of cochlea)
  Genetic
    Hearing loss alone
      Familial progressive: bilateral; autosomal dominant
      Otosclerosis[b]
      Presbycusis
    Hearing loss with other abnormalities (syndromes)
      Alport's: hematuria, nephritis, renal failure
      Mucopolysaccharidoses: Hurler's, Hunter's
      Klippel-Feil: skeletal defects
      Refsum's: retinitis pigmentosa, ichthyosis,
        neuropathy
      Alstrom's: retinitis pigmentosa, diabetes, obesity
      Paget's: osteitis deformans
      Richards-Rundle: ataxia, hypogonadism
      Neurofibʮromatosis type 2
      craniofacial dysostosis
      Sylvester's: optic atrophy, ataxia
      Cockayne's: cachectic dwarfism, retinal
        degeneration
  Nongenetic (all these may be just hearing loss)
    Infections:
      Bacterial
      Viral: measles (rubeola), mumps, influenza, chickenpox
      Syphilis[b]
    Ototoxic poisons: aminoglycosides, erythromycin, polymyxin,
    Cisplatin, loop diuretics, quinine, neomycin
    Neoplastic disorders:[b] leukemia, ear and brain tumors
    Trauma:
      Acoustic (i.e., noise)
      Temporal bone fractures
      Labyrinthine fistula[b]
    Metabolic:
      Hypothyroidism   Diabetes mellitus
      Meniere's disease[b]
    Neurologic disease: multiple sclerosis
    Autoimmune disease[b]
    Vasculitis[b]

[a]CHARGE, coloboma, heart disease, atresia choamae, retaided growth and development and/or CNS anomalies, genital hypoplasia, and ear anomalies and/or deafness.

[b]Potentially retrievable, treatable. The clinician may be unable to determine whether a specific patient's hearing loss is acquired, or congenital with delay in diagnosis. At least 427 syndromes involve hearing loss (2).

(Adapted from ref. 1, with permission).

the stars in the night sky? At following-on visits, query again about aunts, uncles, grandparents, and cousins. Construct the family tree. A maternal transmission pattern of heritable hearing loss may be related to a multitude of different mitochondrial defects, including the mitochondrial 1555 mutation that accounts for a number of cases of aminoglycoside-induced deafness (3). On numerous occasions, diagnosis-making familial factors have come to the author's attention at follow-on visits. Families guard their privacy, and time is required to cultivate their trust and demonstrate the empathy and understanding that allow and facilitate discovery of the family history.

Verify the results of government-mandated newborn screening tests, as well as maternal rubella and congenital cytomegalovirus infection (CMV) titers. Encourage the family to make a scrapbook of all the child's hearing tests and to bring it for review at each clinic visit. Are the data consistent? Know that two problems may coexist in a child's ear. Manning et al. (4) report a 1% concurrence of sensorineural hearing loss in children with tympanostomy-tube placement.

In patients with microtia or atresia, inquire about swellings (even intermittent) and drainage. Congenital squamous epithelial cysts (cholesteatomata) are sneakily common in such ears.

Physical Examination

In addition to the general otolaryngic examination with microtympanoscopy, the child seems best served by a focused general physical examination done by an otolaryngologist interested in and knowledgable of hearing loss in children. Do pneumatic tympanoscopy routinely. Induced dizziness may suggest a perilymphatic fistula. Note the child's receptive and expressive verbal language. Unusual facies? Heterochromia or synophrys or dystopia canthorum may suggest Waardenburg's syndrome (5). Is the head circumference normal?

Laboratory Tests and Electrocardiogram

Although an abundance of laboratory tests need to be considered, rarely are "fishing expeditions" warranted, rather laboratory tests are appropriate if the history or physical examination prompt a specific concern (6). For example, if the results of newborn and maternal screening tests cannot be obtained, then serologic tests for syphilis and thyroid-stimulating hormone level may be needed. If the history reveals a family member with Bright's disease and hearing loss, then complete urinalysis and serum creatinine need checking. Poor speech discrimination scores raise concern for syphilis. Hearing losses attributable to autoimmune disorders are apparently rare in children, but searching for the 69-kd inner ear antigen is probably appropriate if the sensorineural hearing loss is fluctuating or worsening (Table 2). Kenna and Neault (6) report that complete blood count, urinalysis, blood urea nitrogen, creatinine, electrocardiogram, sedimentation rate, rapid plasmin reagin, and the fluorescent treponemal antibody test were not helpful in evaluating their 127 patients. Although congenital CMV infection may account for nearly 40% of congenital hearing impairment, the role of CMV cannot be known unless viral shedding in the first weeks of life is documented (7).

One rare but potentially lethal autosomal recessive syndrome should be sought in deaf–mute children for whom the etiology of the hearing loss is undetermined. Electrocardiography is needed to identify the long QT interval of the Jervell and Lange-Nielsen syndrome. Patients with Jervell and Lange-Nielsen syndrome are at risk for sudden

TABLE 2: Workup for a Child with Fluctuating or Progressive Sensory Hearing Loss

Laboratory Test	*Suspected Etiology*
Complete blood count	Acute myelogenous leukemia
Fluorescent treponemal antibody test	Syphilis
Thyroid function test	Thyroid dysfunction
Lipid profile	Hyperlipidemia
Glucose	Diabetes mellitus
Erythrocyte sedimentation rate	Vasculitis
Toxicology	Ototoxic drugs and chemicals
69-kd inner ear antigen	Autoimmune disorder
Ophthalmology consultation	See Table 3
Computed tomography of temporal bones	Large vestibular aqueduct or perilymphatic fistula scenario

(Data from ref. 8.)

death from malignant ventricular arrhythmias (9). The age of onset of syncope varies. The arrhythmias appear to be related to heightened autonomic tone and may occur with exercise, excitement, or anxiety.

In patients with microtia or atresia, look for fullness which may herald an enlarging cholesteatoma. Look for functional integrity of the facial nerve, remembering that palsy in lowering of the bottom lip (asymmetric crying facies) is found ipsilateral to some microtia or atresia ears. New-onset facial palsy, even partial, should prompt computed tomography of the temporal bones.

Consultants (Input from other Specialities)

Ophthalmologic consultations are helpful in children with sensorineural hearing loss (10). The identification and attention to myopia or hyperopia are important to the child. Leguire et al. (11), in a study of 505 hearing-impaired and deaf students in Ohio, found that more than 20% had a refractive error, more than 20% had a retinal abnormality, and

TABLE 3: Correlation of Ophthalmologic Findings and Hearing Loss

Eye Problem	Examples	Youngest Age for Clinical Detection
Strabismus	Crouzon's disease Mobius', Apert's Turner's, Noonan's, and postmeningitic syndromes	Birth
Hypertelorism	Crouzon's disease, Apert's and Waardenburg's syndromes	Birth
Eyelid coloboma	Goldenhar's, Treacher Collins, and CHARGE syndromes	Birth
Microphthalmos	Congenital rubella, trisomy 13 and 18, fetal alcohol syndrome	Birth
Cornea	Thinning, megalocornea, keratoconus in osteogenesis imperfecta	Birth
Cornea	Intersitial keratitis of syphilis or Cogan's syndrome	Childhood
Cornea	Clouding in mucopolysaccharidoses	Childhood
Iris	Pupil abnormalities in congenital syphilis, Waardenburg's syndrome	Any
Iris	Heterochromia (complete or segmental), or brilliant sapphire blue	Birth
Lens	Cataract in congenital rubella	Birth
Optic atrophy	Congenital syphilis	Childhood
Cherry red spot in fundus	Gangliosidosis	Infancy
Macular pigmentary degeneration	Mucopolysaccharidoses	Infancy
Retinitis pigmentosa	Usher's, Alstrom's, Laurence-Moon, and Refsum's syndromes	Late childhood
Coloboma of retina	CHARGE association	Birth
Coloboma of choroid	Thalidomide, trisomy 13	Late childhood
Chorioretical scars	Congenital syphilis, toxoplasmosis, rubella, CMV	Birth or early infancy
Vasculitis	Polyarteritis nodosa Wegener's granulomatosis, Takayasu's arteritis, Behcet's syndrome	Childhood
Interstitial keratitis	Cogan's syndrome (13)	Childhood

CMV, cytomegalovirus.

(Adapted from ref. 12, with permission.)

about 8% had strabismus. The prevalence of ocular abnormalities generally increased with the severity of the hearing loss. The association of eye abnormalities and hearing loss is summarized in Table 3. Notwithstanding these data, Kenna and Neault (6) report that ophthalmologic consultation revealed only occasional myopia and hyperopia, and that only one patient had Usher's syndrome (Table 4), in their series of 127 children.

PEARLS AND PERILS

When to refer a patient with hearing loss to the medical geneticist
1. The patient seems to have a syndrome (e.g., Waardenburg's, CHARGE, Usher's) (See Table 1).
2. At least one family member (first and/or second degree) has the same pattern of hearing loss.
3. The shape of the audiogram (cookie-bite, ascending) suggests genetically determined hearing loss (Table 5).

TABLE 4: Minimal Criteria for the Diagnosis of Usher's Syndrome

Test	Usher Type 1	Usher Type 2
Bruininks-Oseretsky[a]	Fail	Pass
Ice-water calorics	No nystagmus	Brisk nystagmus
Hearing loss	Sensorineural, severe to profound	Sensorineural, mild to severe, no progression
Ophthalmoscopy[b]	Pigmentary degeneration	Pigmentary degeneration
Electoretinogram	Retinal dystrophy	Retinal dystrophy

[a]Specifically, the balance subtest.
[b]In the absense of pigmentary degeneration by ophthalmoscopy, an electroretinogram must be obtained.
(From ref. 14, with permission.)

TABLE 5: Classification of the shapes of Audiograms Exhibiting Sensorineural Hearing Loss[a]

Shape	Definition, Characteristics
Flat	Thresholds for 0.25, 0.5, 1, 2, 4, 6, and 8 kHz differ by <10 dB
Sloping sharply, high frequency	Mean of thresholds at 4, 6, 8 kHz is >25 dB the mean of thresholds at 0.5, 1, and 2 kHz or difference in thresholds between any two octave frequencies is >25 dB
Sloping gently, high frequency	Mean of thresholds at 4, 6, and 8 kHz is 10–24> the mean of thresholds at 0.5, 1 & 2 kHz
Corner (residual)	Responses to pure tone stimuli only at ≤1 kHz and ≥80 dBHL
U ("cookie-bite")	The thresholds for the middle frequencies are ≥15 dB worse than the thresholds for lower and higher frequencies
Ascending	The thresholds for low frequencies are ≥10 dB than the thresholds for high frequencies

[a] A person is considered to have symmetry of pure tone audiometric thresholds if the two ears have the same shape of audiograms and the bilateral difference in mean thresholds across the frequeny range is <15 dB.
(Adapted from ref. 15, with permission.)

TABLE 6: Approximate Probability of a Child Having Congential Hearing Loss

Parents' Hearing from Infancy	First-Degree Relative with Congenital Loss	First Child
Both normal	No	1 : 1,000
Both impaired	No	1 : 10
One normal, one impaired	No	1 : 20
Both normal	Yes	1 : 100

(Adapted from ref. 16, with permission.)

The medical geneticist can be a valuable consultant to the hearing-impaired child. Some generalizations can be made about the risks of congenital hearing loss (Table 6). Beyond generalizations about nonsyndromic hearing loss (Table 7), the geneticist is best equipped to counsel the family on a case by case basis. Syncope and long QT syndrome prompt consultation with a cardiologist. Only about 6% of patients with the long QT problem have deafness (Jervell and Lange-Nielsen syndrome), and 94% have normal hearing (Romano-Ward syndrome). A patient with neural hearing loss should have a consultation with a neurologist.

PEARLS AND PERILS

Reasons to do computed tomography (CT) of the temporal bones

1. When a mass lesion (tumor) is suspected in the temporal bone.
2. Suspected retrocochlear tumor; do CT with contrast.
3. At age 18 months in preparation for cochlear implant or bone-anchored hearing aid; do scans immediately in case of meningitis (see Chapter 19B)
4. Before atresia surgery.
5. Fluctuating or progressive hearing loss.
6. When needed to work up etiology of sensorineural hearing loss:
   a. If parents are planning more children and desire to know the risks of next child being hearing impaired.
   b. If patient has nonsyndromic familial hearing loss.

TABLE 7: Nonsyndromic Sensorineural Hearing Loss[a]

Hearing Loss	Autosomal Dominant	Autosomal Recessive
Occurrence rate	About 80%	About 18%
Degree	Mild	Severe
Intrafamily variability in degree	Much	Little
Incidence of shapes of audiograms	Flat or sharply or gently sloping in about the same proportions; although rare, both the cookie-bite and ascending shapes are highly suggestive of autosomal dominant hearing loss	Most are corner, a few slope sharply

[a] Counseling of family members is better based on the specific family's condition rather than on group information. Of all hereditary hearing impairment patients, about two-thirds are nonsyndromic, and about one-third have an identifiable syndrome. Nonsyndromic hereditary sensorineural hearing impairment is typically bilateral, and about 2% of such impairments are X-linked (probably mitochondrial). The various types of nonsyndromic hearing losses vary by the age at which the hearing loss starts, by how rapidly the hearing deteriorates, by the ultimate severity of the hearing loss, and by the presence/absence of vestibular dysfunction.

(Adapted from ref. 15, with permission.)

Imaging Studies

In contrast to the low yield of laboratory studies, imaging studies are often of both diagnostic and therapeutic usefulness in the care of children with hearing loss. In the series of Kenna and Neault (6) of 42 patients with unexplained sensorineural hearing loss, 10 had abnormal temporal bone computed tomography: 6 had large vestibular aqueduct; 3 had Mondini-type deformity, and 1 had cochleae lacking bony partitions.

PEARLS AND PERILS

Reasons to obtain hearing assessments on first-degree relatives (biologic parents, full siblings)

1. To identify unrecognized hearing loss.
2. To help the family members understand the rigors of testing.

Hearing Assessment of Parents and Siblings

Audiologic studies should be performed on each parent and sibling. It often helps with the child's diagnosis and always makes the family more sympathetic to the patient undergoing repeated testing.

PEARLS AND PERILS

Potentially treatable causes of sensory hearing loss

1. Syphilis.
2. Perilymphatic fistula.
3. Hypothyroidism (if diagnosed extremely early).
4. Leukemic infiltrates (e.g., granulocystic sarcoma of acute myelogenous leukemia).
5. Cochleotoxics (e.g., aspirin, ethacrynic acid, gentamicin, quinine).
6. Autoimmune disease.
7. Vasculitis (e.g., Cogan's syndrome).

Potentially treatable causes of neural hearing loss

1. Cerebellopontine angle cysts and tumors.
2. Inflammation (e.g., meningitis, syphilis, multiple sclerosis). Note, however, that dexamethasone has not been shown conclusively to improve significantly the audiologic, neurologic, or developmental outcome in children with bacterial meningitis (17).

Focus on the treatable causes. Follow-on assessments, especially historical recapitulation and physical examinations, along with imaging studies, eventually facilitate a diagnosis in most children with hearing loss. As Katz (18) has noted, "Our job is to maximize the individual's potential. Since true potential is too subtle for us to measure, we should always aim high."

 TREATMENT RECOMMENDATIONS

Prevention of Problems

Presumably, for patients with a large vestibular aqueduct, the patient can reduce the risk of worsening hearing by avoiding trauma and radical exercise (19). Noise-induced hearing loss is well described. Perhaps the noise created by suctioning middle ear fluid is potentially damaging (20). Notwithstanding concerns about noise-induced hearing loss, Axelsson et al. (21) surprisingly noted well-preserved hearing in pop/rock musicians, possibly attributable to (a) "training effect," i.e., exposure to loud but not harmful sound levels is associated with increased resistance to subsequent traumatic noise; and/or (b) more or less continuous stapedius muscle contractions.

One problem of unilateral hearing impairment is the difficulty in localizing the source of sound. Therefore, such children especially should be taught to look both ways before crossing a street (22).

Amplification

Although a discussion of hearing aids is beyond the scope of this chapter, a few points should be mentioned. A snugly fitting earmold, which minimizes acoustic feedback, often prompts ceruminous debris accumulation in the ear canal. Otomicroscopy with debris removal during the course of routine visits every few months for these children is a workable solution. A bias of this author is that children are best served if their hearing aids are fitted and attended in the same clinic that provides otologic care. The clinical adage that "a hearing aid mold used in an ear with an open tympanic membrane increases the risk of suppurative otitis" is probably true.

A bone conduction hearing aid is the only feasible amplification for some children, e.g., bilateral ear atresia in a child younger than age 2 years. A bone conduction aid may be the more feasible amplification for a child with persistently draining bilateral chronic otitis media. These comments are offered despite the drawbacks of bone conduction hearing aids: poor acoustic fidelity, poor effective amplification above 3 kHz, and the discomfort of a tight-fitting but aiding device. The bone-anchored hearing aid may have usefulness for some patients (see Chapter 20).

Amplification for children with unilateral aidable hearing loss was rarely advocated a generation ago. However, with the realization that on average such children do poorly in school (23), some sort of amplification is often appropriate. Most commonly, this is a "personal FM trainer" or other assistive device for use in the classroom (22,24).

Surgery

Cochlear implantation for bilaterally profoundly hearing-impaired children as young as 24 months of age was released from investigational status in the United States in 1990. With careful candidate selection, attention to surgical details, mapping, and aggressive rehabilitation, many cochlear implant children perform well in regular school classes.

The results of surgical correction of the hearing loss of congenital aural atresia are better when the deformity is minimal, generally characterized by the following: pinna mildly abnormal, at worse; external auditory canal open to the tympanic membrane; normal size tympanic cavity; and pneumatized mastoid (25). If the malformation is more than minimal, the patient is probably best served by a surgeon trained and experienced in congenital aural atresia. If both ears of a a patient have more than minimal atresia, some otologic surgeons defer attempting surgery until the patient is an adult and meanwhile recommend that the patient use a traditional bone conduction hearing aid or bone-anchored hearing aid (see chapter 20).

Tympanostomy tubes and tympanomastoid surgery are discussed in Chapters 14 and 16.

Pharmacotherapeutics

Few sensorineural hearing losses are treatable by medicine. Writing a drug prescription is more easily accomplished than is identifying the etiologic diagnosis.

TABLE 8: Comparison of Various Educationsl Settings for Hearing-Impaired Children

Feature	Auditory–Verbal	Auditory–Oral	Total Communication	Manual
Type of school	Usually private	Usually private	Public	Public
Parental involvement	Extremely high	Very high	High	High
Difficulty for child	Extreme	High	Average	Average
Graduate's listening–speaking ability	Can be very good	Can be good	Minimal	Nil
Visual cues allowed	None	Some	Many	Exclusively visual

Education for the Hearing-Impaired Child

The otolaryngologist is often asked about educational recommendations for a hearing-impaired child. How much the child can hear with hearing aids is the major otologic factor in recommending an educational setting. Generally, a child with moderate (or milder) hearing loss (see Table 5 of Chapter 12, on hearing assessment), with hearing aid(s) is well served in a regular school classroom. A child with severe (or worse) hearing in the better ear, notwithstanding hearing aids, usually needs a different educational setting (Table 8). The physician should have liaison with the educational settings, e.g., auditory–verbal (10), and should be an advocate for the child.

 ## MANAGEMENT OF COMPLICATIONS

The care of hearing-impaired children is far from an exact science. Despite knowledge, trust, empathy, and abundant data, there are problems. The refusal of assessments and hearing aids and failed follow-up visits often seem to be manifestations of grieving. Feelings for children with hearing loss seem to progress, as Kubler-Ross has described in dealing with other forms of loss, through five stages: (a) denial, (b) anger, (c) bargaining, (d) depression, and (e) acceptance. For children with congenital hearing loss, this stage theory may be meaningful in describing behaviors occurring among families, teachers, and practitioners (26). A psychiatrist and social worker can be invaluable in helping with cochlear implant children.

Hearing loss itself may be nonexistent, e.g., fabricated. Kahn and Goldman (27) report on an infant whose hearing loss was concocted—a case of Munchausen's syndrome by proxy.

 ## REFERENCES

1. Todd NW At-risk populations for hearing impairment in infants and young children. *Int J Pediatr Otorhinolaryngol* 1994;29:11–21.
2. Gorlin RJ, Toriello HV, Cohen MJ Jr, eds. *Hereditary hearing loss and its syndromes.* New York: Oxford University Press, 1995.
3. Prezant TR, Agapian JV, Bohlman MC, et al. Mitochondrial ribosomal RNA mutation associated with both antibiotic-induced and non-syndromic deafness. *Nat Genet* 1993;4:289–294.
4. Manning SC, Brown OE, Roland PS, Phillips DL. Incidence of sensorineural hearing loss in patients evaluated for tympanostomy tubes. *Arch Otolaryngol Head Neck Surg* 1994;120:881–884.
5. Reynolds JE, Meyer JM, Landa B, et al. Analysis of variability of clinical manifestations in Waardenburg syndrome. *Am J Med Genet* 1995;57:540–547.
6. Kenna MA, Neault MW. Pediatric sensorineural hearing loss: evaluation and managed care. *Laryngoscope* 1998 (*in press*).

7. Fowler KB, McCollister FP, Dahle AJ, et al. Progressive and fluctuating sensorineural hearing loss in children with asymtomatic congenital cytomegalovirus infection. *J Pediatr* 1997;130:624-630.

8. Brookhouser PE, Worthington DW, Kelly WJ. Fluctuating and/or progressive sensorineural hearing loss in children. *Laryngoscope* 1994;104:958–964.

9. Komsuoglu B, Goldeli O, Kulan K, et al. The Jervell and Lange-Nielsen syndrome. *Int J Cardiol* 1994;47:189–192.

10. Goldberg DM, Flexer C. Outcome survey of auditory-verbal graduates: study of clinical efficacy. *Am Acad Audiol* 1993;4:189–200.

11. Leguire LE, Fillman RD, Fishman DR, et al. A prospective study of ocular abnormalities in hearing impaired and deaf students. *Ear Nose Throat J* 1992;71:643–646, 651.

12. Peterson RA. In: Jaffe BF, ed. *Hearing loss in children.* Baltimore: University Park Press, 1977;228–240.

13. Podder S, Shepherd RC. Cogan's syndome: a rare systemic vasculitis. *Arch Dis Child* 1994;71:163–164.

14. Smith RJ, Berlin CI, Hejtmancik JF, et al. Clinical diagnosis of Usher syndomes. *Am J Med Genet* 1994;50:32–38.

15. Liu X, Xu L. Nonsyndromtic hearing loss: an analysis of audiograms. *Ann Otol Rhinol Laryngol* 1994;103:428–433.

16. Ruben RJ, Rapin I. In: Alberti PW, Ruben RJ, eds. *Otologic medicine and surgery* New York: Churchill Livingstone, 1988;1665–1694.

17. Wald ER, Kaplan SL, Mason EO Jr, et al. Dexamethasone therapy for children with bacterial meningitis. *Pediatrics* 1995;95:21–28.

18. Katz FA. In: Gerber SE, ed. *The handbook of pediatric audiology.* Washington: Gallaudet, 1996;15–34.

19. Okumura T, Takahashi H, Honjo I, et al. Sensorineural hearing loss in patients with large vestibular aqueduct. *Laryngoscope* 1995;105:289–294.

20. Wetmore RF, Henry WJ, Konkle DF. Acoustical factors of noise created by suctioning middle ear fluid. *Arch Otolaryngol Head Neck Surg* 1993;119:762–766.

21. Axelsson A, Eliasson A, Israelsson B. Hearing in pop/rock muscians: a follow-up study. *Ear Hear* 1995;16:245–253.

22. Brookhouser PE, Worthington DW, Kelly WJ. Unilateral hearing loss in children. *Laryngoscope* 1991;101:1264–1272.

23. Bess FH, Tharpe AM. Unilateral hearing impairment in children. *Pediatrics* 1984;74:206–216.

24. Crandell CC, Samaldino JJ, Flexer C, eds. *Sound-field FM amplification: theory and practical applications.* San Diego: Singular Publishing, 1995.

25. Hough JVD, Baker RS. Congenital aural atresia. In: Gates GA, ed. *Current therapy in otolaryngology—head and neck surgery—4.* Toronto: BC Decker, 1990;3–8.

26. Mencher GT. Counseling families of hearing-impaired children: suggestions for the audiologist. In: Gerber SE, ed. *The handbook of pediatric audiology.* Washington: Gallaudet, 1996;343–351.

27. Kahn G, Goldman E. Munchausen syndome by proxy: mother fabricates infant's hearing impairment. *J Speech Hear Res* 1991;34:957–958.

N.W. Todd: Departments of Otolaryngology and Pediatrics, Emory University School of Medicine, Atlanta, Georgia 30322.

• *Practical Pediatric Otolaryngology*
• edited by Robin T. Cotton
  and Charles M. Myer, III
• Lippincott-Raven Publishers,
  Philadelphia © 1999

14

Diagnosis and Management of Otitis Media with Effusion

Margaret A. Kenna

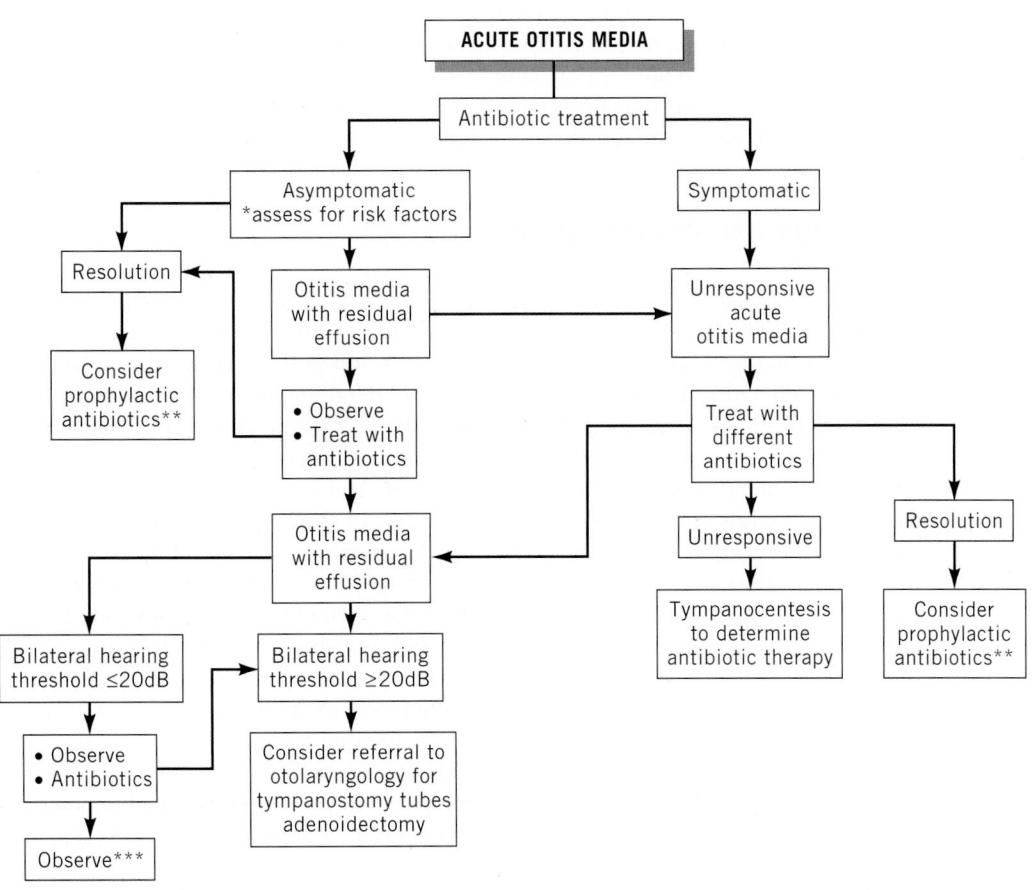

*Risk factors include: age less than 15 months, family history of otitis, male gender, attendance at large day care, occurrence of otitis in previous month.

**After resolution, prophylactic antibiotics can be considered in any child who has had more than 3 episodes of otitis media over a 6-month period.

***Chronic middle ear fluid may lead to tympanic membrane changes, retraction pockets, and ossicular erosion. Even children with only mild hearing loss need to be watched closely for appropriate development of speech and language.

⬤ HISTORICAL BACKGROUND

Otitis media is the most common reason, except for upper respiratory tract infections (URI), for young children to visit the primary care provider; it is also one of the most common infectious diseases of childhood. Prior to the introduction of antibiotics, otitis media was also responsible for very significant morbidity and mortality. For example, in a study by Rosenwasser and Adelman (1) that looked at mortality at the Los Angeles County Hospital in the 5 years (1928 to 1933) preceding the introduction of sulfa, 1 in 40 deaths resulted from intracranial complications of otitis media. Similarly, Courville (2) noted that the death rate from otitis media in 1944 to 1953 was 10% of the rate in 1929 to 1933. Even now, with common use of systemic antimicrobials, morbidity continues to be problematic, and in some parts of the world mortality still occurs (3).

To muddy the waters further, the frequent use of antimicrobials in the treatment of many forms of otitis media is now being questioned due to the increased emergence of resistant bacterial organisms (4). Other controversial areas in otitis media include whether the conductive hearing loss that accompanies the presence of middle-ear effusion has a significant impact on speech and language, and if so, whether surgical or medical therapy is the most appropriate course. In the 12 months from April 1995 to March 1996, 965 articles concerning otitis media were listed on MEDLINE, most dealing with management, demonstrating that these issues continue to be far from clear.

DEFINITION AND CLASSIFICATION

Otitis media means inflammation of the middle ear, without reference to etiology or pathogenesis. The other areas of the temporal bone contiguous to the middle ear, including the mastoid and perilabyrinthine air cells and petrous apex, may become inflamed as well. Otitis media can be further classified into many variants, including acute otitis media without effusion, acute otitis media with effusion, chronic otitis media with effusion, chronic suppurative otitis media with and without cholesteatoma, and atelectasis of the tympanic membrane/middle ear/mastoid. Atelectasis may or may not be associated with a prior clinical history of otitis media. In the (especially older) literature, many other terms have been used to describe these various stages of otitis media. Acute otitis media without effusion may be called myringitis; acute otitis media with effusion may be labeled acute suppurative, purulent, or bacterial otitis media. Otitis media with effusion is also often referred to as serous, mucoid, secretory, glue ear, or, depending on the duration, chronic otitis media. Ears with dry tympanic membrane perforations may also be designated chronic otitis media. Although chronic suppurative otitis media currently refers to a nonintact tympanic membrane with middle-ear otorrhea, in the older literature it also occasionally meant an intact tympanic membrane with chronic middle-ear changes; yet another name for chronic suppurative otitis media is tubotympanitis or chronic purulent otitis media. Finally, adhesive otitis media and atelectasis are often used interchangably, although they are distinct clinical entities (5).

The profusion of terms makes it difficult to read and evaluate the literature with regard to both diagnosis and treatment. In this chapter, *acute otitis media with effusion* implies rapid onset of one of the following: otalgia, fever, otorrhea, recent onset of anorexia, irritability, vomiting, or diarrhea. These symptoms should be accompanied by otoscopic findings of a tympanic membrane that is opaque, often bulging, and limited in mobility on pneumatic otoscopy. Erythema may or may not be present. Very early acute otitis media, or *myringitis*, may not have obvious middle-ear effusion, but rather just a fiery red and sometimes thickened tympanic membrane; this should be distinguished from a normal tympanic membrane in a crying child. *Otitis media with effusion* means middle ear effusion of any duration, and *chronic otitis media with effusion* means a middle ear effusion that persists for 3 months or longer after a diagnosis of acute otitis media, or at least 3 documented months of asymptomatic otitis media with effusion. Actually, "asymptomatic" may be somewhat of a misnomer: although these patients do not have the acute symptoms of pain, fever, irritability, etc., they usually do have hearing loss in the affected ear that is often evident to a parent, teacher, or the patient. These patients may also be somewhat off balance and have tinnitus, symptoms difficult to elicit from a very young child. Chronic suppurative otitis media refers to middle ear otorrhea coming through a nonintact tympanic membrane with a tympanotomy tube and/or perforation. Although there is no "official" time when acute otorrhea becomes chronic, 6 to 12 weeks of continuous drainage is used as a general guide. *Effusion* simply refers to the presence of fluid in the middle ear/mastoid spaces; it can be suppurative, serous, mucoid, or a combination. *Atelectasis* of the middle ear/mastoid refers to collapse of the tympanic membrane. This may be passive and may present without an obvious history of otitis media, or it may be due to apparent negative middle-ear pressure with eustachian tube dysfunction. Adhesive otitis media, often confused with atelectasis, is actually a complication of otitis media. Adhesive otitis occurs as a result of chronic inflammation of the middle ear and mastoid resulting in proliferation of fibrous tissue; this can limit ossicular motion, cause adhesion of a severely atelectatic tympanic membrane to the middle ear, and result in a conductive hearing loss. Finally, *retraction pockets* represent an atelectatic area of the tympanic membrane, and *otorrhea* means drainage of fluid from the middle ear into the external auditory canal.

EPIDEMIOLOGY

As noted above, otitis media is one of the most common reasons for a child to visit the primary care provider's office, and there are indications that the incidence and prevalence is increasing (5). Some of the factors making the diagnosis of otitis media more frequent include increased awareness of the disease, better otoscopic equipment, ready availability of tympanometers in primary care providers' offices and schools, and concern on the part of working parents about keeping children healthy so that they can attend day care and the parents can continue to work. Day-care attendance itself seems to be a factor in the increased occurrence of otitis, due at least in part to increased exposure to multiple respiratory pathogens from the other children (5).

In the Boston study, the occurrence of both recurrent acute otitis media and otitis media with effusion peaked between the ages of 6 months and 13 months of age; similar results have been found in other studies in other countries (5,6). The peak age-specific attack rate occurs between the ages of 6 and 18 months, and if a child has not had otitis before the age of 3 years, he or she is statistically unlikely to develop severe or recurrent disease. A study in Pittsburgh showed that by the age of 2 months, 2% of children had experienced at least one episode of acute otitis media; by 12 months, 34% of children had developed acute otitis; and by 24 months, 59% had developed acute otitis. With regard to middle-ear fluid, 10% had had at least one episode by age 2 months, and by age 12 months 78% had had at least one episode of middle ear fluid. Finally, by age 24 months 92% of children had been diagnosed with at least one episode of middle ear fluid (7). Additionally, after a single episode of acute otitis media the fluid may persist for months. In the Boston study, 70% of children had fluid at 2 weeks, 40% at 4 weeks, 20% at 2 months, and 10% at 3 months, with studies from many other centers supporting these observations (6).

Many factors influence the incidence of otitis media (Fig. 1). Those associated with an increased incidence of otitis include age under 2 years, male gender, certain ethnic backgrounds, various social and economic conditions, attendance at a day-care center, cold-weather season (because of the association with increased URI rates), second-hand smoke, genetic factors, and certain underlying diseases. In many studies, breast feeding is associated with a decreased incidence of otitis media. Children with a first incidence of acute otitis media before age 6 months or otitis media with effusion before age 2 months are statistically at increased risk of further significant otitis media compared with

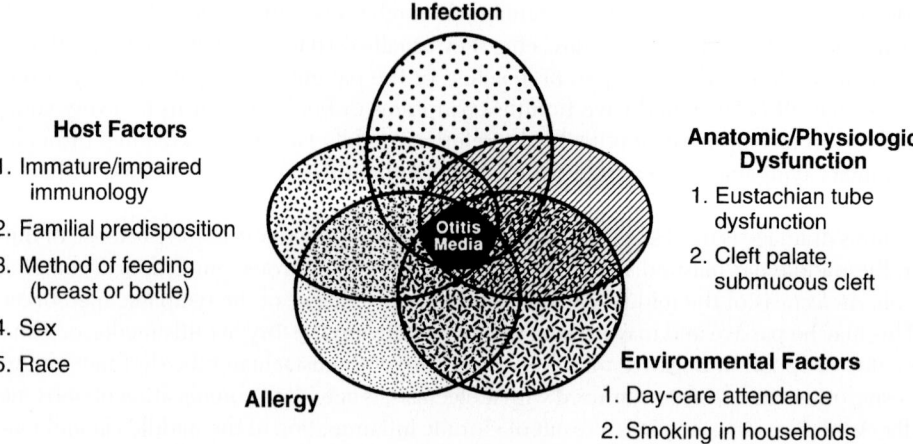

FIGURE 1 Pathogenesis of otitis media: multiple factors. (From Bluestone CD, Stool SE, Kenna MA, eds. *Pediatric Otolaryngology*, 3rd ed. Philadelphia: Saunders, 1996:412, with permission.)

children whose ear disease started later (otitis prone). Children who are Native Americans (Alaskan and Canadian Inuits) and who live in developing areas or in crowded conditions have statistically more middle ear disease than other children. Until recently there was some evidence that African-American children had less ear disease than white children, but a recent study by Casselbrant and coworkers (8) suggests that this is not the case (8). Children whose biologic parents and siblings have/had significant otitis are more likely to have increased episodes and duration of otitis as well. Children in large day-care centers are more likely to have otitis than children in family day care, who are in turn more likely to have otitis than those in home care. Finally, children exposed to second-hand smoke are more likely to have otitis than those who are not.

Because of underlying medical or anatomic conditions some children are more prone to otitis media than others. Children with cleft palate and other midface anomalies, including Down's syndrome, have a much higher incidence of otitis media, especially chronic middle ear effusion, than do other children (9). This is thought to be due at least in part to anatomic and physiologic abnormalities leading to eustachian tube dysfunction. Children with altered immune systems, including hypogammaglobulinemia and human immunodeficiency virus (HIV) disease, and children with ciliary dysfunction are much more likely to have otitis and sinusitis. Finally, there has been some suggestion that gastroesophageal reflux, with reflux into the nasopharynx, may cause or exacerbate otitis media and sinusitis.

PATHOGENESIS

Pathophysiology

Abnormal function of the eustachian tube is the most important factor in the pathogenesis of otitis media. In infants and small children the eustachian tube is shorter, more horizontal, and functionally more immature compared with the adult eustachian tube. When a child gets a URI there may be edema and congestion of the respiratory mucosa, including that of the middle ear, with narrowing of the eustachian tube isthmus; this results in negative pressure in the middle ear relative to the nasopharynx. Therefore, when the tube opens, viruses and bacteria from the nasopharynx are "aspirated" into the middle ear, causing inflammation.

Many other confounding variables affecting eustachian tube function include patulous or functionally/anatomically obstructed tubes, as well as abnormalities of the respiratory mucosa, including allergy, immunocompromise, and ciliary dysfunction. Allergy has long been implicated in the etiology of otitis media, but the exact mechanism remains elusive. Possibilities include inflammatory swelling of the middle ear/mastoid/eustachian tube mucosa; allergic nasal obstruction; or the middle ear mucosa reacting as a "shock organ." However, as large numbers of highly allergic children do not have significant otitis, and many children with significant otitis do not have documented allergy, the relationship is clearly not a simple one.

Children with congenital or acquired (including drug-induced) immunocompromise, although relatively small in number, require special consideration, as they are often more susceptible to infections in general, including otitis media, and are more likely to have unusual organisms. Congenital immune abnormalities include B-cell deficiencies, such as hypogammaglobulinemia and IgA deficiency; T-cell deficiencies, such as DiGeorge's syndrome; combined T- and B-cell deficiencies, including ataxia telangiectasia; phagocyte defects, including Chédiak-Higashi syndrome; and others, including complement deficiencies. Acquired abnormalities include those secondary to neoplasms, inflammatory processes such as acute or chronic infections (e.g., HIV disease) and rheumatoid arthritis, and metabolic abnormalities such as diabetes. Drugs causing immune deficiencies include steroids, chemotherapeutic agents, and antirejection agents used in transplant patients. These severe forms of immune deficiency are uncommon in children; however, many of the significantly otitis-prone children may have "immature" immune systems as documented by poor response to polysaccharide antigen vaccines, including *Hemophilus influenzae* type B (HIB) and the pneumococcal vaccines.

Abnormalities, either physiologic or anatomic, of the palate and associated musculature, especially the tensor veli palatini, may cause or worsen eustachian tube dysfunction. For example, many craniofacial abnormalities, including cleft palate, midface anomalies such as Crouzon's or Apert's syndrome, and Down's syndrome are associated with abnormal skull base and/or palate shapes with resultant eustachian tube dysfunction.

Microbiology

The most commonly identified aerobic pathogens associated with acute otitis media are *Streptococcus pneumoniae* (30% to 50%) and nontypable *H. influenzae* (20% to 30%), followed by *Moraxella catarrhalis* (10% to 20%) and group A streptococcus (1% to 5%) (10). Other bacteria such as *Staphylococcus aureus* and gram-negative enteric organisms, including *Escherichia coli*, *Klebsiella* sp., and *Pseudomonas aeruginosa* are infrequently, although consistently, isolated in a few percent of patients. In neonates and young infants *S. pneumoniae* and *H. influenzae* are still the most commonly isolated pathogens; however, *S. aureus*, group B streptococcus, gram-negative enteric pathogens, and other organisms associated with local and systemic infection are found up to 20% of the time. Infants and children in intensive care settings, especially if the stay is prolonged, and immunocompromised children may also have unusual organisms recovered from their middle-ear fluid. Other bacterial organisms that have occasionally been isolated from middle ear fluid include *Mycoplasma pneumoniae*, *Chlamydia trachomatis*, and *Mycobacterium tuberculosis*. Most recently, a new bacteria, *Alloiococcus otitidis*, has been isolated under very careful culture conditions from chronic middle-ear fluid, and unusual organisms continue to be reported as isolated cases in the literature (11) (Fig. 2).

Although anaerobic bacteria have been isolated in several studies of both acute and chronic otitis media, the consensus is that their role is a minor one. *Peptostreptococcus*, *Fusobacterium* sp., and *Bacteroides* sp. organisms are the most commonly isolated. In chronic suppurative otitis media, however, anaerobes are often found, and sometimes in more abundance than aerobic organisms. The management of these organisms, even when isolated in large numbers, remains unclear in all these various forms of otitis media.

Over the past 10 to 15 years an increasing number of beta-lactamase-producing bacteria have been isolated from the middle ear (10). These include up to 80% of the *H. influenzae* organisms, close to 100% of the *M. catarrhalis* organisms, and many *S. aureus*

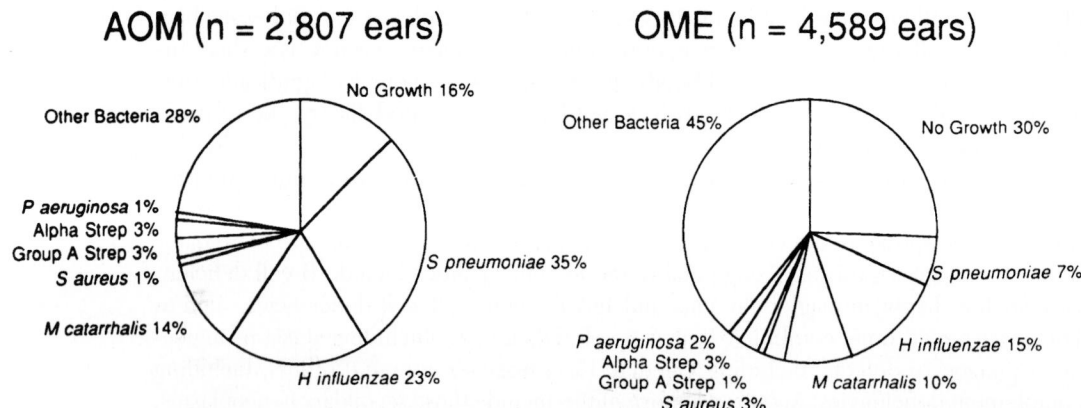

FIGURE 2 Distribution of bacteria (Acute otitis media) in 2807 ears from the Pittsburgh Otitis Media Research Center 1980–1989. (From ref. 5, with permission.)

organisms and anaerobes (Fig. 3). Fortunately, *S. pneumoniae* does not yet make beta-lactamase. However, a significant percentage of the *S. pneumoniae* organisms have become resistant to penicillin and other antimicrobials, the exact percentage varying with the geographic area and the population of patients studied (12). The mechanisms for beta-lactamase and penicillin resistance are different, so different strategies in terms of antimicrobial usage are needed for treatment. Possible clinical factors in the development of bacterial resistance include multiple and prolonged exposures to antimicrobials, including prophylaxis, not taking the entire prescribed course of antimicrobial, and inappropriate administration. This last is now being targeted in the treatment of otitis media.

Recently viruses have gained increasing attention as causative, or copathogenic organisms, along with bacteria, involved in otitis media. Viruses that have been directly isolated from middle ear fluids include respiratory syncytial virus, rhinovirus, influenza virus, adenovirus, enteroviruses, and parainfluenza viruses. Cytomegalovirus and herpes simplex virus have also been isolated, although in a smaller number of cases. Otitis media is also known to accompany viral exanthems, including measles and the Epstein-Barr virus (5).

COMPLICATIONS

The complications of otitis media can be divided into intratemporal and intracranial. The intratemporal complications include hearing loss, which can be either conductive

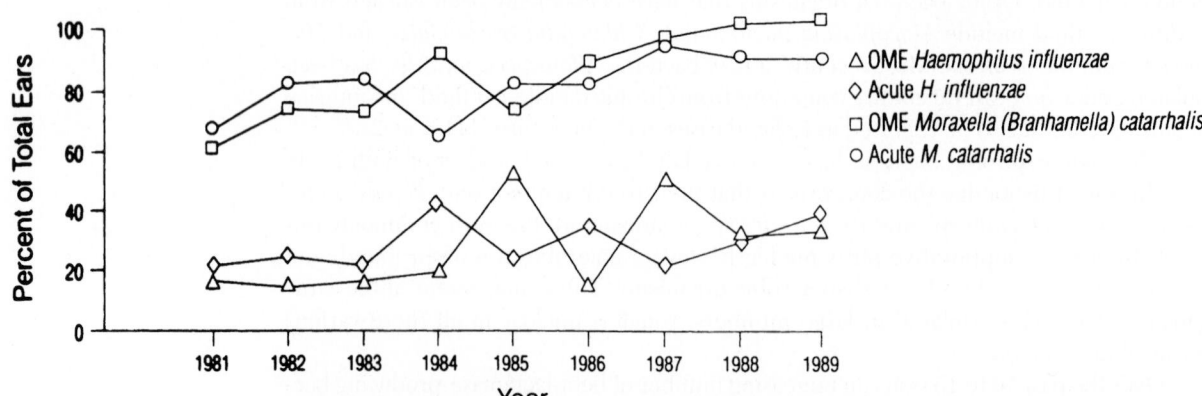

FIGURE 3 Change in the percentage of beta-lactamase-producing strains of *Haemophilus influenzae* and *Moraxella catarrhalis* from patients with acute otitis media and otitis media with effusion (OME) at the Pittsburgh Otitis Media Research Center, 1980–1989. (From ref. 10, with permission.)

(common) or sensorineural (uncommon), perforation of the tympanic membrane, chronic suppurative otitis media, cholesteatoma, retraction pocket, adhesive otitis media, tympanosclerosis, ossicular discontinuity and fixation, mastoiditis, petrositis, labyrinthitis, facial paralysis, and cholesterol granuloma. Conductive hearing loss is extremely common, occurring in most cases of acute or chronic otitis media with effusion and perforated tympanic membranes. Sensorineural hearing loss is fortunately very uncommon, but can occur in the setting of very long-standing chronic suppurative otitis media or secondary to some of the other suppurative complications, including acute mastoiditis, labyrinthitis, and meningitis. Perforation of the tympanic membrane may occur spontaneously due to acute otitis media or may result when a tympanostomy tube falls out and the resulting perforation does not heal. Tympanosclerosis, adhesive otitis, ossicular discontinuity, cholesteatoma, and cholesterol granuloma usually occur secondary to chronic otitis media; tympanosclerosis and cholesteatoma are also known complications of tympanostomy tubes. Fortunately, labyrinthitis, severe mastoiditis, meningitis, petrositis, and facial paralysis are very infrequently seen but can have significant morbidity if they go unrecognized.

There continues to be a lot of controversy about what degree of conductive hearing loss, and for what duration, may have an effect on speech, language, and cognitive development, both short- and long-term, in children with otitis media (13). Since conductive hearing loss is one of the complications of otitis media that significantly guides both the medical and surgical management of the disease there has been a lot of research on how important this hearing loss is. The clinical studies in this area are especially difficult to compare because the outcomes (short- and long-term speech, language, and cognitive ability) can be evaluated using so many different methods. Additionally, the study populations are often not comparable, with a wide range of subjects varying from mainly white middle-class children to severely disadvantaged minority children. Recently, some studies have started to focus on the longer term aspects of hearing and central auditory processing brought about by long-term effusion and conductive hearing loss; since these types of more sophisticated evaluations can only routinely be performed on children over the age of 5, it is difficult to know how soon some of these effects may have started.

Despite the variance in study design and results, enough data exist that both the American Academy of Pediatrics (through their Committee on Early Childhood, Adoption, and Dependent Care) and the Agency for Health Care Policy and Research (through their clinical guidelines) feel that there is growing evidence of correlation between middle-ear effusion with hearing impairment and delays in speech, language, and cognitive development. If the effusion has persisted for 3 months or longer, hearing should be assessed and communication skills evaluated. Clinicians must then decide for themselves on a course that is best for the child in the current situation, being cognizant that too long a period of watchful waiting could be detrimental to the child (14–16).

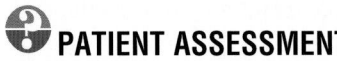

PATIENT ASSESSMENT

History

The two mainstays of diagnosis of otitis media are history and physical examination. The most common symptoms of acute otitis media with effusion are sudden onset of otalgia, otorrhea, fever, irritability, and lethargy, followed less commonly by anorexia, nausea, vomiting, diarrhea, and headache. Fever is present in up to two-thirds of children with acute otitis media, but fevers over 40°C are uncommon and may represent bacteremia or other complications. Older children may also complain of hearing loss, tinnitus, and vertigo; small children may not be able to complain about these specific things but may be off-balance or appear to not be hearing (17). Children with relatively asymptomatic otitis media with effusion may complain of, or seem to have, hearing loss. Some children with subacute otitis media with effusion may not have sudden onset of symptoms but may complain of intermittent otalgia, imbalance, and hearing loss. Children with acute otitis media and some children with chronic otitis media with effusion may appear to be sicker at night or during naps, with frequent awakenings and pain: the eustachian tube is less functional when the child is lying down. Some children have truly asymptomatic otitis media with effusion; fluid is seen on otoscopy and is frequently only suspected due to hearing loss. Children with draining ears, especially if the problem is chronic, may have little or no pain and may sleep well but may still complain of hearing loss and occasional low-grade fevers. Children with tympanic membrane perforations are usually asymptomatic except for hearing loss, unless they get water in their ears, when they may have significant discomfort. Finally, children with atelectasis of the tympanic membrane are also usually asymptomatic, although many of these children will have hearing loss as well.

Physical Examination

The normal tympanic membrane is gray and translucent (like waxed paper) with normal mobility on pneumatic otoscopy. Middle-ear landmarks that may be seen through a normal tympanic membrane include the short process of the malleus, the incudostapedial joint, and very occasionally the chorda tympani. In small and mobile children the malleus is the most frequently seen landmark. In acute otitis media the tympanic membrane is opaque, often bulging, may be thickened and erythematous, and has very limited mobility; the middle ear landmarks are obscured. Uncommonly bullae may be seen on the tympanic membrane when the disease is very acute and can be present either with or without effusion. Acutely perforated tympanic membranes are usually erythematous, and thickened and have otorrhea draining through them that can be purulent, serous, or mucoid. In otitis media with effusion the tympanic membrane may be opaque but is less likely to be erythematous. Air/fluid levels or bubbles may be seen, indicating at least intermittent aeration of the middle ear. If the tympanic membrane is opaque then it usually has limited mobility with obscured landmarks, but if there are bubbles or an air/fluid level the tympanic membrane motion may be fairly normal and the malleus may be seen. The tympanic membrane may be in a relatively normal position or may be retracted but is usually not bulging. The color of the tympanic membrane reflects the middle-ear contents and may be opaque and white, or amber; less commonly the tympanic membrane may appear almost dark blue, the sign of a "glue ear." Although many older texts emphasize the presence of the "light reflex" on the tympanic membrane in an otherwise normal ear, this reflex may be absent in entirely normal ears and present in ears with middle-ear effusion; therefore, it is not helpful in making a diagnosis of otitis media. In tympanic membranes with perforations the perforation can be of any size and location within the tympanic membrane, may rarely be multiple, and there may be tympanosclerosis within the remaining tympanic membrane. If the perforation is large the ossicles may be clearly seen. In atelectasis the tympanic membrane is often thinned out and transparent, draped over the promontory and the ossicles; it may move when negative pressure is applied with the pneumatic otoscope. In tympanic membranes with a significant amount of tympanosclerosis the uninvolved portion can be very atelectatic and look more like retraction pockets. However, retraction pockets are more often seen in tympanic membranes that are relatively normal and, although they can occur anywhere, usually occupy the site of an old tympanostomy tube or are found in the posterior/superior aspect of the tympanic membrane in patients with ongoing eustachian tube dysfunction.

Although middle-ear effusion is often described as serous (thin and watery), mucoid/secretory (thick and viscous), purulent (pus-like), or clear (which rarely may represent a cerebrospinal fluid leak rather than inflammation), the description of the type of fluid is most accurately made if there is otorrhea or fluid is obtained at myringotomy, as an intact tympanic membrane may be thickened or diseased, obscuring the view of the middle ear. Treatment decisions cannot be made solely on the basis of what type of fluid the observer thinks is in the middle ear, for example, serous fluid is not always sterile and may be present in acute otitis media, for which antibiotics would often be indicated.

Hearing Evaluation

The most common complication of otitis media is conductive hearing loss, which may result from middle-ear effusion, eustachian tube dysfunction, or pathology resulting from inflammation. Every child with recurrent otitis media and/or ongoing eustachian tube dysfunction should have their hearing checked. The evaluation of hearing in a child with otitis media is really twofold; audiometric evaluation to test the peripheral hearing and impedance audiometry to evaluate the stiffness of the tympanic membrane and middle-ear system. The audiometric technique used to test the child varies with the age and maturity of the child. Although otacoustic emissions (OAEs) are often used for hearing screening in the newborn nursery, this is not a good technique to clarify the hearing status in a child with otitis media, as one of the main causes of OAE failure is middle-ear fluid. In infants under the age of 6 months, auditory brainstem response (ABR) testing gives the most accurate thresholds and may be able to distinguish a conductive from a sensorineural loss. However, ABR testing is time consuming and expensive, so it is usually reserved for further diagnostic evaluation in infants and young children who fail OAE testing, with greater than expected losses obtained with behavioral testing, or if a loss persists after resolution of middle-ear disease. ABR testing may also be of great value in children who are unable to participate in behavioral testing due to age or level of disability, or in young children when asymmetric hearing loss is suspected but ear-specific testing cannot be carried out due to the child's age.

PEARLS AND PERILS

1. Although the diagnosis of otitis sounds straightforward, it is not. The clinical signs and symptoms of otitis are similar to those of many other common childhood conditions and illnesses, including URI without otitis, teething, and viral gastroenteritis. Therefore repeated diagnoses over the phone based on symptomatology alone do not always provide an accurate picture of the true incidence of otitis in that child.

2. Otitis is also both over- and underdiagnosed by examiners who may not be fully aware of what to look for, and who are often being "leaned on" by parents to make a diagnosis that can be medically treated.

3. Pneumatic otoscopy must always be utilized to examine the tympanic membrane, as middle-ear fluid may or may not be obvious on visualization alone. In most crying children the tympanic membrane will be somewhat hyperemic due to increased prominence of the blood vessels; this must be distinguished from acute otitis media so that treatment is appropriately prescribed.

4. On the other hand, an episode of acute otitis may be resolved both clinically and on examination (redness and bulging gone), but middle-ear fluid may still be present; parents of these children may be told that "the ears are clear," although fluid may still be there.

5. Along the same lines, children with asymptomatic chronic middle-ear fluid may fail a screening hearing test, only to be told by an examiner that "the ears are normal"; further investigation may, however, reveal abnormal tympanograms, a conductive hearing loss, and definite middle-ear fluid when the ears are examined by someone familiar with the physical findings associated with otitis media with effusion.

TYMPANOGRAM TYPES AND VARIANTS RELATED TO CLINICAL FINDINGS

	TYMPANOGRAM TYPES	COMMON VARIANTS	PRESUMPTIVE DIAGNOSIS OF TYMPANIC MEMBRANE MIDDLE EAR CONDITION
1.	NORMAL	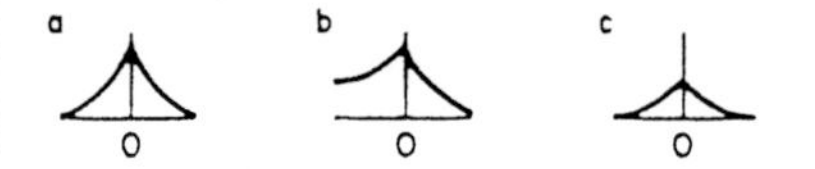	NORMAL
2.	HIGH COMPLIANCE (NORMAL PRESSURE)	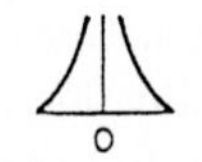	FLACCID TYMPANIC MEMBRANE OR OSSICULAR DISCONTINUITY
3.	NEGATIVE PRESSURE (NORMAL COMPLIANCE)	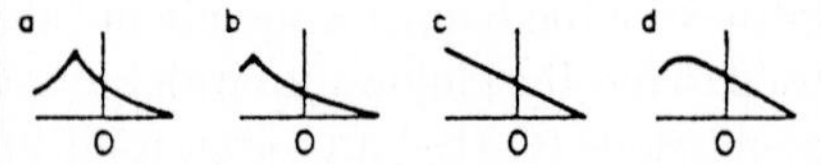	HIGH NEGATIVE PRESSURE WITH OR WITHOUT MIDDLE EAR EFFUSION
4.	HIGH NEGATIVE PRESSURE AND HIGH COMPLIANCE	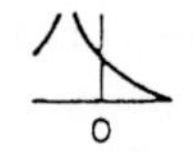	FLACCID TYMPANIC MEMBRANE AND HIGH NEGATIVE PRESSURE (OR OSSICULAR DISCONTINUITY AND HIGH NEGATIVE PRESSURE)
5.	HIGH POSITIVE PRESSURE		HIGH POSITIVE PRESSURE WITH OR WITHOUT MIDDLE EAR EFFUSION
6.	LOW COMPLIANCE	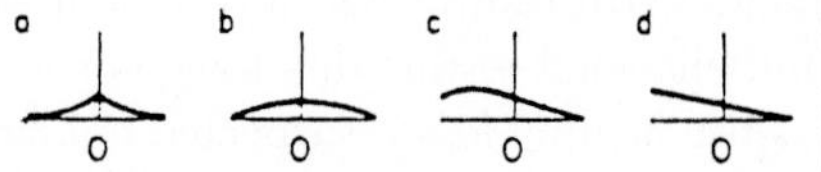	MIDDLE EAR EFFUSION, &/OR THICKENED TYMPANIC MEMBRANE, &/OR OSSICULAR FIXATION &/OR ADHESIVE OTITIS MEDIA

FIGURE 4 Tympanogram types related to presumptive conditions of the middle ear. (From Bluestone CD, Klein JO. *Otitis media in infants and children*. Philadlephia: Saunders, 1988:86, with permission.)

Since most children do not develop very frequent or persistent otitis media until 6 months of age or older, behavioral testing is the standard technique. Behavioral observation audiometry (BOA) is used for infants from age 6 months to 1 year and provides an estimation of hearing, especially for the better hearing ear. Visual reinforcement audiometry (VRA) is used for toddlers aged 1 to 2 years and also gives results for the better hearing ear. Although BOA and VRA can document hearing loss, they do not differentiate between conductive and sensorineural hearing loss. Play audiometry can be used with cooperative children over the age of 2 years and can provide both ear-specific data and air and bone conduction thresholds, needed to distinguish between conductive and sensorineural losses. Conventional audiometry can be employed in most cooperative children older than 5 years of age.

Immitance audiometry includes tympanometry, which measures the amount of sound reflected by the tympanic membrane and middle-ear structures and is a graphic representation of compliance changes as the ear canal pressure is varied from –200 to +200mm H_2O (some machines can provide more pressure). Various tympanometric patterns are associated with normal examinations, middle-ear fluid, retracted tympanic membranes, tympanic membrane perforations/patient tympanotomy tubes, and stiff tympanic membrane/middle-ear systems (as in otosclerosis). Any tympanometric pattern should always be correlated with pneumatic otoscopy and other audiometric data (Fig. 4). Two other aspects of immitance audiometry are the middle-ear muscle reflex (acoustic reflex) and equivalent ear canal volume. These studies, especially the acoustic reflex, are often used by experienced audiologists for further determination of hearing loss and middle-ear dysfunction.

Acoustic reflectometry uses a hand-held instrument placed next to the opening of the child's external ear canal and provides an 80-dB sound source that varies from 2,000 to 4,500 Hz in a 100-msec period; the instrument then measures the total level of reflected and transmitted sound. This device has been found to be useful by some investigators, but not as helpful by others, in screening for middle-ear fluid. Some of this difference in experience may be due to varying techniques by the instrument user, including right versus left hand and angle of the instrument with the ear canal. Currently, acoustic reflectometry is not widely used in the diagnosis of otitis media.

Other techniques that are, or have been used, in the evaluation of eustachian tube dysfunction include sonotubometry, manometry, and tympanometry using various pressure-changing maneuvers. These studies are available in research settings and are not routinely used in evaluation of the child with otitis media (5).

TREATMENT RECOMMENDATIONS

Rationale

There are several reasons to treat otitis media: to avoid complications, to treat symptomatic disease effectively, to "wait out" the URI season, and to buy time until the child's eustachian tube function and immune system have matured. Management options should be matched to the patient's pattern of otitis: recurrent acute otitis media that clears in between episodes, recurrent acute otitis media with persistent fluid in between acute episodes, and chronic middle ear fluid with few acute symptoms. In many cases, medical therapy will work well in the first, and sometimes the second, pattern but is often ineffective in the third.

Acute otitis media has a spontaneous resolution rate of about 60% to 80% (18). Possible reasons for this include drainage of middle-ear contents down the eustachian tube or perforated tympanic membrane, natural clearing by the body's local or systemic immune system, or acute otitis that occurred as a result of viruses or some noninfectious process. Therefore, some investigators have felt that no initial antimicrobial therapy is indicated for acute otitis media, rather, agents to control the symptoms of pain and fever should be given and the child watched closely. If the child is not significantly better after a few days, then antimicrobial therapy can be initiated. However, several studies suggest that the resolution rate is higher if antimicrobials are given from the beginning, and the complication rate may be lower as well. Some studies that have evaluated middle-ear fluid several days into an acute infection have found that *S. pneumoniae* is often the cause of persistent otitis. Since *S. pneumoniae* is also associated with a large number of the complications secondary to otitis media, nontreatment in the acute stage is at least worrisome. Based on all these factors, routine nontreatment of symptomatic acute otitis media is not advocated.

The routine treatment of asymptomatic middle-ear fluid is at least as controversial. The child with asymptomatic middle-ear fluid typically has a viral URI and the fluid is noted incidentally on physical examination; the tympanic membrane is often dull but not red or bulging, and serous fluid or bubbles are noted behind it. Although the parents may have noted decreased hearing, the child has no other symptoms. In this child, watchful waiting may be entirely appropriate. The key here is whether the child is truly asymptomatic (no fever, pain, etc.) and has reliable caretakers to make sure that the child returns for follow-up and/or to report if the child develops symptoms consistent with acute otitis media. However, this type of middle-ear fluid is not necessarily sterile, with bacterial organisms documented 30% to 70% of the time by conventional culture techniques and 77% by the polymerase chain reaction (19). Several months of documented middle-ear fluid is cause for concern, and treatment should be strongly considered.

Medical Therapy

The mainstay of otitis media management is medical therapy using antimicrobials. The choice of drug is based on the presumed pathogen, age of the patient, (e.g., in children under the age of 2 months sulfa should not be used routinely), duration of disease, what other antimicrobials have been used recently for otitis, and the presence of any drug allergies. In the otherwise normal patient who probably has one of the three major bacterial organisms as a cause for the otitis, amoxicillin still remains the antimicrobial of choice in the treatment of a first, or infrequent, episode of acute otitis media. It is inexpensive, the side effects are few and well known, and children will usually take it. If the child has a prompt response to therapy with resolution of otalgia, fever, and irritability and the parents feel that the child is clinically well, then follow-up with the primary care provider can be in 2 to 4 weeks (20). The person doing the follow-up must remember that, in many cases, there will be persistent middle-ear fluid after the antimicrobial is completed (Fig. 5). In many studies, including those in the United States and Scandinavia, there was persistent fluid after an episode of acute otitis media in 40% of patients at 4 weeks, 20% at 8 weeks, and 10% at 3 months. Additionally, the younger the patient the more likely the fluid is to persist. Many practitioners are inclined to prescribe further antimicrobial therapy at this point if they see middle-ear fluid; however, in the truly asymptomatic patient with this fluid it is also quite reasonable to observe these children closely to see if the fluid resolves on its own, and consider initiating another course of medical therapy only if the patient develops recurrent symptoms or does not have resolution on their own within 2 to 3 months.

In the patient who does not have significant improvement in the signs and symptoms of acute disease within 2 to 3 days, then there are three options. The first is to continue the current regimen, perhaps at a higher dosage, for a few more days to see if there is symptomatic improvement. If there is no improvement, then the second or third options should be considered. The second option would be to change to another antimicrobial that provides either better or more selective coverage of the suspected bacterial organism(s), including consideration of those bacteria that are beta-lactamase producing or penicillin resistant. Since it is often not possible to accomplish both goals with one antimicrobial, the clinician should be familiar with the bacterial resistance patterns in the community and should base empiric therapy on that.

The third option is most frequently used if the patient with acute otitis media is "toxic," with high fever, severe lethargy, and other significant symptoms. In this situation, acute tympanocentesis or myringotomy with culture of the middle-ear contents may be indicated. Empiric systemic therapy should still be started after cultures are obtained but may need to be changed based on the susceptibility patterns of the isolated organism. Tympanocentesis may also be indicated if an unusual organism is suspected, such as in a very young or immunocompromised child, prior to starting antimicrobial therapy.

In the patient with only occasional acute otitis media that responds promptly to medical therapy, including resolution of middle-ear fluid, other management is seldom necessary. However, if the child has very frequent episodes of otitis, over three episodes in

FIGURE 5 Persistence of middle-ear effusion after onset of acute otitis media with effusion. (Adapted from Teele DW, Klein JO, Rosner BA. Epidemiology of otitis media in children. *Ann Otol Rhinol Laryngol* 89:5, 1980.)

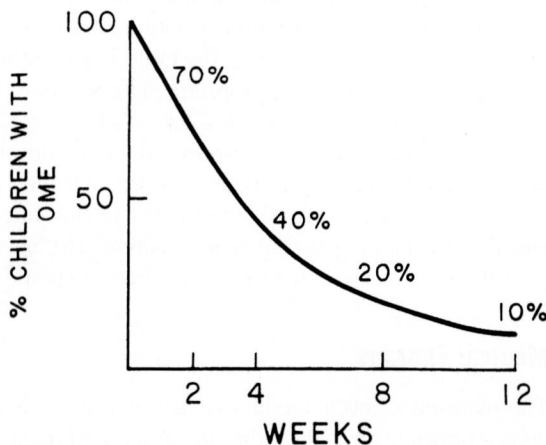

6 months or four episodes in a year, then other management options should be considered. Until recently, long-term antimicrobial prophylaxis was often used very effectively in many children. However, with the rise in resistant organisms the enthusiasm for this treatment method has, understandably, dropped off. Amoxicillin and sulfisoxazole are the most commonly used agents, with many of the others being used in allergic children or if the others fail. Commonly, prophylaxis is given during the winter months and can often be stopped during the summer, when URIs are less common. Short-term prophylaxis in children either with or without middle-ear fluid is practical if the parents are trying to keep the child healthy over a holiday or vacation, or until an upcoming surgical procedure (including tympanostomy tube placement.) If a child has frequent breakthrough episodes of otitis while on prophylaxis then it is not working and other options should be considered.

In children with recurrent acute otitis media who have persistent fluid in between episodes, the goal of therapy is to prevent further acute symptoms as well as clear the fluid. Again, antimicrobial therapy is the mainstay of treatment, and the choice of antimicrobials is similar to the scenario with recurrent acute otitis media alone. If the symptoms of recurrent acute disease are controlled with medical therapy, but there is persistent middle-ear fluid for 3 months or longer, then the treatment becomes the same as for chronic middle-ear fluid.

Treatment should be considered for chronic otitis media with effusion that has persisted for 3 months or longer, especially if the disease is bilateral, very symptomatic, and associated with significant conductive hearing loss (especially if sensorineural hearing loss is also present) and if there are significant tympanic membrane changes, such as deep retraction pockets, or middle ear changes, such as adhesive otitis or ossicular involvement. If the disease has been quite symptomatic then antimicrobials, and occasionally steroids, may already have been tried. If not, a trial of one or two antimicrobials that would be used for acute otitis media can be considered. However, the resolution rate, based on multiple studies using different antimicrobials, is not as high as for acute otitis media.

Multiple other medications have been tried or suggested for chronic otitis media with effusion. Decongestants, both systemic and intranasal, continue to be frequently used in children with otitis media, despite several clinical trials demonstrating lack of efficacy. Similarly, antihistamine–decongestant combinations are frequently prescribed for children with otitis; again, however, there is no evidence that they change the clinical course or promote resolution of middle-ear fluid. There is some evidence that eustachian tube dysfunction without middle-ear fluid may be helped by these agents, and there may be improvement in nasal symptoms in children with allergic rhinitis. Although these drugs, both singly and in combination, are ubiquitous on pharmacy shelves, they may have side effects and are not recommended for the treatment of otitis media (5).

Steroids, both systemic and topical, have gained wide interest in the treatment of chronic middle-ear fluid. Multiple studies have been performed with varying results; the studies are difficult to compare due to lack of uniformity in steroid type, dosage, route of administration, and duration of effusion before steroid use. Some studies included antimicrobial use and others did not; many studies were not controlled for the presence or absence of allergy. The potential side effects of steroids, especially those used systemically, weighed against their uncertain efficacy, make routine use of steroids to treat chronic otitis media with effusion difficult to recommend (18).

Other nonsurgical strategies that have been suggested in the management of chronic otitis media with effusion include mucolytics, allergy management, and eustachian tube inflation. As previously noted, in some patients it is likely that there is a relationship of otitis media to allergy; however, otitis as the only manifestation of allergy is unusual. If the patient has definite signs and symptoms of allergy other than otitis then pursuit of allergy diagnosis and management may be warranted (21).

Valsalva's maneuver daily or politzerization weekly may help to resolve effusion secondary to barotrauma or from infrequent acute serous otitis media; however, there is very little evidence to support their use in patients with long-standing middle-ear effusion due to chronic eustachian tube dysfunction. A few studies have attempted to evaluate autoinflation using devices that provide "feedback" to the patient (i.e., the device provides some indication of how much air is being delivered by either inflation of a balloon or a ball rising in a chamber). These studies have failed to show long-term improvement, however, in middle-ear effusion. Limiting factors include the need to be at last 3 years old to use these devices and differing durations and documentation methods for the middle-ear fluid (22,23).

Surgical Therapy

Three basic surgical procedures are routinely used for the diagnosis and treatment of otitis media. The first, tympanocentesis and/or myringotomy, is generally used to relieve extreme otalgia and/or to obtain middle-ear fluid for culture. Tympanocentesis may be followed by myringotomy if wide drainage of the middle ear is desired. Both procedures can be performed at the bedside, in the outpatient clinic, or in the operating room. In the acutely ill infant and small child tympanocentesis can be performed under no or local anesthesia or with mild systemic sedation; the older child is more comfortable if local or general anesthesia is utilized. If a tube is to be inserted after the myringotomy then local (or general) anesthesia should be used for the whole procedure. If general anesthesia is required for the myringotomy then strong consideration should be given to tube insertion at the same sitting, especially if there is a strong past history of otitis or an intratemporal complication is present. If the tympanocentesis is being performed to obtain middle-ear cultures, the ear canal should be thoroughly cleaned of cerumen and then isopropyl alcohol instilled for 1 minute prior to tapping the ear; the ear canal can also be cultured after the alcohol is removed but before the tympanocentesis is performed; this helps sort out organisms that may be considered contaminants.

Tympanostomy tube insertion is used for both the treatment of recurrent acute otitis media (with or without effusion) and chronic otitis media with effusion. In addition, a tube may be inserted urgently as part of the treatment of some complications of otitis media, such as acute mastoiditis or facial nerve dysfunction. In recurrent acute otitis media, tube insertion may be indicated if the child has had four episodes of otitis in 6 months, or six episodes in a year, or more, and there is no indication that the child is improving on medical therapy; if the patient has failed prophylaxis; or if recurrent acute otitis is accompanied by chronic fluid. Less commonly, children with severe multiple antimicrobial allergies may need tubes as an alternative to medical therapy.

In children with chronic middle-ear fluid, tympanotomy tubes should be considered to restore hearing and avoid the possible complications of chronic otitis media. Tympanostomy tube insertion should be considered in those children who have had bilateral middle-ear fluid for 3 months or longer, or unilateral fluid for 6 months, and who are refractory to medical, including antimicrobial, therapy. Other factors to be considered include the degree and laterality of hearing loss, the presence of clinical symptoms (otalgia, fever), and the presence of a tympanic membrane retraction pocket or suspected ossicular erosion. Tympanostomy tube insertion should be considered sooner if underlying sensorineural hearing loss is present or the child has significant speech, language, and/or learning delays that would be affected by any degree of hearing loss. If a possible source of fever needs to be eliminated in a medically complex child, (e.g., immunocompromised patients, transplant patients) then early tube insertion should also be considered.

In the patient with minimal conductive hearing loss and air–fluid levels or bubbles, the decision to insert a tube may be more difficult, as the indications may not seem as strong. In a reliable patient without sensorineural hearing loss, speech and language problems, and clinical symptoms of otitis, cautious observation could be employed. If the hearing loss worsens, symptoms other than hearing loss develop, or the tympanic membrane becomes very retracted or retraction pockets form, then insertion of a tympanotomy tube would still be indicated.

Adenoidectomy has long been advocated as an adjunct procedure in the management of otitis media, especially chronic otitis media with effusion. The results of studies looking at the effectiveness of adenoidectomy to prevent otitis media with effusion vary widely, with some showing modest to good effects and some showing no improvement at all. Shortcomings and variations in design and methods make them somewhat difficult to compare. These factors include (a) nonstandard definition of otitis media, including duration; (b) concurrent surgical procedures (usually tonsillectomy); (c) control for adenoid size; (d) varying adenoidectomy technique; (e) measurement of nasal and eustachian tube function not routinely performed; and (f) presence or absence of environmental allergy. In several prospective randomized trials involving children with chronic otitis media with effusion, a modest but positive effect of adenoidectomy was demonstrated with regard to recurrent chronic middle ear fluid. In the studies by both Gates et al. (24) and Paradise et al. (25), time to recurrence of effusion, duration of effusion, and need for further myringotomy was improved in the adenoidectomy groups. Based on these and many other studies, adenoidectomy can be recommended, especially in a slightly older child who is having a second set of tubes placed for chronic middle-ear fluid. The efficacy of adenoidectomy without myringotomy (with or without tympanotomy tube placement) has not been extensively studied. Gates and his group, based on their data, recommended adenoidectomy with myringotomy but without tube insertion at least partly due to their rate of purulent otorrhea through the tubes. However, when otitis recurred after surgery it recurred sooner in the group that had adenoidectomy and myringotomy than in the group that had the same procedure plus tube insertion.

Fewer studies have evaluated the usefulness of adenoidectomy in the management of recurrent acute otitis media. Paradise (25) and his group in Pittsburgh did look at this as part of a large study involving adenoidectomy for children who had already had one set of tubes placed and who now were eligible for a subsequent set. The number of episodes of acute otitis were slightly less in the adenoidectomy group than in the control group (28 vs 35%).

With regard to tonsillectomy either with or without adenoidectomy, no study has demonstrated any efficacy in the prevention of otitis over adenoidectomy alone, although there is much anecdotal evidence that tonsillectomy helps. Currently, tonsillectomy for otitis should only be considered (if at all) if adenoidectomy alone has not helped and there are other indications for tonsillectomy, such as sleep apnea or recurrent pharyngitis, in addition to the otitis media.

MANAGEMENT OF COMPLICATIONS

The management of complications often involves both medical and surgical therapy. Identification of the bacterial pathogen is highly desirable, and middle-ear cultures should be obtained early in the course of treatment. If possible, middle-ear cultures should be obtained before antimicrobial therapy; obviously, many of these children will already have been on therapy, but cultures will help direct more appropriate or different antimicrobials. For acute otitis unresponsive to medical therapy tympanocentesis/myringotomy with or without tympanostomy tube insertion is often indicated

PREVENTION

Many strategies have been suggested for the prevention of recurrent acute otitis media. These include antimicrobial prophylaxis, allergy control, tonsillectomy and/or adenoidectomy, vaccination, the administration of immunoglobulins, and changing possible environmental contributors. Antimicrobial prophylaxis has been shown to be effective in preventing new episodes of acute otitis media. Amoxicillin/ampicillin and sulfisoxazole have been studied the most, although many other antimicrobials have been used in clinical studies. In general, in these studies younger children benefited more than older children, and the effect on the duration of middle-ear effusion was found to be insignificant. Prophylaxis can be considered in children who have had three or more episodes of recurrent acute otitis media in 6 months or four or more episodes in a year. Additionally, children with recurrent acute otitis media being considered for tympanostomy tube placement and who have not tried prophylaxis would be possible candidates. Also, children who had their first episode of acute otitis media during the first 6 months or life, and who have siblings with severe and recurrent otitis media (otitis prone), might be good candidates for prophylaxis. If the child, even on prophylaxis, experiences prolonged asymptomatic middle-ear fluid, then treatment of this fluid should be considered, as in all cases of chronic otitis media with effusion (5).

Allergy management may help if a specific allergen(s) can be identified. Allergy identification and possible modification of the environment, however, should not be done at random but in concert with an allergist or primary care provider, especially if major dietary changes (e.g. stopping all milk products) are contemplated. If definite allergies that, may be contributing to otitis are identified, specific additional treatment of the otitis, either medically or surgically, may still be needed, as allergy management is often a long-term plan that may take a while to have its full effect. Likewise, if intravenous gamma-globulin is recommended for proven or suspected immunoglobulin deficiency, specific medical or surgical management of the otitis may be needed while waiting for the immunoglobulins to have an effect or for the child's own immune system to mature.

Changes in possible contributing environmental factors include removing possible allergens, prolonging breast feeding, removing the child from day care, and preventing exposure to second-hand cigarette smoke. Although a direct cause-and-effect relationship between second-hand cigarette smoking and otitis media has been difficult to document consistently, there are enough other health hazards associated with cigarette smoking to make banning smoking around small children advisable. There is some anecdotal evidence that feeding an infant in an upright or semi-upright position, and not allowing the infant to fall asleep in a supine position with a bottle in his/her mouth, may also help prevent otitis media.

Vaccines could provide an intriguing method of prevention. Until now, however, vaccines directed against the main offending bacterial pathogens have not been very effective. Most of the vaccine research has been aimed at *S. pneumoniae* and nontypable *H. influenzae*; although the *HIB* vaccine has been extremely successful in preventing meningitis, epiglottis, and soft tissue infections due to this specific organism, it has had very little effect on otitis, as less than 10% of *H. influenzae* otitis is due to the type B strain. A vaccine against both *S. pneumoniae* and *H. influenzae* would be especially welcome, as they both have developed extensive and complicated resistance patterns, making the correct choice of antimicrobial more challenging. To date, the 23 valent *S. pneumoniae* vaccine has not proved very immunogenic in children under the age of 6 years; however, several studies are under way using conjugate vaccines, similar to the HIB vaccine, to boost the immune response in patients of all ages. Despite the shortcomings of the current pneumococcal vaccine, it is still recommended for children with impaired immune responses to polysaccharide antigens, as side effects are very uncommon and children may derive some benefit.

As viruses are now not uncommonly isolated from middle-ear fluid, the question of vaccination against these viruses has been raised. Recently, an article in *Archives of Pediatrics and Adolescent Medicine* showed that children aged 6 to 30 months who had received the influenza vaccine had 32% fewer episodes of acute otitis media than those who did not (26). This is potentially exciting news and hopefully will be supported by future studies.

SUMMARY

Otitis media is very common, but the diagnosis and management are not always straight-forward. Factors adding to the controversy about treatment include an increased awareness of the role of viruses, emergence of resistant bacterial organisms, frequent introduction of new antimicrobials, and the difficult-to-measure effects of otitis media with effusion on speech, language, and behavior. This means that the medical care provider must always be aware of both current research and the needs of each individual child when planning and recommending treatment for their pediatric patients.

PEARLS AND PERILS

1. Acute otitis media occurs in two-thirds of all children by the age of 3 years.
2. Beta-lactamase-producing and penicillin-resistant organisms must be considered when devising treatment.
3. Day care, smoking, male gender, and family history of otitis media are risk factors.
4. Pneumatic otoscopy is still the gold standard for diagnosis.
5. Otitis media is both over- and underdiagnosed, especially by inexperienced examiners.
6. "Asymptomatic" otitis media effusion is usually associated with conductive hearing loss.
7. Complications can still occur in children who have been appropriately treated, so resistant organisms must always be considered.

REFERENCES

1. Rosenwasser H, Adelman N. Otitic complications. *Arch Otolaryngol* 1957;65:225–234.
2. Courville CB. Intracranial complications of otitis media and mastoiditis in the antibiotic era. *Laryngoscope* 1955;65:31–46.
3. Berman S. Otitis media in developing countries. *Pediatrics* 1995;96:126–131.
4. Paradise JL. Managing otitis media: a time for change. *Pediatrics* 1995;96:712–715.
5. Bluestone CD, Klein JO. Otitis media, atelectasis, and eustachian tube dysfunction. In: Bluestone CD, Stool SE, Kenna MA, eds. *Pediatric otolaryngology*, 3rd ed. Philadelphia: WB Saunders, 1996: 388–582.
6. Teele DW, Klein JO, Rosner B, Greater Boston Otitis Media Study Group. Epidemiology of otitis media during the first seven years of life in children in greater Boston: a prospective cohort study. *J Infect Dis* 1989;160:83–94.
7. Casselbrant ML, Mandel EM, Rockette HE, Bluestone CD. Incidence of otitis media and bacteriology of acute otitis media during the first two years of life. Recent Advances in Otitis Media. Proceedings of the Fifth International Symposium. New York: Decker, 1993:1–3.
8. Casselbrant ML, Mandel EM, Kurs-Lasky M, Rockette HE, Bluestone CD. Otitis media in a population of black American and white American infants. *Int J Pediatr Otorhinolaryngol* 1995;33:1–16.
9. Pappas DG, Flexer C, Shackelford L. Otological and habilitative management of children with Down syndrome. *Laryngoscope* 1994;104:1065–1070.
10. Bluestone CD, Stephenson JS, Martin LM. Ten-year review of otitis media pathogens. *Pediatr Infect Dis J* 1992; 11[Suppl 8]: S7–11.
11. Bosley GS, Whitney AM, Pruckler JM, et al. Characterization of ear fluid isolates of *Alloiococcus otitidis* from patients with recurrent otitis media. *J Clin Microbiol* 1995;33:2876–2880.
12. Rodriguez WJ, Schwartz RH, Akram S, Khan WN. *Streptococcus pneumoniae* resistant to penicillin: incidence and potential therapeutic options. *Laryngoscope* 1995;105:300–304.

13. Roberts JE, Burchinal MR, Medley LP, et al. Otitis media, hearing sensitivity, and maternal responsiveness in relation to language during infancy. *J Pediatr* 1995;126:481–489.

14. Bluestone CD, Klein JO. Intratemporal complications and sequelae of otitis media. In: Bluestone CD, Stool SE, Kenna MA, eds. *Pediatric otolaryngology*, 3rd ed. Philadelphia: WB Saunders, 1996; 583–635.

15. Bluestone CD, Klein JO. Intracranial suppurative complications of otitis media and mastoiditis. In: Bluestone CD, Stool SE, Kenna MA, eds. *Pediatric otolaryngology*, 3rd ed. Philadelphia: WB Saunders, 1996; 636–645.

16. Stool SE, Berg AO, Berman S, et al. *Otitis media with effusion in young children*. Clinical Practice Guideline, Number 12. AHCPR Publication No. 94–0622. Rockville MD: Agency for Health Care Policy and Research, Public Health Service, U.S. Department of Health and Human Services, July 1994.

17. Casselbrant ML, Furman JM, Rubenstein E, Mandel EM. Effect of otitis media on the vestibular system in children. *Ann Otol Rhinol Laryngol* 1995;104:620–624.

18. Rosenfeld RM. What to expect from medical treatment of otitis media. *Pediatr Infect Dis J* 1995;14:731–737.

19. Post JC, Preston RA, Aul JJ, et al. Molecular analysis of bacterial pathogens in otitis media with effusion. *JAMA* 1995;273:1598–1604.

20. Hathaway TJ, Katz HP, Dershewitz RA, Marx TJ. Acute otitis media: who needs posttreatment follow-up? *Pediatrics* 1994;94:143–147.

21. Bernstein JM. Role of allergy in eustachian tube blockage and otitis media with effusion: a review. *Otolaryngol Head Neck Surg* 1996;114:562–568.

22. Chan KH, Cantekin EI, Karnavas WJ, Bluesone Cd. Autoinflation of eustachian tube in young children. *Laryngoscope* 1987;97:668.

23. Blanshard JD, Maw AR, Bawden R. Conservative treatment of otitis media with effusion by autoinflation of the middle ear. *Clin Otolaryngol* 1993;18:188–192.

24. Gates GA, Avery CA, Prihoda TJ, et al. Effectiveness of adenoidectomy and tympanostomy tubes in the treatment of chronic otitis media with effusion. *N Engl J Med* 1987;317:1444.

25. Paradise JL, Bluestone CD, Rogers KD, et al. Efficacy of adenoidectomy for recurrent otitis media in children previously treated with tympanostomy-tube placement: results of parallel randomized and nonrandomized trials. *JAMA* 1990;263:2066.

26. Clements DA, Langdon L, Bland C, Walter E. Influenza A vaccine decreases the incidence of otitis media in 6–30 month old children in day care. *Arch Pediatr Adoles Med* 1995;149: 1113–1117.

M.A. Kenna: Department of Otology and Laryngology, Harvard Medical School, and Children's Hospital, Boston, Massachusetts 02115.

• *Practical Pediatric Otolaryngology*
• edited by Robin T. Cotton and Charles M. Myer, III
• Lippincott-Raven Publishers, Philadelphia © 1999

The Child With Vertigo

Susan Snashall

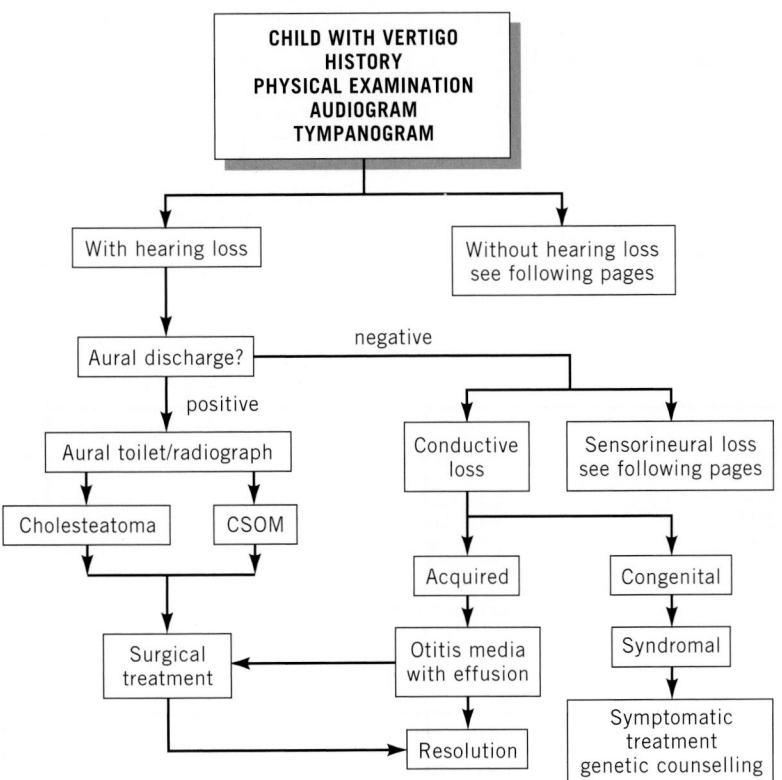

continued on next page

continued

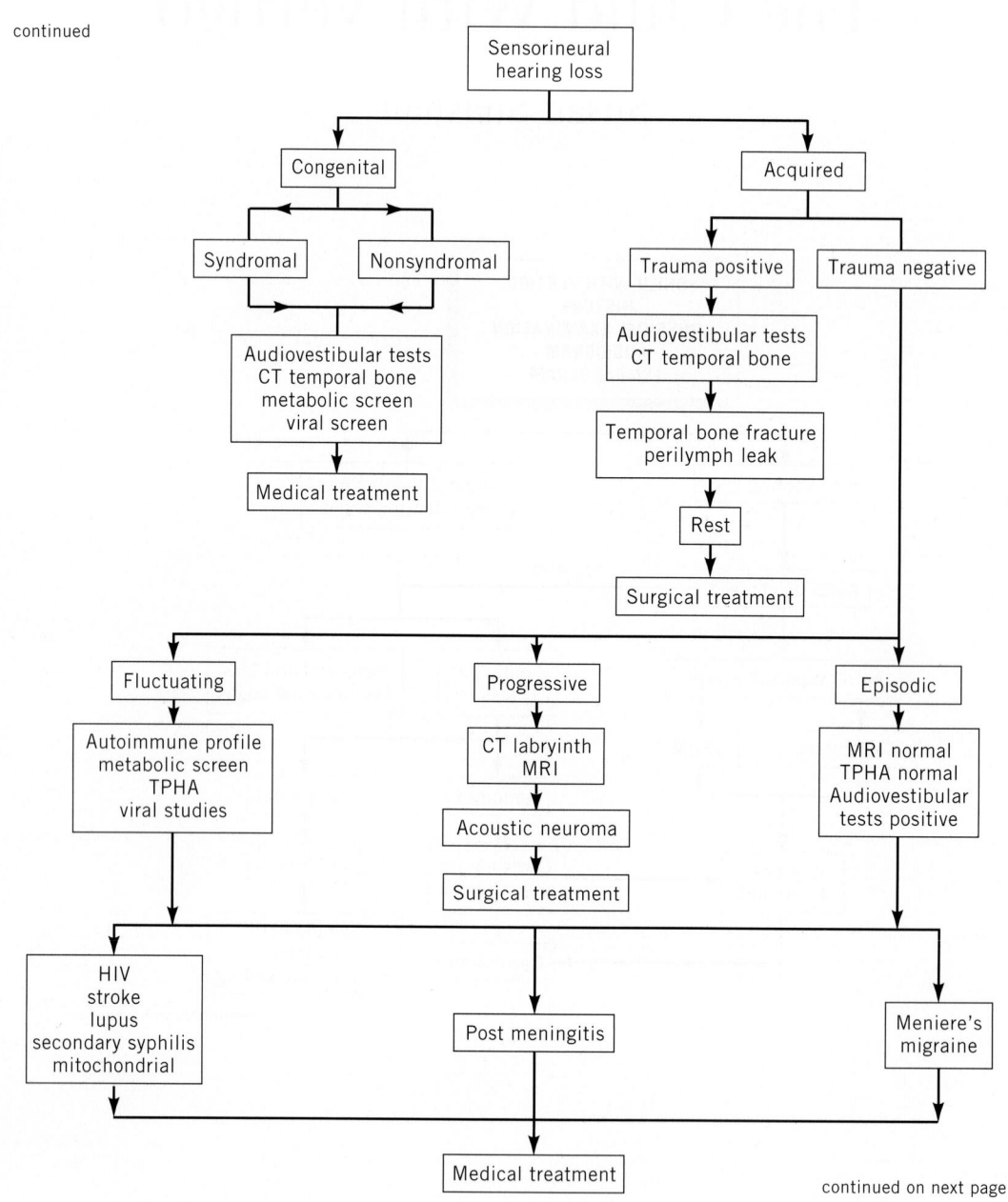

continued on next page

continued

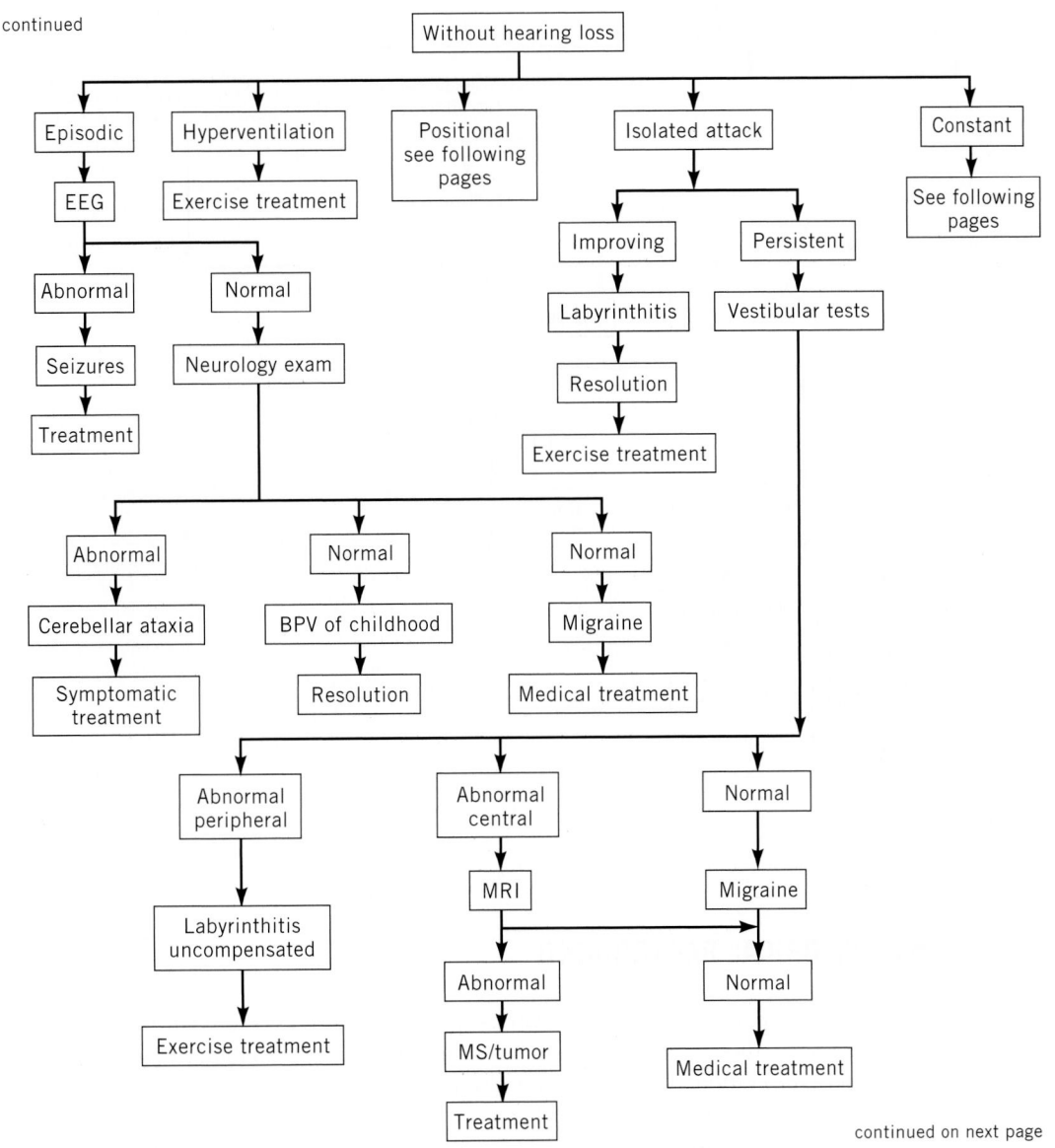

Without hearing loss

Episodic → EEG

Hyperventilation → Exercise treatment

Positional
see following
pages

Isolated attack

Constant → See following pages

Abnormal → Seizures → Treatment

Normal → Neurology exam

Improving → Labyrinthitis → Resolution → Exercise treatment

Persistent → Vestibular tests

Abnormal → Cerebellar ataxia → Symptomatic treatment

Normal → BPV of childhood → Resolution

Normal → Migraine → Medical treatment

Abnormal peripheral → Labyrinthitis uncompensated → Exercise treatment

Abnormal central → MRI → Abnormal → MS/tumor → Treatment

Normal → Migraine → Normal → Medical treatment

continued on next page

continued

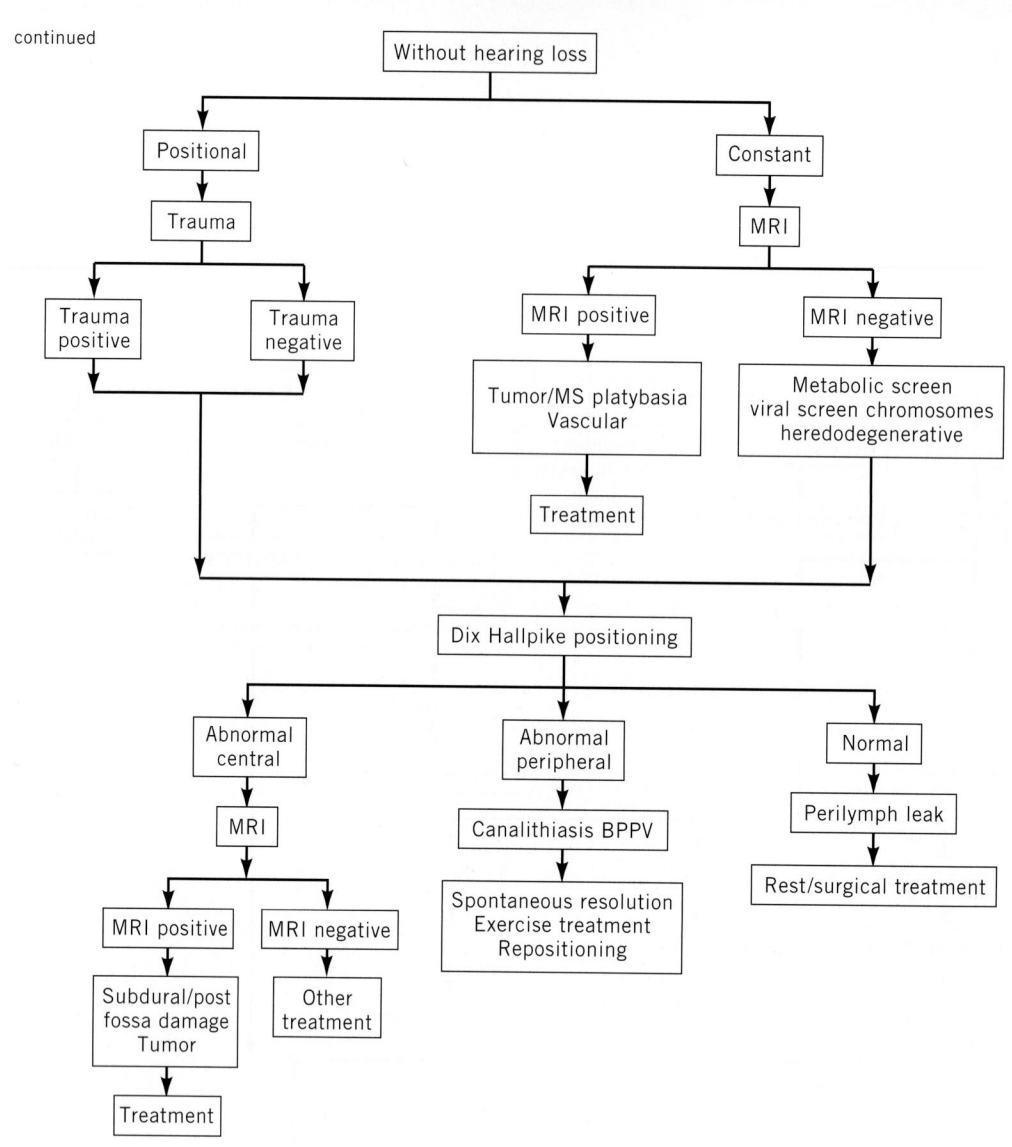

⊗ HISTORICAL BACKGROUND

Vestibular deficit in association with congenital deafness was recognized as early as 1882 (1). Since then, a number of studies have documented vestibular function in deaf children (2,3). *Vestibular dysfunction* is also recognized in a number of syndromes such as Down's, Waardenburg's, Usher's, Hurler's, Stickler's, Pendred's, and Alport's. Childhood Meniere's disease was initially recognized by Brain (4), although reported numbers remain small (5,6). Perilymph fistula has been recognized as a cause of vertigo associated with a stepwise deterioration in hearing in children with congenital defects of the temporal bone (7). Otitis media with effusion is a common but poorly documented cause of vertigo in small children (8). The differential diagnosis of vertigo in children has been classified (9–11). Gates (11) recognized the rapid recovery of children after labyrinthine failure. Although uncommon, benign paroxysmal positional vertigo has been described in children (12).

The recognition of *vertigo without hearing loss or ear disease* in young children began with Basser's (13) classic description of benign paroxysmal vertigo of childhood. Since then a number of other migraine-related causes of childhood episodic vertigo have been described (Table 1–3): benign paroxysmal torticollis (14); basilar artery migraine (15,16); and classical migraine (17,18). Seizure disorders are an important cause of ver-

TABLE 1: Differentiating Between Central and Peripheral Vertigo

	Peripheral	*Central*
Positional vertigo	Latent period	Immediate
	Duration <20 sec	Duration >30 sec
	Adapts	Does not adapt
	Nystagmus inhibited	Nystagmus present
	Fixed direction	Direction changing
Nonpositional episodic vertigo	Prodromal symptoms	No warning
	Vegetative symptoms	Few other symptoms
	Full recovery	Amnesia for attack
Ataxia	Short-lived in attack	Progressive, loss or arrest of motor skills
	Well between attacks	Neurologic signs

tigo in this age group (19). Central vertigo may be due to a hereditary degenerative disorder (20), familial cerebellar ataxia (21), or tumors of the posterior fossa (see Table 2). Lead exposure has been demonstrated to give rise to imbalance in children (22).

PEARLS AND PERILS

Physiologic vertigo syndromes

1. Due to sensory mismatch
2. Family history of migraine
3. Motion sickness
4. Visual vertigo
5. Height vertigo

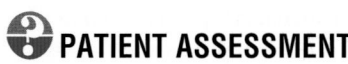

PATIENT ASSESSMENT

History

An *acute attack of vertigo* is a frightening experience for a child, but the nature of the problem may not be recognized if the child is unable to describe the symptom (see Table 4). Vertigo should be suspected if an infant lies face down wedged against the side of the

TABLE 2: Causes of Central Vertigo

1. Seizures
   Vertiginous epilepsy
   Aura of grand mal
2. Congenital abnormalities of the skull base
3. Infections
   a. Meningitis
   b. Encephalitis
   c. Cerebellar abscess
4. Trauma
5. Neoplasia
6. Heredodegenerative disorders
7. Acute intermittent familial cerebellar ataxia
8. Acute cerebellar ataxia
9. Demyelination

TABLE 3: Causes of Peripheral Vertigo—With and Without Ear Symptoms

With ear symptoms
    Disorders of the middle ear
        Otitis media with effusion
        Cholesteatoma
        Acute suppurative otitis media
    Disorders of the inner ear
        Viral labyrinthitis
        Congenital malformations
        Congenital hearing loss
        Meniere's disease
        Trauma
        Perilymphatic fistula
        Ototoxicity
Without ear symptoms
    The migraine continuum
        Benign paroxysmal vertigo of childhood
        Benign paroxysmal torticollis
        Basilar artery migraine
        Classical migraine
    Labyrinthine and eighth nerve disorders
        Vestibular neuronitis
        Benign positional vertigo

crib with the eyes closed, not wanting to be moved. Sudden falling or tipping over, clinging for support, and inability to sit or walk unaided, with crying, nystagmus, pallor, and sweating are indicative of vertigo. In an infant, more persistent vertigo may present as torticollis. Vertigo should also be suspected if a child becomes afraid of the dark or is unwilling to get out of bed after the acute phase of an illness has passed. Descriptions such as "the skies are falling" or "the world is going round" may be obtained. Accompanying headache should be suspected if the attack is accompanied by persistent screaming and pulling their own hair.

Additional accompanying symptoms to be established are ear symptoms, such as discharge, ear pain, tinnitus, hearing loss, hyperacusis, and other symptoms such as visual disturbance, vomiting, photophobia, rash, alteration in mood or level of consciousness, amnesia for the attack, sensory or motor deficits, and bizarre movements.

The attacks may be isolated or episodic. If the attack is isolated, preceding events are recorded including head injury, however minor (perilymph fistula); barotrauma, i.e. straining or coughing; and febrile illness. If the attack occurs immediately after febrile illness, labyrinthitis is likely. If it occurs 7 to 10 days after febrile illness, cerebellar ataxia is more likely. If the attack is episodic, the pattern is established including age of onset, duration of attack, frequency and periodicity, and precipitating and alleviating factors. *Episodic vertigo must be distinguished from other causes of "funny turns" in children.*

PEARLS AND PERILS

Differential diagnosis of episodic vertigo from other paroxysmal disturbances

1. Breath-holding spells
2. Seizures
3. Recurrent syncope
4. Infantile spasms
5. Night terrors
6. Hypoglycemia
7. Psychosomatic dizziness
8. Hyperventilation

TABLE 4: Characteristic Features of the Childhood Pathologic Vertigo Syndromes

Benign paroxysmal vertigo of childhood
    Age of onset 1–3 years
    Age of spontaneous resolution 3–8 years
    Family history of migraine
    Followed by classical migraine in teenage years
    Duration of attack seconds to minutes
    Complete resolution in minutes
    Good memory for and description of attack
    Fearful, may cry out in attack
    Drops to ground or clings for support
    Pallor, nystagmus, no warning
    Random attacks, can be more than once a day, or none for months, at any time or activity.
Basilar artery migraine
    Age of onset 10 months and onwards
    Spontaneous resolution may take place, or change to another form of migraine
    Preceded by change in mood/yawning for up to 1 day
    Often at night or after sleep
    Vertigo causes an unwillingness to be moved
    Accompanied by screaming and pulling hair (headache)
    Pallor, sweating, nystagmus, vomiting
    Duration hours, followed by sleep
    Attacks periodic or grouped
Vertiginous epilepsy
    Age of onset any time in childhood
    May have an aura, or vertigo may constitute the aura
    Falls to the ground, does not cling for support
    Amnesia for attack, dazed afterwards, not fully aware of surroundings
    Electroencephalogram abnormal
Meniere's disorder
    Any age, but prevalence increase with age
    May go into remission, with change in presentation with time
    Often bilateral and fluctuating from ear to ear.
    Accompanied by hearing loss and tinnitus (bees in ears)
    Pale, nauseated, and ataxic in attack
    Duration hours to days
    Unwell before attack

Persistent vertigo and dysequilibrium due to vestibular dysfunction must be distinguished from ataxia due to central nervous system disease. Dysequilibrium may result in delayed acquisition of motor milestones, fear of open spaces such as the playground, and poor performance in, and fear of, the dark or keeping the eyes closed. Children usually adapt extremely quickly to persistent vestibular deficit, and the possibility may thus be easily overlooked.

PEARLS AND PERILS

Consequences of bilateral vestibular failure

1. Symptomless, therefore unrecognized
2. Children adapt, therefore no disability
3. Adaptation by use of proprioception and vision
4. Swimming underwater can be dangerous
5. Skiing in whiteout can be difficult
6. Usher's and Refsum's syndromes can progress to loss of vision, hearing, and vestibular function
7. Beware vestibular failure in congenital/early-onset progressive deafness

Family history should include migraine; seizures; hearing loss, tinnitus, or vertigo; episodic ataxia; renal, endocrine, or metabolic disorders; and syndromes with aural manifestations. *Past history* should include head injury; infections, including mumps, meningitis, perinatal; ototoxic drugs, including those in utero; and ear disease/operations.

General health and *development* includes congenital malformations, motor milestones, language development, cognitive, visual, and hearing status, motion sickness, headaches, personality, ear disease, intercurrent illness, and exposure to toxic chemicals. *Social history* is relevant in terms of interpersonal relationships at home and school, school performance, and anxiety.

Physical Examinations

The ear is examined for congenital defects and the tympanic membrane in particular for evidence of otitis media with effusion, perforation, and chronic suppurative otitis media. Tuning forks may establish the nature of any hearing loss in children over the age of 6 years.

A neurologic examination must include the cranial nerves, cerebellar function, tone and reflexes, and a full examination of eye movements for pursuit, convergence, saccades, nystagmus, and the cover test for latent strabismus. Visual pursuit tasks are best accomplished in preschool children if the target captures their interest. This is achieved by replacing the conventional target (such as a pencil) with a small toy. Static and dynamic balance and coordination are examined by having the child hop, kick a ball, jump with two feet together, stand on a cushion and across a beam, run, heel–toe walk, get up from sitting on the floor, and march on the spot, with the eyes closed. Encouragement is required for eyes-closed tests such as Romberg and Unterberger's tests. The Dix-Hallpike positioning test is particularly important in children as it is important to distinguish the uncommon benign paroxysmal positional vertigo from central positional vertigo due to brainstem tumors in this age group.

The vestibuloocular reflex to rotation is examined with eyes open and fixed on a target. An infant younger than 6 weeks is rotated in the examiner's arms around the perimeter of a circle (Farmer's test). The eyes open and deviate in the direction of rotation. Older infants are seated on the caregiver's lap, and children are seated directly on a chair; postrotation nystagmus is observed as for adults, except that children may inhibit the response more effectively.

Visual acuity is assessed, ophthalmoscopy undertaken and any heterochromia observed. Development is assessed with particular attention to speech and language, motor milestones, and primitive and righting reflexes. A general medical examination is performed with attention to stature, pigmentation, and goiter.

Investigations

In many instances it is possible to reach a diagnosis on the basis of careful history and examination. Most causes of vertigo in childhood are not associated with any abnormality on investigation, which can be unproductive if not used selectively.

Auditory Tests

Age-appropriate hearing assessment is done by behavioral play audiometry in sound field (age 2 to 4 years) or pure tone earphone audiometry. Tympanometry with stapedius reflexes can establish middle-ear function and recruitment of loudness. Age-appropriate speech discrimination is determined by toy tests (ages 2 to 4 years); junior word lists in sound field (ages 5 to 6); and earphones (from age 7 years). Otoacoustic emissions are a useful objective measure of cochlear function. Auditory brainstem evoked potentials take longer but are an essential objective measure of the integrity of the auditory nerve and brainstem pathways.

Vestibular and Balance Tests

As with hearing assessment, it is possible to conduct vestibular and balance investigations on children providing the environment, the time available, and the test routine are adjusted to the concerns and capabilities of the child. Useful investigations are as follows:

1. *Fitzgerald Hallpike bithermal caloric test*, measuring the response as the maximum slow-phase velocity with eyes open in the dark, as children easily inhibit their responses by visual fixation.
2. *Vestibuloocular reflex* elicited by rotation tests recording the response with eyes open in dark. This test can be achieved with very young children sitting on the caregiver's lap.
3. *Eye movements* may recorded by *electrooculography*. Eyes-closed recordings cannot be used as children exhibit a high degree of random eye movements behind closed lids, even with mental alerting. Other methods of recording eye movements in the absence of fixation, such as infrared video-photography, can be extremely useful. For optokinetic tests a full-field stimulus is essential. An intermittent light source will improve attention for pursuit tracking. Stability of gaze for recording spontaneous nystagmus is improved with proprioceptive clues. Removal of fixation is accomplished by recording responses with eyes open in the dark, as this minimizes the artifact due to excessive random eye movements in this age group. All measurement of eye movements must be interpreted in the light of age-related normal data, as immaturity can be confused with central vestibular abnormalities. Age-related rotational and caloric results from birth until the age of 15, when adult patterns are established, are available (23,24).
4. Static and dynamic platform posturography give valuable information regarding truncal ataxia and instability in children from the age of three years. Postural stability improves considerably between the ages of 3 and 8 years and is not fully mature until 18 years. Results in children must therefore be compared with age-matched normal controls. Normal children exhibit much greater intersubject variability than adults so that the database at each age must be large enough to allow for variability. Posturography is a sensitive tool for demonstrating differences between groups or documenting response to treatment in an individual. The change in postural control with age is also well documented in children (25).

Other Tests

Electroencephalography and *electrocardiography* should be undertaken whenever there is any suspicion of fits or faints. *Urinalysis* should be done for protein and red blood cells. *Thyroid* and *renal function tests* and random *glucose* are required. *Computed tomography* of the petrous temporal is needed to demonstrate subtle congenital defects of the labyrinth. *Magnetic resonance imaging* is required to exclude tumors, vascular malformations, and multiple sclerosis. *Ophthalmology* for both establishing visual fields and acuity for rehabilitation and for detecting syndromes affecting both the labyrinth and the eye. *Microbiology* for congenital syphilis, human immunodeficiency virus, Borrelia, infectious mononucleosis, and viral studies.

TREATMENT RECOMMENDATIONS

Author's Preferred Method

Treatable causes of childhood vertigo are middle-ear disease, central nervous system tumors, and migraine. Middle-ear disease is described elsewhere in this volume. Tumors of the cerebellopontine angle including acoustic neuroma and congenital cholesteatoma are also dealt with elsewhere. The otologist may wish to initiate treatment for basilar artery migraine as described below, but if this initial approach is unsuccessful the condition is best managed by a pediatric neurologist, as are other central causes of vertigo.

Vertigo usually resolves spontaneously in children, either because the disorder itself is self-limiting (benign paroxysmal vertigo of childhood) or because children adapt rapidly to vestibular deficit. Recurrent episodic vertigo causes anxiety for the parents, and the children themselves may develop a fear of falling. School-age children can develop illness behavior following an episode of vertigo from which they have recovered. Some children react disproportionately to the sensation of imbalance and vertigo, insisting that they be carried or pushed in a wheelchair/buggy. Teenagers may fear the presence of an undiagnosed brain tumor. Although most children with vertigo require no specific treatment, there are a few in whom the rehabilitative challenge is even greater than that of adults.

The first step in treatment is a full explanation of the cause and mechanism of the condition. This should include an age-appropriate explanation to the child. The explanation should include the prognosis and likely time course of the condition. For those children with one of the varieties of migrainous vertigo an exclusion diet may be beneficial. Avoidance of chocolate, cheese, and citrus fruit can abolish attacks in some children.

Vestibular sedatives are rarely required, but if used they should only be antihistamines as these are safe in children. Phenothiazine derivatives such as prochloperazine can cause tardive dyskinesia. Beta-histine is sometimes beneficial in secondary endolymphatic hydrops associated with congenital deafness. It is not as satisfactory in improving vestibular symptoms due to childhood Meniere's disease. Salt restriction is difficult for children as so many of their favorite foods are processed, but this approach should be tried for endolymphatic hydrops. Beta-blockers and other antimigraine therapy may be required for basilar artery migraine in older children, but younger children should be treated with antihistamines only.

Vestibular rehabilitation exercises administered by a physiotherapist can be vital in restoring the confidence of a child in whom vertigo has precipitated an anxiety reaction. These can be made into a game such as juggling. Advice on leisure and sporting activities is vital if children with vestibular failure are to be kept safe while leading a full life. They should not dive into murky water. Hyperventilation control may be required for some anxious children. Ongoing support and monitoring is useful for children with episodic disease as the explanations may need reinforcement if remission of symptoms is delayed.

PEARLS AND PERILS

1. Be positive: children adapt rapidly.
2. Avoidance diet is useful in migraine.
3. Antihistamine-based vestibular sedatives are safe.
4. Do not use prochlorperazine in children.
5. Meniere's disease does not respond well to treatment.

MANAGEMENT OF COMPLICATIONS

Psychological Management

A minority of children react adversely to vertigo and develop school avoidance, or even become confined to a wheelchair. The instability experienced in open spaces by someone with vertigo can make the school playground a very difficult place, sowing the seeds of agoraphobia. These psychological complications of vertigo require skilled sympathetic handling. A full explanation of why such environments as the playground create instability may be sufficient, but referral to a psychologist may be required.

Multidisciplinary Approach

A child easily becomes confused by conflicting advice and may play one party off against another to obtain sympathy. It is vital that good communications exist between hospital and school, and between professionals of different disciplines. The parents and the child must be included within the rehabilitative team.

Awareness of Potential Danger

Dangerous disorientation may arise in children with bilateral vestibular failure who are in situations in which proprioception and vision are not available. Diving into murky water can result in drowning, even if the child is a good swimmer. As vestibular deficit is symptomless, caregivers must be aware of the possibility that the child may have no vestibular function. Children born hearing impaired, or who have lost hearing and vestibular function from meningitis or a viral infection, may have no obvious balance defect in normal activities.

PEARLS AND PERILS

1. Psychological sequelae can be severe.
2. Career and sports guidance is required.
3. If adaptation does not occur, review diagnosis.
4. Peripheral vertigo gets better; central vertigo gets worse.

✳ REFERENCES

1. James W. The sense of dizziness in deaf mutes. *Am J Otol* 1882;4:239–254.
2. Brookhouser PE, Cyr DG, Beauchaine KA. Vestibular findings in the deaf and hard of hearing. *Otolaryngol Head Neck Surg* 1982;90:773–777.
3. Enbom H, Magnusson M, Pyykkö I. Postural compensations in children with congenital or early acquired bilateral vestibular loss. *Ann Otol Rhinol Laryngol* 1991;100:472–478.
4. Brain WR. Vertigo: neurologic, otologic, circulatory and surgical aspects. *BMJ* 1938;2:605–608.
5. Sade J, Yaniv E. Ménière's disease in infants. *Acta Otolaryngol* 1984;97:33–37.
6. Filipo R, Barbara M. Juvenile Ménière's disease. *J Laryngol Otol* 1985;99:193–196.
7. Supance JS, Bluestone CD. Perilymph fistulas in infants and children. *Otolaryngol Head Neck Surg* 1983;91:663–671.
8. Blaney AW. The dizzy child. *Proc Ir Otolaryngol Soc* 1983; 55–61.
9. Eviatar L, Eviatar A. Vertigo in children: differential diagnosis and treatment. *Paediatrics* 1977;59:833–838.
10. Curless RG. Acute vestibular dysfunction in childhood, central versus peripheral. *Childs Brain* 1980;6:39–44.
11. Gates GA. Vertigo in children. *Ear Nose Throat J* 1980;59:358–365.
12. Eadie MJ. Paroxysmal positional giddiness. *Med J Aust* 1967;1:1169–1173.
13. Basser LS. Benign paroxysmal vertigo of childhood. *Brain* 1964;87:141–152.
14. Dunn DW, Snyder CH. Benign paroxysmal vertigo of childhood. *Am J Dis Child* 1976;130:1099–1100.
15. Ouvrier R, Hopkins I. Occlusive disease of the vertebro-basilar arterial system in childhood. *Dev Med Child Neurol* 1970;12:186–192.
16. Golden GS, French JH. Basilar artery migraine in young children. *Paediatrics* 1975;56:722–726.
17. Eviatar L. Vestibular testing in basilar artery migraine. *Ann Neurol* 1981;9:126–130.
18. Kuritzky A, Ziegler DK, Hassenien R. Vertigo, motion sickness and migraine. *Headache* 1981;21:227–231.
19. Alpers BJ. Vertiginous epilepsy. *Laryngoscope* 1960;70:631–637.

20. Menkes JH. *Textbook of child neurology*. Philadelphia: Lea & Febiger, 1985.
21. Hill W, Sherman H. Acute intermittent familial cerebellar ataxia. *Arch Neurol* 1968;18: 350–357.
22. Bhattacharya A, Shukla R, Dietrich K, Bornschein R, Berger O. Effect of early lead exposure on children's postural balance. *Dev Med Child Neurol* 1995;37:861–878.
23. Tibbling L. The rotatory nystagmus response in children. *Acta Otolaryngol* 1969;68:459–467.
24. Kenyon GS. Neuro-otological findings in normal children. *J R Soc Med* 1988;81:644–648.
25. Woollacott MH. Posture and gait from newborn to elderly. In: Ambland B, Berthos A, Clarac F, eds. *Posture and gait. Development, adaptation and modulation.* International Congress Series 812. Amsterdam: Excerpta Medica, 1988:3–12.

S. Snashall: Department of Audiological Medicine, St. George's Hospital, London SW17 OQT, United Kingdom.

• *Practical Pediatric Otolaryngology*
• edited by Robin T. Cotton and Charles M. Myer, III
• Lippincott-Raven Publishers, Philadelphia © 1999

16

Surgical Considerations in Chronic Otitis Media

William P. Potsic

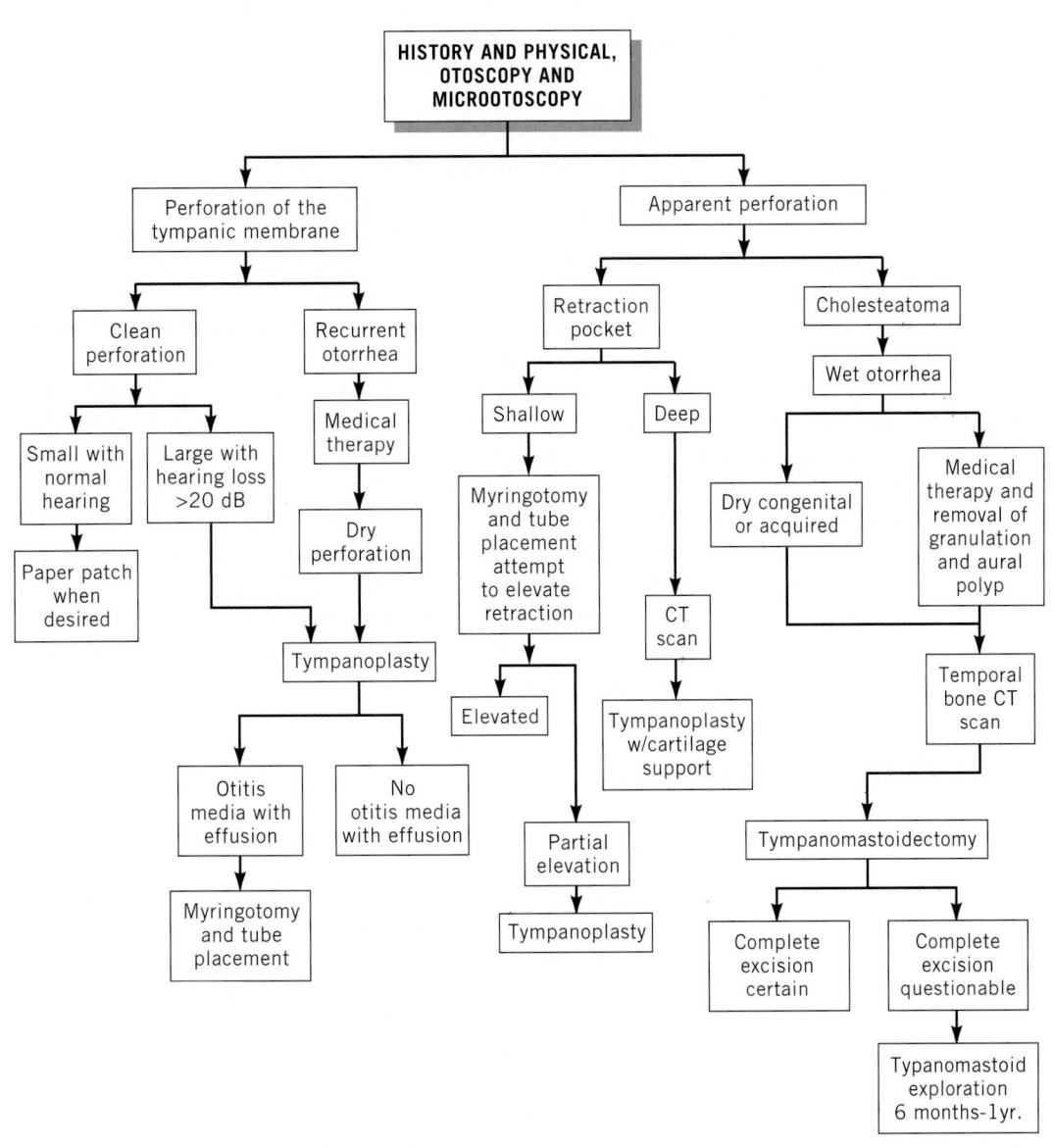

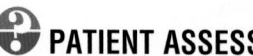 HISTORICAL BACKGROUND

Over the years, there has been a smoldering controversy about the nature and management of chronic suppurative otitis media (CSOM) in children. The pathogenesis of CSOM in children was suspected to be different from that in the adult, primarily based on the observations of clinicians who had greater difficulty managing children, as well as achieving the results expected in their adult patients. This belief was fueled by success rates for tympanoplasty in children that varied widely and were generally reported to be poorer for children than adults. However, recent reports in the literature have dispelled this concern (1,2). Even though differences in the management of CSOM between children and adults do exist, proper technique and appropriate expectations can yield success rates for tympanoplasty in children comparable to those in adults. If success is defined as an intact tympanic membrane at specified intervals following surgery, then results may be as good or better in children than in some adult series (1,2). This is also true of anterior–superior perforations of the tympanic membrane, which are the most difficult perforations to close in all age groups. Although the past reasons for this difficulty are not entirely clear, with the appropriate technique, an otolaryngologist can expect success rates for anterior–superior perforations in children equal to tympanoplasty for perforations in any location of the tympanic membrane (3).

In addition to concerns about tympanoplasty results, it was believed that cholesteatomas behave differently in children than adults because they tend to be more extensive at diagnosis and have a higher rate of recidivism (4,5). It is difficult to assess how cooperation on the part of the child impacts on the early or late detection of cholesteatoma, as well as how postsurgical management has been affected by concerns about the ease of postoperative management. However, subsequent reports have shown that with appropriate management, using second surgical procedures, cholesteatoma in children can also yield success rates comparable to those expected for adults (6,7). This is also true for children who require ossicular reconstruction to restore hearing after cholesteatoma surgery (8). This more accurate information has taken much of the mystery out of managing CSOM in children. It permits the otolaryngologist to take a rational approach to treatment, to be critical of our technique, and not to blame the disease or age of the patient for our results. Appropriate modifications in management and reasonable expectations for the treatment of CSOM can result in consistent outcomes for children. This chapter presents a plan for the management of CSOM in children that has evolved over years of experience and that has produced consistent outcomes for a difficult management problem in patients of any age.

PATIENT ASSESSMENT

Signs and Symptoms of CSOM

The most common symptom of CSOM is hearing loss. It is conductive and may vary from mild to moderate. Young children often take no notice of hearing loss, and older children rarely complain of it, especially if they have normal hearing thresholds in the opposite ear. Parents may not be aware of the hearing difficulty but may be alerted by ear-preferred behavior such as consistently switching the phone to the "good" ear. Even then, the hearing loss is frequently first identified on a primary care or school screening examination. Even screening examinations may miss mild hearing losses associated with CSOM, and the hearing may approach normal in the presence of significant disease. A perforation of the tympanic membrane may be small, a retraction pocket may not impede ossicular mobility, and a cholesteatoma may conduct sound to the ossicular chain. When hearing loss is the only sequela of CSOM, detection and assessment of the disease process is frequently and inadvertently delayed.

The most common sign of CSOM is purulent otorrhea that is either recurrent or persistent despite medical therapy (4). The otorrhea is most often mucopurulent but may be blood tinged. The quantity and quality of the otorrhea is of little significance, but recurrence or persistence indicates a chronic inflammatory process such as chronic infection or the presence of a cholesteatoma. Otorrhea does not go unnoticed by the child or the caretaker, but if the otorrhea stops, it does not guarantee that underlying predisposing pathology is *not* present.

Other signs and symptoms that are seen less frequently are a sensation of fullness, ear pain, facial nerve weakness or paralysis, middle ear granulation, or an aural polyp. Unfortunately, compared with children who have signs and symptoms, an equal number have none until the hearing deficit is detected by audiologic examination. This makes the inspection of the tympanic membrane by the primary medical caregiver the most important method of diagnosing CSOM in the pediatric patient. Congenital cholesteatomas (epithelial cysts behind an intact tympanic membrane) are most frequently found by otoscopy and are often completely asymptomatic. Fortunately primary care physicians almost always include otoscopy in their well child examinations. However, routine otoscopy may not detect early subtle disease, and middle-level providers (advanced practice nonphysician providers), who are assuming a larger role in primary care, may not be as adept at otoscopy, especially in the young child. The impact of managed care, specifically primary care capitation, on the incidence and severity of CSOM at diagnosis remains to be evaluated.

Otoscopy and Microotoscopy

The otolaryngologist is expected to perform a complete examination and visualize all parts of the tympanic membrane in every child examined. It is essential in the diagnosis of CSOM because most often what is seen defines the disease process and the strategy for future evaluations and therapy. To visualize the ear adequately in a child, the skin, cerumen, and any secretions must be cleared from the external canal and surface of the tympanic membrane. This often requires gentle suction. It is easily performed in a cooperative, older child, but young children may require immobilization in a restraint, sedation, or (rarely) a general anesthetic.

Even after clearing the visual obstructions, the full extent of the disease may not be apparent until completing a period of medical therapy to reduce inflammation, edema, granulation tissue, and secretions. Pneumatic otoscopy with the application of negative pressure on the surface of the tympanic membrane may temporarily evert a retraction pocket (early cholesteatoma), indicating that fibrous adhesion to the middle-ear structures has not yet taken place. This maneuver, which is usually associated with mild to moderate pain, is required if the limits of the retraction pocket are not visible.

By microotoscopy, the otolaryngologist can assess the structural changes in the tympanic membrane architecture and is usually able to determine what, if any, surgical procedure is required to alleviate the disease process. However, other assessment methods may be helpful to define the extent of the disease not visible at the tympanic membrane or in the middle ear.

Other Assessment Methods

Ear-specific audiometry by behavioral testing is possible and essential prior to undertaking any surgical intervention, unless it is either unavailable or imprudent to delay therapy to obtain it. If behavioral testing is *not* feasible, brainstem evoked responses should be obtained. Bone and air conduction thresholds provide information about residual hearing and may suggest the presence of ossicular discontinuity. This provides a framework to set long-term expectations with the child's caregiver.

Impedance audiometry is of limited value in the presence of a perforation or cholesteatoma. However, it may be of real use to assess the opposite ear that is free of disease to predict future eustachian tube function.

PEARLS AND PERILS

1. What you see at otoscopy and microotoscopy defines the disease.
2. Adequate preparation by debridement and medical therapy may be required for complete assessment.
3. Audiologic assessment is essential to define hearing status and may indicate extent of disease.
4. Computed tomography provides a road map for surgical strategy.
5. Complaints by children with CSOM may be absent.
6. Hearing loss from CSOM is often identified first by routine screening audiometry.
7. Chronic or recurrent otorrhea through a tympanostomy tube may be a warning sign of cholesteatoma.
8. Delay in detection causes more extensive disease and more difficult management.

Mastoid radiographs are of little value for modern pediatric otology, and computed tomography (CT) is not required for uncomplicated perforations of the tympanic membrane. However, CT is helpful to assess the anatomy of the mastoid, as well as the extent of a retraction pocket or cholesteatoma. CT findings rarely change the treatment strategy but are essential to plan the surgical strategy based on the extent of disease and to avoid surgical complications from anatomic variations.

 TREATMENT RECOMMENDATIONS

Medical Management

Medical management of CSOM consists of cleaning the ear canal, tympanic membrane, and exposed portions of the middle ear. This can be done with loose cotton swabs or, preferably, by suction with otologic suctions and microscopic visualization. If purulent secretions are present, broad-spectrum, topical steroid-containing antimicrobial drops are applied three times daily for 10 days. The drops should contain antibiotics that are effective against multiple gram-negative organisms, specifically *Pseudomonas*, organisms. These often contain one antibiotic or combinations of neomycin, polymyxin, gentamycin, tobramycin, or ciprofloxacin with either hydrocortisone or dexamethasone. There are no controlled, prospective studies to validate the concern that these preparations may be ototoxic when topically applied to the middle ear in children. This author prescribes ophthalmic preparations, because they cause less discomfort when they are applied to the inflamed middle-ear mucosa, providing greater compliance in children. In addition, a broad-spectrum oral antimicrobial effective against beta-lactamase-producing organisms should be taken simultaneously. Frequent mechanical cleansing is helpful until mucopurulence is absent.

If the otorrhea does not subside or recurs shortly after completion of the therapeutic course, a culture of the middle-ear secretions is obtained for bacteria, fungus, and antimicrobial sensitivities. Occasionally a predominant culture of fungus (usually *Candida albicans* or *Aspergillus*) is present. The antifungal agent clotrimazole (drops) may be used two times daily for 7 days.

If bacteria predominate and culture- and sensitivity-directed oral and topical antimicrobial coverage is not possible, intravenous antibiotic therapy is employed. Intravenous antibiotic therapy is also indicated in the presence of facial nerve weakness and impending or existing intracranial complications of otomastoid infection. If possible, this author prefers to achieve a dry ear even if cholesteatoma is present prior to surgical intervention. However, occasionally the infection may be only reduced and not eliminated, and the surgical procedure must be undertaken to eliminate the source of the organisms.

Surgical Therapy

Perforation of the Tympanic Membrane

The controversies over the timing of surgery based on age have been eliminated by the publications demonstrating comparable results in children and adults. The timing of surgery has become a decision based on the child's otologic condition, functional goals, and long-term expectations.

Small perforations of the tympanic membrane are usually residual from a tympanostomy tube. If the perforation is dry and the hearing is normal, it is wise to follow the child closely (4 to 6-month intervals) until the opposite ear no longer requires a tube. After the tube extrudes from the opposite ear and remains free of fluid, retraction of the tympanic membrane, and recurrent infection for 4 to 6 months, the perforation may be closed by a patch myringoplasty. Using general anesthesia, the edge of the perforation is denuded of epithelium by cauterization with 30% trichloracetic acid (Fig. 1). A small paper patch is placed on the lateral surface of the tympanic membrane (Fig. 2). The patch separates in 2 to 3 weeks, with a closure rate that approaches 90%. Instead of a paper patch, the perforation may be plugged with fat, Gelfoam, or fibrous tissue with the expectation of equally good results. Paper patching is fast, easy, effective, and does not require obtaining a tissue plug.

Tympanoplasty to close a large persistent perforation can be successfully performed in children of any age. In my experience, there is no significant difference in short-term healing rate at any age and only a small difference in long-term repeat perforation rates for children under 6 years of age. Other considerations such as the size of the perforation, quadrants involved, or condition of the opposite ear are not significant (1). The timing of a tympanoplasty should be based on the child's disease state and functional goals. A tympanoplasty is indicated in a child with a persistent perforation for longer than 6 months who is having recurrent otorrhea or who has a conductive hearing loss of 20 dB or greater.

After a tympanoplasty, a child may develop otitis media with effusion requiring a tympanostomy tube. This is easily done by placing the tube in the healed tympanic membrane. If eustachian tube function is suspected of being poor at the time of surgery a tube

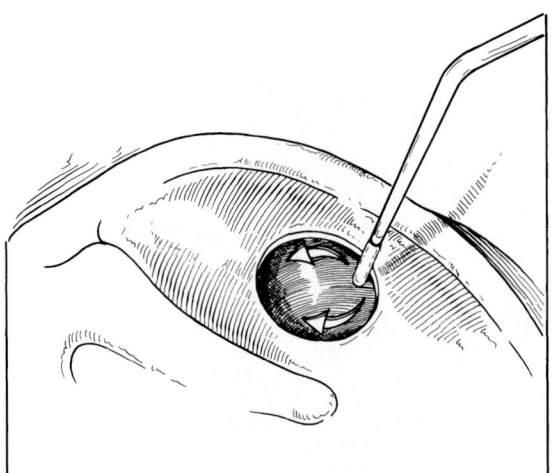

FIGURE 1 The edge of a small perforation may be cauterized with trichloracetic acid using an applicator.

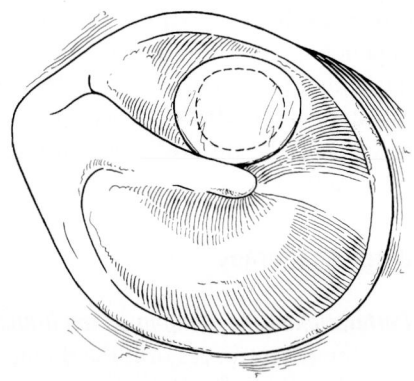

FIGURE 2 A small paper patch is placed on a small perforation that has been prepared using trichloracetic acid.

can be placed in the tympanic membrane remnant or the fascia graft. The author's preference, however, is to let the ear heal and place the tube later if an effusion is present. This approach converts CSOM with a 20 dB or greater conductive hearing deficit to otitis media effusion (OME) managed by a tympanostomy tube and normal hearing. This is by far a better functional result to achieve improved health, as well as academic and psychosocial goals.

The author performs all tympanoplasties in children through a postauricular incision in the postauricular crease (Fig. 3). This provides maximum exposure of the tympanic membrane in all quadrants, allowing access through the same incision to the temporalis fascia for grafting. It also provides immediate access to the bone of the ear canal, as well as the mastoid if unexpected disease extends beyond the perforation.

The two most important maneuvers for successful tympanoplasty surgery, after adequate exposure of the surgical field, are removal of the epithelial edge of the perforation and careful placement of the graft. With a pick, a rim of tissue that includes the epithelium is released (Fig. 4) and removed with a cup forceps (Fig. 5). To facilitate graft healing, a rim of mucosa is scraped from the undersurface of the circumference of the remnant with a reverse microtab knife (Fig. 6). I use a rectangular temporalis fascia graft positioned medial to the malleus and supported in the middle ear with Gelfoam that is saturated with antibiotic ototopical solution (Fig. 7). The lateral surface of the tympanic membrane remnant, temporalis fascia graft, and tympanomeatal flap are covered with moistened Gelfoam. The remainder of the external meatus is also packed with Gelfoam moistened by antibiotic solution. The postauricular incision is closed using absorbable subcutaneous and subcuticular sutures.

Special consideration should be given to anterior–superior perforations, which are common in children and frequently occur following extrusion of tympanostomy tubes. In

FIGURE 3 An incision is used for all tympanoplasties in children.

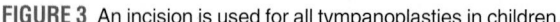
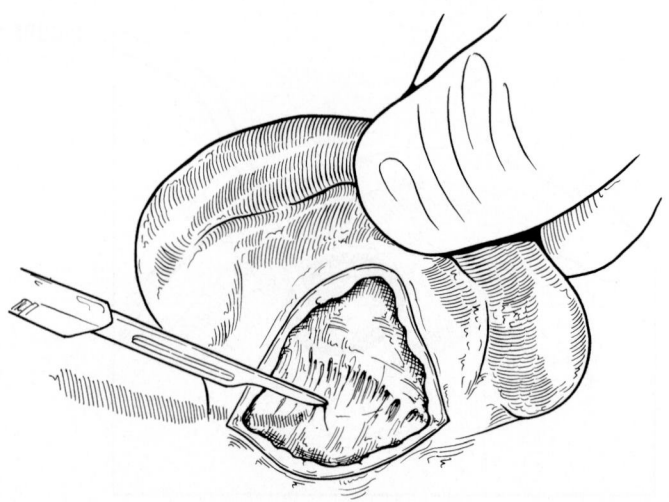

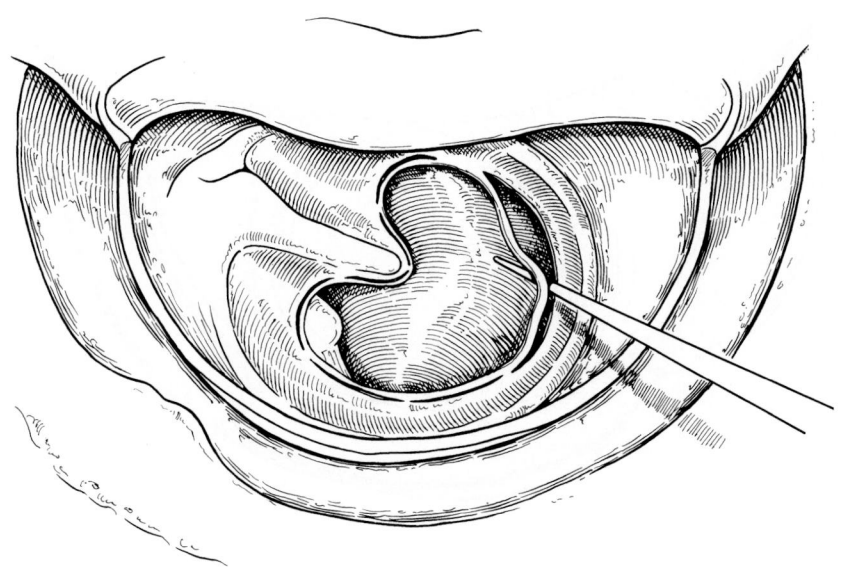

FIGURE 4 The rim of epithelium is released from the edge of the perforation with a pick.

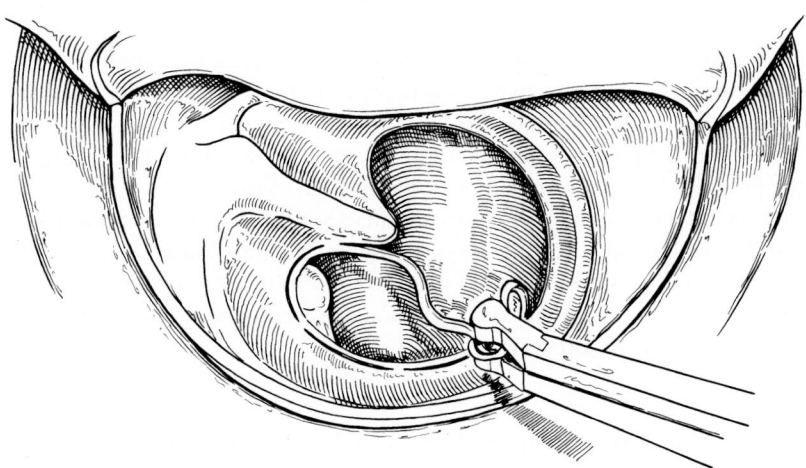

FIGURE 5 The released rim of epithelium is removed with a cup forceps.

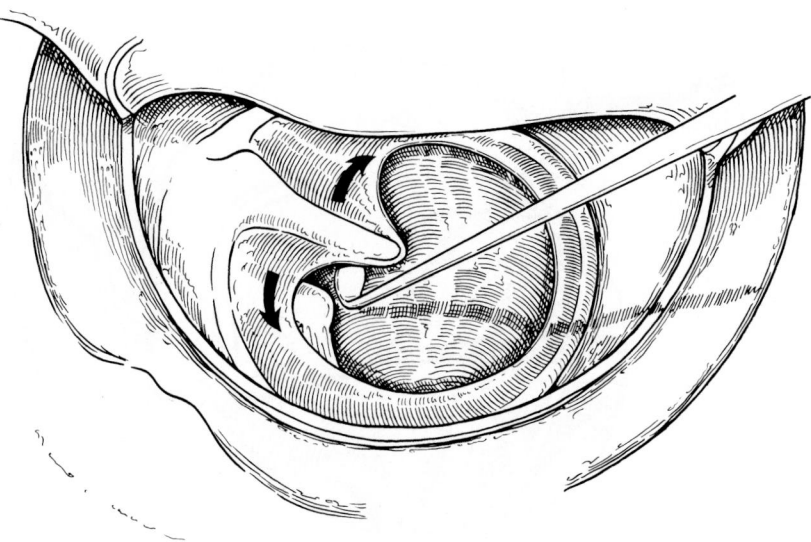

FIGURE 6 Mucosa is scraped from the undersurface of the tympanic membrane remnant to facilitate graft healing.

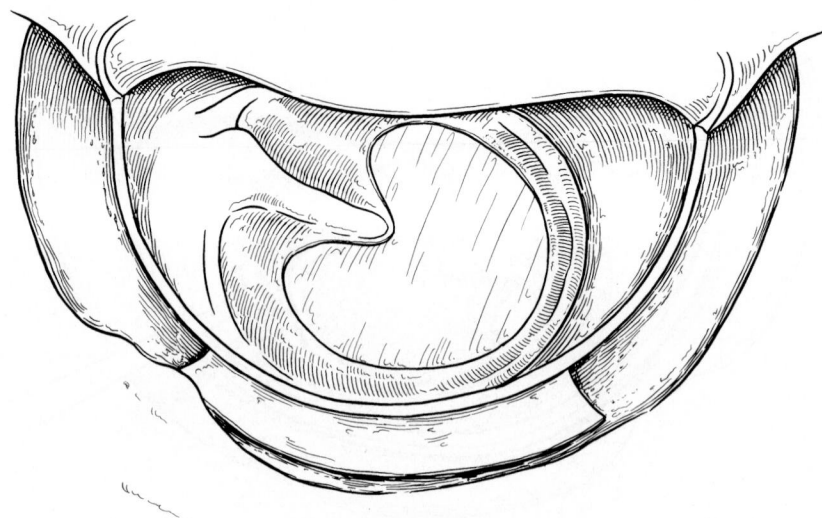

FIGURE 7 The temporalis fascia graft is positioned medial to the malleus and tympanic membrane remnant in contact with rim of the perforation.

this circumstance, it has been believed that the success rate of tympanoplasty is reduced for any number of postulated reasons. However, with appropriate technique, the author's group has achieved a 98% immediate healing rate in children for anterior–superior perforations (3).

After the standard postauricular approach, the tympanic membrane remnant is released in part or completely from the malleus as needed (Fig. 8). The anterior annulus is elevated, and the rectangular temporalis fascia graft is placed medial to the anterior annulus (9), medial to the tympanic membrane remnant, and lateral to the malleus (Fig. 9). This technique provides firm anterior and posterior fixation of the graft.

Attention to detail and careful technique produces surgical results in children that are excellent and provides control of infection, as well as functional hearing results. Although children may be less cooperative and may have more frequent upper respiratory infections (URI's) and poor eustachian tube function, this should not dissuade the otolaryngologist from providing optimal care.

Cholesteatoma

The management of cholesteatoma in children has been clouded by the impression that cholesteatoma is more aggressive and invasive and requires a more radical treatment

FIGURE 8 The tympanic membrane is released from the malleus to get exposure of the anterior–superior perforation.

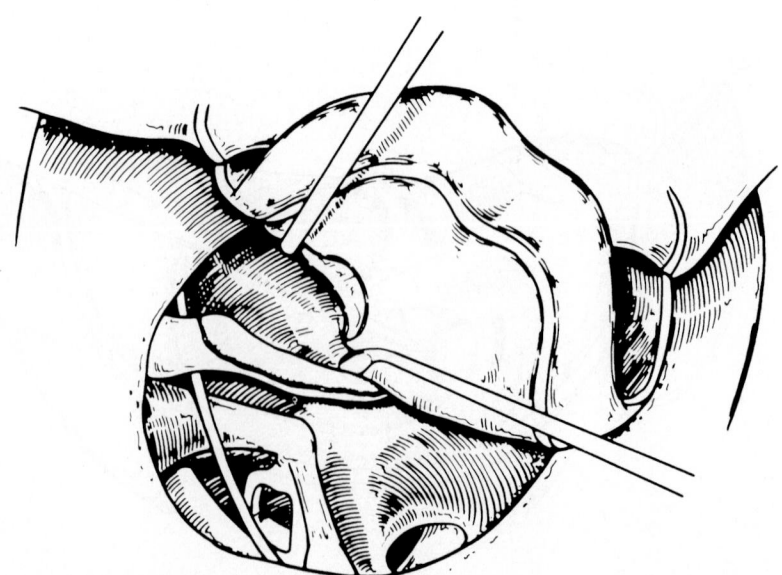

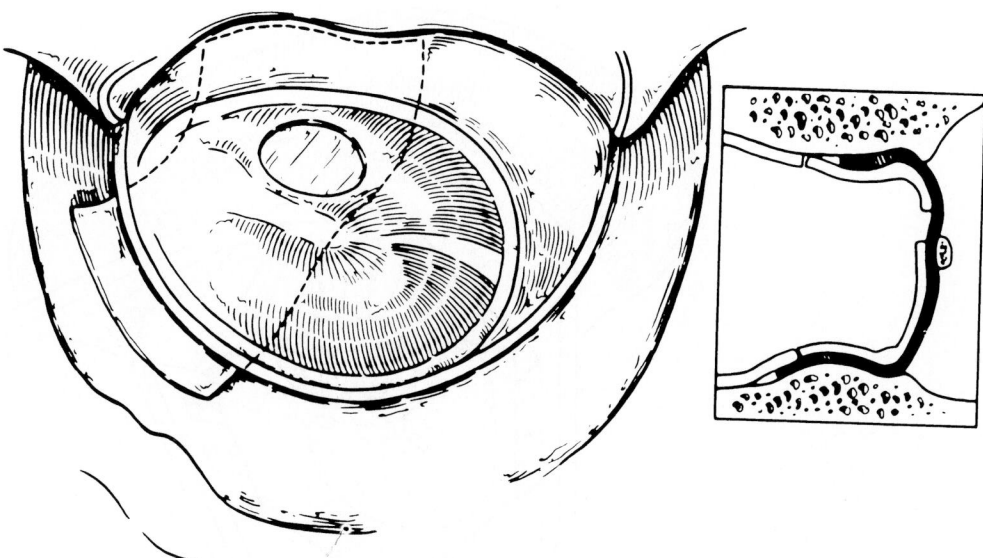

FIGURE 9 The graft is placed to provide anterior and posterior fixation for anterior–superior perforations.

strategy to achieve the desired goals. Attempts to find a single-stage operation that would avoid the inconvenience of continued care of children who are less cooperative and prevent recurrence or residual disease have been unsuccessful. It is the author's impression that the surgeon who takes care of children must adapt the surgical approach and postoperative management to eradicate disease and conserve hearing. The author is aware of no single operation that will dependably do so in all cases of childhood cholesteatoma. In the changing and growing child, one can expect to encounter the need for revision surgery and second-look procedures.

With this in mind, the author's preferred approach to cholesteatoma in children is to perform a closed, intact canal wall procedure with excision of the cholesteatoma and to perform reconstructive procedures as needed. The timing of the reconstruction (at the first operation or at a second stage) is a matter of surgical judgment. Intact canal wall procedures have proved to be effective methods for eradicating disease and preserving hearing when adequate follow-up includes judicious second-look tympanomastoidectomy especially when the surgeon is uncertain that every remnant of cholesteatoma has been excised. When a second-look procedure is planned, the author usually waits 6 months to 1 year to allow cholesteatoma to demarcate and perform the ossicular reconstruction if the ear is safe to do so.

At the first procedure all cholesteatoma and whatever structures are involved must be removed. All or a portion of the ossicular chain may need to be taken out with the cholesteatoma. The appropriate ossicular reconstruction can then be performed when the ear is safe, i.e., no likelihood of residual or recurrent disease. If large portions of bone are removed from the posterior external canal, these can be reconstructed with conchal cartilage. The author performs all tympanomastoid surgery for cholesteatoma through a standard postauricular incision placed in the postauricular crease (Fig. 10) and also uses a facial nerve monitor for these cases. Cholesteatoma is dissected from the middle-ear structures and from all involved areas of the mastoid. Bone may need to be removed with cutting and diamond burrs from the posterior and posterior–superior portions of the external canal to expose cholesteatoma medial to the bony annulus. This medial exposure of the facial recess may be extended to the hypotympanum if needed (Fig. 11). The facial recess may also be opened from the mastoid side as well. This exposure may be extended into the hypotympanum and superiorly to remove the bridge of the fossa incudis completely (Fig. 12). Hypotympanic extension requires sacrifice of the chorda tympani nerve. When this is required, it has usually been sacrificed in re-

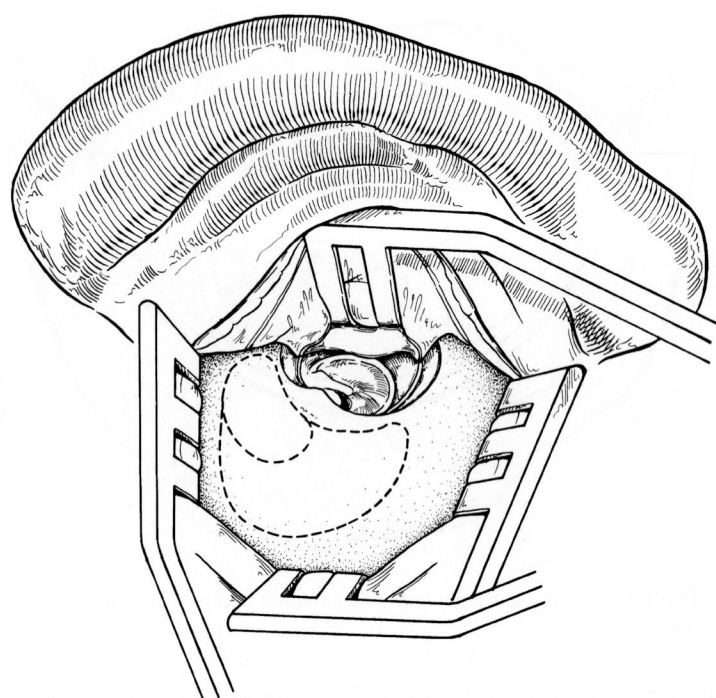

FIGURE 10 Mastoid exposure for tympanomastoid surgery in children.

moving cholesteatoma from the middle ear. It is extremely rare for children to complain of dysgeusia following removal of the chorda tympani nerve. If a large portion of the external canal needs to be removed, it can be reconstructed with conchal cartilage covered with a thick fascia graft (Figs. 13, 14). This is done before placing a thinner temporalis fascia graft for tympanic membrane reconstruction (Fig. 15). If ossicles have been eroded or removed and ossicular reconstruction is required, I perform this at the second procedure. The decision to perform a second-look operation is a matter of judgment but typically is indicated for extensive cholesteatoma, when the facial recess is deeply invaded and the sinus tympani contains cholesteatoma. Ossicular erosion that requires removal of epithelium from the ossicular chain, erosion of the ossicles, or the need to remove one or more ossicles to remove the disease completely should also suggest the need for a second-look procedure (9).

The sinus tympani is the most difficult region of the middle ear to reach in cholesteatoma surgery. For surgeons who are anchored to their chairs behind the patient, it may be impossible to visualize directly. This author has been disappointed with

FIGURE 11 Medial exposure of the facial recess may be needed for cholesteatoma exposure.

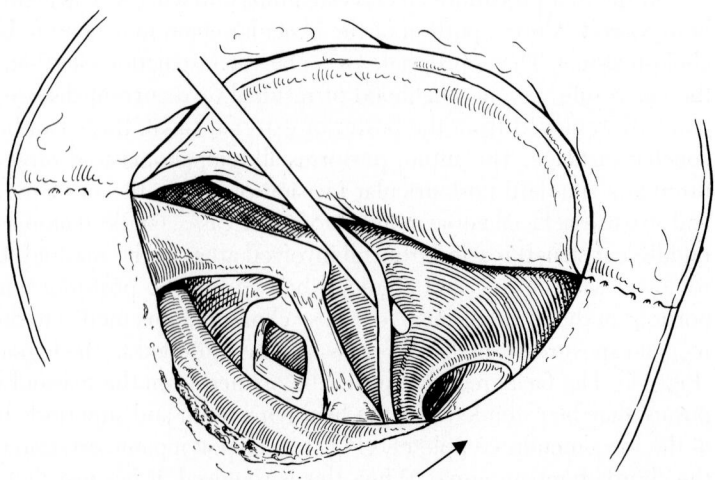

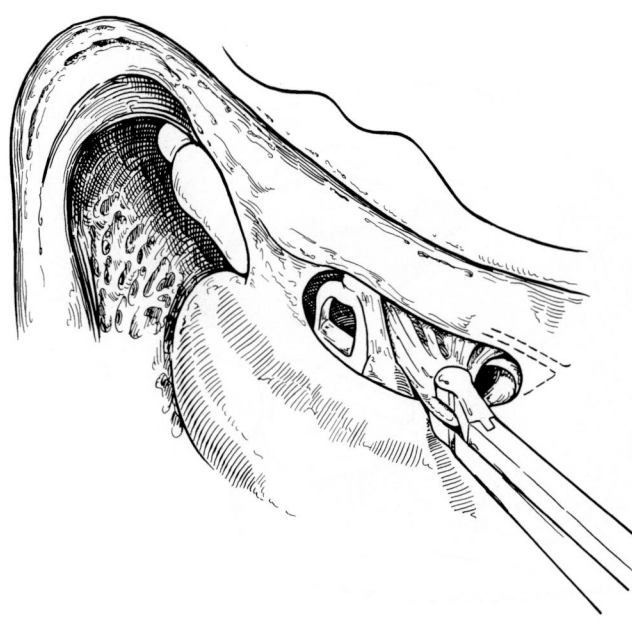

FIGURE 12 An intact canal wall facial recess approach may be needed and can be extended inferiorly or superiorly.

indirect views using a mirror or telescope to inspect the sinus tympani, a place where blood frequently pools and suction cleaning is difficult. For direct visualization, the surgeons must move to the top of the patient or to the opposite side. Removal of the bone from the anterior–superior portion of the external meatus even into the base of the zygoma can facilitate a direct view. This adds a small amount of time and some minimal inconvenience for the surgeon and nurse but is very rewarding in terms of removing middle-ear disease.

Once the decision has been made to perform a second-look procedure, it should be done 6 months to 1 year after the initial operation. The physician should apply the same

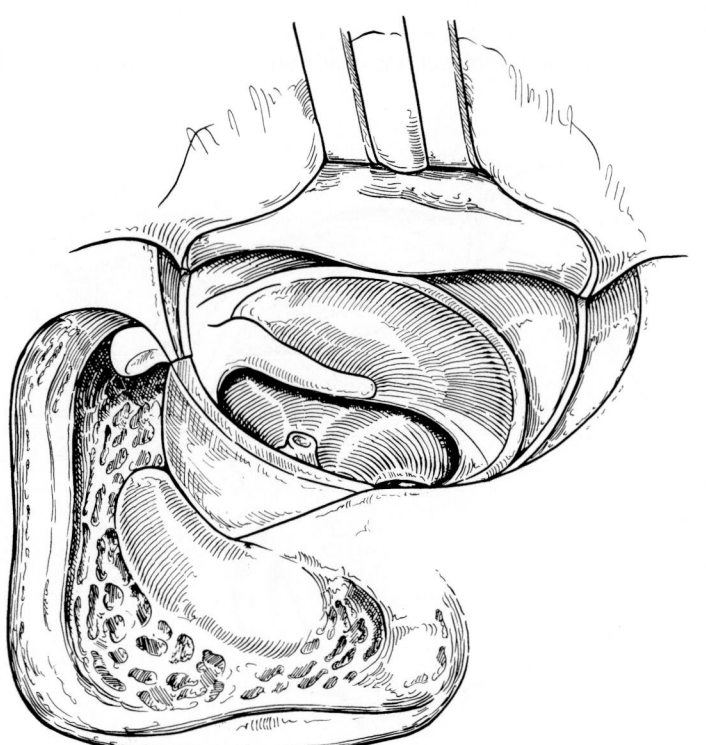

FIGURE 13 Conchal cartilage is used to reconstruct bony canal wall defects.

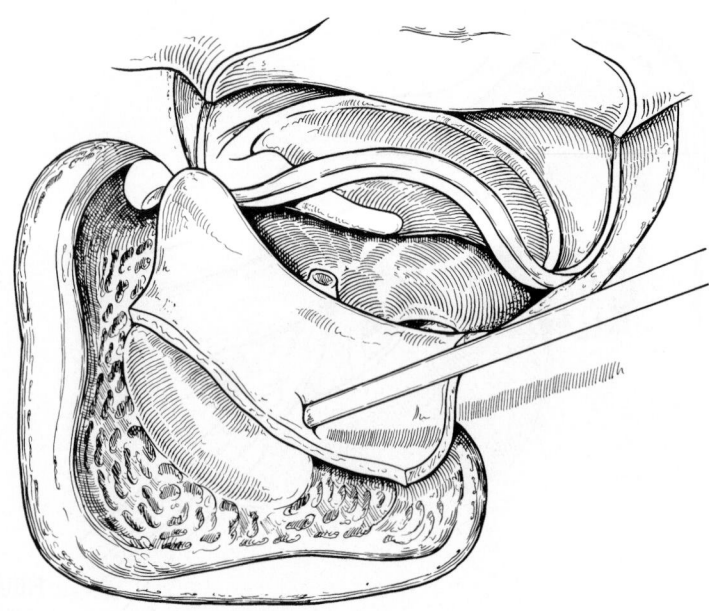

FIGURE 14 Thick fascia is used to cover the cartilage to graft a canal wall defect.

surgical principle of maximum exposure, visualization of all the previously involved areas, and excision of any residual cholesteatoma. The author is usually able to do this well with minimal incisions and telescopic visualization. Residual cholesteatoma may be found in 30% or more of children requiring a second-look procedure (6,7). When a monolocular cholesteatoma is found, it may be removed easily and confidently, but when large irregular sheets of epithelium are present, a third procedure (second tympanomastoid exploration) is required.

The need to be certain that there is no residual or recurrent cholesteatoma by reoperation does not represent a failing of the intact canal wall operation. It is simply what is required to achieve a disease-free, safe ear with structural integrity and serviceable hearing for 70 or 80 more years of the child's life.

The author has not completely done away with the classically described open procedures of modified radical and radical mastoidectomy in all patients. A surgeon may need

FIGURE 15 Thin temporalis fascia is positioned to reconstruct the tympanic membrane in tympanomastoid procedures.

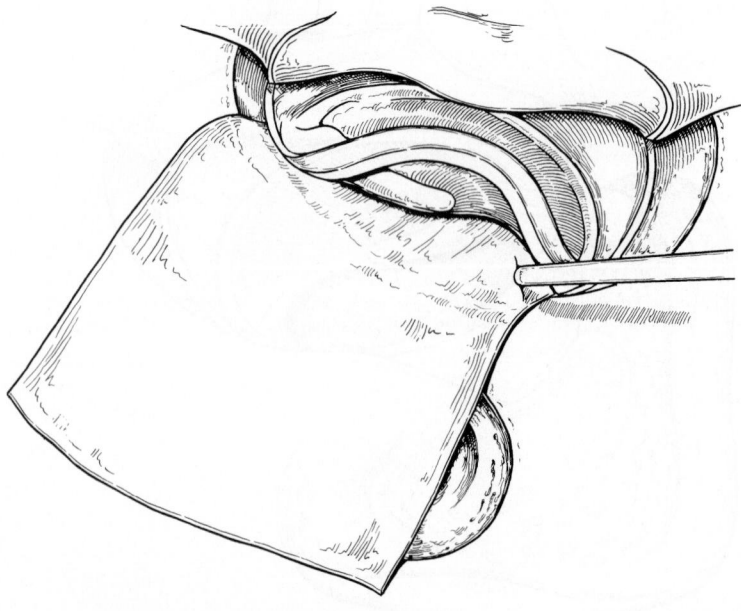

to employ these procedures to control extremely extensive disease or when other closed procedures either fail or are not within reach. This may be the case in patients with recurrent disease who require revision after another surgeon performed the first operation. The authors's experience is that open cavities are rarely free of management problems in children. There is often retention of debris, granulation tissue formation, and intermittent, although frequent, otorrhea. Many of these children eventually require at least minor revision of their open tympanomastoid architecture. This reaffirms my belief that no single procedure can resolve all present and future problems in children.

Atelectasia of the Middle Ear

The author considers atelectasis of the middle ear with retraction of the tympanic membrane as part of the management continuum of cholesteatoma. It has a full spectrum of presentation from mild, fully visible retraction pockets without keratin debris to severe retraction and adhesion to bony structures of the middle ear. The long process of the incus and promontory are most frequently involved. As the retraction extends posteriorly and interiorly into the facial recess, squamous debris collects to form frank cholesteatoma (10,11). Although retraction of the tympanic membrane is most frequently seen posteriorly and superiorly in the pars flaccida and pars tensa, it may occur in any portion of the tympanic membrane and extend deeply into the middle ear and mastoid.

Early management by myringotomy and tube placement is the best technique to avoid deep retraction and cholesteatoma formation. Shallow pockets without severe structural changes in the fibrous layer of the tympanic membrane are easily reversed by placing a tube. Even moderate to severe retractions that appear to be irreversibly adherent to the middle-ear structures may be completely or partially reversed by myringotomy and tube placement, as well as elevation of the retracted tympanic membrane with suction. Care should be taken to peel the epithelial casts of the surface of the retraction pocket to prevent stenting of the concavity by the dry squamous material.

When small portions of the tympanic membrane are involved and the retraction pockets cannot be elevated, the involved tissue should be resected through a standard postauricular tympanomastoid approach as for any cholesteatoma. All epithelium must be removed from the involved areas of the middle ear and a medially placed temporalis fascia graft used to reestablish the structural integrity of the tympanic membrane. A Gelfilm sheet is positioned medial to the graft to prevent adhesion to the bony middle-ear structures. A tympanostomy tube may be used to equalize middle-ear pressure during the healing process.

In cases of recurrent atelectasis or severe retractions in which the surgeon suspects that the fibrous portion of the tympanic membrane has lost its elasticity, more rigid support is required. This is particularly true when eustachian tube dysfunction is likely to persist for several years. Resection of the entire retraction pocket with all of its epithelial elements must be accomplished. This may require sacrifice of the chorda tympani nerve, as well as removal of portions or all of the ossicles. Support is provided by placing conchal cartilage pieces between the middle-ear structures and the temporalis fascia graft (12). Tragal cartilage may also be used to provide the structural integrity to prevent future retraction (Fig. 16). The author uses conchal cartilage because it is accessible through the postauricular incision, thinner, and easier to cut to the desired shape. Gelfoam should be placed between the cartilage sheets and the promontory to prevent adhesions that reduce tympanic membrane mobility.

If resection of all epithelium elements has been questionable, an exploration of the middle ear is warranted 6 months to 1 year later to be certain no residual disease is present. This is particularly necessary because the conchal cartilage graft prevents visualization of the middle ear through the tympanic membrane. A period of ventilation with a tympanostomy tube may also be helpful to facilitate the healing process.

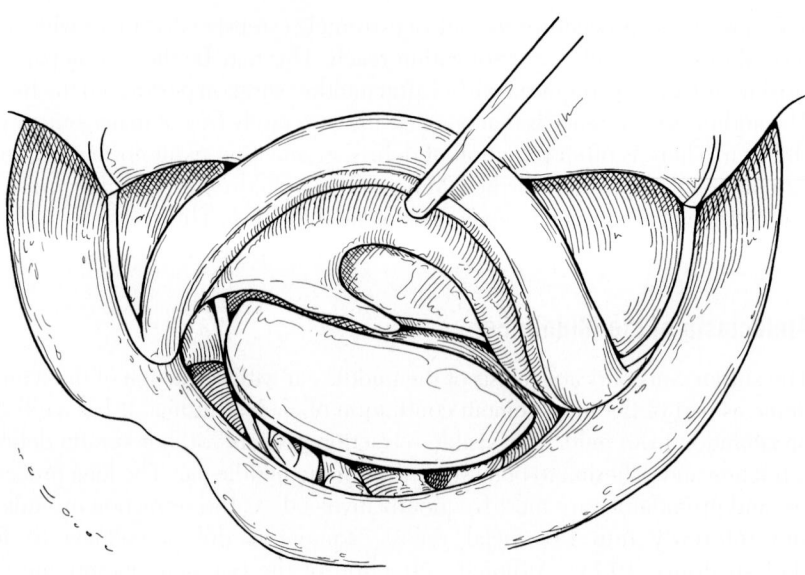

FIGURE 16 Conchal cartilage is placed in the middle ear to provide structural integrity and prevent retraction after tympanoplasty for atelectasis.

PEARLS AND PERILS

1. Medical therapy controls infection and reduces inflammation to facilitate surgery.
2. Surgery of CSOM has a high success rate in children and should not be delayed due to age.
3. Middle-ear atelectasis is best treated early by myringotomy and tube placement to avoid cholesteatoma.
4. Cholesteatoma must be completely removed from involved structures prior to reconstruction.
5. A second-look operation may be required, as well as treatment of concurrent conditions, i.e., OME.
6. Delaying a cholesteatoma surgery in children causes extensive disease.
7. Although closed techniques are preferred for primary surgery, open techniques may be needed for revision.
8. In CSOM, there is no single-stage operation that cures all ills.
9. Delay of treatment of middle-ear atelectasis leads to cholesteatoma.

🔱 MANAGEMENT OF COMPLICATIONS

Granulation Tissue and Aural Polyposis

Granulation tissue and aural mucosal polyps that are at the level of the tympanic membrane or extend into the external meatus are a sign of underlying disease, either a retained tympanostomy tube or cholesteatoma. There may be considerable resolution after 7 to 10 days of oral antibiotic and topical antibiotic and steroid drops.

If granulation or an aural polyp cannot be effectively and comfortably removed in the office, the procedure should be performed using general anesthesia. This permits complete removal of the tissue and an adequate examination of the middle ear prior to definitive surgery. After the polyp is removed, a period of medical therapy will often reduce infection and inflammation in preparation for surgery, as well as provide an opportunity to obtain a computed tomography scan of the temporal bone.

The surgeon should always keep in mind the rare but occasional possibility of malignancy presenting as granular or polypoid tissue in the external meatus.

Ossicular Erosion

Ossicular erosion is common in the presence of large cholesteatoma in children. Depending on the surgeon's preference, a variety of ossiculoplasties may be performed, and a wide variety of prostheses are available. The author's preference is to perform a myringoincudopexy whenever the incus remains intact and is articulated to the stapes. When only the stapes or stapes footplate is left after removal of cholesteatoma, a tragal cartilage-covered partial or total ossicular replacement prosthesis made of Plasti-Pore has been effective in children (Figs. 17 and 18) (8). Such prostheses, with a Plasti-Pore shaft and hydroxyapatite head, may avoid the need for a cartilage cover, but long-term follow-up data are not yet available in children.

Tympanosclerosis

Tympanosclerosis is frequently encountered in the tympanic membranes of children undergoing tympanoplasty surgery. Although it is tempting to remove large sheets of the material prior to placing a graft, it is unnecessary to do so. Tympanosclerotic plaques only need to be removed at the edge of the perforation to denude the epithelium adequately enough to stimulate healing. Hard tympanosclerosis may need to be cut with a sharp knife or scissors to rim the perforation, which presents a minor technical problem but does not reduce the success rate.

Tympanosclerosis in the middle ear may impede ossicular mobility. This material must be carefully removed to release the ossicles. This rarely occurs in children, but the pediatric otologic surgeon must be prepared for this eventuality, including the occasional need to perform a stapedectomy or drill out a stapes footplate.

Intracranial Complications

Fortunately, intracranial complications of CSOM are rare in children. However, occasional epidural abscess, brain abscess, meningitis, otitic hydrocephalus, venous thrombosis, and abducens nerve paralysis are seen.

With the advent of the modern antibiotic era, these complications are treated primarily by culture-specific intravenous antibiotic therapy, capable of crossing the blood–brain barrier, and eliminating the focus of the tympanomastoid infection surgically. Otosurgical management consists of elimination of the infected areas of the mastoid by mastoidectomy, drainage of adjacent abscesses when possible, and following the infection to the petrous apex, if necessary. Cholesteatoma management and adequate drainage of the middle ear are also essential.

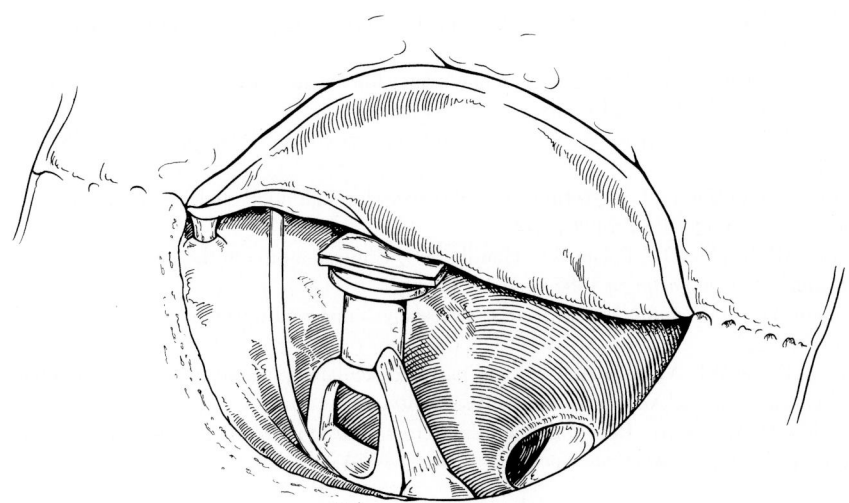

FIGURE 17 A partial ossicular replacement prosthesis may be used with a cartilage cover for partial ossicular reconstruction.

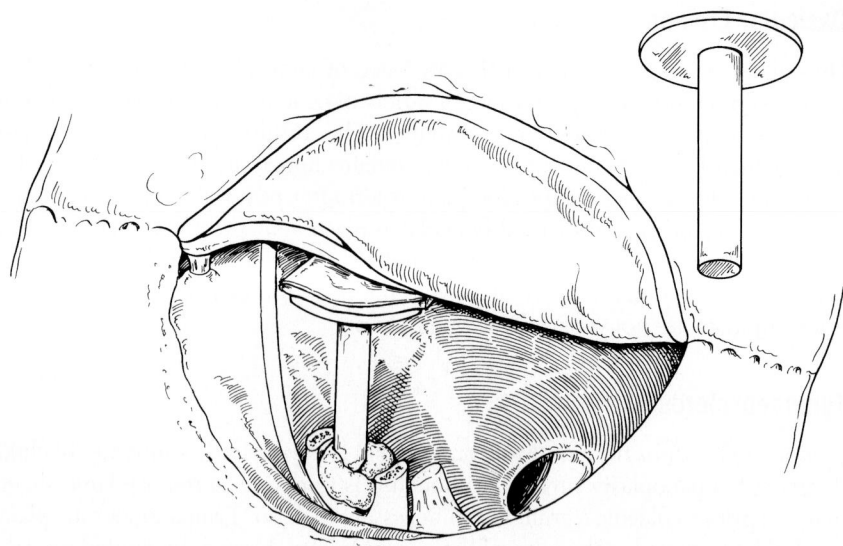

FIGURE 18 A total ossicular replacement prosthesis may be used with a cartilage cover when only the stapes footplate remains after cholesteatoma removal.

Neurosurgical drainage of an epidural and brain abscess may be needed. Medical management of increased cerebrospinal fluid pressure with diuretics and steroids in conjunction with a cerebrospinal fluid shunt may be required to prevent headache, visual changes, and cranial nerve palsies (sixth nerve). Surgical therapy is guided by computed tomography of the temporal bone and magnetic resonance imaging findings in the brain and cerebral vasculature.

Venous thrombosis may be extensive and may include the petrosal veins, transverse sinus, sigmoid sinus, and jugular vein. In addition to the methods for management of the complications of increased intracranial pressure mentioned, the role of anticoagulation is still being debated, and the new frontier of interventional radiography using direct application of intravascular thrombolytic enzymes may have promise. Following venous thrombosis the signs and symptoms of headache, papilledema, visual changes, and sixth nerve palsy may take weeks to months to resolve. Likewise, recanalization of thrombosed vessels may also take months.

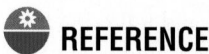 **REFERENCES**

1. Kessler A, Potsic WP, Marsh RR. Type 1 tympanoplasty in children. *Arch Otolaryngol Head Neck Surg* 1994;120:487–490.
2. Podoshin L, Fradis M, Malatskey S, Ben-David J. Type I tympanoplasty in children. *Am J Otol* 1996;17:293–296.
3. Potsic WP, Winawer MR, Marsh RR. Tympanoplasty for the anterior-superior perforation in children. *Am J Otol* 1996;17:115–118.
4. Glasscock ME, Dickins JRE, Wiet R. Cholesteatoma in children. *Laryngoscope* 1981;91: 1743–1753.
5. Vartiainen E, Nuutinen J. Long-term results of surgery for childhood cholesteatoma. *Int J Pediatr Otorhinolaryngol* 1992;24:201–208.
6. Wetmore RF, Konkle DF, Potsic WP, Handler SD. Cholesteatoma in the pediatric patient. *Int J Pediatr Otorhinolaryngol* 1987;14:101–112.
7. Brackmann DE. Tympanoplasty with mastoidectomy: canal wall up procedures. *Am J Otol* 1993;14:380–382.
8. Kessler A, Potsic WP, Marsh RR. Total and partial ossicular replacement prosthesis in children. *Otolaryngol Head Neck Surg* 1994;110:302–303.
9. Rosenfeld RM, Moura RL, Bluestone CD. Predictors of residual-recurrent cholesteatoma in children. *Arch Otolaryngol Head Neck Surg* 1992;118:384–391.

10. Ruah CB, Schachern PA, Paparella MM, Zelterman D. Mechanisms of retraction pocket formation in the pediatric tympanic membrane. *Arch Otolaryngol Head Neck Surg* 1992;118: 1298–1305.

11. Akyildiz N, Abkay C, Özgïrgïn ON, Bayramoglu Ï, Sayin N. The role of retraction pockets in cholesteatoma development: an ultrastructural study. *ENT J* 1993;72:210–212.

12. Poe DS, Gadre AK. Cartilage tympanoplasty for management of retraction pockets and cholesteatomas. *Laryngoscope* 1993;103:614–618.

W. P. Potsic: Department of Otorhinolaryngology—Head and Neck Surgery, University of Pennsylvania, The Children's Hospital of Philadelphia, Philadelphia, Pennsylvania 19104.

• *Practical Pediatric Otolaryngology*
• edited by Robin T. Cotton
  and Charles M. Myer, III
• Lippincott-Raven Publishers,
  Philadelphia © 1999

Aural Rehabilitation for Hearing-Impaired Children

Gayle P. Riemer & Jodi K. Paetsch

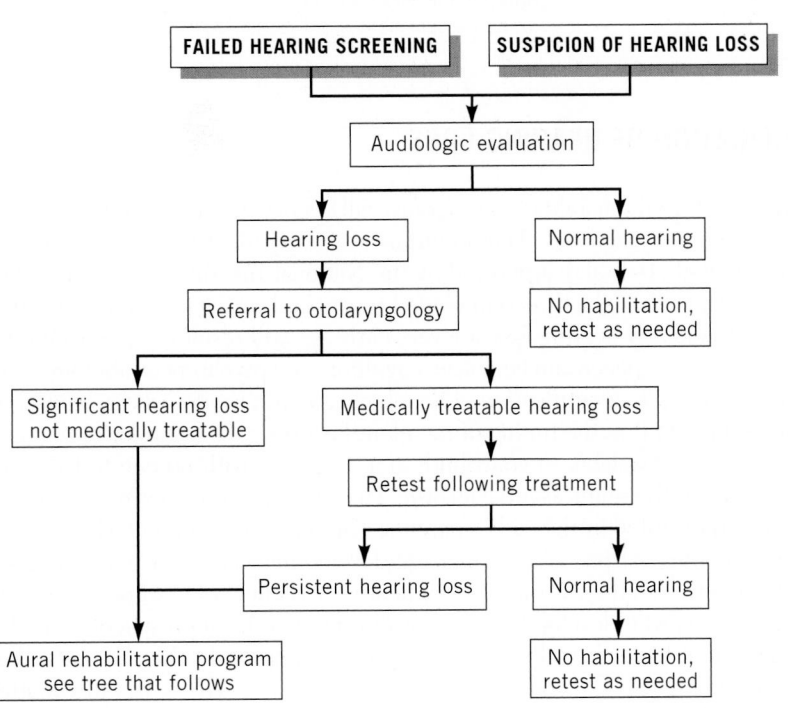

continued on next page

continued

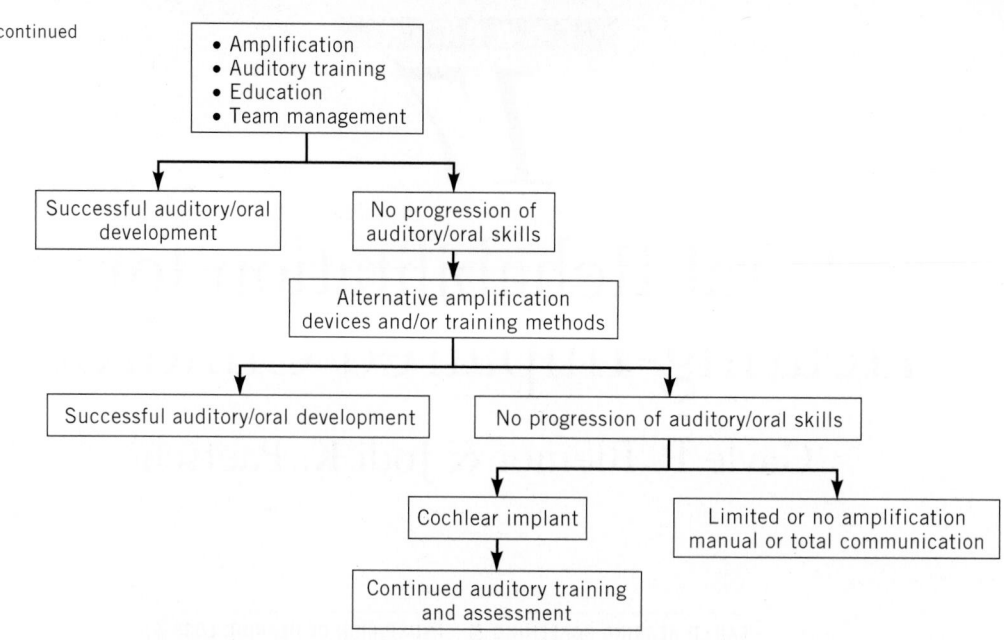

IDENTIFICATION OF HEARING LOSS

The best of aural rehabilitation programs will begin with early identification and proceed with accurate diagnoses. The importance of early identification of hearing loss is well documented (1–4) and supported by the National Institute of Health's 1993 Consensus Statement (5), which recommended universal hearing screening for newborns. The failure to identify hearing loss at a very early age will result in significant effects on the development of speech and language, cognition, and psychosocial abilities. Even with intensive therapy, late identification of hearing loss may have devastating consequences.

Just as important as the timing of the identification is the accuracy of the diagnosis. Multiple tools are available to contribute to a diagnosis, with no one test method currently considered the quintessential answer. The single most overlooked testing method is the input contributed by the child's parents. The voice of any parent who questions the auditory responses or speech and language development of his or her child should be heard. Even if we see the day of universal hearing screening of newborns, there will still be those children who develop hearing loss during the critical preschool years. If a parent suspects that his or her child is not responding appropriately to sounds, there is a definite possibility that the child could have a hearing loss. Of course, it will often be a treatable, conductive loss, but even mild hearing losses can contribute to delayed development. Any parental concern about hearing loss, at any age, should result in a referral to an audiologist for an audiologic evaluation.

Audiologists have available a whole battery of tests for identification of hearing loss. No single test should be used to diagnosis hearing impairment, and no treatment program should begin without a compilation of test results. Identification through the Infant Hearing Screening and Assessment Program (as mandated by the State of Ohio) (6) is a result of a failed evoked potential screening. The auditory brainstem response (ABR) is currently accepted as the high-risk screening method of choice with a 35 dB hearing level (HL) response to a click stimulus used as pass criteria. As the statewide committee moves toward universal screening, we expect to see otoacoustic emissions incorporated into the program. A two-stage universal screening program would be an excellent combination of these two tools (7).

Failure of an initial screening should always result in the referral to an audiologist for diagnostic testing. At this point, the test battery usually begins with a threshold ABR (for infants or hard-to-test populations) or a behavioral audiologic evaluation. The ABR testing should include threshold evaluations for low-frequency tone pips (500 Hz), mid-high-frequency clicks, and high-frequency tone pips (4,000 Hz). This will provide an "audiogram" derived from the evoked potential thresholds. This audiogram must be confirmed with behavioral testing as much as possible. Even young infants (under 6 months) can be tested with behavioral observation audiometry to attempt to confirm the ABR results. Conversely, older infants and children whose behavioral audiometry results suggest a significant hearing loss may need to have an ABR to confirm those findings.

Additional tools available to confirm the hearing loss include acoustic reflex testing and otoacoustic emissions. Acoustic reflex threshold testing is difficult to correlate with true hearing sensitivity thresholds, but certainly the presence or absence of reflexes can be diagnostically helpful. The presence or absence of otoacoustic emissions can also be used as a confirmation of hearing loss, bearing in mind that otoacoustic emissions will be absent for any hearing loss greater than approximately 30 dBHL. Although prediction of hearing thresholds may not be as accurate with these test methods, they can provide useful information about the function of the peripheral auditory system. Use of these tests in conjunction with the evoked potentials and behavioral results will help the audiologist to document the case of the neurologically impaired child who has no evoked potential responses but has peripheral hearing sensitivity and may not require the use of amplification.

Input from the parents, teachers, caregivers, or therapists who provide service to the child may contribute invaluable information regarding the child's ability to respond to different types of auditory stimuli. This information can help to confirm or deny any electrophysical findings or behavioral test results. This sharing of information is also critical to the success of the aural rehabilitation program, as all the people involved with the child come to an agreement on the diagnosis and planning.

PEARLS AND PERILS

1. Parental concern should always be considered a valid reason for referring a child for an audiologic evaluation.
2. If a parent does not feel that the baby or child is responding appropriately to sounds, there is a good chance that the child may have a hearing loss.

TEAM APPROACH TO AURAL REHABILITATION

Once a child has been identified as hearing impaired, there are many people who will contribute to his or her care and development. First and always, the child's family must function as a member of the team. By virtue of spending the most time with the hearing-impaired child, the family (usually the parents) has a lot of information to contribute about the child's abilities and appropriateness of care. Who the other members of this team will be depends on each individual case. The clinical audiologist, aural rehabilitation audiologist, otolaryngologist, and speech pathologist make up the primary members of the team. Many of the hearing-impaired children we follow will have multiple problems, and their care may include occupational and/or physical therapists, nurses, and physicians from other specialities. School-aged children will also have classroom teachers, school speech pathologists, and an educational audiologist functioning on the team. Psychological or social issues for the child or family may necessitate the inclusion of a psychologist or social worker.

The team approach may be formalized for some hearing-impaired children. Referral to the Hearing Impaired Clinic at Children's Hospital Medical Center in Cincinnati, Ohio, will provide the family with the opportunity to meet with multiple team members (as appropriate) in one place, at one time. This will serve to bring together the multiple disciplines for discussion and to provide coordinated recommendations for the parents.

A less formal and more on-going team approach will put much more responsibility on the parents and require more efforts at communication among the professionals. Interdisciplinary meetings can facilitate this communication. Another valuable tool is the parent notebook, used to record progress, concerns, and test results for the hearing-impaired child. Follow-up activities for the parents to complete are entered into the notebook after each therapy session. This helps the parent carry over the therapy goals into the home environment. This notebook can be carried from appointment to appointment and/or from home to school to serve as both a communication system and means for the parents to keep reminders of the recommendations made. Again, this is successful in the hands of a responsible family.

As a final note on the team approach, it is important for all members of the team to keep in mind that the child is the focus of the team. Communication and recommendations should be based on the needs of the child and not reflect a "hidden agenda," through which any one discipline has plans pertaining to personal or professional goals. For example, the need to include as many children as possible in a particular program for financial gain should not affect decision making, or a personal bias for or against the appropriateness of using sign language with hearing-impaired children may not best serve the individual child's needs. Personalities and personal gain should not affect the child's care.

PEARLS AND PERILS

1. Beware of the professional with the "hidden agenda" who may not have the child's needs foremost in mind.
2. The services the child receives need to be designed specifically for him or her, not to fit the financial, social, or professional needs of the people involved in his or her care.

AMPLIFICATION

The early identification of hearing loss is important but effective only if amplification and aural rehabilitation are also off to an early start. Getting hearing aids on the hearing-impaired child as quickly as possible will serve multiple purposes. Of course, the early opportunity to optimize residual hearing is the goal, but early amplification also gives the parents a sense of effectiveness and inclusion. The hearing aids for an infant or young child are ultimately the parents' responsibility and getting them actively involved in the rehabilitation process can begin with hearing aid use and care. Many parents use these activities as an outlet for their intense need to contribute to their child's care.

Because the speed of the hearing aid fitting is important, the flexibility of the fitting is also integral to success. Options for fitting (body style hearing aids versus behind-the-ear or in-the-ear hearing aids versus personal FM systems, etc.) should be discussed with the parents and presented as potentially changing over time. At our institution, newly identified hearing-impaired infants with moderate or greater hearing losses have earmold impressions taken at the first hearing aid evaluation appointment (usually within days of the diagnostic evoked potential testing). Infants with poor head control may be given the opportunity to rent a body-style hearing aid that can be coupled to their earmolds with long tubing and snap connectors (to reduce feedback). Older infants are more often fit with behind-the-ear hearing aids.

Years ago, the fitting of infants and young children with hearing aids was more art than science. Choices were made based on experience with particular hearing aids and similar hearing loss configurations. Audiologists today have the means to make hearing aid fitting a science, even with minimal cooperation from the "client." The old tool of measuring functional gain by testing the child in sound field (with speech and tonal stimuli) can still provide behavioral information that is useful in determining the appropriateness of the fit. For example, testing that reveals a very narrow dynamic range (little loudness difference between what appears to be a comfortable listening level and what is obviously an uncomfortable or painful level) will indicate the need for prescription of a hearing aid that incorporates automatic gain control.

Electroacoustic measurements are another old tool that remain useful when fitting hearing aids on infants and children. Knowing the precise output characteristics of the hearing aid (via an electroacoustic test box) will help the clinician and parents monitor the appropriateness of the fitting and the need for repair, modification, or replacement.

We take a step closer to science now with the addition of probe microphone measurements. The placement of a probe microphone directly in the ear canal allows us to measure the output of the hearing aid as it is modified by the characteristics of that individual's ear canal. Not only can we measure the actual gain but we can also learn what modifications will protect the child's ears from excessive output. Probe microphone measurements do require some level of cooperation on the child's part, but even infants can often be quieted or distracted for the few seconds it takes to obtain a measurement. If extensive comparative measurements are not realistic, obtaining real ear-to-coupler differences to compare the ear canal resonance with the electroacoustic measurements (Fig. 1) is a fast and simple way to confirm the appropriateness of the fitting. This and any other probe microphone measurements obtained can also be used to help determine the need for earmold modifications to shape the response or control the output of the hearing aids.

Parents and therapists can make their contribution to determining appropriate amplification by monitoring a child's behavior at home or at school. Behavioral changes may alert the parents to changes in the child's hearing or function of the hearing aids. A child's rejection of a hearing aid fitting may be just behavioral (as in the case of the child who pulls out his or her earmolds for attention), but it may also indicate that the amount of

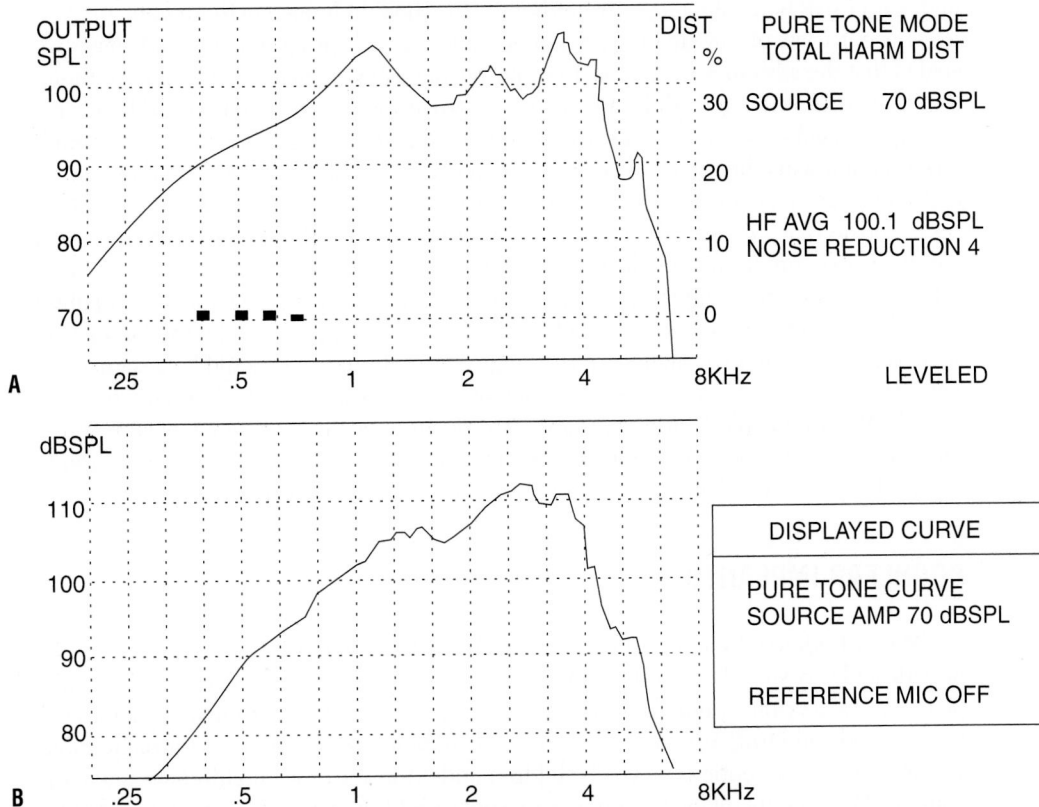

FIGURE 1 A: Output characteristics of a hearing aid as measured in a 2cc coupler. **B:** Output characteristics of the same hearing aid as measured in an ear canal with a probe microphone. These "Real Ear-to-Coupler" differences should be used to determine the desired output characteristics in a hearing aid fitting.

gain or the frequency response for the hearing aid may be inappropriate. A child's inability to respond to certain environmental sounds or certain aspects of speech may also indicate that he or she is not receiving optimal amplification.

Try as we might, there are some hearing-impaired children who do not receive adequate benefit from traditional amplification. Alternative devices may be recommended for short-term use (as when included in a precochlear implant evaluation period) or as a long-term alternative to traditional hearing aids. A vibrotactile device is recommended to provide vibratory information coded from a speech or environmental signal. The vibrotactile stimulus is most often used in a therapy situation to work on detection of sound or discrimination of durational cues. As used in a preimplant therapy situation, the device can train the child to perform tasks that will be performed postimplant to evaluate detection and discrimination.

For those children who have residual hearing only in the low frequencies and do not demonstrate benefit from traditional hearing aids, a frequency transpositional hearing aid may be a viable alternative. This type of hearing aid actually compresses the speech signal into the low-frequency range, giving the user input from all speech-spectrum signals but in the range of usable hearing. The transpositional hearing aid will typically have multiple controls to vary the output for each individual's needs. Use of this type of hearing aid will require a significant effort to "get used to it" and auditory training to maximize its use.

The advent of programmable hearing aids has provided adult users with multiple amplification options within one hearing aid. Because they require user input for acceptable modifications, programmable hearing aids are difficult to fit on children. So much depends on user preference in various acoustic environments that young children cannot usually provide the subjective information necessary to set the programs. The older, cooperative hearing-impaired child, however, may find the multiple programs highly useful as he or she moves from therapy to school to home environments.

Recent trials of amplifying very young children with programmable aids have revealed that the advantages available to sophisticated listeners may be of benefit to them, too. If older children and adults are gaining improved speech recognition and better listening in speech-in-noise situations, it would logically follow that young children would, too. Programmable hearing aids can offer better performance with less sound distortion and more high-frequency gain. The fitting of hearing losses of unusual configurations (i.e., "cookie-bite," reverse slope, or severe recruitment) can be less frustrating when a highly flexible, programmable hearing aid is used. Choices for output limiting are more varied, and multiple memory hearing aids offer alternative programs for even a baby's use. The different programs can be adjusted for use during periods of close interaction such as cradling, nursing, singing, or reading. A different program could be designed for periods of excessive background noise such as traffic noise, grocery shopping, or large crowds. Programmable hearing aids also provide an opportunity for enhanced involvement by parents in the habilitation process. The multiprogram instruments allow parents and professionals to collaborate in observing a child's auditory responses.

COCHLEAR IMPLANTS

When traditional amplification or even the new advances in amplification do not provide auditory stimulation sufficient for developing speech and language, cochlear implants can be a viable option. Children over the age of 18 months are currently approved by the Food and Drug Administration for implantation if they meet the criteria in Table 1. There are also exceptions in which children under the age of 18 months have been implanted. The preimplant evaluation on very young children generally cannot include formal standardized tests of auditory skills. Preimplant auditory training should include comparative trials with conventional hearing aids, tactile hearing aids, and FM systems (coupled with the personal hearing aids). The same specific therapy activity and the Ling

TABLE 1: Cochlear Implant Criteria for Children[a]

Profound sensorineural hearing loss in both ears

18 months through 17 years of age

Little or no useful benefit from hearing aids (<30% speech discrimination ability in the best aided condition)

No medical contraindications

High motivation and appropriate expectations for the child and family

Placement in an educational program that emphasizes development of auditory skills after implantation

[a]Criteria courtesy of Cochlear Corporation, Denver, Colorado.

Six Sound Test can be used to compare performance. Poor performance with all devices would certainly suggest candidacy.

A cochlear implant is a surgically implanted device (Fig. 2), but the surgery itself is a minor part of the success of a child who has been implanted. Appropriate selection of candidates is crucial, and the rehabilitation process following implantation is the key to success.

Aural rehabilitation after implantation involves conscientious "mapping" of the speech processor and "turning on" of the electrodes. Multiple visits are required, especially for the inattentive or very young child. Like the setting of hearing aids for very young children, the concept of mapping needs to be a flexible one that may depend somewhat on behavioral findings outside the clinic. Again, the information obtained from the child's parents is as important as the test findings in the clinic.

The single most important factor for cochlear-implanted children is the auditory training that follows for years. Learning to listen with an implant is much like a newborn learning to talk. It may take months or years for the young child to make obvious use of the information/stimulation he or she gets from the implant. For some children, the process may need to begin at so simple a level as detection of sound versus absence of sound. The attachment of meaning to the information will occur much later. The parents need to be trained to maximize the home environment for their child's listening. Working with

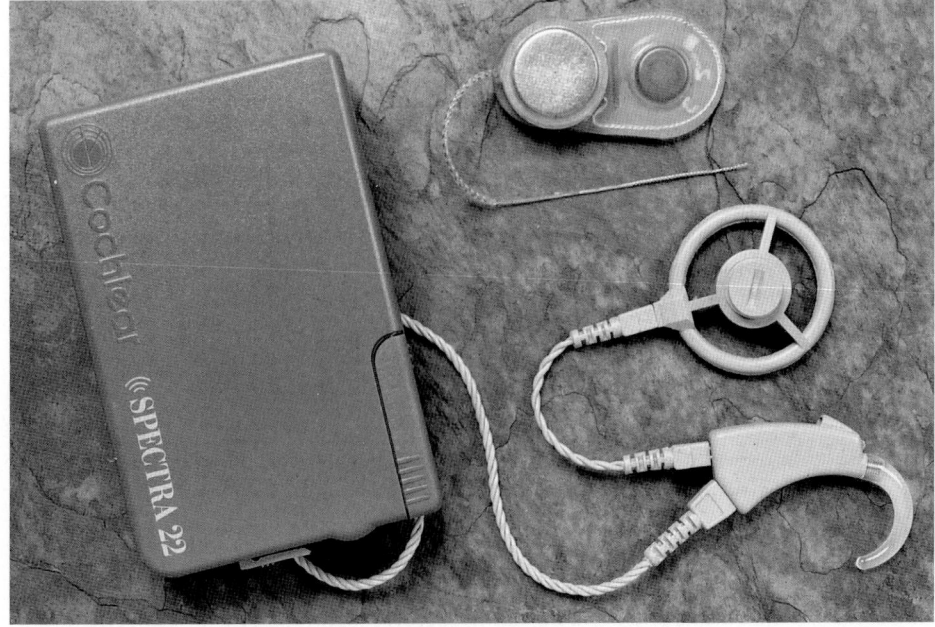

FIGURE 2 Cochlear implant device including speech processor (about the size of a deck of cards), postauricular headset, and internal components.

a parent-centered aural rehabilitation audiologist on a program of specific listening activities will provide the parents with the skills they need to be their child's best teacher.

USE OF NO AMPLIFICATION

One additional option facing parents of profoundly hearing-impaired children is the use of no amplification. Certainly, a trial of amplification is recommended for all hearing-impaired children, but when amplification does not appear to be providing benefit and other options (tactile hearing aids, FM systems, frequency transpositional hearing aids) have been attempted, the use of no devices at all is an option. There are a significant number of parents who choose this option for their child, relying on a manual communication system. In some cases, the parents feel very strongly that their child should feel part of a deaf community that chooses to communicate through sign language. Other strong feelings against cochlear implantation may include not wanting to "change" their child, feeling that an implant will give the child the message that he or she is not "OK" just the way he or she is, or just not wanting to make the decision for their child. Allowing a child to reach the age of, say 12, however, when he or she can make a thoughtful choice for or against cochlear implantation may not be truly practical. The preschool years are widely accepted as the critical learning period for making the most use of auditory input and language learning.

The amplification options and choices that parents make for their child have a considerable impact on the child's educational placement—and vice versa. What educational programs are available in their community may influence their choice. If there are no follow-up services nearby for aural rehabilitation therapy after cochlear implant, an implant may not be the best choice for that child. If there is a large deaf community that uses sign language to communicate and the best academic program available is a total communication or manual one, the parents might easily choose this option for their child. Conversely, if access to the surgeon, aural rehabilitation audiologist, and auditory/oral educators is within the family's grasp, the parents might consider amplification or implantation the best option.

What option is best for the profoundly hearing-impaired child? Should professionals insist on the option they know to be best for the child? Should we actively pursue the reluctant cochlear implant candidate? No. It is up to the professionals involved to provide the parents with all the information they need to make the best choice they can for their hearing-impaired child.

AUDITORY TRAINING

Children identified as having an educationally significant hearing loss can usually benefit from training to maximize their residual hearing and develop listening skills. Children who derive benefit from amplification, a tactile device, or a cochlear implant are referred for aural rehabilitation therapy. At Children's Hospital Medical Center, this therapy takes the form of parent-centered sessions designed to train the parents as much or more than training the child. The therapist promotes an auditory learning environment that will hopefully lead to natural speech and language development. Parents are usually directly involved in the therapy sessions or observing through a one-way glass if their presence prohibits the child's full cooperation.

During the therapy sessions, the parent actually participates in the listening activity, frequently taking turns with the child. In this way, the parent can serve as a role model for the child to follow. The parent will also gain experience with the activity, easing carryover to the home environment. Sessions generally last 50 minutes with an additional 10 minutes at the end for discussion and planning for activities to do at home. Most parents choose to use the parent notebook format to record recommendations and activities, as well as progress notes to share with other professionals. This helps the therapist by reducing the number of contacts needed with the other professionals: many of their questions can be answered by reading the entries in the parent notebook.

Periodic hearing aid check appointments with the clinical audiologist are also recommended for the children enrolled in aural rehabilitation therapy. The children return for clinical evaluation every 1, 3, 6, or 12 months (depending on the age of the child and/or the stability of the hearing loss). The hearing aid check includes electroacoustic analysis of the hearing aids, unaided and aided behavioral thresholds, speech recognition testing, tympanometry (to rule out otitis media that might affect behavioral thresholds), and probe microphone measurements. Ample time is also allowed for counseling and coordinating the clinical audiology findings and services with the other members of the child's "team."

Children enrolled in aural rehabilitation therapy progress through a hierarchy of goals, beginning with simple detection of sound. The amount of time spent on each goal varies widely, depending on the degree of hearing loss, age of identification, cognitive abilities, etc. Each child is an individual, and no two children will progress at the same rate. Monitoring for progress can be formalized, however, with the use of an auditory skills checklist (see chapter Appendix). Periodic evaluation (usually every 3 months) can reveal which skills are mastered, which may be emerging, and which are yet to be developed. Consideration should be made for the progress at home or in school in addition to what is observed in therapy.

A sample favorite aural rehabilitation activity is called the *Surprise Box.* Toys or objects of varying pitch and loudness are hidden inside and presented auditorily one at a time. (Care must be taken that the child cannot see the object at all!) Some good objects to use in the box are: a bicycle horn, a squeak toy, metal spoons, a pocket-sized tape recorder with taped sounds, keys, a glass and spoon, and a jar of coins. Young children may indicate that they heard the sound by localizing, changing facial expression, or even pointing to an ear if trained to respond this way. The reward for responding is, of course, getting to see the surprise object. Older preschoolers may learn to recognize the sounds and choose the object that was used to make the sound. A chip or sticker hidden on the bottom of the stimulus item can be a fun visual reward to discover when choosing the correct item. More advanced children can be asked to associate the sound they hear from one of the surprise objects with other familiar sounds ("Name two things at home that sound like this").

A tried and true tool for evaluating how hearing-impaired children are making use of their residual hearing is the Ling Six Sound Test, originally published as the Five Sound Test (8). Behavioral responses (spontaneous or as a trained response) to the sounds "Mm, Ah, Oo, Ee, Ss, Sh" can provide considerable information about the child's ability to hear across the speech frequency range. This is a useful supplement to the aided behavioral audiogram obtained by the clinical audiologist. The Six Sound Test can confirm or deny that a child is able to hear the high-frequency sounds especially necessary for speech recognition.

There is a decided advantage to seeing hearing-impaired children frequently for aural rehabilitation therapy. Periodic hearing aid checks provide limited opportunities to discuss the child's progress or issues that are affecting development. Weekly therapy sessions give the therapist the opportunity to provide on-going counseling and repeated teaching. The parents will be better equipped to make appropriate choices for their child if they get more information, more often, and have the comfort level to discuss their concerns openly.

The aural rehabilitation therapist, therefore, functions as a vital member of the child's "team." The therapist is constantly gathering information that can help modify the child's environment or help with educational planning. The behavior of the child during therapy, for example, may help the parents to realize that the child's attention span is quite brief or that placement in a program based on total communication may be appropriate. The need for hearing aid modifications may become clear if therapy reveals poor detection of certain speech sounds. The need for a return to audiologic and medical evaluation may surface when the therapist notices a significant change in the child's responsiveness.

PEARLS AND PERILS

1. If you teach the parent how to foster auditory skills, the potential is greater for these skills to be maximized in their natural environment.
2. The more enthusiastic a parent is toward auditory training, the greater the chances are for a hearing-impaired child to succeed in a listening world.

TRANSITION TO INDEPENDENCE

There must come a time when the hearing-impaired child needs to make the transition to independence from aural rehabilitation therapy. How do we decide, however, when all the "special attention" is no longer necessary? Certainly, age is a factor to consider—independence from aural rehabilitation therapy may evolve along the same pathway as adolescent independence. There are other factors to consider, though. The hearing-impaired child may make such rapid progress through the therapy goals that listening skills catch up and he or she achieves age-appropriate skills. Dismissal from therapy for this child is a simple concept, and the transition to dependence on traditional educational settings is a proud and joyous one.

Much more difficult is the decision that aural rehabilitation therapy is no longer appropriate because, despite the dedicated therapist and the hard-working family, the child has not made significant progress. This may apply in the case of the developmentally delayed child whose cognitive deficits, when coupled with a profound hearing loss, make great strides improbable. It may also apply in the case of the very profoundly hearing-impaired child, who, even with the use of powerful hearing aids, does not even achieve sound detection. If this family does not elect to have a cochlear implant for their child, alternative rehabilitative methods should be recommended as an option.

Care must be taken that the dismissal from aural rehabilitation is not viewed as a failure but rather a transition to an alternative method. If a child is not making progress in aural rehabilitation therapy, enrollment solely in a program that incorporates much more visual and tactile input (including sign language) may be appropriate. Considerable contact with the other members of the child's "team" should be made before this recommendation for dismissal is made. The child's speech pathologist should be particularly helpful in comparing the child's progress with developing communication skills to his or her progress with developing listening skills. Input from the family is absolutely crucial to this decision-making process, but they too must be given all the available information from the various professionals, so that they can make an informed decision with which they feel comfortable.

CONCLUSIONS

Helping the child with a hearing impairment to become the best communicator he or she can be is the primary goal of the professionals who work with the child and family. Aural rehabilitation focuses on trying to get the child with a hearing impairment to reach his or her own maximum auditory potential through teaching the parents to create an auditory learning environment and promote the child's listening skills. Auditory training, amplification, and education are actually explorations of what the child can do or will someday be able to do. Together the health-care professionals, educators, and parents learn to nurture the child's auditory development and to follow his or her communication lead as decisions are made on the child's behalf.

REFERENCES

1. Levitt H, McGarr NS, Geffner D. *Development of language and communication skills in hearing-impaired chidren.* ASHA Monographs Number 26. Rockville, MD: American Speech-Language-Hearing Association, 1987.
2. Northern JL, Downs MP. *Hearing in children,* 4th ed. Baltimore, MD: Williams & Wilkins, 1991.
3. American Academy of Audiology. *Audiol Today* 1988;8–9.
4. American Speech-Language-Hearing Association. *ASHA* 1988;90.
5. National Institutes of Health. *Early identification of hearing loss in infants and young children: Consensus Development Conference on Early Identification of Hearing Loss in Infants and Young Children.* Bethesda, MD: National Institutes of Health, 1993.
6. Riemer G, Farrer S. In: Bess FH, Hall JW, eds. *Screening children for auditory function.* Nashville, TN: Bill Wilkerson Press, 1992.
7. White KR, Maxon AB, Behrens TR, Blackwell PM, Vohr BR. In: Bess FH, Hall JW, eds. *Screening children for auditory function.* Nashville, TN: Bill Wilkerson Press, 1992.
8. Ling D. *Foundations of spoken language for hearing-impaired children.* Washington, DC: Alexander Graham Bell Association for the Deaf, 1988.

G. P. Riemer and J. Paetsch: Department of Audiology, Children's Hospital Medical Center, Cincinnati, Ohio, 45229-3039.

• *Practical Pediatric Otolaryngology*
• edited by Robin T. Cotton and Charles M. Myer, III
• Lippincott-Raven Publishers, Philadelphia © 1998

Auditory/Verbal Skills Checklist

Auditory Skill (Awareness → Discrimination → Recognition → Comprehension)	Pre	3 mo	6 mo	9 mo	12 mo
Relies on hearing aids					
Shows awareness of loud environmental sounds					
Shows awareness of voice					
Shows awareness of soft environmental sounds					
Detects voice on telephone					
Perceives spatial relations through listening					
Discriminates between speech and nonspeech sounds					
Discriminates environmental sounds					
Discriminates singing from talking					
Discriminates between loud and soft voice					
Recognizes individuals' voices					
Associates own name with self					
Pattern recognition: one- versus three-syllable word sets					
Pattern recognition: one- versus two-syllable word sets					
Pattern recognition: two- versus three-syllable word sets					
Pattern recognition: one- versus two- versus three-syllable word sets					
Recognizes one-syllable words in a closed set					
Recognizes one-syllable words in an open set					
Recognizes two-syllable word strings in a closed set					
Recognizes two-syllable word strings in an open set					
Recognizes three-syllable word strings in a closed set					
Recognizes three-syllable word strings in an open set					
Comprehends environmental sounds					
Comprehends prosodic cues					
Understands frequently heard phrases/sentences					
Follows one-step directions					
Follows two-step directions					
Follows three-step directions					
Understands most of what is said during daily routines through audition alone					
Acquires information incidentally through audition alone					

key　✽　has skill
　　　E　emerging skill
　　　—　does not have skill

continued

Verbal Skill	Pre	3 mo	6 mo	9 mo	12 mo
(Random vocalizations → Meaningful utterances → Prosodics → Intelligible verbalizations)					
Engages in vocal play					
Total communication (TC) with unintelligible vocalizations					
Vocalizes for attention					
Vocalizes on demand					
Uses intonation in speech/vocalizations					
TC with intelligible vocalizations					
Uses casual phrases					
Monitors pitch and intensity of own voice					
Talks in simple sentences with consistent verb usage					
Self-corrects language error					

key   ✼ has skill
        E emerging skill
        — does not have skill

Congenital and Acquired Facial Paralysis

Rick A. Friedman

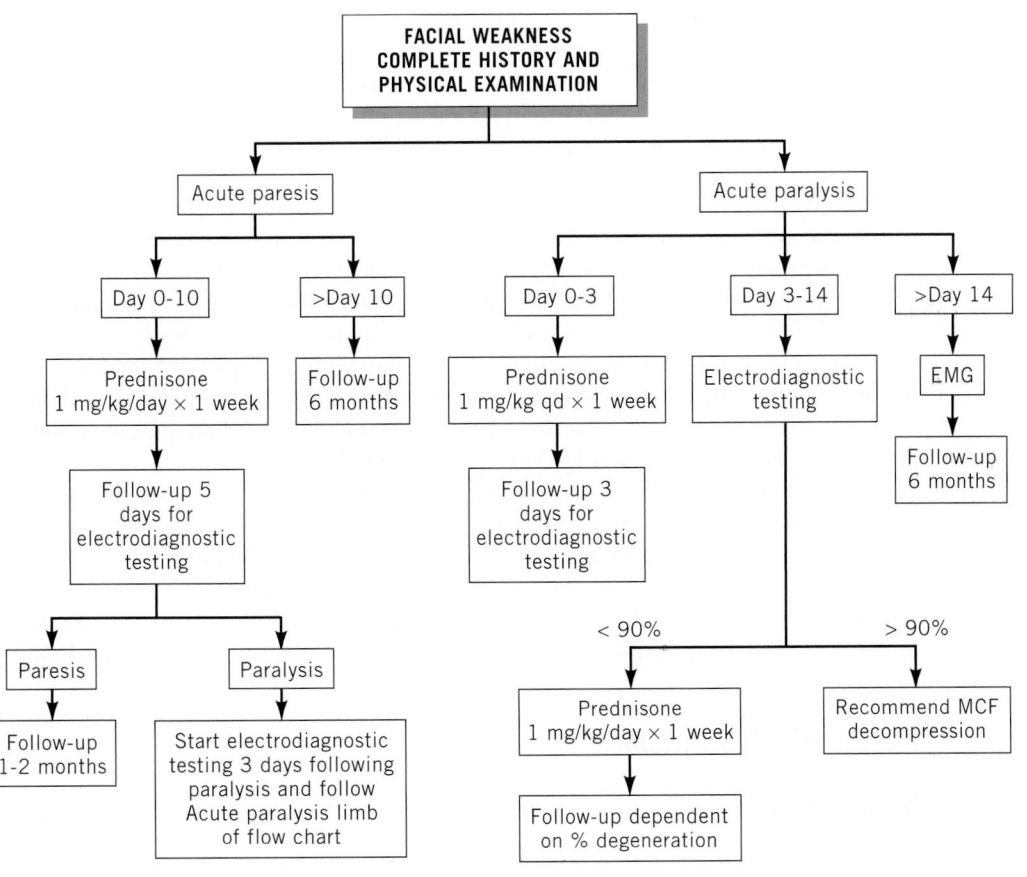

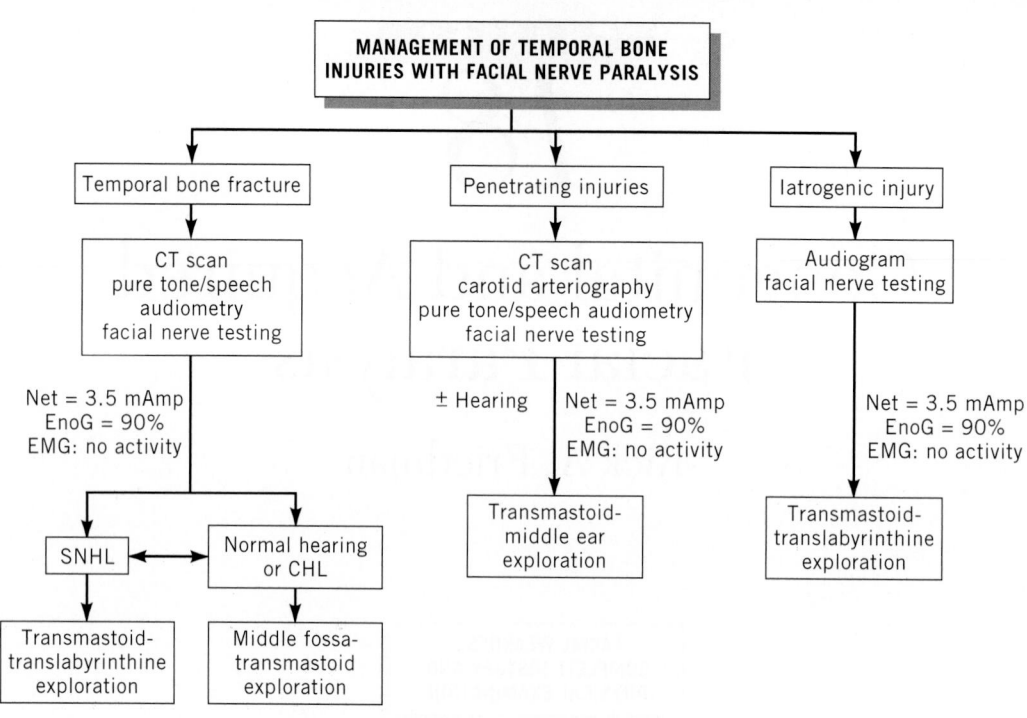

Facial expression, although not unique to humans, is a fundamental part of our ability to convey our thoughts and feelings. The evolutionary significance of facial expression is best exemplified by the stirring of emotions elicited by the face of a crying child or the newborn's first smile. Although cranial nerve dysfunction of any type leads to some form of debility, facial nerve dysfunction in children brings with it unique functional and emotional difficulties. In addition to the risks of excessive ocular exposure and poor ability to feed, the emotional impact of facial weakness may interfere with the parent's ability to bond, or in older children, may lead to unfair ridicule by peers.

The anatomy of the facial nerve in its course through the temporal bone places it at significant risk for injury during the course of a lifetime. Furthermore, although many of the diseases that affect the adult facial nerve affect children in the same manner, a closer look at the pediatric population reveals several anatomic and pathologic factors that singularly affect this group. This chapter presents a review of the anatomy of the facial nerve, as well as the diagnosis and management of facial nerve disorders in children.

FACIAL NERVE ANATOMY

Blood Supply

The facial nerve derives its blood supply from three sources: one from the vertebrobasilar system and two from the external carotid artery (1). The proximal facial nerve is supplied by the labyrinthine branch of the anterior inferior cerebellar artery, a branch of the basilar artery. The petrosal artery, a branch of the external carotid artery, originates from the middle meningeal artery and enters the facial hiatus in the middle cranial fossa where it supplies the labyrinthine and tympanic segments of the nerve. The third source, the stylomastoid artery, typically derives from the postauricular artery and supplies the vertical segment of the nerve.

Functional Considerations

The facial nerve is the nerve of the second branchial arch; it provides motor innervation to the muscles derived from the second arch mesoderm. The facial nerve can be divided into five populations of fibers, which subserve different functions: (a) *special visceral efferent fibers* that provide the innervation to the muscles of facial expression, the stapedius muscle, the posterior belly of the digastric muscle, the stylohyoid muscle, and the auricularis and occipitalis muscles; (b) *special visceral afferent fibers* that provide taste sensation from receptors located on the anterior two-thirds of the tongue and the soft palate via the chorda tympani and greater superficial petrosal nerves, respectively; (c) *general visceral efferent fibers* that supply parasympathetic preganglionic input destined for the pterygopalatine ganglion and ultimately influencing nasal and lacrimal secretion and sublingual and submandibular salivary gland function via the greater superficial petrosal and chorda tympani nerves, respectively; (d) *general visceral afferent fibers* from the nose, palate, and pharynx; and (e) *somatic sensory fibers* conveying the sensations of touch, pressure, pain, and temperature from the external auditory canal and proprioception from the innervated muscles (1).

Corticobulbar Tracts

Many of the motor cranial nerves are supplied by crossed and uncrossed supranuclear fibers in the corticobulbar tracts (Fig. 1). The motor nucleus of the facial nerve is unique in that the efferent fibers to the upper face (forehead) are supplied by both crossed and uncrossed supranuclear tracts; however, the lower facial efferent fibers are only innervated by crossed corticobulbar fibers. As such, supranuclear facial nerve disorders, such as cerebrovascular accidents, affect the lower face on the contralateral side and spare the

FIGURE 1 Upper and lower motor neuron tracts of the facial nerve.

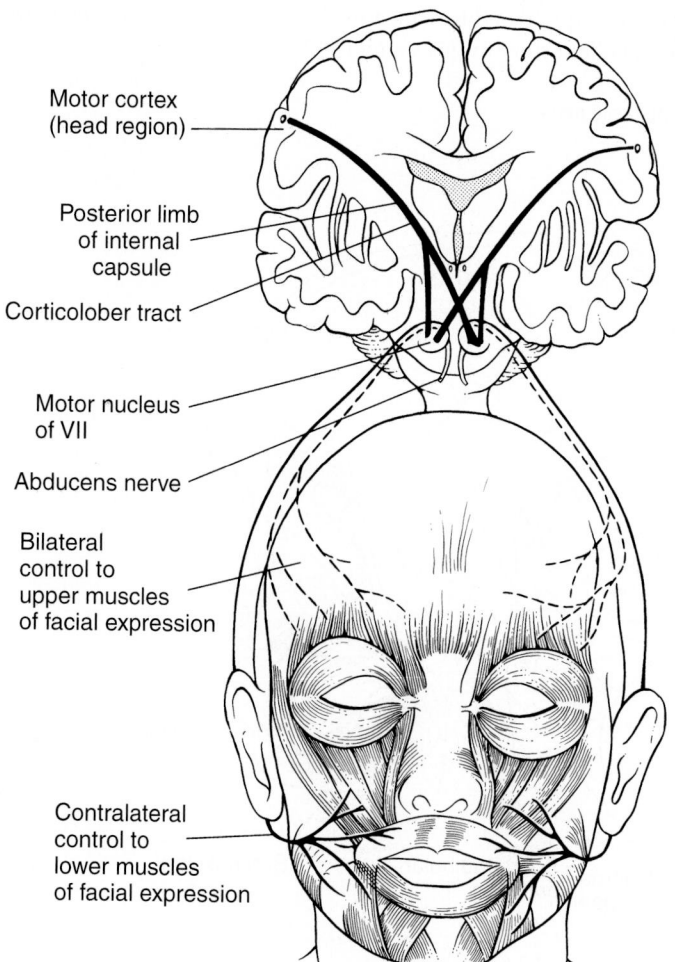

Motor cortex (head region)

Posterior limb of internal capsule

Corticolober tract

Motor nucleus of VII

Abducens nerve

Bilateral control to upper muscles of facial expression

Contralateral control to lower muscles of facial expression

forehead. Supranuclear lesions often spare facial movements associated with emotion, unlike lesions of the periphery. These anatomic factors provide important information for clinical diagnosis.

Facial Nerve Nuclei

There are three nuclei that transmit and receive impulses from the various divisions of the facial nerve. The *motor nucleus*, as described in the previous section, is located in the caudal pons and receives supranuclear input and houses the cell bodies of the motor neurons supplying the muscles of the second branchial arch. The *superior salivatory nucleus* lies superior to the motor nucleus and is the site of the cell bodies of the parasympathetic preganglionic fibers that innervate the seromucinous glands of the nose and palate and the sublingual and submandibular glands. Lastly, the *nucleus solitarious,* located in the medulla, receives the various sensory fibers of the facial nerve.

Intracranial and Intratemporal Facial Nerve

After leaving the motor nucleus, the facial motor fibers course dorsally and loop over the sixth nerve nucleus (Fig. 2). The motor and sensory fibers leave and enter the brain at the pontomedullary junction between the olive and the pyramid. The sensory and autonomic fibers travel in the nervus intermedius (nerve of Wrisberg), which is situated caudal to the motor fibers of the facial nerve and rostral to the eighth cranial nerve. At this point, the course of the nerve is often divided into five anatomic segments:

1. The *intracranial segment* traverses the cerebellopontine angle (CPA) approximately 24 mm before entering the internal auditory meatus. It is intimately associated with the anterior inferior cerebellar artery in this segment (2).

FIGURE 2 Neuroanatomy of the facial nerve.

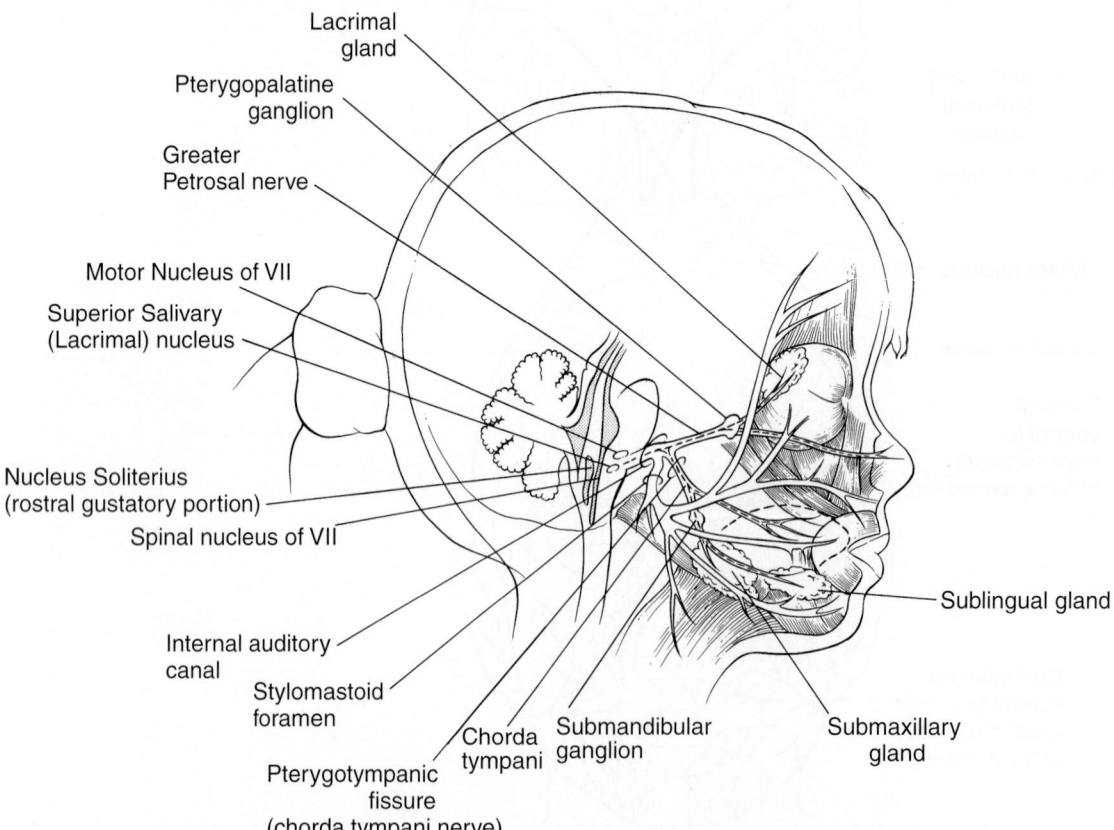

2. The *internal auditory canal segment* is 7 to 8 mm in length and is situated anterosuperiorly. It is separated from its close association with the auditory nerve in the fundus of the canal by the transverse crest. This segment terminates at the nervi facialis (meatal foramen), where it enters the fallopian canal.

3. The *labyrinthine segment* is the shortest and most confined segment, measuring approximately 3 to 4 mm. This portion of the nerve rises superiorly and anteriorly from the fundus to curve posterior and lateral to the cochlea, lying less than 1 mm from the basal cochlear turn (3). This segment ends at the geniculate ganglion. As this is the narrowest portion of the bony canal, traumatic and inflammatory lesions associated with edema are likely to compress the nerve in this segment. The greater superficial petrosal nerve can be identified in this region.

4. The *tympanic segment* measures approximately 12 to 13 mm and traverses the middle ear in a posteroinferior direction between the lateral semicircular canal above and the oval window below. It can be identified in the middle ear by its relationship to Jacobson's nerve and the cochleariform process (4). The nerve can be located by tracing Jacobson's nerve superiorly toward the cochleariform process where the facial nerve lies immediately superior to the latter structure. Bony dehiscences in the fallopian canal occur with regularity, most commonly in the tympanic segment in the area of the oval window. Several developmental aberrations in the intratympanic course have been identified (5). The facial nerve has been described coursing superior to the lateral semicircular canal and through the arch of the superior semicircular canal. Aberrancies in the proximal nerve including bifurcation anterior to the oval window and direct vertical descent from the geniculate ganglion often occur in association with anomalies of the stapedial footplate.

5. The vertical segment or *mastoid segment* begins at the second genu and continues downward in the posterior tympanum a distance of 15 to 20 mm to its point of exit at the stylomastoid foramen. The nerve courses laterally in its descent and can often be identified lateral to the tympanic annulus in the lower half of its course through the mastoid (6). Aberrancies in the course of the facial nerve through the mastoid can occur (5). A more posteriorly placed second genu, bifurcation distal to the second genu, and an abnormal medial or lateral course have been identified. The chorda tympani nerve typically arises 5 mm proximal to the stylomastoid foramen (5). Its origin can vary substantially and can even be found extratemporally entering the mastoid through a separate canaliculus.

Extratemporal Facial Nerve

The extratemporal facial nerve in children younger than 2 years old is quite superficial and often immediately subcutaneous. As the squamous portion of the mastoid bone and the tympanic ring develop, the facial nerve gradually assumes its adult position.

The proximal extratemporal facial nerve can be identified superior to the posterior digastric belly, approximately 8 mm medially along the tympanomastoid suture line. Other useful landmarks include the tragal pointer and the posterior facial vein. The main trunk is approximately 1 cm anteroinferior and 1 cm medial to the pointer, and it always lies superficial to the posterior facial vein.

After leaving the stylomastoid foramen, the facial nerve sends motor branches to the posterior digastric, the stylohyoid, the auricular muscles, and the occipitalis. After traveling approximately 2 cm, the nerve bifurcates within the substance of the parotid gland at the *pes ansurinus*. Here, the temporofacial and the cervicofacial divisions are identifiable and give rise to the temporal, zygomatic, buccal, marginal mandibular, and cervical branches. There are a number of peripheral anastomoses, especially between the zygomatic and buccal branches (7). Within the substance of the parotid gland, the facial nerve is covered by two densely adherent layers of fascia: the parotid–masseteric and the superficial musculoaponeurotic system (SMAS) (8). Anterior to the parotid, overlying the masseter muscle, the nerve is covered only by the SMAS. All the muscles of facial expression are innervated from their deep surface except for the buccinator and mentalis muscles (9). Unlike its course inferior to the mandibular angle in the adult, the marginal mandibular division overlies the mandible in children and is subject to injury in this more vulnerable position.

🟦 PATIENT ASSESSMENT

All diagnosis begins with a careful history. The essentials of the history of the present illness in pediatric facial nerve dysfunction will depend on the age at onset and the circumstances surrounding the problem. History taking will be difficult in very young children, and associated symptoms may only be inferred from the child's behavior or from an observant parent.

When considering facial nerve dysfunction in children, it is helpful to classify the diseases affecting the nerve as congenital, infectious, inflammatory, neoplastic, and traumatic (Table 1). Each of these categories will have unique circumstances and symptoms surrounding their presentation. For example, as described in subsequent sections, congenital facial paralysis can be divided into developmental and traumatic subtypes. A maternal and family history will be most helpful for delineating the causes of developmental facial nerve dysfunction. Maternal illness or exposures and family history of developmental disorders may suggest the etiology of the facial nerve dysfunction. A detailed birth and perinatal history can help to diagnose a traumatic etiology for a congenital paralysis. For example, intrauterine trauma, prolonged labor, and forceps delivery may all be etiologic factors gleaned from a thorough history.

In the older child, a complete account of the symptoms can usually be obtained. A history of recent trauma to the head or face, or surgery of the brain or temporal bone will be easily elicited from the child and his/her parents. The onset, duration, and associated neurotologic symptoms must be ascertained at the time of history taking. A gradual onset over weeks to months associated with progressive dysfunction and facial twitching is suggestive of a neoplastic process affecting the facial nerve. A sudden onset with fever, otalgia, and otorrhea suggests an otogenic source. Associated neurootologic symptoms of dizziness, hearing loss, tinnitus, and vertigo suggest disease at the level of the inner ear or the CPA from either an infectious, inflammatory, or neoplastic process. After careful history taking, a likely etiologic classification can be made that is substantiated by a careful neurootologic examination.

In addition to a complete neurootologic examination, a detailed evaluation of the symmetry, distribution, and degree of facial nerve dysfunction must be recorded. Involvement of only the lower face, as described earlier, may suggest a central process affecting facial movement. This must not be confused with a peripheral lesion affecting only the lower division of the nerve. Similarly, weakness in all areas of innervation sug-

TABLE 1: Pediatric Facial Nerve Disorders

Congenital	Infectious	Inflammatory	Neoplastic	Traumatic
Acquired	Lyme disease	Kawasaki disease	*Benign*	Intratemporal
Forceps	Mononucleosis	Wegener's disease	Neuroma	Iatrogenic
Maternal pelvic or sacral pressure	Otitis media	Melkersson-Rosenthal syndrome	Hemangioma	Temporal bone fracture
Developmental	Ramsay Hunt syndrome		*Malignant*	Extratemporal
Oculo-auriculovertebral spectrum			Rhabdomyosarcoma	Iatrogenic
Möbius' syndrome	Bell's palsy	Chloroma	Laceration	
CULLP			Parotid tumors	

CULLP, congenital unilateral lower lip palsy.

TABLE 2: House-Brackmann Facial Nerve Grading Scale

Degree of Injury	Grade	Definition
Normal	I	Normal symmetric function in all areas
Mild dysfunction	II	Slight weakness noticable only on close inspection; complete eye closure with minimal effort; slight asymmetry of smile with maximal effort; synkinesis barely noticable; contracture or spasm absent
Moderate dysfunction	III	Obvious weakness but not disfiguring; may not be able to lift eyebrow; complete eye closure and strong but asymmetric mouth movement with maximal effort; obvious but not disfiguring synkinesis, mass movement, or spasm
Moderately severe dysfunction	IV	Obvious disfiguring weakness; inability to lift brown; incomplete eye closure and asymmetry of mouth with maximal effort; severe synkinesis, mass movement, or spasm
Severe dysfunction	V	Motion barely perceptible; incomplete eye closure, slight movement of corner of mouth; synkinesis, contracture, and spasm usually absent
Total paralysis	VI	No movement; loss of tone; no synkinesis, contracture, or spasm

gests a lesion at the level of the facial motor nucleus or more peripherally. The House-Brackmann scale provides a standardized method of assessment and reporting of patients with facial nerve dysfunction (10) (Table 2).

After thorough head and neck examination, attention must be directed to a careful neurologic examination. In addition to the cranial nerves, peripheral motor and sensory function, as well as cerebellar, testing may aid in determination of the site of the lesion. Lesions of the facial nucleus without other sequelae of lower brainstem dysfunction are extremely rare. Lesions of the posterior cranial fossa or CPA affect the mid- and lower cranial nerves and cerebellum, much of which can be delineated by careful examination.

Further laboratory, radiographic, and physiologic testing is tailored to the findings in the history and physical examination. Each of the sections that follow will describe the additional studies needed to assist in diagnostic evaluation.

NEUROPHYSIOLOGY OF FACIAL NERVE INJURY

Sunderland (11) provided a classification scheme for injury based on the microanatomy of the facial nerve (Fig. 3 and Table 3). Peripheral nerves, such as the facial nerve, typically have a layered architecture (Fig. 4). Each axon is surrounded by a lipid membrane called the axolemma. Surrounding the axolemma of the facial nerve is a myelin sheath, which is a spiraled lipid layer of the overlying Schwann cell's membrane. Each fiber is encased within a fibrous sheath called the endoneurium. Multiple fibers arranged in fascicles are compartmentalized by the perineurium. The entire group of fascicles is ensheathed in epineurium, completing the formation of the peripheral nerve. The motor fibers of the facial nerve, unlike somatic peripheral motor nerves, undergo a transition in the CPA from a central nerve with myelin derived from oligodendroglia, to a peripheral myelinated nerve, with a sheath derived from Schwann cells. This region, called the Obersteiner-Redlich zone, possesses a tenuous blood supply and is considered one of the critical areas for potential injury during CPA surgery (12).

According to Sunderland's classification, there are five degrees of facial nerve injury. First-degree injury, also called *neuropraxia*, occurs most commonly from a traumatic or inflammatory compression injury resulting in the inability to conduct an action potential

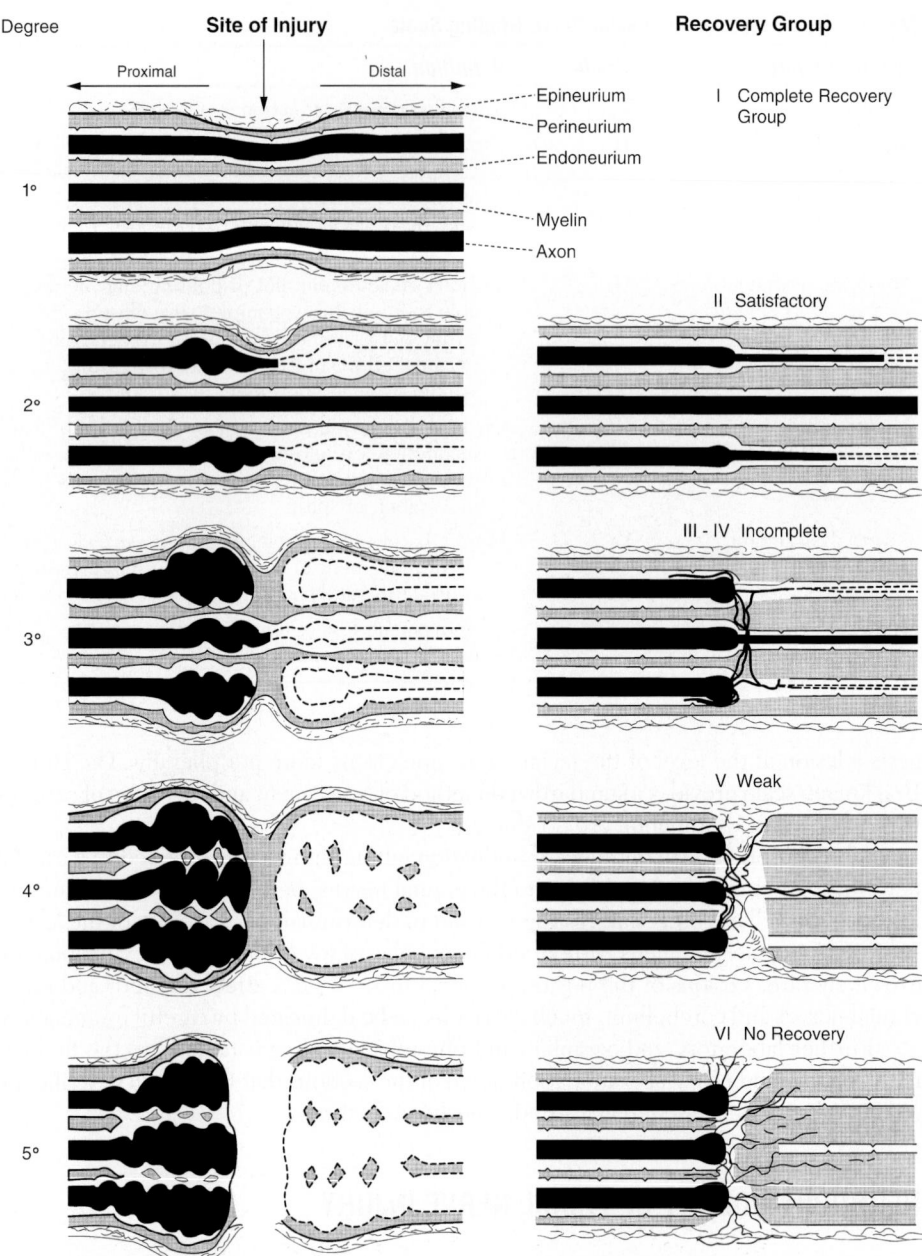

FIGURE 3 Relationship of degree of injury to its microanatomy and prognosis (Adapted from ref. 63, with permission.)

across the site of injury. This type of injury does not result in antegrade axonal degeneration (wallerian degeneration) and will conduct an electrical stimulus distal to the site of injury. First-degree injuries generally have excellent prognoses with return of function within days to weeks and few if any permanent sequelae.

Second-degree injury, *axontemesis*, results from traumatic or inflammatory compression of the nerve to such a degree that wallerian degeneration occurs. These injuries respond to an electrical stimulus distal to the injury for up to 3 to 5 days. After that time, wallerian degeneration results in axonal loss, and the nerve will no longer stimulate distally. This type of injury has a favorable prognosis, although the time course of recovery is more protracted than that of a first-degree injury. The endoneurial tubules are preserved; hence, the ultimate outcome is similar to that in neuropraxic injuries.

Third-, fourth-, and fifth-degree injuries all involve the perineural connective tissue to some degree, and all are considered forms of *neurotmesis*. A third-degree injury results in disruption of the endoneurium. As a result of disruption of the endoneurial

TABLE 3: Neuropathology and Spontaneous Recovery Correlated with Degree of Facial Nerve Injury

Degree of Injury	Pathology of Injury	EEMG Response	Neurobiology of Recovery	Clinical Recovery Begins	Spontaneous Recovery (Result 1 Year Postinjury)[a]
1°	Compression; damming of axoplasm; no morphologic changes (neurapraxia)	Normal	No morphologic changes noted	1–4 weeks	Grade I—complete: without evidence of faulty regeneration
2°	Compression persists; increased intraneural pressure; loss of axons, but endoneurial tubes remain intact (axonotmesis)	25% of normal	Axons grow into intact empty myelin tubes at a rate of 1 mm/day, which accounts for longer period for recovery in 2° injuries compared with 1°; less than complete recovery is due to some fibers with 3° injury	1–2 months	Grade II—fair: some noticable difference with volitional or spontaneous movement; minimal evidence of faulty regeneration
3°	Intraneural pressure increases; loss of myelin tubes (neurotmesis)	0–10% normal	With loss of myelin tubes, new axons have opportunity to get mixed up and split, causing mouth movement with eye closure (synkinesis)	2–4 months	Grade III–IV—moderate to poor; obvious incomplete recovery to crippling deformity, with moderate to marked complications of faulty regeneration
4°	Above, plus disruption of perineurium (partial transection)	No response	In addition to problems caused by 2° and 3° injuries, the axons are blocked by scarring, which impairs regeneration	4–18 months	Grade V—motion barely perceptible
5°	Above, plus disruption of epineurium (complete transection)	No response	Complete disruption with a scar-filled gap presents insurmountable barrier to regrowth of axons and neuromuscular reanastomosis	Never	Grade VI—none

[a]Classification by grades I–IV modified from ref. 10.

EEMG, evoked electromyography.

(From ref. 63, with permission.)

tubules, regenerating axons may enter and travel down aberrant pathways, resulting in abnormal patterns of reinnervation. This aberrant reinnervation results in mass movement or *synkinesis*. Although third-degree injuries will often regenerate spontaneously, the time course to recovery can be several months to a year, and the outcome is often only satisfactory. Fourth-degree injuries result in disruption of the perineurium surrounding bundles of nerve fibers. Fifth-degree injuries are complete transections of the nerve including the epineurium. These latter two degrees of injury most often require surgical repair for any hope of recovery.

PROGNOSTIC TESTING

Topognostic testing of the fibers of the nervus intermedius has not proved to be accurate either in site of lesion testing or prognostication (13). Electrical testing of the facial nerve, although controversial, has been shown to provide prognostic information and can aid in the management of a variety of facial nerve disorders.

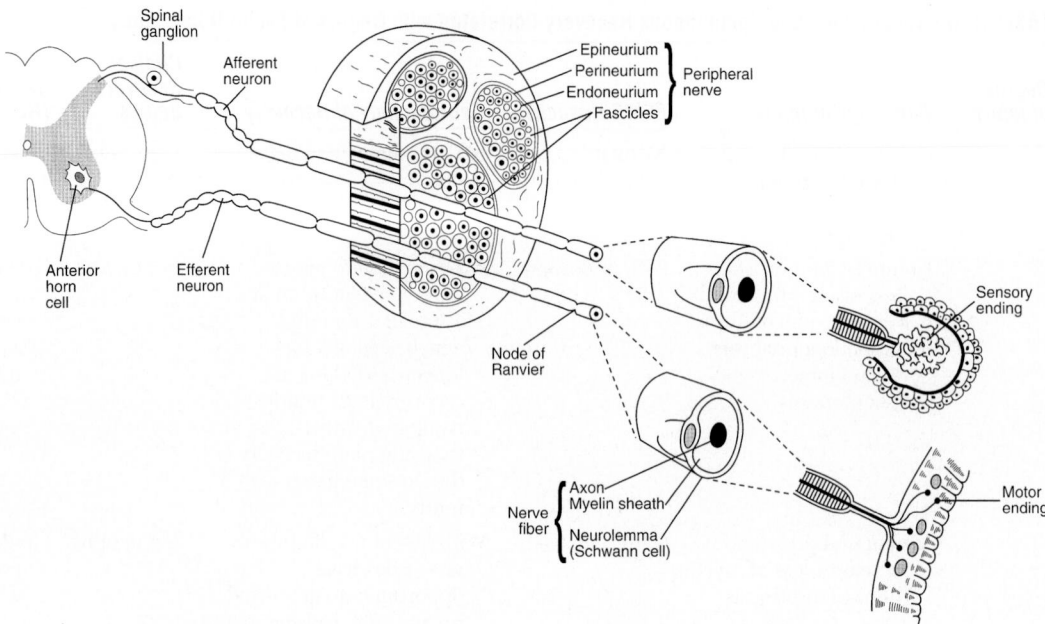

FIGURE 4 Microanatomy of a peripheral nerve. (Adapted from ref. 76, with permission.)

The nerve excitability test (NET), maximal stimulation test (MST), electroneurography (ENOG), and electromyography (EMG) are the most commonly utilized electrophysiologic tests in patients with facial nerve disorders. There are several limitations to electrodiagnostic testing. The NET, MST, and ENOG may be falsely positive for 72 to 96 hours postinjury, until wallerian degeneration has occurred. Furthermore, denervated muscle may be electrically silent on EMG early in the course of disease, but detection of fibrillation and polyphasic reinnervation potentials, elements essential to predicting outcome, do not appear for 10 to 14 days after injury. These tests are associated with some patient discomfort and may require sedation when performed on children. Despite these limitations, electrodiagnostic tests have demonstrated utility in the pediatric population (14).

Nerve Excitability Test

The NET assesses the difference in threshold for excitability of the diseased facial nerve compared with the normal side. Using a Hilger nerve stimulator with bipolar electrodes, the facial nerve branches are stimulated first on the normal side and then on the involved side. An excitability threshold difference of greater than 3.5 mA is considered significant and indicates a more severe degree of injury with a poorer prognosis for recovery (15).

Maximal Stimulation Test

This test is similar to the NET in its use of the Hilger stimulator and its subjective comparison of the normal with the involved side. It differs in that it utilizes maximal stimulation (5 mA) and assesses the extent of facial motion to stimulation. The maximally stimulated motion is described as equal, diminished, or absent in comparison with the normal side. Results of the MST have been found to be more reliable than those of NET (15). First-degree injuries demonstrate normal symmetry. More extensive injuries, depending on the number of fibers involved, demonstrate varying degrees of reduced motion. Analysis of the MST demonstrated that when the response was equal, 12% of the patients had incomplete recovery compared with 73% when the response was diminished (15).

Electroneurography

ENOG is a measure of the evoked compound action potential (CAP) generated by maximal stimulation of the facial nerve at the stylomastoid foramen and measured peripherally at the nasolabial fold. Individual peripheral branches can also be tested. Popularized by Fisch and Esslen, this test provides a quantitative measure of the difference in amplitude of the CAP between the normal and the involved sides of the face. The degree of amplitude reduction correlates with the number of degenerated facial nerve fibers. The degree and rate of degeneration provide prognostic information and it is for this reason that serial ENOG is recommended (16).

Fisch (16) has established guidelines for surgical management of facial nerve disorders based on the degree and time course of degeneration. Facial nerve exploration and decompression for traumatic injuries and weakness associated with acute otitis media without resolution with conservative treatment is recommended for patients with greater than 90% CAP amplitude reduction within 6 days. For patients with Bell's palsy and greater than 90% amplitude reduction within 2 weeks, surgical decompression is felt to result in more rapid recovery and fewer long-term sequelae (16).

Despite its usefulness as a guide to therapy, ENOG has potential pitfalls. There is often tremendous variability on ENOG testing: Control patients with normal facial function bilaterally may demonstrate as much as 25% amplitude reduction. The variability probably stems from technical problems including electrode placement, pressure, skin resistance, and stimulating current (17). There are clinical situations in which the CAP will be absent or diminished, suggesting a poor prognosis despite ongoing regeneration or even clinically evident function. This phenomenon, called desynchronization, is due to the regeneration of nerve fibers with differing impulse velocities, precluding the measurement of a CAP (17). ENOG, in conjunction with EMG, is helpful in sorting out these patients as they will probably demonstrate motor unit potentials or polyphasic reinnervation potentials, as described below.

Electromyography

EMG, used for many years as a diagnostic aid in neuromuscular diseases, provides useful prognostic information in disorders of the facial nerve as well. A completely denervated muscle is electrically silent early on in the disease process. After 2 to 3 weeks, the denervated facial muscle will demonstrate fibrillation potentials and no voluntary motor unit potentials. By contrast, cases of incomplete or resolving injury will demonstrate voluntary motor unit potentials and/or polyphasic potentials characteristic of reinnervation. These findings would obviate the need for surgical intervention and suggest a good prognosis for recovery of function. Additionally, patients with desynchronization will demonstrate motor unit potentials on EMG clarifying the abnormal ENOG. The limitation of this technique is the time required for these potentials to become manifest.

CONGENITAL FACIAL PARALYSIS

Congenital facial paralysis has an incidence of 0.23% to 7% of live births (18–22). These patients can be broadly grouped into two categories: traumatic and developmental (Table 1). Traumatic injuries are felt to result from delivery, but intrauterine positioning may play a role in the pathogenesis (20,22,23,24). Developmental facial nerve anomalies imply failed embryogenesis due to either teratogens, genetic defects, or a combination. Distinguishing these two entities has significant prognostic and therapeutic implications. For example, traumatic facial nerve dysfunction has an excellent prognosis for spontaneous recovery, whereas developmental anomalies by definition are unlikely to resolve (18). Furthermore, some traumatic injuries require immediate surgical intervention, whereas the management of developmental facial nerve dysfunction can be undertaken in a nonemergency fashion.

These two entities can often be distinguished by careful history taking, physical examination, and the results of electrophysiologic and radiographic studies (18,25). A history of maternal illness, a familial disorder, or teratogen exposure would support a developmental anomaly. By contrast, a difficult labor in a primipara would support a traumatic etiology. Physical examination can corroborate the history. Associated developmental anomalies, including other cranial neuropathies, cardiopulmonary defects, or craniofacial abnormalities, would suggest a developmental process; severe cranial molding, forceps impressions, or surrounding ecchymoses are consistent with trauma.

High-resolution computed tomography (CT) scans of the temporal bone may aid in the diagnosis by demonstrating injuries to the facial nerve, or developmental anomalies of the otic capsule and second branchial arch structures. Early electrodiagnostic testing can provide important information about the etiology of congenital paralysis. Facial nerve conduction studies are typically abnormal in the first few days of life in children with developmental dysfunction, in contrast to traumatic paralyses (18,25). The differentiation may be obscured in intrauterine compression as these children may demonstrate abnormal electrophysiology, incorrectly suggesting a developmental basis. Finally, auditory brainstem evoked response may assist in determining the etiology of congenital facial paralysis (25). Abnormalities of interwave latencies and the relative amplitudes of waves I and V have been demonstrated in some patients with developmental anomalies (18).

Birth Trauma

There is much debate in the literature about the mechanisms underlying acquired congenital facial paralysis. One large study concluded that forceps did not contribute to a greater incidence of paralysis and that the causative factor was pressure on the nerve from the mother's sacral prominence during labor (24). Several recent reports identify forceps delivery as a causative factor in facial nerve compressive injuries (22,23).

Conservative management of traumatic injuries to the facial nerve in the newborn is warranted as the prognosis for complete recovery is excellent. Surgical management is indicated when the paralysis is immediate and complete, is associated with radiographic evidence of nerve impingement or transection, and demonstrates electrophysiologic evidence of significant degeneration on ENOG (more than 90% CAP amplitude reduction) within 6 days of injury (16).

Developmental Factors

A developmental etiology for congenital facial paralysis should be suspected in children with other identifiable developmental anomalies. The most common associated malformations are those of the maxilla including clefts of the palate and hypoplasia of the maxilla (18,26). Malformations of the pinna, microtias, are occasionally associated with facial nerve dysfunction (26).

The vast majority of developmental facial palsies are associated with the oculo-auriculo-vertebral spectrum (Goldenhar's syndrome and hemifacial microsomia), Möbius' syndrome, and congenital unilateral lower lip palsy (CULLP). The oculo-auriculo-vertebral spectrum is a heterogenous disorder characterized by varying degrees of facial asymmetry including maxillary and mandibular hypoplasia, microtia, and vertebral anomalies (27). Other manifestations of the disease include blepharoptosis, epibulbar dermoids, central nervous system anomalies, and cardiac, pulmonary, and gastrointestinal developmental abnormalities. Approximately 10% to 20% of affected children display involvement of the facial nerve. Although these phenotypic abnormalities have been noted in families and children of diabetic mothers and mothers exposed to teratogens, the mechanisms underlying the abnormal development are unknown.

Möbius' syndrome, in its classic form, consists of facial diplegia and bilateral abducens nerve palsy (27). The manifestations are variable, and the facial nerve dysfunction can be unilateral without other cranial neuropathies (25). The mechanisms involved are controversial. Brainstem developmental defects, muscular hypoplasia, and a combination of these have been reported in affected individuals (28). Thalidomide exposure has been associated with a Möbius phenotype. Complete paralysis is rare in this disorder.

CULLP, also known as the asymmetric crying face, is a focal weakness of the lower lip depressors (29). This abnormality is felt to arise from a deficiency of the depressor anguli oris muscle in association with a brainstem abnormality (25). This disorder can occur in isolation, but it is frequently associated with other developmental anomalies. A strong association with cardiac developmental abnormalities has been described, and the disorder has been termed the *cardiofacial syndrome* (29).

Fortunately, most developmental facial nerve disorders are segmental and incomplete. Congenital paralyses associated with nerve or muscle agenesis or brainstem defects may be rehabilitated with microneurovascular free muscle transfer (30). This procedure is often two-staged and involves cross-facial nerve grafting utilizing the sural nerve, followed by free muscle transfer, usually the gracilis muscle, after nerve ingrowth to the involved side. Early success has been observed in one-half to two-thirds of patients treated in this fashion (30).

INFECTIOUS DISEASES

Lyme Disease

Lyme disease is the most prevalent tick-borne illness in the United States. It is caused by the spirochete *Borrelia burgdorferi*, which is transmitted by the bite of a tick in the *Ixodes ricinus* complex. This disease was first reported in the United States in 1977 when a small epidemic of juvenile arthritides occurred in the town of Lyme, Connecticut.

Much like another spirochetal illness, syphilis, Lyme disease occurs in three stages. The first stage, occurring within days to weeks of the tick bite, is heralded by the appearance of a characteristic rash, erythema chronicum migrans. The rash is characterized by a migrating pattern with central clearing.

In the second stage, meningoencephalitis, cardiac conduction defects, and polyneuropathies become manifest. Unilateral or bilateral facial nerve paralysis has been reported in 10% to 60% of cases of Lyme disease associated with meningoencephalitis (31). Facial nerve involvement in Lyme disease can occur without meningoencephalitis and in some instances may be the only alerting sign of the disease, presenting prior to or in the absence of a skin rash (31). The third stage is similar to the tertiary stage of syphilis and includes neuropsychiatric disorders and encephalopathy.

Although the paralysis is usually unilateral, Lyme disease is felt to be the most common cause of bilateral facial paralysis (31). There is evidence that bilateral involvement is more common in children and occurs more often in boys (31,32).

The mechanism of facial nerve dysfunction is unclear. As with Bell's palsy, there is speculation about direct infection of the nerve versus inflammatory edema and compressive neuropathy. Like Bell's palsy, facial nerve dysfunction in Lyme disease is not always complete. Sixty percent of patients in one series had complete paralysis (31). Unlike Bell's palsy, the facial nerve dysfunction in Lyme disease is more often bilateral and displays a more rapid and complete rate of recovery. Well over 90% of patients obtain good recovery (House grade I or II). Patients with bilateral involvement appear to be at greater risk of delayed and incomplete recovery.

The diagnosis of Lyme disease can be corroborated by laboratory evaluation. Indirect immunofluorescence detection of serum immunoglobulin M (IgM) and immunoglobulin G (IgG) antibodies to the organism can be helpful, although they do not correlate with disease severity. Elevated antibody titers in the cerebrospinal fluid of affected patients, primarily those with signs and symptoms of meningoencephalitis, can be helpful in the diagnosis.

The mainstay of treatment for Lyme disease is systemic antibiotics. Tetracycline and, in children, amoxicillin have demonstrated efficacy in the prevention of progression of disease. Neither antibiotics nor steroids have demonstrated significant benefit for facial nerve outcomes, as all patients have excellent prognoses. At present, there does not appear to be a role for surgery in the treatment of this disease. In summary, Lyme borreliosis must be suspected in any child with unilateral, and especially bilateral, facial nerve dysfunction presenting in the summer months and associated with a tick bite or rash. It must be kept in mind that it is probably etiologic in many cases without associated symptoms and signs (33).

Infectious Mononucleosis

Infectious mononucleosis, caused by the Epstein-Barr virus, a member of the herpesvirus family, is characterized most commonly by pharyngotonsillitis and cervical lymphadenopathy. Infectious mononucleosis is a systemic disease with the potential for widespread manifestations. Neurologic manifestations, although uncommon, do occur. These manifestations include lymphocytic meningitis, encephelomyelitis, polyneuritis, and mononeuritis. Unilateral and bilateral facial nerve paralysis has been infrequently reported. Infectious mononucleosis associated with a granulomatous mastoiditis and facial nerve paralysis has been reported (34).

In most cases the mechanism of facial nerve dysfunction is unknown. The course of the disease is similar to that of Bell's palsy, with complete resolution in most patients. The diagnosis is suggested by atypical lymphocytes in the peripheral blood and the demonstration of heterophile antibodies in the serum. Patients under the age of 10 years frequently demonstrate false-negative results when tested for heterophile antibodies, and the diagnosis in this group rests on clinical suspicion. As few reports exist in the literature on the treatment of facial paralysis in infectious mononucleosis, and the prognosis for good return of function is favorable, management of potential complications is all that is recommended.

Otitis Media

Acute and chronic otitis media are associated with facial nerve paralysis. Acute otitis media is more often associated with facial nerve paralysis in young children. Older children and adults are more at risk for facial nerve dysfunction as a complication of chronic otitis media.

Facial nerve involvement by acute infection of the middle ear does not only occur with coalescent mastoiditis. The facial nerve is often dehiscent in the area of the oval window and is vulnerable to the acute inflammatory process. If is felt that the nerve is subjected to venous stasis and inflammatory edema, which lead to compression within the bony confines of the fallopian canal. By contrast, facial nerve dysfunction in chronic disease most often results from direct invasion by cholesteatoma or granulation tissue.

The different mechanisms proposed for facial nerve dysfunction in acute and chronic otitis media dictate different methods of management. As the cause of facial paralysis in acute infection is felt to be inflammatory edema, initial management consists of wide myringotomy and paracentesis for culture, followed by the institution of antibiotics on an empiric basis until specific organisms have been identified. Intravenous antibiotic coverage for pneumococcus, *Hemophilus influenzae*, and *Moraxella catarrhalis*, such as an augmented penicillin or second-generation cephalosporin would be sufficient. The vast majority of children improve with this approach. Children failing to improve and demonstrating progressive denervation on ENOG (more than 90% decrease in CAP) should undergo mastoidectomy and facial nerve decompression.

Facial nerve dysfunction in chronic otitis media, resulting from direct compression or invasion by cholesteatoma and/or granulation tissue, requires surgery. Treatment consists of tympanomastoidectomy with facial nerve decompression. It is generally recommended that the sheath of of the nerve not be opened. Deeply invasive granulation tissue or cholesteatoma present difficult management problems. Open cavity techniques with exteriolazation of disease provide an option, especially in extensively invasive cholesteatoma, which might otherwise require facial nerve resection and grafting.

Herpes Zoster

Herpes zoster oticus (Ramsay Hunt syndrome) is an unusual cause of facial paralysis in children. The patients typically present with otalgia and unilateral facial weakness. This disease, unlike Bell's palsy, is often a polyneuritis, and patients may present with other complaints including facial hypesthesias, hearing loss, tinnitus, dizziness, and dysphagia. Grouped vesicles on an erythematous base often appear early in the disease and are usually found on the concha or posterosuperior canal wall. Vesicles can also appear on the soft palate and in the oral cavity.

The diagnosis is largely based on clinical presentation. A Tzanck smear of virally infected cells taken from a vesicle may show characteristic intranuclear inclusions. Neurootologic evaluation including pure tone and speech audiometry and ENOG may be helpful in establishing baseline deficits and in deciding on appropriate rehabilitation. Although enhancement of the facial nerve on magnetic resonance imaging (MRI) has been demonstrated in many patients with Ramsay Hunt syndrome, it is of unknown significance. Therefore, the routine imaging of affected patients is not recommended.

The facial nerve dysfunction in this patient population is often of rapid onset and severe in degree. In general, the prognosis for complete recovery is poorer than in patients with Bell's palsy. Medical management of this disease with acyclovir has demonstrated promising results. Intravenous acyclovir at a dose of 10 mg/kg every 8 hours has been associated with diminished viral replication and shedding, as well as more favorable return of facial nerve function (35).

Bell's Palsy

Bell's palsy, the most commonly diagnosed form of facial palsy in children, is a diagnosis of exclusion. Although described as idiopathic for many years, many feel that this is a viral neuropathy induced by reactivation of latent herpes simplex virus (HSV). In a recent study employing molecular biologic techniques, HSV type 1 DNA was identified in the endoneurial fluid of 79% of patients with Bell's palsy (36). The mechanism of injury to the facial nerve is the subject of debate. Inflammatory edema with compression of the nerve at the meatal foramen is one purported pathophysiologic mechanism (37). In support of this theory, the meatal foramen is the narrowest portion of the fallopian canal, and a region of tenous blood supply to the facial nerve. Virally induced neuritis with autoimmune demyelination is another proposed mechanism (38). Supporting this view is histopathologic evidence of lymphocytic infiltration of the entire nerve associated with degeneration of the myelin sheath (39).

Bell's palsy can be recurrent in up to 15% of patients, lending further support to the latent viral reactivation hypothesis. Its association in families, and with diabetes mellitus, suggests the possibility of other pathophysiologic mechanisms (40). A spectrum of neural injury occurs in this disease, from neuropraxia to axonotemesis, with its attendant wallerian degeneration.

Patients typically present with an abrupt onset of unilateral facial weakness occurring over 1 to 2 days, often associated with a recent viral illness (38). Many patients report retroauricular pain and hyperacusis. The facial paresis can progress to paralysis over 1 to 7 days. The physical examination demonstrates unilateral weakness and no other cranial neuropathies. The presence of polyneuropathy suggests a diagnosis other than Bell's palsy. Confirmation of this diagnosis rests on a thorough search for known causes of facial nerve dysfunction including complete neurootologic examination and bimanual palpation of the ipsilateral parotid gland.

The diagnostic evaluation for patients with Bell's palsy is largely electrophysiologic. Audiometry and vestibular testing are reserved for patients with symptoms and by definition suggest a diagnosis other than Bell's palsy. As in Ramsey Hunt syndrome, facial nerve enhancement on MRI scan has been detected in some patients with Bell's palsy, often lasting for weeks after the return of function. The MRI findings do not provide prognostic information, and routine scanning of patients with Bell's palsy is not recommended.

The natural history of Bell's palsy is quite favorable. Approximately 85% of patients will experience good recovery (House grade I or II) regardless of therapy. The other 15% of patients will usually have some return of function within 6 months, but this will be complicated by synkinesis or spasm (41).

Electrodiagnostic testing is an essential element in the management of Bell's palsy, providing prognostic information and guiding therapy. ENOG and EMG are the primary testing modalities. These tests are not performed until 48 to 72 hours after the onset of paralysis and are not employed in patients with paresis. Patients with paresis only can generally be assured of complete functional return. As stated previously, the time course and degree of dysfunction identified on serial ENOG provide significant prognostic information. Patients with a rapid and complete paralysis are at risk for incomplete recovery with synkinesis (16) (Fig. 5). Patients demonstrating greater than 90% reduction in the CAP amplitude within 2 weeks have only a 50% chance of complete recovery.

As opinions regarding the etiology of Bell's palsy vary, so do opinions regarding its management. Patients seen within the first 10 days with paresis are placed on a 2-week tapering dose of prednisone beginning with a dose of 1 mg per kilogram. These patients are followed up within 5 days and only undergo electrical testing if they have progressed to complete paralysis. Those presenting with paresis after the tenth day are reassured of a favorable prognosis and followed up after several months.

Patients presenting with paralysis within 3 days of onset are placed on prednisone and undergo serial electrodiagnostic testing after the third day. Those presenting after 3 days but less than 2 weeks with complete paralysis undergo immediate testing. Patients presenting after 2 weeks can undergo EMG testing for prognostic purposes. Patients with complete paralysis who demonstrate less than 90% degeneration on ENOG are treated with prednisone and observed. Those patients demonstrating greater than 90%

FIGURE 5 Prognosis for facial nerve recovery. (Adapted from ref. 63, with permission.)

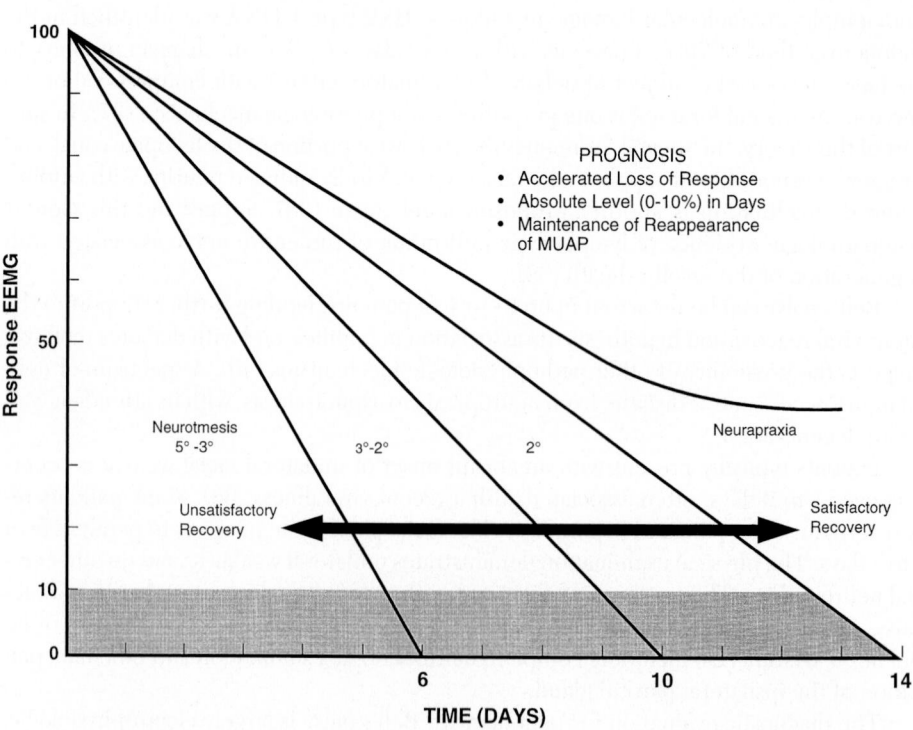

degeneration on ENOG within 2 weeks and no evidence of voluntary potentials on EMG are treated with prednisone and counseled about the option for surgery. The procedure consists of a middle cranial fossa decompression of the facial nerve from the meatal foramen to just beyond the geniculate ganglion. The medical and surgical management of Bell's palsy suffers from a paucity of well-controlled studies. There is literature supporting and refuting a beneficial effect of steroids on the natural history of Bell's palsy (42). There is also ample debate in the literature on the effects of surgery on the natural history of Bell's palsy (15,42). Until concrete conclusions are reached by well-controlled studies, the patient and parents must be well informed of the issues, and therapeutic decisions must be made in a cooperative manner.

INFLAMMATORY DISEASES

Kawasaki Disease

There are a variety of inflammatory lesions that primarily affect the temporal bone and its structures, including the facial nerve. Kawasaki disease, an idiopathic inflammatory disease of children, is most commonly associated with high fevers, injection and desquamation of the oral cavity epithelium and conjunctiva, cervical adenitis, erythema and desquamation of the extremities, and coronary arteritis with aneurysm formation. Like other vasculitides, this disorder is rarely associated with mononeuropathies including facial paralysis (43). The facial nerve dysfunction typically resolves with treatment of the primary disease with aspirin.

Wegener's Granulomatosis

Wegener's granulomatosis, another idiopathic inflammatory disease, is occasionally seen in children. This disease is characterized by necrotizing vasculitis of the upper and lower respiratory tract and necrotizing glomerulonephritis. Involvement of the temporal bone most commonly manifests as a serous otitis media with an associated conductive hearing loss. Facial nerve palsy has been reported to occur in approximately 3% of affected patients (44). Treatment of this disease often includes cyclophosphamide and prednisone. Successful management of patients with limited Wegener's disease has been reported with the use of trimethoprim/sulfamethoxazole (45).

Melkersson-Rosenthal Syndrome

Melkersson-Rosenthal syndrome is also known as orofacial granulomatosis. This clinical entity is defined by recurrent or persistent orofacial swelling, tongue plication, and facial nerve paralysis (46). Most patients manifest facial swelling in two or more locations, with the lips and buccal mucosa most frequently involved. Recurring unilateral or bilateral facial paralysis is found in approximately 20% of patients (46). Histopathologic findings include inflammatory infiltrates, perivascular monocytic infiltration, and noncaseating epithelioid granulomas with multinucleated Langhans' type giant cells. Although the vast majority of patients with facial weakness recover, there is some evidence in the literature supporting middle fossa–transmastoid total facial nerve decompression for the prevention of recurrence (47).

TUMORS

Approximately 5% cases of facial paralysis in children are associated with a neoplasm (48). A variety of lesions, both intrinsic and extrinsic, can involve the facial nerve from the CPA to the periphery. Tumors affecting facial nerve function should be suspected in

TABLE 4: Factors Suggesting Facial Nerve Tumor

Recurrence	Progression	Duration	Associated symptoms
Ipsilateral	Beyond 3–4 weeks	Paralysis beyond 6 months	Twitching Other cranial neuropathies Long tract sign

patients with facial paralysis that does not resolve after 6 months, facial paralysis that continues to progress beyond 3 weeks, recurrent ipsilateral paralysis, facial twitching, and paralysis associated other cranial neuropathies or long tract signs (Table 4) (48). Rapidly progressive facial paralysis in the presence of a CPA lesion is highly suggestive of a malignancy (49).

The two most common tumors of the facial nerve in children are facial neuromas and hemangiomas. The presentation of these tumors is often nonspecific. Tumors involving the nerve within the internal auditory canal often present with hearing loss and are easily confused with acoustic neuromas. Tumors presenting in the middle ear may be associated with conductive hearing loss. Patients with facial neuromas do not necessarily present with facial weakness (50). By contrast, hemangiomas of the facial nerve, which have a predilection for the geniculate region, often present with early facial nerve paresis (51).

The diagnosis can be clarified with imaging. Facial neuromas of the internal auditory canal cannot be distinguished from acoustic neuromas on MRI, and the diagnosis can only be made at operation. Facial neuromas of the tympanic segment often demonstrate a "beads on a string" appearance with remodeling of the fallopian canal. Facial nerve hemangiomas enhance much the same as neuromas on T_1-weighted gadolinium-enhanced MRI. High-resolution CT scanning may demonstrate the characteristic "honeycomb" appearance of hemangiomas due to the frequent intratumoral calcifications (52).

The management of these benign lesions of the facial nerve can be difficult. In general, resection of the tumor with either primary anastomosis or cable grafting results in a House grade III or IV functional outcome. Children with normal facial function and only mild degrees of hearing loss can be followed with the knowledge that progressive hearing loss is likely. In children presenting with facial nerve dysfunction, a surgical approach is recommended, particularly when significant dysfunction is evidenced on examination and electrical testing (CAP less than 50%) (53). Prolonged delay of resection after the onset of facial nerve paresis is associated with poorer postoperative facial nerve function (50).

The surgical approach to tumor resection is dictated by the location of the tumor and the degree of hearing loss. Small tumors in the region of the geniculate ganglion in patients with good hearing can be most easily approached through the middle cranial fossa. Larger tumors with extension into the internal auditory canal and posterior fossa, in the face of poor hearing, can most easily be managed through the translabyrinthine approach. After tumor resection, the facial nerve is repaired either by rerouting and primary anastomosis, or by interposition grafting utilizing the greater auricular or sural nerves (54).

Malignant lesions of the temporal bone are uncommon in children. Rhabdomyosarcoma, the most common sarcoma of the head and neck in children, does occur in the temporal bone and is associated with facial nerve paralysis (55). Childhood leukemias (chloromas) can infiltrate or compress the facial nerve in the temporal bone (56). Parotid malignancies must also be considered in the differential diagnosis of lesions associated with facial paralysis. Mucoepidermoid carcinoma, the most common malignancy of the parotid gland in children, is associated with facial nerve paralysis secondary to direct infiltration (57). Rhabdomyosarcoma and chloroma are often treated with chemotherapy, radiation therapy, or a combination. Surgery is reserved for tissue diagnosis. Parotid malignancies are managed surgically with postoperative radiation therapy when indicated. Facial nerve resection is recommended when frank invasion is noted intraoperatively. Immediate repair with interposition grafting is successful even in cases undergoing postoperative radiotherapy (58).

TRAUMATIC INJURIES OF THE INTRATEMPORAL FACIAL NERVE

Iatrogenic Injuries

A multitude of diseases of the head and neck can affect the facial nerve either directly or indirectly. Many factors unique to the facial nerve, including its long and occasionally variable course, its limited blood supply, and its intimate relationship to a variety of structures in the head and neck, place it at risk for postoperative dysfunction. Lesions of the CPA in children, most commonly acoustic neuromas, are often intimately related to the facial nerve in the internal auditory canal. Larger tumors often displace and attenuate the nerve, making postoperative dysfunction unavoidable.

The intratemporal facial nerve is at risk of injury during otologic surgery. Although the facial nerve has a typical course through the temporal bone, areas of natural or disease-induced dehiscence or extensive infectious or neoplastic disease of the middle ear and mastoid may place the nerve at significant risk for injury. Congenital anomalies of the tubotympanum, such as aural atresias, are often associated with aberrancies in the course of the facial nerve.

Injury to the facial nerve in otologic surgery occurs most commonly in the tympanic segment (59). Several key landmarks in this region may help to orient the surgeon in extensively diseased ears. For example, as described previously, identification of the horizontal semicircular canal and the oval window niche provide significant information about the course of the facial nerve near the second genu. More proximally, the cochleariform process, the semicanal of the tensor tympani, and the course of Jacobson's nerve all provide useful clues as to the position of the fallopian canal in the protympanum and epitympanum (4).

Although early studies on the timing of facial nerve repair suggested waiting 21 days for optimal recovery of the nerve cell body, recent data reveal no detrimental effect of immediate repair (60,61). Disruption of the facial nerve in the CPA during tumor removal should be repaired intraoperatively. Nerve injury during translabyrinthine surgery can most easily be repaired by nerve rerouting and either direct anastomosis or interposition grafting (54). The nerve endings should be trimmed back atraumatically, and the closure must be tension free. There is no demonstrable difference between epineurial and perineurial anastomoses. However, these anastomoses should be performed with the minimally required number of 9.0 or 10.0 monofilament nylon sutures under the operating microscope. Nerve injury during the middle fossa approach often requires juxtaposing the severed ends within the fallopian canal. The anastomosis can be reinforced with fibrin glue or microfibrillar collagen (Avetin). Repair of injuries to the facial nerve within the internal auditory canal through the middle cranial fossa can be challenging and often one is only able to juxtapose the severed nerve and support the anastomosis with a bed of microfibrillar collagen (Avetin).

Repair of facial nerve injuries during tympanomastoid surgery should also be undertaken at the time of operation. Nerve repair by direct anastamosis or interposition grafting has been recommended for injuries of 50% or more of the nerve's diameter (60). The severity of these injuries is often difficult to assess completely during surgery and is often more extensive than it appears. Failure to identify these significant injuries leads to poor long-term facial recovery, whereas early identification and repair often leads to satisfactory results (House grade III to IV) (59).

The best results for primary repair or interposition grafting have been noted when they are performed within 30 days. Primary anastamosis and interposition grafting should not be performed beyond 1 year (48). After 1 year and prior to 2 years, hypoglossal–facial anastamosis or hypoglossal–facial jump grafting provides useful rehabilitation (62). Patients with complete paralyses seen beyond the 2-year period can be rehabilitated with temporalis muscle transfer (63).

Temporal Bone Fractures

In a review of facial palsy after head injury, Potter (64) found a 1% incidence of facial nerve injury in 2,712 cases. Virtually all the cases of facial nerve palsy were associated with skull base fractures. The incidence of facial nerve injury in children, like the incidence of temporal bone fracture in general, is highest in the younger age group. Facial nerve paralysis in adults is seen in 10% to 18% of longitudinal fractures and 30% to 50% of transverse fractures (65). The incidence of facial nerve injury in pediatric temporal bone trauma is lower than that of adults, occurring in 6% to 32% of temporal bone fractures. The lower incidence is felt to be due to decreased ossification and hence greater resistance to deformation.

The mechanisms of injury to the facial nerve are different for longitudinal and transverse fractures. Fisch (66) found transection of the nerve in 100% of the transverse fractures. By contrast, the pathology in the group of longitudinal fractures revealed intraneural hematoma in 50%, bony impingement in 17%, and complete transection in 26%. He concluded that lesions of the facial nerve in temporal bone fractures, particularly longitudinal, were the result of traction on the greater superficial petrosal nerve. In support of this, a postmortem pathologic study of a longitudinal fracture identified demyelinization and swelling of the facial nerve beginning at the meatal foramen, the narrowest portion of the fallopian canal (67). It was concluded that the delayed paralysis in this case was not due to injury at the fracture site, but to traction of the greater superficial petrosal nerve leading to edema and entrapment of the nerve at the meatal foramen. This proposed mechanism helps to explain the overwhelming incidence of perigeniculate lesions of the facial nerve associated with temporal bone fractures (68).

The treatment of facial nerve injuries in pediatric temporal bone fractures is similar to that in adults and is equally controversial. The decision to proceed with surgical decompression is based on the neurologic status of the patient, the onset and severity of the paralysis, the radiographic findings, and the results of electrical testing. Coker et al. (68) describe an algorithm for the management of temporal bone fractures complicated by facial paralysis that includes high-resolution CT (axial and coronal views) of the temporal bone, audiometric evaluation, and electrical testing with either nerve excitability or ENOG (68).

In general, the prognosis for spontaneous recovery of posttraumatic facial paralysis in children is quite favorable. In a review of 70 cases of traumatic facial paralysis, 34 of which were delayed, 32 of the 34 (94%) delayed-onset palsies recovered spontaneously (69). In a similar review, 94% of patients with delayed-onset facial paralysis recovered (House grade I) without surgical intervention (70). May (63) advocates surgical exploration in cases of immediate-onset paralysis without response on maximal stimulation within 5 days of injury and evidence of fracture or bony impingement on high-resolution CT. Lambert et al. (71) and Coker et al. (68) recommend surgery based on the results of electrical testing. Early exploration is indicated if, after a fracture, more than 90% degeneration of facial nerve fibers is demonstrated on ENOG within 6 days of the onset of the palsy (17). Lambert et al. (71) like Fisch (66), recommend decompression in cases of delayed paralysis within 6 months if no evidence of regeneration is present on EMG.

As stated previously, the timing of surgery is also a controversial issue. McCabe (60) recommended delaying repair of facial nerve paralysis in temporal bone fracture for 21 days, the amount of time necessary for the nerve cell body to push axoplasmic filaments across the nerve gap. More recent work suggests that the optimum time for repair is dictated by the overall condition of the patient.

The approach to repair is primarily dictated by the status of the hearing. Patients with nonservicable sensorineural loss undergo decompression via the transmastoid–translabyrinthine approach. Those patients with normal hearing or conductive loss undergo the middle cranial fossa–transmastoid approach. In cases of edema or hematoma, decompression is facilitated by removing the bone of the fallopian canal and slitting the epineural sheath at the injured site (66). Partial transections greater than one-third to one-half the diameter, as well as complete transections, should be repaired either by rerouting and direct anastamosis, or by interposition grafting. Moderate to severe dysfunction (House grade III to IV) is the likely outcome in cases requiring grafting.

The role of steroids in the management of traumatic facial nerve injury is undefined. There are no randomized prospective trials available that demonstrate efficacy. Therefore, at the present time, no specific recommendations can be made for the use of steroids in traumatic facial nerve injury.

TRAUMATIC INJURIES OF THE EXTRATEMPORAL FACIAL NERVE

The extratemporal facial nerve is vulnerable to injury in children less than 2 years old undergoing tympanomastoid surgery. The postauricular incision must be modified in these young children to avoid incising the nerve in its subcutaneous course. This can often be accomplished by extending the incision posteriorly as it approaches the developing mastoid tip. Additionally, dissection of the mastoid periosteum under the otologic microscope facilitates neural preservation.

Postoperative facial nerve dysfunction is a common sequela of parotid surgery, with the vast majority being only temporary in nature (72). Hemangiomas and lymphangiomas often interdigitate with the fine branches of the nerve within the parotid gland. Careful identification of the nerve at the stylomastoid foramen utilizing the landmarks described will help prevent injury to the proximal extratemporal facial nerve. Dissection within the substance of the parotid gland is facilitated by magnification, meticulous hemostasis, and delicate dissection. The marginal mandibular and temporal branches are the two most commonly injured segments in surgery of the parotid gland. Although injuries to these branches are associated with some morbidity, injury to the buccal branches appears to result in the greatest overall morbidity due to speech and masticatory dysfunction.

Extratemporal injuries of the facial nerve, whether traumatic or iatrogenic, should be explored as soon as possible, taking advantage of the ability to stimulate electrically and localize the distal segment within the first 48 to 72 hours (73). In contaminated wounds, exploration and tagging of the distal segments at the time of debridement is a useful option, with repair at a later date. Ideally, these injuries should be repaired within 30 days for the best possible outcome (73). There is evidence for improved outcome with repair of facial nerve lesions as far out as their insertion into their respective muscles (73).

✛ MANAGEMENT OF COMPLICATIONS

The major morbidity associated with facial paralysis is to the eye. Dryness and exposure can lead to vision-threatening keratitis. When evaluating a child with facial nerve paralysis, close attention to the child's ability to close the eye completely, the presence of a satisfactory Bell's phenomenon, and the presence or absence of tearing are essential. Although Schirmer testing allows a quantitative assessment of basal and stimulated lacrimation, provision of artificial tears and nighttime lubricants is an essential first step in the management of all patients with facial nerve dysfunction. The acronym BAD provides a useful way of identifying children at risk for ocular complications (48). An absent *B*ell's phenomenon, *a*nesthesia of the cornea, and *d*ryness individually and in combination are indicators of children at risk.

Management of the ocular complications of facial nerve paralysis should follow a graded approach and should include ophthalmologic consultation (74). The initial management, as stated previously, is ocular lubrication. Specifically, artificial tears should be instilled every hour during the day, and lubricating ointments should be instilled at bedtime. Carboxymethyl-cellulose 1% (Celluvisc, Allergan, Irvine, CA) is a viscous, preservative-free ointment that protects the eye during sleep. Additional protection during the day and at night can be provided by the use of a moisture chamber. Taping the eye closed should be avoided as the paralyzed orbicularis oculi muscle cannot maintain complete closure, placing the cornea at risk for abrasion. The use of permanent tarsorrhaphy is discouraged as the palpebral adhesions are cosmetically unfavorable and difficult to revise.

Passive reanimation of the upper eyelid with gold-weight implantation is an excellent means of providing eye closure for patients with permanent paralysis requiring additional ocular protection. The procedure is reversible and can be used for patients with good long-term prognoses. Palpebral spring implants provide an active closing mechanism that, unlike the gold weight, ensures lid closure irrespective of the patient's position (74). The potential complications of this technique are greater than that of the gold weight, and the spring should be reserved for more complicated cases.

Children with more permanent paralysis may suffer from paralytic ectropion and epiphora. These patients require lower lid repositioning in addition to reanimation of the upper eyelid. The lateral tarsal strip provides tightening and repositioning of the eyelid. These lower lid shortening procedures alone do not always result in adequate or long-lasting improvement. Lengthening of the posterior lamella with an autogenous hard-palate mucosal spacer has resulted in improved cosmetic and functional results when used alone or in combination with lid-shortening procedures (75).

✸ REFERENCES

1. Gulya AJ, Schuknecht HF. *Anatomy of the temporal bone with surgical implications.* New York: Parthenon, 1995.
2. Martin RG, Grant JL, Peace D, Theiss C, Rhoton AL Jr. *Neurosurgery* 1980;6:483–507.
3. Redleaf MI, Blough RR. *Ann Otol Rhinol Laryngol* 1996;105:323–326.
4. Sheehy JL. *Otolaryngol Clin North Am* 1974;7:493–503.
5. Nager GT, Proctor B. *Otolaryngol Clin North Am* 1991;24:531–553.
6. Litton WB, Krause CJ, Anson BA, Cohen WN. *Laryngoscope* 1969;79:1584–1604.
7. Hollinshead WH. *Anatomy for surgeons.* New York: Harper & Row, 1982.
8. Mitz V, Peyronie M. *Plast Reconstr Surg* 1976;58:80–88.
9. Baker DC, Conley J. *Plast Reconstr Surg* 1979;64:781–795.
10. House JW, Brackmann DE. *Otolaryngol Head Neck Surg* 1985;93:146–147.
11. Sunderland S. *Nerve and nerve injuries*, 2nd ed. London: Churchill Livingstone, 1978;88–89, 96–97, 133.
12. Sekiya T, Moller AR. *Neurosurgery* 1987;67:244–249.
13. May M, Klein SR, Taylor FH. *Laryngoscope* 1985;95:406–409.
14. Eavey RD, Herrmann BS, Joseph JM, Thornton AR. *Arch Otolaryngol Head Neck Surg* 1989;115:600–607.
15. May M, Harvey JE, Marovitz WF, Stroud M. *Laryngoscope* 1971;81:931–938.
16. Fisch U. *Am J Otol* 1984;5:494–498.
17. Gantz BJ, Holliday M, Gmuer AA, Fisch U. *Ann Otol Rhinol Laryngol* 1984;93:394–398.
18. May M, Fria TJ, Blumenthal F, Curtin H. *Otolaryngol Head Neck Surg* 1981;89:841–848.
19. Falko NA, Erickson E. *Plast Reconstr Surg* 1990;85:1.
20. Smith JD, Crumley R, Harker L. *Otolaryngol Head Neck Surg* 1981;89:1021–1024.
21. Alberti PjjW, Biagioni E. *Laryngoscope* 1972;82:1013–1020.
22. Kumari S, Bhargava SK, Choudhury P, Ghosh S. *Indian Pediatrics* 1980;17:917–922.
23. McLellan MS, Vautier T. *Am J Obstet Gynecol* 1973;117:572–574.
24. Hepner WR Jr. *Pediatrics* 1951;8:494–497.
25. Harris JP, Davidson TM, May M, Fria T. *Arch Otolaryngol* 1983;109:145–151.
26. Bergstrom L, Baker BB. *Otolaryngol Head Neck Surg* 1981;89:336–342.
27. Gorlin RJ, Cohen MM Jr, Levin LS. *Syndromes of the head and neck.* New York: Oxford University Press, 1990.
28. Pitner SE, Edwards JE, McCormick WF. *J Neurol Neurosurg Psychiatry* 1965;28:362–374.
29. Pape KE, Pickering D. *J Pediatr* 1972;81:21–30.
30. Aviv JE, Urken ML. *Arch Otolaryngol Head Neck Surg* 1992;118:909–912.
31. Clark JR, Carlson RD, Pachner AR, Sasaki CT, Steere AC. *Laryngoscope* 1985;95:1341–1344.
32. Christen HJ, Bartlau N, Hanefeld F, Eiffert H, Thomssen R. *Acta Paediatr Scand* 1990;79:1219–1224.

33. Puhakka HJ, Laurikainen E, Viljanen M, Meurman O, Valkama H. *Acta Otolaryngol* 1992;492:103–106.
34. Michel RG, Pope TH Jr, Patterson CN. *Arch Otolaryngol* 1975;101:486–489.
35. Dickins JRE, Smith JT, Graham SS. *Laryngoscope* 1988;98:776–779.
36. Murakami S, Mutsuhiko M, Nakashiro Y, Doi T, Hato N, Yanagihara N. *Ann Intern Med* 1996;124:27–30.
37. Fisch U, Esslen E. *Arch Otolaryngol* 1972;85:355–341.
38. Adour K. *Otolaryngol Clin North Am* 1991;24:663–673.
39. Liston SL, Kleid MS. *Laryngoscope* 1989;99:23–26.
40. Pitts DB, Adour KK, Hilsinger RL Jr. *Laryngoscope* 1988;98:535–540.
41. Brackmann DE, Shelton C, Arraiga MA. *Otologic surgery.* Vol. 2, Philadelphia: WB Saunders, 1994.
42. May M, Klein SR, Taylor FH. *Laryngoscope* 1984;95:406–409.
43. Kleinman MB, Passo, MH. *Pediatr Infect Dis J* 1988;7:301.
44. Macias JD, Wackym PA, McCabe BF. *Ann Otol Rhinol Laryngol* 1993;102:337–341.
45. DeRemee RA. *Arthritis Rheum* 1988;31:1068–1072.
46. Cleary KR, Batsakis, JG. *Ann Otol Rhinol Laryngol* 1996;105:166–168.
47. Graham MD, Kemink JL. *Am J Otol* 1986;7:34–37.
48. Paparella MM, Shumrick DA, Gluckman JL, Meyerhoff WL. *Otolaryngology,* Vol. 2, 3rd ed. Philadelphia: WB Saunders, 1991.
49. Brackmann DE, Bartels LJ. *Otolaryngol Head Neck Surg* 1980;88:555–559.
50. O'Donoghue GM, Brackmann DE, House JW, Jackler RK. *Am J Otol* 1989;10:49–54.
51. Shelton C, Brackmann DE, Lo WWM, Carberry JN. *Otolaryngol Head Neck Surg* 1991;104:116–121.
52. Lo WWM, Brackmann DE, Shelton C. *Ann Otol Rhinol Laryngol* 1989;98:160–161.
53. Brackmann DE, Shelton C, Arraiga MA. *Otologic surgery.* Philadelphia: WB Saunders, 1994.
54. Brackmann DE, Hitselberger WE, Robinson JV. *Ann Otol* 1973;87:772–777.
55. Feldman BA. *Laryngoscope* 1982;92:424–440.
56. Lilleyman JS, Antonion AG, Sugden PJ. *Scand J Hematol* 1979;22:87–90.
57. Callender DL, Frankenthaler RA, Luna MA, Lee SS, Goepfert H. *Arch Otolaryngol Head Neck Surg* 1992;118:472–476.
58. McGuirt WF, Welling DB, McCabe BF. *Laryngoscope* 1989;99:27–34.
59. Green JD, Shelton C, Brackmann DE. *Otolaryngol Head Neck Surg* 1994;111:606–610.
60. McCabe BF. *Laryngoscope* 1972;82:1891–1896.
61. Barrs D. *Laryngoscope* 1991;101:835–848.
62. May M, Sobol S, Mester SJ. *Otolaryngol Head Neck Surg* 1991;104:818–825.
63. May M. *The facial nerve* New York: Thieme, 1986.
64. Potter JM. *J Laryngol Otol* 1964;78:654.
65. McHugh HE. *Ann Otol Rhinol Laryngol* 1959;68:855.
66. Fisch U. *Laryngoscope* 1974;84:2141–2154.
67. Grobman LR, Pollak A, Fisch U. *Otolaryngol Head Neck Surg* 1989;101:404–408.
68. Coker NJ, Kendall KA, Jenkins HA, Alford BR. *Otolaryngol Head Neck Surg* 1987;97:262–269.
69. Turner JWA. *Lancet* 1944;1:156.
70. McKennan KX, Chole RA. *Am J Otol* 1992;13:167–172.
71. Lambert PR, Brackmann DE. *Laryngoscope* 1984;94:1022–1026.
72. Conley J. In: Brackmann DE, ed. *Neurological surgery of the ear and skull base.* New York: Raven, 1982:93–98.
73. May M, Sobol S, Mester SJ. *Laryngoscope* 1990;100:1062–1067.
74. Seiff SR, Chang J. *Otolaryngol Clin North Am* 1992;25:669–690.
75. Kersten R, Kulwin DR, Levartovsky S, Tiradellis H, Tse DT. *Arch Opthalmol* 1990;108:1339–1343.
76. Ham AW. *Histology,* 9th ed. Philadelphia: JB Lippincott, 1985:109.

R.A. Friedman: House Ear Clinic, Inc., Los Angeles, California 90057.

• *Practical Pediatric Otolaryngology*
• edited by Robin T. Cotton and Charles M. Myer, III
• Lippincott-Raven Publishers, Philadelphia © 1999

19A

Controversies in Cochlear Implantation: Ethical Issues

Annelle Hodges & Thomas J. Balkany

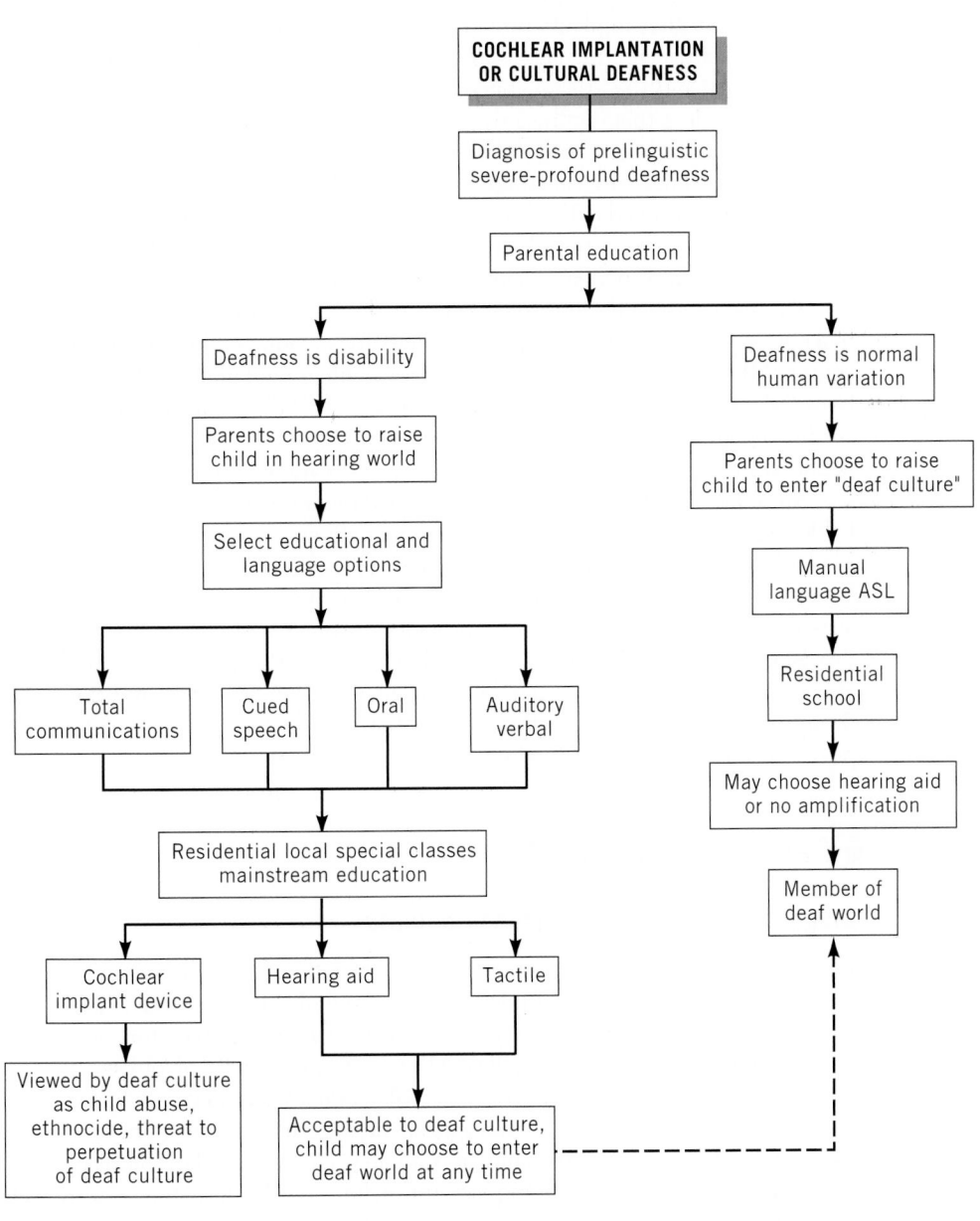

🌀 HISTORICAL BACKGROUND

Cochlear implants have been available as a treatment for profound deafness for approximately 15 years. Data collected on hundreds of postlinguistically deafened patients during this period show that for most of this group, word understanding without visual cues is possible, and communication is enhanced in nearly everyone who receives a cochlear implant. Recently reported data show that adult cochlear implant users are able to understand an average of 78% open set sentence materials with no visual information (1). Cochlear implants are now a widely accepted and effective treatment for profound sensorineural deafness in adults who lose hearing after developing oral language.

The use of cochlear implants in children has not yet received the same level of acceptance. Those who have questioned implantation of children include physicians, educators, audiologists, parents, and members of the deaf community. Their concerns have rightfully included the unknown effects of long-term electrical stimulation; the risks involved in any surgical procedure from anesthesia, infection, or medical incompetence; the uncertainty that implants provide adequate auditory information for the development of oral language; the increased risks in children from otitis media and its potential complications; and the ethical concerns surrounding a decision to perform an invasive surgical procedure that significantly alters an individual's relationship to his or her world. Since clinical trials began with children in 1986, cochlear implants have proved to be safe and effective. Major surgical complications have been few, and fears related to middle-ear disease have proved to be unfounded. In addition, children who receive adequate rehabilitation have demonstrated repeatedly that cochlear implants do in fact provide sufficient auditory information to allow the development of oral language abilities.

The major question left unanswered is thus an ethical one: Who has the right to make a decision regarding cochlear implants for a young child? This question is at the center of the ethical controversy in pediatric cochlear implantation. This issue pits members of the deaf community and hearing supporters of deaf culture against those who favor full integration of deaf individuals into mainstream culture and also generates heated debate over the rights of individuals versus preservation of deaf culture.

After identification of profound childhood deafness, parents enter a sometimes bewildering maze in which their goal is to obtain, digest, and analyze information from all available sources. Enactment of Public Law (PL) 99-457 in the United States was intended to ensure that such information, as well as the appropriate services were readily available. Even with the assistance provided through programs established under the provisions of PL 99-457, obtaining complete and impartial information on options available for deaf infants and their families remains a problem, and the education of deaf children continues to be based on the personal bias and degree of charisma of the individual providing counseling to the family.

🌀 PATIENT ASSESSMENT

Diagnosis of Profound Childhood Deafness

It is well accepted that 1 of 1,000 infants is born with a significant hearing loss. Identification programs aimed at identifying these congenitally deaf children as early as possible have focused on screening neonates for high-risk factors and recommending audiometric evaluation, such as auditory brainstem response (ABR) or otoacoustic emission (OAE) for those who exhibit one or more risk factors. Such programs have received verbal support from professional organizations such as the American Speech and Hearing Association, the American Academy of Audiology (AAA), and the American Academy of Otolaryngology but are not yet in place throughout the United States. In addition, such programs are estimated to reach only 50% of the children who are congenitally hearing impaired and will reach none of the additional 30% who lose their hearing during the first years of life (2). Early identification, whether through large-scale neonatal screening or more aggressive pediatric care, is the first step toward more effective education and parenting of deaf children.

Parental Education and Decision Making

Once a child is identified, there is frequently very little in place for assisting parents in making the necessary decisions. Deafness is a strange and foreign concept to most people, and parents are understandably looking for someone with the knowledge to guide them. In spite of early identification and intervention mandates established by PL 99-457, the low incidence of profound hearing loss often means that few if any options are offered. The local school official, who is often relied on as the "expert," can easily sway parents based on his or her own bias. This bias is often influenced by what is available in the school system, most often a "total communication" approach. Unless the parent has the means and motivation to pursue additional information, he or she may remain unaware that other options exist such as auditory–verbal speech, American sign language (ASL), traditional oralism, or verbotonal or cued speech. On the other hand, as happens to many parents, they may bounce from one professional to another, being told one thing by one group and something entirely different by another. As a result, a child may be switched from methodology to methodology as parents attempt to sort through the "guidance" they are being given.

Opposing Philosophies of Deafness

In spite of the communication and educational methodologies available for deaf children, there are in reality two idealogies. The first is based on the belief that deafness is a disability. Disability is defined as "the failure to achieve an expected state of function" (3) or a condition that produces a "limitation of functional ability" (4). If the philosophy is adopted that deafness is a disability, then the parent makes a decision to provide whatever means are available to overcome the inherent limitations and enable the child to take an active and productive role in mainstream society. This means that the parent will choose to raise and educate the child as part of the hearing world, making development of oral language and communication skills necessary. Adoption of this philosophy leads parents to obtain the best amplification available and to pursue educational options that include oralism, cued speech, or auditory verbal communication. Full integration into the culture and lifestyle of his or her own family is the ultimate goal for these children. Commitment to this philosophy while seeking to provide the best auditory input for the profoundly deaf child today ultimately brings these parents to explore the cochlear implant option. The implant may or may not be appropriate, but it must be considered a viable option.

The second philosophy is based on a belief that deafness is not a disability but rather a normal human variation. Adherents of this philosophy believe that deafness overrides the ties of the family and automatically places the child into a separate social structure, that of deaf culture. As such, the deaf child has no disability to overcome, but should instead be allowed to maximize the benefits of his or her deafness. This choice leads parents to reject the notion that oral language is desirable. Amplification may or may not be pursued. The main thrust of this philosophy is that the child's language be manual (i.e., ASL), the natural language of the deaf. The child is raised to take his or her place in deaf society with as little interaction as necessary with the hearing world. The task of raising the child into deaf culture may be left to other deaf adults or proponents of deaf culture in residential school settings. Participation in deaf culture is highly satisfying and rewarding to its members. Here they find the ease of communication, common experience, and social interaction that is not easily attainable in hearing culture. Parents who select this option for their children do not seek cochlear implants.

The Compromise

Total communication (TC) was developed as a compromise between those favoring oral communication and those favoring manual communication. In theory, TC makes use of all modalities, i.e., sign, gesture, speech reading, and auditory input to promote rapid development of communication. Since ASL has no spoken correlate, teachers who claim to sign and speak simultaneously most often use a form of Pidgen Sign together with broken English. As a result, children in TC programs are often fluent in neither English nor ASL and are caught somewhere in the middle.

Children who are educated orally, as well as those educated in TC programs, may as adults participate in deaf culture. They may even choose to become part of the deaf world, rejecting participation in hearing society. These individuals may or may not continue to use their hearing aids, which are an acceptable although not vital option in deaf society. However, those individuals who have cochlear implants find themselves ridiculed and rejected (5). They are forced to give up use of the device and hide its existence to be accepted into deaf culture. Children who attend residential schools have been found to have a nonuse rate exceeding 75% (6), much greater than that of children in mainstream settings.

Whether deafness is viewed as a disability or as a difference is clearly a matter of perspective. Proponents of the belief that deafness is a disability point to studies such as that conducted by the California Department of Rehabilitation, which associates deafness with the lowest educational levels, the lowest family income, the lowest percentage working, the lowest in professional technical jobs, and the poorest self-assessment of well-being when compared with other disabilities (7). That deafness is a disability is further supported by its costs to society, including in the United States $121.8 billion a year in the cost of education, $2.5 billion a year in lost workforce productivity, and over $2 billion annually for the cost of equal access, Social Security disability income, and other entitlements of the disabled (8). Educating a child in a residential setting has been estimated to cost approximately $429,000 during his or her school tenure, compared with $9,000 in a regular classroom (9), yet the product of such a costly education has an average reading level at the third grade and is employed in a low-level position if at all. On the other hand, proponents of deafness as a normal human variation blame such statistics on the educational system, which tries to force deaf children to become hearing rather than educating them appropriately in their native language of ASL. They hold that if interpreters are made available, then the deaf are employable and that with the appropriate technical assistance, deaf persons can become more self-sufficient. Unfortunately, there are significant costs associated with these types of benefits, and the equity of providing such extras for individuals who do not consider themselves handicapped may be questioned by other workers.

Cochlear Implant Evaluation

As defined by medical and audiologic guidelines, the pediatric cochlear implant evaluation includes: (a) audiologic evaluation, (b) medical evaluation, (c) radiologic evaluation, (d) a hearing aid trial period, and (e) assessment of the educational setting. Audiologic evaluation establishes the presence of bilateral profound sensorineural hearing loss. Medical evaluation confirms that the child is able to undergo the surgical procedure. Radiologic evaluation determines that a cochlea is present and provides information necessary for surgical planning. The hearing aid trial period proves that traditional forms of amplification are inadequate for the development of oral language abilities. Finally, an assessment of the educational environment ensures that the child will receive the necessary rehabilitation in a supportive atmosphere. Every cochlear implant team member knows the vital importance of counseling parents about the risks and limitations associated with the procedure, as well as the patience and long-term commitment necessary for maximum success. In the enthusiasm most implant team members have for the potential of the device, informing parents fully of all their options may be overlooked.

When any child is brought to a cochlear implant center for evaluation, it should be the responsibility of someone on the implant team to assess the parents' level of knowledge and understanding of their options. Success with a cochlear implant is highly dependent on the attitudes of both the parents and the school. Maximum achievement with a cochlear implant requires total commitment by both to a belief that the ability to function in the hearing world (or to be able to move back and forth) is more desirable than choosing to exist solely within the deaf community. Maximum achievement also requires a belief that cochlear implants can provide sufficient auditory input to enable a deaf child to achieve such a goal. Finally, maximum achievement requires a different set of expectations—that the child use the available auditory information both at home and at school. Competence in any language be it oral English, Spanish, or ASL requires immersion and consistent use.

Members of cochlear implant teams who recognize the potential that implants offer must be concerned with implanting only those children who are likely to succeed; otherwise, the cochlear implant rather than the circumstances is viewed as the reason for failure. To implant a child whose parents have not been fully apprised of both options and who have not made a committed decision toward integration of their child into the hearing world is to jeopardize the future reputation of cochlear implants. Such statistics as a 75% nonuse rate among children in residential schools have been taken out of context and used as proof that cochlear implants do not work, when in fact what this proves is that the residential setting is inappropriate for children with cochlear implants. Just as important as a reliable audiogram and a sufficient hearing aid trial is a fully informed, knowledgable and committed parent. As part of each child's assessment as a potential cochlear implant recipient, the parents should be fully educated with regard to their options. This means introducing them to both the good and bad aspects of each philosophy. The ease of communication and sense of belonging enjoyed by members of the deaf community should be stressed. Parents should be exposed to successful members of the deaf community and allowed to see how these deaf persons interact with each other and with hearing individuals. From these deaf individuals, parents can learn that it is not necessary to hear and speak to have a satisfying and productive life. They should also be provided with the statistics that show the low levels of educational achievement and poor economic outlook experienced by many within the deaf population. They should be made aware of the numbers of manually compared with orally educated deaf persons dependent on public assistance. They should also have the opportunity to meet deaf adults who have selected the alternative option and live their lives as part of the hearing world. Although full integration may sound like a desirable goal, many deaf individuals can speak of the frustration, isolation, and work required to cope in hearing society. In short, it is necessary that the parents see first hand the successes and failures within both camps and only then make the decision that they truly feel is in the best interest of their child.

A 15-year-old boy who has attended a residential school, whose primary affiliation is with the deaf community, who has never used or has abandoned use of amplification and whose language is sign language is quite a different implant prospect than the child who has received auditory–verbal therapy since identification, who would not think of being without his hearing aids, and who struggles to use every bit of the limited auditory input available to him. Once the child reaches midteens, parents become aware that the end of schooling is in sight, and the responsibility for the child will be returned to them. It is not unusual for parents to inquire about cochlear implantation at this time. Even if a nonaural child was willing to go along with the implantation, his potential for success with the device is limited by several factors. First, sound has no meaning for him. With a cochlear implant, sound would be present but would be meaningless noise. Sorting out the meaningful from the meaningless would require years of intensive training and motivation. Second, since his language is ASL, which has no spoken correlate, it would require learning an entirely new language based on an arbitrary sound system for which he has no reference. Being past the critical age for language learning makes that task all the more difficult. Third, his peer group will be made up of other deaf students at the residential school (or contained classroom), where the use of auditory prostheses of any type is not encouraged, and, in keeping with deaf world values, cochlear implants are taboo. To implant this child would be to cut him off from his main support system and leave him isolated from both the hearing and deaf worlds. Success with a cochlear implant is not an impossibility, but the overwhelming odds are that this child will become a nonuser. Diane Brackett (10) has developed an excellent and applicable hierarchy of factors that affect progress with a cochlear implant. While she developed the categories as guidelines for (re)habilitative training, her explanations can be useful in guiding parental expectations as part of the preimplant counseling process.

If forced to select one factor on which to base the decision for or against recommending implantation of an older child, our implant team would choose exposure to sound. A 6-year-old who has never worn a hearing aid merits a red flag. This is an indication that the parent has no control over the child and/or no real commitment to development of oral language. There is no child who cannot be trained to wear a hearing aid just as he or she is trained to wear shoes and socks. Most parents who are committed enough to ensure that the child has well-fitting and -working hearing aids—which he or she uses regularly—are also likely to make sure that the child receives training to use the input. It is highly unlikely that the child will derive no benefit at all from a hearing aid, and even a little consistent sound experience gives the child a better chance with the implant. Without that experience, candidacy at 6 years of age would be highly questionable. By 11, and certainly by 15, a prelinguistically deafened child who has had no consistent exposure to sound would be an inappropriate cochlear implant candidate. However, we have had remarkable success with implants in 13-, 14-, and 15-year-olds, who, while receiving minimal benefit from hearing aids, made use of every bit of auditory information available to them. It is our experience that fewer and fewer children whose parents are dedicated to development of oral language are waiting until a child is 6 or 11 or 15 to explore the implant option. Still, each child has individual circumstances, and black and white guidelines are difficult to establish.

As implant team members we often find it difficult to turn away any potential implant candidate. We see so many positive outcomes that we get caught up in wanting all deaf individuals to derive the same benefits. We become concerned with denying a candidate for reasons based on anything other than the audiogram, because all other reasons are subjective judgments. We often approach the decision by rationalizing that "even if he or she does not benefit, at least we did not deny him or her the opportunity," and against our better judgment, we may condemn a child and an implant to a failed relationship. Moreover, as things change, it may soon no longer be within the power of the implant team members to turn down a patient. At the recent National Institutes of Health Consensus Conference, deaf adults spoke out for the right to make that decision for themselves. Because of the lack of rigid guidelines, it may even now be the case that if one center finds candidacy not to be an appropriate choice, parents will search until they find a program that will approve the child's candidacy. Adequately informed and knowledgable parents are the only safeguard against potentially harmful choices.

ETHICAL DECISION MAKING

Since the treatment option referred to here is the cochlear implant, the focus of this section will be on the process of ethical decision making in selection of this option. Two important questions arise regarding this process: (a) Who should decide for the child? and (b) According to what standards should the decision be made?

Who Should Decide for the Child?

The Medical–Legal View

In our social and legal structure, the family is viewed as the core unit, and the parents are responsible for that unit. It is, furthermore, "the right of parents to raise their children according to the parents' own standards and values and to seek to transmit those standards and values to their children" (11). In their book, *Deciding for Others: The Ethics of Surrogate Decision Making*, Buchanan and Brock state (11): "There must be a clear locus of authority or decision making will lack coherence, continuity and accountability." It is the parents (or, in their absence, a legal guardian) who has authority for all aspects of a child's life and can provide this continuity and accountability. Parents will usually do a better job of deciding what is best for their child than anyone else for several reasons. First, parents care more deeply for their children than do strangers. Parents know their children better than anyone else and are more concerned with their welfare. Because they are involved in all aspects of the child's life, not simply the choice of a cochlear implant, parents have a more complete picture of the child, his or her role within the family, and therefore what is best for the child within the family structure. It is also true that parents must bear the consequences and are financially responsible for decisions made about their children (12).

Parental rights to make health-care decisions for children, while broad, are not unlimited. For instance, a decision to forgo treatment for a disability or a dangerous but treatable disorder might appropriately be regarded as neglect. The exercise of a parent's judgment is rarely constrained, and only in extreme cases of neglect is parental judgment overridden.

The Deaf Community View

The most vehement objection to the use of cochlear implants in children is currently being raised by certain deaf individuals within the deaf community, who further define themselves as belonging to the "deaf world" (13). They see a distinction between themselves and other deaf individuals based on their affirmation that deafness is in fact a normal human variation and is not a deficit or a medical condition requiring treatment. They express the same type of militant pride in their deafness as others might express in their ethnic origins.

Sociologists who have studied the deaf community explain that membership in that community is not based on one's audiometric configuration but must be achieved through meeting several criteria (14). First and foremost is the exclusive use of ASL for communication. Second, one must have the shared experiences of deafness. Finally, the individual must identify him or herself with the deaf community. More often than not, these three characteristics have their roots in the educational experience. It is within the isolation of special programs or residential schools that ASL becomes the primary link to other human beings. The other human beings who share the language and the same sense of physical and social separation from the hearing world are also deaf. Within the deaf community, everything from deaf beauty pageants to deaf Olympic competition to social clubs is provided for members, effectively reducing the need to interact with the hearing world and creating an interdependent and tightly knit community. So strong is the hold of the deaf community that "to be a part of the deaf community, you have to associate with the deaf all the time. . . . not only social: any part of your everyday life. Then you can become part (of the community)" (14) and further, "some individuals may participate in activities of the deaf community, but are not members. They are tolerated, though they are not accepted. . . . audiologically they are deaf, socially they are not" (14). Strong identification with the deaf world comes not through family tradition or values as does normal development of cultural mores, but rather through horizontal acculturation by individuals whose relationships are based solely on their deafness (5).

Deaf children from hearing families who are educated in the mainstream or in schools which emphasize development of oral language do not necessarily meet the three criteria that qualify them as members of the deaf world. Without the shared experience of physical and social isolation from hearing individuals, exclusive use of ASL, and socialization solely with other deaf individuals, the deaf community does not play the same central role in their lives as they become adults. Ties may be formed with hearing family members and coworkers in addition to other deaf persons. Ninety percent of deaf children have two hearing parents, and 97% have at least one hearing parent. Should these parents opt to keep the child at home and educate him or her in a local school, there is a significantly increased chance that child will not develop the commitment to his or her deafness required by members of the deaf world. This has the potential to reduce drastically the number of individuals who meet the criteria of the deaf world, thereby threatening the continuation of that culture and its language. If cochlear implants can provide sufficient auditory information to enable a child to be successfully educated in the mainstream and to fit more comfortably into the lifestyle of a hearing family, that threat becomes even stronger.

As viewed by hearing individuals, the idea that anyone would oppose an advance that could provide expanded opportunity for any child is difficult to fathom. Activists within the deaf community argue that the belief that hearing and oral language are desirable puts hearing parents in a conflict of interest with the deaf child and renders the parent unfit to make a decision for or against cochlear implantation. According to these deaf activists, this decision should be made by a culturally deaf adult (who is usually no relation of the child). Members of the deaf community who support this view use several arguments on which they base the opinion that they, and not the parents, should decide if a child is to have a cochlear implant.

Arguments of the Deaf Community

Deaf Children Are De Facto Members of the Deaf Community

According to a recent presentation by Lane and Bahan (13), children born deaf are already on a course that should not be altered. As stated by Dr. Marina McIntire (13), "It has been argued that hearing parents have the right to raise youngsters who are linguistically and culturally like themselves. We disagree." It is a common belief among members of the deaf world that all deaf children "belong" to the deaf community and should be "given over" by their hearing parents to take their places in deaf society. The usual values taught in families and passed from parent to child, generation to generation (vertical acculturation), should instead be taught by culturally deaf adults (horizontal acculturation).

This translates, as described by Harlan Lane in the *Mask of Benevolence* (5), into the belief that hearing parents cannot make decisions for their own deaf child because they don't "really know the patient" and "are in a conflict of interest with their own child." Specifically related to the question of cochlear implants, Roz Rosen, president of the National Association of the Deaf, stated that "hearing parents are not qualified to decide about implants" (16), again indicating that the decisions for deaf children should be made within the deaf community.

Cochlear Implant Proponents Are Serving Self-Interests

A second argument used by the deaf community is that the doctors, teachers, audiologists, and others who favor cochlear implants are serving their own self-interest and that they are in the business to make money off deaf people or "hapless parents" (17). The strategy used by the deaf community to support this concept is the spreading of misinformation among both the deaf and sympathetic hearing communities. Some of the information is blatantly false, such as the statements by Dr. Yerker Andersson (18), president of the World Federation of the Deaf, who wrote how a certain surgeon was "eager to use his skills on 17 deaf individuals. Three died due to complications and one became mentally ill. The rest were failures." Other statements are simply supposition, such as the claim by the director of the Bureau of Deaf Services in Missouri that cochlear implants "would be truly debilitating in the mental health sense" (15) and the surgical description given by Harlan Lane (5), who is neither a surgeon nor an auditory physiologist, in which he states that "the exquisitely detailed microstructure of the inner ear is often ripped apart as the electrode weaves its way, crushing cells and perforating membranes" (5).

Still other information fed to the public shows ignorance of the available scientific data such as the position paper developed by the National Association of the Deaf in which it is affirmed that "there is no evidence of material benefit. . . .there is no evidence of enhancement of speech perception, English or greater educational success with cochlear implants" (19). There is in fact a growing body of research results that prove otherwise. Waltzman et al. (20), at New York University, reported on 91 children with cochlear implants, 14 of whom were congenitally or prelinguistically deafened. All these children had received a cochlear implant prior to the age of 3 and had been followed for periods of 2 to 5 years. All these children now use oral language as their primary means of communication and attend regular schools. The Glendonald Auditory Screening Procedure evaluates word and sentence recognition in an auditory-only open set (no picture or written choices available) condition. After 2 years, the 10 subjects with 2 years of implant experience who completed this test had a mean score of 86% word understanding. For those subjects with 3 to 4 years of experience, the mean score rose to 96%. Children who had used their cochlear implants for 4 to 5 years averaged 99% on the Iowa Sentences Test, an open set evaluation of sentence understanding in the auditory-only condition.

Several other published studies (21–23) support these results and show that children can in fact benefit significantly from cochlear implants. In a study of 54 implanted children at Iowa University, after 4 years of implant use, 82% of the children achieved open set word recognition. In a report out of Indiana University, 61 implanted children attained an average of 63% open set understanding. Fifty-five of these children were either congenitally or prelinguistically deafened. These and other studies show that children, even congenitally deafened, have much to gain from cochlear implants if implanted at a young age.

Finally, some statements made by opponents are simply sensationalistic rhetoric. A comparison of a cochlear implant to a mouse placed under the skin with its tail fed into the cochlea (24) and likening the implant to Nazi medical experimentation on helpless children (25) are both meaningless statements intended only to create a vivid negative image.

This type of adverse publicity by deaf advocates and deaf activists has resulted in misunderstanding and distrust of the cochlear implant and members of the medical community by deaf individuals. Several letters from Gallaudet college students (15) illustrate both the lack of understanding and the negative attitude toward the implant fostered by the deaf community (quotes are taken directly from letters as they appear):

"I read few articles about how cochlear implant. For deaf people died from cochlear implant. It was explained about how cochlear implant affected to brain damage."

"I feel that cochlear implants are wrong because it makes the recipient a robot with wires sticking out of their head."

"I may not aware of cochlear implant much but I do have a strong against it"

"My hearing loss is sensorineural. I know it can not be help by cochlear implant."

Cochlear Implants Are a Tool to Destroy Deaf Culture

The term "genocide" has been applied to the use of cochlear implants by members of the deaf world (12). It is claimed that the implant is one more attempt by hearing people to do away with the deaf. This concept is supported by the "new ethics" of politically correct science which claims that "if research or technology affects a community, it must benefit the community or it is unethical" (26). If the 90% of deaf children whose parents can hear receive cochlear implants that enable them to participate in mainstream culture, deaf culture will surely be affected. According to this ethic, the deaf community could justifiably consider cochlear implants unethical. In this same vein, research aimed toward the prevention and treatment of conditions that may result in deafness such as cytomegalovirus infection or meningitis, or even something as basic as adequate prenatal care, could be considered unethical by the deaf community since these also have the potential to affect its membership. When questioned, certain deaf world supporters would not deny holding such beliefs (13). This view of ethical action is at odds with the traditional view that parents are expected to act in the best interests of their child and physicians are to act in the best interests of their patients without regard to the beliefs of any special interest group such as the deaf community (3).

A "Victimized Minority"

To increase political power, and further discredit medical and educational professionals, deaf leaders categorize themselves as members of a "victimized minority." Discrimination is evidenced by the attempts to teach deaf children to speak and force them to adapt to the hearing world, thereby denying them their deafness. Surgery to provide hearing to a deaf baby is likened to a procedure intended to turn an Asian into an Occidental, or a black person white (12). Such arguments confuse the concept of restoration of function with cosmetic homogeneity and are demeaning both to persons with handicaps and to those who have suffered real discrimination (12).

According to What Standards Should the Decision Be Made?

There are three well-established standards for making surrogate decisions: advanced directive, substituted judgment, and best interest. If an advanced directive has been established by the patient, such as a living will or a specific nomination of surrogate, that should be meticulously followed. If none is available, a family member should make decisions on the basis of substituted judgment. (Using knowledge of the patient, the surrogate does what he believes the patient would do under the circumstances if he or she were competent.) Harlan Lane and Ben Behan (15) suggest that substituted judgment should be the guiding ethical principle in the decision for a child to have (or not to have) a cochlear implant. They claim that the decision should be made as the child would make it if he or she were an adult and that as a deaf adult he or she would clearly opt not to have a cochlear implant. This statement does not acknowledge the many deaf individuals who do not choose to be associated with the deaf world and who use hearing aids and oral communication. It is obviously impossible to determine what any child will be like as an adult, and saying that a child should not have an implant as a child because he or she will not want it as an adult is an unfair and restrictive assumption. It is impossible for anyone to predict, and unacceptable in our society for anyone to predetermine, what a child will become as he or she grows into an adult.

It is the third standard, that of best interest, which is most applicable to children. It is the parents' responsibility to make decisions according to their understanding of what is in the best interest of their child.

According to Buchanan and Brock (11) two underlying ethical values should guide those who are in a position to make decisions for others: (a) respect for self-determination (autonomy) and (b) concern for well-being (beneficence). The underlying ethical values of autonomy and beneficence apply to the child as represented by the parents.

In foreseeing the desire for influence of outside groups, Engelhardt (3) states, "This principle of autonomy provides moral grounding for public policies aimed at defending the innocent." In exercising autonomy for their children, parents act within the rights of their children, which include freedom of choice, respect for the individual, and free informed consent to make decisions on behalf of their child. Englehardt (3) defines free choices as "being unrestrained by prior commitments or justified authority and being free from coercion." Associated with the right of self-determination is the right of privacy. The courts, as well as legal scholars and ethicists, concur that the rights and interests of self-interest groups should be strictly excluded from decisions concerning the best interests of individual children (11). Interference from outside groups deprives families of their right of privacy. Parents exercise free informed consent on behalf of their children. "Others do not have the right to intervene in their . . . actions" (3). When deaf activists maintain that parents are in conflict of interest with their own children and attempt to impose the collective will of leaders of deaf culture on parents, they ignore the family's right to privacy and self-determination and attempt to override family autonomy.

The ethical value of beneficence is in simplest terms a prudent effort to do good and avoid evil (3). Advocates of deaf culture claim that making cochlear implants available to deaf children is tantamount to "genocide" for deaf culture. The question that arises is whether these individuals are more concerned with their culture than honoring the value of beneficence as it applies to an individual child.

As applied to an individual child, beneficence ensures a child's "right to an open future" (11). Children have a clear interest in maintaining functional abilities. The ability to hear not only has communicative value, but also provides auditory enjoyment and is important to safety. Deaf children also have an interest in their future educational and employment opportunities and interpersonal relationships (12). It has already been noted that educational and employment expectations for deaf persons are much less than those for their hearing peers. And since 99.8% of the population of the United States cannot communicate in ASL (27), the opportunities for personal relationships are substantially restricted.

SUMMARY

Clearly there exist two distinctly opposing views on the cochlear implant. Proponents of cochlear implants believe that deafness is a disability and that everything possible should be done to enable the deaf individual to live the least restrictive existence with the greatest degree of freedom and opportunity possible. Those who favor implants also favor the use of traditional amplification for those who benefit, as well as the development of written and spoken English. This group believes that being able to hear is a more favorable condition than being deaf and that being able to communicate effectively gives one an advantage in our society. No proponent of cochlear implants believes that the surgery should be mandatory for all deaf people. It is a choice to be made based on the deaf individual's own wish to integrate as fully as possible into mainstream culture. When that person is a child who is unable to make that decision on his or her own, it is believed that ethically, the decision should be made by informed parents. Proponents of cochlear implants include both hearing and deaf persons.

The opposing view is held by deaf activists and their hearing supporters. These individuals do not see cochlear implants as a medical advance similar to corneal transplants, which allow the blind to see, or neural stimulators now being developed, which may enable the paralyzed to use their limbs. They view the cochlear implant as a tool, not to increase opportunity for deaf persons, but rather as weapon to decrease their numbers and threaten their way of life.

Members of the American deaf community are closely linked by their use of ASL and their separation from the hearing culture. They have a well-developed social structure; for individuals who are often isolated from their own families and communities by their language barrier, this community provides the sense of belonging desired by all human beings. The support they receive from other members of the deaf community and the enjoyment they derive from deaf social clubs, deaf theatre, deaf bowling leagues, and other aspects of deaf culture allow them to have the type of emotionally fulfilling life every person wants. Many individuals find complete satisfaction in the deaf community and have no desire to integrate into mainstream society. They have no interest in obtaining a cochlear implant, and cochlear implant proponents support this as an acceptable personal choice. This group of individuals feels that as hearing persons, the parents have a conflict of interest which makes them ethically inappropriate to make the decision to have a deaf child implanted.

At this point in time, the two sides have reached an understanding regarding deaf adults who choose cochlear implants. Most of the adults who choose implants are postlinguistically deafened and were never participants in the deaf community. When these persons benefit from cochlear implants, the deaf community is not threatened. However, the question of implanting children remains an unresolved issue. Proponents of implants feel the decision should be left up to the parents, and traditional medical ethics support this view. Members of the deaf community argue that the decision should be made by culturally deaf adults because it is the deaf community which is ultimately affected by the decision. A new school of politically correct ethical thought supports this view.

Neither cochlear implant team members nor culturally deaf adults can determine with complete accuracy which children will decide as adults that they wish to associate only within the deaf community, and which others will desire different opportunities. There are likely to be implanted children who grow up to reject the implant and resent those who made the decision for an implant. On the other hand, there are just as likely to be deaf children who do not get implants and as adults see successful implant users, leading them to question why they were denied the same opportunity.

To minimize these types of experiences, several steps must be taken. First, implant supporters must continue to improve the device, to study and report outcomes objectively, and to make the information widely available to both the hearing and deaf communities. Implant supporters must evaluate and determine those factors that result in the greatest degree of success for implanted children and identify those that are likely to lead to failure. Deaf education must be improved so that undereducation and underemployment no longer plague the deaf. There should be no place for spreading of disinformation either for or opposed to the implant, since those who persist in doing so may harm those they wish to help. Members of the deaf community may wish to welcome individuals with cochlear implants (who are in reality still deaf) for participation in the deaf community. Allowing added diversity into the deaf community could serve to enlarge and strengthen rather than destroy it, as some fear. Finally, we must all recognize that it is a parental right to decide for the child. It is the parents who are responsible for the child and are also the people legally and morally most concerned with the child's best interest. It is they who will live with the consequences of any decision, be it good or bad. Cochlear implant proponents and members of the deaf community must work together to educate the parent on the benefits and limitations involved with either choice and then allow them to make the decision most appropriate for their child and their family circumstances.

REFERENCES

1. Clinical Bulletin, Cochlear Corporation, April 1994:1–8.
2. Hearing and Hearing Loss Packet. Bethesda, MD: NIDCD Information Clearing House, 1994.
3. Englehardt HT. *The foundation of bioethics*. New York: Oxford University Press, 1986.
4. Boorse C. On the distinction between disease and illnesses. *Phil Public Affairs* 1975;5:61.
5. Lane H. *The mask of benevolence*. New York: Vintage Books, 1993.
6. Rose DE. Letter to the Editor. *Am J Otol* 1994;15:813–814.
7. Harris JP, Anderson JP, Novak R. An outcome study of cochlear implants in deaf patients. *Arch Otolaryngol Head Neck Surg* 1995;121:398–404.
8. NIH. Early identification of hearing impairment in infants and young children. National Institutes of Health Consensus Statement. 1992;11:1–12.
9. Johnson JL, Mank GW, Takekawa KM, et al. Implementing a statewide system of services for infants with hearing disabilities. *Seminars in Hearing* 1993;14:105–118.

10. Brackett D. Rehabilitation/education strategies for children with cochlear implants. *Cochlear Clin Bull*, November, 1991.

11. Buchanan AE, Brock DW. *Deciding for others: the ethics of surrogate decision making.* Cambridge: Cambridge University Press, 1989.

12. Balkany TJ, Hodges AV, Goodman KW. Ethics of cochlear implantation in young children. *Otolaryngol Head Neck Surg* 1996;114:748–755.

13. Lane H, Bahan B. Ethical dilemmas in cochlear implants in children. Presented at the VIth Biennial Symposium on Cochlear Implants in Children, Miami Beach, FL, February, 1996.

14. Higgins PC. *Outsiders in a hearing world.* Beverly Hills, CA: Sage Publications, 1988.

15. Letters to the William House Cochlear Implant Study Group, September, 1993 (on file).

16. Coffey R. *Caitlin's story on 60 Minutes.* Bicultural Center News 1992;53:3.

17. Silver A. Cochlear implant: surefire prescription for longterm disaster. TBC News 1992;53:4–5.

18. Andersson Y. Do we want cochlear implants? World Fed Deaf News 1994;1:3–4.

19. National Association for the Deaf Position Paper on American Sign Language. Bicultural Center News 1994;67:2.

20. Waltzman SB, Cohen NL, Gomolin RH. Long term results of earlier cochlear implantation in congenitally and prelingually deafened children, *Am J Otol* 1994;15:9–13.

21. Gantz BJ, Tyler RS, Woodworth GG. Results of multichannel cochlear implants in congenital and acquired prelingual deafness in children: a five year follow-up. *Am J Otol* 1994;15:1–7.

22. Miyamoto RT, Osberger MJ, Robbins AM, Myers WA, Kessler K. Prelingually deafened children's performance with the Nucleus multichannel cochlear implant. *Am J Otol* 1993;14:437–45.

23. Lusk RP, Jenison V, Stoe B, Fears B. Speech perception in congenitally deaf children with cochlear implants. *(in press)*.

24. Pollard R. Psychological risks in childhood cochlear implantation. Times Union, Rochester, NY, January 18, 1993.

25. Solomon A. Defiantly deaf. *New York Times Magazine*, August 28, 1994:38–68.

26. Pollard RQ. Cross cultural ethics on the conduct of deafness research. *Rehabil Psychol* 1987;37:87–99.

27. Padden CA. American sign language. *Gallaudet Encyclopedia of Deaf People and Deafness.* Washington D.C., 1987;343–53.

A. Hodges: Department of Otolaryngology, University of Miami, Miami, Florida 33101. • T.J. Balkany: Departments of Otolaryngology, Neurological Surgery, and Pediatrics, University of Miami, and University of Miami Ear Institute, Miami, Florida 33136.

• *Practical Pediatric Otolaryngology*
• edited by Robin T. Cotton and Charles M. Myer, III
• Lippincott-Raven Publishers, Philadelphia © 1999

19B

Controversies in Cochlear Implantation: Technical and Surgical Considerations

Richard T. Miyamoto & Karen Iler Kirk

Cochlear implantation is a therapeutic option for profoundly deaf children and adults. However, as with any evolving technology, controversy exists regarding a number of technical and surgical issues.

In general terms, cochlear implants are electronic devices that consist of an electrode array, which is surgically implanted into the cochlea; an external unit, consisting of a microphone that picks up sound energy and converts it to an electric signal; and a signal processor that modifies the signal, depending on the processing scheme in use. The processed signal is amplified and compressed to match the narrow electrical dynamic range of the ear. The typical response range of a deaf ear to electrical stimulation is on the order of only 10 to 20 dB, and even less in the high frequencies. Transmission of the electrical signal across the skin from the external unit to the implanted electrode array is most commonly accomplished by the use of electromagnetic induction or radiofrequency transmission. The critical residual neural elements stimulated appear to be the spiral ganglion cells or axons. Damaged or missing hair cells of the cochlea are bypassed.

MULTICHANNEL PROCESSING STRATEGIES

Multichannel, multielectrode cochlear implants use place coding to transfer frequency information in addition to accurately providing time and intensity information. Three types of multichannel cochlear implants are presently available in the United States. The Nucleus 22-channel cochlear implant has received Food and Drug Administration (FDA) approval for use in both adults and children and is currently the most commonly used multichannel system. (Over 15,000 Nucleus devices have been implanted worldwide.) The Nucleus implantable electrode array consists of platinum–iridium band electrodes placed in a silastic carrier (1). Several generations of speech processors have been employed with the Nucleus multichannel cochlear implant. Until recently, all the Nucleus speech processors used a feature-extraction scheme in which selected key features of speech were presented to the central auditory system through the implanted electrode array. An early speech processing strategy, the F0F1F2 strategy, primarily conveyed vowel information, including the first and second formant frequencies and their amplitudes, as well as voice pitch. A later coding scheme, the MULTIPEAK strategy, presented these acoustic features along with additional information from three high-frequency spectral bands. The aim of the MULTIPEAK scheme was to present additional cues that would aid in the perception of consonants. The current speech processing strategy provided to all who receive the Nucleus 22-channel implant is the Spectral Peak (SPEAK) strategy implemented in the Spectra 22 processor. This strategy uses a vocoder in which a filterbank consisting of 20 filters covering the center frequencies from 200 to 10,000 Hz is employed. Each filter is allocated to an active electrode in the array. The filter outputs are scanned, and the electrodes that are stimulated represent filters which contain speech components with the highest amplitude. Depending on the acoustic input, the number of spectral maxima detected (and thus the number of electrodes stimulated) on each scan cycle can vary from one to ten, with an average of six per cycle. The rate at which the electrodes are stimulated varies adaptively between 180 and 300 pulses/sec.

The Clarion multichannel cochlear implant has recently received FDA approval for both adults and children. The Clarion multichannel cochlear implant has an eight-channel electrode array that utilizes a radial bipolar configuration through electrode pairs positioned adjacent to the osseous spiral lamina in a 90° orientation (2). The Clarion multichannel cochlear implant offers two types of speech processing strategies: compressed analog (CA) and continuous interleaved sampling (CIS). Both strategies represent the waveform or envelope of the speech signal (3). The Clarion CA strategy first compresses the analog signal into the restricted range for electrically evoked hearing and then filters the signal into a maximum of eight channels for presentation to the corresponding electrodes. Speech information is conveyed via the relative amplitudes and the temporal details contained in each channel. The CIS strategy filters the incoming speech into eight bands and then obtains the speech envelope and compresses the signal for each channel. Stimulation consists of interleaved digital pulses that sweep rapidly through the channels at a rate of 833 pulses/sec when using all eight channels for a maximum pulse rate of 6,664 pulses/sec ($8 \times 833 = 6,664$). With the CIS strategy, rapid changes in the speech signal are tracked by rapid variations in pulse amplitude. The pulses are delivered to consecutive channels in sequence to avoid channel interaction. More than 90% of Clarion multichannel cochlear implant recipients use the CIS speech processing strategy (4).

The MED-EL Combi 40-Cochlear Implant system utilizes the CIS strategy, which provides both spectral and temporal resolution. Up to eight active electrodes can be utilized. The electrode array used has the capability of deep insertion into the apical regions of the cochlea (5). The MED-EL has the capacity to provide the most rapid stimulation rate of any of the currently available implants (maximum of 12,000 biphasic pulses/sec) (6).

PEARLS AND PERILS

Summary of Controversies
Device issues:
1. The ideal speech coding strategy is yet to be defined. (CIS and SPEAK are the latest versions.)
2. The ideal intracochlear electrode configuration is not known.
3. The advantages of high stimulation rates are yet to be demonstrated (The MED-EL is currently the fastest implant device.)

Patient issues:
1. The ideal lower age limit for cochlear implantation remains to be determined.
2. How much residual hearing can be present in an appropriate candidate?
3. The advantages of cochlear implantation in congenitally and early deafened adolescents need to be defined.

DEVICE ISSUES REQUIRING FURTHER REFINEMENT

The ideal intracochlear electrode configuration is yet to be defined. There is currently no preoperative measure to quantitate or to localize the remaining neural elements to be stimulated. In addition, the precise pathways through which electrical currents flow through the cochlea are not known. For this reason, the unique features of the electrode array of each of the currently available devices have attractive characteristics. The longitudinal array of 22 electrodes incorporated in the Nucleus device allows electrical current to be spread over a wide distribution in common ground, or the current can be more localized using the various bipolar configurations. Ineffective or subjectively unpleasant electrodes can be programmed out. The Clarion electrode is designed to wrap tightly around the modiolus, placing the electrodes in close proximity to the neural elements. The radial bipolar orientation is theoretically more beneficial in achieving channel separation. The MED-EL electrode has the capability of the deepest insertion. This is theoretically advantageous if the optimum neural population is in the cochlear apex, as is often the case in temporal bone studies.

Device stimulation speed may prove to be a key variable. High stimulation rates are necessary to represent the rapid fluctuations in the acoustic speech stream. The MED-EL is the fastest cochlear implant commercially available in the United States and has the capability of incorporating advanced CIS strategies using extremely rapid stimulation rates.

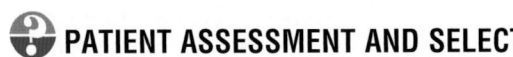 **PATIENT ASSESSMENT AND SELECTION**

The selection of cochlear implant candidates is a complex and ever evolving process that requires careful consideration of many factors. Current selection criteria are as follows:

1. Age 18 months and above
2. Profound bilateral sensorineural hearing loss
3. No appreciable benefit from hearing aids
4. No medical contraindications
5. High motivation and appropriate expectations
6. Enrollment in program that emphasizes development of auditory skills

Age Considerations

A trend toward earlier cochlear implantation in children has emerged in an attempt to ameliorate the devastating effects of early auditory deprivation. Electrical stimulation appears to be capable of preventing at least some of the degenerative changes in the central auditory pathways (7).

A lower age limit of 2 years has been applied during the FDA clinical trials. However, because the development of speech perception, speech production, and language competence normally begins at a very early age, implanting congenitally or neonatally deafened children under age 2 years may have substantial advantages. When the etiology of deafness is meningitis, progressive intracochlear ossification may occur, which can preclude standard electrode insertion. A relatively short time window exists during which this advancing process can be circumvented. Impending intracochlear ossification may serve as another incentive to consider implantation before the age of 2 years.

Lowering the age of implantation to less than 2 years remains controversial. The audiologic assessment in this population remains extremely challenging. As with older children, profound deafness must be substantiated and the inability to benefit from conventional hearing aids demonstrated. In addition, special consideration must be given to the small dimensions of the temporal bone and to the potential for problems from postoperative temporal bone growth.

The feasibility of implantation earlier than the currently accepted age of 2 years is substantiated by developmental anatomy. The cochlea is adult size at birth, and by age 1 year, the facial recess and mastoid antrum, which provide access to the middle ear for electrode placement, are adequately developed. For these reasons, extension of implant candidacy to the 1- to 2-year age group is feasible and in selected cases desirable. No upper age limit is applied as long as the patient's health status will permit an elective surgical procedure. The age at implantation in the Indiana University Cochlear Implant Program spans a range from 16 months to 87 years.

Pediatric Cochlear Implantation

Pediatric cochlear implant recipients can be loosely divided into three main categories, which significantly affect the anticipated outcomes when this technology is applied.

1. *Postlingually deafened children.* Children who become deaf at or after age 5 are generally classified as postlingually deafened. Even though these children have developed many aspects of spoken language before the onset of their deafness, they demonstrate rapid deterioration in the intelligibility of their speech once they lose access to auditory input and feedback. Early implantation can potentially ameliorate this rapid deterioration in speech production and perception abilities. However, a postlingual onset of deafness is an infrequent occurrence in the pediatric population. If this were to be the only category for which cochlear implants positively impacted deaf children, there would be limited applicability for this technology in children.
2. *Congenitally or early-deafened young children.* Congenital or early acquired deafness is the most frequently encountered type of profound sensorineural hearing loss. The acquisition of communication skills is a difficult process for these children. Whether sufficient acoustic input can be provided by cochlear implantation to perceive a speech signal linguistically is the focus of a comprehensive longitudinal study.
3. *Congenitally or early-deafened adolescents.* When cochlear implantation is considered in adolescence or young adulthood for a patient who has had little or no experience with sound because of congenital or early-onset deafness, caution must be exercised, for this group has not demonstrated high levels of success with electrical stimulation of the auditory system.

Audiologic Assessment

Audiologic evaluation is the primary means of determining suitability for cochlear implantation. Both unaided and aided thresholds using conventional amplification are determined. A period of experience with a properly fitted hearing aid coupled with training in an appropriate aural (re)habilitation program is necessary. Hearing aid performance can then be compared with normative cochlear implant performance.

Children who have been the most obvious candidates for a cochlear implant are those who have demonstrated no response to warble tones in the sound field with appropriate hearing aids, or responses suggestive of vibrotactile rather than auditory sensation, i.e., aided responses at levels greater than 50 to 60 dB hearing level (HL) in the lower frequencies with no responses above 1,000 Hz.

Not all children with profound sensorineural hearing losses are implant candidates. Many children with pure-tone thresholds between 90 and 100 dBHL with residual hearing through at least 2,000 Hz demonstrate closed and open set speech recognition skills that are superior to multichannel implant users.

Sufficient receptive and expressive abilities to allow the child to learn to make a conditioned response will assist in accurately estimating the child's auditory potential and, if accepted as an implant candidate, will ultimately assist in device setting and permit the child to begin the extensive (re)habilitation program.

Medical Assessment

The medical assessment includes the otologic history and physical examination. Radiologic evaluation of the cochlea is performed to determine whether the cochlea is present and patent and to identify congenital deformities of the cochlea. High-resolution, thin-section computed tomography (CT) scanning of the cochlea remains the imaging technique of choice (8). Intracochlear bone formation resulting from labyrinthitis ossificans can usually be demonstrated by CT scanning. However, when soft tissue obliteration occurs following sclerosing labyrinthitis, CT may not image the obstruction. In these cases, T_2-weighted magnetic resonance imaging (MRI) is an effective adjunctive procedure providing additional information regarding cochlear patency. The endolymph/perilymph signal may be lost in sclerosing labyrinthitis. Intracochlear ossification is not a contraindication to cochlear implantation but can limit the type and insertion depth of the electrode array that can be introduced into the cochlea. Congenital malformations of the cochlea are likewise not contraindications to cochlear implantation. Cochlear dysplasia has been reported to occur in approximately 20% of children with congenital sensorineural hearing loss (9). Several reports of successful implantations in children with inner-ear malformations have been published (10–14). A thin cribriform area between the modiolus and a widened internal auditory canal is often observed (15). This is believed to be the route of egress of cerebrospinal fluid (CSF) when it occurs during surgery or postoperatively. A CSF gusher has been reported in several cases. Temporal bone dysplasia may also be associated with an anomalous facial nerve, which may increase the surgical risk.

The precise etiology for the deafness cannot always be determined but is identified whenever possible. However, stimulable auditory neural elements are nearly always present regardless of cause of deafness (16). Two exceptions are the Michel deformity, in which there is a congenital agenesis of the cochlea, and the small internal auditory canal syndrome, in which the cochlear nerve may be congenitally absent.

Routine otoscopic evaluation of the tympanic membrane is performed. An otologically stable condition should be present prior to considering implantation in children. The ear proposed for cochlear implantation must be free of infection, and the tympanic membrane must be intact. If these conditions are not met, medical and/or surgical treatment prior to implantation is required.

Because children are more prone to otitis media than adults, justifiable concern has been expressed that a middle-ear infection could cause an implanted device to become an infected foreign body, requiring its removal. Of even greater concern is that infection might extend the electrode into the inner ear, resulting in a serious otogenic complication such as meningitis or further degeneration of the central auditory system. To date, although the incidence of otitis media in children who have received cochlear implants parallels that seen in the general pediatric population, no serious complications have occurred in our patients.

TREATMENT RECOMMENDATIONS

Surgical Implantation

Cochlear implantation in both children and adults requires meticulous attention to the delicate tissues and small dimensions. Skin incisions are designed to provide access to the mastoid process and coverage of the external portion of the implant package while preserving the blood supply of the postauricular skin. The incision employed at the Indiana University Medical Center has eliminated the need to develop a large postauricular flap. The inferior extent of the incision is made well posterior to the mastoid tip to preserve the branches of the postauricular artery. From here, the incision is directed posteriosuperiorly and then directed superiorly without a superior anterior limb. In children, the incision incorporates the temporalis muscle to give added thickness. A pocket is created for positioning the implant induction coil. Well anterior to the skin incision, the periosteum is incised from superior to inferior, and a posterior periosteal flap is developed. At the completion of the procedure, the posterior periosteal flap is sutured to the skin flap, compartmentalizing the induction coil from the skin incision. A bone well tailored to the device being implanted is created, and the induction coil is fixed to the cortex with a fixation suture or periosteal flaps.

Following the development of the skin incision, a mastoidectomy is performed. The horizontal semicircular canal is identified in the depths of the mastoid antrum, and the short process of the incus is identified in the fossa incudis. The facial recess is opened using the fossa incudis as an initial landmark. The facial recess is a triangular area bounded by (a) the fossa incudis superiorly, (b) the chorda tympani nerve laterally and anteriorly, and (c) the facial nerve medially and posteriorly. The facial nerve can usually be visualized through the bone without exposing it. The round window niche is visualized through the facial recess approximately 2 mm inferior to the stapes. Occasionally, the round window niche is posteriorly positioned and is not well visualized through the facial recess or is obscured by ossification. Particularly in these situations, it is important not to be misdirected by hypotympanic air cells. Entry into the scala tympani is best accomplished through a cochleostomy created anterior and inferior to the annulus of the round window membrane. A small fenestra slightly larger than the electrode to be implanted (usually 0.5 mm) is developed. A small diamond burr is used to "blue line" the endosteum of the scala tympani, and the endosteal membrane is removed with small picks. This approach bypasses the hook area of the scala tympani allowing direct insertion of the active electrode array. After insertion of the active electrode array, the round window is sealed with small pieces of fascia.

PEARLS AND PERILS

1. An otologically stable middle ear should be present prior to cochlear implantation. (Chronic perforations should be closed by standard tympanoplasty techniques; cholesteatomas must be controlled prior to implantation; ideally, tubes should be removed prior to implantation, so a normal tympanic membrane is present at the time of implantation.)
2. Ears with Mondini deformities are appropriate for implantation, but gushers should be anticipated and controlled if they occur.
3. Cochlear ossification following meningitis is not a contraindication to implantation.
4. A variety of skin incisions may be used, but meticulous care of the soft tissues is always imperative.
5. The active electrode should be introduced into the cochlea through a cochleostomy anterior to the round window to bypass the hook end of the cochlea.
6. Leave the facial nerve bone covered in the facial recess if possible.

Special Surgical Considerations

In cases of cochlear dysplasia, a CSF gusher may be encountered. The senior author prefers to enter the cochlea through a small fenestra and tightly pack the electrode at the cochleostomy with fascia. The flow of CSF has been successfully controlled in this way.

In patients with severe malformations of the labyrinth, the facial nerve may follow an aberrant course. In these cases, the most direct access to a common cavity deformity may be by a transmastoid labyrinthotomy approach. The otic capsule is opened posterosuperior to the second genu of the facial nerve, and the common cavity is entered directly. Four patients have been treated in this way with no vestibular side effects (17).

In cases of cochlear ossification, our preference is to drill open the basal turn and create a tunnel approximately 6 mm in length and partially insert a Nucleus electrode. This allows implantation of 10 to 12 active electrodes, which has yielded very satisfactory results. Gantz et al. (18) has described an extensive drill-out procedure to gain access to the upper basal turn. The benefits of this extended procedure are under investigation. Steenerson et al. (19) has described the insertion of the active electrode into the scala vestibuli in cases of cochlear ossification. This procedure has merit. However, the scala vestibuli is frequently ossified when the scala tympani is completely obliterated.

PERFORMANCE RESULTS IN CHILDREN

The assessment of speech perception abilities in children with cochlear implants has relevance in both the clinical and research domains. Speech perception assessment is clinically important because it allows the clinician to evaluate whether and to what degree improvement has occurred. This, in turn, influences decisions about adjustments that are made to the patient's speech processor program. The results of assessments are also useful in determining goals for aural rehabilitation training. From the research perspective, speech perception assessment yields empiric data regarding the benefits that can be derived from a cochlear implant and allows a comparison of the effectiveness of different sensory aids in this population. This information is also crucial in establishing cochlear implant candidacy criteria.

Postlingually deafened adults use the information transmitted by a cochlear implant to compare with previously stored representations of spoken language. Pediatric implant users, on the other hand, must rely on the same information to develop these representations first. Because of this, perceptual skills develop over a relatively long time course in prelingually deafened children (20–22). Substantial improvements in closed set word recognition usually did not occur in prelingually deafened children until after they had used their multichannel implants for more than 1 year, and improvements in open set speech recognition occurred after an even longer period of device use.

Performance With Multichannel Implants

The research design most commonly applied to evaluate implant speech perception benefit in children is a within-subject design wherein the subject serves as his or her own control in the pre- and postimplant conditions. The largest studies of this nature have been conducted as part of the FDA clinical trials of the Nucleus multichannel implant in children (23). After 12 months of multichannel implant use, Staller et al. (23) reported mean scores of 39% ($n = 84$) on a closed set word identification test, 23% ($n = 42$) on a test of open set sentence recognition, and 12% ($n = 25$) on a test of a test of open set, monosyllabic word recognition. Examination of individual data revealed that 13% of the subjects demonstrated significantly above chance closed set word identification before implantation, whereas, postoperatively, 62% of the subjects achieved this level of performance. Preoperatively, the subjects showed no open set speech recognition, but 12 months after implantation, 45% of the subjects recognized one or more words in sentences administered in an open set.

Pediatric implant performance is also reported in terms of clinically descriptive categories of benefit. Geers and Moog (24) developed a classification system that describes performance along a hierarchy of speech perception abilities: (1) no pattern perception, (2) consistent pattern perception, (3) inconsistent word identification, (4) consistent word identification, and (5) open set word recognition. Staller et al. (23) reported that the percentage of children reaching category 3 and above (i.e., closed or open set word recognition) increased from 12% to 80% postoperatively, and roughly half of the subjects demonstrated open set speech recognition and were assigned a category rating of 5. Osberger et al. (25) developed a similar classification scheme, modified to describe performance on the tests in their assessment battery, and reported that roughly one-half of the subjects demonstrated open set speech recognition after they had used their implants for an average of 2 years.

The time course over which perceptual skills emerge varies depending on the population under study. Postlingually deafened children who receive a cochlear implant are quite different from those of children with congenital or prelingually acquired deafness (26–28). Postlingually deafened children must map the new signals from the implant onto an existing base of auditory and linguistic knowledge, and most of these children show rapid progress in their listening skills within the first 6 months to 1 year of cochlear implant use. However, most children who receive a cochlear implant are either congenitally deaf or acquire their hearing loss early in life before speech and language skills are established. These children must use the signal provided via a cochlear implant to develop perceptual and expressive representations of spoken language. The ability to understand and to produce speech develops over a relatively long time course in children with prelingual hearing loss and may not be accomplished by all children in this group. Therefore, it is important to follow these children over an extended period to determine the eventual communication benefits to be obtained from cochlear implant use.

Speech perception abilities emerge in an overlapping fashion, rather than sequentially. On average, children with the Nucleus cochlear implant are able to recognize words from a closed set of responses at significantly better than chance levels only after about 1.5 years of device use (25,26,28,29). Mean scores for open set speech understanding through listening alone show gradual improvements within the first 2 years of device use and increase to approximately 40% by 4 years after implant (30). Substantial auditory–visual enhancement is seen prior to the time that children demonstrate closed or open set speech understanding in the auditory-only modality. Across all tasks, mean group scores increase over time, even up to 5 years after implant (28,29), suggesting that learning takes place over an extended time course. Finally, studies of children implanted at very early ages (less than 6 years) suggest that high levels of speech perception performance may be obtained by many of these children (31,32).

Variables Affecting Performance With Multichannel Cochlear Implants

Large individual differences among implanted children have been documented on speech perception measures. Some children demonstrated relatively high levels of speech recognition, whereas others perceived primarily prosodic speech information from their devices (23,25). Age at onset of deafness, duration of deafness before implantation, and educational setting are the independent variables most often examined to explain such performance differences. Studies by Staller et al. (23,26) reported that two factors, age at onset of deafness and duration of deafness, were significantly related to speech perception performance in children who used the Nucleus multichannel cochlear implant. They found that subjects with later onset and shorter duration of deafness performed better on measures of speech perception than did subjects with early onset of deafness but relatively long duration of deafness at the time of implantation.

The effect of age at onset of deafness on speech perception skills was examined by Osberger et al. (27) in children who received a single- or multichannel cochlear implant. No significant differences in the mean postoperative speech perception scores as a function of age at onset of deafness unless the subjects were postlingually deafened (i.e., onset of deafness at or after age 5) were found. Subjects with postlingual deafness achieved significantly higher speech perception scores on all measures than did the subjects with prelingual deafness (i.e., congenital or acquired deafness). In a more recent study that included only children with multichannel implants (i.e., Nucleus device) with prelingual deafness who were implanted before age 10, the results showed no significant difference between the speech perception scores of a group of subjects with congenital deafness and the mean scores of a second group of subjects with deafness acquired before age 3 years (33). The finding of a similar performance in children with both congenital and early acquired deafness is probably influenced by the secondary effects of meningitis (i.e., neurologic problems and cochlear ossification) on the performance of the children with acquired deafness. These results indicate that children who are born deaf have the potential to derive the same benefit from multichannel implants as do children who had some exposure to spoken language before the onset of their deafness from meningitis.

The postimplant performance of children with postlingual deafness (i.e., onset of deafness at age 5 or later) differs from that of children with prelingual deafness in several important respects. Children with relatively late onset of deafness typically show rapid and marked improvement in speech perception abilities with an implant (20,27). As noted earlier, speech perception performance improves very gradually in prelingually implanted children.

A significant relationship between the communication method used by the child and performance on speech perception measures has been shown by several investigations. In these studies, more children who used oral communication achieved higher levels of implant performance than did children who used total communication (i.e., signs plus speaking and listening) (25). The relationship between communication mode and implant performance is less clear in other studies. For example, Miyamoto et al. (33) found that children who used oral communication obtained significantly higher scores on only 2 of the 13 speech perception measures in their study. Additional research is needed to clarify this issue.

Comparison of Cochlear Implants, Hearing Aids, and Tactile Aids

Children with profound hearing impairments demonstrate a wide range of auditory capabilities (34). A within-subject research design is influenced by this variability, confounding the evaluation of various sensory aids. Therefore, the establishment of a control group is desirable. Using the results of previous investigators as a guide, Osberger et al. (35) developed a descriptive system to classify the range of hearing levels in children with profound hearing impairments. Hearing aid users were divided into three groups based on the unaided better ear pure-tone thresholds at 500, 1,000, and 2,000 Hz. Subjects classified as *Gold* hearing aid users demonstrated pure-tone thresholds of 90 to 100 dBHL at two of the three frequencies (with none of the thresholds greater than 105 dBHL). *Silver* hearing aid users demonstrated hearing levels of 101 to 110 dBHL at two of the three frequencies, whereas *Bronze* hearing aid users demonstrated two of three thresholds greater than 110 dBHL. Using this approach, the Gold hearing aid users were viewed as setting the "gold standard of performance" for children with profound hearing impairments because children with this amount of residual hearing developed the most intelligible speech. At the other end of the continuum were Bronze hearing aid users, who appeared to respond to auditory stimuli on the basis of vibrotactile sensation. To date, most children who have received implants would be classified as Bronze hearing aid users. The unaided pure-tone thresholds of the Silver hearing aid users were intermediate to those of the other two groups.

The benefits of multichannel cochlear implantation in prelingually deafened children can be demonstrated only by comprehensive longitudinal studies. Valid performance trends may be not become apparent for 1 to 3, or even more years, postoperatively. Studies in our laboratory have documented the ability of deaf children who were unable to even detect sound with conventional hearing aids preoperatively (Bronze hearing aid users) to achieve scores with their multichannel implants that were comparable to those of the Gold hearing aid users on most tests (except on a test of open set speech recognition).

The intermediate group of children, classified as Silver hearing aid users (i.e., pure-tone thresholds between 100 and 105 dBHL), clearly might derive more benefit from multichannel implants than from continued use of only hearing aids. Extension of implant candidacy to this group and even to selected Gold hearing aid users is the target of future research. Improved implant technology and earlier implantation promise to widen the candidacy window.

An important issue in sensory aid research with profoundly deaf children has been determination of the benefits derived from noninvasive alternatives to cochlear implants, such as tactile aids. The results of a recent study by Miyamoto et al. (36) demonstrated that children who used multichannel implants derived substantially more speech perception benefit from their devices than did children who used multichannel tactile aids. The performance of two groups of subjects who either received a Nucleus implant or a multichannel vibrotactile aid (Tactaid 7) were compared. There were ten subjects in each group, matched on the basis of age at onset of deafness, age fit with a multichannel device, and nonverbal intelligence. Subjects were tested on a battery of speech perception measures in the predevice interval and at one postdevice interval (i.e., after an average of roughly 1 1/2 years of device use). The results revealed that the scores of the implant users improved significantly between the pre- and postdevice intervals on all measures. Moreover, the scores of the Nucleus users were significantly higher than those of the Tactaid users on all measures. By contrast, the scores of the tactile aid users showed negligible change over time except on a test that evaluated open set recognition of phrases with both auditory *and* visual cues. The results suggested that children learned to recognize words and understand speech without lip reading with a multichannel implant, whereas children who used a multichannel tactile aid demonstrated evidence of speech recognition only if tactile cues were combined with visual ones.

Speech Production

Although the primary role of a cochlear implant is to make speech sounds accessible auditorily, cochlear implants also serve as aids to speech production. Osberger et al. (37) have demonstrated that profoundly hearing-impaired children's phonetic repertoires increase after receiving a multichannel cochlear implant. Improvements in the production of consonant and vowel features that are typically difficult for children with profound hearing losses to master have been documented (i.e., high vowels, diphthongs, alveolar consonants, and fricatives). Improvements in speech productions have also been documented by Tobey et al. (38).

Children who are postlingually deafened or those who are implanted at an early age generally demonstrated large improvements in speech, whereas those with early onset of deafess who are not implanted until adolescence typically show more limited improvements in speech production performance.

The scores for the implanted subjects showed gradual improvement over time. After 2.5 years of cochlear implant use, the average speech intelligibility of the implanted subjects began to exceed that of the Silver hearing aid users. After 3.5 to 4 years of device use, the average intelligibility of the implant users was 40%, which is approximately 20% higher than that of Silver hearing aid users. Most of the children in this study were not implanted until they were 5 to 8 years old. Further studies are under way to examine changes in speech intelligibility in children who were implanted at a younger age.

CONCLUSIONS

Controversial issues regarding cochlear implant technology and cochlear implant surgery require continuous reevaluation. Only through careful longitudinal studies of the performance of pediatric cochlear implant recipients will many of these issues be resolved.

ACKNOWLEDGMENTS

This work was supported in part by research grants 2 RO1 DC 00064-06, RO1 DC 00423, and KO8 DC 00126-02 from the National Institute on Deafness and Other Communication Disorders, National Institutes of Health.

REFERENCES

1. Clark GM, Blamey PJ, Brown AM, et al. The University of Melbourne Nucleus multi-electrode cochlear implant. *Adv Otol Rhinol Laryngol* 1987;38:1–181.

2. Schindler RA, Kessler DK, Rebscher SJ, Yanda JL, Jackler RK. The UCSF/Storz multichannel cochlear implant: patient results. *Laryngoscope* 1986;96:597–603.

3. Wilson BS, Finley CC, Lawson DT, Wolford RD, Eddington DK, Rabinowitz WM. Better speech recognition with cochlear implants. *Nature* 1991;352:236–237.

4. Schindler RA, Kessler DK, Barker, M. Clarion patient performance: an update on the clinical trials. *Ann Otol Rhinol Laryngol* 1995;104(Suppl 166):269–272.

5. Gstoettner WK, Baumgartner WD, Franz P, Hamzavi J. Cochlear implant deep-insertion surgery. *Laryngoscope* 1997;107:544–546.

6. Hochmair ES. Clinically relevant aspects of the high-rate CIS-speech coding strategy for cochlear implants. Abstracts of the First Asia Pacific Symposium on Cochlear Implant and Related Sciences. Abstract 19, p 47, 1996.

7. Matsushima JI, Shepard RK, Seldon HL, Xu SA, Clarl GM. Electrical stimulation of the auditory nerve in deaf kittens: effects on cochlear nucleus morphology. *Hear Res* 1991;56:133–42.

8. Yune HY, Miyamoto RT, Yune ME. Medical imaging in cochlear implant candidates. *Am J Otol* 1991;12[Suppl]:11–17.

9. Jensen S. Malformation of the inner ear in deaf children. *Acta Radiol* 1969;286[Suppl]:1–97.

10. Mangabeira-Albernaz PL. The Mondini dysplasia: from early diagnosis to cochlear implant. *Acta Otolaryngol* 1983;95:627–631.

11. Miyamoto RT, Robbins AM, Myres WA, Pope ML. Cochlear implantation in the Mondini inner ear malformation. *Am J Otol* 1986;7:258–261.

12. Jackler RK, Luxford WM, House WF. Sound detection with the cochlear implant in five ears of four children with congenital malformations of the cochlea. *Laryngoscope* 1987;97[Suppl 40]:15–17.

13. Silverstein H, Smouha E, Morgan N. Multichannel cochlear implantation in a patient with bilateral Mondini deformities. *Am J Otol* 1988;9:451–455.

14. Tucci DL, Telian SA, Zimmerman-Phillips MS, Zwolen TA, Ceyon PR. Cochlear implantation in patients with cochlear malformations. *Arch Otolaryngol Head Neck Surg* 1995;121:833–838.

15. Schuknecht HF. Mondini dysplasia: a clinical and pathological study. *Ann Otol Rhinol Laryngol* 1980;89[Suppl 65]:3–23.

16. Hinojosa R, Marion M. Histopathology of profound sensorineural deafness. *Ann NY Acad Sci* 1983;405:459–484.

17. McElveen JT, Carrasco VN, Miyamoto RT, Lormore KA, Brown C. Surgical approaches for cochlear implantation in patients with cochlear malformations. Presented at the Vth International Cochlear Implant Conference, New York City, May 1997.

18. Gantz BJ, McCabe BF, Tyler RS. Use of multichannel cochlear implants in obstructed and obliterated cochleas. *Otolaryngol Head Neck Surg* 1988;98:72–81.

19. Steenerson RL, Gary LB, Wynens MS. Scala vestibuli cochlear implantations for labyrinthine ossification. *Am J Otol* 1990;11:360–363.

20. Fryauf-Bertschy H, Tyler RS, Kelsay DM, Gantz BJ. Performance over time of congenitally deaf and postlingually deafened children using a multichannel cochlear implants. *J Speech Hear Res* 1992;35:913–920.

21. Miyamoto RT, Osberger MJ, Robbins AM, et al. Longitudinal evaluation of communication skills of children with single- or multichannel cochlear implants. *Am J Otol* 1992;13:215.

22. Waltzman SB, Cohen NL, Gomolin R, et al. Long-term results of early cochlear implantation in congenitally and prelingually deafened children. *Am J Otol* 1994;14[Suppl 2]:9–13.

23. Staller SJ, Dowell RC, Beiter AL, Brimacombe JA. Perceptual abilities of children with the Nucleus 22-channel cochlear implant. *Ear Hear* 1991;12[Suppl]:34S–47S.

24. Geers AE, Moog JS. *Early speech perception test.* St. Louis, MO: Central Institute for the Deaf, 1990.

25. Osberger MJ, Miyamoto RT, Zimmerman-Phillips S, et al. Independent evaluation of the speech perception abilities of children with the Nucleus 22-channel cochlear implant system. *Ear Hear* 1991;12[Suppl]:66S–80S.

26. Staller SJ, Beiter AL, Brimacombe JA, et al. Pediatric performance with the Nucleus 22-Channel Cochlear Implant System. *Am J Otol* 1991;12[Suppl]:126.

27. Osberger MJ, Todd SL, Berry SW, et al. Effect of age at onset of deafness on children's speech perception abilities with a cochlear implant. *Ann Otol Rhinol Laryngol* 1991; 100:883–888.

28. Gantz BJ, Tyler RS, Woodworth GG, Tye-Murray N, Fryauf-Bertschy H. Result of multichannel cochlear implants in congenital and acquired prelingual deafness in children: five year followup. *Am J Otol* 1994;15:1–7.

29. Miyamoto RT, Osberger MJ, Todd SL, et al. Variables affecting implant performance in children. *Laryngoscope* 1994;104:1120–1124.

30. Miyamoto RT, Kirk KI, Robbins AM, Todd S, Riley A. Speech perception and speech production skills of children with multichannel cochlear implants. *Acta Otolaryngol* (Stockh) 1996;116:240–243.

31. Waltzman SN, Cohen NL, Gomolin R, Shapiro WH, Ozdamar S, Hoffman R. Long-term results of early cochlear implantation in congenitally and prelingually deafened children. *Am J Otol* 1994;15[Suppl]:9–14.

32. Miyamoto RT, Kirk KI, Robbins AM, Todd S, Riley A, Pisoni DB. Speech perception and speech intelligibility in children with multichannel cochlear implants. *Adv Otorhinolaryngol* 1997;52:198–203.

33. Miyamoto RT, Osberger MJ, Robbins AM, et al. Prelingually deafened children's performance with the Nucleus multichannel cochlear implant. *Am J Otol* 1993;14:437–445.

34. Boothroyd A. Auditory perception of speech contrasts by subjects with sensorineural hearing loss. *J Speech Hear Res* 1984;27:134–144.

35. Osberger MJ, Maso M, Sam L. Speech intelligibility of children with cochlear implants, tactile aids, or hearing aids. *J Speech Hear Res* 1993;36:186–203.

36. Miyamoto RT, Robbins AM, Osberger MJ, et al. Comparison of tactile aids and cochlear implants in children with profound hearing impairments. *Am J Otol* 1995;16:8–13.

37. Osberger MJ, et al. Analysis of the spontaneous speech samples of children using a cochlear implant or tactile aid. *Am J Otol* 1991;12[Suppl]:151–164.

38. Tobey EA, Angelette S, Murchison C. Speech production performance in children with multichannel cochlear implants. *Am J Otol* 1991;12[Suppl]:165–173.

R.T. Miyamoto: Indiana University School of Medicine, and Riley Hospital, Indianapolis, Indiana 46032. • K.I. Kirk: Department of Otolaryngology—Head and Neck Surgery, Indiana University School of Medicine, Indianapolis, Indiana 46032.

• *Practical Pediatric Otolaryngology*
• edited by Robin T. Cotton and Charles M. Myer, III
• Lippincott-Raven Publishers, Philadelphia © 1999

Bone-Anchored Hearing Aids and Ear Prostheses

David W. Proops

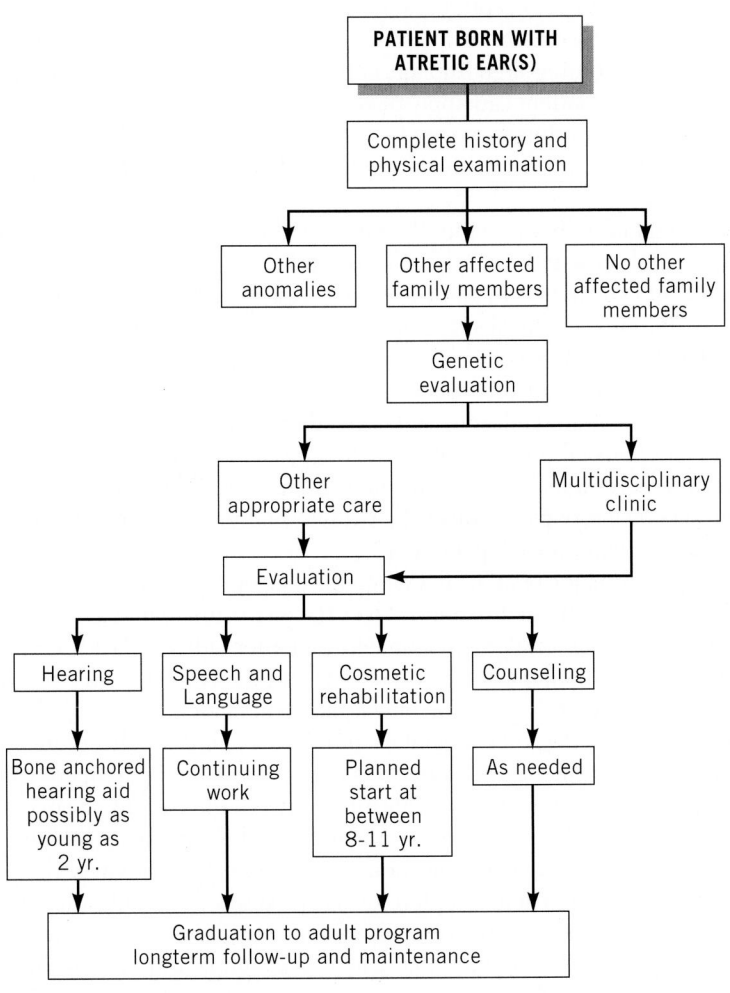

HISTORICAL BACKGROUND

Children born with congenital ear abnormalities produce enormous feelings of guilt in their parents. This is translated into anxiety to do something, and the physician may be put under great pressure by the naturally distraught family. Two approaches have traditionally been used (sometimes coordinated but rarely so). First, an otologist would attempt a middle-ear reconstruction, and then a plastic surgical approach would be made later to reconstruct the pinna.

The results of such treatment have not been generally successful, and middle-ear reconstructions have been particularly prone to operative complications with later restenosis and otorrhea (1,2). The problems were so great that Bellucci (3) stated in 1981 that surgery should not be attempted if the contralateral ear was normal. In 1977, Branemark et al. (4) announced the use of titanium implants in the treatment of the edentulous jaw. The discovery that titanium would form permanent nonfibrous union with bone opened up huge opportunities for prosthetic rehabilitation because of the stable fixation offered.

Soon the extraoral applications of this technique were reported by Tjellström et al. in 1983 (5). The first obvious application was for the prosthetic rehabilitation of those with missing ears, from surgical, traumatic, or congenital causes. The results of this technique are now widely used and form the simplest and most reliable method of rehabilitation (6).

The bone-anchored hearing aid is an ingenious combination of the bone-conducting hearing aid and the osseointegrated implant. Direct bone conduction was introduced by Tjellström et al. in 1980 (7) and is achieved by using a skin-penetrating coupling, from an osseointegrated implant in the mastoid bone, to an impedance matched transducer that the patient can apply or remove at will. The absence of interposed soft tissue (direct bone conduction) gives better quality sound, requires less energy, and offers much greater comfort (8). Results with the bone-anchored hearing aid have been reported (8–12).

Osseointegration thus provides the method whereby two major issues for those with congenital ear abnormalities can be addressed: hearing, by the use of a bone-anchored hearing aid, and cosmetics, by the use of an osseointegrated retained prosthesis. Three professional groups are involved: audiologists, maxillofacial prosthetists (anaplastologists), and otologists. When one recognizes that these children may also have speech and language delay, then the team expands to include speech therapy (pathology); finally, as these children are often syndromic and have other craniofacial abnormalities, clinical genetics and maxillofacial surgery may be included. The management of congenital ear abnormalities requires a team approach, and thus, it is sensible to organize joint clinics, so all the professional groups can meet the patients and their families and together formulate a treatment plan for each patient (13).

The first and major benefit of a clinic for congenital ear problems is that it allows new patients to meet treated patients. Over the years, the team has been impressed by the patient's or parents' excitement at meeting another individual with a similar problem. One of the major difficulties that our patients and their parents suffer is the feeling of isolation. They feel that they are the only afflicted individuals in the world.

The second advantage of congenital ear deformity clinics is that there are patients at various stages of treatment, which permits both patients and parents to gain a sense of orderliness and planned treatment. This often reduces the patient's or parental pressure for immediate action. The most important and overwhelming benefit of this clinic, however, is the guiding principle of education: in this context education of the parent by the patient. All patients seen and accepted for our program do so only after they have met, in private, another patient with a similar problem who has completed treatment. It is an understanding within the program that when they complete treatment the patients and parents will be asked to discuss their progress and results with the next patient. Doctors, technologists, and audiologists can talk endlessly with the patients, but the level of understanding of what is being said remains woefully low. It is often said that one picture is worth a thousand words. For the patient to see a completed prosthesis, with or without a bone-anchored hearing aid in position, is often the very best form of explanation that any new patient can require. A space is set aside in the clinic for old patients to meet new patients on their own. Privacy is important because there is considerable embarrassment about the congenitally deformed ear. It is vital that neither the surgeon or any member of the team be present during this discussion, so that there can be no pressure from the enthusiast. Before the decision to embark on the treatment is made, a time for reflection is necessary and the patient and relatives are encouraged to go away and think about what they have seen and heard.

The sequence of events can be summarized as follows:

1. Referral to the clinic
2. Attendance at the clinic with the whole team present
3. Surgical/audiologic and prosthetic assessment
4. New patients meet old patients in privacy
5. Team discussion/acceptance on the program
6. Stage one surgical procedure: placement of fixtures
7. Stage two: 3 months later, skin penetration/placement of abutments/thinning of flap
8. Stage three: fitting of prosthesis, or bone-anchored hearing aid, or both
9. Rehabilitation and review
10. Planned replacement program for both prosthesis and bone-anchored hearing aid (an assumed life of 2 years for the prosthesis and 3 to 5 years for the bone-anchored hearing aid)

PATIENT ASSESSMENT AND TREATMENT

To illustrate the algorithms of management, three cases will be used:

1. A child with nearly normal pinnae but with atretic ear canals, unable to wear a conventional hearing aid and at present aided by a conventional bone-conducting hearing aid.
2. A child with a unilateral atretic ear and normal hearing in the unaffected ear.
3. A child with severe Treacher Collins syndrome with bilateral atretic ears, cleft palate, and a maximum conductive hearing loss.

PEARLS AND PERILS

1. Hearing is rarely a worry in unilateral aural atresia.
2. In bilateral aural atresia, the hearing should be addressed before cosmesis.
3. Devise a plan for long-term management.
4. Complete management requires a multidisciplinary team.

Case 1

A 1-year-old male child was referred to a pediatric otolaryngologist after having failed several community hearing assessments. The parents are concerned with his apparent hearing loss, and his mother has noticed that his ear canals are very narrow. Pediatric audiology detects a conductive hearing loss, but bone conduction brainstem electric response audiometry confirms normal cochlear function. Otoscopy reveals narrow blind-ended external auditory meatuse, so a diagnosis of bilateral aural atresia is made. A computed tomography scan is not performed, as it will not contribute to short-term decision making and will subject the child to unnecessary radiation exposure and probably a general anesthetic.

The child is reviewed in a multidisciplinary clinic comprising audiology, otology, speech therapy (pathology), and clinical genetics specialists. The following treatment plan is formulated:

1. Fit the child with a conventional bone-conducting hearing aid immediately.
2. Monitor speech and language progress.
3. Offer genetic advice and counseling to the parents.

4. Undertake an evaluation for suitability for a bone-anchored hearing aid at 2 years plus.
5. Evaluate the options for otosurgical management of the meatal stenosis at between 5 and 7 years.

Case 2

A 2-year-old girl is brought in by her parents with unilateral aural atresia. She was also noted to be short necked and to hold her head tilted toward the affected ear. Her parents had noticed mild facial asymmetry made worse when she smiles or cries, and the mother also noted a white lesion on the globe of her eye on the affected side. The parents' greatest concern is the reaction of others to their daughter's absent ear; they wish something to be done before she starts attending kindergarten. Pediatric audiology confirms a complete conductive hearing loss in the affected ear, and otoscopy confirms a normal contralateral ear but a severe atresia of the affected ear with a linear cartilage-containing ear remnant situated more anteriorly and inferiorly than the normal ear. There is no sign of an external auditory canal. A clinical diagnosis of Goldenhar syndrome is made (Fig. 1).

The child is reviewed in a multidisciplinary clinic, comprising otology, audiology, speech therapy (pathology), clinical genetics, and maxillofacial surgery specialists. A treatment plan is formulated to:

1. Confirm the diagnosis of Goldenhar syndrome and offer the parents genetic counseling
2. Reassure the parents that although the child is monaural, the hearing in the unaffected ear is normal and at the moment nothing need be done about hearing except close monitoring of the normal, unaffected ear
3. Discuss the implications of the incomplete facial palsy and epibulbar dermoid neither of which will be amenable to or need intervention except explanation
4. Discuss the shortening of the mandibular ramus and possible consequences on the dentition; mention the possibility of distraction techniques of the mandibular ramus and the timing of such procedures if required
5. Investigate the palatal function on the affected side and discuss the possibility of nasal regurgitation of fluids and possible hypernasality of speech
6. Discuss the option for cosmetic rehabilitation of the affected ear, including the "do nothing" option, plastic surgical reconstruction techniques, or the use of osseointegrated retained prostheses; both surgical techniques are unlikely to be offered until the child is at least 8 years of age and later if possible.
7. Address the parents' huge guilt head on; this naturally manifests in anxiety as to the the way the child is seen by others needs and offer appropriate support; this is a classic case of "manage the parents first and the child afterwards."

Case 3

The neonatologists request an opinion on a recently born male child with severe Treacher Collins syndrome (Fig. 2). The child is intubated because of respiratory distress and has absent ears and a cleft palate. The first imperative is the airway; trials of extubation fail, and thus a tracheostomy is performed to secure the airway so that the child can be removed from the pediatric intensive care unit. The child is referred to the cleft palate team, a feeding plate is fitted, and plans are made for the closure of the cleft palate.

Simultaneously, the child is referred to the congenital ear problems clinic and assessed by otology, audiology, maxillofacial surgery, speech therapy (pathology), and clinical genetics. A treatment plan is formulated:

1. Pediatric audiology is conducted including bone conduction brainstem evoked response audiometry to evaluate the cochlear function and a conventional bone con-

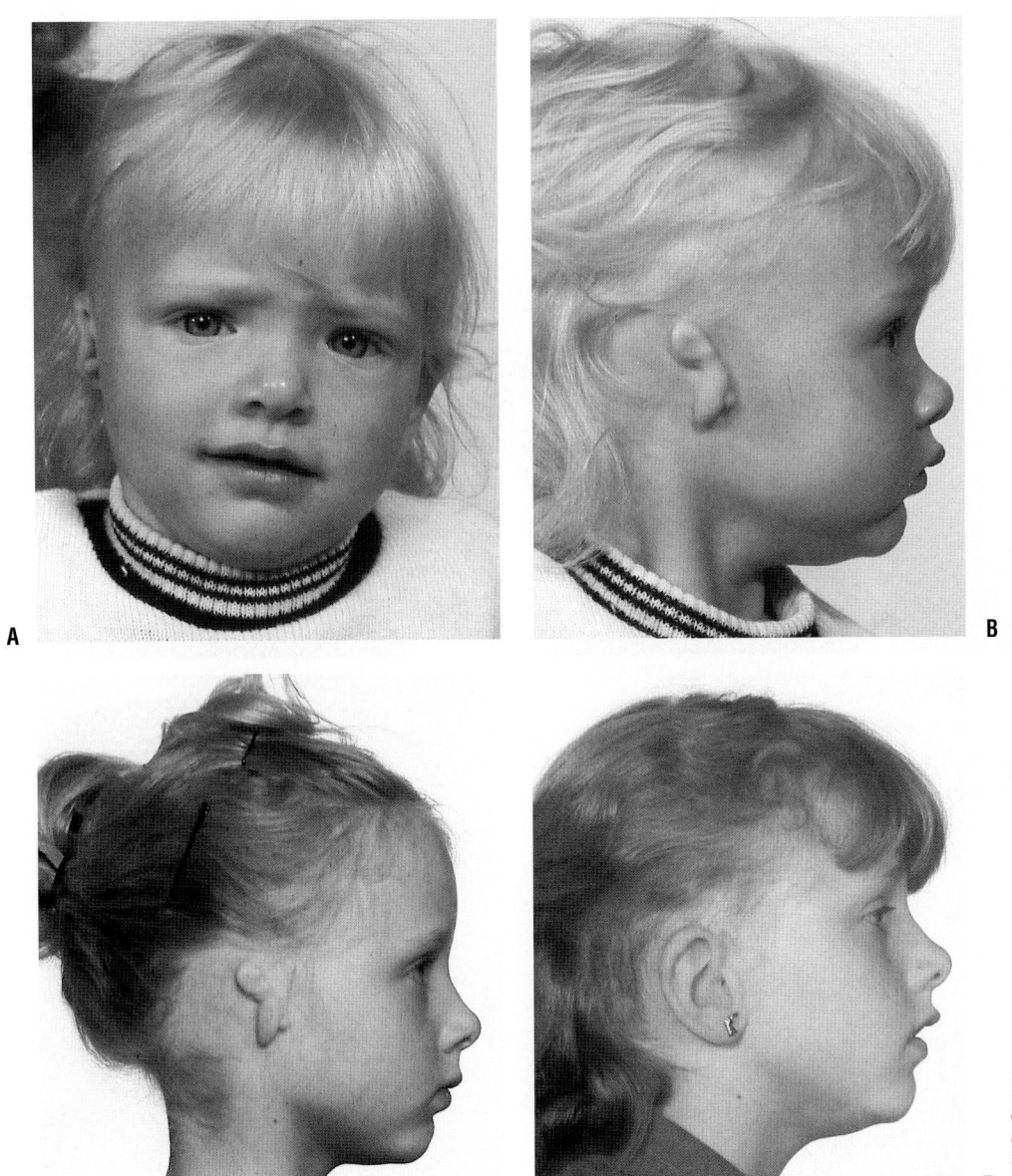

FIGURE 1 A,B: A 2-year-old child with Goldenhar syndrome and right atretic ear. **C, D:** Pre- and postoperative view with auricular prosthesis.

ducting hearing aid is fitted as soon as possible. The parents are counseled as to long-term aid and the provision of a bone-anchored hearing aid as soon as possible and hopefully as young as 2 years.

2. Speech therapy involvement early on because the child has four distinct but compounding problems: (a) the tracheostomy, which may be maintained for a moderate term, so the child must be helped and encouraged to vocalize; (b) the cleft palate, which will pose particular problems for the speech therapist; (c) the severe conductive hearing loss, which will have an inevitable affect on speech and language development; and (d) the retracted mandible and crowded tongue, which produce a particular pattern of sound systems and require superspecialist advice.

3. Clinical genetic advice is vital early on to answer the parental questions.

4. Long-term management of facial problems should be jointly decided by the otologist, maxillofacial surgeon, patient, and parents. Auricular prostheses will most likely be offered using osseointegration at around 10 years. Mandibular advancement and maxillary augmentations will most likely take place in the late teens.

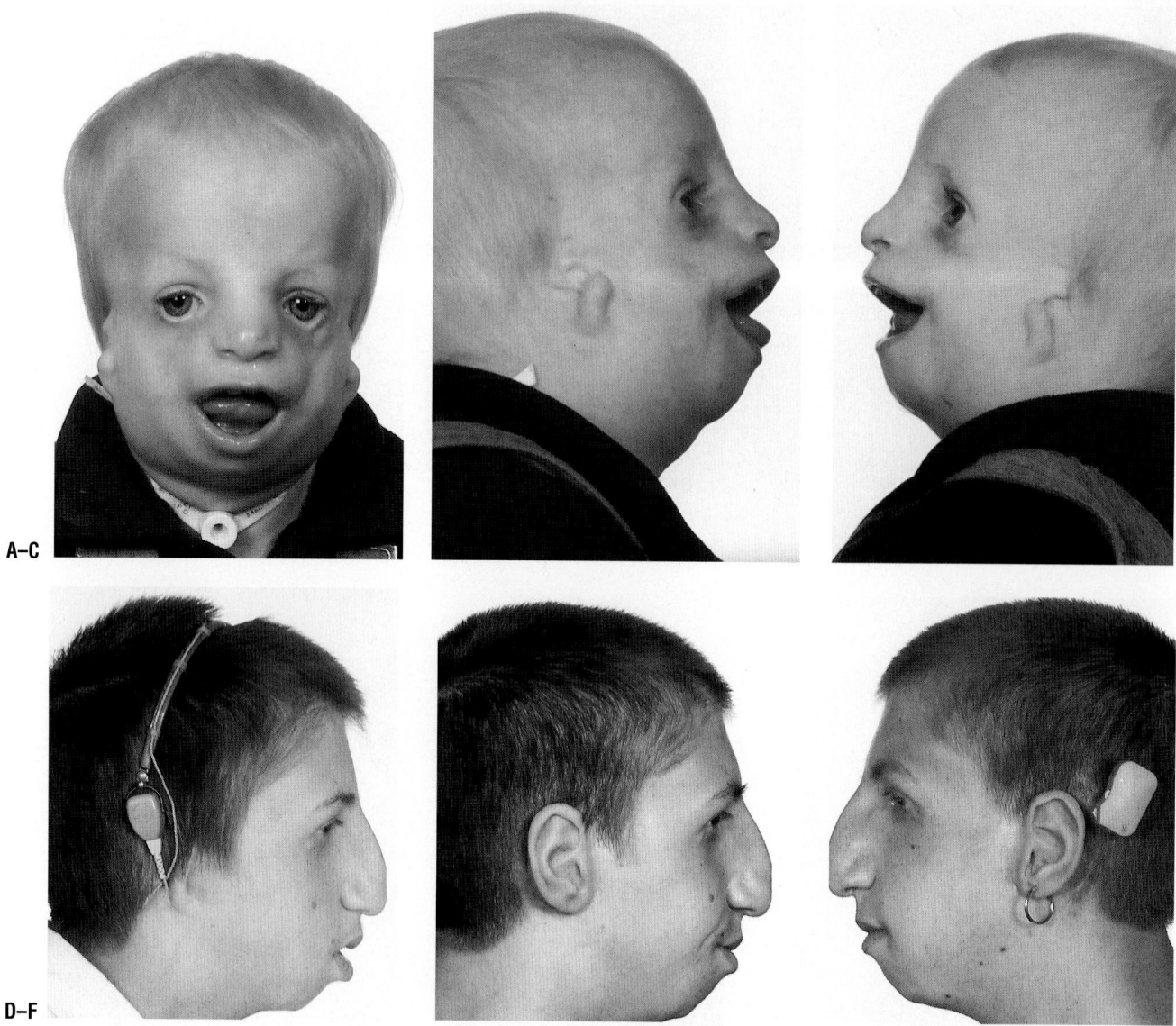

FIGURE 2 A–C: Child with severe Treacher Collins syndrome, tracheostomy, and bilateral absent ears. **D–F:** Young teenager with severe Treacher Collins syndrome who has been rehabilitated with bilateral auricular prostheses and a bone-anchored hearing aid.

🔅 MANAGEMENT OF COMPLICATIONS

Once the decision to use osseointegration as the basis of the rehabilitation process, then the complications fall into three categories: operative difficulties, failure of integration, and soft tissue reactions.

PEARLS AND PERILS

1. Manage the parents and then manage the child.
2. A consistent and positive approach must be taken with patients and parents.
3. Multidisciplinary clinics allow all the relevant professionals to make a contemporaneous contribution and formulate an agreed treatment plan.
4. Long-term management must form part of the assessment.

Operative Difficulties

In young children, there may not be a great thickness of calvarial bone. This problem has been addressed in various ways, the simplest being to continue to drill guide holes until adequate bone is located. If there is still only 2 mm of bone, then the fixture can be left proud and the flange fixture packed around with bone chip, or alternatively, the proud fixture can be covered with Gortex membrane, which is osteoneogenic. Recently, however, satisfactory results have been obtained by placing the fixture to full depth, displacing the dura. Inadvertent entry to the lateral venous sinus need not cause alarm as the bleeding is easily stopped with a soft tissue plug.

Failure of Integration

This may be primary when the fixture fails to become integrated and is presumably due to a failure of technique. Late loss of previously well-integrated fixtures is very disturbing and much more common with a bone-anchored hearing aid than with a prosthesis. The overall fixture failure rate in the Birmingham series is 10.1%, but the young and syndromic patients have a higher loss. This can be obviated by placing two fixtures and only loading one, thus leaving a sleeper to be used if necessary.

Soft Tissue Reactions

The importance of thinning the subcutaneous tissues and producing immobility of the skin surrounding the skin penetrating implant is paramount (14). Regular cleaning is vital to maintain the health of surrounding skin, and the ability to cope with this regular hygiene should be a major determinent when offering this therapy. Generally, this is not a major problem with children who have parents habituated to the responsibility of hygiene for their children.

PEARLS AND PERILS

1. Skull thickness problems can be overcome by planning and experience.
2. Plan placement and use templates.
3. Some fixture failures are inevitable and can be salvaged by using sleepers.
4. Successful soft tissue management depends on good surgical reduction and meticulous patient hygiene.

CONCLUSIONS

Bone-anchored hearing aids and prostheses have made a dramatic improvement in the management of children with congenital ear defects. The key to success in this work is a focused multidisciplinary team undertaking this work regularly in a planned and long-term fashion. This work should not be undertaken by the occasional dabbler. The primary guiding principle should be to benefit the patients, and management of parental guilt is the key to successful long-term care.

Congenital ear abnormalities account for 1 in 10,000 new births. This means that these patients are best treated in a small number of centers based on a large population. The ability to work in teams whose members offer each other mutual respect is vital, and the outcomes are then rewarding for all concerned.

● REFERENCES

1. Fenner T, Wachter I, Fisch U. Atresia auris congenita, Probleme und Resultate des Operation therapie. In: *Aktuelle probleme der otorhinolaryngologie.* Besn: Verlag Hans Hubert, 1981.

2. Colman BH. *Congenital deformities of the ear.* Chicago: The International Otology Workshop, 1976.

3. Bellucci RJ. Congenital aural malformations: diagnosis and treatment. *Otolaryngol Clin North Am* 1981;14:95–124.

4. Banemark PI, Hanson BO, Adell R, Breine U, Lindström J, Hallew O. Osseointegrated implants in the treatment of the edentulous jaw. *Scand J Plast Reconstruct Surg* 1997; (Suppl)II:11–16.

5. Tjellström A, Rosenhall U, Lindström J, Hallam O, Albrektsson T, Branemark PI. Five year experience with skin penetrating implants in the temporal bone. *Acta Otolaryngol* 1983;95:568–575.

6. Tjellström A, Jacobbson M, Albrektsson T, Janson K. Use of tissue integrated implants in congenital aural malformations. *Adv Otol Rhinol Laryngol* 1988;40:24–32.

7. Tjellström A, Hakannson B, Ludström J. Analysis of the mechanical impedance of bone anchored hearing aids. *Acta Otolaryngol* 1980;89:85–92.

8. Tjellström A, Ganstrom G. Long term follow up with the bone anchored hearing aid: a review of the first 100 patients between 1977–1985. *Ear Nose Throat J* 1994;73:112–114.

9. Cremers CWRJ, Snik AFM, Beynon AJ. Hearing with the bone anchored hearing aid (BAHA) compared to a conventional bone conducting hearing aid. *Clin Otolaryngol* 1992;17:275–279.

10. Mylanus EAM. The bone anchored hearing aid: clinical and audiological aspects. Thesis, Proesfchrifa Nijmegen, Netherlands, 1994.

11. Proops DW. The Birmingham bone anchored hearing aid programme: surgical methods and complications. *J Laryngol Otol* 1996;Supp. 7–12.

12. Powell, RH, Burrell SP, Cooper HR, Proops DW. The Birmingham bone anchored hearing aid programme paediatric experience and results. *J Laryngol Otol* 1996 (Suppl): 4–29.

13. Stevenson DS, Proops DW, Wake MJC, Deadman MJ, Worrollo SJ, Hobson JA. Osseointegration implants in the management of childhood ear abnormalities: the initial Birmingham experience. *J Laryngol Otol* 1993; 107:502–509.

14. Holgers KM, Tjellström A, Bjursten LM, Erlandsson BE. Soft tissue reaction around percutaneous implants: a clinical study of the soft tissue conditions around skin penetrating implants for bone anchored hearing aids. *Am J Otol* 1988;9:56–59.

D.W. Proops: Department of Otolaryngology, University Hospital, Birmingham B15 2TH, United Kingdom.

• *Practical Pediatric Otolaryngology*
• edited by Robin T. Cotton
  and Charles M. Myer, III
• Lippincott-Raven Publishers,
  Philadelphia © 1999

Audiometric Screening

Gayle P. Riemer

Audiometric screening is based on the same principles that govern the screening guidelines for any other condition: identification and prevention. The purpose of pediatric audiometric screening is to identify which children need further audiologic assessment. According to the American Speech-Language-Hearing Association (ASHA), audiometric screening is also preventative because "if a hearing disorder, impairment, or disability is detected and treated early, potential hearing-related problems can be prevented or ameliorated" (1).

When considering audiometric screening, you must consider first what condition is being screened and what can be done to completely diagnose and treat the condition. Are the tools for accurate diagnosis available, and once the condition is identified, are there treatment resources that are available and effective? Does the condition, if left untreated, represent a significant burden to the individual and society?

The appropriateness of screening for hearing disorders is well documented (1–4). The incidence of hearing disorders is great enough to warrant screening (Table 1) (4), and treatment is effective (see Chapter 17). Who, then, should perform hearing screenings? According to the AHSA guidelines (1), it should be audiologists with the Certificate of Clinical Competence (CCC-A) from ASHA and state licensure where applicable or support personnel under the supervision of an audiologist.

PEARLS AND PERILS

"Professional accountability and liability refer to the responsibility of the audiologist who develops, implements, and supervises the screening program to ensure appropriate patient care in all activities. These guidelines recommend that an audiologist be responsible for program accountability. Other personnel may perform the screening procedure." (1).

Consider, then, if you are going to screen for auditory disorders, what population you will be screening, which specific disorders you wish to rule out, and what screening tools have the sensitivity and specificity to identify those at risk. ASHA recommends the screening of all children, birth through 18 years, for any hearing impairment that may adversely affect the development of the auditory nervous system or the social, emotional, cognitive, and academic development (1).

NEWBORN HEARING SCREENING

The definition of hearing impairment is any hearing threshold level greater than 20 decibels (dBHL), including unilateral or bilateral, sensorineural or conductive loss. The

TABLE 1: Estimated Number of Infants with Hearing Impairment in Two Populations: Infants with No Known Risk Factors and Infants at High Risk

Category	Number Born Annually	Prevalence	Total Number of Hearing Impaired
No known risk	3,600,000	3 : 1,000	10,800
At high risk	400,000	30 : 1,000	12,000
Total	4,000,000	5.7 : 1,000	22,800

newborn screening tools available at this time, however, most reliably detect hearing impairments of greater than 30 dBHL. This is viewed as sufficient to rule out peripheral hearing disorders that will most adversely affect communication, development, and education (1,2).

The 1993 National Institutes of Health consensus statement recommended a two-stage screening process for identification of hearing loss in infants: initial screening using evoked otoacoustic emissions (EOAEs) and second-stage screening using auditory brain stem responses (ABRs) for those who fail the EOAE test. ASHA's 1997 *Guidelines for Audiologic Screening*, however, go on to recommend screening "using one or two recommended physiologic measures" (1). Throughout the United States, programs exist that utilize EOAEs, ABRs, or both effectively and research continues to support their use (5–8). The following information was adapted from the 1997 ASHA guidelines (1).

The recommended procedures are as follows:

1. ABRs
   a. Use either operator-controlled or automated ABRs.
   b. Note that the recommended stimulus conditions include presentation of air-conducted click stimuli to each ear at 35 dB normalized hearing level (nHL) or lower, with a stimulus rate upper limit of 37 per second.
   c. Alternating polarity may be appropriate in screening applications when the presence or absence of wave V is the only criterion used to determine a pass/refer outcome.
   d. For automated ABRs, the number of repetitions will be determined automatically by the manufacturer's protocol. For operator-controlled ABRs, a minimum of 1,000 repetitions is required under optimal recording conditions to yield reliable screening results. In less optimal recording conditions, more repetitions may be required.
   e. Wave V amplitude is enhanced in the neonate when a high-pass filter of 30 Hz is used and if an electrode montage of F_z–nape of neck rather than F_z–ipsilateral ear configuration is used.
2. Otoacoustic emissions
   a. Otoacoustic emission screening protocols vary. Either transient evoked (TEOAEs) or distortion product otoacoustic emissions (DPOAEs) may be appropriate for neonatal screening.
   b. For TEOAEs, the suggested stimulus conditions are broad-band clicks presented at 50 to 80 per second at 80 dB sound pressure level (SPL).
   c. For DPOAEs, the suggested stimulus conditions are f2/f1 = 1.2, with f2 at 2, 3, and 4 kHz; L2 = 55 dB SPL; L1 = 65 dB SPL.
   d. Remove the probe if a response is not seen, and inspect for debris before reinserting. Alternatively, the probe should be removed and visual inspection with an otoscope should be performed before the probe is reinserted.

An ABR should be considered a "pass" if a reliable evoked response is present at 35 dBHL or lower. The EOAE result should be considered a "pass" if an acceptable signal-to-noise ratio or reproducibility is reached. More stringent pass/refer criteria are anticipated as research in the use of otoacoustic emissions continues.

Behavioral screening procedures are not recommended as accurate predictors of hearing impairment for neonates or very young infants (3). Likewise, the screening of only high-risk newborns (as many states still mandate) will identify only slightly more than half of the infants who are born with significant peripheral hearing loss (4) (see Table 1).

INFANT, TODDLER, AND PRESCHOOL HEARING SCREENING

While the identification of peripheral hearing losses greater than 30 dBHL is appropriate for newborns, the older infant or preschool child with even minimal hearing loss should be identified and referred for habilitative services. The accepted definition for hearing impairment as greater than 20 dBHL and screening for hearing loss that exceeds 20 to 30 dBHL should be adhered to. The most effective frequencies to be screened are 1,000, 2,000, and 4,000 Hz. There are accurate screening tools available to meet these criteria, but the ASHA guidelines (1) do suggest that screening of preschoolers age 7 months through 2 years be performed by audiologists who hold the Certificate of Clinical Competence from ASHA and state licensure where applicable. Older preschoolers, ages 3 to 5 years, should be screened by either audiologists or support personnel who work under the supervision of audiologists.

Any preschooler who has not passed a newborn hearing screening should be screened. Preschoolers who have previously passed a newborn screening should be rescreened if they have indicators associated with progressive, fluctuating, or acquired hearing loss (3). Indicators listed in the ASHA guidelines (1) include the following:

1. Parent/care provider or health-care provider expresses concerns regarding hearing, speech, language, or developmental delay based on observation or standardized developmental screening;
2. Craniofacial anomalies, including those with morphologic abnormalities of the pinna and ear canal;
3. Birth weight less than 1,500 g (3.3 lb);
4. Hyperbilirubinemia at a serum level requiring exchange transfusion;
5. Ototoxic medications, including but not limited to chemotherapeutic agents or aminoglycosides, used in multiple courses or in combination with loop diuretics;
6. Bacterial meningitis and other infections associated with sensorineural hearing loss;
7. Apgar scores of 0 to 4 at 1 minute or 0 to 6 at 5 minutes;
8. Mechanical ventilation lasting 5 days or longer;
9. Stigmata or other findings associated with a syndrome known to include sensorineural or conductive hearing loss;
10. Head trauma associated with loss of consciousness or skull fracture;
11. Family history of hereditary childhood sensorineural hearing loss;
12. In utero infection, such as cytomegalovirus infection, rubella, syphilis, herpes, and toxoplasmosis;
13. Recurrent or persistent otitis media with effusion for at least 3 months;
14. Neurofibromatosis type II or neurodegenerative disorders; and
15. Anatomic disorders that affect eustachian tube function.

Care should be taken to have those children monitored who are at risk for progressive or fluctuating sensorineural or conductive hearing impairment (at least every 6 months until age 3 years and regular intervals after that, depending on the risk factor) (3).

By the *developmental* age of 7 months, most infants can be conditioned using visual reinforcement audiometry (VRA) with sounds presented either through headphones (conventional or insert) or in a soundfield (where the sounds are presented through speakers mounted in a sound-treated test room). By the *developmental* age of 2½ years, most toddlers can be conditioned to respond under headphones by using conditioned play audiometry. The ASHA guidelines (1) suggest using 30 dBHL as a pass/refer criterion for VRA and 20 dBHL as a pass/refer criterion for conditioned play audiometry.

VRA requires a setup of an audiometer with at least one speaker and headphones, as well as at least one toy, preferably two, that can be lighted or animated as the "reinforcer" to a response. The response observed is typically a head turn toward the reinforcer. If the infant or child will not cooperate for testing using headphones (conventional or insert), soundfield localizations are considered a valid screening procedure. It should be noted, however, that a unilateral hearing loss may not be ruled out completely unless some responses are obtained under headphones.

Conditioned play audiometry involves the use of a toy (often a can of blocks or set of stacking rings) and an audiometer. The child is asked to respond with an action ("put the block in the can") each time a stimulus is heard.

Older infants and preschoolers who are unable to cooperate for VRA or conditioned play may require an ABR or EOAE screening to rule out a hearing loss. EOAEs may prove particularly useful because ABR testing in older infants and children may require sedation in order to obtain accurate results. EOAEs require that the child remain quiet and calm, whereas an evoked potential evaluation like ABR is accurate only when the infant or child lies still and relaxed with eyes closed throughout.

PEARLS AND PERILS

The following are examples of screening "tools" that are *not recommended* (1):
1. Noncalibrated signals, such as rattles, music boxes, noisemakers
2. Nonconditioned behavioral procedures, such as behavioral observation audiometry
3. Signals that lack frequency specificity, such as music, broadband noise
4. Speech stimuli in lieu of frequency-specific stimuli

HEARING SCREENING FOR SCHOOL-AGE CHILDREN

School-age children who have not been previously identified as hearing impaired, and therefore are not receiving regular audiologic management, should have a hearing screening if, according to the ASHA guidelines, any of the following indicators are present:

1. Parent/care provider, health-care provider, teacher, or other school personnel have concerns regarding hearing, speech, language, or learning abilities;
2. Family history of late- or delayed-onset hereditary hearing loss;
3. Recurrent or persistent otitis media with effusion for at least 3 months;
4. Craniofacial anomalies, including those with morphologic abnormalities of the pinna and ear canal;
5. Stigmata or other findings associated with a syndrome known to include sensorineural or conductive hearing loss;
6. Head trauma with loss of consciousness; and
7. Reported exposure to potentially damaging noise levels or ototoxic drugs.

Screening procedures for school-age children can be very similar to adult procedures, with a simple behavioral response to a stimulus (such as raising a hand or pushing a response button). Frequencies to be screened should include, at least, 1,000, 2,000, and 4,000 Hz. Many screening programs also include 500 Hz but care should be taken to ensure that the environment is quiet enough that there is not too much low-frequency ambient noise to screen accurately at this frequency. The intensity used for screening should be 20 dBHL at all frequencies (1).

Screening programs for school-age children should be performed or supervised by certified and licensed audiologists (1). In the opinion of this author, many school programs and pediatrician offices employ nurses or supportive personnel who are quite adept at hearing screening, but personnel employed in this capacity should, at least initially, be trained by certified, licensed audiologists.

If a school-age child does not pass a hearing screening, a rescreening should be performed within the same screening session. Failure to respond at 20 dBHL at 1,000, 2,000, and 4,000 Hz means that the child should be referred to an audiologist for a diagnostic assessment.

The use of EOAEs as a screening tool for school-age children is only in the research stages. EOAEs are sensitive to both hearing impairment and middle-ear disorders, so it shows some promise as a screening tool. Pass/refer criteria do not yet exist but the sensitivity and specificity make EOAEs a potential cost-effective tool for the future (9).

SCREENING FOR OUTER- AND MIDDLE-EAR DISORDERS

Primary-care practitioners should regularly screen for these disorders as part of well-care visits. Infants and children under the care of a physician for known outer- or middle-ear disorders should not participate in other organized screening programs for these disorders.

There are many existing programs, however, that do screen for these disorders in conjunction with their hearing screening protocols for preschool and school-age children. Screenings should be conducted by certified audiologists or support personnel under the supervision of certified audiologists. For these programs, the following procedures are recommended by the ASHA guidelines (1):

1. When possible, obtain a case history through verbal report of parent or guardian.
2. Visually inspect the ears to identify risk factors for outer- and middle-ear disease and to ensure that no contraindications exist for performing tympanometry (e.g., drainage, foreign bodies, tympanostomy tubes).
3. As training and scope of practice permit, use a lighted otoscope or video-otoscope to examine the external ear canal and tympanic membrane for obvious obstructions or structural defects.
4. As training and scope of practice permit, perform tympanometry with a low-frequency (220-, 226-Hz) probe tone and a positive to negative air pressure sweep.

Referral criteria, as suggested by the ASHA guidelines (1), are as follows:

1. Ear drainage is observed.
2. Visual identification of previously undetected structural defect(s) of the ear occurs.
3. Ear canal abnormalities such as obstructions, impacted cerumen or foreign objects, blood or other secretions, stenosis or atresia, otitis externa, and perforations or other abnormalities of the tympanic membrane are apparent.
4. Tympanometric equivalent ear canal volume is greater than 1.0 cm^3 accompanied by a flat tympanogram (i.e., there is no admittance peak) to select those at risk for tympanic membrane perforation. Do not refer if a tympanostomy tube is in place or if a perforation of the tympanic membrane is under management of a physician.
5. Follow-up tympanometric screening test results (at 6 to 8 weeks) are outside the test criteria presented in Table 2 (1).

Universal screening for middle-ear disease is not as widely accepted as screening for hearing impairment, but a 1994 panel of the U.S. Department of Health and Human Services (10) recommended that identification and treatment of outer- and middle-ear disorders are critical. Failure according to the above-mentioned screening criteria should result in immediate referral to the primary-care physician.

TABLE 2: Recommended Initial Tympanometric Screening Test Criteria

Infants[a]	One Year to School Age[b]
$Y_{tm} < 0.2$ mmho	$Y_{tm} < 0.3$ mmho[c]
or TW > 235 daPa	or TW > 200 daPa

mmho, millimho; daPa, decapascal; TW, tympanometric width; Y_{tm}, peak admittance.

[a]Infants: Roush, Bryant, Mundy, Zeisel, and Roberts, 1995 (16).

[b]Older Children: Nozza, Bluestone, Kardatzke, and Bachman, 1992; 1994 (17).

[c]For children > 6 yr, when using ± 400 daPa for compensation of ear canal volume, $Y_{tm} < 0.4$ mmho is the recommended criterion.

SCREENING FOR CENTRAL AUDITORY PROCESSING DISORDERS

There are no universal screening programs for central auditory processing disorders (CAPDs) known to this author. Most children at risk for CAPDs are referred for audiologic assessment by parents, teachers, physicians, or other professionals who identify a child with learning problems that appear to involve poor auditory skills. Central auditory processing is best defined as "what we do with what we hear" (11), which is a very global, but very essential element to communication and education. One would think this aspect of audition would be at least as critical as peripheral hearing sensitivity. Screening for this should be part of any developmental assessment, but problems arise in trying to design tools that can accurately screen for CAPDs.

The best "screening" for CAPDs lies in the hands of the audiologist who receives a referral for evaluating the child who "doesn't hear very well" but demonstrates an intact peripheral auditory system. The child who has difficulty with age-appropriate test strategies or has difficulty localizing in a soundfield may be a young child at risk for CAPD. Parent and teacher complaints that the child just does not respond appropriately, does not do well in the presence of background noise, or has trouble following directions are red flags that this child may be at risk. Pediatric audiologists frequently test preschoolers who are referred because their speech is delayed and they have a history of otitis media. Some of these children are certainly at risk for CAPD (12), and some should be monitored over time to consider intervention when appropriate.

Bellis (13) presented a list of indicators that can be used to screen children for CAPD referral. Any combination of indicators would certainly warrant referral to a pediatric audiologist for a central auditory processing evaluation:

- Behaves as if peripheral hearing loss is present, despite normal hearing.
- Demonstrates significant scatter across subtests within domains assessed by speech-language and psychoeducational tests, with weaknesses in auditory-dependent areas.
- Verbal IQ scores often lower than performance scores.
- Requires high degree of external organization in the classroom.
- Exhibits difficulty following multistep directions.
- Exhibits poor reading and spelling skills.
- May refuse to participate in class discussions or respond inappropriately.
- May be withdrawn or sullen.
- Exhibits a positive history of chronic otitis or other otologic or neurologic sequelae.
- May exhibit poor singing and music skills.
- Fine- or gross-motor skills may be deficient.

There are also formal screening tools that have been developed for use with school-age children who are at risk for CAPD. Two standardized tests, the SCAN: A Screening Test for Auditory Processing Disorders (14) and the Selective Auditory Attention Test (SAAT) (15), are designed to quickly screen for CAPDs. Both of these tests should be administered by audiologists. The best screening for CAPDs, however, continues to be a thorough case history and a team approach with the parents and other professionals who work with the child.

PARENT AND CHILD EDUCATION

A key component of any screening program should be providing education about the disorder. Educational materials should be provided that address the importance of identifying the disorder, the likelihood of any given child having the disorder, and what follow-up is available for the child if a disorder is identified. The best screening tool of all has always been the parents who suspect their child may have a hearing problem. Providing education (which may be as simple as brochures in their doctor's office or community awareness programs) may be one effective way to get infants and children to the screening programs that are available.

PEARLS AND PERILS

"At present, 70 percent of children with acquired hearing impairments are initially identified by parents. *Parental concern about hearing should be sufficient reason to initiate prompt formal hearing evaluation*" (2).

SUMMARY

Failure to identify significant hearing loss at a very early age will result in potentially severe effects on a child's ability to communicate, develop, learn, and relate to others. The results of delaying identification are costly to society and may be irreparable. The goal of any audiometric screening program is to identify the auditory disorder before the effects of the disorder have serious long-term consequences. Early identification through universal newborn screening is only part of our responsibility. We must also diligently look for the hearing disorders that are acquired later or whose subtleties manifest themselves later (like CAPDs).

Researchers in the field of audiology have provided us with the tools we need to identify hearing disorders but they still have a long way to go. Efforts still need to be made to design tools that are as simple and as cost-effective as they can be to ensure widespread use.

⚙ REFERENCES

1. *Guidelines for audiologic screening.* Rockville, MD: American Speech-Language-Hearing Association, 1997.
2. NIH Consensus Statement. *Early identification of hearing loss in infants and young children* [review]. Bethesda, MD: National Institutes of Health, 1993;11(1):1–24.
3. Joint Committee on Infant Hearing: position statement. *ASHA* 1994;36.
4. Northern JL, Hayes D. *Audiology Today* 1994;6(2).
5. White KR, Vohr BR, Behrens TR. *Semin Hearing* 1993;14:18–29.
6. Norton SJ. *Am J Otol* 1994;15:4–12.
7. Mason JA, Herrmann KR. *Pediatrics* 1998;101(2).
8. Jacobson JT, Jacobson CA, Spahr RC. *J Am Acad Audiol* 1990;1:187–195.
9. Nozza RJ. In: Martin FN, Clark JG, eds. *Hearing care for children.* Needham Heights, MA: Allyn and Bacon, 1996.
10. *Otitis media with effusion in young children (clinical practice guideline, no. 12).* Rockville, MD: Agency for Health Care Policy and Research, Department of Health and Human Service 1994.
11. Katz J, Stecker N, Henderson D. *Central auditory processing.* St. Louis, MO: Mosby–Year Book, 1992.
12. Chermak G, Musiek F. *Central auditory processing disorders: new perspectives.* San Diego, CA: Singular Publishing, 1997.

13. Bellis T. *Assessment and management of central auditory processing disorders in the educational setting.* San Diego, CA: Singular Publishing, 1996.

14. Keith RW. *A screening test for auditory processing disorders.* New York: Psychological Corporation, 1986.

15. Cherry R. Selective auditory attention test. St. Louis, MO: Auditec, 1980.

16. Roush J, Bryant K, Mundy M, Zeisel S, Roberts J. *J Am Acad Audiol* 1995;6:334–338.

17. Nozza RJ, Bluestone CD, Kardatzke D, Bachman RN. *Ear and Hearing.* 1992;13(6):442–453.

G. P. Riemer: Department of Audiology, University of Cincinnati, Children's Hospital Medical Center, Cincinnati, Ohio 45229-3039.

• *Practical Pediatric Otolaryngology*
• edited by Robin T. Cotton
  and Charles M. Myer, III
• Lippincott-Raven Publishers,
  Philadelphia © 1999

22

Imaging of the Ear in Children

Peter D. Phelps

The technical principles that apply to imaging in adults apply equally for the demonstration of head and neck lesions in infants and children. Optimum spatial and density resolution with lowest possible level of patient irradiation and freedom from movement artifacts must be achieved. Limitation of radiation dose is particularly important in this age group, and limitation of patient movement is hard to obtain. The role of computed tomography (CT) is established and will remain so, although many examinations require sedation or general anesthesia to ensure stillness. Magnetic resonance imaging (MRI) involves no irradiation and is increasingly used, although its main application is for intracranial diseases.

The middle and inner ears are fully developed at birth, but the temporomandibular joint and mastoid process are not. Postnatal changes in the temporal bone consist of growth and pneumatization of the mastoid process and alteration in the shape of the tympanic ring. Prior to full ossification of the petrous pyramid, the dense bone of the labyrinthine capsule can be clearly identified on plain mastoid views, enabling gross developmental abnormalities to be identified without the need for sectional imaging. In the middle ear, the ossicles can be shown, and in the neonate even the narrow spaces within them. The mastoid antrum is fully formed at birth, but further pneumatization posteriorly only occurs during the first decade of life with the development of the mastoid process. It is still not clear how much the variable extent of this pneumatization is due to genetic factors and how much to interference from disease processes. Plain lateral oblique mastoid views show the extent of pneumatization which can also be assessed on the standard views.

IMAGING TECHNIQUES

Plain X-Rays

The following are the usual plain film projections used to examine the petromastoid:

1. *Perorbital view*. This should be done in the posteroanterior (PA) position if possible. The orbitomeatal line is at right angles to the film, and the tube is angled 5 to 10° caudally, centering between the orbits. The petrous pyramids are thus projected through the orbits and a good view of the internal auditory meatus (IAMs) obtained (Fig. 1).
2. *Lateral oblique view*. The head is placed in true lateral position and the tube angled 15° caudally to prevent superimposition of the two mastoid processes (Fig. 2).
3. *Oblique PA view (Stenvers projection)*. The whole length of the petrous bone is placed parallel to the x-ray film with the incident ray passing at right angles to it. This view should demonstrate the petrous tip, the IAM, the superior and lateral semicircular canals, the middle-ear cleft, and the mastoid antrum (Fig. 3).

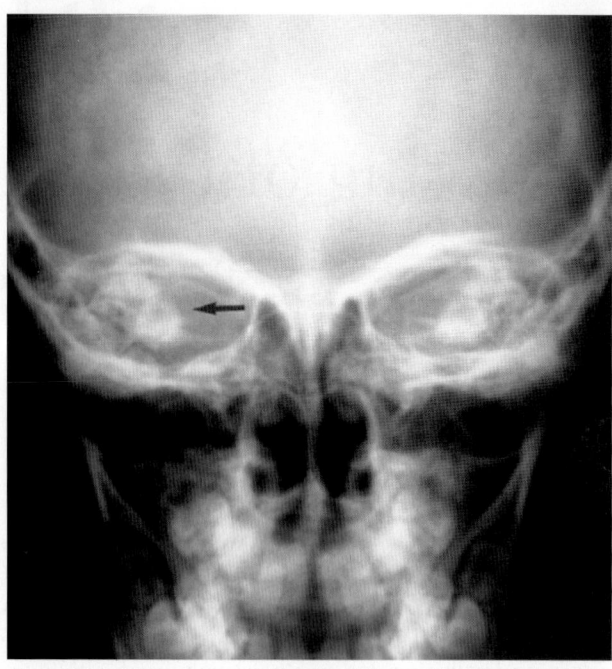

FIGURE 1 Perorbital view. The arrow indicates the internal auditory meatus (IAM).

Plain mastoid views are, however, rarely indicated, are inferior to CT and are no substitute for adequate clinical assessment of the eardrum in inflammatory ear disease.

Computed Tomography

Short scan times, good bone detail, and superior demonstration of soft tissue abnormalities have now made CT the investigation of choice in most cases. It is essential, therefore, that the pediatric radiologist have a sound knowledge of cross-sectional anatomy of the petrous temporal bone. While four or five 2-mm axial sections are sufficient for most examinations, thinner (1-mm) slices may be required to study specific areas, such as the oval window or incudostapedial joint (Fig. 4). However, care should be taken to limit radiation dose to the eyes by careful positioning. A few of the more relevant axial sections

FIGURE 2 Lateral oblique view showing a well-pneumatized mastoid. The arrows indicate the plates of bone underlying the dura and the sigmoid sinus.

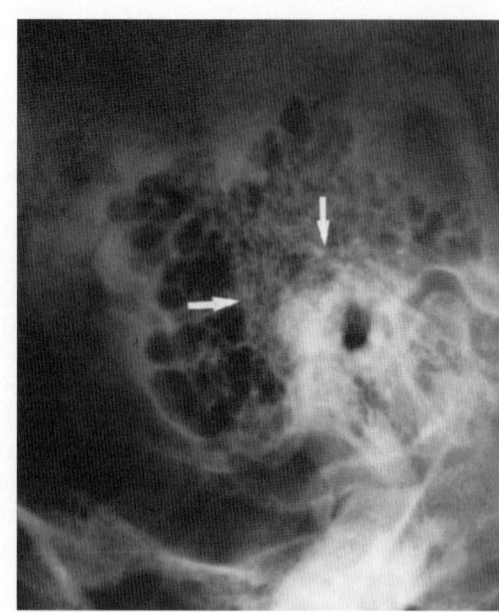

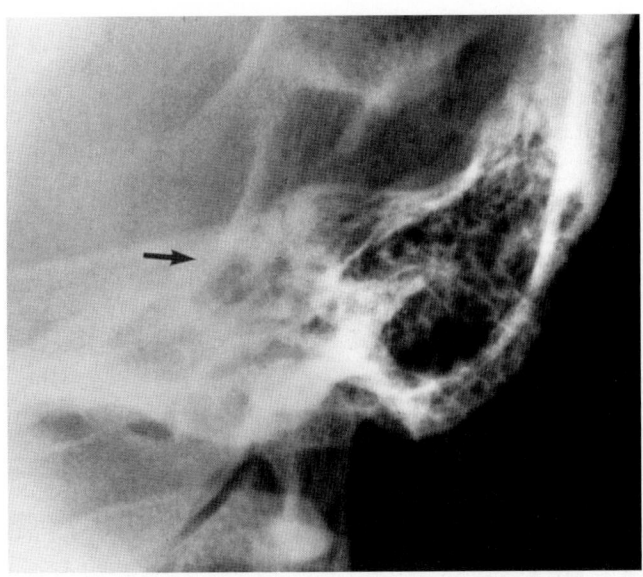

FIGURE 3 The Stenvers view. The arrow indicates the IAM.

are illustrated here (Fig. 5), but as the important anatomic features do not differ significantly from those of the adult, a study of works listed in the References is recommended. Supplementary views in the coronal plane should be obtained when necessary with the patient either in the chin-up or head-hanging position (Fig. 6).

Adequate imaging of all structures can usually be obtained by axial and coronal CT including the course of the facial nerve. Reformatted lateral views in the sagittal plane are useful for showing disruption of the ossicles and the descending facial nerve canal (Fig. 7). The course of the vestibular aqueduct, especially if this is enlarged, is also best shown in the sagittal plane; for this we use pretargetted scout views made in the axial projection to define the plane of the vestibular aqueduct (Fig. 8).

PEARLS AND PERILS

A large jugular fossa and bulb with well-corticated bony margins should not be mistaken for an expansile tumor, but MRI and magnetic resonance angiography (MRA) may rarely be needed to confirm.

FIGURE 4 A routine lateral scout view showing the scan planes for an examination in the axial projection.

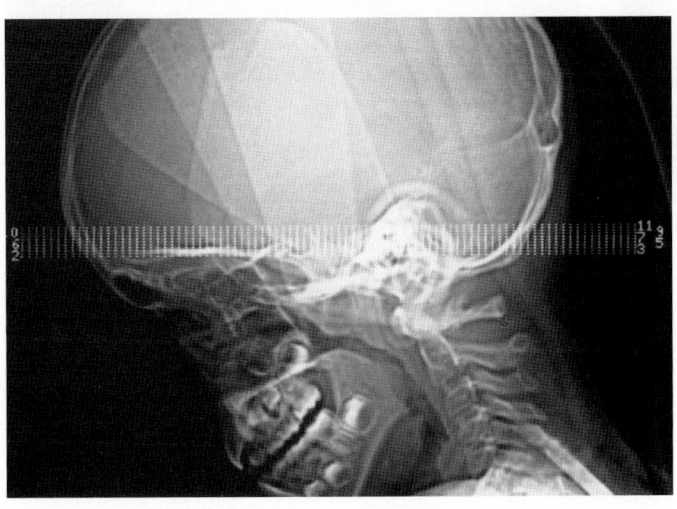

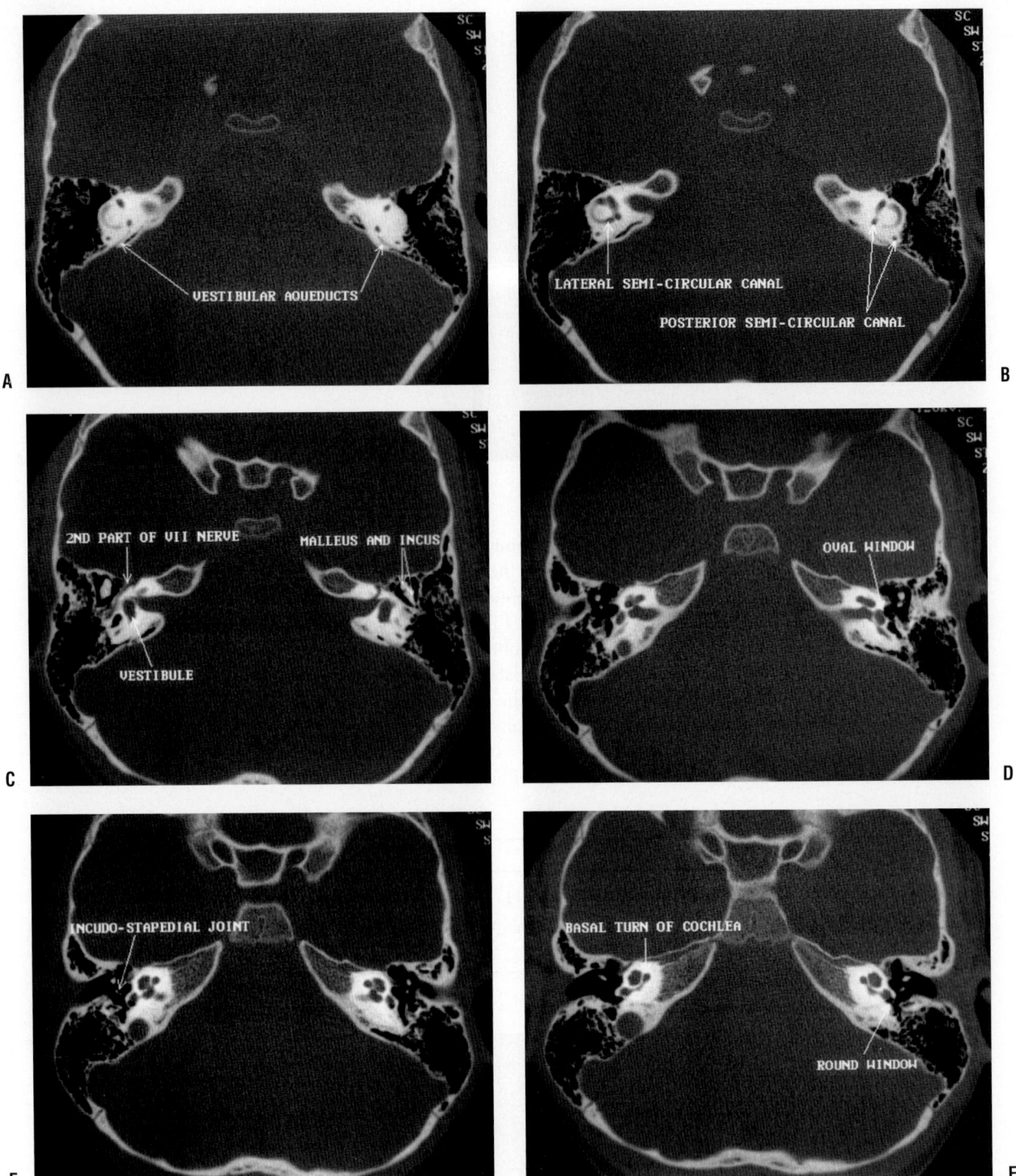

FIGURE 5 A–F: Six sections in the axial plane from highest to lowest showing some of the most important structures demonstrated.

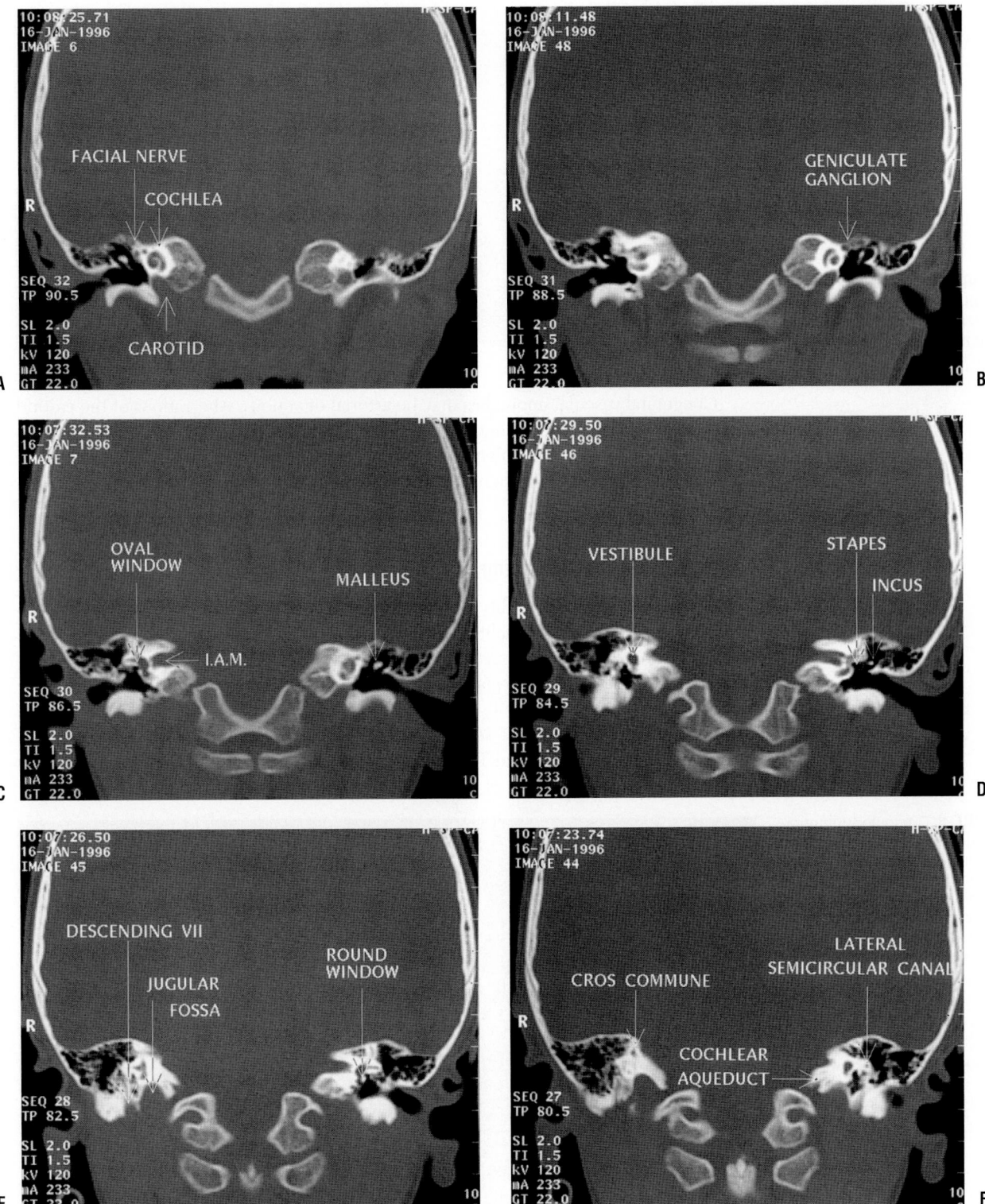

FIGURE 6 A–F: Six sections in the coronal plane showing some of the most important structures demonstrated from anterior to posterior.

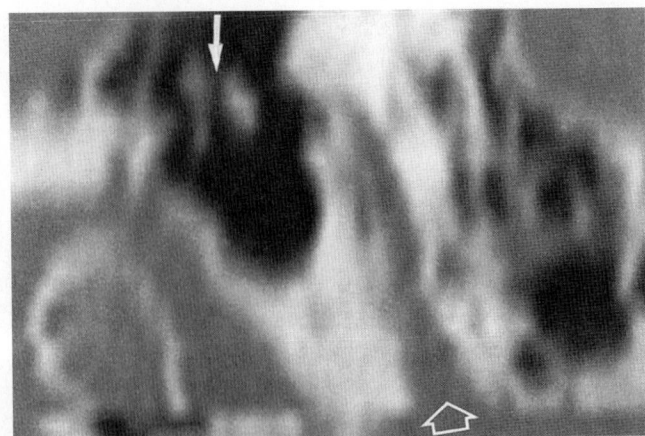

FIGURE 7 Reformatted sagittal section showing the descending part of the facial nerve canal. The *open arrow* points to the stylomastoid foramen. The *small arrow* indicates a slight traumatic disruption between malleus and incus.

Congenital vascular anomalies may be arterial or venous. Aberrations of the carotid artery do not usually present in childhood, but a large jugular bulb can cause problems at any age. The large vein, sometimes with one or more diverticula, may extend into the middle ear cavity with or without a bony covering or may encroach on inner ear structures (Fig. 9).

Magnetic Resonance Imaging

Besides its multiplanar capability and freedom from artifacts, MRI gives a better demonstration of soft tissue abnormalities than CT and is now the investigation of choice for most intracranial lesions and masses in and below the skull base. As air and bone give essentially no MR signal, the normal middle ear is not defined adequately. The fluids of the labyrinth give high signal on T_2-weighted sequences and nerves in the IAM, and the cerebellopontine angle can be seen as well as the facial nerve in its whole length. The original MR examinations used T_1-weighted spin-echo sequences showing intermediate

FIGURE 8 Computed tomography demonstration of a large vestibular aqueduct. The reformatted sagittal sections from multiple axial images show that the width of the descending limb of the vestibular aqueduct measures 6.0 mm in its midportion.

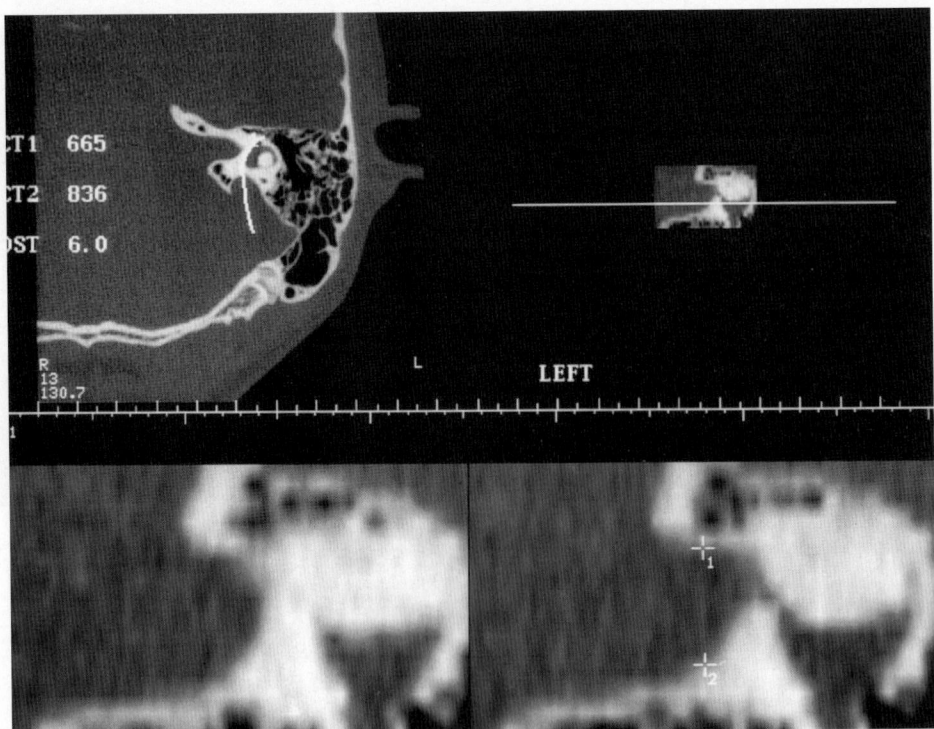

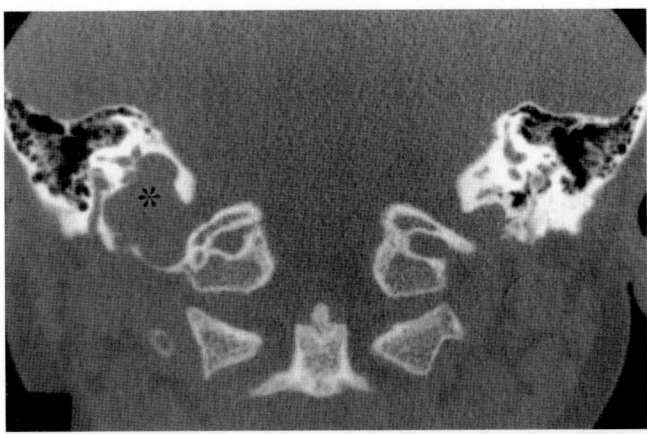
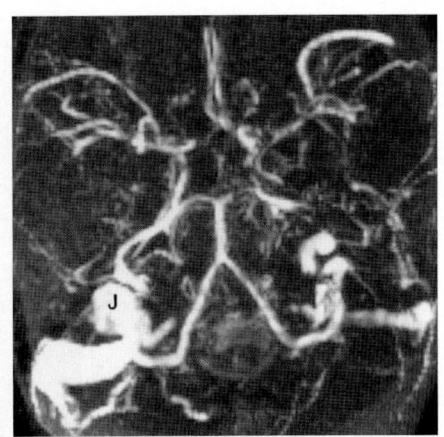

A   B

FIGURE 9 A: A large jugular fossa in a 4-year-old child. The child suffered from progressive unilateral sensorineural hearing loss. The large jugular bulb (*asterisk*) appears to encroach on the labyrinth of the inner ear and is very close to the descending portion of the facial nerve. However, the fossa has well-corticated margins. **B:** Magnetic resonance angiography demonstrates the large jugular bulb (*J*) with very little flow on the opposite side.

signal from the nerves and fluids in the inner ear and high signal from the marrow fat in the petrous apex (Fig. 10). The routine precontrast T₁-weighted images provide sharp depiction of the fatty and fascial planes of the deep neck and skull base. By providing clear definition of these planes, a pathologic process can easily be detected as an infiltrating lesion extending into and distorting these normal anatomic boundaries. A T₂-weighted sequence takes longer but shows the fluids in the inner ear and the cerebrospinal fluid (CSF) as high signal.

Fast Spin Echo

Fast spin echo (FSE) is a new fast scanning method that uses spin echoes and altered k-space filling. It is designed to provide more conventional spin-echo type contrast in shorter times. This is done by use of a frequency-encoding gradient, which means that up to 16 times as much k-space (collection of raw data) can be filled compared with a traditional spin echo, by which one line of k-space is generally completed between radiofrequency pulses (relaxation time). In the FSE pulse sequence, the initial 90° pulse is followed by the acquisition of 16 echoes. Each echo is acquired with a different phase-

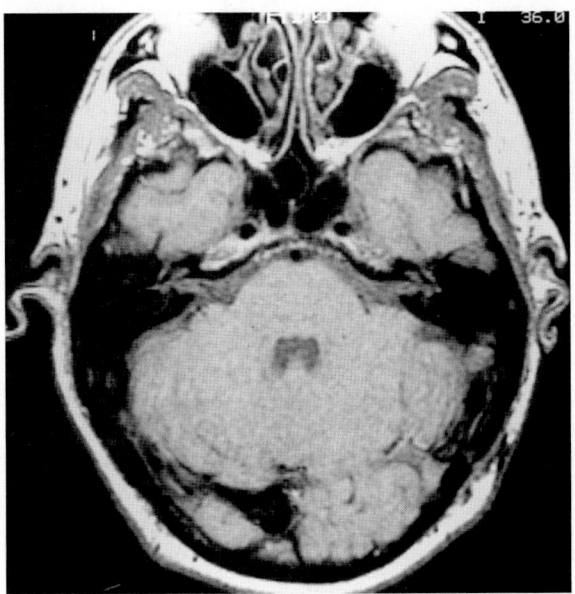

FIGURE 10 Axial T₁-weighted section through the posterior cranial fossa at the level of the IAMs.

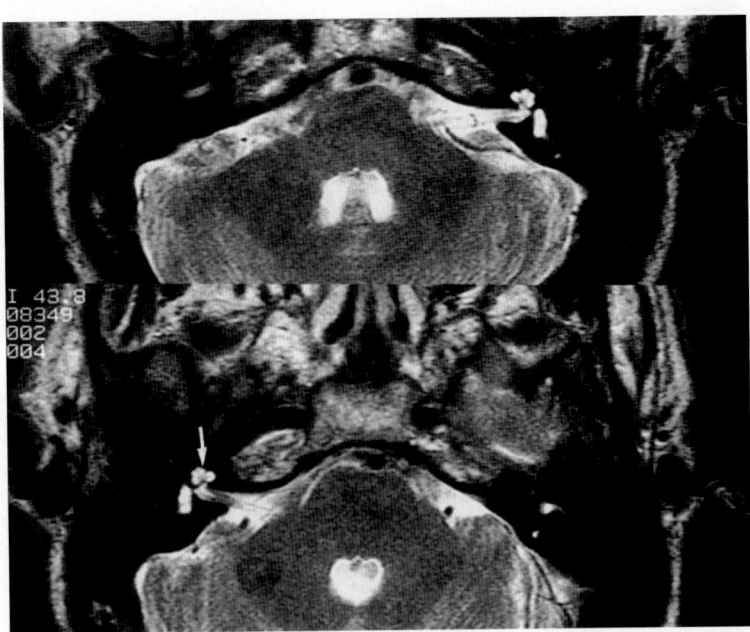

FIGURE 11 Two axial T$_2$-weighted sections at the level of the IAMs. Note the VIIth and VIIIth cranial nerves and the coils of the cochlea (*arrow*).

encoded gradient. The total acquisition time is greatly reduced with FSE, permitting a greater number of phase-encoding steps to be made. The matrix size can therefore be increased with improved spatial resolution while still maintaining an acceptable examination time. Thus, the latest MR equipment can give bone detail almost on a par with CT: 2-mm sections and good contrast among bone, soft tissues, and fluids of the inner ear. The normal cranial nerves in the IAM are clearly seen surrounded by the high-signal CSF (Fig. 11).

PATIENT ASSESSMENT (CONGENITAL EAR DEFORMITIES)

Congenital ear abnormalities have many and varied types and present a wide range of clinical problems, the commonest of which is hearing loss. The defect producing the deafness may in any one individual involve any or all of the parts of the hearing mechanism, namely, the external, middle, or inner ears or the central neural connections, and may be unilateral or bilateral.

In some cases, a family history of deafness, a history of maternal rubella during pregnancy, neonatal asphyxia or jaundice, or identification in the neonatal period of a deafness-associated abnormality, e.g., external ear deformities or Treacher Collins syndrome, may alert the clinician to the possibility of the presence of deafness, but more commonly the deafness is identified only as a result of a hearing screening program.

The essential management of such cases lies in the fields of audiology and special education, but this management may be influenced or modified as a result of the assessment by imaging. How, when, and if to image in the assessment of the congenitally deaf child is a complex and difficult problem. The patient often needs a general anesthetic or at least good sedation for the examination. As many as one-half of the cases of profound deafness in childhood are thought to be due primarily to acquired causes. It is virtually impossible to distinguish between congenital and rapid-onset deafness in the neonate. Moreover, some congenital aberrations, such as a dilated vestibular aqueduct and some bone dysplasias, are associated with progressive hearing loss. The most important assessment of the deaf child is a continuous clinical evaluation between the ages of 1 and 3 years, when the normal speech process develops. Failure to develop normal speech is often the first indication of hearing deficiency.

Until recently, radiology provided the only objective assessment of abnormalities of hearing, albeit only in a small group of patients with structural deformities of the bony hearing apparatus. Electrocochleography, auditory brainstem response, and impedance audiometry are now established as reliable objective means of assessing hearing impairment in this important age group. Ideally, the various types of objective audiometry and sophisticated radiologic techniques should be available on the same premises. Electrophysiology and radiology are complementary investigations in selected cases.

Congenital Deafness

Important information on the state of both inner and middle ears can be obtained. For the inner ear, the state of the bony labyrinth and IAM, minor or severe deformity with no cochlear function, probable better hearing side, risk of CSF fistula and route, and suitability for cochlear implantation should be determined. For the middle ear, the feasibility of surgery for improved sound conduction, most favorable ear for exploration or aiding, size of middle-ear cavity and state of ossicles, and surgical hazards—aberrant facial nerve, carotid artery, jugular bulb—should be determined. Three periods of infancy and childhood can be considered:

Up to 3 months of age. Any infant with external deformity of the ears or with syndromic features known to have a high incidence of deafness such as Treacher Collins hemifacial microsomia, or Klippel-Feil syndromes should have CT, only a few sections being required. This should be done even with unilateral lesions because of the high incidence of occult abnormalities detectable by radiology in the "good" ear.

"Difficult period" (6 months to 4 years). This is the age at which the deafness is usually discovered; the requisite degree of immobility usually cannot be achieved without some form of sedation. Radiology is not required in minor or moderate degrees of deafness when there is no external or relevant syndromic deformity, nor is it required at this age for unilateral atresias with normal hearing in the other ear. Exploratory surgery is not normally undertaken for unilateral atresias, and radiology can be left until the third period. Deafness associated with suspected CSF otorrhea or rhinorrhea or with meningitis calls for full radiologic evaluation of the temporal bones. Patients with severe deafness and no speech may have severe labyrinthine deformities, some of which may be associated with a CSF fistula and may require CT demonstration.

"Age of Reason" (4 years and over). In this period, assessment is by pure-tone audiometry and radiology.

Radiologic Examination

Plain films are of little value due to overlap of bony structures but may occasionally be useful to exclude gross abnormalities, to show the extent of pneumatization, or to assess the position of an implant. Best results are obtained by sectional imaging, especially high-resolution CT in two planes or by MRI.

Assessment for Surgery

Assessment of the middle-ear cavity is best made by CT, which will show whether or not the cavity contains air. Unfortunately, it is not possible to tell by "tissue characterization" whether soft tissue density in the cavity is due to fluid, mesenchymatous glue, soft tissue, or cholesteatoma, but only by experience and indirect signs such as bone erosion.

MR is now the imaging investigation of choice for sensorineural hearing loss to show lesions of the inner ear or central connections. This examination is best performed with T_2-weighted fast spin-echo thin sections initially, but T_1 sections before and after contrast enhancement, as well as the 3 D Fourier transformation-constructive interference in steady state (3DFT-CISS) sequences described by Casselman et al. (1) for the study of the labyrinth and IAM, may be required. However, these MR sequences will usually require a general anesthetic in young children.

Inner-Ear Deformities

Congenital malformations of the bony labyrinth, IAM, and vestibular aqueduct vary widely in severity from minor anomalies with normal cochlear function to severe deformities that preclude any level of hearing whatever may be suggested by audiologic assessment.

Traditionally, two common eponyms need to be defined:

1. *Michel defect*. Complete lack of development of any inner ear structures (2).
2. *Mondini defect*. A cochlea with one and a half turns and the apical coil replaced by a distal sac (3). Mondini's case also had very large vestibular aqueducts and endolymphatic sacs. Some hearing is usually present, but deafness may be progressive. True Mondini deformity is not associated with a spontaneous CSF fistula.

Line drawings of some examples of labyrinthine deformities are shown in Figure 12. A primitive sac with one or more appendages is commoner than a Michel deformity.

The semicircular canals may be missing or dilated in varying degrees, but the commonest labyrinthine ear anomaly, namely, a solitary dilated dysplastic lateral semicircular canal (Fig. 13), is often associated with normal cochlear function. Dilation of the vestibular aqueduct often accompanies minor abnormalities of the bony cochlea and vestibule and congenital hearing loss. The deafness may be fluctuant or progressive, suggesting that endolymphatic hydrops is also a feature. Minor head trauma seems to be a precipitating feature of progressive hearing loss. However, of more relevance than a demonstration of the bony outlines of the vestibular aqueduct is an appraisal of the soft tissue contents, namely, the endolymphatic duct and sac (4). This can now be made by thin-section high-resolution MRI (Fig. 14).

FIGURE 12 Line drawings based on sectional imaging of various congenital structural malformations of the inner ear.

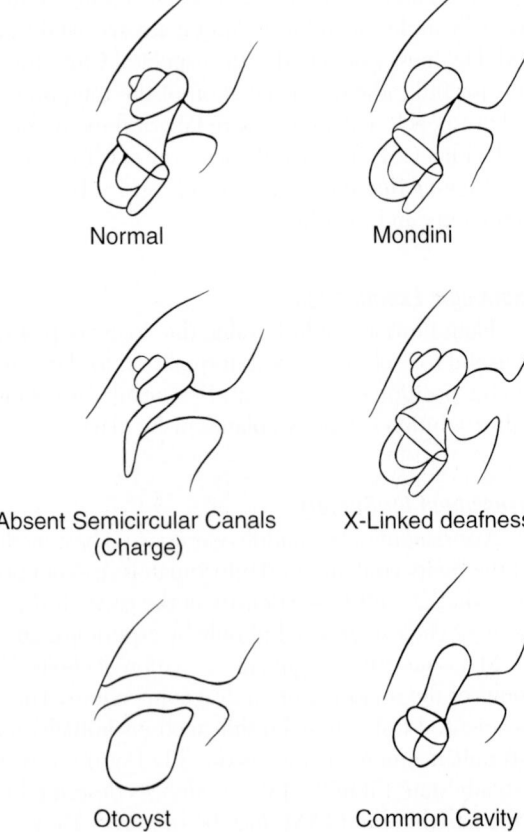

Normal

Mondini

Absent Semicircular Canals (Charge)

X-Linked deafness

Otocyst

Common Cavity (Cock)

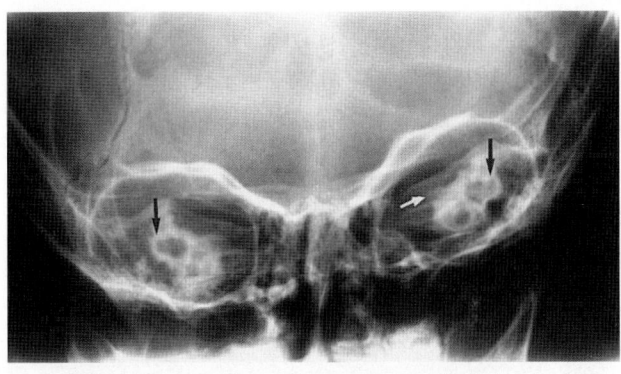

FIGURE 13 Plain perorbital view of an infant showing dilated dysplastic lateral semicircular canals (*black arrows*). This anomaly may be associated with normal cochlear function if there are no other abnormalities of the labyrinth, but note, in this case, there is a narrow IAM on the left (*white arrow*).

Anomalies of the IAM include the bulbous type, which is usually of no significance unless associated with X-linked deformity (5) (Fig. 15); unusual direction, which is the result of skull base malformations; and very narrow or double IAMs, which usually indicate severe or total deafness.

Inner-Ear Lesions Associated With Cerebrospinal Fluid Fistula

Congenital CSF fistula into the middle-ear cavity is a rare but potentially fatal condition that is frequently misdiagnosed. When the fistula occurs spontaneously, it usually presents in the first 5 and 10 years of life as:

1. CSF rhinorrhea if the eardrum is intact. CSF passes down the eustachian tube causing a nasal discharge.
2. CSF otorrhea if there is a perforation in the eardrum or if myringotomy has been performed for presumed serous otitis media.
3. Attacks of meningitis that are usually recurrent. At times, meningitis is the sole presenting manifestation of a CSF fistula.

Deafness is usually severe or complete, but it is difficult to diagnose and assess, especially in a young child. It is frequently unrecognized if unilateral. The conductive and sensorineural components of the deafness are also hard to define.

Spontaneous CSF fistulas from the subarachnoid space into the middle-ear cavity may be classified as perilabyrinthine or translabyrinthine. The *translabyrinthine group* is nearly always associated with anacusis, severe labyrinthine dysplasias, and a route via the IAM. The labyrinthine deformity is more severe (Fig. 16) than the type classically described by Mondini, and evidence of a dilated cochlear aqueduct in these cases is also unconvincing. The cochlea is an amorphous sac that lacks a modiolus or central bony spiral. No proper basal turn can be recognized as in a true Mondini deformity, and there is a

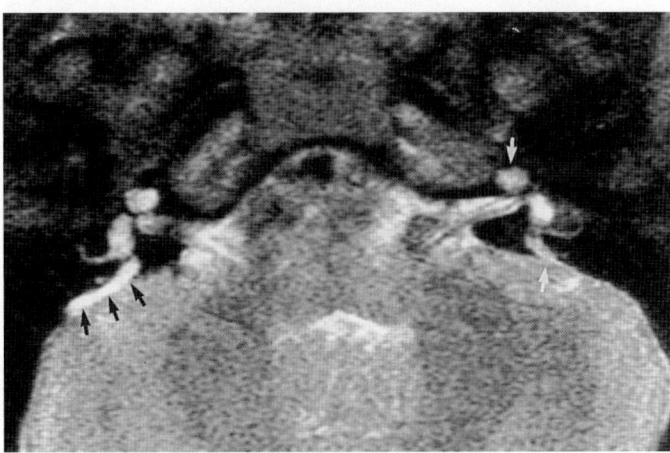

FIGURE 14 Axial fast spin-echo section of a 7-year-old child with bilateral Mondini cochlea and large vestibular aqueduct dysplasia (*white arrows*). However, note the large endolymphatic sac and ducts on one side (*black arrows*) and the normal cranial nerves in the IAM.

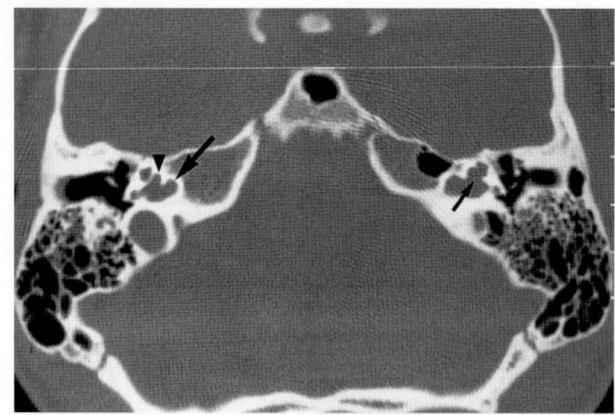 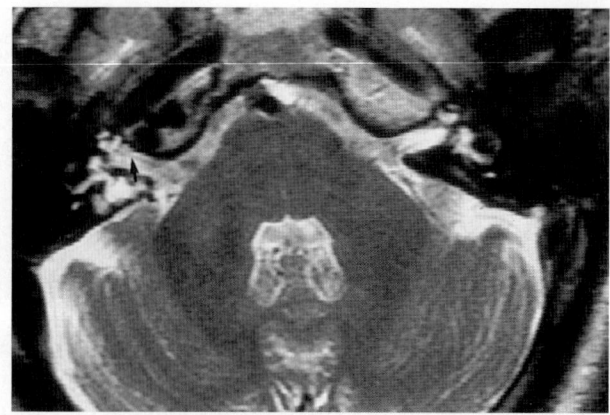

A   B

FIGURE 15 X-linked ear deformity. Axial CT section **(A)** and fast spin-echo **(B)**. **A:** The basal turn of the cochlea is indicated by the *arrowhead*, the IAM by the *large arrow*, and the deficient bone between the two by the *small arrow*. **B:** The *arrow* points to the cochlear nerve.

wide communication between the cochlear sac and the vestibule, which is itself abnormal and enlarged. The semicircular canals may be dilated in varying degrees, especially the lateral. The labyrinthine malformation is usually accompanied by a defective stapes—usually a hole in the footplate—and the exit route of CSF into the middle ear is via the oval or, less commonly, the round window. This "common cavity" lesion was the first described in 1838 by Cock in a child who died of otogenic meningitis (6).

PEARLS AND PERILS

1. Severe congenital dysplasia of the labyrinth with a fistulous communication with the subarachnoid space is a most important cause of meningitis and should be recognized on a CT examination on any child with anacusis who has an attack of meningitis.
2. This "common cavity" malformation first described by Cock in 1838 is different from the deformity described by Mondini.

FIGURE 16 The "common cavity" lesion shown by axial CT. There is indentation between the sac representing the cochlea (*C*) and vestibule (*V*). The *open arrow* points to the tapering IAM. Note the normal labyrinth on the other side. This patient nearly died from otogenic meningitis before the abnormal inner ear was packed. A hole in the footplate of the stapes was found at operation.

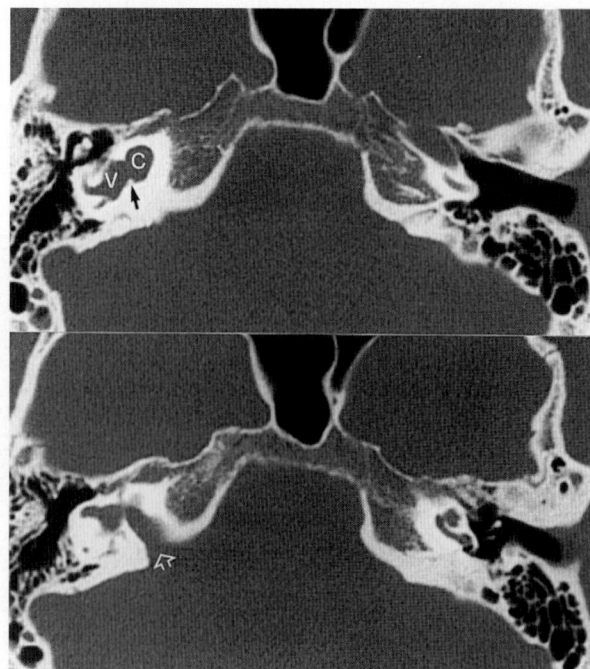

Perilabyrinthine fistulas are extremely rare and usually associated with normal hearing. Bone defects around the labyrinth may be shown by high-resolution CT, but contrast medium or radionuclide studies may be necessary to show the site. Sensorineural deafness or two unexplained attacks of meningitis make a CT study of the temporal bone mandatory.

Middle-Ear Deformities

Most unilateral atresias of the external auditory meatus have associated deformity of the pinna but no other congenital abnormality. The mastoid is normally formed with good pneumatization, and the middle-ear cavity is of relatively normal shape. A patient with good surgical prospects is illustrated in Figure 17. There is rarely complete absence of the middle ear, even in the most severe deformities and usually at least a slit-like hypotympanum can be shown lateral to the basal turn of the cochlea. The middle-ear cavity may be reduced in size by encroachment of the atretic plate laterally, by a high jugular bulb inferiorly, or by descent of the tegmen superiorly. In hemifacial microsomia and mandibulofacial dysostosis, the attic and antrum are typically absent or slit-like, being replaced in varying degrees by solid bone or by descent of the tegmen (Fig. 18). If the middle-ear cavity is air containing, its shape and contents are relatively easy to assess. Frequently, however, the middle ear in congenital abnormalities contains undifferentiated mesenchyme, a thick glue-like substance radiologically indistinguishable from soft tissue or retained mucus. Thin bony septa may divide the middle ear cavity into two or more compartments.

Facial Nerve

The next most important structure from a surgical point of view is the facial nerve. The main problem is variation in the course of the nerve. The course of the second and third

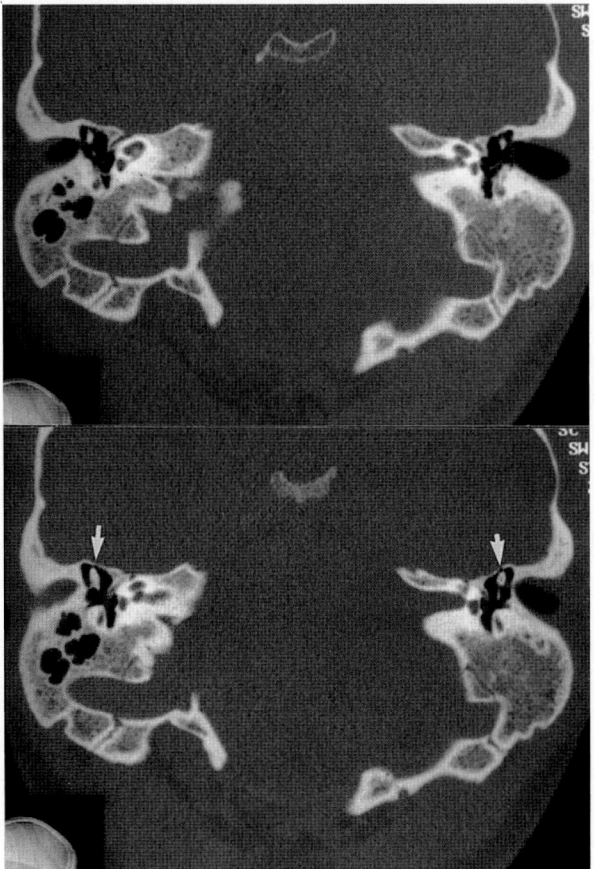

FIGURE 17 Axial CT scan showing minor deformities of the ossicles on each side with fusion of the malleus and incus but a normal incudostapedial region.

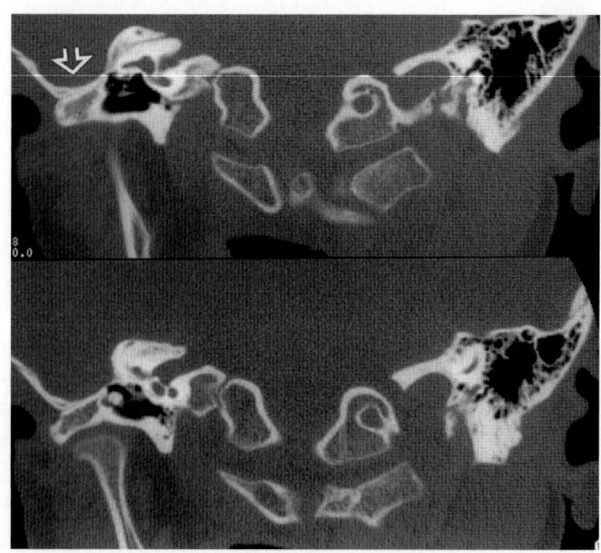

FIGURE 18 Coronal CT section of typical hemifacial microsomia with depression of the tegmen to below the level of the lateral semicircular canal (*open arrow*). Note the deformity of the temporomandibular joint and the ossicular mass.

parts is dependent on normal development of the branchial arches, the facial nerve being the nerve of the second arch. If, during development, the external pharyngeal groove of the first branchial arch is active and atresia is due only to maldevelopment of the tympanic ring, then the second and third parts of the facial canal follow a relatively normal course. In major atresias, when the external pharyngeal groove is not active, then development of malformations is much worse. The temporomandibular joint may abut directly onto the mastoid process.

The greater the deformity the more marked the tendency for the facial nerve to follow a more direct route into the soft tissues of the face (Fig. 19A). Exposed facial nerves in the middle-ear cavity are the most common abnormalities recorded at surgery for congenital malformations. Usually the fallopian canal is dehiscent, but the descending segment may also be exposed, and overhanging of the facial ridge with absence of the second genu is a usual finding in the Treacher Collins syndrome, making access to the oval window difficult. A short vertical segment of the facial canal and high stylomastoid foramen mean that the nerve turns forwards in the cheek in a high position.

In the preoperative radiologic assessment, the descending facial canal and its relationship to other structures must be demonstrated, preferably in both coronal and sagittal sections. Axial CT sections will show the descending canal in cross section, and identification is less certain. Grossly displaced nerves that cross the middle-ear cavity are more difficult to identify even by CT. Bifurcation of the descending portion is far more common in children with congenital malformations.

PEARLS AND PERILS

Although bone-anchored hearing aids have meant that few surgical explorations are now undertaken for congenital atresias, nevertheless aberrations in the course of the facial nerve can still be a hazard for implant procedures, especially when the exit from the skull is high and anteriorly placed.

Ossicles

A normal ossicular chain is rarely found where there is atresia of the external ear, but complete absence of the ossicles is unusual. In most cases, some vestige of the ossicular chain is evident. The ossicles are often thicker and heavier than normal or, less fre-

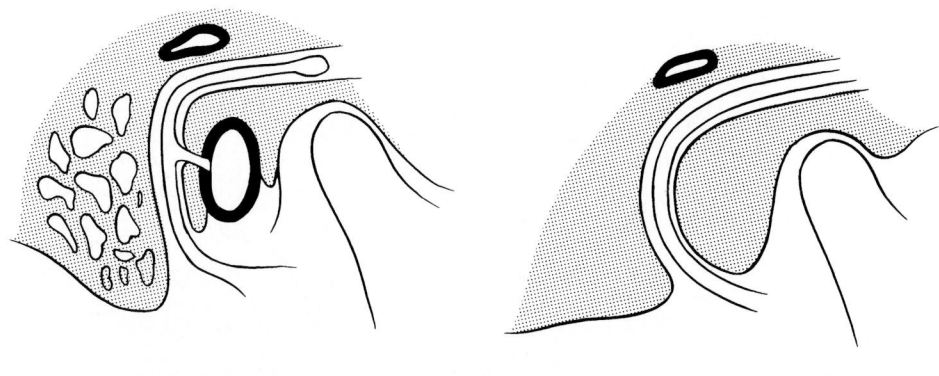

A   Normal   Congenital Atresia

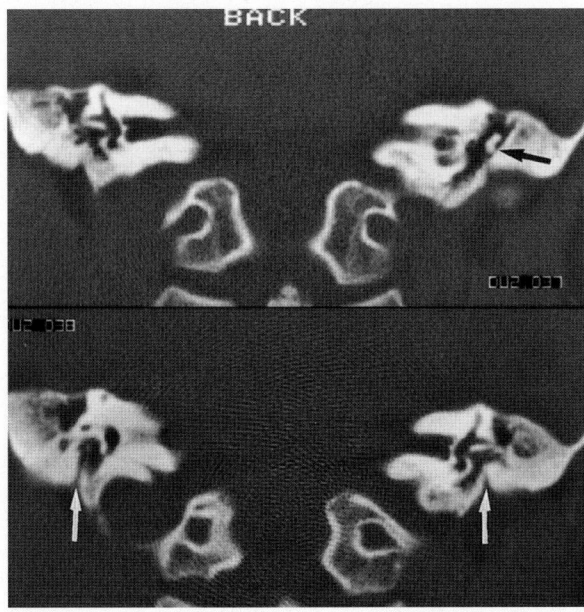

B

FIGURE 19 A: Diagram based on sagittal sections showing the typical abnormal route of the facial nerve in congenital atresia. **B:** Two coronal CT sections showing the anterior position of the descending facial nerve canal at the level of the oval and round windows (*white arrows*). The *black arrow* points to an ossicular mass.

quently, thin and spidery. They may be fixed to the walls of the middle ear cavity by bosses of bone, but the more usual deformity discovered at surgery is a fusion of the bodies of the malleus and incus. The ankylosis varies in degree and may be bony or fibrous. The radiologic definition of this ossicular union is difficult but is, in any case, not of great practical importance, and an irregular lump of bone in the middle ear cavity usually represents an ossicular mass (Fig. 19B). Because of the partial or complete replacement of the tympanic membrane by a bony plate, the handle of the malleus is the part of the chain most often abnormal and most easily recognized by imaging. The handle of the malleus is often bent toward the atretic plate to which it may be fixed, and this gives the typical L-shaped appearance to the ossicular mass. A slit-like attic so typical of Treacher Collins syndrome or an overhanging facial ridge may obstruct the free movement of the ossicular chain.

External Auditory Meatus

In congenital deformities of the external ear, the external auditory meatus may be narrow, short, or completely or partially atretic, or it may run in an abnormal direction. It often slopes up toward the middle ear, and in such cases, it may be curved in two planes, becoming more horizontal at its medial end. The obstruction in atresia may be due to soft tissue or bone, but usually both are involved. The tympanic bone may be rarely hyperplastic, deformed, or absent.

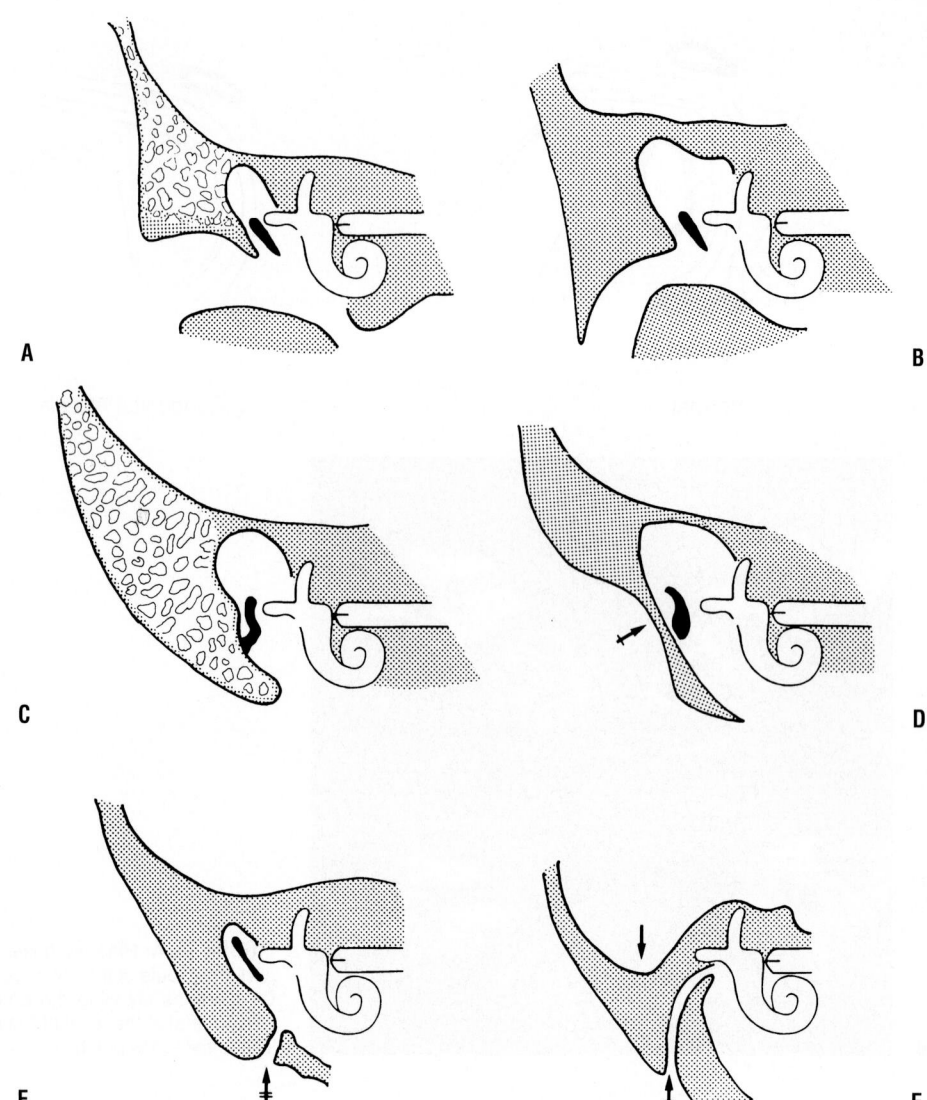

FIGURE 20 Congenital deformities of the middle and external ear. (From ref. 12, with permission.)

The so-called atretic plate may be composed partly of a deformed tympanic bone and partly of downward and forward extension of squamous temporal and mastoid, in which case it may be pneumatized.

Figure 20 gives a diagrammatic representation of some of the congenital structural abnormalities of the middle and external ears shown by coronal section imaging.

Syndromes

A full account of syndromes with structural deformities of the petrous bone is given in *Diagnostic Imaging of the Ear* (7), and only a few of the most common and important syndromes are considered here.

Characteristic small cochleae are a feature of the familial brancho-oto-renal syndrome (Fig. 21), Mondini cochlea and large vestibular aqueduct in Pendred syndrome, and absent semicircular canals in the CHARGE association, which is derived from the acronym *coloboma of the eye, congenital heart disease, choanal atresia, retarded growth, genital hypoplasia, and ear abnormalities. Structural deformities of both inner and middle ears can be demonstrated by CT.

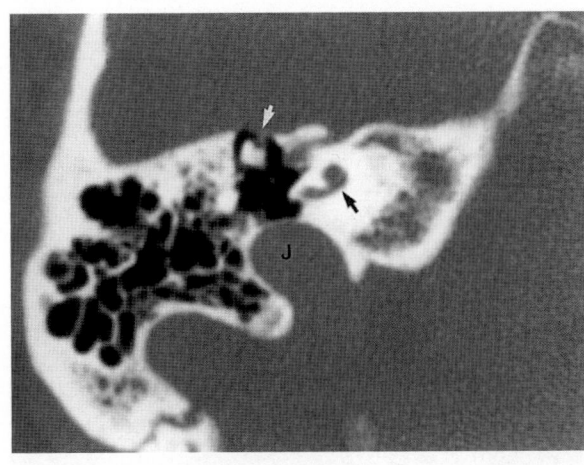

FIGURE 21 Axial CT of the petrous temporal bones of a typical case of brancho-oto-renal syndrome. Note the smaller than normal cochlea with reduced number of turns (*black arrow*), the ossicular mass attached to the anterior wall of the middle ear cavity (*white arrow*), and the large jugular bulb (*J*).

Hemifacial Microsomia

The ear lesions are usually bizarre and severe. The pinna is often represented by a small tag. Meatal atresia and middle-ear abnormalities are almost constant findings (Figs. 18 and 22), and there may be gross descent of the tegmen to, or even below, the level of the lateral semicircular canal. Occasionally, some degree of hypoplasia of external ear structures, particularly the tympanic bone, occurs, but the mastoid is hypoplastic and unpneumatized. The middle-ear cavity is usually small, being encroached on by the low tegmen and thick atretic plate. The ossicles, in such cases, are absent or hypoplastic and malformed, and may be displaced laterally, far from the oval window. The condition is not always unilateral. The bones of the skull base are often affected. If bilateral, there is always considerable asymmetry between the two sides, and this distinguishes the syndrome from Treacher Collins syndrome, with which it has often been confused in the past. A nonfamilial condition, craniofacial microsomia, is the most common of the otocraniofacial syndromes.

Treacher Collins Syndrome

The middle-ear abnormalities in Treacher Collins syndrome are symmetric and characteristic, although they may vary in severity. The mastoid is unpneumatized, and the attic

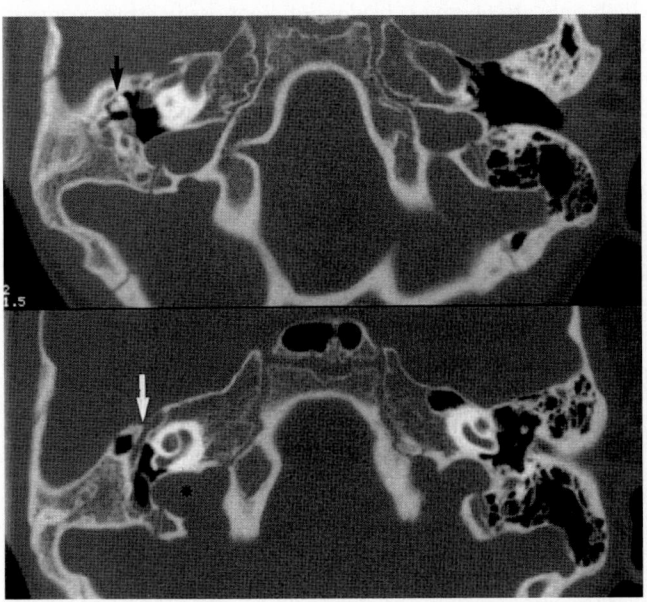

FIGURE 22 Facial microsomia. Axial CT section showing minor dysplasia on the left but more severe dysplasia on the right with laterally placed ossicular mass (*black arrow*) and marked overhang of the facial nerve (*white arrow*). The *asterisk* indicates the jugular bulb.

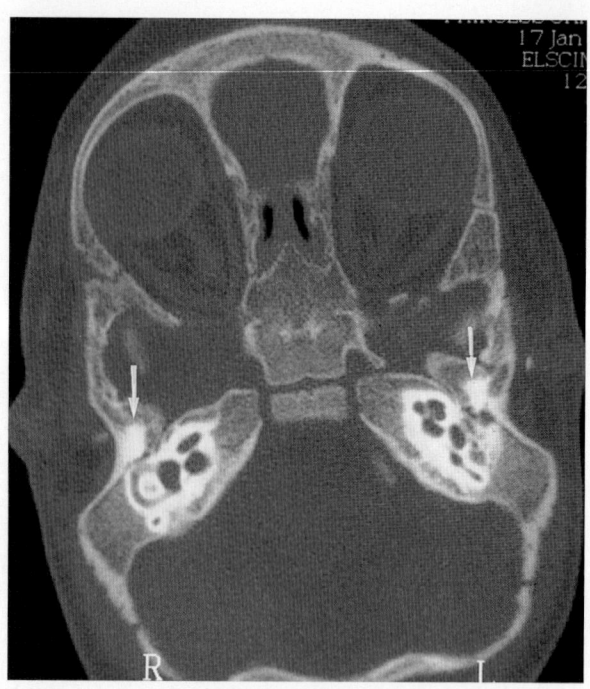

FIGURE 23 Axial CT section of typical Treacher Collins syndrome. There are normal inner ears but grossly deficient middle ears with large masses of bone representing the ossicles (*arrows*).

and antrum often reduced to slit-like proportions (Fig. 23). Atresia of the external auditory meatus is a less constant feature. Ossicular abnormalities are common, and the facial nerve follows a more direct path. The prospects for surgery in cases of Treacher Collins syndrome are not good due to the general hypoplasia.

Osseous Dysplasias

Deafness is a common childhood feature of rare congenital generalized bone dysplasias. Only a brief account of the radiologic features of osteogenesis imperfecta and of the dysplasias with increased bone density is given here. Deafness in osteogenesis imperfecta tarda may be conductive, sensorineural, or mixed. The radiologic appearances consist of demineralization of the labyrinthine capsule indistinguishable from otospongiosis, but, in contrast to otospongiosis, which only affects the capsule, deficient ossification occurs in other sites in the petrous pyramid (Fig. 24).

A group of uncommon genetic disorders, such as osteopetrosis and craniometaphyseal and craniodiaphyseal dysplasias, is characterized by increased skeletal density and

FIGURE 24 Osteogenesis imperfecta. Coronal CT section showing areas of rarefied bone around the cochlea (*arrows*).

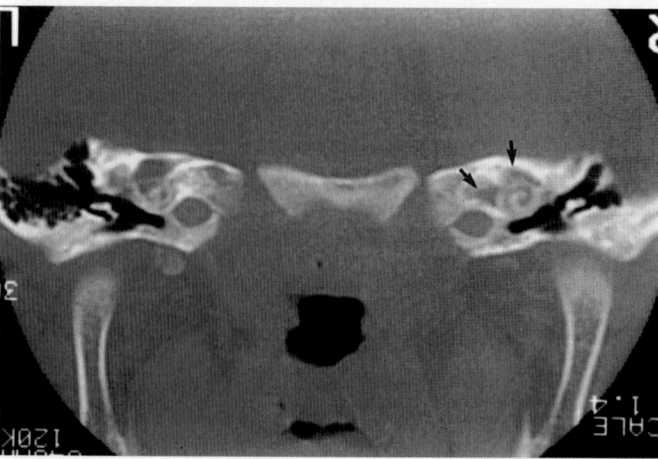

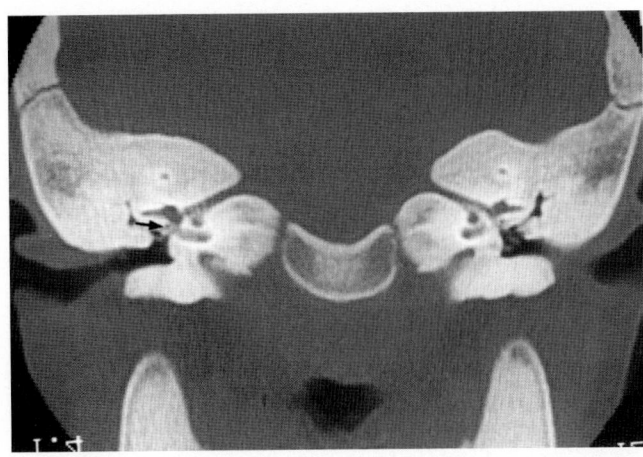

FIGURE 25 Congenital osseous dysplasia. The labyrinth is virtually normal, but the IAMs and middle ears are grossly narrowed. The *arrow* points to the second part of the facial nerve canal.

abnormalities of bone modeling, involving the calvaria and skull base. A variety of neurotologic symptoms may result, secondary to bony encroachment on the cranial foramina. Sectional imaging of the petrous temporal bones shows generalized sclerosis and narrowing of the IAMs, but densitometry studies have shown that only the surrounding periosteal bone becomes sclerosed. The otic capsule is the densest bone in the body and cannot become denser. Encroachment by bosses of bone in the attic may also be revealed (Fig. 25).

CONCLUSIONS

To some extent, the emphasis in congenital ear deformity imaging has changed in recent years. A demonstration of the abnormal structural anatomy is indicated in any severely deaf child or infant, especially one with an ear abnormality, a syndrome (e.g., Klippel-Feil) in which there is an incidence of temporal bone deformity, or a history of deafness associated with meningitis. This will usually be by CT initially to demonstrate the osseous anatomy, although the success of bone-anchored hearing aids has meant that surgical exploration of a deformed middle ear is usually only carried out now for minor ossicular dysfunction. If the hearing loss can be shown to be sensorineural in type rather than conductive, there is a good case for using MRI initially to assess the inner ear and central connections. This also applies to the prospects of cochlear implantation for congenital deformities: The common cavity type of lesion (8,9) would seem less suitable than a more minor deformity that is without risk of a CSF gusher (10,11).

PEARLS AND PERILS

1. Beware the narrow IAM for cochlear implant candidates and try to confirm the presence of a cochlear nerve with MRI.
2. The true Mondini deformity of either the cochlear or the large vestibular aqueduct type would seem eminently suitable for a cochlear implant (9).
3. Implanting common cavity lesions is more controversial, but some good results are claimed despite the initial inevitable flood of CSF at operation (7,8).

REFERENCES

1. Casselman JW, Kuhweide R, Ampe W, Meeus L, Steyaert L. Pathology of the membranous labyrinth: comparison of T1- and T2-weighted and gadolinium-enhanced spin-echo and 3DFT-CISS imaging. *AJNR* 1993;14:59–69.

2. Michel. Mémoire sur les anomalies congénitales de l'oreille interne. *Gazette Med Strasbourg* 1863;4:55–58.

3. Mondini C. Anatomica surdi nati sectio. Bononiensi scientarium et artium institute atque academia commentarii. *Bononiae* 1791;VII:419–428.

4. Harnsberger HR, Dahlen RT, Clough S, Gray SD, Parkin JL. Advanced techniques in magnetic resonance imaging in the evaluation of the large endolymphatic duct and sac syndrome. *Laryngoscope* 1995;105:1037–1041.

5. Phelps P, Reardon W, Pembrey M, Bellman S, Luxon L. X-linked deafness, stapes gushers and a distinctive defect of the inner ear. *Neuroradiology* 1991;33:326–330.

6. Phelps PD, Michaels L. The common cavity congenital deformity of the inner ear. *J Otorhinolaryngol Relat Spec* 1995;57:228–231.

7. Phelps PD, Lloyd GAS. *Diagnostic imaging of the ear.* 2nd ed. London: Springer Verlag, 1990.

8. Miyamoto RT, Robbins AJM, Myres WA, Pope ML. Cochlear implantation in the Mondini inner ear malformation. *Am J Otol* 1986;7:258–260.

9. Molter DW, Pate BR, McElveen JT. Cochlear implantation in the congenitally malformed ear. *Otol Head Neck Surg* 1993;108:174–177.

10. Silverstein H, Smouha E, Morgan N. Multichannel cochlear implantation in a patient with bilateral Mondini deformities. *Am J Otol* 1988;9:451–455.

11. Jackler RK, Luxford WM, House WF. Sound detection with the cochlear implant in five ears of four children with congenital malformations of the cochlea. *Laryngoscope* 1987; 97:15–17.

12. Phelps PD, Lloyd GAS, Sheldon PWE. Congenital deformities of the middle and external ear. *Br J Radiol* 1977;50:714–727.

P.D. Phelps: The Royal National Throat, Nose and Ear Hospital, London WC1X 8DA, United Kingdom.

• *Practical Pediatric Otolaryngology*
• edited by Robin T. Cotton
  and Charles M. Myer, III
• Lippincott-Raven Publishers,
  Philadelphia © 1999

Section Editor
Scott C. Manning

23

Allergic Rhinitis

Gail G. Shapiro

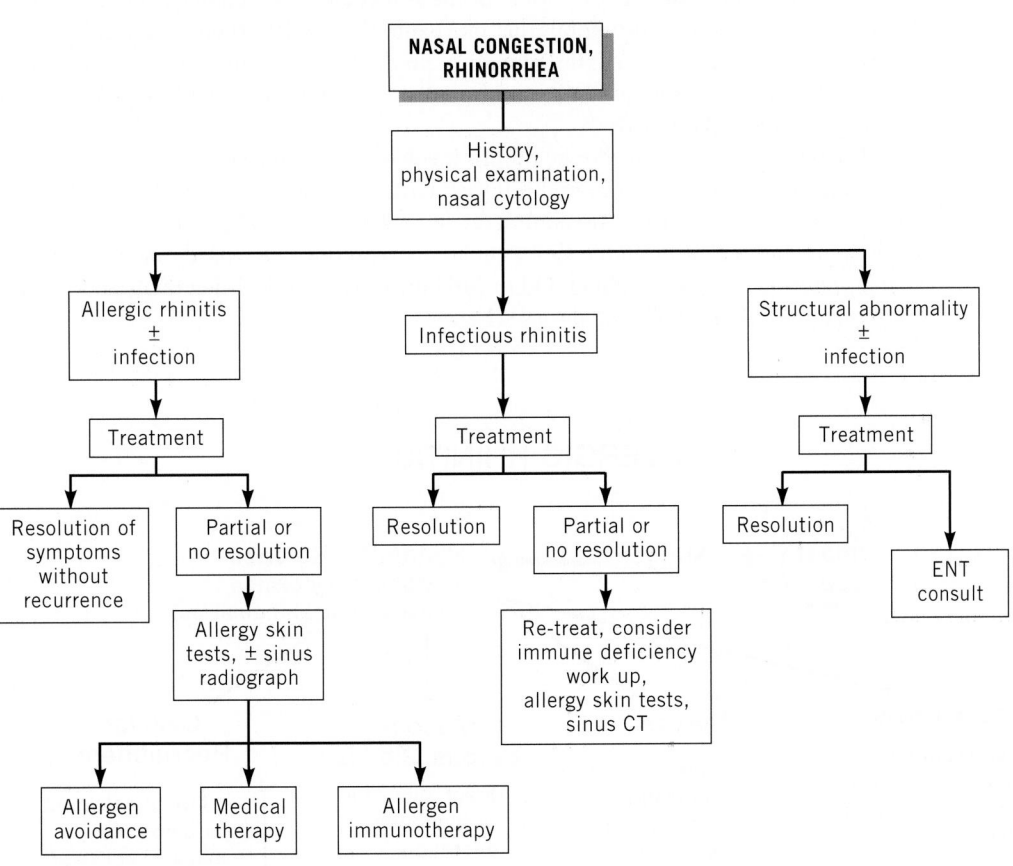

HISTORICAL BACKGROUND

Chronic rhinitis is a common childhood problem, with allergic rhinitis being the most common cause of chronic nasal congestion in children. The number of children affected is huge when one considers that 20% or more of the population is allergic and that nasal manifestations are the most common way that allergy makes itself known. Allergic rhinitis accounts for 3% of all visits to the doctor's office (1). The easily recognized symptoms of allergic rhinitis are nasal stuffiness and rhinorrhea, but nasal disease appears to impact other systems. The incidence of middle-ear disease may be higher in allergic children than in others (2). Allergic nasal insufflation has been documented to cause negative middle-ear pressure in allergic subjects (3). The incidence of chronic sinusitis seems to be higher in allergic children (4). In children with asthma, treatment with nasal corticosteroids can decrease bronchial hyperresponsiveness, suggesting that nasal disease can exacerbate pulmonary disease (5–7). There is arguable evidence that chronic nasal congestion may be a factor in facial development, prolonged mouth breathing leading to altered use of facial musculature with subsequent deviations in growth from what normal nasal use would have engendered (8).

The pathophysiology of allergic rhinitis involves antigen–antibody interaction followed by the release of inflammatory mediators (9). Patients with allergic rhinitis produce immunoglobulin E (IgE), which is directed toward specific allergens in the environment, for example, dust mites, pet dander, molds, and pollens. This IgE is bound to mast cells of the nasal mucosa. After this process of sensitization has occurred, subsequent exposure to allergen molecules results in a binding of mast-cell-bound IgE and allergen. This results in influx of calcium and release of preformed mediators such as histamine from the mast cell. This occurs within minutes; other mediators are produced and released in the hours that follow. Some of these mediators are chemoattractants for inflammatory cells such as eosinophils that move into the nasal epithelium and submucosa. These cells produce additional inflammatory products and augment cellular migration. Thus, the immediate release of chemical mediators is followed by a late-phase inflammatory reaction in the mucosa.

The pathophysiology of allergic rhinitis involves membrane edema, increased mucus secretion, and stimulation of neural reflexes. Histamine causes vasodilation with subsequent edema and stimulates the neuronally mediated sneeze reflex. Histamine also acts directly and indirectly through reflex stimulation to produce increased mucus and serous gland secretion and nasal itching. Other inflammatory chemicals augment and prolong these manifestations of allergic disease (Fig. 1).

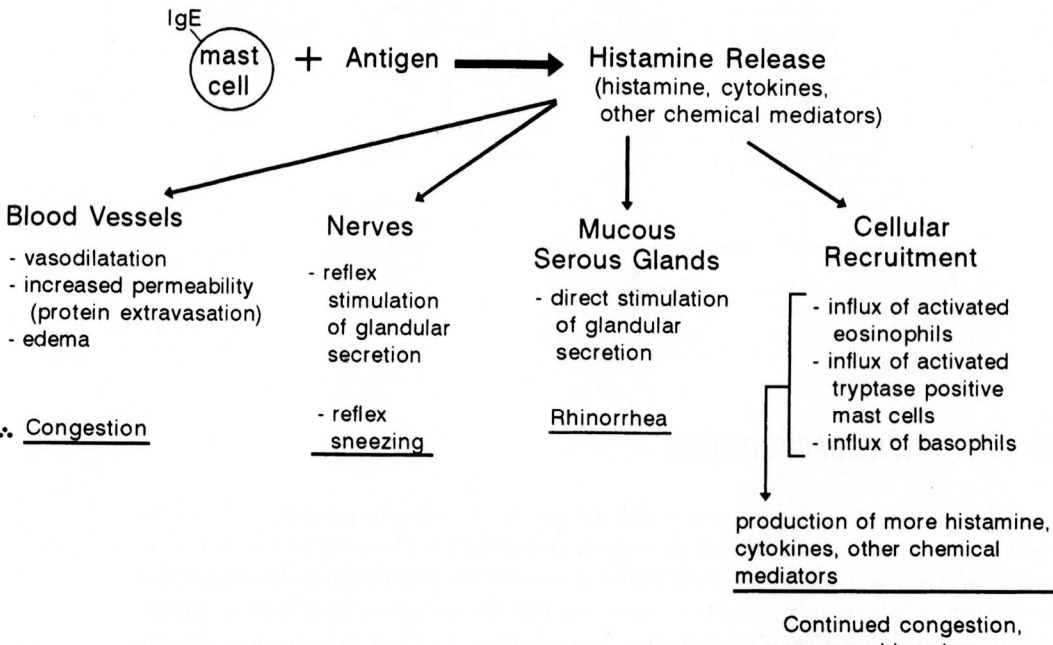

FIGURE 1 This schematic diagram shows how mediator release following mast cell activation causes nasal inflammation. Blood vessels, nerves, and mucosal glands are stimulated by mast cell products. In addition, the influx of inflammatory cells such as the eosinophil will prolong and augment the inflammatory reaction that creates the clinical entity we recognize as allergic rhinitis.

Although allergic rhinitis is the most common cause of chronic nasal airway obstruction in children, it is not the sole cause. By means of a thorough history, appropriate physical examination, and directed laboratory assessment, one can decide on the likelihood of allergic rhinitis versus infectious rhinitis (which may be superimposed on allergic rhinitis) versus structural abnormalities that may cause nasal obstruction, including hypertrophied adenoid tissue, severe nasal septal deviation, and nasal polyps. Occasionally, children may show nonallergic eosinophilic rhinitis or nonspecific vasomotor rhinitis, the causes of which are unknown.

PATIENT ASSESSMENT

The usual features of allergic rhinitis are nasal congestion, rhinorrhea, sneezing, and nasal itching. Some patients complain of feeling that they have an ongoing cold. Some experience itching of the palate or ear as a result of common cranial nerve innervation of the nose and ear canal. Young children may habitually rub their nose or make strange facial gestures to overcome nasal pruritus. Dark periorbital circles called allergic shiners may indicate chronic lymphatic and venous stasis in the periorbital region secondary to chronic airway edema, although sinusitis and hereditary factors may also cause this darkened appearance, which is often attributed to allergic disease. There may be a history of being sick more than other children with related conditions, such as frequent otitis or sinusitis. The patient may be experiencing other allergic diseases, such as asthma, atopic dermatitis, or food allergy.

History

The family history may support a suspicion of allergic disease. Prospective studies show that if one parent expresses allergy in such forms as atopic dermatitis, allergic rhinitis, or asthma, there is a 38% to 58% chance that his or her child will be allergic. If both parents are allergic, the likelihood of a child also being allergic is 60% to 80% (10).

It is helpful to explore cause and effect relationships. Does the congestion seem worse at the home of a caregiver who has pets? Is the problem year round, as with dust mite, mold, and animal allergy, or is it seasonal, as with pollen allergy? Younger children are most likely to have allergic rhinitis secondary to perennial allergens, such as dust mites, molds, and pets, since it takes a number of years to have enough exposure to elicit pollen-related symptoms. By age 5, pollen-induced rhinitis is common, and it certainly can occur in the younger child. Pollen-induced rhinitis in a child without concomitant perennial allergen sensitivity is unusual. Food allergy is an uncommon cause of allergic rhinitis, though rhinitis may be one aspect of food reactivity, for example, one of the symptoms during an anaphylactic reaction to a food.

It can be very difficult to prove cause and effect because of the dual nature of allergic inflammatory reactions. Whereas patients may experience symptoms of rhinitis within minutes of an allergen exposure, the subsequent cascade of events leads to an augmented reaction hours after the initial insult. Thus, a patient may notice mild discomfort when around a pet and then have severe nasal obstruction several hours later, when the inciting agent is no longer in the environment. Additionally, if the inciting allergen is present on an ongoing basis, the continual liberation of allergic mediators and recruitment of inflammatory cells, which then produce more inflammatory chemicals, soon leads to chronic swelling and rhinorrhea, for which the timetable of events is impossible to sort. It is common to hear that a child is stuffy all the time and that the family is certain the family cat is unrelated to the problem, since the child is never worse when close to the cat. Actually, it is quite likely that an allergic child could be experiencing chronic symptoms from chronic exposure to an allergen like cat, even though there are no dramatic acute symptoms after so much exposure.

In addition to allergens, irritants may be causative agents by augmenting inflammatory processes in the airway (11). It is important to inquire about tobacco smoking in the home. It is also valuable to assess other aggravants, such as wood stove-related pollutants, chlorine vapors at swimming pools, and paint fumes or construction dust related to remodeling at home or at school.

Physical Examination

The physical examination may be dramatic or unimpressive, depending on whether there has been a recent acute exposure or chronic ongoing exposure. Signs and symptoms of acute allergen exposure include sneezing, nose rubbing, and clear nasal discharge. With time, the patient may show periorbital darkening, i.e., allergic shiners. There may be edema of the bulbar conjunctiva, sometimes so severe as to produce a gelatinous layer over the eye. The hard palate may show petechiae; these result from negative pressure exerted by the tongue as the patient attempts to scratch the itchy palate, usually producing unique clucking noises in the process. Between exposures, the patient may be asymptomatic. Congestion and sniffing may be low grade but constant when the exposure is chronic.

The typical appearance of the allergic nasal vault is swollen, pale pink mucosa overlying the turbinates along with thin, colorless secretions. This prototypical appearance, however, is frequently replaced by a less classic one. The nasal vault may look normal; the mucosa may be erythematous; secretions may be turbid. These deviations may occur because at the time of the examination the patient is asymptomatic, has an upper respiratory infection, or has a distinctive pattern of disease.

Children with chronic nasal disease may experience eustachian tube dysfunction presumably due to edema around the tube's orifice. It is common to see retracted or scarred tympanic membranes, middle-ear ventilating tubes, or middle-ear effusions in patients presenting with allergic rhinitis, a nonspecific finding considering the large number of children with ear problems independent of nasal disease. Sinus disease also may be more likely in allergic children. When one encounters nasal purulence and membrane erythema, consider an infectious etiology either secondary to allergic rhinitis or independent of it.

The child with allergic rhinitis is likely to show other signs of allergic disease. It is valuable to check for atopic dermatitis. The chest examination may reveal expiratory wheezing or rhonchi suggesting bronchial hyperresponsiveness or frank asthma. Since cough may be a chief complaint in patients with both allergic rhinitis and asthma, it is important to pay attention to this possibility of pulmonary involvement.

The microscopic evaluation of nasal secretions often provides valuable information in making a diagnosis (12). The patient blows his or her nose into plastic wrap, or a swab can be used to obtain the specimen. The secretions are wiped onto a glass slide, which is then heat fixed and stained with Hansel's stain. The presence of more than 5% eosinophils/field suggests allergic rhinitis (Fig. 2). However, less common problems such as nonallergic rhinitis with eosinophilia and nasal polyposis (with or without concomitant allergic rhinitis) cannot be discounted. The absence of eosinophils does not rule out allergy. During an infectious episode in particular, it is common for neutrophils to dominate. A predominance of polymorphonuclear cells suggests infectious rhinitis (Fig. 3), most likely related to a viral syndrome if the condition is acute, or, if more long-standing, to bacterial rhinosinusitis. If there are watery secretions that yield few cells, vasomotor rhinitis is quite likely, although it is possible that the patient has allergic rhinitis but is currently asymptomatic.

Differential Diagnosis and Entering the Decision Tree

With the information gleaned from the history, physical examination, and evaluation of nasal secretions, one can pass to the first branch points of the decision tree. The differ-

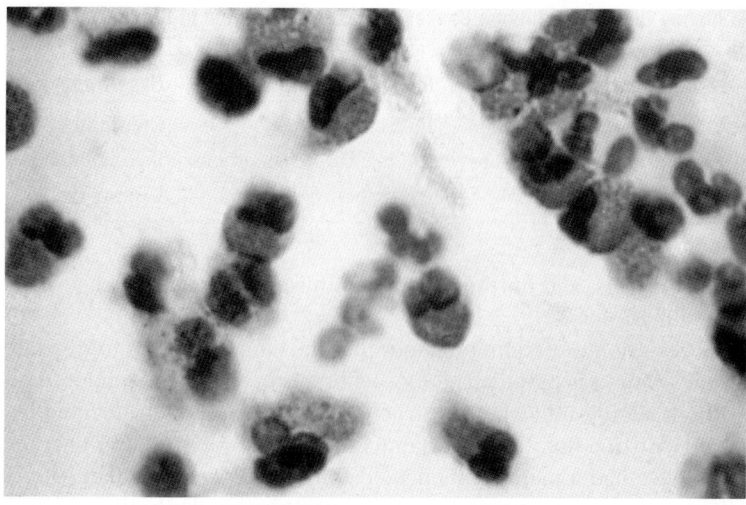

FIGURE 2 The presence of 5% to 10% or more eosinophils in nasal secretions highly suggests allergic rhinitis. Eosinophils stain distinctly with eosin and methylene blue, making them easy to separate from other cells in the nasal secretions.

ential diagnosis of rhinitis in children includes a number of conditions besides allergic rhinitis. Infectious rhinitis secondary to unrecognized sinusitis brings nonallergic children to the allergist's office rather frequently. Of course, allergic children may also develop this problem and may be more prone to sinusitis than the average child due to chronic inflammation in the nasal airways that impedes normal clearance of infection. Nonallergic rhinitis with eosinophilia resembles allergic rhinitis identically on examination; however, allergy testing is negative, and the etiology of the nasal disease is unknown. This problem is uncommon prior to puberty. Vasomotor rhinitis is nasal membrane edema and mucus hypersecretion of unknown etiology, but it is probably due to autonomic imbalance in the nasal airway. Secretions tend to be thin, watery, and acellular on microscopic examination. This diagnosis is actually much more common in middle-aged adults than in children. Nasal polyposis is another inflammatory disorder of unknown origin but is sometimes associated with allergic rhinitis. Nasal polyps in children recall the diagnosis of cystic fibrosis, which is the most common cause of this problem in childhood. Rhinitis medicamentosa refers to nasal membrane inflammation secondary to overuse of vasoconstrictive nose sprays. Structural problems, including septal deviations, unilateral choanal atresia, tumors, and foreign bodies, are unusual causes of chronic rhinitis in children. Adenoidal hypertrophy is a common cause of upper airway congestion that can be confused with allergic rhinitis. A very static congestion free of rhinorrhea, not fluctuat-

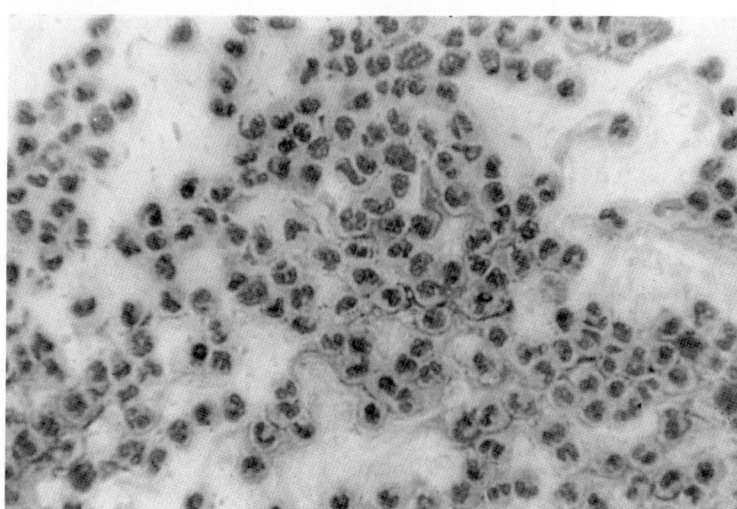

FIGURE 3 During a viral or bacterial upper respiratory infection, it is common to see a preponderance of neutrophils in the nasal secretions. If the infection has been short lived, the likelihood of it being viral is great. As the duration extends past a week to 10 days, the likelihood of bacterial involvement increases.

TABLE 1: Comparison Among the Most Common Causes of Nasal Obstruction in Children

	Allergic Rhinitis	*Infectious Rhinosinusitis*	*Adenoid Hypertrophy*
History of symptoms	Intermittent or constant	Intermittent	Constant
Nasal examinations	Edema, clear secretions	Edema, turbid secretions	Unremarkable
Nasal secretions	>5% eosinophils	>90% neurophils	Unremarkable

ing with environmental changes, and unresponsive to antihistamines and decongestants suggests an adenoid problem.

In day to day practice, the most common issues that the clinician needs to separate are whether the patient's rhinitis is based on allergy, whether there is an infectious etiology along with or without allergy, and whether structural issues, most likely adenoid hypertrophy, are involved (see decision tree). Certainly, the history, physical examination, and nasal cytology will have had a major influence, leading the search in a likely direction. More diagnostic testing may be necessary at this juncture to clarify the situation (Table 1).

Allergy Skin Testing

Allergy skin testing plays an important role in distinguishing allergic rhinitis from other diagnostic possibilities. The decision to perform skin tests or to treat allergic rhinitis empirically depends on the chronicity and severity of the problem. For some situations, brief courses of antihistamines or decongestants will provide satisfactory relief so that in-depth evaluation is unnecessary. In performing skin testing, extracts of common aeroallergens are applied to the epidermis in such a way as to reproduce the interaction of environmental allergen and mast-cell-bound IgE that occurs in the nose. Initial testing is usually carried out by an epicutaneous method: prick, puncture, or scratch

FIGURE 4 Extracts of common allergens are applied to the skin with a simple needle, which is used to lift the skin and bring the allergen in contact with mast cells in the epidermis. This is the prick puncture technique.

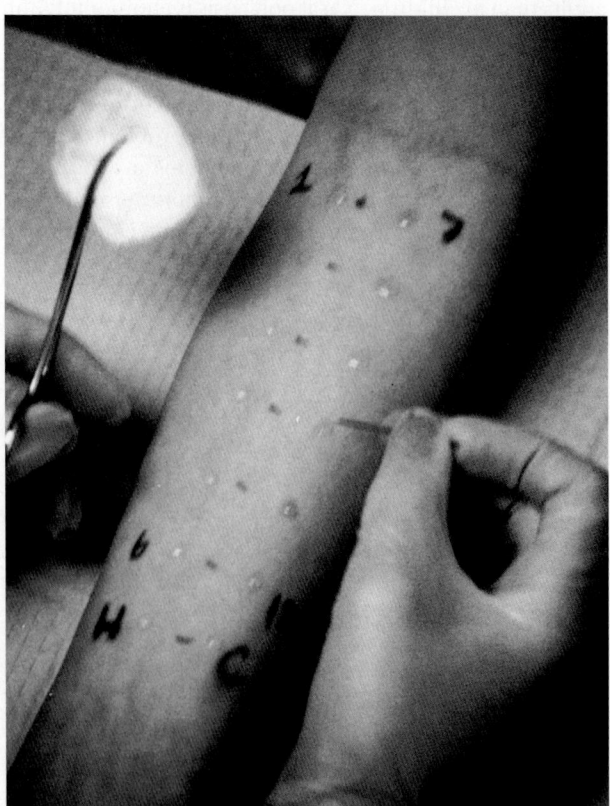

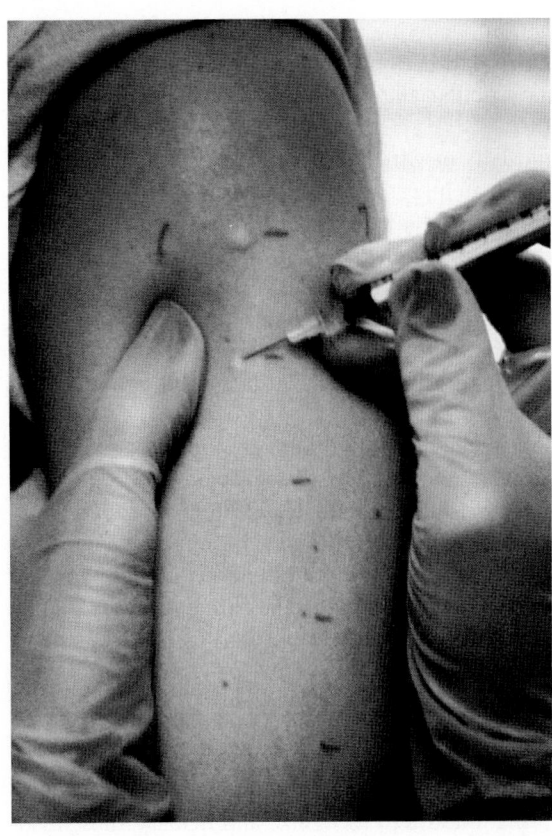

FIGURE 5 Intradermal skin testing is more sensitive but less specific than prick puncture testing.

(Figs. 4 and 5). A drop of an extract of each allergen in question is applied to the skin, and a needle is used to pierce the skin superficially, enough to bring antigen and mediator-containing cells into contact. Within 15 to 20 minutes, a wheal and flare will appear if significant amounts of histamine are released (Fig. 6). There is good correlation between positive epicutaneous skin testing to inhaled allergens and clinical symptoms on exposure. Because this testing is not always adequately sensitive, intradermal skin testing may be needed. A small quantity of allergen is directly injected into the epi-

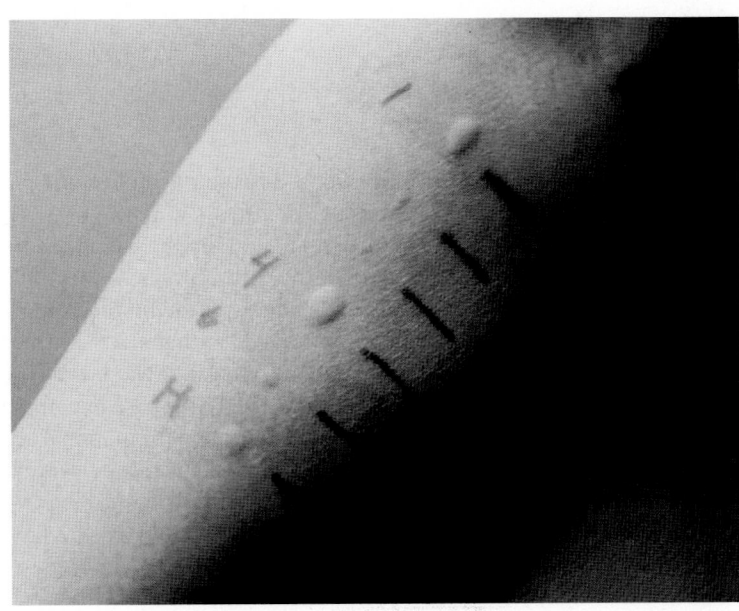

FIGURE 6 A wheal and flare will appear within 15 to 20 minutes of testing if a person is sensitive to an allergen that has been applied. At numbers 1 and 4 on the arm, one can see a positive reaction that is comparable to the reaction evoked by the histamine control (*H*).

dermis. Again, a wheal and flare reaction occurring within 15 to 20 minutes of exposure indicates allergic reactivity. The correlation between positive intradermal test and actual symptoms from exposure to a particular allergen is less commanding than epicutaneous reactions.

An alternative approach to diagnosis is in vitro measurement of allergen-specific IgE. The patient's serum is incubated with an inert carrier material coated with allergen. Serum IgE to specific allergen will react with the allergen–carrier complex to form an IgE–allergen–carrier complex that can be radiolabeled and then quantitated. The prototype of this is the radioallergosorbent test (RAST). In general, such in vitro methods are more costly and less sensitive than skin testing and are rarely preferable. Because total serum IgE is elevated in only about one-half of allergic rhinitis patients, determination of total IgE is helpful when the level is higher than the normal range but not when it is within the normal range.

Since allergic rhinitis often exists in association with other conditions that it actually may instigate, certain diagnostic tests relating to these problems may be important in the patient's evaluation. Cough may be due to irritation of cough receptors secondary to allergic rhinitis or may be related to asthma, a situation that may require spirometry for clarification. Eustachian tube dysfunction may be associated with nasal inflammation and may be evaluated with audiometry and tympanometry. Chronic rhinitis may be related to sinus disease, which may require imaging studies of the sinuses.

PEARLS AND PERILS

1. Allergic rhinitis often coexists with other health problems, particularly middle-ear disease, sinusitis, and asthma. Failure to recognize and manage these associated problems will lead to a less than optimal outcome.
2. Many patients who present with possible allergic rhinitis do not actually have allergic disease. A fairly comprehensive evaluation that includes history, physical examination, nasal cytology, and skin testing may be just as valuable in determining future therapy if it is negative as if it is positive. If such a workup is negative, chronic sinusitis is a likely diagnosis that deserves consideration.
3. Chronic sinus disease may masquerade as allergic rhinitis, as may other forms of nasal disease which are discussed in the differential diagnosis that are not as common as allergic rhinitis and sinusitis.

 # TREATMENT RECOMMENDATIONS

Nonpharmacologic Intervention

The common allergens provoking allergic rhinitis are housedust mites, molds, animal proteins, and pollens. Insect antigens (especially from cockroaches) are important in certain parts of the United States. It is unusual to see isolated allergic rhinitis secondary to food allergy, although rhinitis may accompany atopic dermatitis and gastrointestinal manifestations of allergy (13). It is uncommon to see pollen allergy in the first few years of life, probably because pollen seasons are relatively short-lived, so that several exposures are needed to deliver enough immunologic information to sensitize the host. The most effective therapy is avoidance of the inciting allergens (14,15). In the case of animal exposure, this may represent severe sacrifice. One must weigh the patient's emotional attachment to a pet against the degree of disease involvement and relief through other modalities. Since allergic rhinitis can exacerbate bronchial hyperresponsiveness, the possibility that asthma may be a sequela of continued antigen exposure should also be factored into the equation when deciding how aggressive to be in counseling about environmental control.

Among the most important allergens for childhood allergic rhinitis is the dust mite (14,15). Housedust mites are ubiquitous microscopic creatures that feed off human skin scales. They thrive in climates with high relative humidity, and they avoid ambient daylight. They tend to be abundant in stuffed furniture, mattresses and carpets, where they leave fecal particles that are more antigenic than the mites themselves.

Dust mites do not survive extremes of boiling and freezing and do not proliferate in dry conditions, requiring at least 50% relative humidity to survive. Their viability may be drastically reduced by such measures as decreasing moisture, removing carpets, and encasing mattresses and pillows in covers that are either vinyl or coated with impermeable layering. Hot water washing of bedding on a 1- to 2-week basis appears to be helpful. Placing stuffed toys that cannot be washed in a hot dryer or freezer may be helpful, although little firm data exist to validate these measures. Acaricides (dust mite killers) are probably valuable but are not well studied. Benzyl benzoate powder is commercially available for application to carpets every 6 months. Tannic acid solution (3%) is also available commercially for application to carpets and upholstery every 1 to 3 months. Although it does not kill mites, tannic acid appears to denature mite and pet antigens, rendering them nonimmunogenic.

Mold avoidance also involves measures to decrease household humidity. Heating and cooling systems should be checked to eliminate mold reservoirs. A layer of heavy plastic (Visqueen) in the crawl space of a home will decrease moisture problems and mold growth. A dehumidifier may be necessary at times. An application of liquid laundry bleach removes mold growth on window frames and bathroom tiles. When houses are built on concrete slabs without basement or crawl space, the chances of mold problems are high, since the concrete serves as a wick transporting moisture from the ground into the carpeting.

Pollen avoidance is extremely difficult because pollens are so widespread at certain times of year. Keeping doors and windows closed and using air conditioning effectively filters most pollen from the home. This is not helpful, however, for individuals with outdoor-oriented lifestyle. Similarly, it is impractical where air conditioning is unnecessary for temperature control. High-efficiency filters (electrostatic precipitators and high-efficiency particulate air HEPA filters remove particulate matter, including pollens, mold spores, and mites. They, too, are most effective if doors and windows are kept closed. The correlation between high-efficiency filter use and control of rhinitis symptoms is unclear (Table 2).

Although environmental control is the theoretic ideal for managing allergic rhinitis, it is difficult to institute and to sustain. The impressive improvement seen in many patients who have accomplished such preventive measures encourages one to continue providing these recommendations. Nevertheless, complicated lifestyles involving such confounding factors as rental homes, dual-parent custody of children, and day-care settings are important factors that force the use of other approaches in addition to attempting to improve the environment.

TABLE 2: Environmental Control Suggestion

Exposure	Intervention
Airborne irritants	Avoid tobacco smoke, wood stoves, noxious fumes
Dust mites	Remove carpet if possible; if not, use acacaricides: 　1. Tannic acid solution 3%: spray on carpets and stuffed furniture every 6 months (denatures mite and pet antigen but does not kill mites). 　2. Benzyl benzoate: spread on carpets every 2–3 months (denatures antigen and kills mites with repeated use). Place zippered plastic cover on mattress and box spring cover. Wash pillow, blankets, and sheets in hot water weekly.
Mold	Decrease humidity in home to <50% relative humidity. Apply bleach-containing cleaners to visible mildew.

Pharmacologic Intervention

Antihistamines

Antihistamines are first-line therapy for allergic rhinitis. They competitively inhibit the allergic mediator histamine at its receptor sites. Although there are both H1 and H2 receptors in the tissues of the upper airway, H1 receptors are most relevant to allergic rhinitis. Antihistamines block both the vasodilation that results from stimulation of the blood vessels by H1 receptor–histamine interaction and the mucous gland hypersecretion and sneezing that result from reflex initiation consequent to the stimulation of H1 receptors in proximity to sensory nerves by histamine. In terms of symptomatic benefit, antihistamines are most effective for diminishing nasal itch and hypersecretion but do not effectively decrease mucous membrane edema.

The classic or so-called first-generation antihistamines are classified on the basis of chemical structure. Familiarity with a representative drug from each of several classes allows alternation between them if tachyphylaxis or adverse side effects makes an alternate choice necessary. Not uncommonly, a patient will respond to a drug within the same family as the now-inadequate agent, pointing out the scanty scientific basis for the practice of shifting antihistamine families (Table 3).

Although they are considerably more expensive than the first-generation drugs, the newer, nonsedating antihistamines are very valuable therapeutic agents for allergic rhinitis (16). Besides avoiding drowsiness for most patients, they also prevent the decreases in reaction time that patients may not consciously recognize but that can cause suboptimal performance of fine motor tasks and maneuvers requiring fast reflex reactions (16). These agents are not officially approved by the Food and Drug Administration (FDA) for children under age 12, but terfenadine has been approved in a liquid formulation in Canada and has been used by younger children for years. Loratadine will soon be available in a liquid form for children 6 years and older. The nonsedating antihistamines terfenadine, astemizole, and loratadine do not cross the blood–brain barrier very well and are known to be nonsedating. A newer agent in terms of U.S. usage is cetirizine, a relatively nonsedating metabolite of hydroxyzine.

The nonsedating antihistamines have peculiarities that distinguish them from each other. Astemizole differs from the other agents in having a slow onset of activity and long half-life. It may take a week to see its peak effect and a month or more before its activity is totally gone. This makes it a poor choice for as-needed use but a good one for known

TABLE 3: Classification of Commonly Used Antihistamines

Class	Generic Name	Trade Name	Suggested Dose for Children (mg/kg/24 hr)	Suggested Dose for Adults
Ethanolamine	Diphenhydramine hydrochloride	Benadryl	5.0	25–50 mg q.i.d.
	Carbinoxamine maleate	Clistin	0.8	4–8 mg q.i.d.
Ethylenediamine	Tripelennamine hydrochloride	PBZ	5.0	25–50 mg q.i.d.
Alkylamine	Chlorpheniramine maleate	Chlor-Trimeton, Teidrin	0.35	4 mg q.i.d.
	Brompheniramine maleate	Dimetane	0.35	4 mg q.i.d.
	Triprolidine hydrochloride	Actidil	0.18	2.5 q.i.d.
Phenothiazine	Promethazine hydrochloride	Phenergan	0.5	12.5–25 mg q.i.d.
	Methdilazine	Tacaryl	0.3	16–32 mg q.i.d. (as b.i.d. or q.i.d.)
Piperazine	Hydroxyzine hydrochloride	Atarax, Vistaril, Durrax	2.0	10–20 mg q.i.d.
Piperidine	Cyproheptadine hydrochloride	Periactin	0.25	4–20 mg q.i.d.
Miscellaneous	Terfenadine	Seidane	—	60 mg b.i.d.
	Astemizole	Hismanal	—	10 mg q.d.
	Loraradine	Claritin	—	10 mg q.d.
	Cetirizine	Zyrtec	—	10 mg q.d.

seasonal exacerbations. Astemizole must be discontinued at least a month prior to allergy skin testing, or the histamine-induced wheal and flare will be suppressed, compared with 24 to 72 hours for most antihistamines. Terfenadine and loratadine are effective in less than an hour and retain clinical efficacy for 12 and 24 hours, respectively. Cetirizine has a similar rapid onset and 24-hour duration of effect. Although it is usually nonsedating, clinical trials submitted for its FDA approval were judged to show enough sedative potential to obviate its receiving the nonsedating imprimatur.

The metabolism of the nonsedating antihistamines terfenadine, astemizole, and loratadine by the P450 enzyme system of the liver results in certain problems of drug interaction. Terfenadine and astemizole but not loratadine or cetirizine can cause prolongation of the QT interval and cardiac arrhythmia if blood levels become elevated, as when there is competitive inhibition of their breakdown because of concomitant use of agents such as macrolide antibiotics and quinolines. Cetirizine does not undergo extensive hepatic metabolism.

Decongestants

The oral decongestants phenylpropanolamine, phenylephrine, and pseudoephedrine are alpha-adrenergic agents capable of producing nasal mucous membrane vasoconstriction adequate to reduce edema. Theoretically, they should enhance the effectiveness of antihistamines. Their drawback is the incidence of such adverse effects as irritability and insomnia.

There are currently a large number of combination products containing both antihistamine and decongestant. Clinical trials have shown the benefit of combination products compared with placebo but have failed to show clear benefit of the combination over the individual constituents (17–19). Although fixed-combination preparations are convenient and increase compliance, they prevent individualized dose adjustments. However, because little is currently known about dose–response relationships of many of these preparations, they remain practical and popular. The pseudoephedrine-containing product with loratadine is an interesting example of the problems with dose adjustments and multiple constituents. Loratadine alone is available as a 10-mg tablet for once a day use. Since there is no 24-hour-duration decongestant, loratadine with pseudoephedrine contains 5 mg of loratadine and is available as a 12-hour product.

Topical decongestants are poor choices for treating chronic rhinitis. With repeated use, they tend to cause less sustained decongestion, leading both to overuse and to rebound vasodilation with increased congestion. This iatrogenic congestion is known as rhinitis medicamentosa.

Cromolyn

Cromolyn in a 4% solution is an alternative to antihistamines as primary therapy for treatment of allergic rhinitis. It is formulated as a nasal spray and may act by preventing mast cell mediator release. Cromolyn is effective only as a prophylactic agent and must be used regularly rather than after symptoms occur. Clinical trials support the value of cromolyn compared with placebo when it is used as one spray per nostril six times a day (20,21). After an initial 1 to 2 weeks of this therapy, less frequent use at two to three times a day may be adequate. Adverse effects are uncommon and benign. These include transient sneezing, nasal stinging and headache.

Corticosteroids

Intranasal administration of corticosteroids is an extremely effective therapy for allergic rhinitis. It may be used for brief intervals when the previously mentioned agents inadequately control symptoms. More and more, physicians are prescribing intranasal corticosteroids as primary therapy because of their safe profile and superior efficacy in many patients. Corticosteroids appear to diminish the activation of inflammatory cells that contribute to inflammatory rhinitis, while also inhibiting the production and release of inflammatory mediators (22). Clinical trials comparing intranasal corticosteroids with placebo for seasonal and perennial rhinitis consistently show favorable results for the active preparation (23–25).

Aside from dexamethasone spray, the intranasal corticosteroids are highly active topically and are very poorly absorbed from the mucosa. The portion that is swallowed and absorbed from the gastrointestinal tract is rapidly metabolized to an inactive form. These new preparations have greatly improved the safety of long-term topical therapy. They are commonly used for several weeks during rhinitis exacerbations, although longer treatment periods may be needed during pollen seasons and for especially severe, chronic, perennial rhinitis. Often therapy with antihistamines and decongestants is continued. Customary dosing with these preparations involves one or two actuations per nostril once or twice a day. This is usually well tolerated, most complaints relating to nasal stinging and nosebleeds, which remit when use of the drug is discontinued. Perforation of the nasal septum is extremely uncommon but reported (26–29). Intranasal corticosteroids have been reported to be associated with disseminated varicella in two patients, so that immunization should be offered to patients who have not had clinical chickenpox (30). Some of these products have been approved for use in children aged 6 and older (Table 4).

In clinical practice, intranasal steroids are now being used in very young children who are intolerant of oral agents or who have particularly chronic rhinitis. As with many interventions for young children, it is unlikely that pharmaceutical firms will sponsor the sorts of evaluation that are needed to gain FDA approval. In view of the apparently benign nature of intranasal corticosteroids used properly, as well as their effectiveness, the risk–benefit ratio weighs toward using them in the lowest effective dose and for the shortest period needed for youngsters over 2 to 3 years with difficult rhinitis. Since beclomethasone is the least potent agent available and has the longest use record worldwide, it is probably the best agent to use for very young children. A typical dose would be one puff per nostril twice daily. Systemic corticosteroid therapy is rarely needed for allergic rhinitis. In patients who have severe involvement that appears refractory to other therapy, a short course of oral, short-acting steroid (e.g., prednisone or methylprednisolone) is helpful. Long-term use puts the patient at risk for a long list of steroid-induced adverse effects, which may well be more worrisome than the initial rhinitis. Intramuscular steroid injection has produced unsightly keloid formation and subcutaneous fat atrophy. Injection of steroids into the turbinates has been associated with blindness due to intraarterial embolization of the mixture (31).

Deciding Between Antihistamines and Intranasal Steroids for Primary Therapy

Conventionally, antihistamines have been the mainstay of initial pharmacologic therapy for allergic rhinitis. Decongestants have been added to shrink swollen membranes. Intranasal steroids have been used when patients have been refractory to other therapy. The high benefit to risk ratio of today's intranasal steroids make them an attractive choice to be considered earlier than in the past. Added to their good safety record

TABLE 4: Intranasal Corticosteroids

Chemical Name	Trade Name	Usual Dosage (puffs/side)[a]	FDA Approval Age (years)
Beclomethasone	Beconase, Vancenase	1–2 b.i.d.	≥6
Budesonide	Rhinocort	2 b.i.d. or 4 q.d.	≥6
Dexamethasone	Dexacort	1–2 b.i.d. or t.i.d.	≥6
Flunisolide	Nasaret	2 b.i.d.	≥6–14
Fluticasone	Flonase	2 q.d. or 1 b.i.d.	≥12
Triamcinolone	Nasacort	2 b.i.d. or 4 q.i.d.	≥12

[a]Base initial adult dosage. Lower end of dosage range pertains to children.

(From ref. 39, with permission.)

are comparative trials of antihistamine versus intranasal steroid that almost always favor the latter for control of nasal disease (32–34). When significant ocular involvement, pruritus, and headache exist, combination therapy with antihistamine, decongestant, and intranasal steroid leads to the best response (9).

Immunotherapy

Immunotherapy, also called desensitization or hyposensitization, involves the injection of allergens into an immunologically sensitive individual for the purpose of building tolerance to those allergens. Many studies attest to its usefulness, provided that appropriate patients are selected and that appropriate allergenic extract and dosing are used (35). Immunotherapy should be reserved for those allergic patients who continue to have recalcitrant disease after optimal avoidance measures and pharmacologic intervention have been attempted. These children may suffer from sensitivity to pollens that are present much of the year, or they may be in day-care settings, thus reducing the impact of environmental control measures in the home. Children under age 5 are rarely appropriate candidates for immunotherapy since their allergic sensitivity is quickly changing, pollen sensitivity is unlikely to be a major issue, and the trauma of injection therapy for the very young child is potentially substantial (36).

Prior to initiating immunotherapy, one should confirm the patient's sensitivity to allergens by skin testing. Only clinically significant allergens with such skin test verification should be added to the treatment mixture. Therapy is usually confined to housedust mite, pollen, and mold allergies. While avoidance is preferable, standardized cat antigen for immunotherapy is now commercially available. Therapy is usually initiated at a concentration of allergenic extract orders of magnitude less than that which produces a 5-mm wheal on prick skin testing. Frequently, this is a 1:100,000 concentration. Patients receive 0.05 ml of this concentration, and, with subsequent injections once or twice weekly, advance to 0.5 ml. They then begin receiving injections with the next higher concentration and progress as before, eventually reaching the 1:100 concentration level. A maintenance dose (usually 0.2 or 0.3 ml) is then selected and given every 2 to 4 weeks. There are many variations of this schedule, but all follow the principle of gradual progression from a dilute to a concentrated antigen mixture.

PEARLS AND PERILS

1. Environmental control is a key element for optimal results. Medication alone is less likely to give the best outcome for this chronic condition.
2. Antihistamines and decongestants have been traditional first-line therapies, but intranasal steroids are now moving into this position. All these therapies entail possible adverse effects, and their use must be monitored.
3. Although intranasal steroids are usually effective and benign, one can detect subtle alterations in endocrine function with their use. These changes are rarely clinically significant. Also, an association between intranasal steroid and severe varicella has led to FDA warnings about possible immunosuppression. These issues underscores the need to follow patients who take these medications for chronic therapy.
4. Nonsedating antihistamines are usually effective and well tolerated. Drug interactions with terfenadine and astemizole can lead to adverse effects, specifically QT interval prolongation and subsequent arrhythmia.

Although the benefits of immunotherapy are often achieved in the first year, most patients receive it for 3 to 5 years. After this time, many of those who have responded seem to retain symptomatic benefit even when this therapy is discontinued. Responsiveness appears to relate to production of IgE blocking antibodies, downregulation of IgE production, and decreased releasability by mediator-containing cells (25,37).

Physicians who administer immunotherapy must be prepared to treat anaphylaxis (38). Although patients are most at risk as they progress to higher antigen doses, anaphylaxis is to some degree unpredictable. Life-threatening reactions occur most commonly immediately after immunotherapy injections. For this reason, patients should remain in the clinic for 30 minutes after each injection so they can be observed for possible systemic complications. Quite commonly, patients experience local reactions at the injection site. If a large immediate or late-phase local reaction occurs, the dose should be decreased and then advanced slowly if reactions diminish.

🔆 MANAGEMENT OF COMPLICATIONS

Before jumping to the area of medication complications, it is important to discuss environmental control complications. It is common to find that noble measures at home are undone by a second home where there is little concern for allergens. The physician needs to be directive to all caregivers concerning such issues as dust mite and pet avoidance when these are appropriate. This may take a special session with a part-time custodial parent or day-care person, but this is usually a worthwhile investment.

Antihistamines come in a wide variety of types and have a wide range of potentially adverse effects. The most commonly encountered ones are drowsiness, excessive dryness, gastrointestinal upset, and urinary retention. Drug interactions pose a problem with terfenadine and astemizole, which are largely metabolized in the liver and whose half-life can be enhanced by use in conjunction with macrolide antibiotics and quinolines.

Decongestants can cause excessive dryness. They may create a feeling of anxiety and irritability, as well as insomnia. They are often used only in the morning and are omitted from a nighttime medication regimen.

Intranasal corticosteroids may quite commonly cause nasal crusting and bleeding. The use of over-the-counter saline nose spray prior to using the steroid can be very helpful. Rarely, nasal septal perforation can occur if the intranasal steroid jet repeatedly impacts the same area of the septum and erodes it over time. This is associated with gross overuse and misdirecting the spray to the midline. The risk of disseminated varicella with intranasal steroid is extremely small; however, a case report describes two instances of this association and raises the possibility of cause and effect. Neither of these cases was fatal (30).

PEARLS AND PERILS

1. Patients usually respond well to rhinitis medications. Failure to respond well suggests concomitant problems including infectious rhinitis (sinusitis) and/or asthma.
2. There are many choices and combinations of therapy. Some trials of various combinations may be made before satisfactory results are realized.
3. Do not overlook allergen immunotherapy as an option for patients with allergic disease.

An important management issue that might be considered to be a complication is the frequent tendency to attribute all of a patient's upper airway symptomatology to allergic rhinitis without recognizing concurrent infection. The incidence of bacterial sinus disease in children is high and perhaps higher still in allergic children. An increase in rhinorrhea and cough that fails to remit after 1 or 2 weeks may represent an exacerbation of allergic disease or sinusitis. As the decision tree recommends, an examination of the patient and an evaluation of the nasal secretions may lead one to empiric treatment of sinusitis.

The presence of cough in a patient with allergic rhinitis poses a management issue. Cough can be secondary to pharyngeal irritation and posterior nasal drainage-related allergic rhinitis. Alternatively, cough can be related to asthma, a frequent concomitant problem in allergic children. Failure to appreciate this possibility leads to inadequately treated pulmonary disease and often overtolerated rhinitis. The use of office spirometry and/or home peak flow monitoring of airway function can clarify the situation in children over 5 years. Since younger children cannot perform these tests, the physician must use clinical judgment, as well as a trial of asthma therapy in certain situations.

✴ REFERENCES

1. Kaliner M, Lemanske R. Rhinitis and asthma. *JAMA* 1992;268:2807–2829.
2. Fireman P. Nasal allergy: a risk factor for middle ear disease. *Ann Allergy* 1987;58:395–400.
3. Skoner DP, Doyle WJ, Chamovitz A, Fireman P. Eustachian tube obstruction after intranasal challenge with house dust. *Arch Otolaryngol* 1986;112:840–842.
4. Shapiro GG, Virant FS, Furukawa CT, Pierson WE, Bierman CW. Immunologic defects in patients with refractory sinusitis. *Pediatrics* 1991;87:311–316.
5. Aubier M, Levy J, Clerici C, Neukirch F, Herman D. Different effects of nasal and bronchial glucocorticosteroid administration on bronchial hyperresponsiveness in patients with allergic rhinitis. *Am Rev Respir Dis* 1992;146:122–126.
6. Corren J, Adinoff AD, Buchmeier AD, Irvin CG. Nasal beclomethasone prevents the seasonal increase in bronchial responsiveness in patients with allergic rhinitis and asthma. *J Allergy Clin Immunol* 1992;90:250–256.
7. Watson WT, Becker AB, Simon FE. Treatment of allergic rhinitis with intranasal corticosteroids in patients with mild asthma: effect on lower airway responsiveness. *J Allergy Clin Immunol* 1993;91:97–101.
8. Trask G, Shapiro PA. In: David G. Tinkleman, ed. *Childhood rhinitis and sinusitis.* New York: Marcel Dekker, 1990:217–229.
9. Naclerio R. Allergic rhinitis. *N Engl J Med* 1991;325:860–869.
10. Zeiger RS, Heller S, Mellon MH, et al. *Pediatr Allergy Immunol* 1992;3:110.
11. Koenig JQ, Williams PV. Nonallergenic environmental factors. In: Bierman CW, Pearlman DS, Shapiro GG, Busse WW, eds. *Allergy, asthma, and immunology from infancy to adulthood.* Philadelphia: WB Saunders, 1996:124–133.
12. Lee HS, Majima Y, Sakakura Y, Shinogi J, Kanaguchi S, Kim BW. Quantitative cytology of nasal secretions under various conditions. *Laryngoscope* 1993;103:533–537.
13. Sampson HA, Metcalfe DD. Food allergies. *JAMA* 1992;268:2840–2844.
14. Rakes GP, Platts-Mills TA. Principles of avoidance. In: Bierman CW, Pearlman DS, Shapiro GG, Busse WW, eds. *Allergy, asthma, and immunology from infancy to adulthood.* Philadelphia: WB Saunders, 1996:195–207.
15. Evans R. Environmental control and immunotherapy for allergic disease. *J Allergy Clin Immunol* 1992;90:462–468.
16. Simons FE, Simons KJ. Second-generation H1-receptor antagonists. *Ann Allergy* 1991;66:5–16.
17. Henauer S, Seppey M, Huguenot C, et al. Effects of terfenadine and pseudoephedrine, alone and in combination in a nasal provocation test and in perennial rhinitis. *Eur J Clin Pharmacol* 1991;41:321–324.
18. Blockhuys S, Janssens M. *Allergy* 1992;49:319–323.
19. Bronsky E, Rogers C, Altman L, et al. A comparison of acrivastine + pseudoephedrine, chlorpheniramine + pseudoephedrine, and placebo in the treatment of perennial allergic rhinitis. *J Allergy Clin Immunol* 1987;79:191.
20. Handelman N, Friday GA, Schwartz HJ. Cromolyn sodium nasal solution in the prophylactic treatment of pollen-induced seasonal allergic rhinitis. *J Allergy Clin Immunol* 1977;59:237–242.
21. Chandra RK, Heresi G, Woodford G. Double-blind controlled crossover trial of 4% intranasal sodium cromoglycate solution in patients with seasonal allergic rhinitis. *Ann Allergy* 1982;49:131–134.
22. Cohan RH, Bloom FL, Rhoades RB, et al. Treatment of perennial allergic rhinitis with cromolyn sodium. Double-blind study of 34 adult patients. *J Allergy Clin Immunol* 1976;58:121–128.

23. Turkeltaub PC, Norman PS, Johnson JD, et al. Treatment of seasonal and perennial rhinitis with intranasal flunisolide. *Allergy* 1982;37:303–311.
24. Norman PS, Creticos PS, Tobey R, et al. Budesonide in grass pollen rhinitis. *Ann Allergy* 1992;69:309–316.
25. Ruhno J, Anderson B, Denburg J, et al. A double-blind comparison of intranasal budesonide with placebo for nasal polyposis. *J Allergy Clin Immunol* 1990;86:946–953.
26. Kaliner M, Lemanske R. Rhinitis and asthma. *JAMA* 1992;268:2807–2829.
27. La Force C, Davis V. *J Allergy Clin Immunol* 1985;75:186.
28. Soderberg-Warner ML. Nasal septal perforation associated with topical corticosteroid therapy. *J Pediatr* 1984;105:840–841.
29. Schoelzel EP, Menzel ML. Nasal sprays and perforation of the nasal septum [letter]. *JAMA* 1985;253:2046.
30. Abzug MJ, Cotton MF. Severe chicken pox after intranasal use of corticosteroids. *J Pediatr* 1993;123:577–578.
31. Mabry RL. Practical applications of intranasal corticosteroid injection. *Ear Nose Throat J* 1981;60:506–510.
32. Beswick KBJ, Kenyon GS, Cherry JR. A comparative study of beclomethasone dipropionate aqueous nasal spray with terfenadine tablets in seasonal allergic rhinitis. *Curr Med Res Opin* 1985;9:560–567.
33. Bernstein DI, Creticos PS, Busse WW, et al. Comparison of triamcinolone acetonide nasal inhaler with astemizole in the treatment of ragweed-induced allergic rhinitis. *J Allergy Clin Immunol* 1996;97:749–755.
34. Jordana G, Dolovich J, Briscoe MP, et al. Intranasal fluticasone propionate versus loratadine in the treatment of adolescent patients with seasonal allergic rhinitis. *J Allergy Clin Immunol* 1996;97:588–595.
35. Creticos P. Immunotherapy with allergens. *JAMA* 1992;268:2834–2839.
36. Ownby DR, Adinoff AD. The appropriate use of skin testing and allergen immunotherapy in young children. *J Allergy Clin Immunol* 1994;94:662–665.
37. Norman PS. Immunotherapy of IgE-mediated disease. *Hosp Prac* 1990;25:81–92.
38. Position Statement, American Academy of Allergy and Immunology. *J Allergy Clin Immunol* 1994;93:811–812.
39. Abramowicz M, ed. *Med Lett* 1995;37:50.

G.G. Shapiro: Department of Pediatrics, University of Washington, Seattle, Washington 98105.

- *Practical Pediatric Otolaryngology*
- edited by Robin T. Cotton and Charles M. Myer, III
- Lippincott-Raven Publishers, Philadelphia © 1999

24

Medical Treatment of Rhinosinusitis in Children

Evelyn A. Kluka

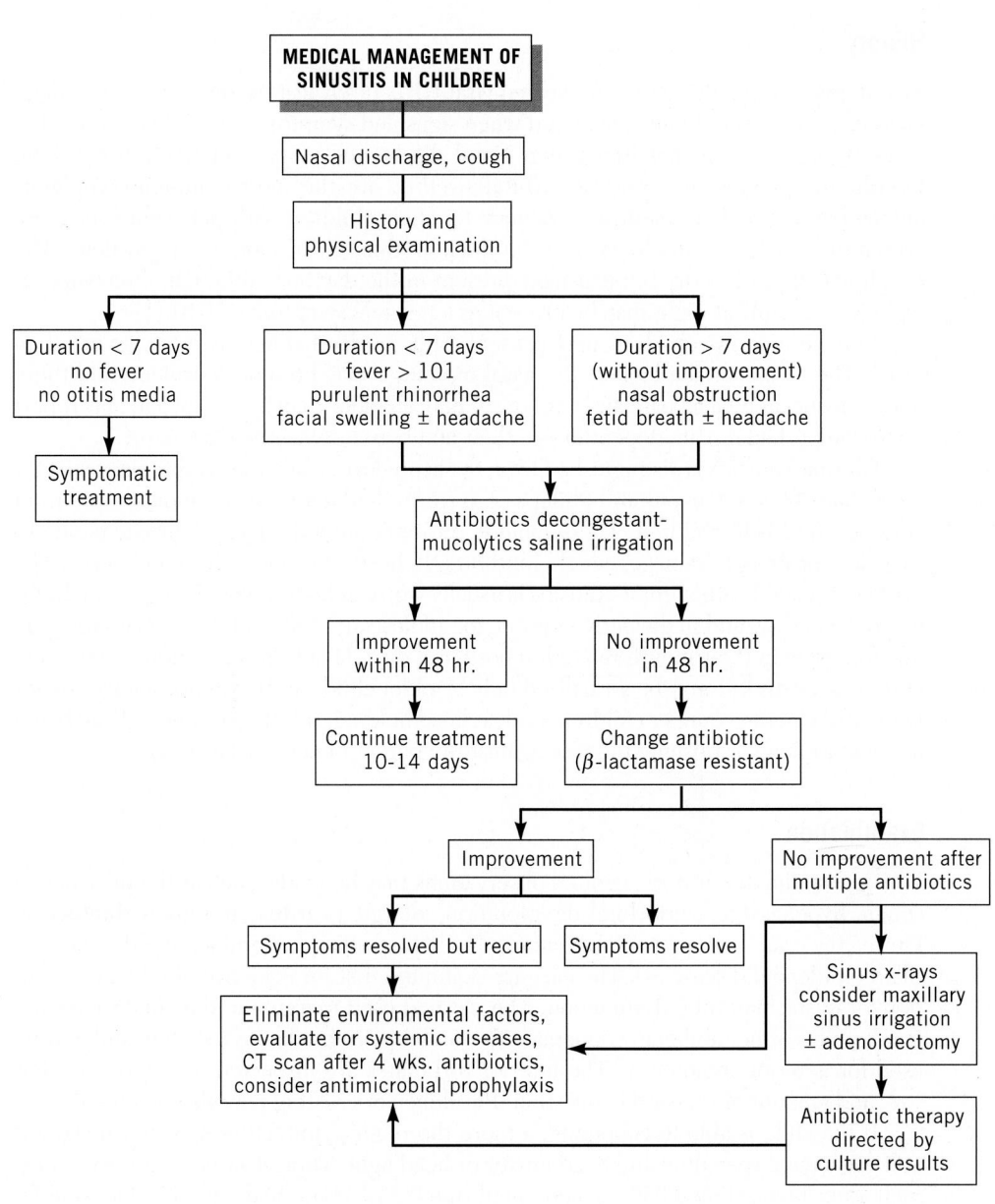

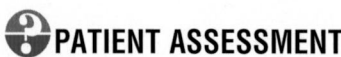HISTORICAL BACKGROUND

Increasing interest in pediatric sinusitis has arisen in the past decade secondary to several factors. Great strides in understanding the pathophysiology of sinusitis have resulted in rapid accumulation of knowledge that applies directly to diagnosis and management. Improved sinus imaging via computed tomography (CT) and magnetic resonance imaging (MRI) has enhanced awareness, and advances in endoscopic techniques have provided additional tools in management. Finally, the growing number of children in the day-care setting has led to an increase in the incidence of viral upper respiratory infection (URI), known to be an important etiologic factor in the development of sinusitis.

PATIENT ASSESSMENT

History

Symptoms accompanying uncomplicated viral URIs rarely last beyond 7 days. The diagnosis of sinusitis should be considered when signs and symptoms of a cold continue beyond 10 days and are not improving. Nasal discharge, cough, low-grade fever, fetid breath, and painless morning periorbital swelling are the most common complaints among parents seeking medical assistance for their children with persistence of these symptoms. The nasal discharge may be thick or thin, clear, cloudy, or purulent. The cough may be wet or dry but is usually present in the daytime, although often worse at night. Cough only at night may be present as a residual symptom of URI (1).

Less commonly, children may present with a cold that seems more severe than usual. The fever may be higher, the nasal discharge may be more purulent, and there may be associated facial pain and swelling. Children older than 5 years of age may report headache or dental pain, depending on their ability to localize the discomfort.

Chronic sinusitis is distinguished from the acute form when the symptoms persist for more than 30 days. Parsons and Phillips (2) have studied the most common symptoms of chronic sinusitis in children. These include purulent nasal discharge, chronic nasal obstruction, postnasal drainage, cough, fetid breath, headache, and behavior changes. The cough associated with chronic sinusitis is usually worse at bedtime or during the night for younger children and in the early morning for adolescents. Older children may complain of a foul taste in their mouth related to postnasal drip. Headaches are more common in chronic sinusitis but may be verbalized only by older children. It is important to look for nonverbal clues in younger children, such as head holding, rubbing of cheeks, head banging, hair pulling, or pushing the face against the parent or cool surfaces (3).

Examination

While obtaining the history, general observations may be made, such as the presence of cough, hyponasality, periorbital discoloration, allergic pruritus, and gross rhinorrhea. During the examination, special attention should be paid to concomitant middle ear, tonsillar, or adenoid disease (4). The ears are examined first for evidence of infection, effusion, or eustachian tube dysfunction. The method used to examine the child's nose depends on his or her ability to cooperate. The otoscope is familiar to the child and may be used for anterior rhinoscopy. The inferior turbinates are inspected in regard to color, size, and amount of mucosal congestion. Purulence or crusting may also be noted.

If the child is able to cooperate, a more thorough examination may be carried out utilizing a nasal speculum and head mirror or head light. Topical vasoconstrictive agents such as oxymetazoline 0.05% or neosynephrine 0.25% combined with 4% lidocaine facilitate the nasal examination in a child. The septum is inspected for deviation. The head is then extended and middle turbinates identified. Erythema or polypoid mucosa should be noted, as well as the presence of concha bullosum. Attention is then directed to the middle meatus for evidence of narrowing, purulence, or polyps. Polyps in young children are highly suggestive of cystic fibrosis (5). Nasal endoscopy with the rigid or flexible scope may improve visualization in this area and also allows inspection of the adenoid pad.

The oral cavity and oropharynx are examined for tonsillar hypertrophy, erythema or lymphoid hyperplasia of the posterior pharyngeal wall, and the presence of a postnasal discharge. Finally, inspection of the facial soft tissues and cervical lymph nodes is made for the presence of edema or inflammation. Transillumination of the sinuses has not been particularly useful in children.

Imaging

Radiography is often helpful in determining the absence or presence of sinus disease. Standard radiographic projections include an anteroposterior, a lateral, and an occipitomental view. The most common view used as screening tool for sinusitis is the occipitomental view, which is taken after tilting the chin 45° from the horizontal and allows evaluation of the maxillary sinuses. The anteroposterior view is optimal for the ethmoid sinuses, and the lateral view allows visualization of the frontal and sphenoid sinuses.

Much has been written regarding the inadequacy of plain sinus x-rays in the ability to predict presence or absence of chronic sinusitis (6,7). Plain films are more helpful in the diagnosis of acute sinusitis in the presence of opacification or an air–fluid level. However, an air–fluid level is an uncommon radiologic finding in children less than 5 years of age. In the absence of air–fluid level or complete opacification of the sinuses, measuring the degree of mucosal swelling may be useful. If the width of the sinus mucous membrane is 4 mm or greater, the sinus is likely to contain pus or yield a positive bacterial culture (1). An advantage of plain radiography is the cost and the ability to obtain these films without the use of sedation. It is generally agreed, however, that sinus x-rays are not helpful in children less than 1 year of age.

When considering the diagnosis of chronic or recurrent sinusitis, CT has proved to be superior to plain sinus x-rays. Coronal thin-section images offer excellent delineation of pathology in the ostiomeatal complex, which is now felt to be the critical region in the pathophysiology of recurrent sinus disease (8). Axial images are useful for the evaluation of periorbital complications and is often the view obtained in children less than 4 years of age. CT scanning most often involves the use of sedation in children. The position of the patient for coronal scanning may precipitate airway obstruction in the younger sleeping child.

PEARLS AND PERILS

1. The diagnosis of acute sinusitis is considered when symptoms of URI persist beyond 10 days and are not improving, or when symptoms are more severe than usual.
2. Symptoms that persist more than 30 days suggest the diagnosis of chronic sinusitis and include purulent nasal discharge, nasal obstruction, postnasal drainage, fetid breath, headache, behavior changes, and cough.
3. Careful examination for accompanying eustachian tube dysfunction and adenotonsillar hypertrophy must be performed in addition to the nasal examination. Anterior rhinoscopy utilizing the otoscope may be the least intimidating method when examining small children.
4. CT is the radiographic imaging modality of choice but should be obtained after adequate medical treatment. Coronal sections are preferred but may be difficult to obtain in children less than 4 years of age.

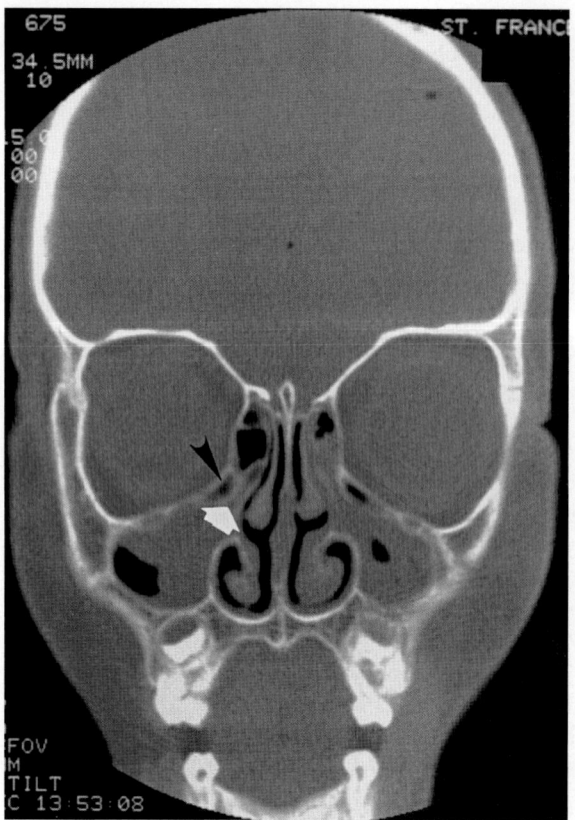
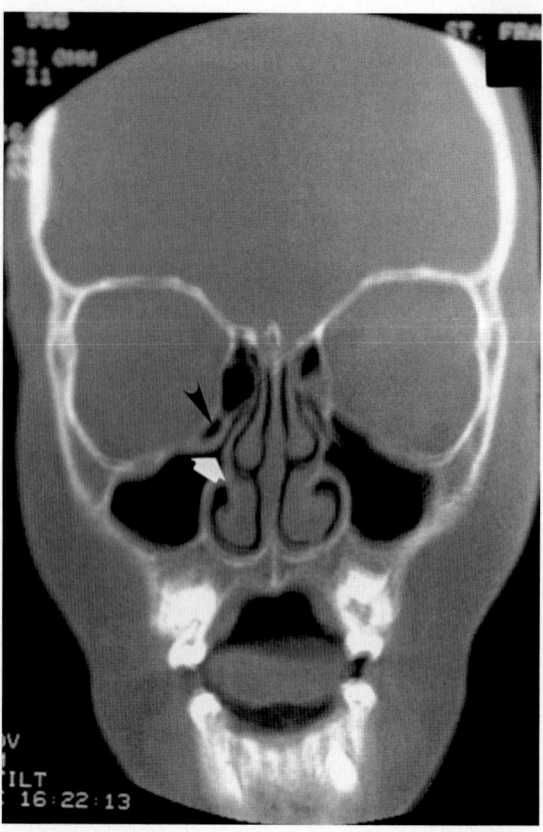

FIGURE 1 **A:** Coronal computed tomography (CT) of paranasal sinuses of child prior to maximal medical therapy. *Black arrow* points to Haller cell; *white arrow* indicates narrow ostiomeatal complex. **B:** Coronal CT of same patient after treatment. Although movement artifact is present, anatomy is more clearly seen after treatment.

MRI has several limitations in the evaluation of inflammation of the paranasal sinuses (9). These include high cost, long imaging times, and the inability to display bony landmarks, which is of particular importance to the endoscopic surgeon. CT scanning offers the advantage of resolution of soft tissue and bone and is the radiologic modality of choice. The scan is most often obtained only after the patient has undergone extensive evaluation and medical treatment (Fig. 1).

🌑 TREATMENT RECOMMENDATIONS

Establish Patency of the Ostiomeatal Complex

Technologic advances have improved our understanding of the pathophysiology and treatment of sinus disease. Primary among the evolving tenets of sinusitis pathophysiology is that the ostiomeatal complex is a key to normal sinus function and that its continued patency is very important to sinus health (Fig. 2).

Blockage of the sinus ostia appears to initiate the cycle of events leading to sinusitis (Fig. 3). Ostial obstruction creates an increasingly hypoxic environment within the sinus, and microbiologic flora may be increasingly anaerobic. Retention of secretions results in inflammation and bacterial infection within the cavity. As airflow and drainage remain blocked, secretions stagnate, obstruction becomes more severe, and ciliary and epithelial damage become more pronounced. Only by ensuring ostial patency and proper aeration and drainage can the cycle be interrupted (10).

Treatment of acute and chronic sinusitis generally includes the use of antimicrobial agents but also involves measures attempting to decrease sinonasal edema. This involves the local use of saline irrigation either commercially available or prepared at home. The

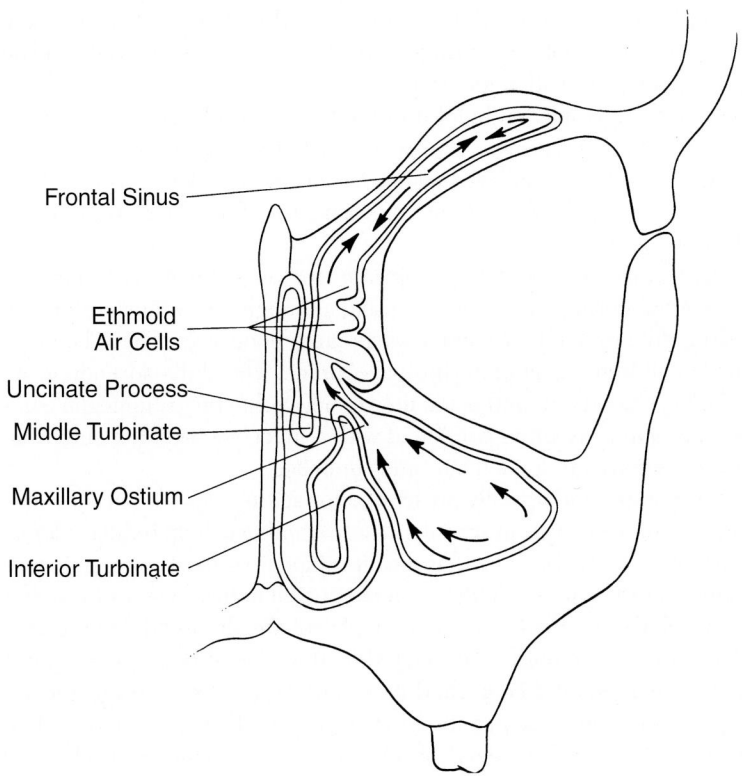

Frontal Sinus

Ethmoid
Air Cells

Uncinate Process

Middle Turbinate

Maxillary Ostium

Inferior Turbinate

FIGURE 2 Anatomy of ostiomeatal complex. Arrows show direction of mucociliary flow through maxillary and frontal sinuses.

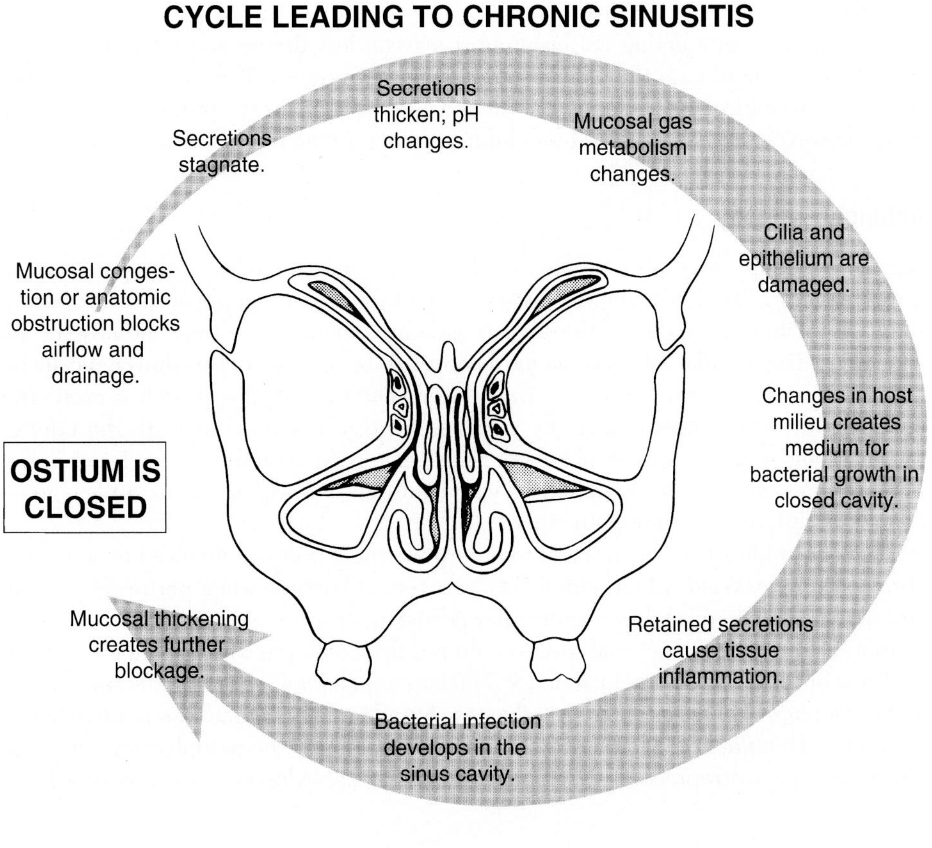

CYCLE LEADING TO CHRONIC SINUSITIS

FIGURE 3 Cycle leading to chronic sinusitis. (Modified from ref. 10, with permission.)

Secretions thicken; pH changes.

Secretions stagnate.

Mucosal gas metabolism changes.

Cilia and epithelium are damaged.

Mucosal congestion or anatomic obstruction blocks airflow and drainage.

OSTIUM IS CLOSED

Changes in host milieu creates medium for bacterial growth in closed cavity.

Mucosal thickening creates further blockage.

Retained secretions cause tissue inflammation.

Bacterial infection develops in the sinus cavity.

mixture commonly consists of 1 pint water, 1 teaspoon salt, and 1/2 teaspoon baking soda. Administration is through a spray bottle or syringe, and it is helpful to cleanse debris from the nose, as well as to decongest swollen membranes.

Topical nasal decongestants may be helpful in the treatment of acute sinusitis but are appropriate for only short-term use. The two agents most commonly used are oxymetazoline hydrochloride 0.05% and phenylephrine hydrochloride 0.125%, 0.25%, or 0.5%. Use after 3 days may make the patient vulnerable to rebound rhinitis and may have a negative effect of ciliary stasis.

Systemic decongestants are more appropriate for long-term use. Phenyl-propanolamine or pseudophedrine are commonly used, although the author prefers the use of pseudoephedrine. Reports of behavioral changes and mood swings have been reported from parents of children taking phenylpropanolamine. The alpha-adrenergic action of these agents reduce blood flow and maintain patency within the ostiomeatal complex. These oral decongestants are often combined with a mucolytic agent, guaifenisin, in an attempt to thin secretions and to facilitate sinus drainage.

Topical corticosteroids are not typically prescribed for acute sinusitis, but they may be helpful in treating chronic or recurrent sinusitis. These agents can help reduce edema, inflammation, and hyperreactivity. Beclomethasone dipropionate is most commonly prescribed by the author because younger children tolerate it well in the aqueous form, but other available agents include dexamethasone sodium phosphate, flunisolide, fluticasone propionate, and triamcinolone acetonide. Although the safety and effectiveness of most of these agents have not been established in children younger than 6 years of age, the author has selectively prescribed their use in patients even younger than 1 year of age. Use of these agents is usually preceded by the use of saline irrigations to mechanically clear the mucosa.

Systemic steroids are not typically prescribed by the author in treatment of acute or chronic sinusitis. Classic antihistamines are helpful in the treatment of allergic rhinitis, but they have no role in the treatment of sinusitis. Negative effects include mucosal drying and the thickening of sinus secretions, thereby hindering mucociliary flow and clearance.

The newer nonsedating antihistamines may be less drying and cause less ciliary motility impairment than the older generation antihistamines. Their use may therefore be helpful in children with allergic rhinitis and chronic sinusitis symptoms. Most of these drugs, however, are not approved for children younger than 6 years of age.

Antibiotic Therapy

Antibiotic therapy is empiric because of the relative inaccessibility of the paranasal sinuses to culture. To determine the bacteriology of sinusitis, a sample of sinus secretions must be obtained from one of the sinuses without contamination from the nose or nasopharynx. The maxillary sinus is the most accesible, but culture of this sinus typically requires the use of general anesthesia in children. The transnasal approach is used after sterilizing the nasal mucosa with 4% cocaine. A trocar is passed beneath the inferior turbinate and a sinus aspirate obtained. Sinus aspiration should be considered in immunosuppressed patients or in children who fail to show a response to multiple courses of antibiotics based on empiric therapy.

Several studies have been made to determine the pathogens involved in acute and chronic sinusitis. Wald (11) reported 70% recovery of bacteria when performing maxillary sinus aspiration on children with either persistent or severe symptoms and abnormal sinus radiographs. The bacterial species cultured from children with presumed acute sinusitis in order of prevalence included *Streptococcus pneumoniae*, *Moraxella catarrhalis*, and *Hemophilus influenzae*. The *H. influenzae* found in sinus aspirate was nontypable, in contrast to *H. influenzae* type b, which frequently colonizes the nasopharynx. Only one anaerobe, a peptostreptococcus, was isolated, and no staphylococci were recovered.

In 1981, Brook (12) published a study in which he evaluated 40 children with respiratory symptoms that had lasted more than 3 weeks. In 50% of these patients, specimens for culture were obtained at the time of sinus surgery. Bacteria were isolated from 37 of the 40 patients and were most commonly anaerobic gram-positive cocci, such as staphylococci and streptococci. Also recovered to a large extent were the *Bacteroides* species, especially *B. melaninogenicus*, and fusobacteria. Aerobes were isolated in approximately 38%. The most common aerobes were streptococci and staphylococci. *Hemophilus* species were isolated from only four patients.

By contrast, Muntz and Lusk (13) reported the bacteriology of tissue cultures taken from the ethmoid bullae of children undergoing endoscopic sinus surgery. They found that the principal aerobic organisms isolated were alpha-hemolytic streptococcus (23%), *Staphylococcus aureus* (19%), *M. catarrhalis* (7%), and *H. influenzae* (7%). Anaerobic organisms were isolated in only 7% of cases. The authors concluded that antibiotic therapy for chronic sinusitis should cover beta-lactamase-producing organisms, with special emphasis on *S. aureus*. The anaerobic bacteria identified were sensitive to the broad-spectrum antibiotics that the patients were receiving, and those organisms were not cultured in high concentrations.

Antimicrobial therapy of acute sinusitis should be directed toward *S. pneumoniae*, *M. catarrhalis*, and *H. influenzae*. Amoxicillin is an acceptable first-line agent for treatment of uncomplicated acute sinusitis and is recommended in a dosage of 40 mg per kilogram of body weight per day in three administrations. It is effective in most uncomplicated cases and is inexpensive, with relatively few side effects. The major disadvantage of amoxicillin is its susceptibility to beta-lactamase-producing organisms. Approximately 75% of *M. catarrhalis* and 30% of *H. influenzae* are beta-lactamase producers (5). Also of concern is the emergence of resistant strains of *S. pneumococcus*. This is thought to be due to overzealous antibiotic use (14), or transmission of resistant organisms in the daycare environment (15,16).

Alternative therapy includes the use of erythromycin (30 to 50 mg per kilogram per day) combined with sulfisoxizole (150 mg per kilogram per day). This combination provides good coverage for the spectrum of acute sinusitis but has disadvantages of bitter taste, as well as frequent administration, three to four times daily. Trimethoprim–sulfamethoxizole, another combination agent, allows twice-daily dosing but provides inadequate coverage of group A streptococcus.

Amoxicillin with potassium clavulanate is an excellent alternative to amoxicillin, providing coverage of beta-lactamase-producing organisms and anaerobic bacteria. The major disadvantage of this agent is the high potential for gastrointestinal intolerance. The author has noted decreased complaints of diarrhea when prescribing the newly formulated twice-daily dosing at 45 mg per kilogram per day based on the amoxicillin component.

Cephalosporins have provided appropriate treatment of acute and chronic sinusitis. First-generation cephalosporins lack coverage of gram-negative organisms and are therefore infrequently used for the treatment of sinusitis in children. Second-generation cephalosporins, however, have gained widespread use. Cefaclor (20 to 40 mg per kilogram per day) may be administered two to three times daily but may be susceptible to beta-lactamase-producing organisms. Newer agents offer better beta-lactamase stability and may therefore replace its use. Cefuroxime–axetil (30 mg per kilogram per day) provides excellent coverage but in suspension form is unpalatable to children. Other broad-spectrum cephalosporins include cefpodoxime (10 mg per kilogram per day), cefprozil (30 mg per kilogram per day), and loracarbef (30 mg per kilogram per day). All offer twice-daily dosing. Once-daily dosing is offered by cefixime and ceftibuten, but these are indicated only as second-line agents due to their relative lack of susceptibility to *S. pneumoniae*.

Clarythromycin and azithromycin are macrolide antibiotics now available in suspension form. They offer a broad spectrum of activity against gram-positive and gram-negative organisms and provide excellent tissue concentration. Their use in the treatment of sinusitis in children is relatively new.

Clindamycin should be considered for the patient with chronic sinusitis who has failed to respond to treatment with the augmented penicillins or broad-spectrum cephalosporins, especially when resistant *S. pneumoniae* is suspected. It provides good anaerobic coverage and may also be useful when patients exhibit multiple antibiotic allergies. It is available as a suspension and apparently is only rarely associated with diarrhea and colitis in children (17).

Empiric treatment of sinusitis has been 10 to 14 days. The author uses the approach of continuing the antibiotic an additional 7 days beyond the time the patient becomes asymptomatic. If the initial antibiotic prescribed fails to bring about improvement in symptomatology within 48 hours of administration, a change to a broader spectrum antibiotic is considered.

The duration of treatment of chronic sinusitis with antimicrobial agents is somewhat controversial. Most would agree, however, that a minimum of 4 weeks with a broad-spectrum antibiotic would be indicated.

Antibiotic prophylaxis is considered for patients with chronic recurrent sinusitis. Amoxicillin 20 mg per kilogram daily or sulfisoxazole 30 mg per kilogram twice daily are the two commonly used schedules of chemoprophylaxis. This is especially indicated for patients with known immunodeficiencies.

Immunodeficiencies

Patients with primary or secondary immunodeficiencies are usually identified with a history of frequent otitis media, pneumonia, and sinusitis. Serum IgG, IgA, IgM, and IgE are usually quantitated, as well as IgG subclasses. Ability to respond to polysaccharide capsular antigens of *S. pneumoniae* is evaluated and nonresponders identified. These patients are typically under the care of pediatric allergy immunologists and may be considered candidates for gamma-globulin replacement if overall health is impaired and if infections continue in spite of antibiotic prophylaxis.

The efficacy of pneumococcal vaccine in preventing recurrent acute otitis media in young children is currently being studied. Mixed results have precluded the recommendation for universal vaccination of children. As our understanding of the vaccine and the clinical significance of efficacy increases, these data may be helpful in making recommendations for vaccination in prevention of recurrent acute sinusitis.

Environmental Factors

The environments of children with chronic recurrent or persistent infections should be evaluated for potential causes. Utilization of day-care facilities is associated with an increased number of respiratory illnesses in children. Although use of these facilities may not be avoided completely, parents are encouraged to seek out cleaner and less populated day-care environments in an attempt to decrease exposure to potential viral and bacterial pathogens.

Primary or secondary cigarette smoke predisposes some children to frequent respiratory infections. Cessation of smoking should always be encouraged, but if this is not possible, parents should be made aware of the secondary effect on their children. Attempts should be made to discontinue smoking in houses and automobiles, and parents should be educated about covering their own clothing and hair while smoking outside.

Sinonasal Allergies

Environments also pose problems for children with sinonasal allergies. It is important to distinguish allergic from infective symptomatology. Factors suggesting allergy are itching mucous membranes of the upper aerodigestive tract, clear rhinorrhea, and other remote symptoms of allergy, such as eczema and food intolerance (18). Symptoms suggestive of infection are purulent anterior rhinorrhea or postnasal drainage, pharyngitis, and production of purulent sputum. Symptoms that are common to allergy and infection are nasal congestion, stuffiness, fluctuating rhinorrhea, sneezing, cough, behavioral changes, and headaches with facial pain or pressure. These two disorders are, however, known to coexist.

PEARLS AND PERILS

1. Decrease sinonasal edema with the use of saline irrigation and systemic decongestant–mucolytics. Do not use topical decongestants beyond 3 days and avoid the use of antihistamines.
2. Empiric therapy is directed toward the most common sinus pathogens. Consider changing antibiotic to broader spectrum when initial therapy fails to bring about improvement in 48 hours.
3. Antimicrobial therapy should continue for 10 to 14 days in acute sinusitis and 3 to 4 weeks when treating chronic sinusitis.
4. Attempts should be made to avoid aggravating environmental factors, such as potential allergens, secondary cigarette smoke, and day-care facilities.

Decreasing allergic mucosal edema may help prevent secondary infection of the sinuses. A careful history is obtained and avoidance of potential allergens encouraged. Antihistamines alone or combined with decongestants are prescribed as first-line therapy. Topical steroids inhibit both the early- and late-phase inflammatory responses and as a result are very useful in treatment of allergic rhinitis. Cromolyn sodium is helpful when exposure to a known allergen or seasonal rhinitis is anticipated. It is applied topically and is approved for children of all ages.

When pharmacotherapy fails to effect improvement, consideration is given to specific allergy testing. Knowledge of specific triggering allergens may aid in avoidance therapy or possibly determine the need for desensitization.

The association of asthma and sinusitis in patients with reactive airway disease is noteworthy. The premise of this association is that sinus mucosal disease effects bronchial hyperreactivity (19). Cough is frequently noted in patients with asthma and radiographically diagnosed sinusitis. Investigators have suggested that antibiotic treatment of sinusitis in hard-to-treat cases of asthma resolves symptoms of asthma.

Cystic Fibrosis

Aggressive treatment of sinus disease is also advocated for patients with cystic fibrosis. Paranasal sinus involvement in cystic fibrosis is initiated by blockage of sinus ostium by thickened sinus secretions, but secondary events occur that cause damage to the mucosal lining (20). Hypoxia, carbon dioxide retention resulting in ciliary injury, mucosal edema, and inflammation with bacterial colonization are the events responsible for the mucosal damage.

In a study on the bacteriology of maxillary sinus in cystic fibrosis patients, bacterial colonization was found to occur in over 95% of cases (21). The predominant organisms isolated were *Pseudomonas aeruginosa*, *H. influenzae*, and anaerobes. The antimicrobial agents chosen should therefore have significant antipseudomonal activity. Currently, this may require the use of intravenous antibiotics until the patient is of an age to receive oral ciprofloxacin therapy. This drug has not yet been approved for children or adolescents less than 18 years of age.

Treatment is not based strictly on radiographic findings of pan-opacification of the paranasal sinuses because this is an almost universal finding in these patients. The clinical features of sinusitis, when they do occur, are usually more severe than those in non-cystic fibrosis patients. Nasal obstruction, purulent rhinorrhea, postnasal drainage, mouth breathing, halitosis, and snoring are the common complaints in younger children. Older children and adolescents may also complain of headache.

Nasal polyps may be present on examination and may initially be treated with topical nasal steroids. Steroid nasal sprays may also be used postoperatively after functional endoscopic surgery in an attempt to prevent recurrence of nasal polyposis.

Primary Ciliary Dyskinesia

Infants and children with a history of chronic otitis media, chronic sinusitis, and chronic bronchitis or bronchiectasis should be evaluated for primary ciliary dyskinesia. Also known as immotile cilia syndrome, this disease causes structural or functional abnormalities of the ciliated pseudostratified columnar epithelium lining the nose, nasopharynx, and paranasal sinuses. It may be associated with Kartagener's syndrome (sinusitis, situs inversus, bronchiectasis, and male infertility), but diagnosis is usually confirmed by biopsy of inferior or middle turbinate mucosa or tracheal mucosa.

Patients diagnosed with primary ciliary dyskinesia and frequent recurrent sinusitis may be administered antibiotic prophylaxis, but in the chronic state, they may require surgical intervention via inferior meatal antrostomies.

✸ REFERENCES

1. Wald E. *Ann Otol Rhinol Laryngol* 1992;101:37–41.
2. Parsons D, Phillips S. *Laryngoscope* 1993;103:899–903.
3. Parsons DS, Wald E. *Otolaryngol Clin North Am* 1996;29:11–25.
4. Manning SC. *Otolaryngol Clin North Am* 1993;26:623–638.
5. Arjmand EM, Lusk RP. *Am J Otolaryngol* 1995;16:367–382.
6. McAlister WH, Lusk RP, Muntz HR. *AJR* 1989;153:1259–1264.
7. Lazar RH, Younis RT, Parvey LS. *Otolaryngol Head Neck Surg* 1992; 107:29–34.
8. Zinrech SJ, Kennedy DW, Rosenbaum AE, Gayler RW, Kumar AJ, Stammberger H. *Radiology* 1987; 163:769–775.
9. Diament MJ. *J Allergy Clin Immunol* 1992;90(3 Pt 2):442–444.
10. Kennedy DW, Gwaltney JM, Jones JG. *Ann Otol Rhinol Laryngol* 1995;104(10 Pt 2):22–30.
11. Wald E. *J Allergy Clin Immunol* 1992;(3 Pt 2):452–456.
12. Brook I. *JAMA* 1981;246:967–969.
13. Muntz HR, Lusk RP. *Arch Otolaryngol Head Neck Surg* 1991;117:177–181.
14. Tan TQ, Mason EO Jr, Kaplan SL. *Pediatrics* 1993;90:928–933.
15. Reichler MR, Allphin AA, Breiman RF, et al. *J Infect Dis* 1992;166:1346–1353.
16. Henderson FW, Gilligan PH, Wart K, Goff DA. 1988;157:256–263.
17. Randolph MF, Morris KE. *Clin Pediatr* 1977;16:772–775.
18. Cook PR, Nishoka GJ. *Otolaryngol Clin North Am* 1996;29:39–56.
19. Ott NL, O'Connell EJ, Hoffmans AD, Beatty CW, Sachs MI. *Mayo Clin Proc* 1991; 66:1238–1247.
20. Hui Y, Gaffney R, Crysdale WS. *Eur Arch Otorhinolaryngol* 1995;252:191–196.
21. Shapiro ED, Milmoe GJ, Wald ER, Rodnan JB, Bowen AD. *J Infect Dis* 1982;146:589–593.

E.A. Kluka: Department of Otolaryngology, Louisiana State University Medical School, New Orleans, Louisiana 70112.

• *Practical Pediatric Otolaryngology*
• edited by Robin T. Cotton and Charles M. Myer, III
• Lippincott-Raven Publishers, Philadelphia © 1999

Surgical Therapy for Sinusitis and Its Complications

Scott C. Manning

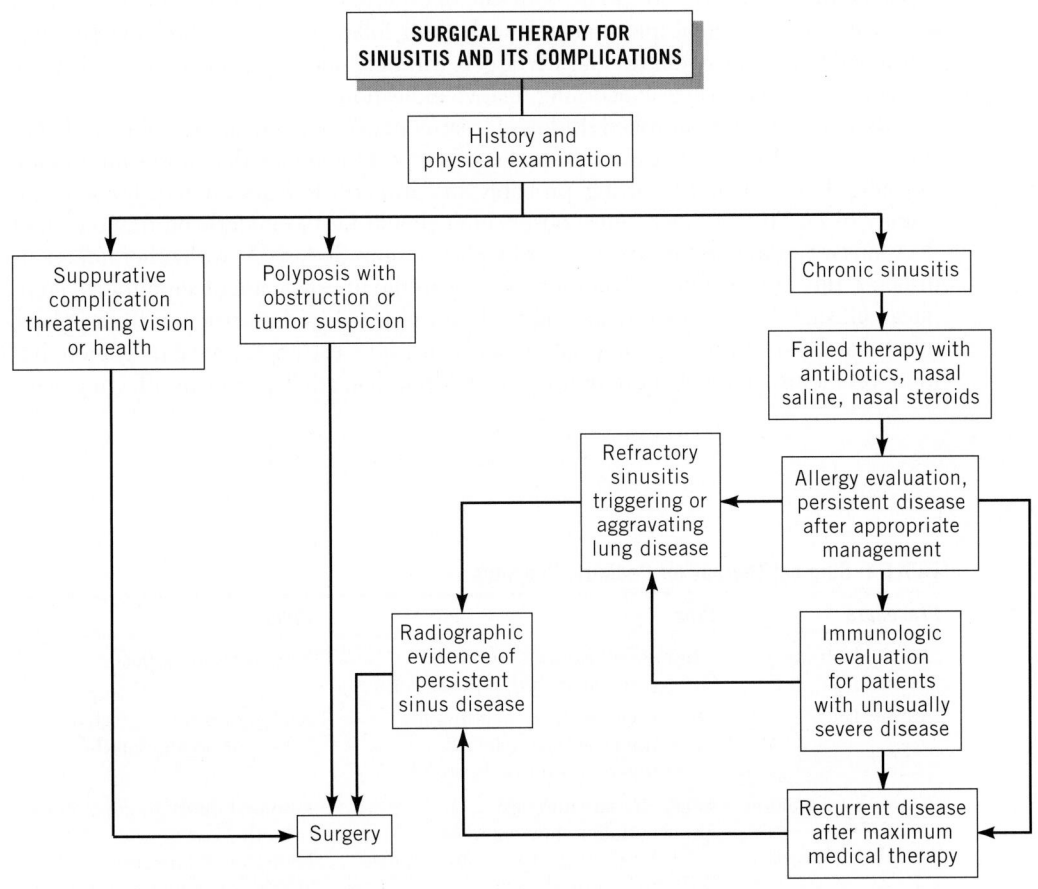

∿ HISTORICAL BACKGROUND

The concept of pediatric sinusitis as a distinct clinical entity is relatively new, and some primary caregivers still discount the notion that sinusitis can be distinguished from rhinitis in young children. The development of computed tomography (CT) and magnetic resonance imaging (MRI) along with the introduction of rigid endoscopes has improved diagnostic capability and is increasing awareness of pediatric sinusitis. Also, the rise in day-care attendance in young children over the past 15 years has probably increased both the real incidence of sinusitis and the social pressure for effective treatment.

For the last 30 years, the most common surgical procedures for chronic rhinosinusitis in young children have been adenoidectomy and maxillary sinus lavage or inferior meatus antrostomy, often performed in conjunction (Table 1 and Fig. 1). A few prospective studies have examined the efficacy of adenoidectomy in relieving pediatric sinusitis symptoms with findings of a moderate treatment effect in some series (1). Controlled studies of maxillary sinus lavage have shown no or only temporary benefit, and retrospective reviews of inferior meatus antrostomy have shown both a high rate of closure and a limited treatment effect (2). Thus, it was with great enthusiasm that many otolaryngologists embraced endoscopic techniques introduced in the mid- to late eighties with their promise of a more physiologic approach, leading to better long-term results. The new surgical techniques arrived at a time when pediatric primary care physicians were struggling with large numbers of day-care children with chronic rhinorrhea and with increasing numbers of children with asthma and other chronic diseases who were experiencing growing morbidity from sinusitis. In this environment, many surgeons were able to amass large series of pediatric endoscopic sinus surgery cases, and early published reports found the procedures to be both safe in experienced hands and effective at least as measured by parental questionnaire with short follow-up (3,4). Other practitioners continued to manage pediatric sinusitis largely without endoscopic sinus surgery, leading to the present controversy concerning relative indications (5).

Both prospective controlled studies of treatment efficacy and radiographic studies of the incidence of sinus disease at different ages support the notion that most sinus disease in young children is self-resolving, probably due primarily to maturation of systemic immunity (6,7). This common-sense observation should be the underlying framework of decisions regarding surgical treatment of pediatric sinus disease. As with other infectious diseases, the strongest indication for surgery is in the unusual case of suppurative complication, such as sinusitis threatening health or vision. Fixed obstruction from polyps, other masses, or severe septal deviation may constitute a strong surgical indication, but these problems are much more unusual in children than adults. Sinusitis affecting over-

TABLE 1: Surgical Therapy for Pediatric Sinusitus

Procedure	Pros	Cons
Adenoidectomy	? Removes bacterial source One prospective study showing efficacy	Not always beneficial
Antral lavage	May provide culture material for treatment guidance in immunocompromised patients	No long-term (6 months) benefit documented
Nasal antral window (NAW) (*inferior meatus*)	Relatively safe and easy Animal studies show increased incidence of sinusitis with window through natural ostium	Potential injury to developing teeth High rate of closure Studies question long-term benefits
Caldwell-Luc approach	Good visualization of maxillary sinus	May lease to permanent sinus hypoplasia with facial and dental abnormalities ? Mucosal disease is rarely "irreversible" in children
Endoscopic ethmoidectomy (*middle meatus NAW*)	Concept of ostiomeatal unit as site of sinus obstruction Better visualization of anatomy ? More "physiologic"	No prospective controlled studies documenting efficacy More difficult in children May require second visit to operating room

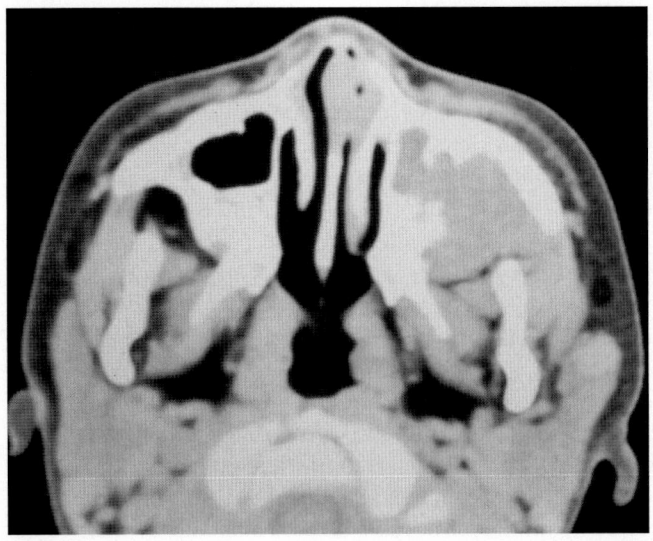
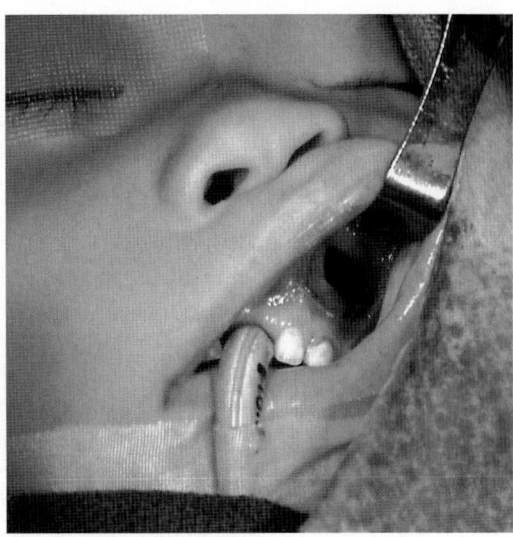

A   B

FIGURE 1 **A:** A 4-year-old boy with a painful expanding left cheek. Computed tomography (CT) demonstrates destructive lesion of the left maxilla. **B:** Caldwell-Luc approach for biopsy, which confirmed a diagnosis of histocytosis. The patient was treated successfully with low-dose radiation.

all health in patients with asthma, cystic fibrosis, or immunodeficiency is a growing problem, and studies are beginning to support the concept that sinus surgery can be of benefit in some situations. Chronic sinusitis truly refractory to medical management and significantly affecting quality of life in otherwise healthy people is difficult to define, and as yet there are no comparison studies proving improved efficacy of endoscopic sinus surgery over other treatment modalities in these patients (Table 2).

 PATIENT ASSESSMENT

Radiographic Diagnosis

In general, sinus radiographs are indicated for documentation of presence or absence of suppurative complications, to confirm resolution or persistence of disease after medical therapy, and to provide an anatomic road map for planned surgery. Plain films, such as Water's view radiographs, are relatively insensitive when compared with CT but may be useful for confirming clinical diagnoses or for ruling out severe disease. CT in the coronal plain without contrast is the imaging modality of choice for documenting sinus dis-

TABLE 2: Relative Indications for Pediatric Sinus Surgery

Suppurative complications	Fixed obstructions	Sinusitis aggravating pulmonary disease	Chronic sinusitis
Stronger .... _Weaker_			
Medial subperiosteal orbital abscess	Refractory polyps (CF, AFS)	Asthma	Impact on quality of life, school attendance
Complicated sphenoid or frontal sinusitis	Antrochoanal polyp	Cystic fibrosis	Persistent mucosal disease in sinus outflow tracts on CT after maximum medical therapy
	Inverted papilloma Other suspected tumor	Immunodeficiency	

CF, cystic fibrosis; AFS, allergic fungal sinusitis; CT, computed tomography.

ease with its advantages of bone resolution and detailed imaging of the sinus outflow tracts through the middle meatus anteriorly and sphenoethmoidal recess posteriorly. The newer generations of high-speed scanners have made sinus CT much more practical for young children, and limited screening scans of six to eight images can be obtained relatively inexpensively and quickly. Axial views with and without contrast should be requested in addition to coronal views whenever orbital or intracranial disease is suspected to obtain the greatest sensitivity in detecting pathology. MRI carries the disadvantage of no bone resolution, but it may be helpful in limited situations, such as documenting epidural or intraparenchymal disease in patients with frontal sinusitis and neurologic findings. The unusual finding of central sinus signal absence on MRI along with CT evidence of irregular central high signal and peripheral mucosal inflammation is diagnostic of allergic fungal sinusitis.

The fundamental principle underlying endoscopic sinus surgical technique is that mucosal or bony anatomic obstruction of sinus outflow tracts through the middle meatus or (less commonly) the sphenoethmoidal recess leads to upstream infection and a cycle of continued inflammation and obstruction. Limited opening of the sinus drainage tracts should therefore be expected to be of benefit in cases of fixed anatomic or irreversible mucosal obstruction. The problem in applying this logic to young children is that studies show that major bony anatomic abnormalities are unusual in children and that most sinus mucosal disease is self-resolving in the pediatric age group. Specific anatomic findings implicated in sinus obstruction in adults such as choncha bullosa, Haller's cell, paradoxical middle turbinate, septal deviation, and large bulla ethmoidalis are found in inverse proportion to age in studies of sinus CT, and no studies have demonstrated strong associations between these findings and an increased incidence of sinusitis at any age. The finding of a small or "hypoplastic" maxillary sinus is possibly associated with an increased incidence of mucosal disease in that sinus (Fig. 2). The author's own study of head CT and MRI findings in children assessed for non-sinus-related problems showed an overall incidence of 60% with sinus image mucosal inflammation, which was strongly associated with history or physical findings of viral upper respiratory infection in patients under age 3 years (8). Other imaging studies have shown that the overall incidence of sinus mucosal inflammation drops off significantly after age 7 or 8, again supporting the idea that most sinus disease in children is eventually self-resolving.

Image findings of mucosal inflammation at one point in time must be interpreted in the light of physical findings and history and do not in themselves constitute an indication for surgery. CT can confirm certain diagnoses, such as medial subperiosteal orbital abscess or antrochoanal polyp, and can strongly support other diagnoses, such as cystic fibrosis, in patients with total maxillary opacification with widened infundibulae and medial bowing of the lateral nasal walls (Fig. 3). For the more common problem of refractory disease in otherwise healthy patients, CT is best utilized after maximum medical

FIGURE 2 CT demonstrating hypoplastic maxillary sinuses in a 9-year-old with chronic maxillary sinusitis. Note the concavity of the lateral nasal walls in the middle meatus, which makes surgical middle meatus antrostomy technically challenging.

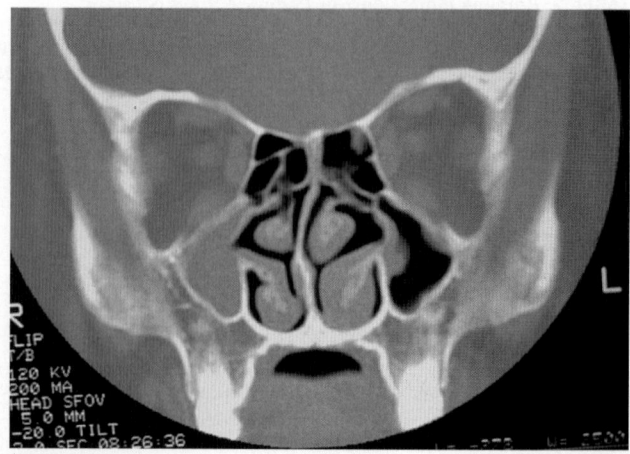

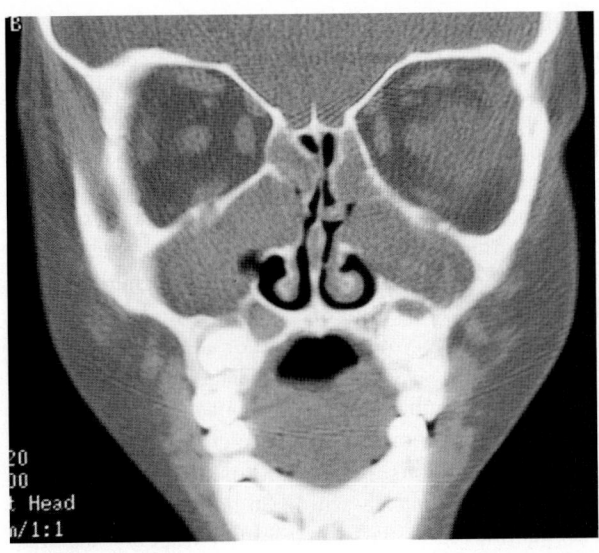

FIGURE 3 A 10-year-old child with cystic fibrosis. CT demonstrates maxillary opacification with medial bowing of the lateral nasal walls. Note previous inferior meatus antrostomies.

therapy in order to document any significant persistent disease that may represent true "irreversible" mucosal inflammation. The adult controversy of whether or not to operate ever on patients with radiographically normal sinuses after medical treatment of recurrent sinusitis is now spilling over to the pediatric age group. The author's view is that surgery cannot improve on anatomically normal sinuses, as evidenced by our most sensitive imaging techniques.

The issue of the potential effect of sinus surgery on facial growth is pertinent to the topic of radiographic diagnosis, since radiographs have shown subsequent sinus hypoplasia in patients undergoing surgery at a young age. Maxillary Caldwell-Luc procedures with stripping of mucosa can definitely lead to maxillary hypoplasia, and patients requiring an external ethmoidectomy approach to orbital inflammation at a young age have been shown to develop imaging evidence of ethmoid hypoplasia. Whether these sinus changes can impact on facial appearance is another matter, and to date no studies have confirmed an effect in humans. An animal study of endoscopic anterior ethmoidectomy surgery in piglets has demonstrated a measurable effect on subsequent facial growth (9). The same authors document that sinus surgical specimens from children under age 9 usually contain immature woven bone as opposed to mature lamellar bone from older patients. Since the anterior ethmoid region is a significant facial growth center, concerns remain about the potential impact of even limited surgery on facial growth in very young patients.

TREATMENT RECOMMENDATIONS

Suppurative Complications of Sinusitis

Medial Subperiosteal Orbital Abscess

Suppurative complications are defined as spread of infection beyond the anatomic boundaries of the sinus, and they constitute the strongest potential indications for surgery. Medial subperiosteal abscess is the most common extrasinus infectious complication in the pediatric age group, arising from direct or perivascular spread of ethmoid infection. By contrast, preseptal or eyelid inflammation in young children arises secondary to cutaneous infection (such as secondary infection of chickenpox lesions) or from hematogenous seeding during episodes of bacteremia. Preseptal cellulitis is characterized by the absence of orbital signs, such as chemosis or proptosis, and the treatment consists of systemic antibiotics alone. In the past, *Hemophilus influenzae* type B (HIB) bacteremia was by far the most common cause of preseptal cellulitis; the incidence of this disorder has decreased considerably since the development of the HIB vaccine. The incidence of medial subperiosteal abscess appears to have dropped also since introduction of the HIB vaccine, and the average age of these patients in the author's practice seems to be increasing. In contrast to older series, a significant percentage of patients diagnosed with medial subperiosteal abscess at present are older than age 5, with a history consistent with allergic rhinitis and with surgical findings of ethmoid polyps, which presumably act as a predisposing condition through ethmoid obstruction.

The diagnosis of medial subperiosteal orbital abscess is made when a child presents with periorbital cellulitis and orbital signs, such as chemosis, proptosis, and gaze restriction. Usually, a recent history of upper respiratory infection and/or allergy exacerbation can be elicited. Physical examination will also reveal at least ipsilateral evidence of sinusitis such as middle turbinate edema and erythema with purulent middle meatus secretions. The initial treatment consists of intravenous antibiotics such as cefuroxime, appropriate for the usual pediatric sinus pathogens. At the author's institution, CT is performed when the patient fails to improve clinically within 36 hours or when orbital signs progress. Decreasing visual acuity or progressive orbital fixation are grave signs indicating possible intraconal (orbital or intraperiosteal) extension of infection and should trigger immediate radiographic evaluation and ophthalmologic consultation.

When CT confirms a medial orbital inflammatory mass effect adjacent to ethmoid infection with medial bowing of the periorbital layer in a patient unresponsive to medical therapy, then surgical drainage is indicated (Fig. 4). Traditionally, external ethmoidectomy approaches have been utilized, but many pediatric sinus surgeons are now reporting excellent results with endoscopic techniques (10). By definition, these patients have highly inflamed ethmoid mucosa, and a slow, careful approach to endoscopic ethmoidectomy with frequent pauses for oxymetazoline-soaked gauze packing to achieve hemostasis and visualization is necessary. When ethmoid mucosa has been completely removed, the surgeon should be able to visualize the dehiscence in the lateral ethmoid wall (Fig. 5). Gentle pressure on the globe while viewing the lamina papyracea endoscopically should demonstrate medial prolapse of the smooth white periorbital through the dehiscence; at this point, the abscess can be presumed to be adequately drained. No attempt is made to incise periorbita when the diagnosis is subperiosteal abscess. Fortunately, intraconal orbital inflammation is rare in the pediatric age group, and these cases are managed at the author's institution with external techniques in conjunction with ophthalmologic surgeons. The advantages to endoscopic management of

FIGURE 4 **A:** A 5-year-old girl with progressive chemosis, proptosis, and cellulitis despite intravenous antibiotics. **B:** CT coronal view shows right medial subperiosteal abscess. More posterior views show ipsilateral sinusitis. The patient was managed with endoscopic ethmoidectomy and direct drainage of the subperiosteal space.

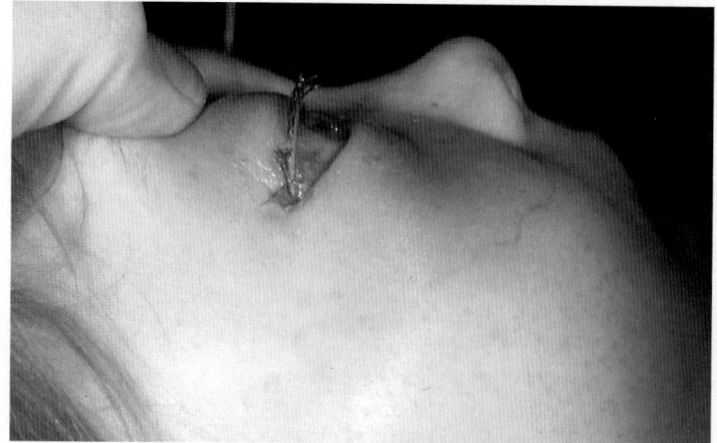

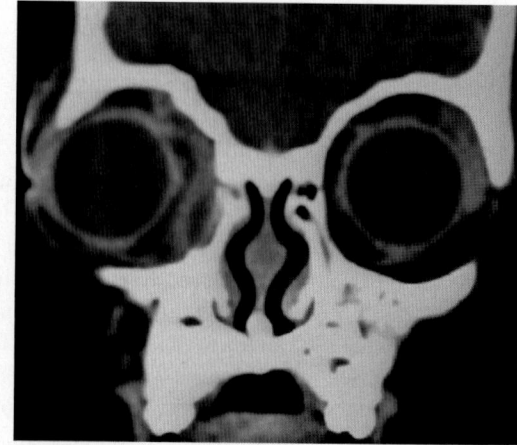

A

B

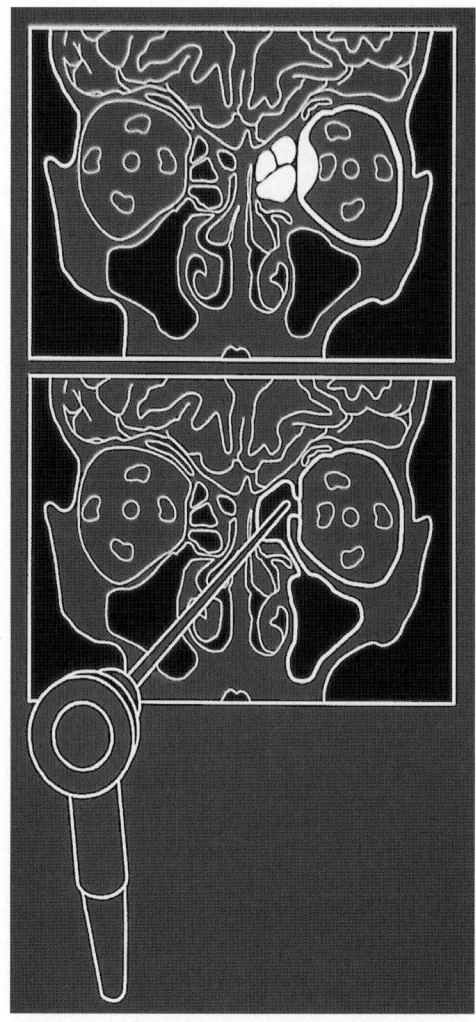

FIGURE 5 Schematic of left ethmoidectomy infection with adjacent left medial sub-periosteal orbit abscess. An endoscopic ethmoidectomy is carried out with subsequent visualization of periorbita through the dehiscence in the lamina papyracea.

medial subperiosteal abscesses include avoidance of a facial scar and more rapid resolution of symptoms with shorter hospitalization. The technique represents a natural broadening of pediatric endoscopic surgery but is appropriate only for experienced pediatric sinus surgeons.

Intracranial Complications

Under age 3, congenital heart disease is the most common predisposing condition in cases of brain abscess, but in older children, ear and sinus infection remains the principle source of intracranial suppurative process other than meningitis. Sphenoid and frontal sinus diseases predominate as sources of brain abscess and epidural and subdural empyema because of proximity to middle and anterior cranial cavities, respectively, but are often not suspected initially in patient evaluation. A recent 10-year review of rhinogenic pediatric intracranial suppurative processes from the Children's Medical Center of Dallas, Texas, revealed two deaths from subdural empyema with panencephalitis and ten other cases of frontal epidural or subdural empyema with two associated intraparenchymal frontal abscesses (11). Most patients were young adolescents with small developing frontal sinuses and CT evidence of pansinusitis at presentation. One theory proposes that actively developing frontal sinuses contain more vascular routes for potential spread of infection to the frontal epidural space. Predisposing conditions included a recent history of upper respiratory infection and a history of sudden pressure change, such as diving or a visit to a water slide park. Initial neurologic symptoms were subtle in cases of anterior

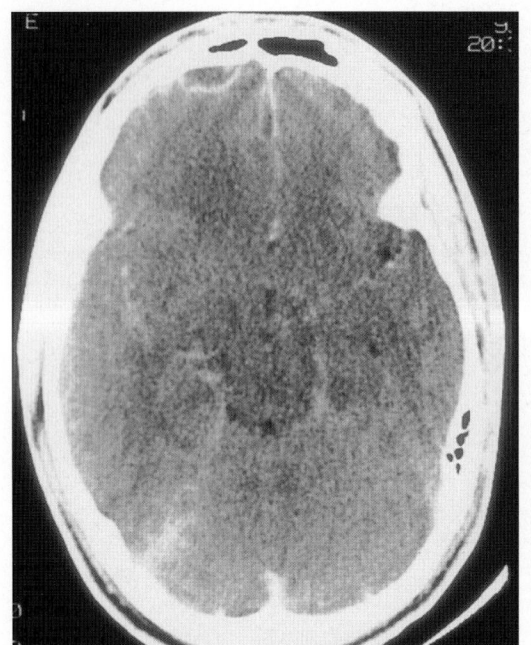
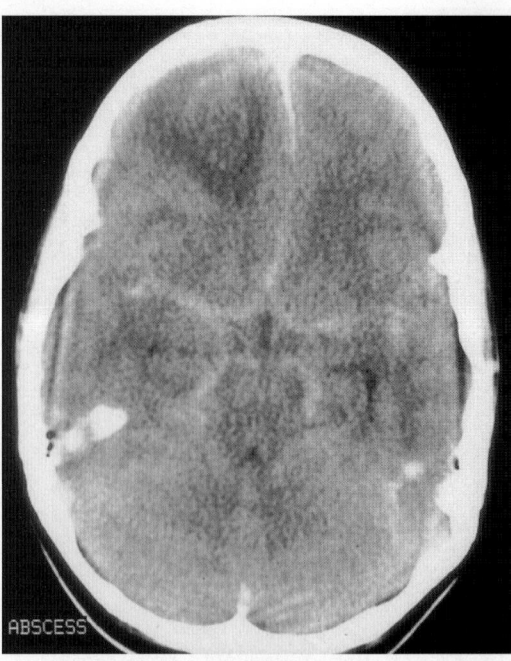

FIGURE 6 A: A 13-year-old boy with fever, forehead swelling and lethargy 2 days after swimming and diving with a cold. Axial CT shows small frontal sinuses with adjacent left epidural empyema. **B:** More superior views show a left frontal lobe abscess. The patient underwent frontal sinus cranialization and drainage of the epidural space. He required a subsequent direct drainage procedure for a coalescing left frontal lobe abscess despite intravenous antibiotics.

cranial fossa processes and included retroorbital or vertex headache and lethargy. Focal signs were rare.

CT utilizing contrast and including axial views is the imaging modality of choice for suspected intracranial spread of inflammation (Fig. 6). Treatment consists of intravenous broad-spectrum antibiotics, including coverage of gram-negative enteric organisms, and appropriate neurosurgical drainage procedures. At our institution, infected sinuses are usually drained endoscopically at the time of the neurosurgical procedure. Small frontal sinuses adjacent to frontal epidural empyema collections can be managed with cranialization via the frontal craniotomy with takedown of the posterior wall and obliteration of the nasofrontal ducts. Unfortunately, the Dallas review showed that even after successful therapy, patients with intracranial suppurative complications of sinusitis may be left with permanent neurologic sequelae, such as learning disabilities.

Occasionally, children undergoing CT evaluation because of severe or persistent headache will be found to have sphenoid or frontal sinus opacification without evidence of intracranial inflammation. These patients should be managed initially with intravenous broad-spectrum antibiotics but may require surgical drainage for refractory disease. Depending on the age of the patient and the experience of the surgeon, endoscopic techniques can be utilized for direct sphenoidotomy or opening of the frontal recess in these unusual cases.

Polyposis

Nasal polyps represent epithelial proliferation secondary to inflammation (12). True polyps are relatively unusual in young children, and a physical finding of polypoid tissue within the nasal cavity in a child should raise suspicion for foreign body, cystic fibrosis, or tumor. True polyps usually appear as pale, fleshy masses arising from the middle meatus and are most often bilateral (Fig. 7). As with adults, bilateral polyposis may be associated with allergic rhinitis or aspirin sensitivity syndrome (polyposis, asthma, aspirin sensitivity, and sinusitis). Persistent disease with nasal airway obstruction and/or recurrent sinusitis constitutes an indication for imaging and surgery (13) (Fig. 8).

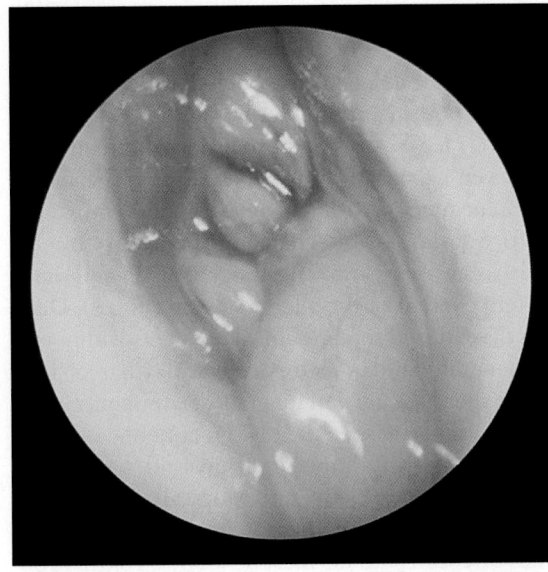

FIGURE 7 Right nasal cavity with mass of polypoid mucosa in the middle meatus. Surgery confirmed the diagnosis of allergic fungal sinusitis.

Tumors   Rhabdomyosarcoma originating from the nasopharynx or maxillary sinus is a rare origin of unilateral nasal mass in very young children. These lesions appear denser and more vascular on examination than true polyps and may be associated with ipsilateral pain, middle ear effusion, maxillary expansion, and cervical adenopathy. Diagnosis is based on imaging findings of rapid expansion with bone destruction and on biopsy. The treatment remains primarily chemotherapy and radiation with surgery usually confined to the role of diagnosis. A unilateral nasal mass in an adolescent male with nasal obstruction and epistaxis defines the clinical diagnosis of nasopharyngeal angiofibroma. The diagnosis is confirmed by imaging findings of a vascular mass arising in the nasopharynx with widening of the pterygomaxillary fissure. In most institutions, therapy is surgical excision via either a transmaxillary/transpalatal, facial degloving, or LeFort 1 approach. Recently, a few surgeons have reported successful endoscopic removal of small angiofibromas with decreased blood loss and reduced hospitalization times.

FIGURE 8   **A:** A 10-year-old boy with right-sided nasal obstruction. Endoscopic view of right nasal cavity showing pale polypoid mass extending from under the middle turbinate through the middle meatus and into the posterior inferior nasal cavity. **B:** CT scan shows right maxillary mass extending in through the right middle meatus into the right nasal cavity. More posterior views showed extension through the choanal opening, confirming the diagnosis of antrochoanal polyp. Patient was treated with endoscopic excision of the polyp.

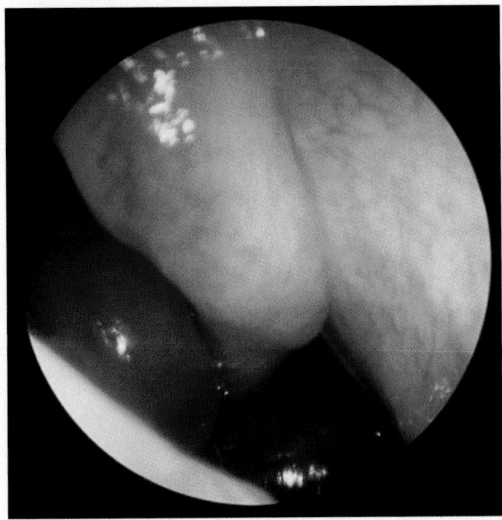

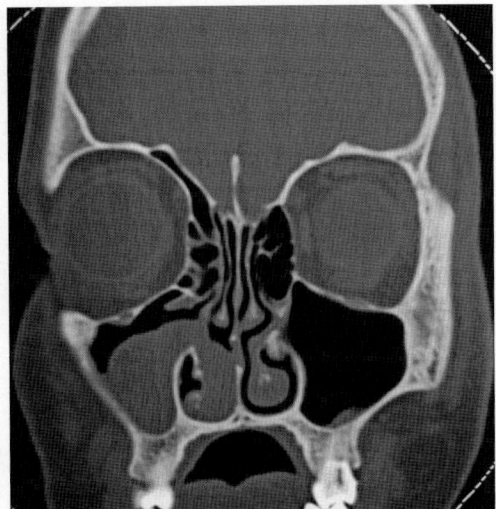

A   B

Allergic Fungal Sinusitis   Allergic fungal sinusitis is a disease that is increasingly recognized in warmer, humid areas of the United States. Patients are most commonly teenagers and young adults, but children as young as age 6 have been described with the disease. Patients present with an area of polyposis most commonly centered unilaterally in the middle meatus. At times, patients may have associated expansion of the ethmoid with blunting of the medial canthus or even expansion of the maxilla. A CT scan will demonstrate peripheral areas of hypertrophic mucosa within involved sinuses with a central area of irregular higher density. MRI will show a very characteristic pattern of high peripheral signal from the inflamed mucosa and very low central signal on T_1 and signal void on T_2 imaging due to the high protein content of the allergic mucin (Fig. 9). Diagnosis is confirmed by histologic findings of scattered septate fungal elements within mucinous debris comprised of sheets of degenerated inflammatory cells with Charcot-Leyden crystals. The disease represents a true allergy to inhaled fungi most commonly in the dematiaceous family, such as *Bipolaris* or *Curvularia* species (14). Treatment consists of complete removal of all mucinous debris along with drainage of involved sinuses. Patients are treated with perioperative oral steroids and postoperative topical nasal steroids, and all patients are also treated with appropriate immunotherapy for other inhalant allergies. The disease has a high recurrence rate, and patients must be followed closely. Because of growing evidence that this represents a true allergy rather than an infection, we do not treat with antifungal drugs at our institution.

Foreign Body   The most common cause of persistent unilateral rhinorrhea in young children is intranasal foreign body. Especially between the ages of 2 to 4, children may explore body cavities with materials such as pieces of sponge, paper, beads, and pebbles. In unusual cases, patients with psychiatric or neurologic disorders are capable of hoarding remarkable numbers of household items within their nasal cavities. The diagnosis is usually made with rhinoscopy after suctioning of purulent secretions. Long-standing foreign bodies may be surrounded with granulation and even calcifications. A hand-held operating head otoscope or a microscope, with an assistant providing head restraint, and proper instruments, such as blunt right-angled hooks, are vital for successful office removal. A history of unilateral rhinorrhea since birth indicates the possibility of unilateral choanal atresia. Careful rhinoscopy including a flexible fiberoptic examination can easily confirm this diagnosis.

FIGURE 9   A: A 14-year-old patient with chronic nasal obstruction. CT scan demonstrates expansile sphenoid mass with speckled central areas of high attenuation. **B:** T_1-weighted MR image demonstrates peripheral enhancement with central signal loss. Endoscopic ethmoidectomy and sphenoidotomy demonstrated thick central mucin. Histology and culture confirmed allergic fungal sinusitis.

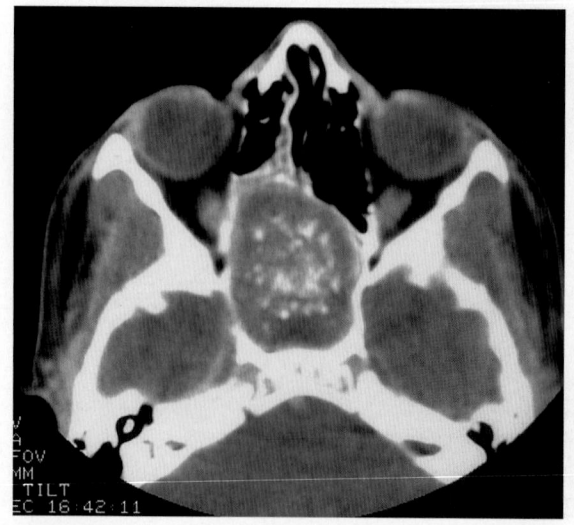 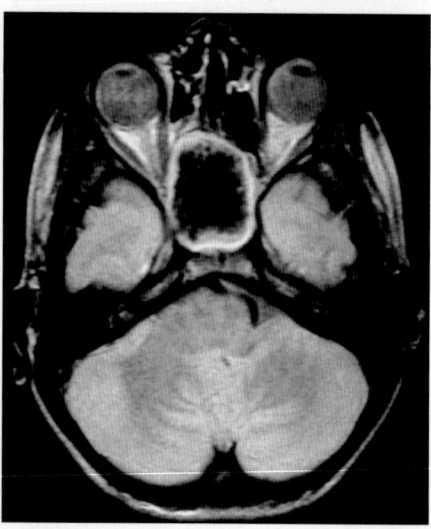

Sinusitis Impacting Pulmonary Status and Overall Health

Impaired sinus and nasal function can potentially have a negative impact on underlying pulmonary disease via aerosolized secretions or, of probably greater importance, via loss of normal filtering of antigen-sized particles. Refractory sinusitis is commonly associated with immunoglobulin E (IgE)-mediated inflammatory processes, such as allergic rhinitis and asthma, and also with primary immunodeficiency, such as IgG subclass deficiency. Early viral illnesses in genetically predisposed patients may be an etiologic common pathway through suppression of T-cell regulatory function.

Cystic Fibrosis

Cystic fibrosis (CF) is the most common inherited lethal disease of whites, with an estimated 1 in 50 heterozygous carrier rate in white populations. Over 500 mutations effecting the CF transmembrane conductance regulator gene (determining chloride ion channel function) have been identified in recent years, bringing the hope of future effective gene therapy (15). Close to 100% of children with a diagnosis of CF will have radiographic evidence of sinus mucosal abnormalities by age 1 year and an estimated 20% to 40% of patients will eventually develop nasal polyps on physical examination. Therefore, a finding of nasal polyposis in a pediatric patient should prompt diagnostic evaluation for CF, including sweat chloride testing.

Recently, cases have been described of older, previously health children with nasal polyposis and/or histologic evidence of inspissated mucus glands after sinus surgery and mildly elevated or borderline sweat chloride values. Subsequent blood analysis then demonstrated genetic evidence of cystic fibrosis. At present we are not able to predict the long-term phenotypic expression of many CF compound heterozygous genotypes, and some patients with carrier state alone may have phenotypic expression of severe chronic sinusitis at some point in their life.

Sinus surgery in CF patients is considered for polyposis with nasal airway obstruction refractory to topical steroids, or for symptomatic recurrent sinusitis appearing to aggravate underlying pulmonary status (Fig. 10). Retrospective studies of CF patients after sinus surgery have generally found symptom improvement by questionnaire but no evidence of improvement in pulmonary function (16). Postsurgical imaging invariably shows persistent mucosal thickening within maxillary sinuses even after adequate drainage of inspissated mucus with evidence of central sinus aeration (17). Some authors have described a natural history of worsening of sinus disease to a peak at about age 8 to 12 followed by gradual improvement in the later teenage years. Thus, families of CF patients undergoing sinus surgery at our institution are advised that future sinus procedures for recurrent disease may be required at least through the early teenage years.

Surgical bleeding represents a greater potential problem for CF patients because of their high degree of mucosal inflammation and because of vitamin K malabsorption. This author routinely checks prothrombin and partial thromboplastin values prior to surgery

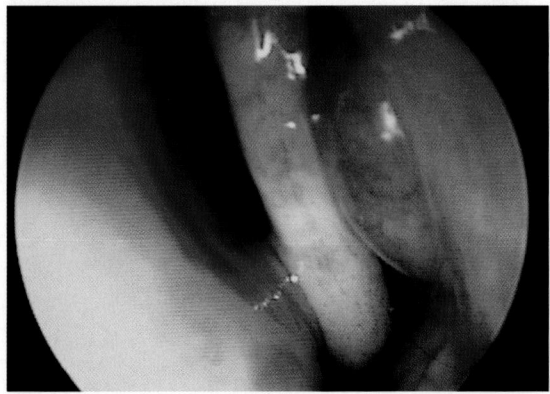

FIGURE 10 A 6-year-old girl with cystic fibrosis with a history of worsening sinusitis aggravating her pulmonary status. Endoscopic view of left nasal cavity demonstrates fleshy polypoid mass in the left middle meatus lateral to the middle turbinate.

even if the patient is taking vitamin K supplements. Surgery is not undertaken until coagulation profiles are normal. Oral steroids are administered at a dose of 0.5 to 1.0 mg per kilogram per day of prednisone or equivalent beginning 1 week prior to surgery. The goal is to decrease mucosal inflammation and thereby reduce both surgical bleeding and postsurgery edema. Topical steroids are resumed as oral steroids are tapered over 3 to 5 days in the postsurgical period.

Asthma

Asthma appears to be doubling in incidence approximately every 20 years in industrialized societies, perhaps due, in part to increasing outdoor and indoor air pollution. Anecdotally, upper respiratory infection may trigger or aggravate symptoms and signs of asthma, and parents and primary care physicians increasingly seek better solutions to the problem of recurrent sinusitis in these patients. Logically, normal nasal mucociliary clearance is vital in the mitigation of childhood IgE-mediated antigen-triggered asthmatic inflammation, and several authors have described improvements in asthma management after successful medical or surgical treatment of sinusitis (18). The author's study of 14 steroid-dependent asthmatic children demonstrated a reduction in sinusitis symptoms in 13 patients and an improvement in asthma management evidenced by a reduction in school days missed and in hospitalization days in 11 patients after endoscopic surgery for chronic sinusitis. Interestingly, the sickest patients, in terms of hospitalization days in the year before surgery, experienced the greatest improvement in the year after surgery. Pulmonary function tests varied widely over time for each patient, and no case demonstrated improved tests after surgery.

Pediatric patients with asthma constituted the largest single percentage of sinus surgery cases in many tertiary pediatric centers. A decision for surgery is based primarily on radiographic evidence of persistent disease after aggressive medical management (Fig. 11). In the author's practice, patients with definite polyposis or polypoid degeneration of middle turbinate and/or ostiomeatal complex mucosa are treated with perioperative steroids, as with CF patients. Asthmatic patients constitute special anesthetic challenges as the stress of induction or surgery can trigger bronchospasm.

Immunodeficiency

All children have a relative physiologic immunodeficiency, as immune function does not mature to adult levels until about age 12. By age 7, most children have reached approximately 90% of adult levels of specific immunoglobulins, and this fact may explain in part why many difficult cases of chronic rhinorrhea improve spontaneously by then. The author uses age 7 as a general reference point in decision making to help sort out true "chronic" sinusitis from rhinorrhea more likely to resolve on its own. Under age 7, ade-

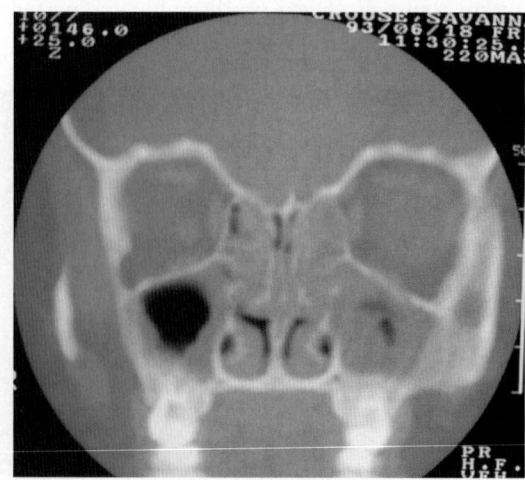

FIGURE 11 A 9-year-old girl with severe steroid-dependent asthma. CT demonstrates persistent maxillary and ethmoid disease after 3 months of broad-spectrum antibiotics.

noidectomy and occasionally maxillary sinus lavage are the author's primary sinus surgical procedures for medical failures.

When a patient appears unusually refractory to medical therapy and especially if sinusitis is associated with pulmonary disease, then true primary immunodeficiency is considered. In fact, some immunologists consider sinusitis to be the most common manifestation of immunodeficiency even in the absence of a history of pneumonia or bronchitis. Initial evaluation of these patients includes measurement of total immunoglobulins and IgG subclasses. A laboratory with age-appropriate normative data is necessary because of the steady maturation in immunoglobulin quantities. The most common immunodeficiency discovered in the evaluation of pediatric patients with chronic sinusitis is IgG2 deficiency, and it is often associated with vaccine hyporesponse (usually assessed with pneumococcal vaccine by measuring before and 1-month after vaccination antibody titers). Management of these patients is primarily medical, including prophylactic antibiotics and aggressive allergy treatment. Consistent low total immunoglobulin defines the entity of common variable hypogammaglobulinemia, and these patients are usually sicker with reactive airway disease and/or recurrent pneumonia and bronchitis. Surgery for immunodeficiency patients is usually considered an adjunct to medical therapy when symptomatic children demonstrate imaging evidence of persistent disease. By itself, surgery is unlikely to result in sustained improvement for these patients (19).

Patients with acquired immunodeficiency constitute special diagnostic and therapy challenges. Neutropenic patients during chemotherapy for lymphoreticular malignancies are at risk both for severe bacterial sinusitis and for invasive fungal infection. Patients with neutrophil counts below 2,000 with spiking fevers while treated with broad-spectrum antibiotics should be evaluated for sinusitis with rhinoscopy and imaging studies. Findings of pale, insensate middle turbinate or septal mucosa with adjacent areas of excoriation precede the classic black ischemic necrosis description of invasive fungal infection and should prompt immediate biopsy for culture and histopathologic examination. The most common organism causing invasive disease in neutropenic cancer and transplant patients is *Aspergillus*, and systemic amphotericin B remains the mainstay of treatment. At the author's institution, serial endoscopic debridement of devitalized tissue is replacing open maxillectomy surgical approaches for these patients. The prognosis for cases of invasive fungal disease remains poor unless the underlying immunodeficiency can be reversed.

Acquired immunodeficiency syndrome (AIDS) patients present occasional dilemmas with regard to surgical intervention for sinusitis. Obviously, systemic antibiotics are the primary treatment modality, and most severe problems of sinus diseases arise in the later advanced stages of disease. The author has performed sinus surgery on AIDS patients for treatment of suppurative complications, such as medial subperiosteal orbital abscess and for drainage of thick maxillary mucopus in symptomatic patients whose disease is otherwise stable (Fig. 12).

Chronic Sinusitis

Chronic sinusitis is the most common potential surgical indication the clinician faces, and it is also the most difficult entity to define. Many authors define chronic as 3 months of unresolving symptoms, but this seems to be a relatively uncommon situation in most pediatric practices. A far more common situation is that of at least partial resolution of sinusitis symptoms while taking antibiotics with recurrence of symptoms shortly after antibiotics are discontinued. A more practical definition of chronic sinusitis might then be three or more cycles of recurrent symptoms despite aggressive medical management, possibly including short courses of prophylactic antibiotics continuing after symptom resolution.

Clinicians are often confronted with the situation of concerned parents anxious about the expense of antibiotics, doctor visits, and missed time from work while, paradoxically, the child seems otherwise healthy and happy. A few minutes devoted to putting

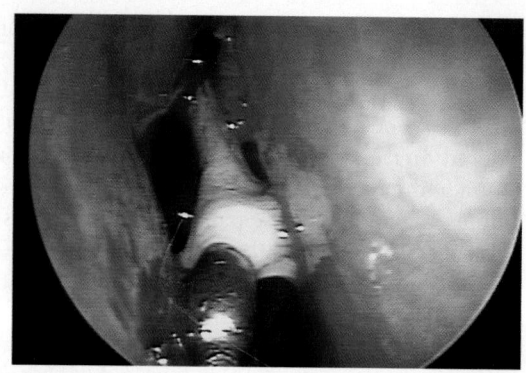

FIGURE 12 An 11-year-old girl with Down syndrome and AIDS after transfusion during open heart surgery at age 3. Endoscopy view of right nasal cavity during endoscopic ethmoidectomy. The metal suction tip inferiorly is removing thick mucopus from the right middle meatus.

things into perspective for the parents can pay large dividends in terms of formulating a rational, effective treatment plan. The author starts with the notion that chronic sinusitis is multifactorial and therefore, much to everyone's disappointment, there is no one single treatment solution (Table 3). The author also emphasizes the concept that most young children will improve spontaneously over time due to maturation of systemic immunity. It makes sense to start with relatively safe and inexpensive options, such as twice-daily nasal saline lavage, and proceed potentially to topical cromolyn and/or topical steroids with the goal of diminishing mucosal inflammation and breaking cycles of infection. Smaller day care, dust reduction measures, and allergy evaluation fit into the first half of the treatment hierarchy. When these measures fail, more expensive and invasive treatment options can be added to the list such as immunotherapy when indicated by documented sensitivities. Surgery is considered at the end of the treatment list after less invasive treatments fail to produce results. For young children, adenoidectomy is my first surgical consideration for chronic sinusitis with the goal of improving nasal breathing and reducing a potential source of upper respiratory tract infection. Endoscopic opening of the sinus outflow tracts is generally only considered in older children with CT evidence of persistent disease and a history of sinusitis significantly impacting quality of life via missed time from school, chronic cough, etc. The author explains to parents that surgery can only alter anatomy, and it does not impact on allergies, immunodeficiency, or exposure to viruses. The realistic goal of surgery in chronic sinusitis patients therefore is to re-

TABLE 3: Hierarchy of Treatment Options for Pediatric Chronic Sinusitis

Less Intensive . . . .*More Intensive*

Smaller day care (*reduce viral exposure*)
    Dust reduction in home
        Daily nasal saline lavage
            Nasal cromolyn sodium
                3–4 weeks of broad-spectrum antibiotic
                    Topical nasal steroids
                        Age-appropriate allergy testing and immunotherapy
                        Antibiotic prophylaxis
                            Adenoidectomy (*young patients*)
                            Antral lavage
                                Endoscopic ethmoidectomy and
                                  antrostomy
                                  Intravenous gamma-globulin
                                    (*documented
                                      immunodeficiency
                                      threatening health*)

TABLE 4: Trends in Endoscopic Sinus Surgery

Focusing indications through better understanding of natural history of pediatric chronic sinusitis

Perioperative steroids for patients with polyposis

More limited, less traumatic approach (cutting forceps, microdebriders)

Less packing and stenting, fewer routine postoperative "debridement" procedures

Expanded horizons—orbit, frontal sinus, tumors

duce the frequency and severity of sinusitis by improving sinus ventilation and drainage. It is not a cure, and surgical results are much better when medical treatment such as saline and allergy management are continued.

Endoscopic sinus surgical techniques were first introduced into the United States in the mid-1980s; by the late 1980s, several reports appeared in the literature supporting the idea that the technique was both safe and effective (at least in the short term) for pediatric chronic sinusitis (Table 4). Lusk's group (20) reported that 80% of children without other systemic disease experienced dramatic improvement in chronic sinusitis symptoms after endoscopic sinus surgery, as evidenced by parental questionnaire. Stankiewicz (21) more recently found less treatment effect by sinus surgery, with 38% of parents reporting that their children were "cured" after surgery and 55% reporting some improvement. Of interest, Stankiewicz reported that 50% of pediatric patients undergoing endoscopic nasal examination after surgery showed that at least one maxillary ostia had closed. This finding naturally raises the possibility that factors other than improved sinus drainage were responsible for the patient's perceived improvement. Surgical intervention can carry a strong placebo effect, and parents may be more likely to follow medical treatment regimens after investing in surgery. Interestingly, Stammberger, one of the pioneers of endoscopic surgical techniques, reports that less than 2% of his thousands of cases in Europe have been children and that the majority of those patients had specific diagnoses, such as CF, antrochoanal polyp, or orbital abscess (20).

Rosenfeld (22) recently reported the results of a "stepped protocol" with a prospective cohort of 41 children with radiographically documented chronic sinusitis. All patients were treated initially with at least 3 weeks of broad-spectrum antibiotics; treatment failures then had adenoidectomy (if adenoids were "present") or endoscopic ethmoidectomy and antrostomy (if adenoids were "absent"). The sinus surgery cohort had more overall systemic disease such as asthma and allergic rhinitis and more severe initial symptomatology. A posttreatment caregiver survey showed that endoscopic sinus surgery was highly effective in reducing major symptoms but did not eliminate all symptoms. Specifically, rhinorrhea was often not resolved. This study offers support to the "real world" logic of reserving more invasive therapy for sicker patients who fail less intensive initial treatment.

PEARLS AND PERILS

1. The natural history of chronic sinusitis in most young children is toward spontaneous resolution.
2. Imaging findings of sinus mucosal inflammation are extremely common in young children even without a history of sinusitis symptoms and must be interpreted in the light of clinical history and signs.
3. Sinus surgery at a young age may affect future facial growth.
4. The logical treatment approach is for a "stepped protocol" of medical therapy first, then less invasive surgical procedures such as adenoidectomy, with more invasive direct sinus drainage procedures reserved for the small minority of treatment failures with sinusitis affecting overall health.

SURGICAL METHOD

Informed Consent

Proper informed consent is important not only from a medicolegal standpoint but also from the standpoint of putting the option of surgical therapy into perspective. A discussion of potential for injury to surrounding structures, such as the eye and brain, can help both parents and the surgeon decide whether or not the patient has truly failed aggressive medical management and is now a candidate for surgery. For patients with chronic sinusitis, the author also emphasizes during the informed consent discussion that the goal of surgery is to reduce the frequency and severity of sinusitis and to provide a window of opportunity for better medical management but that it is not by itself a cure.

Preoperative Preparation

Patients with polyposis or significant polypoid mucosal degeneration are usually placed on a dose of oral prednisone or steroid equivalent at 1 to 2 mg per kilogram per day beginning 5 to 7 days prior to surgery. The goal is to reduce inflammation and surgical bleeding and to diminish surgical edema. The steroids are continued for 3 to 5 days postoperatively and then rapidly tapered. Asthmatic patients are managed aggressively with bronchdilator therapy and steroids when appropriate to minimize pulmonary complications. Patients with a history consistent with possible bleeding disorder, such as those with CF, are evaluated with preoperative coagulation screens.

Endoscopic Ethmoidectomy: Middle Meatus Antrostomy

Oxymetazoline-soaked pledgets are placed into the nasal cavities for 10 minutes prior to the procedure. The author generally does not inject lidocaine. The turbinates and lateral nasal walls are then inspected with a 4.0-mm telescope assessing for areas of inflammation and anatomic abnormalities. If the middle meati are inaccessible because of a severely deviated septum, a conservative septoplasty is performed first (unusual in children). If the uncinate is very horizontal and blocking access to the bulla ethmoidalis, the author starts the ethmoidectomy by performing an uncinectomy with sickle knife and straight forceps (Fig. 13). If the bulla is easily seen, the author starts by opening the bulla and visualizing the lamina papyracea. The advantage of seeing the lamina first lies in reducing the odds for inadvertent penetration of the orbit in the anterior ethmoid, which is very narrow in young children. Dissection is brought anteriorly through facial recess cells and aggar nasi cells if diseased, with care taken to avoid trauma to the frontal nasal duct. Dissection posteriorly through the basal lamella (horizontal attachment of the middle turbinate) into posterior ethmoid cells is performed depending on extent of disease. Diseased mucosa and polyps are carefully removed from involved cells including any Haller's or Onodi's cells and from the lateral recess (between bulla and fovea and lamina). In performing posterior ethmoidectomy, care is taken not to take down all horizontal attachment of middle turbinate, to keep the turbinate in a stable medial position. A smaller 2.8-mm telescope is sometimes necessary for work in the narrow ethmoid of young children, but it delivers an exponential decrease in light and optics. The anterior head of the middle turbinate is excised if it is significantly polypoid and blocks the ethmoid. Similarly, the posterior–inferior portion of the middle turbinate is removed if necessary for access to the sphenoid.

With the lamina papyracea well visualized, any remaining uncinate process is removed with a right-angled ball seeker or back-biting forceps. The natural ostium of the maxillary sinus is then located high in the middle meatus with the ball seeker or curved suction by following diseased mucosa. The ostium is enlarged principally by removing bone (the posterior fontanelle) back to the inferomedial orbit (Fig. 14). Hypertrophic mucosa are also removed from the inferior ostium with careful preservation of the nasolacrimal duct.

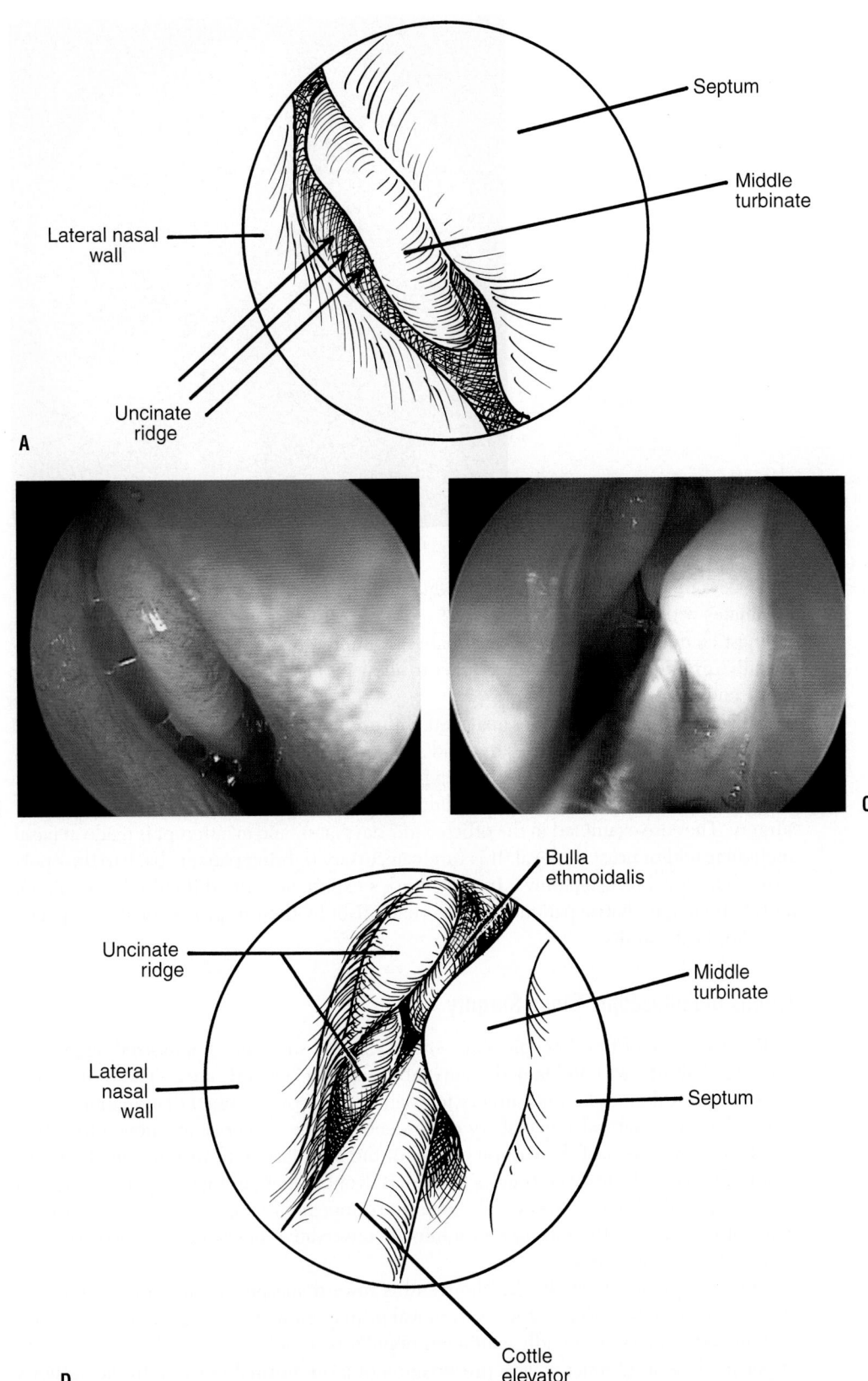

FIGURE 13 A, B: 4.0-mm 0° telescope view of right middle meatus. **C, D:** Middle turbinate retracted laterally revealing uncinate ridge and bulla ethmoidalis. Ethmoidectomy is begun with removal of the uncinate (if it is obstructing visualization of the bulla) or with first opening the bulla (if the uncinate ridge is small).

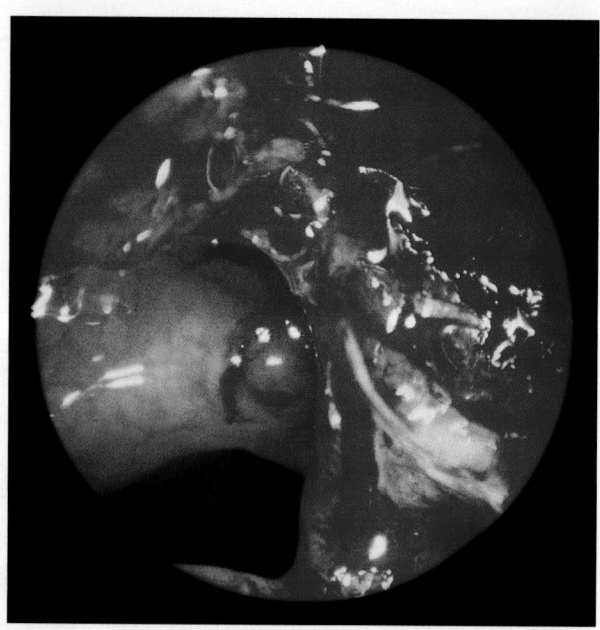

FIGURE 14 A 4-mm 0° telescope view of right nasal cavity. The orbital floor is seen through a right middle meatus antrostomy after removal of the posterior fontanelle.

Occasionally, older pediatric patients will have extremely hypertrophic inferior turbinates with a significant degree of fixed nasal obstruction. This problem appears to be most common with teenaged asthmatics. A limited turbinoplasty via cautery or conservative excision is sometimes necessary to allow for nasal breathing and for subsequent saline and topical steroid therapy.

Bleeding during surgery is managed with oxymetazoline-soaked packs and careful bipolar cautery. The author tries to avoid any postoperative packing or stenting by minimizing operative bleeding and by keeping the middle turbinate as stable as possible. Patients are instructed to resume nasal saline lavage and topical nasal steroids the day after surgery. They are examined in the office 5 to 7 days later, and an attempt is made at nasal suctioning and/or crust removal. It is rarely necessary to bring patients back to the operating room for a "crustectomy." In the author's experience, the difficulty in examining and suctioning pediatric patients is more than offset by their improved healing capacity compared with adults.

Trends in Endoscopic Sinus Surgery

In the early years of endoscopic sinus surgery, many surgeons emphasized aggressive opening of all sinuses and blamed recurrent disease on "missed" areas. The trend lately has been toward more limited surgery focused on areas of mucosal inflammation within the pathways of natural mucociliary coalescence. Some surgeons are now advocating avoiding enlargement of the natural ostium of the maxillary sinus or removal of any anterior ethmoid cells, to avoid trauma to the nasofrontal duct (although these are the two most commonly diseased areas). These authors appear to be coming full circle to the point of no surgery (the ultimate in minimal conservative operating) for pediatric patients with chronic disease.

From a technical standpoint, the trend is toward sharper, cleaner dissection with cutting forceps rather than extensive removal of mucosa with pulling instruments. Suction microdebriders are rapidly gaining in popularity as an elegant method for removal of polypoid diseased mucosa with preservation of more normal mucosa. In the author's experience, the microdebrider instruments reduce operative bleeding and lead to faster recovery of polyp patients, especially those with CF. They are ideal instruments for defining normal anatomy in patients with extensive polyposis having revision surgery as they preserve normal structures, such as the middle turbinate, while removing diseased mucosa. Better nasal drills with slim profiles are being developed by several companies and will improve the ease of choanal atresia and endoscopic orbital procedures.

As surgeons become more comfortable within the tighter confines of the pediatric nose, the horizons of endoscopic techniques are expanding. As mentioned previously, many surgeons now utilize endoscopic approaches instead of external ethmoidectomy for drainage of medial subperiosteal orbital abcesses. Reports are appearing more frequently of endoscopic approaches to chronic frontal disease including removal of the midline frontal sinus floor via a small superior septectomy (23). Inverted papillomas and even nasopharyngeal angiofibromas are being excised endoscopically with increasing frequency.

PEARLS AND PERILS

1. Adequate informed consent puts surgery into perspective.
2. Perioperative steroids are used for patients with polyps.
3. Oxymetazoline is used for hemostasis.
4. The anterior ethmoid is narrow in children. Carefully deflect the uncinate medially away from the lamina and remove or start in the bulla.
5. Dissection should be sharp. Preserve mucosa and middle turbinate stability. Avoid packing.
6. Use a microdebrider for hypertrophic mucosa and polyps.

⊕ MANAGEMENT OF COMPLICATIONS

Complications are best avoided through preoperative planning and careful technique. A common plantiff attorney strategy in litigated cases of surgical complications is to focus on the original operative indications. Obviously, every effort should be made to document valid indications in the patient record prior to any surgical procedure. CT of relevant sinus anatomy is a necessary antecedent to endoscopic procedures.

General Complications

The most common reported complications after sinus surgery are formation of adhesions between the middle turbinate and the lateral nasal wall. Adhesions are inevitable to a certain degree and probably do not usually result in significant ethmoid obstruction. They can be minimized, however, by sharp minimal dissection with cutting instruments, by maintaining turbinate stability, and by avoiding postoperative packing. Nasal lacrimal duct injuries can occur via vigorous removal of bone anterior to the ostium of the maxillary sinus, usually with a back-biting forceps. These injuries appear to have become less common as surgeons have emphasized more conservative ostium enlargement principally via removal of bone posteriorly to the ostium. Significant bleeding can be reduced by obtaining a preoperative bleeding history and by careful dissection in the areas of the anterior ethmoid artery (transverse ridge behind the nasofrontal duct) and the sphenopalatine branches (posteroinferior middle turbinate and sphenoid face). Perioperative steroids for patients with significant polypoid mucosa can help reduce both bleeding and postoperative adhesions by minimizing mucosal inflammation and edema.

Orbit

The most common orbital complication is probably laceration of periorbita with prolapse of orbital fat. This usually occurs in the narrow anterior ethmoid, often in the course of performing an uncinectomy. The fat prolapse can hamper visualization and interfere with completion of the procedure and can cause postoperative medial orbital ecchymosis. If unrecognized, removal of orbital fat could lead to rectus muscle injury or to intraorbital hemorrhage with the potential for blindness. When fat prolapse is suspected, gentle pressure on the globe while visualizing the area in question should demonstrate any break in the periorbita. Alternatively, gentle traction of prolapsed fat should result in motion of the medial canthal area. If the diagnosis is still in doubt, a carefully excised small sample can be sent for frozen section.

If intraorbital bleeding occurs with rapid onset of orbital signs such as proptosis and chemosis, all ethmoid packing should be removed and an intraoperative ophthalmologic consultation should be obtained. An external ethmoidectomy approach for ligation of the ethmoid arteries and partial orbital decompression should be undertaken, with a lateral canthotomy reserved for continued signs of increasing orbital pressure with disc ischemia. Medical measures include head of bed elevation, topical ice, and intravenous steroids and manitol. Rarely, intraconal evacuation of an orbital hematoma by the ophthalmologist may be required.

Cerebrospinal Fluid Leak

The two most common locations for inadvertent penetration of the dura during sinus surgery are the medial fovea (which slopes inferiorly toward the cribiform plate) and the area just superior to the face of the sphenoid. If a small cerebrospinal fluid leak is noted during the case, an attempt can be made to repair it with a free septal mucosal graft, which is held in place with nasal packing for 3 to 5 days. For large defects, a lumbar drain is placed, and the defect is closed with temporalis fascia and muscle or abdominal fat.

PEARLS AND PERILS

1. Start with valid indications
2. Complications are better avoided than treated.
3. Postoperative scarring can be minimized with atraumatic technique and avoidance of packing.

SUMMARY

The strongest indications for sinus surgery in the pediatric age group are treatment of suppurative complications of sinusitis and of fixed obstruction such as polyps refractory to medical treatment. The most common indication in the author's practice is sinusitis refractory to medical therapy aggravating or triggering lung disease. Chronic sinusitis is a difficult entity to define in children, and surgery may be a useful adjunct when medical therapy is unsuccessful and imaging demonstrates significant persistent mucosal disease. The realistic goal of surgery in these patients is to break a cycle of persistent disease and to reduce the frequency and severity of future episodes.

REFERENCES

1. Takahashi H, Fujito A, Honjo I. *Am J Otolaryngol* 1989;10:208–213.
2. Muntz HR, Lusk RP. *Arch Otolaryngol Head Neck Surg* 1991;117:179–181.
3. Lazar RH, Younis RT, Gross CW. *Head Neck Surg* 1992;14:92–98.
4. Gross C, Gurucharri M, Lazar R, Leng T. *Laryngoscope* 1989;99:272–275.
5. Poole MD. *Ear Nose Throat J* 1992;71:622–623.
6. Otten FWA, Aarem A, Grote JJ. *Clin Otolaryngol* 1992;17:32–33.
7. Van der Veken PJ, Clement PAR, Buissert TH, Desprechins B, Kaufman L, Derde MP. *Am J Rhinol* 1992;6:45–58.

8. Manning SC, Biavati MJ, Phillips DL. *Int J Pediatr Otorhinolaryngol* 1996;37:65–74.

9. Mair EA, Bolger WE, Breisch EA. *Arch Otolaryngol Head Neck Surg* 1995;121:729–736.

10. Manning SC. *Arch Otolaryngol Head Neck Surg* 1993;119:789–791.

11. Liu JH, Manning SC, Biavati MJ. (submitted).

12. Coste A, Rateau JG, Roudot, Thoraval F, et al. *Arch Otolaryngol Head Neck Surg* 1996;122:432–436.

13. Triglia JM, Dessi P, Cannoni M, Pech A. *Int J Pediatr Otorhinolaryngol* 1992;23:125–131.

14. Manning SC, Mabry RL, Schaefer SD, Close L. *Laryngoscope* 1993;103:717–721.

15. Farrell PM, Koscik RE. *Pediatrics* 1996;97:524–527.

16. Duplechain JK, White JA, Miller RH. *Arch Otolaryngol Head Neck Surg* 1991;117:422–426.

17. Jones JW, Parsons DS, Cuyler JP. *Int J Pediatr Otorhinolaryngol* 1993;28:25–32.

18. Manning SC, Wasserman RL, Silver R, Phillips DL. *Arch Otolaryngol Head Neck Surg* 1994;120:1142–1145.

19. Lusk RP, Polman SH, Muntz HR. *Arch Otolaryngol Head Neck Surg* 1991;117:60–63.

20. Lund VJ, Neifens HJ, Clement PAR, Lusk R, Stammberger H. *Int J Pediatr Otorhinolaryngol* 1995;32[suppl]:S21–S35.

21. Stankiewicz JA. *Otolaryngol Head Neck Surg* 1995;113:204–210.

22. Rosenfeld RM. *Arch Otolaryngol Head Neck Surg* 1995;121:729–736.

23. Close LG, Lee NK, Leach JL, Manning SC. *Ann Otol Rhinol Laryngol* 1994;103:952–958.

S.C. Manning: Department of Otolaryngology, University of Washington School of Medicine, Children's Hospital and Regional Medical Center, Seattle, Washington 98105-0371.

• *Practical Pediatric Otolaryngology*
• edited by Robin T. Cotton and Charles M. Myer, III
• Lippincott-Raven Publishers, Philadelphia © 1999

26

Epistaxis

Bradley F. Marple

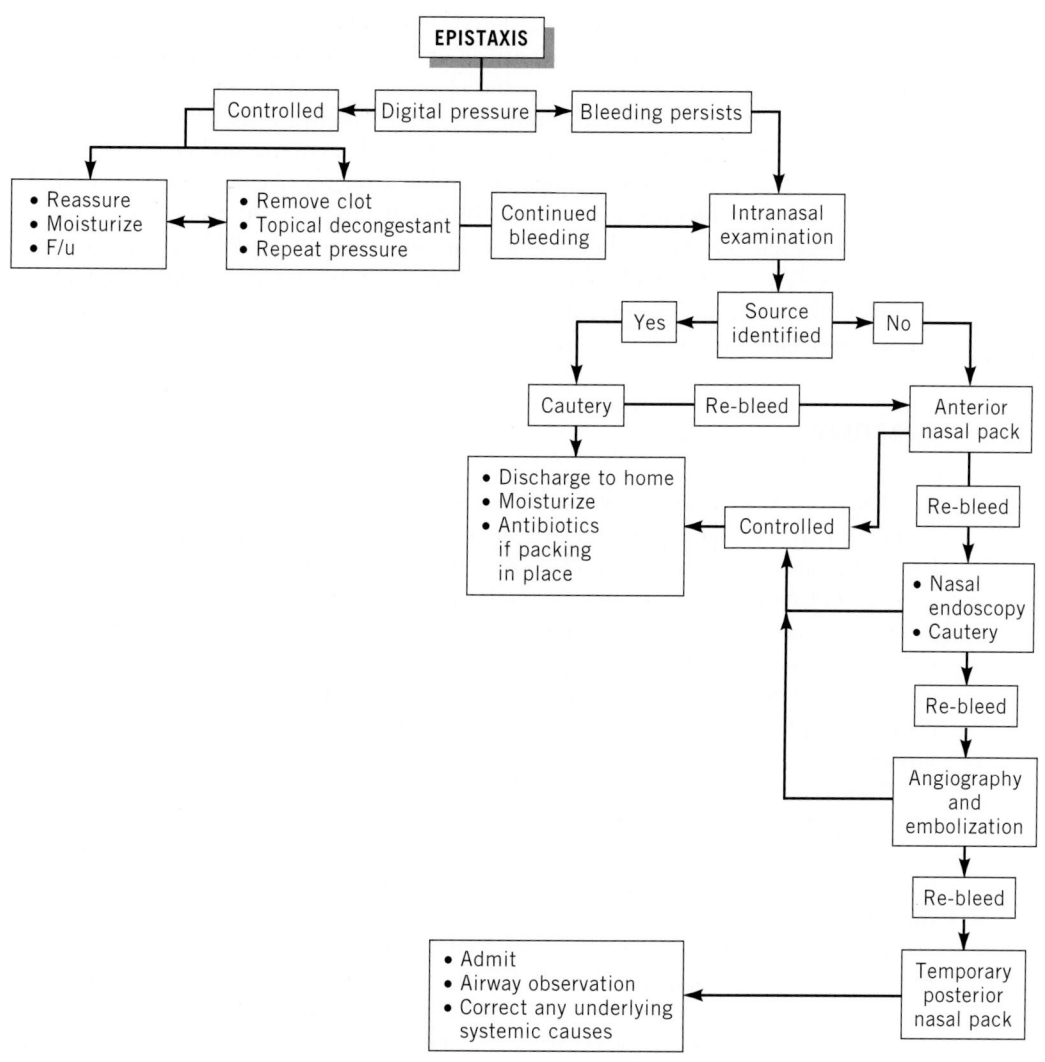

OVERVIEW

Epistaxis has been referred to as the albatross of otolaryngology. Few otolaryngologists relish such cases, but most recognize epistaxis as a significant and common problem. Estimates suggest that 7% to 14% of the U.S. adult population has experienced at least one nosebleed (1), and the incidence among the pediatric population is not significantly different. A study of 1,218 children ranging from 11 to 14 years old revealed a 6% incidence of epistaxis (2). For many adults, recurrent epistaxis first presents as a problem during childhood. When interviewed, 50% of adult patients with recurrent epistaxis complain of onset of symptoms during their childhood years. Most cases of epistaxis in children occur after the age of 2 years. However, occasional cases of epistaxis occur in the neonate and infant, frequently due to trauma at birth (3).

In both the adult and pediatric age groups, nosebleeds are rarely life-threatening; however, catastrophic complications occur on occasion. Fatalities may occur as a result of aspiration, hypotension, or cardiac arrhythmia. Moreover, although epistaxis is usually idiopathic or related to an upper respiratory tract infection, it may herald the presence of underlying systemic disease. With this in mind, careful consideration should be given to each case.

In general terms, nosebleeds within the pediatric and adult populations are similar, but some differences do exist. Trauma and inflammation are leading causes of epistaxis in both groups, with the most common source being the anterior nasal septum (Kiesselbach's plexus) (1). Posterior nosebleeds are exceedingly rare among children, most likely because of the lack of degenerative vascular changes in this population (4). Epistaxis in both groups occurs most commonly during the winter months when relative humidity is at a low point, rendering nasal mucosa more susceptible to drying and ulceration (5).

Pediatric emergencies often require an additional degree of compassion and bedside diplomacy. When a child has a significant nosebleed, family emotions can play a role in the treatment scheme. The sight of blood from the nose of a child often produces a reaction from the patient, as well as his or her parent, that is often out of proportion to the severity of the problem. The practitioner is charged with the task of calming the patient and parents, while controlling the hemorrhage and evaluating its etiology.

ANATOMY

The nasal cavity is the portion of the respiratory tract least protected from the environment. Extreme changes of temperature and humidity, as well as exposure to particulate matter and microbial insults, challenge the nose on a daily basis. The intricate relationship between the macroanatomy and microanatomy of the nose accounts for its protection and maintenance of homeostasis for the lower respiratory tract. Interruption of this balance risks trauma to the overlying mucosa and bleeding from its rich submucosal vascular plexus. As a result, it is easy to appreciate that each anatomic component of the nose plays a significant role in the development and subsequent treatment of a nosebleed.

The mucosal lining of the nose consists predominantly of pseudostratified columnar ciliated epithelium (respiratory epithelium) with interspersed goblet cells, which lie atop a basement membrane. The lamina propria, lying below the basement membrane, is filled with a rich network of arterioles, venules, capillaries, and venous lakes. Blood flow through this vascular plexus facilitates thermoregulation and humidification of inspired air and is regulated by both the parasympathetic and sympathetic arms of the autonomic nervous system. Seromucinous glands, located deeper within the lamina propria of the nasal mucosa, secrete a low-viscosity mucus. These secretions combine with those of mucosal goblet cells to form a protective blanket of mucus that overlies the nasal mucosa and is continuously circulated via ciliary activity. Any pathologic process that causes interruption of mucociliary flow or mucus production leads to drying and ulceration of underlying mucosa, thus exposing the underlying rich vascular plexus.

The most common site of nasal hemorrhage is Kiesselbach's plexus, located along the anterior aspect of the nasal septum within Little's area (Fig. 1). It is made up of a confluence of terminal vessels originating from both the external and internal carotid arterial systems. Major contributing vessels include the anterior ethmoidal artery, the nasal branch of the superior labial artery, the greater palatine artery, and branches of the sphenopalatine artery. To a lesser extent, branches of the posterior ethmoidal artery may

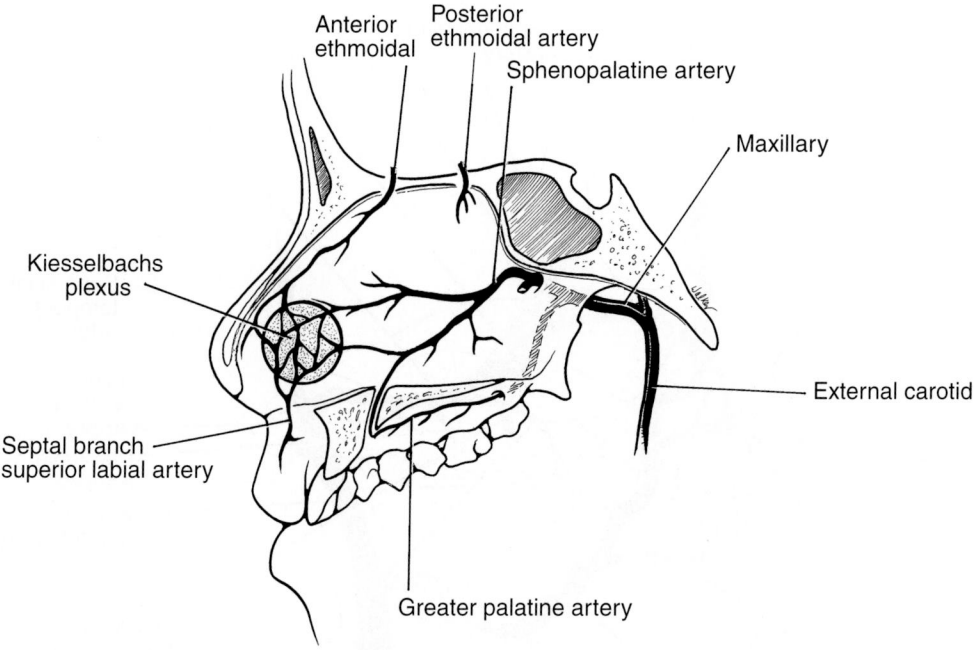

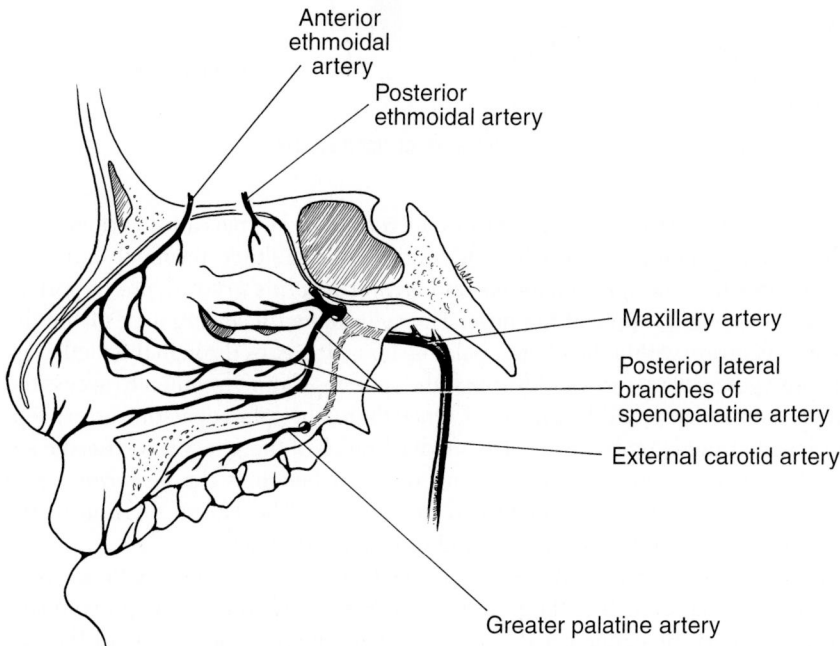

FIGURE 1 Anatomy of the nasal septum and lateral wall. **A:** Nasal septum showing the vascular supply to Kiesselbach's plexus. **B:** Lateral nasal wall—vascular anatomy, turbinates, pediatric profile.

contribute as well. This site's rich vascular anastomoses, coupled with its exposure, doubtless account for it being a prevalent site of hemorrhage.

The majority of the blood supply to the nose is provided by the external carotid system (Fig. 2). The *facial artery* is the most proximal branch of the external carotid artery that provides blood supply to the nose. It crosses the mandible to supply the external part of the face and then terminally divides into several arteries including the *superior labial artery*. The superior labial artery, in turn, gives off a branch that ascends into the nasal vestibule and branches further to supply the caudal nasal septum and the lateral nasal vestibule.

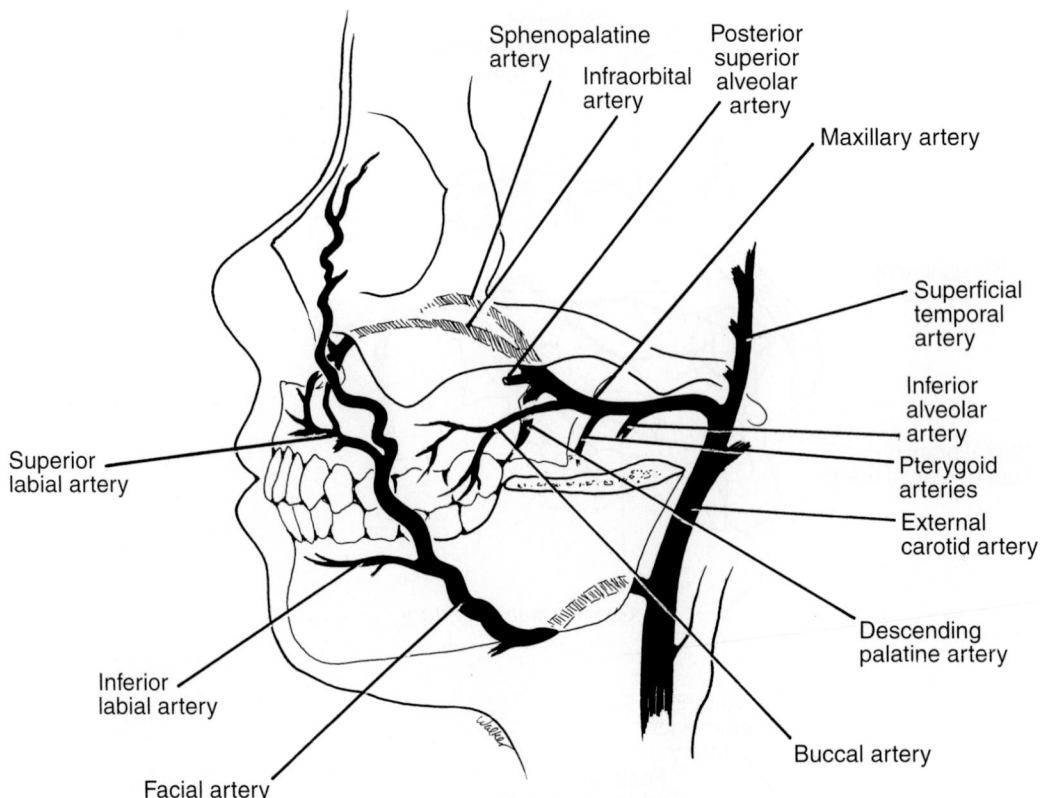

FIGURE 2 External carotid artery contributions to the nasal blood supply.

The *internal maxillary artery*, arising from the terminal external carotid artery, travels into the pterygopalatine fissure where it continues as multiple terminal branches. Two of these branches, the *sphenopalatine* and *greater palatine arteries*, are important contributors to the blood supply of the nose. The *sphenopalatine artery* arises from the internal maxillary artery within the pterygopalatine fossa. It passes through the medial aspect of the pterygomaxillary fossa and through the sphenopalatine foramen to access the nasal cavity posterior to the middle turbinate. Once there, the sphenopalatine artery separates into a medial and lateral division. The medial branch of the artery traverses the anteroinferior sphenoid to the posterior septum where it becomes the *posterior septal artery*, again giving off further branches to the septum. The lateral division of the sphenopalatine artery supplies the lateral nasal wall and turbinates.

The *greater palatine artery*, sometimes referred to as the *descending palatine artery*, also arises as a terminal branch of the internal maxillary artery. It exits the pterygopalatine fossa via the pterygopalatine canal, emerging along the posterior aspect of the secondary palate within the oral cavity. It travels anteriorly within the mucoperiosteum of the hard palate where it ascends through the incisive foramen and provides branches to the inferior nasal septum.

The arterial supply provided by the internal carotid is less direct than that provided by the external carotid system (Fig. 3). There are no branches along the internal carotid artery within the neck. The internal carotid traverses the carotid canal within the petrous portion of the temporal bone. After exiting near the lateral surface of the sphenoid bone, it runs within the cavernous sinus and enters the dura mater lateral to the anterior clinoid process. The first intracranial branch is the *ophthalmic artery*, which travels anteriorly through the superior orbital fissure. The *anterior* and *posterior ethmoidal arteries* originate directly from the ophthalmic artery before exiting through individually named foramina along the frontoethmoidal suture (Fig. 4). Once these foramina are traversed, both arteries again enter the intracranial cavity within the anterior cranial fossa. The *an-*

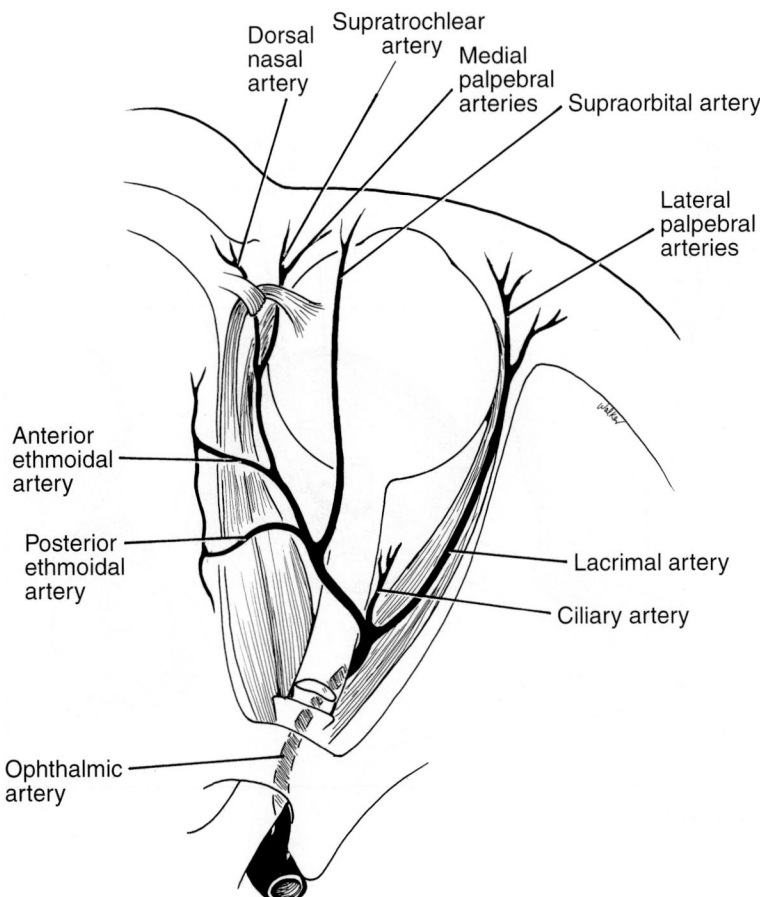

FIGURE 3 Internal carotid artery supply.

terior ethmoidal artery travels ventrally a short distance within the anterior cranial fossa before passing through a beak-like aperture near the crista galli where it enters the nasal cavity. Branches then course to both the medial and lateral nasal wall. The *posterior ethmoidal artery*, the smaller of the two, travels a shorter distance within the anterior cranial fossa. Along the posterior aspect of the cribriform plate, it reenters the roof of the nasal cavity, where it gives branches to the superior nasal septum and posterior ethmoidal sinus cells.

ETIOLOGY

The differential diagnosis of epistaxis is exhaustive, but a systematic approach to the evaluation of an individual patient helps remarkably in arriving at an accurate diagnosis. In broad terms, the cause of a nosebleed can be separated into either a local or systemic cause. A comprehensive history and physical examination commonly provides the first indication of this. Local causes can occur as an isolated event or in a recurrent fashion. The site of bleeding is focal, and frequently, when recurrent, bleeding will occur at the same site. If epistaxis is due to local causes, there should be no signs of systemic bleeding or excessive bruising. Occasionally, a severe posterior nasal hemorrhage will cause bilateral epistaxis due to blood traveling around the posterior nasal septum, while the actual source remains a single site.

Systemic causes are sometimes difficult to differentiate from local causes. A mild form of von Willebrand's disease may initially present as a focal nose bleed that is difficult to control. In other patients, a more overt systemic cause is suggested by multiple

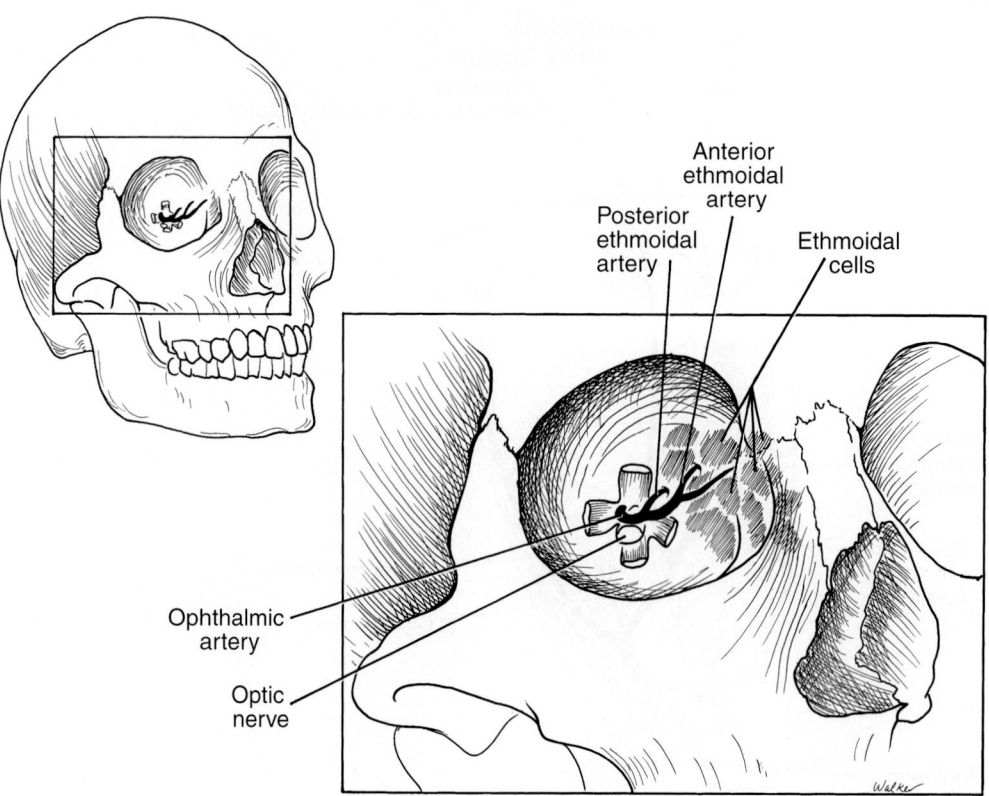

FIGURE 4 Ethmoidal arteries.

sites of hemorrhage, epistaxis in conjunction with oral bleeding, gastrointestinal hemorrhage, or excessive ecchymosis.

Local Causes

Trauma   Trauma to the nose and nasal cavity comes in many forms. Owing to its location on the anterior aspect of the face, the anterior part of the nose is often a ready recipient of blunt trauma. Epistaxis, commonly associated with nasal or facial fractures, can range in severity from mild to severe, sometimes requiring extensive measures for control. In rare cases, following head trauma, epistaxis may represent a more ominous situation than a simple nasal bleed. Pathack (6) reported a case of epistaxis secondary to rupture of an internal carotid artery pseudoaneurysm following head trauma.

Nasal trauma is more often much less overt, rendering it difficult to recognize. Dry air, especially during winter months, is a leading source of nasal trauma. Central heating and air-conditioning systems are notorious for markedly reducing humidity within the home. Drying and crusting within the nasal vestibule may result in ulceration of nasal mucosa with exposure of its underlying vasculature.

Within the pediatric population, digital manipulation (nose picking) is the most common form of trauma to the anterior nasal septum. Even though children's noses are quite small, equally small fingers cause ulceration, laceration, and bleeding of the nasal septum. When this is the case, the site of septal bleeding is commonly on the side of the dominant hand of the child. Modification of this behavior is curative, but sometimes difficult.

Foreign bodies within the nasal cavity are not uncommon among pediatric patients and can go unnoticed for a long period of time. The presence of a foreign body incites a chronic inflammatory response within the adjacent mucosa that is manifested as unilateral purulent rhinorrhea accompanied by a characteristic anaerobic odor. Epistaxis in association with foreign body obstruction of the nose is not uncommon. Diagnosis and removal of the foreign body in the appropriate setting is curative.

Iatrogenic nasal trauma in the form of nasal surgery is uncommon among pediatric patients. Obviously, nasal septoplasty, sinus, or turbinate surgery present a risk of postoperative epistaxis. More commonly, iatrogenic epistaxis is associated with routine pediatric surgical procedures in areas adjacent to the nose (i.e., pharynx or nasopharynx), such as tonsillectomy and adenoidectomy (3).

Deformities of the nasal septum in the form of spurs, deviations, and perforations interrupt the normal flow of air through the nasal cavity. Abnormal regions of turbulence or laminar airflow promote drying and crusting of mucosa, resulting in local ulceration and bleeding. Correction of the septal deformities is normally straightforward and curative. In the case of nasal septal perforations, however, closure can be difficult (7).

Some chemical irritants are recognized for their ability to inflame nasal mucosa, and cause hemorrhage. Common noxious fumes recognized for their capability to induce bleeding include phosphorus, sulfuric acid, ammonia, gasoline, chromates, printer's ink, and glutaraldehyde. Exposure to these chemicals is uncommon within the pediatric population.

Inflammatory   Inflammatory mucosal changes of nasal mucosa are a leading cause of epistaxis in both adult and pediatric populations. An increase in the incidence of nosebleeds during the winter months corresponds with an increased number of viral and bacterial upper respiratory tract infections. The association between nasal mucosal inflammation and epistaxis is multifactorial. Nasal mucosal hypersecretion and stimulation of trigeminally mediated nasal nociceptors occur, causing pain, itching, and a sensation of constant nasal flow. Simultaneously, submucosal venous engorgement causes nasal edema and resultant nasal airway obstruction. Nasal manipulation invariably follows in the form of sniffing, wiping, blowing, and picking, which causes disruption of the already fragile mucosa and initiates bleeding. Concurrent bacterial proliferation may lead to fibrinolysis and to persistence of bleeding. All of these factors combine to increase the susceptibility to recurrent and persistent epistaxis.

The role of allergic rhinitis in pediatric recurrent epistaxis was first noted by Girsh in 1960 (8). Epistaxis among these allergic children was initially attributed to increased digital trauma accompanying nasal pruritis. Since that time, little attention has been given to this association. Murray and Milner (9) revisited the subject by studying 557 consecutive children referred to an allergy clinic. Skin prick test results were compared with questionnaire results to assess the association between allergic rhinitis and recurrent epistaxis. Recurrent epistaxis was noted to be significantly more frequent in patients with both a positive skin test result and a history of allergic rhinitis than in those with a positive skin test result alone or those with neither a positive skin test result nor an allergy history. The etiology of this appears to extend beyond a simple increase in nasal digital trauma. Prostacyclin, generated during allergic reactions, is thought to decrease platelet aggregation. Additionally, decreased platelet aggregation has also been associated with chronic use of antihistamines. Further, tryptase, which is released by basophils during immunoglobulin E (IgE)-mediated allergic reactions, inactivates fibrinogen and causes decreased coagulation (9–12). At any rate, allergic rhinitis appears to play a role in recurrent pediatric epistaxis.

Neoplasms   Any neoplastic process or mass occurring within the nasal cavity may provide a source for bleeding. Meningoceles, encephaloceles, and gliomas are anatomic abnormalities that may be overlooked at birth and during young childhood. Their presence within the nasal cavity can lead to recurrent epistaxis, usually on the side of the lesion. Likewise, rare congenital arteriovenous malformations may give rise to epistaxis.

Recurrent unilateral epistaxis occurring in male patients at the time of puberty is the most common presentation of juvenile nasopharyngeal angiofibroma. This tumor is rare and occurs almost exclusively in the male population. It is richly vascularized, often being supplied by branches of the external carotid artery. Although spontaneous resolution is occasionally observed, surgical extirpation is normally required for treatment. Radiation therapy, potentially associated with later malignant transformation of this otherwise benign tumor, is reserved for nonresectable disease.

Primary malignant tumors of the head and neck during childhood are rare. Many of them, however, present in the region of the nasopharynx. Nasopharyngeal carcinoma and rhabdomyosarcoma are among the most common childhood malignancies of the upper respiratory tract (13). In a review of 29 pediatric patients with nasopharyngeal malignancies studied at Children's Hospital of Philadelphia, approximately half of the neoplasms were found to be rhabdomyosarcoma. Rhabdomyosarcoma was generally found in younger patients, compared to those presenting with nasopharyngeal carcinoma, and was associated with a longer disease-free survival. Other less common malignant tumors that present within the sinonasal tract include lymphoma and sarcoma.

Systemic Causes

Granulomatous Disease   Granulomatous and autoimmune etiologies for epistaxis in the pediatric population are extremely rare. Sarcoidosis, tuberculosis, and polymorphic reticulosis should be considered but are much more common within the adult population. Occasionally, gummatous lesions associated with congenital syphilis will be encountered as a source of epistaxis. Approximately 30 pediatric cases of Wegener's granulomatosis have been reported in the literature. Nasal involvement leads to nasal discharge, stuffiness, and epistaxis. Although the disease is extremely rare, failure to treat yields a very poor prognosis (14).

Coagulopathies   The hemorrhagic disorders that occur in childhood are numerous but are fortunately uncommon. Recurrent epistaxis in childhood may be the manifestation of a such a bleeding disorder. Adult retrospective series report that only 0.7% to 3.5% of patients with recurrent epistaxis actually possess an underlying bleeding disorder (15–17). Katsanis et al. (18) performed a study on 36 children complaining of a history of five or more spontaneous nosebleeds annually, with age-matched control subjects. A comprehensive history was obtained, coupled with coagulation screening tests. Overall, 5.6% of the children were diagnosed with a primary bleeding disorder. However, when historical evidence of severe recurrent bleeding, positive family history, need for use of nasal cautery, or other hemorrhagic events (excluding epistaxis) was coupled with the results of hematologic screening tests, the percentage with primary bleeding disorders diagnosed increased to 17%. It is clear that screening tests such as prothrombin time (PT) and partial thromboplastin time (PTT), bleeding time, and platelet count may be inadequate and misleading when attempting to detect mild forms of bleeding disorders and are only useful when coupled with a thorough history. A clinical suspicion of a primary bleeding disorder, such as von Willebrand's disease, should be further evaluated by methods that include tests specific for von Willebrand's factor antigen and von Willebrand's factor ristocetin cofactor.

Numerous primary hemorrhagic disorders can give rise to epistaxis. Among the most common is von Willebrand's disease. Several variants that range from mild to severe exist. The resultant coagulopathy is a result of decreased platelet aggregation and is caused by a deficiency of a plasma protein necessary for normal adherence of platelets at sites of vascular injury. It occurs more commonly in women than in men and is inherited as an autosomal codominant defect. Classic hemophilia occurs as a result of a factor VIII deficiency. It occurs almost exclusively in the male population due to its X-linked recessive pattern of inheritance. Platelet storage pool deficiency is caused by decreased total platelet adenosine diphosphate and serotonin. This often results in a prolonged bleeding time and abnormal platelet aggregation. This diagnosis depends on specific measurements of platelet adenosine diphosphate and serotonin. Multiple other primary coagulopathies exist, but occur rarely.

TABLE 1: Causes of Thrombocytopenia and Platelet Dysfunction

Lymphoproliferative disease
Myelosuppression (status after bone marrow transplantation)
Idiopathic thrombocytopenic purpura
Congenital rubella
Fanconi's anemia
Isoimmune intravascular coagulation
Disseminated intravascular coagulation
Congenital cavernous hemangioma (Kasabach-Merritt syndrome)

Increasing neonatal survival and treatment of lymphoproliferative diseases have led to an increasing number of patients with secondary coagulopathies (Table 1). Thrombocytopenia can result from a decreased number of bone marrow megakaryocytes, decreased platelet survival, platelet sequestration, or increased platelet consumption. Lymphoreticular malignancies and bone marrow suppression following bone marrow transplantation may lead to a secondary thrombocytopenia that can be corrected by resolution of the underlying disease process. Acute idiopathic thrombocytopenic purpura (ITP) occurs most commonly in children aged 2 to 6, normally following a recent upper respiratory tract infection. Platelet counts drop, resulting in hemorrhagic events. ITP does not occur in a primary form and treatment is directed at correction of the underlying disease. Treatment is not necessary in the absence of hemorrhage. Spontaneous remission is the rule. Disseminated intravascular coagulation results in increased consumption of thrombocytes with resultant thrombocytopenia. Kasabach-Merritt syndrome occurs in the neonatal period. A cavernous hemangioma accompanies thrombocytopenia. Bleeding may occur in the first days of life and the degree of thrombocytopenia does not directly correlate with the size of the hemangioma. In most patients, treatment is not necessary, and the hemangioma will spontaneously regress. Primary acquired hepatic disease leads to inadequate production of coagulation factors X, IX, VII, and II, resulting in defects of the extrinsic coagulation pathway.

Hypertension   Hypertension is rare in the pediatric population but when present, is often severe and may manifest as epistaxis. Any child with hypertension requires a thorough medical evaluation. Aortic coarctation, renal disease, and renal artery stenosis are among the more common causes for hypertension in this age group.

Vessal Wall Disorders   Fragility of submucosal blood vessels normally results from the weakness of the media layer of the arterioles. Two of the more common causes for this include scurvy (vitamin C deficiency) and heredity hemorrhagic telangiectasia (Osler-Weber-Rendu disease). Chronic vitamin C deficiency results in collagen synthesis that is defective. The resulting fragility of blood vessels leads to multiple sites of hemorrhage. It is more common in children than in adults. The disease responds well to repletion of ascorbic acid.

Hereditary hemorrhagic telangiectasia is most commonly diagnosed by the otolaryngologist, owing to its usual initial presentation as epistaxis (19). It is a familial syndrome that is transmitted in an autosomal dominant fashion with variable penetrance, thus affecting male and female members equally. Histologically, dilated subepithelial vessels are the hallmark of the disease. Venules are the most commonly affected vessels and demonstrate decreased muscular and elastic elements within their walls. At times, arteriovenous malformations are formed, occurring in any organ within the body. Manifestations of the disease increase with age, with signs and symptoms rarely identified prior to puberty. Telangiectasias, first noted in the third and fourth decades of life, involve mucosal surfaces within the nasal cavity and along the entire alimentary tract.

Other organs including the brain, liver, pulmonary parenchyma, and bladder may be variably involved.

Recurrent spontaneous epistaxis is the most common symptom. The lack of contractile elements within the vascular walls renders each episode difficult to control. Gastrointestinal bleeding may also be seen in approximately 10% of affected individuals. The severity of the bleeding episodes oftentimes leads to multiple blood transfusions over the course of a lifetime.

Treatment is difficult and, as a rule, temporary. Mild episodes of anterior epistaxis are controlled with anterior nasal packing. Longer-lasting forms of therapy have included the use of systemic estrogen, septal dermoplasty, or recurrent treatment of nasal mucosal telangiectasia with the neodymium:yttrium-aluminum-garnet (Nd:YAG) or argon laser.

PEARLS AND PERILS

1. Most cases of pediatric epistaxis are of anterior origin and easily controlled with local measures.
2. If anterior epistaxis occurs on the side of dominant handedness, then suspect digital trauma.
3. Unilateral epistaxis associated with nasal obstruction and malodorous, purulent rhinorrhea may indicate a foreign body.
4. Allergic rhinitis may contribute to the frequency of epistaxis.
5. Bilateral or recurrent epistaxis, associated bruising, or gastrointestinal bleeding should raise concern of a systemic cause.
6. Hypertension in the pediatric population is rare and may suggest aortic coarctation or renal disease.
7. Juvenile nasopharyngeal angiofibroma most commonly presents as unilateral nasal obstruction and epistaxis in the male population after puberty.

PATIENT ASSESSMENT

Due to the sometimes emergent nature of epistaxis, the initial steps required for control are critical. An initial assessment of the child's blood loss, as well as the circulatory and respiratory status precedes a later, but necessary, complete history and physical examination. The mere sight of blood from a child may elicit a panic-like reaction from not only the child, but also the parents. Care must be taken to objectively assess the quantity of blood lost by the child, because a small amount of blood may appear great to those involved. The otolaryngologist is charged with controlling the immediate problem while calming both the parent and child.

Initial Evaluation

Once immediate control of the hemorrhage is established (see next section), a thorough history and physical examination is performed. Historical factors including recent upper respiratory tract infection, site of hemorrhage, presence of bilateral hemorrhage, and recent trauma must be initially established for further treatment. Recurrent episodes of epistaxis, family history of coagulopathies, and other unrelated hemorrhagic events indicate a possible underlying systemic cause. The medication profile should be surveyed for any medication that might promote a coagulopathy (e.g., frequent antibiotics, acetylsalicylic acid or nonsteroidal antiinflammatory drugs, steroids). If the site of epistaxis is coincident with the dominant handedness of the child, nose picking may be suspected.

The general physical examination should identify possible signs of hypovolemia and excessive blood loss. Early establishment of intravenous access should be instituted if this is suspected. Tachycardia, orthostatic hypotension, altered levels of consciousness, or

TABLE 2: Laboratory Tests

Initial screening
  Hemoglobin
  Hematocrit
  Platelets
  Prothrombin time
  Partial thromboplastin time
  Type and crossmatch of blood type
Additional tests (coagulopathy suspected)[a]
  Bleeding time
  Liver Function tests
  Thyroid Function tests
  Fibrinogen
  Fibrin split products
  D-dimer
  1:1 Dilution of partial thromboplastin time
  von Willebrand's factor antigen
  Ristocetin factor
  Coagulation factor assay

[a]Evaluation of a suspected coagulopathy is individualized and based on historical and physical factors.

pallor may indicate significant blood loss even in the absence of active hemorrhage. Transfusion and volume repletion are infrequently required and should be guided by the status of the patient as well as laboratory information. Abnormal physical findings such as excessive bruising, evidence of gastrointestinal bleeding, splenomegaly, or hematuria suggest systemic disease and warrant a comprehensive evaluation.

Although a general physical examination is warranted, the cornerstone of the physical examination is rhinoscopy. The nose should be adequately decongested and a topical anesthetic applied to allow a thorough examination. The presence of inflammation, nasal airflow obstruction, deviation of the septum, foreign body, or nasal mass should be carefully noted. In most patients, the site of bleeding is encountered along the anterior aspect of the nasal septum within the region of Kiesselbach's plexus, and if this is not the site of bleeding, careful inspection will often reveal either a superior or posterior regional source of hemorrhage. Anterior rhinoscopy, using a nasal speculum, may be supplemented by the use of a nasal endoscope or the operating otomicroscope and a nasal speculum. It is important to note that brisk hemorrhage may obscure the location of a specific bleeding site, and every attempt should be made to control or slow the bleeding prior to examination.

Laboratory tests and radiographic examination may provide further insight into the cause of epistaxis but are more accurate when combined with a thorough history and physical examination (Tables 2 and 3). If the child is actively hemorrhaging or appears hemodynamically unstable, then whole blood or packed red blood cells should be typed, crossmatched, and prepared for use. Complete blood cell count, PT and PTT, liver function tests, and bleeding time are initial tests useful in the initial evaluation of refractory epistaxis, although values may be normal even in the presence of underlying disease. Clinical suspicion of von Willibrand's disease requires specific tests including those for

TABLE 3: Radiology

Radiologic Exam	Utility
Computed tomography	Bone integrity and erosion
Contrast-enhanced computed tomography	Intranasal or nasopharyngeal neoplasm or soft tissue anomaly; bone integrity and erosion
Magnetic resonance imaging	Intranasal or nasopharyngeal neoplasm or soft tissue anomaly
Angiography	Vascular nature of neoplasm; arterial source of hemorrhage

von Willibrand factor's antigen and von Willibrand factor's ristocetin factor. Further hematologic evaluation may be guided by a hematologist.

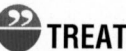 **TREATMENT RECOMMENDATIONS**

Author's Preferred Method

Initial Local Measures

Due to the sensitive nature of the nose and the relative immaturity of the child, sedation is frequently required for adequate examination and treatment of refractory epistaxis. Topical anesthesia can easily be applied in the form of nasal drops or a nasal spray. If sedation is necessary, it should be administered with great care and adequate monitoring. Active nasal hemorrhage and resultant nasopharyngeal drainage of blood may lead to aspiration or respiratory compromise in the presence of an altered sensorium. Oral chloral hydrate is generally regarded as a safe form of sedation when monitored properly, although complications from overdoses have been reported. An initial dose of 25 to 40 mg per kilogram produces a sedative effect, while doses of 50 mg per kilogram often produce a hypnotic effect. While only rarely necessary, general anesthesia in the operating room provides secure control of the airway as well as an optimal setting for careful examination and manipulation of the nose for patients with severe epistaxis.

In many cases, the child may not be actively bleeding at the time he or she is seen by the physician. A thorough examination of the child in this situation not only reassures the child and family, but also will often identify the likely source and facilitate prevention of subsequent episodes of epistaxis. Crusts or clots should be cleaned from the nose and potential bleeding sites identified. If the potential site of hemorrhage is located and appears likely to bleed again, then focal packing or cautery is indicated.

Since the majority of nosebleeds originate from the anterior aspect of the septum, digital pressure is a very effective form of control. The child or parent is instructed to "pinch the nose" between the thumb and forefinger at a point immediately anterior to the frontal processes of the maxilla (Fig. 5). By doing this, the mobile portions of the external nose are compressed against the anterior nasal septum corresponding to Kiesselbach's plexus. Once the hemorrhage is controlled, pressure is maintained for at least 5 minutes as measured by a clock. Having the child hyperextend the neck or assume a

FIGURE 5 Digital control of epistaxis.

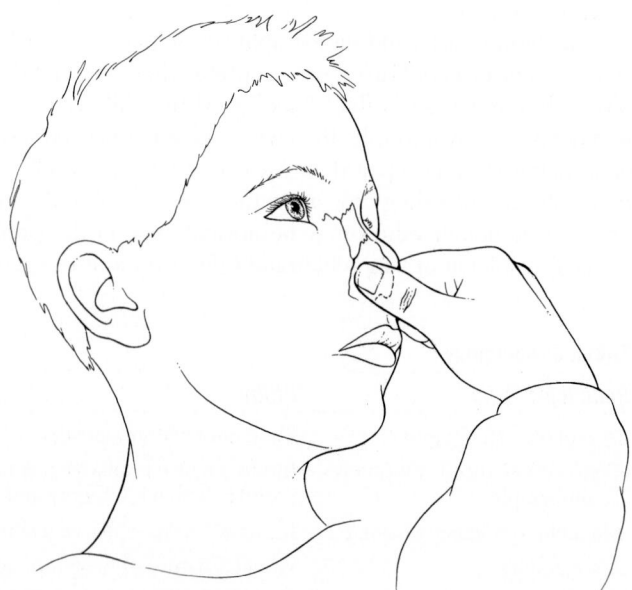

supine position only promotes nasopharyngeal drainage of blood, increasing the risk of aspiration.

If the bleeding continues after an adequate trial of digital pressure, the child is asked to clean the nose of persistent clots by blowing the nose forcefully. Partially congealed blood will often promote local release of local factors, such as tissue plasminogen activator and fibrinogen/fibrin split products, which promote local dissolution of clot and further bleeding (20). If a nose cannot be cleared adequately, then it is necessary for the physician to use suction in the setting of adequate illumination. Once again, this can be facilitated by an operating otologic microscope and nasal speculum, a head mirror and light source, or a fiberoptic nasal endoscope. After the nasal cavities are sufficiently cleaned, then a topical vasoconstrictor is introduced (Table 4) and digital pressure is repeated for 5 minutes.

If local pressure is adequate to control the nosebleed and the history and physical examination do not suggest any underlying pathology, then the child may be released. Concern often exists as to the effectiveness of this treatment. Parents should be counseled to repeat the procedure performed in the clinic if a subsequent nosebleed occurs. Recurrent epistaxis warrants repeat examination by the physician. Prophylactic measures to help prevent further bleeding include increased humidity and local nasal care. Oftentimes, nose picking can be unconscious or occur during sleep. Placing gloves or socks around the hands at night will, at times, be curative. Petroleum jelly applied to the nasal vestibule promotes additional nasal protection. Gelatinous at first, when it reaches body temperature it becomes a thick liquid consistency and is distributed throughout the nose via ciliary transport. It serves to supplement the protective nature of the nasal mucus. The preparation is nontoxic when ingested, as proved by its inventor, Robert Augustus Chesebrough, who attributed his longevity to ingesting a tablespoon of petrolatum daily until his ninety-sixth year (21).

Local Cautery

In the event that pressure and topical vasoconstrictor medications fail to control bleeding, more aggressive therapy should be instituted. If a specific site or area of bleeding is identified, then several measures can be used for control. Direct application of topical vasoconstrictive medications mixed with a topical anesthetic will sometimes be effective. A cotton pledget soaked with 4% lidocaine and 1:10,000 epinephrine may be temporarily placed against the site for a period of approximately 5 minutes. Care should be taken to subsequently remove the piece of cotton to prevent aspiration. Alternatively, a discrete site of bleeding can be treated with cautery in the clinical setting. Most children do not respond well to electrocautery because of the pain and, as such, this is not recommended. More useful is chemical cautery using prepackaged silver nitrate sticks or trichloroacetic acid placed on the tip of a cotton-tipped applicator. Chemical cautery is most effective when the mucosal surface is dried as well as possible. Application should be focally applied only to the area of bleeding (Fig. 6). Widespread application along the nasal septum or bilateral septal application of a cauterizing agent may yeild perforation of the nasal septum.

TABLE 4: Topical Vasoconstrictors

Oxymetazoline
Phenylephrine
Xylometazoline
Naphazoline
4% Cocaine hydrochloride[a,b]

[a]Preparation also provides topical anesthetic properties.

[b]Controlled substance according to Food and Drug Administration; toxicity and potential drug interactions when not used as indicated.

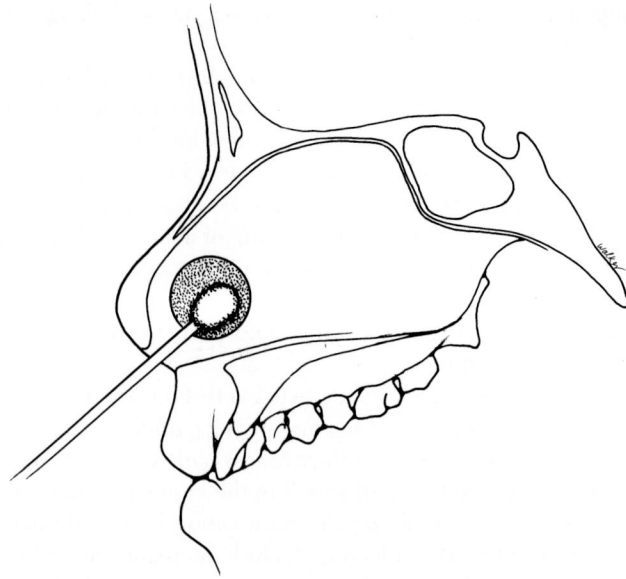

FIGURE 6 Silver nitrate cautery of the septum.

Nasal Packing

Anterior Nasal Packing   Anterior nasal packing constitutes the next level of treatment for control of epistaxis. As with all treatments for nosebleeds, it is most effective when a focal site of bleeding has been identified by physical examination. Various materials are available for packing. Nonabsorbable materials available include long-fiber or rayon cotton, and cotton gauze tape, which are commonly utilized for anterior nasal packs. When used, they should be impregnated with an antibiotic ointment to decrease bacterial proliferation. The disadvantage of using these materials is the need to later remove the pack, which risks subsequent discomfort to the child, as well as trauma to the healing site of hemorrhage. Alternatively, several absorbable materials are available for use (Table 5). These materials come in a variety of forms ranging from a cotton-like preparation to foam-like strips. The preparations are slightly more difficult to handle, owing to their tendency to adhere to instruments and nasal mucosal surfaces, but eliminate the discomfort and risks associated with later removal.

If the specific site of bleeding is identified, then a small focal anterior pack is placed in direct contact with the site, and the remainder of the nasal cavity is left unpacked (Fig. 7). The child is observed; if no other bleeding occurs, then the child may be released to return home. If no specific bleeding site is encountered, however, a more complete anterior nasal pack is required. The absorbable or nonabsorbable packing material is impregnated with small amounts of antibiotic ointment such as mupirocin (Bactroban) and then applied in a systematic fashion from the inferior aspect of the nasal cavity extending to the superior aspect. This procedure can be quite uncomfortable and requires adequate local anesthesia as described previously.

Posterior Nasal Packing   Posterior epistaxis is typically more brisk than anterior epistaxis due to its posterior arterial source. From a practical sense, posterior epistaxis is simply bleeding that cannot be controlled with a well-placed anterior nasal pack. Management

TABLE 5: Absorbable Nasal Packing Materials

Oxidized cellulose (e.g., Surgicel, Interceed)
Absorbable gelatin (e.g., Gelfoam)
Absorbable microfibrillar collagen (e.g., Instat, Avitene)

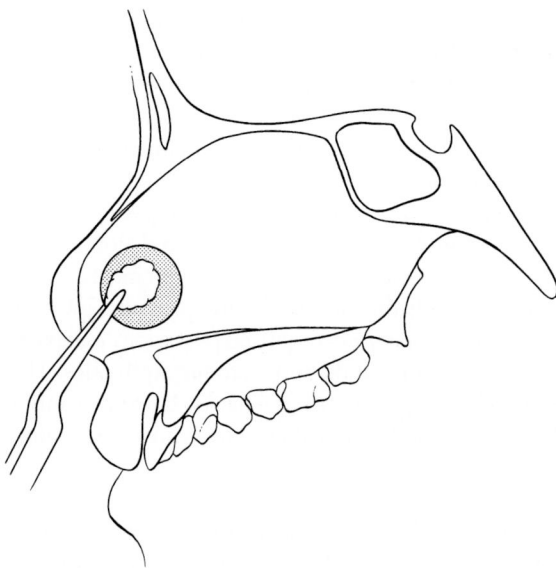

FIGURE 7 Focal nasal packing.

of posterior epistaxis depends, to a great deal, on the preference of the physician treating the patient. The risks and benefits of each form of therapy must be carefully considered with respect to the individual patient, family, and facilities available.

The posterior nasal pack may come in several forms. It functions by providing a direct tamponade of the posterior bleeding sites with a posterior buttress or balloon, and it also functions by providing a solid posterior buttress against which the anterior pack can be placed. The different types of posterior packs include gauze posterior nasal pack, 30-mL Foley catheter posterior nasal pack, and the balloon tampon (e.g., Epistat) (Fig. 8).

Posterior nasal packs have several advantages. They can be placed relatively rapidly under either local or topical anesthesia in either the office setting or emergency department. They will often provide hemostasis until systemic causes can be corrected and will provide time for coagulation if a local cause is present.

Posterior packs also have several disadvantages. They fail to control hemorrhage up to 15% to 30% of the time, necessitating further measures for control. They also present a risk of local ischemic damage to the nose in the form of alar or septal necrosis. In addi-

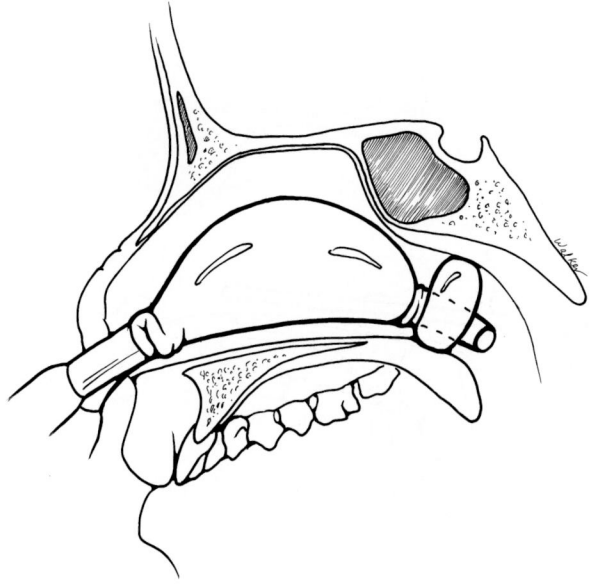

FIGURE 8 Proper position of a manufactured epistaxis balloon. The posterior balloon in the nasopharynx provides an anchor for the anterior balloon to apply pressure to the posterior nasal cavity.

tion to discomfort associated with the packs, patients are at significant risk for the development of acute sinusitis from obstruction of the ostiomeatal complex on the affected side. Cases of toxic shock syndrome associated with nasal packing have been reported in the literature (22). Probably the most significant complication associated with posterior nasal packing is respiratory compromise. This may be particularly problematic in infants or neonates due to obligate nasal respiration, or in patients with underlying pulmonary disease. Hypoventilation and hypoxia associated with posterior nasal packing are well documented (23,24). Large postnasal packs obliterate the nasopharynx and depress the palate, creating an iatrogenic obstructive sleep apnea. Supplemental oxygen must be used with caution as it may depress respiratory drive if the carbon dioxide pressure (pCO_2 is chronically elevated. Currently, it is urged that all patients requiring posterior nasal packing be admitted to the hospital for pulmonary observation and systemic antibiotics. This is particularly true for patients requiring bilateral posterior nasal packs. Extreme caution should accompany the administration of any medication that could cause respiratory depression.

Endoscopic Cautery   Considering the risks and obligate hospitalization of patients undergoing posterior nasal packing, many physicians favor endoscopic evaluation under general anesthesia and cautery of active bleeding sites in lieu of the posterior nasal pack (25). The advantages of this are obvious when this form of therapy is successful. Distal and direct control of bleeding leads to decreased recurrence of episodic epistaxis. The immediate control of the patient's bleeding allows for earlier discharge from the hospital and less discomfort. In patients at risk for pulmonary complications, endoscopic cautery eliminates the potential respiratory embarrassment that accompanies posterior nasal packing.

After general anesthesia is obtained, careful endoscopic examination is performed. At times a nasal septoplasty may be necessary to allow an endoscopic view of the bleeding area around septal deviations (Fig. 9). An insulated bipolar cautery or suction cautery is endoscopically directed to the point of bleeding and focal cautery is applied until the bleeding is controlled. If endoscopic cauterization fails to control the hemorrhage, then a posterior nasal pack can be introduced and the patient prepared for subsequent procedures.

Embolization   An alternative method for control of intractable or recurrent severe epistaxis is that of angiographic embolization (26). Angiography permits identification of the source of hemorrhage, as well as uncommon abnormalities, such as posttraumatic pseu-

FIGURE 9 Endoscopic control of epistaxis.

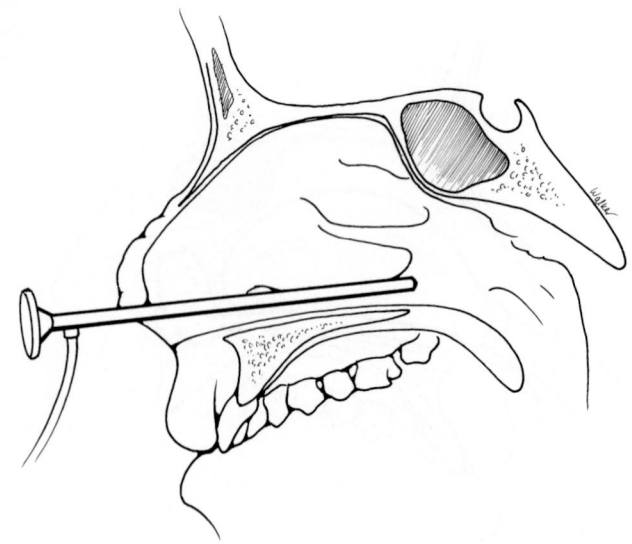

doaneurysms or vascular neoplasms. Embolization is performed using Gelfoam particles, polyvinyl alcohol, or coiled springs. When the procedure is successful, hemostasis is immediate, but this method is limited by the availability of an experienced interventional radiologist as well as by the source of bleeding. Bleeding sources must be limited to branches of the external carotid artery, as embolization of internal carotid artery branches may lead to devastating neurologic complications. Complications such as skin necrosis, cerebrovascular accidents, and hypoesthesias are uncommon.

Special Circumstances

Coagulopathies and the Intensive Care Unit Patient

With advancements in pediatric intensive care, otolaryngologists are increasingly being called on to provide therapy to very ill children in the intensive care unit setting. Epistaxis occurs infrequently within this setting but creates a special set of circumstances that must be considered. Owing to the disease process or its treatment, many of these children have severe thrombocytopenia or coagulopathies. Radiation and chemotherapy may incite a diffuse mucositis, rendering nasal mucosa friable and subject to bleeding. Further, nasal intubation with nasogastric or nasotracheal tubes incites local trauma to the nasal mucosa. Oftentimes, when these children are evaluated, diffuse "mucosal oozing" is encountered. Rapid control of bleeding is necessary in order to prevent further morbidity in an already hemodynamically compromised child.

Anterior and posterior nasal packing are time-honored methods for the control of bleeding in this situation but should be avoided if possible. Preexisting anemia decreases oxygen-carrying capacity and renders the child more susceptible to hypoxia associated with bilateral nasal airway obstruction. Neutropenia, which may accompany various chemotherapeutic treatment protocols, may render the patient more susceptible to bacterial colonization of foreign material within the nasal cavity. For these reasons, it is best to exhaust local conservative measures for control of epistaxis prior to resorting to nasal packing.

Initial management should be similar to that in the clinical setting. The head of the child's bed is elevated to approximately 30 degrees and the nasal cavities are cleared of coagulated blood. A topical anesthetic combined with a vasoconstrictor is applied to the nasal cavity and digital pressure is applied for at least 5 minutes. This may be repeated several times until control is established. If bleeding continues, an intermediate method of epistaxis control can be tried (27). Following maximal vasoconstriction and application of topical anesthetic spray, a 1×4-cm neurosurgical cottonoid is soaked in 0.0125% oxymetazoline. Microfibrillar collagen is coated to one surface of the cottonoid and then gently placed flat against the nasal septum. In cases of bilateral mucosal oozing, an identical cottonoid is situated on the opposite side. Digital pressure is then maintained for at least 5 minutes, after which time hemostasis is normally obtained.

The child is then placed at complete bed rest and the head of the bed is maintained at an elevation of 30 degrees. The cottonoid strips are trimmed and allowed to remain within the nose. Oxymetazoline drops are applied to the pledgets at 8-hour intervals, which serve as a wick to deliver the topical vasoconstrictor to the nasal mucus. Additionally, a systemic decongestant may be of help. It is suggested that gentamicin ophthalmic drops also be placed on the nasal cotton strips in order to prevent nasal infection. The advantages of this technique are less discomfort and improved nasal airflow. The cottonoid strips may be removed from 3 to 5 days after treatment, allowing adequate time for correction of underlying coagulopathies in most patients.

Neoplasms

Immediate control of epistaxis associated with neoplasms progresses in a similar fashion to that of other forms of epistaxis. Local pressure and vasoconstriction are followed in turn by focal anterior packing. Care must be taken with the use of cautery, owing to the possibility of the nasal mass representing a nasal encephalocele. Once hemostasis is obtained, diagnosis of the underlying mass is paramount. Prior to biopsy, a radiologic survey should be performed to evaluate the origin and location of the mass with respect to the skull base. Contrasted computed tomography and magnetic resonance (MR) scans help to assess the vascular nature of the mass, and highly vascular masses should be further evaluated utilizing arteriography. Because vascular nasal masses are often supplied by vessels from the external carotid artery system, embolization may be helpful for control of persistent bleeding. The extent of mucosal disease is best assessed using a gadolinium-enhanced MR scan.

Hereditary Hemorrhagic Telangiectasia (Osler-Weber-Rendu Disease)

This is a recurrent problem due to the nature of this disease. However, young children are rarely affected. Episodes of epistaxis may be encountered during the teen years and are initially relatively easy to control using standard measures. With time this becomes increasingly more difficult and frustrating. All forms of therapy appear to be only temporary. Systemic estrogen has been noted to provide a decrease in the frequency and severity of episodes of bleeding by increasing the media layer of capillaries within the patient. This form of therapy may have an untoward affect, however, on the male patient.

After local forms of therapy become inadequate, alternative forms of therapy are required. Septal dermoplasty was first described by Saunders in the late 1960s (28). The mucosa of the nasal septum and floor of the nose is removed through a lateral alar incision, while leaving the vascular bed of perichondrium intact. A split-thickness skin graft is then applied to the area of resected mucosa. In this manner, mucosal telangiectasias are removed. However, with time, these will recur within the split-thickness skin graft. The Nd:YAG and argon lasers have been used with some success in the treatment of oral and nasal telangiectasias. The laser is used to photocoagulate individual telangiectasias, starting at the periphery and ending at the central feeding vessel of each lesion. Once again, retreatment is necessary and must be repeated on a 3- to 6-month basis.

PEARLS AND PERILS

1. Initial control of epistaxis begins with clearance of intranasal clot and maintainance of digital pressure for 5 minutes "by the clock."
2. Use of a topical anesthetic and decongestant will improve intranasal examination.
3. Batteries of tests to screen for coagulopathies are significantly more accurate when combined with history and physical examination.
4. Petroleum jelly applied to the anterior nasal vestibule controls anterior sources of hemorrhage, as well as protects nasal mucosa from further trauma.
5. Posterior nasal packing may contribute to respiratory embarrassment. Respiratory status should be monitored.
6. Supplemental oxygen may cause respiratory suppression among patients with chronic pulmonary disease and hypercapnea.
7. Cautery of the nasal septum should be used judiciously in order to prevent perforation.
8. Systemic antistaphylococcal antibiotics are used prophylactically while nasal packing is in place to reduce incidence of "toxic shock syndrome."
9. Children in the intensive care unit setting may be neutropenic and anemic due to a variety of factors, rendering them more susceptible to infection and blood loss.

Other Methods

Arterial Ligation

Arterial ligation is an alternative method through which control of persistent or recurrent epistaxis may be provided. Many physicians prefer arterial ligation to the placement of posterior packs, citing the multiple risks associated with posterior packing and the prolonged need for hospitalization while the pack is in place (29).

External carotid artery ligation is the oldest method of ligation and the least effective, owing to its high recurrence rate. The far proximal site of ligation fails to provide control of the rich network of vascular anastomoses present between the internal and external carotid artery system, as well as those from the contralateral carotid system. As a general rule, better hemostasis is provided with more distal arterial control. It is for this reason that the technique has been all but abandoned, except in cases of extreme emergency.

Transantral ligation of the internal maxillary artery provides more distal and, therefore, better control of bleeding (30). Early hypodevelopment of the maxillary antrum must be considered and may render this technique useless in the small child. The procedure is performed through a Caldwell-Luc antrotomy. A mucoperiosteal flap is raised along the posteroinferior antral wall and the bony posterior sinus wall is carefully removed with a chisel, curet, or drill. Care is taken to avoid entering the orbit, which lies immediately superior to this region. After this posterior antral osteotomy is created, the posterior periosteum is incised. The operating microscope is used to identify pulsations corresponding to the arteries of the pterygopalatine fossa. Adipose and connective tissues are partially removed once the artery and branches are identified. Locking hemoclips are then placed around the internal maxillary artery and all identified branches. Elevation of arterial branches with nerve hooks prior to application of hemoclips helps avoid injury to the vidian nerve, which lies in a plane just deep to the internal maxillary artery. After the procedure is complete, nasal packs are removed while the patient is still in the operating room and the nose is carefully inspected for bleeding. Continued bleeding indicates a probable ethmoidal artery source.

Transoral ligation of the internal maxillary artery was first proposed by Maceri and Makielski in 1984 (31). A gingivobuccal incision is made and the buccal fat pad is removed. The attachment of the temporal muscle to the caronoid process of the mandible is identified, and careful blunt dissection reveals the internal maxillary artery as it enters the pterygopalatine fossa. There are several disadvantages to this approach, including the proximal site of ligation of the artery and potential unsightly postoperative change in the contour of the face. This method, however, is most useful in situations when transantral access is prevented, such as severe midfacial trauma or antral neoplasm.

Ligation of the ethmoidal arteries is performed in the event of continued bleeding after internal maxillary artery ligation. The arteries are approached through the orbit and are ligated prior to exiting the orbit through their separate ethmoidal foramina. A Killian-type incision is performed and the medial canthal tendon and nasal lacrimal apparatus are identified and carefully preserved. The periorbita is elevated in a posterior direction along the frontoethmoidal suture. The anterior ethmoidal artery is identified approximately 15 mm posterior to the posterior lacrimal crest. Approximately 10 mm posterior to this site is the posterior ethmoidal artery, which lies from 4 to 7 mm anterior to the optic nerve. Once it is identified, two arterial clips are placed on the anterior ethmoidal artery and the nose is examined. If epistaxis is controlled at this point, there is no need to ligate the posterior ethmoidal artery and risk damage to the optic nerve. If bleeding persists, the anterior ethmoidal artery is divided between the clips, and the posterior ethmoidal artery is clipped. Division or cautery of the posterior ethmoidal artery is avoided in order to minimize risk to the optic nerve (32).

MANAGEMENT OF COMPLICATIONS

Fortunately, complications infrequently accompany the management of epistaxis, but the sequelae of theses complications can be devastating to the patient. Additionally, the severity of the complication is not always proportional to the invasiveness of the treatment, as demonstrated by the disproportionately high number of complications associated with the simple use of nasal packs. By anticipating the potential for these problems, the physician can take prophylactic measures to provide improved protection.

Nasal packs, whether anterior or posterior, interrupt normal nasal and respiratory homeostasis. Simple placement of a foreign body within the nasal cavity results in pain, inflammation, and alteration of normal respiratory function. The resulting edema of the nasal mucosa, the accumulated blood, and the mechanical presence of the pack cause paranasal sinus ostial and eustachian tube obstruction. Acute sinusitis, otitis media, and hemotympanum are frequently encountered while nasal packing is in place and must be treated appropriately (33). The prophylactic use of topical and systemic antibiotics has all but erased reports of complications such as meningitis, sepsis, septic blindness, basisphenoid osteomyelitis, and tetanus that were prevalent during the preantibiotic era.

When left in place, the packing material itself serves as an excellent site for bacterial proliferation, which can yield infectious complications for both the immunocompromised and otherwise healthy patient. Bacteremia was identified in 12% of blood cultures obtained from patients with anterior or posterior nasal packs studied by Herzon (34). Nasal pack material obtained from this same group was almost universally found to be infected. The simple addition of antibiotic ointment on nasal packs yielded fewer anaerobic and gram-negative bacteria but did not completely eradicate the presence of bacteremia.

Toxic shock syndrome from nasal packing was first reported by Thomas et al (22) in 1982 in a patient following rhinoplasty and submucous resection of the nasal septum. First observed following the use of absorbent vaginal tampons, toxic shock syndrome is caused by an endotoxin produced by certain strains of *Staphylococcus aureus*. The pack present within the nose facilitates staphylococcal proliferation even in the presence of topical antibiotic ointments. The current recommendations for protection against infectious complications of nasal packing include the use of topical antibiotic-impregnated packing material in addition to prophylactic, systemic antistaphylococcal antibiotic therapy while the pack is in place (35).

Placement of bilateral nasal packs has been associated with respiratory depression, especially in the presence of bilateral posterior nasal packs. In 1971, Cassissi et al. (24) reported the deaths of three patients who had undergone anterior and posterior nasal packing for posterior epistaxis. Subsequent studies of pulmonary function and arterial blood gases in nasally packed patients revealed significant hypoxia and exacerbation of preexistent pulmonary dysfunction. In the presence of acute anemia, which often accompanies epistaxis, serious tissue hypoxia was noted. Likewise, Taasan et al. (23) described an iatrogenic form of obstructive sleep apnea caused by hypoventilation associated with posterior nasal packs depressing the soft palate and filling the nasopharynx. Severe nocturnal oxygen desaturation was observed in patients while they slept, attempting to breathe past the complete nasopharyngeal obstruction. Current therapy mandates close airway observation in the hospital setting of any patient undergoing posterior nasal packing. Supplemental oxygen is useful for improving hypoxemia. However, care must be used in its administration as it can lead to depression of respiratory drive in patients with chronically elevated carbon dioxide pressures. Sedation must be used with extreme caution as this further depresses respiratory function.

The effect of nasal packing is due, in large part, to pressure that it exerts on nasal mucosa. This can lead to avascular necrosis of underlying tissue with resultant nasal mucosal sloughing, ulceration, or septal perforation. Of special note is the susceptibility of the alar rim of the nose to the anterior nasal buttresses used with posterior nasal packs. Care must be taken to relieve pressure along the nasal ala in order to prevent unsightly cosmetic complications.

CONCLUSIONS

Epistaxis is usually a relatively minor problem that can be resolved in the clinical setting; however, rarely its treatment can be quite challenging. Although uncommon, serious epistaxis and systemic causes occur within the pediatric population from time to time. A systematic approach to the evaluation and treatment will ensure control of hemorrhage while protecting the safety of the child.

✳ REFERENCES

1. Petruson B. Epistaxis: a clinical study with special reference to fibrinolysis. *Acta Otolaryngol Suppl* 1974;317:1–73.
2. Rodeghiero F, Castaman G, Dini E. Epidemiological investigation of the prevalence of von Willebrand's disease. *Blood* 1987;69:454–459.
3. Culbertson MC, Manning S. Epistaxis. In: Bailey B, ed. *Pediatric otolaryngology*. Philadelphia: WB Saunders, 1990:672–679.
4. Shaheen OH. Arterial epistaxis. *J Laryngol Otol* 1975;87:17–34.
5. Jackson K, Jackson R. Factors associated with active refractory epistaxis. *Arch Otolaryngol Head Neck Surg* 1988;114:862–865.
6. Pathak PN. Epistaxis—due to ruptured aneurysm of the internal carotid artery. *J Laryngol Otol* 1972;86:395–397.
7. Fairbanks DNF. Closure of nasal septal perforations. *Arch Otolaryngol* 1980;106:509–513.
8. Girsh LS. Allergic rhinitis: a common cause of recurrent epistaxis in children. *Am J Dis Child* 1960;99:819–821.
9. Murray AB, Milner RA. Allergic rhinitis and recurrent epistaxis in children. *Ann Allergy Asthma Immunol* 1995;74:30–33.
10. Maccia CA, Gallagher JS, Ataman G, et al. Platelet thrombopathy in asthmatic subjects with elevated immunoglobulin E. *J Allergy Clin Immunol* 1977;59:101–108.
11. Schwartz LB. Tryptase—a mediator of human mast cells. *J Allergy Clin Immunol* 1990;86:594–598.
12. Saxena SP, Brandes LJ, Becker AB, et al. Histamine is an intracellular messenger mediating platelet aggregation. *Science* 1989;244:1596–1599.
13. Tom L, Anderson GJ, Womer RB, et al. Nasopharyngeal malignancies in children. *Laryngoscope* 1992;102:509–514.
14. Verschur HP, Struyvenberg PA, van Benthem P, et al. Nasal discharge and obstruction as presenting symptoms of Wegener's granulomatosis in childhood. *Int J Pediatr Otorhinolaryngol* 1993;27:91–95.
15. Okafor BC. Epistaxis: a clinical study of 540 cases. *Ear Nose Throat J* 1984;63:153–159.
16. Evans J. The aetiology and treatment of epistaxis: based on review of 200 cases. *J Laryngol Otol* 1962;76:185–191.
17. Juselius H. Epistaxis: a clinical study of 1724 patients. *J Laryngol Otol* 1974;88:317–327.
18. Katsanis E, Luke K, Hsu E, et al. Prevalence and significance of mild bleeding disorders in children with recurrent epistaxis. *Clin Lab Observ* 1988;113:73–76.
19. Flessa HL. Hereditary hemorrhagic telangiectasia (Osler-Weber-Rendu disease). *Arch Otolaryngol Head Neck Surg* 1977;103:148–151.
20. McKee PA. Disorders of blood coagulation. In: Wyngaarden JB, Smith LH, ed. *Cecil's textbook of medicine*. Philadelphia: WB Saunders, 1985:1053–1056.
21. Panati C. *Panati's extraordinary origins of everyday things*. New York: Harper & Row, 1987.
22. Thomas SW, Baird IM, Frazier RD. Toxic shock syndrome following submucous resection and rhinoplasty. *JAMA* 1982;147:2402–2403.
23. Taasan V, Wynne JW, Cassisi N, et al. The effect of nasal packing on sleep disordered breathing and nocturnal oxygen desaturation. *Laryngoscope* 1982;91:1163–1172.

24. Cassisi NJ, Biller HF, Ogura JH. Changes in arterial oxygen tension and pulmonary mechanics with use of posterior packing in epistaxis. *Laryngoscope* 1971;81:1261–1266.

25. Marcus MJ. Nasal endoscopic control of epistaxis—a preliminary report. *Otolaryngol Head Neck Surg* 1990;102:273–275.

26. Elden L, Montanera W, Terbrugge K, et al. Angiographic embolization for the treatment of epistaxis: a review of 108 cases. *Otolaryngol Head Neck Surg* 1994;111:44–50.

27. Koltai PJ. Nose bleeds in the hematologically and immunologically compromised child. *Laryngoscope* 1984;94:1114–1115.

28. Saunders WH. Septal dermoplasty—ten years experience. *Trans Am Acad Ophthalmol Otolaryngol* 1968;72:153–160.

29. Chandler JR, Serrins AJ. Transantral ligation of the internal maxillary artery for epistaxis. *Laryngoscope* 1965;75:1151–1159.

30. Metson R, Lane R. Internal maxillary artery ligation for epistaxis: an analysis of failures. *Laryngoscope* 1988;98:760–764.

31. Maceri DR, Makielski KH. Intraoral ligation of the maxillary artery for posterior epistaxis. *Laryngoscope* 1984;94:737–741.

32. Friedman WH, Rosenblum BN. Epistaxis. In: Goldblum JL, ed. *Principles and practice of rhinology.* New York: Wiley Medical, 1987:375–383.

33. Pierce DL, Chasin WD. Treatment of epistaxis. *N Engl J Med* 1962;267:768–771.

34. Herzon FS. Bacteremia and local infections with nasal packing. *Arch Otolaryngol* 1971;94:317–320.

35. Fairbanks DN. Complications of nasal packing. *Otolaryngol Head Neck Surg* 1986;94:412–415.

B.F. Marple: Department of Otolaryngology, University of Texas, Southwestern Medical Center, Dallas, Texas 75235–9035.

- *Practical Pediatric Otolaryngology*
- edited by Robin T. Cotton and Charles M. Myer, III
- Lippincott-Raven Publishers, Philadelphia © 1999

Nasal Obstruction in Infancy

Harvey L. Coates

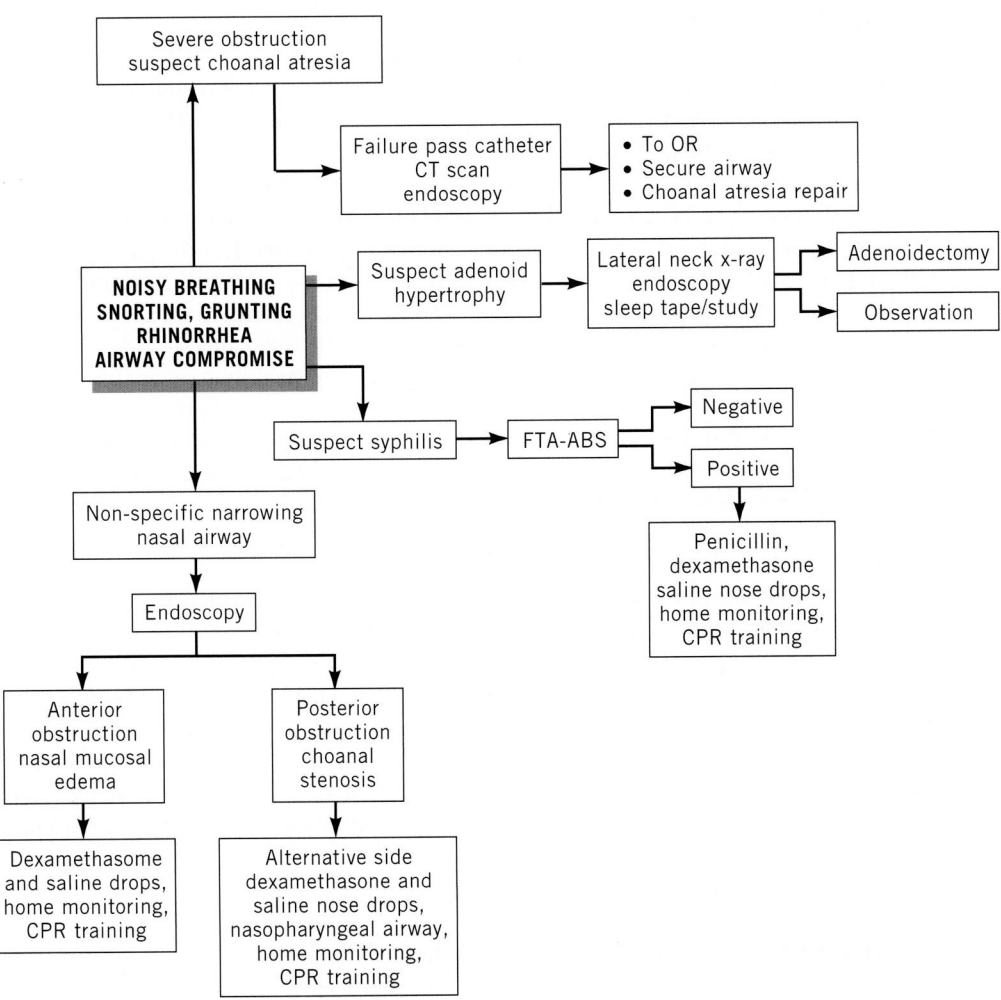

(Adapted with permission from Derkay CS, Grundfast KM. Airway compromise from nasal obstruction in neonates and infants. *Int J Pediatr Otorhinolaryngol* 1990;19:247.)

HISTORICAL BACKGROUND

Nasal obstruction is a common symptom in the neonate and infant. Generally, it is due to inflammation of the nasal mucosa but occasionally may be a characteristic of serious pathology. The neonate is a preferential nasal breather until the approximate age of 2 to 5 months.

Choanal atresia is potentially the most serious of the causes of neonatal nasal obstruction. This condition was first described in 1775 by Roederer, and the first successful procedure for bilateral bony choanal atresia was performed by Carl Emmert in 1851 in Bern. The subsequent historical features of this condition are well described by Pirsig (1). Better diagnostic capabilities with computed tomography (CT) and endoscopy have increased the understanding of choanal atresia and brought to light new clinical entities, such as piriform aperture stenosis.

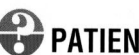 PATIENT ASSESSMENT

History

Maternal and Neonatal

Nasal obstruction may be associated with nasal infections, sleep problems, feeding difficulty, colic, cyanotic attacks, and epiphora (2). Severe nasal obstruction may present with cyclical cyanosis at rest but resolving when the neonate cries. This pattern, especially when there is bilateral obstruction, may be typical of choanal atresia or stenosis and require urgent airway intervention. If introduction of an oral airway relieves the obstruction, then it can be assumed that the level of obstruction is above the hypopharynx.

The history of the infant's nasal obstruction and associated features, as observed by the nursing staff and parents, should be noted to establish whether there is unilateral or bilateral obstruction, nasal discharge, snoring, or cyanosis. In addition, the relationship of the nasal obstruction to crying and feeding should be determined. A family history of atopy may be relevant in the neonate with nasal obstruction reversible by nasal decongestants.

The maternal history regarding medication taken during the pregnancy should be obtained. Mothers taking narcotics, antihypertensives, beta-blockers, and antidepressants may have infants with neonatal nasal obstruction (Table 1).

Infant

The symptoms of cyanotic attacks and cyclical obstruction with crying are seen uncommonly in the infant, but nasal infections, congestion, feeding difficulty, and snoring become more frequent as the infant grows. Exposure to upper respiratory tract infections, especially in day-care centers can lead to repeated nasal infections. The infant with a strong atopic family history may develop the symptomatology of acute seasonal rhinitis or perennial allergic rhinitis, the former manifesting as nasal obstruction, sneezing, and rhinorrhea and the latter presenting as persistent nasal obstruction. Facial signs of typical atopy including "allergic shiners," Dennie's line, transverse nasal crease, broad nasal tip, and circumoral and nasal pallor may develop (Fig. 1).

TABLE 1: Maternal Medications Causing Neonatal Nasal Obstruction

Antihypertensives
Reserpine
Hydralazine
Guanethidine
Methyldopa
Narcotics
Beta-blockers
Propanolol
Antidepressants
Thioridazine
Amitriptyline
Chlordiazepoxide

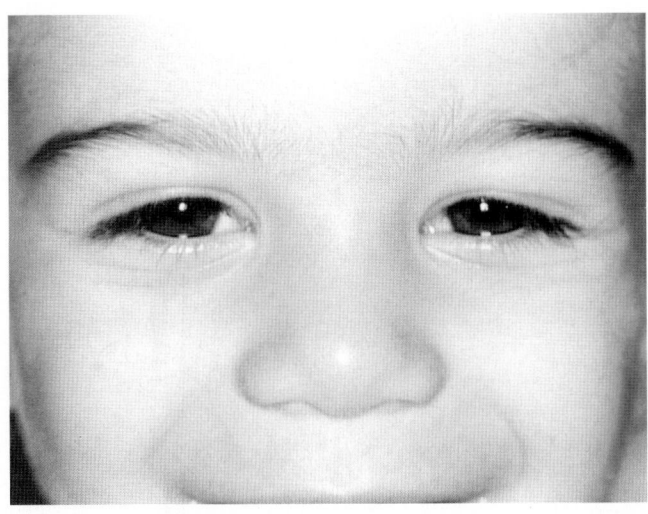

FIGURE 1 Typical allergic shiners and Dennie's line in a 14-month-old infant.

Atopic children, particularly those from the Mediterranean countries, may show signs of lymphoid hypertrophy at a very early age, often before 1 year. The cause is frequently adenoid hypertrophy, or in some children, tonsillar and adenoid hypertrophy. The children may present with snoring, feeding difficulty, obstructive sleep apnea, restless sleep, and perioral cyanosis, with snoring being by far the most common symptom. In fact, it is uncommon to find a child with obstructive sleep disorder (OSD) with no history of snoring.

Physical Examination

Clinical Approach

A thorough examination of the head and neck should be carried out, taking particular note of any abnormalities that could be associated with airway obstruction. These might include craniofacial disorders or Down syndrome, the chronic mouth breathing of adenoid facies, or stigmata of the atopic facies. As up to 30% of infants have some manifestation of atopy, the presence of allergic shiners, Dennie's line, transverse nasal crease or broadened nose, perioral and nasal pallor, and eczema should alert the clinician to this diagnosis. The classic "adenoid facies" with the dull facial appearance, flattened maxillae, open mouth, large dry lower lip, and short upper lip may also have some of the associated features of the allergic facies noted above.

Otologic examination may reveal an associated otitis media with effusion while examination of the teeth and the oral cavity may show early evidence of occlusal abnormalities, macroglossia, palatal abnormalities, tonsillar hypertrophy, or oropharyngeal masses. The infant may demonstrate changed vocal quality, with hyponasality secondary to adenoid hypertrophy being the most common cause. Infants with cleft palate repair and nasal obstruction may produce a complex mixed resonance (hyponasality and hypernasality).

The nasal examination externally may reveal signs of a depressed nasal bridge, nasal pits or masses, or deformity of the cartilaginous septum and nasal tip. Anterior rhinoscopy may be carried out using a head mirror or headlight and elevating the nasal tip. Generally, infants prefer the familiar magnifying fiberoptic otoscope, which can provide an excellent view of the septum, nasal valve, turbinates, and the anterior half of the nasal cavity.

Suctioning of mucus from the nose using a bulb syringe may be necessary. Saline drops may be administered to facilitate suctioning while 0.25% phenylephrine or a similar decongestant will enable comparison of the congested and decongested nasal mucosa.

Evaluation of the nasal airway should include an assessment of the nasal airflow, which is possible by placing a wisp of cotton in front of each naris to determine expira-

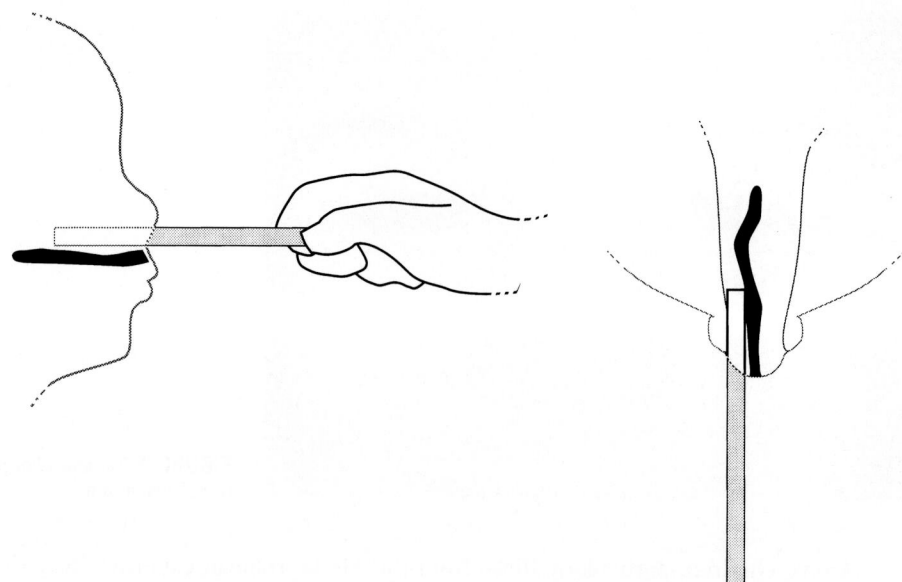

FIGURE 2 Strut testing for neonatal nasal septal obstruction.

tory airflow. This can be carried out also by substituting a mirror and observing the misting from each naris, a rough guide to the presence or absence of total nasal obstruction. In the neonate, assessment must include passage of a soft nasal catheter (5 to 6 Fr gauge) to at least 32 mm to exclude choanal atresia. Smooth plastic struts measuring 6×100 mm (the width and breadth of the normal neonatal nasal cavity) should easily pass the length of the nasal cavity and if their passage is obstructed, it is usually secondary to a septal deviation at 15 to 20 mm from the nares. This procedure is performed normally by nursing staff at the author's neonatal unit and consultation with the pediatric otolaryngologist is sought if there is significant nasal obstruction (Fig. 2).

External or intranasal masses need to be examined carefully to differentiate encephalocele, glioma, and dermoid (Table 2).

Endoscopy   The careful use of either the fiberoptic nasopharyngoscope or straight telescope (Storz-Hopkins 2.7-mm rigid telescope) may enable visualization of the posterior nasal cavity and nasopharynx. The combination solution of lidocaine (Xylocaine) 5% with 0.5% ephedrine is sprayed into the infant's nasal cavity and 5 minutes is allowed to pass for adequate decongestion and anesthesia to occur. The fiberoptic nasopharyngoscope is lubricated with a water-soluble gel and passed gently into the nasal cavity of the infant who is seated upright in the parent's or carer's arms (Fig. 3). Great care must be taken to

TABLE 2: Differential Diagnosis of Encephalocele, Glioma, and Dermoid[a]

Characteristic	Encephalocele	Glioma	Dermoid
Appearance	Bluish, soft Compressible	Reddish-blue solid Noncompressible Telangiectasia	Dimple Hair Solid
Location	Intranasal and external	Intranasal and external	Intranasal and external
Pulsation	Yes	No	No
Cerebrospinal fluid leak	Yes	Rare	Rare
Furstenburg test	Positive	Negative	Negative
Transillumination	Yes	No	No
Cranial defect	Yes	Rare	Rare
Past history	Meningitis	Rare	Local infection

[a]To completely evaluate the posterior nasal cavity and nasopharynx, endoscopy may be performed.

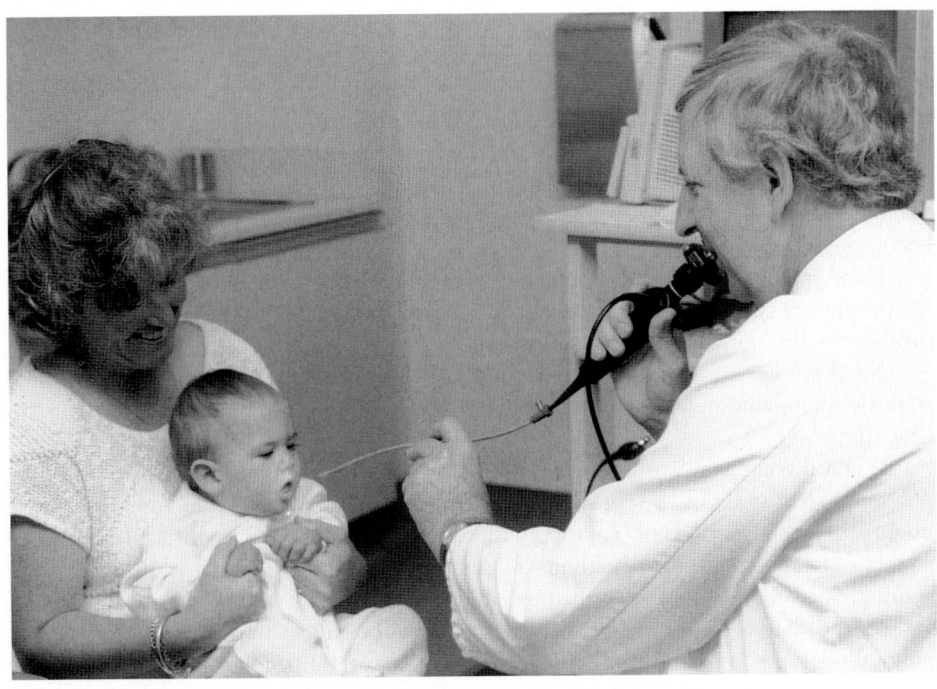

FIGURE 3 Flexible fiberoptic endoscopy of the infant's nose.

avoid traumatizing the delicate mucous membrane of the nasal cavity, and for this reason, the flexible fiberscope is preferred.

Some infants who have significant airway compromise with apneic spells, cyanosis, or severe intercostal retraction may need to be examined in the operating room in a controlled situation, with rigid bronchoscopic options and an anesthesiologist available (Fig. 4).

Investigations

Laboratory

When an infection or an inflammatory origin of nasal obstruction is suspected, a blood cell count with a differential white cell count is a useful adjunct. In the atopic infant, the radioallergosorbent test (RAST) may demonstrate inhalant allergens, such as house dust mite and cat hair, or ingested allergens such as milk, wheat, soya, and egg white. The infant with recurrent upper respiratory tract infections, sinusitis, and recur-

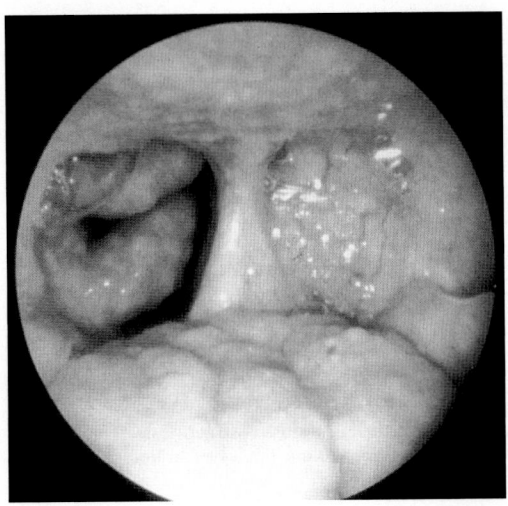

FIGURE 4 Endoscopic appearance of unilateral choanal atresia from nasopharynx. (From Benjamin B. *AAOHNS Home study guide. The Pediatric Airway* 1992, with permission.)

rent otitis media may have an immune deficiency, such as an immunoglobulin G (IgG) subclass deficiency or specific immunoglobulin A (IgA) deficiency.

Cultures of nasal secretions may be helpful despite the lack of correlation between the bacteria isolated from nasal secretions and the organisms that cause sinusitis, such as *Hemophilus influenzae, Streptococcus pneumoniae,* and *Moraxella catarrhalis.*

A high index of suspicion for congenital syphilis as a cause of "snuffles" should be maintained and the appropriate fluorescent treponemal antibody absorption (FTA-ABS) test arranged.

Nasal smears are probably not all that useful in the neonatal and infant group, but in the perplexing case, scrapings for electron microscopy to rule out the immotile cilia syndrome may be contributory to management.

Nasal studies of airway resistance and airway volume using rhinomanometry and acoustic rhinomanometry have been used in infants but their use is not widespread at this time (3).

When the clinician suspects that the infant has clinical features of OSD (Table 3), polysomnography should be considered. Although some normal neonates and premature infants have brief periods of obstructive sleep apnea, infants with significant OSD have a higher incidence of breath-holding spells and fatigue during feeding while awake, and snoring, noisy breathing, and profuse sweating while asleep.

As the diagnosis of OSD in the infant is more subtle than in the older child, polysomnography will confirm the degree of severity of the condition and warn of those children at risk for increased postoperative complications. Polysomnography is possible in the infant in a pediatric sleep laboratory with techniques sensitive to the special needs of the young child and with participation of the parents (4).

Polysomnography monitoring in infants and children may demonstrate the following:

1. Obstructive hypoventilation with hypercarbia
2. One or more obstructive apneas per hour usually with
   a. Arterial oxygen saturation below 90%
   b. Sleep arousal associated with upper-airway obstruction
   c. An abnormal multiple sleep latency test for the infant's age

The polysomnogram helps the clinician differentiate OSD from primary snoring and quantitate, to some degree, the severity of the OSD, especially in those with multiple obstructive apneas and arterial oxygen desaturation (5).

Radiology   Plain paranasal sinus radiographs are useful to exclude maxillary and ethmoidal sinusitis in the infant and to assess the size of the adenoid. The clinician should

TABLE 3: Symptoms of Obstructive Sleep Disorder in the Infant[a]

Snoring
Obstructive sleep apnea
Nocturnal sweating
Restless sleep
Frequent wakening
Abnormal head posture
Paradoxical chest-abdomen motion
Increased respiratory effort
Fatigue while feeding
Failure to thrive

[a]In addition, there may be a history of other associated disorders that can cause obstructive sleep disorder, including Down syndrome, craniofacial abnormalities, achondroplasia, and mucopolysaccharidoses.

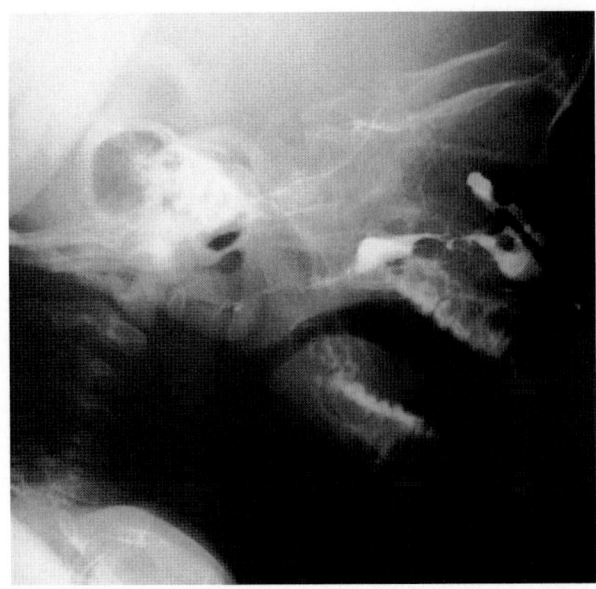

FIGURE 5 Adenoids simulating choanal stenosis.

be careful in assessment of the adenoid size as the lateral radiograph may give a false impression of adenoid hypertrophy if the soft palate is in the posterior position (as in speech or swallowing), or the radiograph has been taken with the neck flexed rather than extended. Similarly, there is not necessarily a correlation between the degree of airway obstruction and adenoid size because of other factors such as turbinate size, tonsillar size, and hypotonia of the lateral and posterior pharyngeal walls (especially in Down syndrome). The author's preferred method is to assess the distance from the posterior wall to the relaxed soft palate and that from the posterior wall to the choanae and to grade the adenoid obstruction on a scale of four. On occasion, adenoid hypertrophy will obstruct the choanae sufficiently to mimic choanal stenosis symptomatically (Fig. 5). Lateral videofluoroscopy is useful in assessing the dynamic function of the soft palate in infants with adenoid hypertrophy and neuromuscular dysfunction in whom adenoidectomy may lead to velopharyngeal incompetence postoperatively.

Ethmoidal and maxillary sinusitis may be seen radiographically as early as 3 to 6 months. Often adenoid hypertrophy and gastroesophageal reflux are associated with sinusitis in this age group.

Contrast radiography of the nasal cavities (choanagram) for assessment of possible choanal atresia (after suction of mucus from the nasal cavity) was a standard examination prior to the advent of CT but is not commonly used today.

In selected patients, CT scanning of the paranasal sinuses, nasal cavity, and nasopharynx is the radiographic investigation of choice (Table 4). Suspected choanal atresia and stenosis, piriform aperture stenosis, dermoids, gliomas, and other nasal and paranasal tumors are optimally assessed using CT (Fig. 6).

PEARLS AND PERILS

1. Remember to exclude maternal medications as cause of nasal obstruction.
2. Fiberoptic endoscopy is the most useful adjunctive procedure for diagnosis.
3. Computed tomography is the investigation of choice for choanal atresia.
4. Polysomnography will help differentiate primary snoring from obstructive sleep disorder.

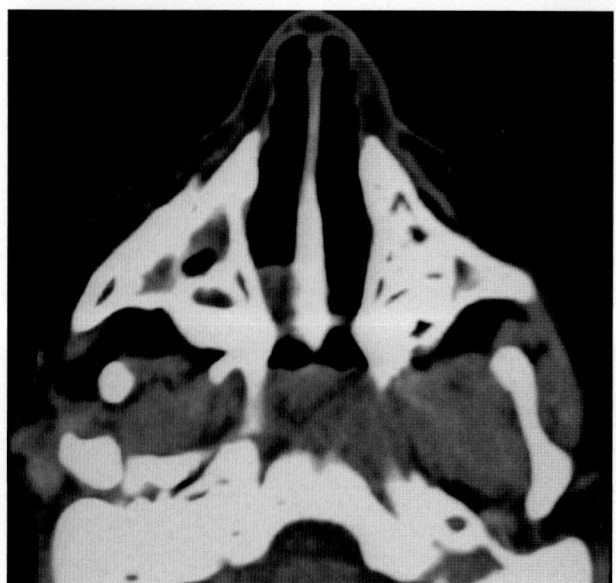

FIGURE 6 Axial computed tomography through the level of the nasal cavity and nasal pharynx. Bilateral mixed bony and membranous choanal atresia is demonstrated with widening of the posterior septum and of the pterygoid areas. The patient was repaired via transnasal drill-out with resection of a portion of the posterior septum.

 ## TREATMENT RECOMMENDATIONS

Congenital Abnormalities

Choanal Atresia

Choanal atresia occurs in 1 in 8,000 live births, with an incidence in female newborns twice that in male newborns. It is believed to be due to a failure of the breakdown of the buccopharyngeal membrane or persistence of epithelial rest cells in the nasal cavities during embryonal development. The atresia, which can be bilateral or unilateral, is either bony or mixed bony and membranous (6) and may be associated with other cranial and extracranial abnormalities (e.g., CHARGE association).

Management of Bilateral Choanal Atresia   The neonate is an obligate nasal breather and airway obstruction secondary to bilateral choanal atresia is a true respiratory emergency requiring urgent management with a taped-in neonatal oropharyngeal airway or McGov-

TABLE 4: Selected Computed Tomography Radiologic Findings[a]

Congenital choanal atresia
Narrowed nasal cavity
Lateral bony obstruction
Medial vomerine bony obstruction
Persistent area of membranous obstruction
Nasal dermoid
Widening of nasal septum
Erosion of contiguous bones
Formation of cyst-like cavity
Increased interorbital distance
Occasionally a cribriform plate bony defect
Congenital dacryocystoceles
Medial canthal cystic mass
Dilated ipsilateral nasolacrimal duct
Intranasal cystic mass

[a]Magnetic resonance imaging does not contribute significantly in the majority of infants with nasal obstruction except where there is a question of soft tissue extension from or into the cranial cavity (e.g., sphenoid meningoencephalocele).

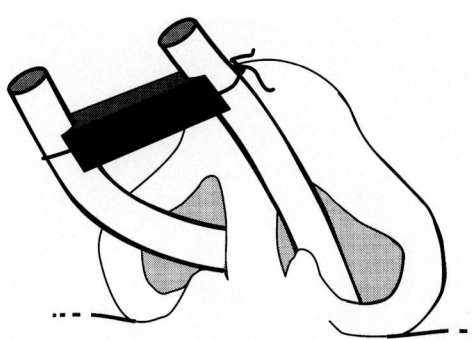

FIGURE 7 Silastic stent with anterior strut to protect the nares.

ern nipple, often with accompanying nasogastric feeding. Occasionally, in the presence of other pathology, definitive surgery is delayed, and either an orotracheal tube or a tracheotomy may be necessary.

Definitive management of bilateral choanal atresia in the neonate is preferably performed by the transnasal route. The neonate may be operated on within the first week of life, using general intubation anesthesia following decongestion of the nasal cavity and using either the operating microscope or rigid telescopes. In either technique, the nasal cavity is decongested with topical application of 0.5% phenylephrine and injection of lidocaine 1% with epinephrine 1:80,000. The choanal bony plate or mixed plate is perforated near its weakest point at the junction of the nasal septum and floor of the nose, using a curved female urethral catheter directed downward into the nasopharyngeal cavity. If this is unsuccessful, then the cutting drill is used under direct vision to perforate the atretic plate and enlarge the defect. The bony plate defect may be enlarged by using either a cutting burr or the microdebrider. The atresia plate is at an oblique angle to the choanae, with the inferior portion of the plate being most anterior. This fact should be noted by the surgeon, to avoid damage to vital structures superiorly and laterally. The safest approach is to concentrate the bony removal at inferior and medial aspects of the choana. The preservation of mucosal flaps as advocated by some authors is virtually impossible when the diamond drill or carbon dioxide laser is used. Drilling or removal of the posterior end of the vomer is essential to help prevent restenosis of the new choanal openings. The author's experience has not included use of the carbon dioxide laser, as suggested by Healy et al. (7), for removal of the membranous and bony atresia plate. When using the diamond burr drill or carbon dioxide laser, one must take great care to use an aural speculum to avoid damage to the nares.

Following establishment of a satisfactory airway bilaterally, the choanae are stented for 4 to 6 weeks using a Silastic endotracheal tube, with an anterior strut separating the two ends of the endotracheal tube (Fig. 7). At the time of removal of the stent, the operated choanal area is examined by a rigid telescope and any granulation tissue is removed or destroyed by diathermy. In view of evidence of a lower incidence of restenosis of the choanae after use of soft stenting with rolled Silastic sheeting for a period of 2 to 3 weeks, as advocated by some authors, this is worth consideration. Serial dilatations of the choanal opening using urethral sounds postoperatively are performed if there is evidence of early restenosis.

The author subscribes to the view held by Pirsig (1), that repair of the choanal atresia by the transpalatal route before the age of 5 years may lead to unacceptable maldevelopment of the upper dental arch with crossbite. Transseptal and transantral approaches are not utilized in this age group.

Management of Unilateral Choanal Atresia   The infant with unilateral choanal atresia may not be diagnosed until quite late and the surgical management is not urgent. Transnasal removal using the methods described for bilateral choanal atresia is done, taking care to remove the posterior portion of the vomer, to avoid restenosis.

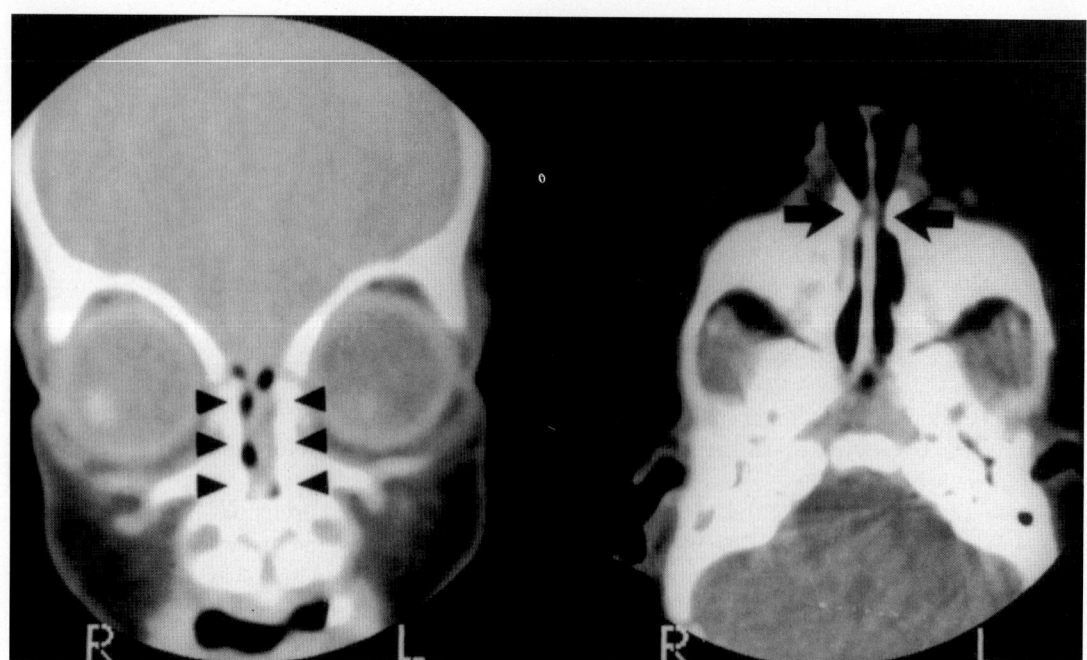

FIGURE 8 Computed tomography scan of congenital nasal piriform stenosis. (From ref. 11, with permission.)

Choanal Stenosis

This condition, which can mimic choanal atresia, may present with airway obstruction, especially with an upper respiratory tract infection. Differentiation from choanal atresia by CT scanning allows conservative management with topical saline or decongestant drops or steroid nasal spray until the nasal cavity enlarges and the symptoms decrease.

Piriform Aperture Stenosis

This uncommon condition caused by overgrowth of the medial aspect of the maxillae causes anterior nasal obstruction with significant changes to nasal airflow. After identification of the classic finding of a shelf-like projection into the posterior vestibule, CT scanning will confirm the diagnosis (Fig. 8). Surgical correction of bilateral stenosis is necessary with a sublabial approach and drilling of the excess bone at the piriform aperture level (8). The mucosa drapes loosely over the newly formed piriform aperture and stenting for several days using soft Silastic tubing is usually adequate to prevent restenosis.

Congenital Dacryocystocele

This rare condition, alternatively known as congenital nasolacrimal duct cyst, presents within the first few weeks of life as unilateral or bilateral swelling with compromise of the airway in more than 50% of infants with nasal extension. CT or magnetic resonance imaging should be performed to rule out intracranial connections and for confirmation of the diagnosis (Fig. 9). Surgical management, if necessary, involves intranasal marsupialization of the cyst (9).

Nasal Malformations

The most common of these deformities, the cleft lip nose, includes a nasal tip deformity, dorsal displacement of the dome, and buckling of the alar cartilage. Primary rhinoplasty at the time of cleft lip repair is the management of choice by the author's cleft palate team. Rarely, absence of the nose or partial absence of the nose with clefting is noted, often in association with other craniofacial deformities, and once again, requires a team approach.

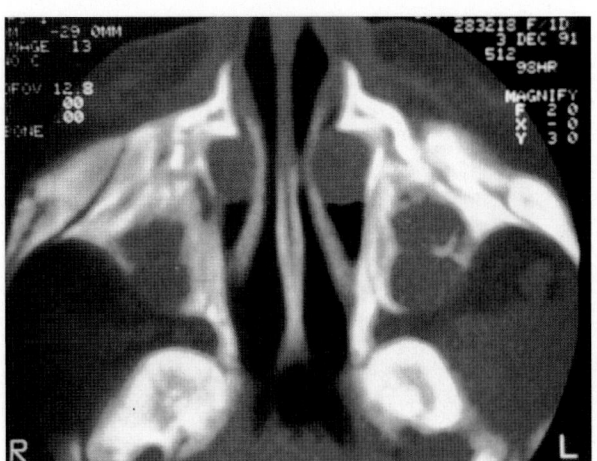

FIGURE 9 Computed tomography scan of congenital dacryocystocele. (From ref. 9, with permission.)

Midline Nasal Masses

Congenital midline masses in the neonate or infant usually include encephalocele, glioma, and dermoid (Fig. 10). Polyps are rarely seen in this age group, even in infants with cystic fibrosis.

The basic rule for midline nasal masses is to never perform a biopsy until one has ascertained whether there is intracranial extension that might cause significant intracranial complications if a biopsy is done. Following CT evaluation, and if there is intracranial extension, neurosurgical consultation should be sought, and removal of the mass may require a neurosurgical or combined approach (Fig. 11). The encephalocele is a herniation

FIGURE 10 **A:** Infant with a left nasal mass and cerebrospinal fluid rhinorrhea after outpatient biopsy at another institution. **B:** Computed tomography demonstrates a left nasal mass appearing to extend through a left anterior cranial fossa dehiscence, consistent with a frontobasal encephalocele. **C:** The surgical specimen after removal via a frontal craniotomy and nasal combined approach. The superior stalk extended through the area of the cribriform plate. The dura was repaired by neurosurgery and olfaction was preserved on the right side.

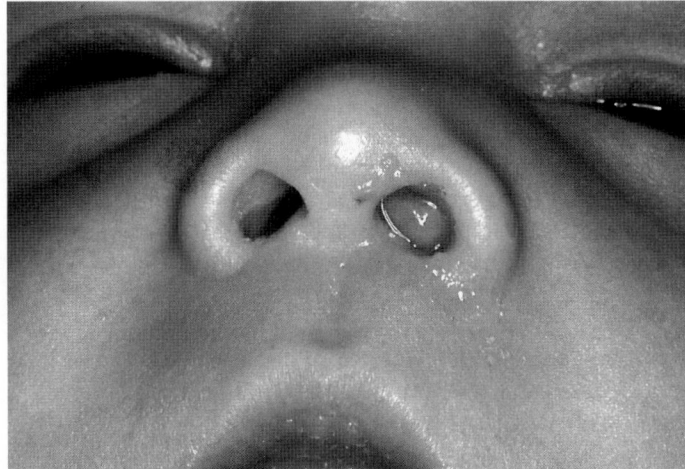

A

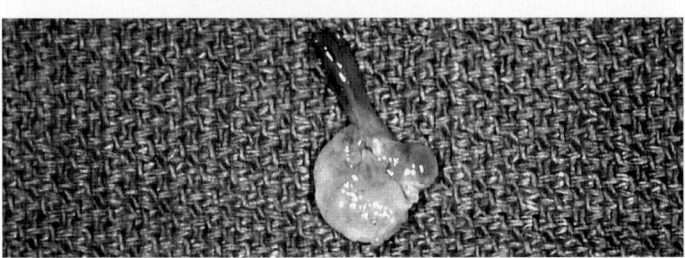

C

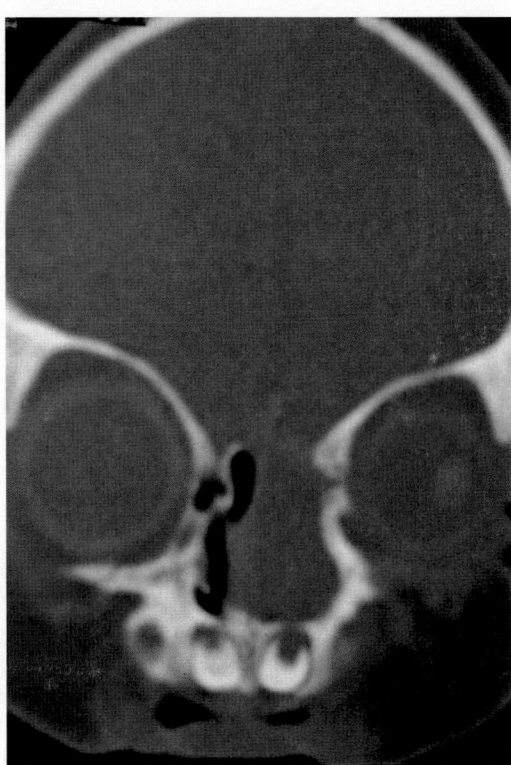

B

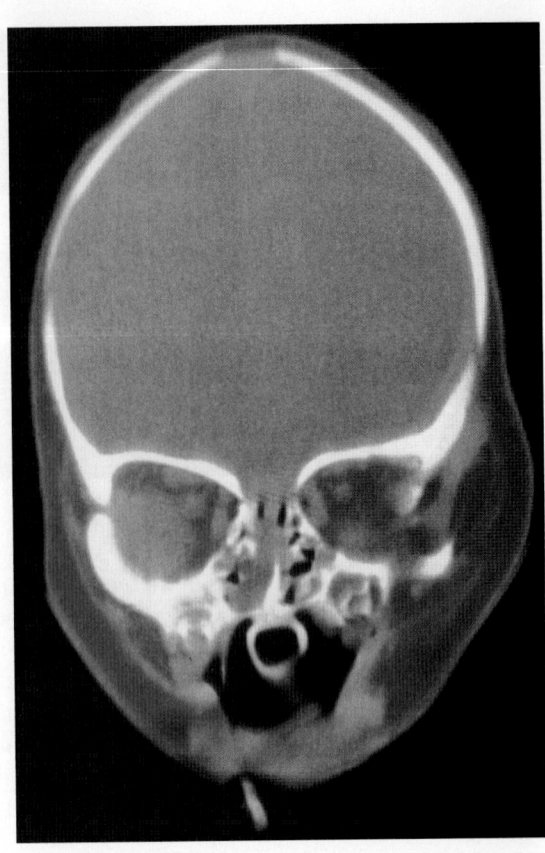

FIGURE 11 Computed tomography scan of a right encephalocele in the nasal cavity.

of meninges with ectopic brain tissue into the nose and may extend over the nasal dorsum or intranasally or both. In glioma, there is either a fibrous connection between the mass and the brain tissue or no connections at all (Fig. 12).

Dermoid cysts containing ectomesodermal elements are usually found in the nasal midline along the dorsum, often with hair protruding from the lesion together with a fistulous tract. CT scanning is crucial for preoperative planning (Fig. 13). The surgical approach can be externally via a midline nasal incision, a bucket handle incision, or through an osteoplastic flap approach. Drilling of the defect in the nasal bone may be necessary to fully remove the lesion and this can best be done using the operating microscope. Intranasal lesions without intracranial extension may be able to be excised under endoscopic control. A simultaneous or nonsimultaneous combined surgical approach is necessary in patients with encephaloceles and a significant bony cranial defect (10).

Teratomas

These congenital masses have all three elements of ectoderm, endoderm, and mesoderm and may contain cartilage, bone, thyroid, or glial tissue. CT examination is, once again, the *sine qua non* for a preoperative assessment.

Inflammation

Upper respiratory tract infection is the most commonly seen cause of nasal obstruction. This viral illness can cause severe airway obstruction in the obligate nasal breather or the infant with an already compromised nasal airway. Management for this ranges from saline nasal drops, to decongestant nasal drops, to suctioning with either a bulb syringe or electric suction in the more severe case. Secondary bacterial infection may warrant antibiotic therapy, and for the patient with persistent nasal obstruction an underlying allergic rhinitis or sinusitis should be considered.

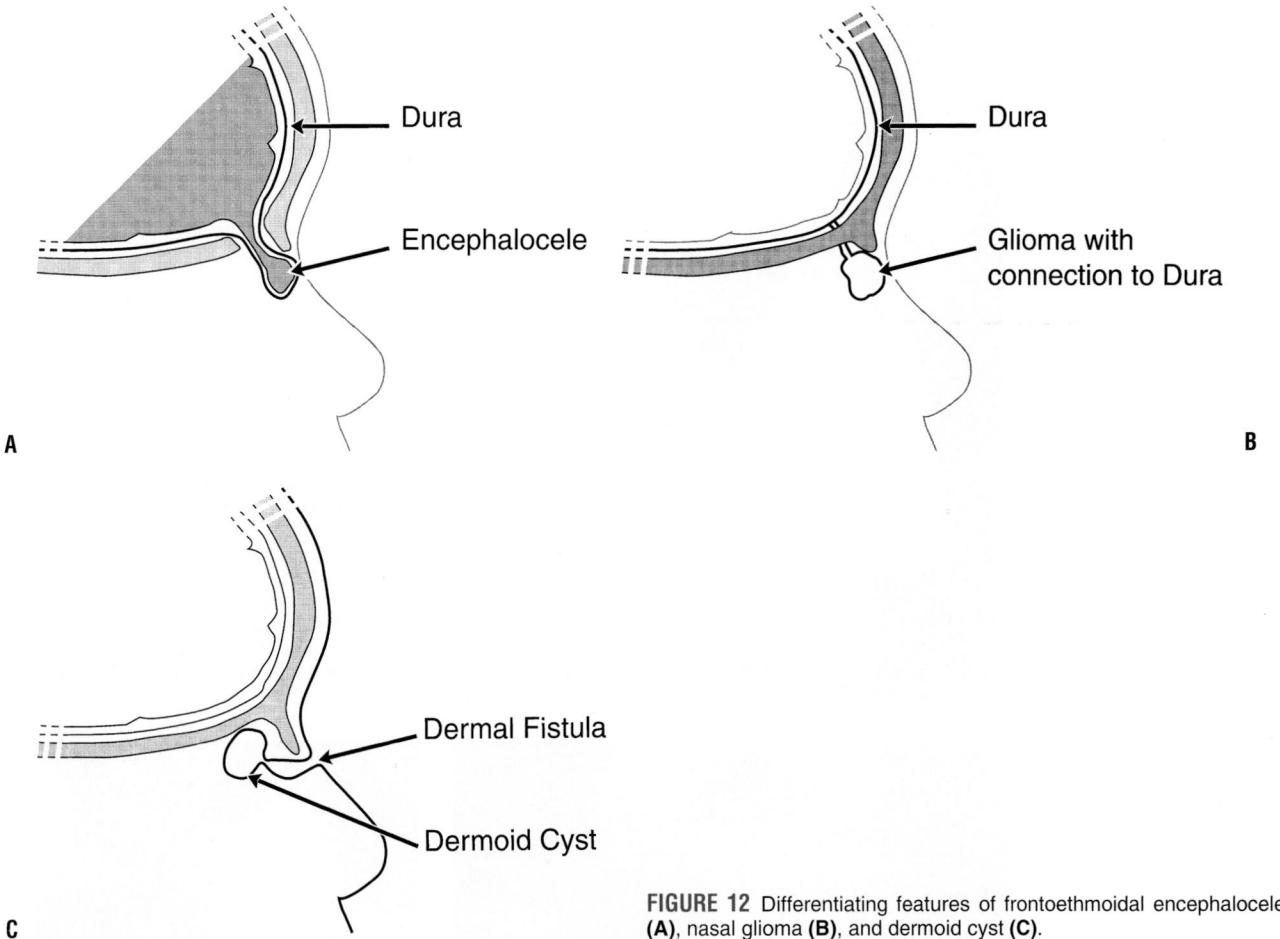

FIGURE 12 Differentiating features of frontoethmoidal encephalocele **(A)**, nasal glioma **(B)**, and dermoid cyst **(C)**.

Allergic rhinitis is a significant cause of nasal obstruction even in the neonate and should be suspected when nasal obstruction persists, when there is a blue or pale turbinate mucosa noted with thin secretions, and when the classic allergic facies is noted in an infant with a family history of atopy. Decongestant or saline nasal drops may be of some help, but cromolyn nasal drops often act within 48 hours of their application, quite different from their action in older children and adults. Occasionally, steroid nasal sprays may be necessary, and on occasion, in the presence of persistent nasal infection, antibiotic-steroid drops may be utilized for 3 to 4 days in the nasal cavity, with excellent results. As with all atopic children, the allergic rhinitis may be accompanied by eczema or asthma, middle-ear effusion, sinusitis, or adenotonsillar hypertrophy. If the problem is more related to the secretions causing obstruction than to nasal congestion, then a nasal antihistamine spray or oral antihistamine-decongestant may be tried. Cow's milk allergy may present in the 1- to 2-month-old infant with excessive mucus production, and this responds to cessation of ingestion of cow's milk (11).

Rhinitis of infancy refers to a constellation of conditions manifested as mucosal edema with airway obstruction. Meconium aspiration, chlamydial infections, gastroesophageal reflux, and idiopathic "vasomotor rhinitis" have all been implicated as causes or associations with this condition. Management involves culturing any purulent secretions, especially for chlamydia, and local measures such as decongestant nasal drops, saline nasal drops, or topical steroid-antibiotic drops. On occasion, systemic steroids may be necessary for a limited period.

The ethmoidal sinuses and maxillary antra can be demonstrated radiologically at birth, and therefore sinusitis is a possibility in the baby and infant. In the presence of persistent nasal infection, radiography should be performed to exclude sinusitis. If sinusitis

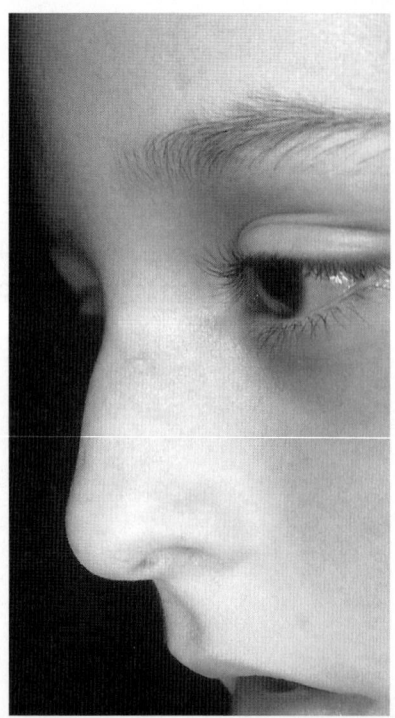

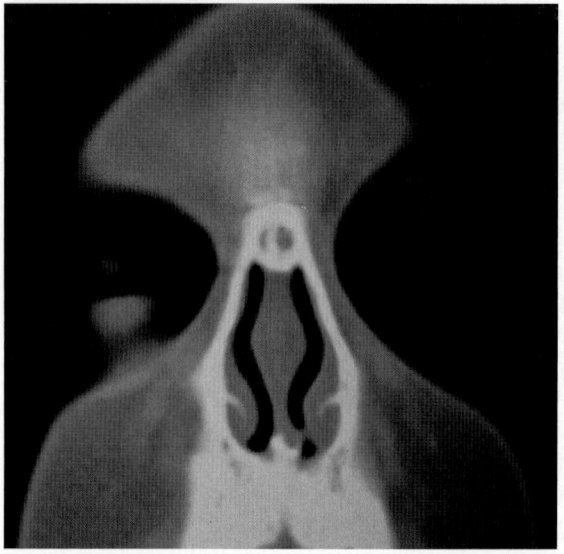

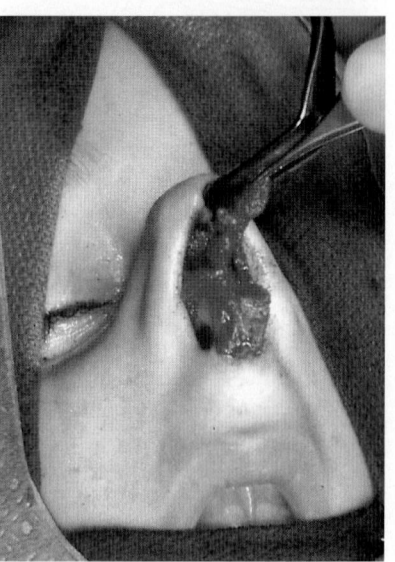

FIGURE 13 A: A 7-year-old boy with a sinus tract in the midline nasal supratip area along with a fibrotic area over the left nasal dorsum at the site of previous recurrent infection. **B:** Computed tomography demonstrates an extension of the tract through the bony dorsum. Other views failed to demonstrate any intracranial extension. **C:** Surgical excision of the dermoid sinus tract and fibrotic cyst area over the dorsum via an open rhinoplasty approach. The sinus tract was followed to the anterior skull base via a midline nasal osteotomy. The sinus tract was excised at the skull base and there was no cerebrospinal fluid connection.

is present, aggressive management with a broad-spectrum antibiotic for 10 to 14 days is warranted, together with local treatment including topical decongestant and subsequent steroid nasal spray. The usual organisms are *H. influenzae, S. pneumoniae,* and *M. catarrhalis.* Broad-spectrum antibiotics, such as amoxicillin, cefaclor, and trimethoprim-sulfamethaxazole, are the usual antibiotics prescribed, but if there are resistant organisms, especially *S. pneumoniae* or *M. catarrhalis,* then an agent such as amoxicillin with clavulanate potassium may be considered. Anaerobic organisms should be suspected when the sinusitis is persistent or chronic.

An inflamed retropharyngeal lymph node from infection of the nose, paranasal sinuses, or nasopharynx may suppurate and form a retropharyngeal abscess with consequent nasal obstruction. The symptoms of stridor, neck stiffness, and dysphagia together with a lateral soft tissue radiograph (in extension) will secure the diagnosis. Drainage under general anesthesia with systemic antibiotic coverage is the appropriate treatment.

Adenoid and adenotonsillar hypertrophy is not an uncommon cause of upper-airway obstruction in infants, and should be suspected in atopic infants with a history of snoring and other features of OSD. In its most severe form, adenoid hypertrophy can cause obstructive sleep apnea and cor pulmonale. The clinician must be aware that nasal obstruction occurs in series and not in parallel; that is, every component from nasal turbinate hypertrophy, septal deformity, adenoid hypertrophy, and tonsillar hypertrophy contributes to the nasal obstruction, and some of these may cause nasal resistance to be sufficiently high to cause significant nasal obstruction and mouth breathing.

Adenoidectomy may be necessary for the infant with OSD, and if the tonsils are moderately large, or tend to flop into the oropharyngeal airway, then consideration of adenotonsillectomy is advisable. Lack of consideration of the tonsillar component occasionally leads to the need for semiurgent tonsillectomy, just days or weeks after the adenoidectomy was performed for ongoing OSD symptoms. Use of the diathermy tonsillectomy technique with meticulous hemostasis together with suction diathermy of the adenoid bed will reduce the blood loss in these infants, and careful postoperative monitoring with oximetry with judicious and sparing use of narcotic analgesics will help prevent postoperative hypoventilation and hypoxia. Dexamethasone given intravenously at the time of surgery for tonsillectomy and adenoidectomy may help reduce postoperative palatal, uvular, and pharyngeal edema. Nursing in a high-care area postoperatively is indicated and some children may require placement of a nasopharyngeal airway postoperatively to bypass the edematous operative site.

The infant who has floppy pharyngeal tissue or a reduced oropharyngeal or nasopharyngeal diameter, such as with Down syndrome, cerebral palsy, and craniofacial disorders, may also demonstrate a degree of nasal obstruction, not seemingly consistent with the degree of obstruction visible on clinical inspection or radiographically.

Cautery or submucosal diathermy is generally not a good idea in this age group as it can lead to total nasal obstruction postoperatively with subsequent risks of airway problems. If the turbinates are prominent, then in this age group, an out-fracture of the inferior turbinates will cause less nasal congestion in the postoperative period.

Congenital syphilis (snuffles) may present in a fashion similar to sinusitis if there are no other classic signs of the disease, and subsequently may be accompanied by nasal ulceration and blood-stained discharge. A high index of suspicion of this disease will enable its diagnosis to be considered.

Iatrogenic

Maternal medication (see Table 1) may cause nasal congestion in neonates and infants, and a careful history will exclude this as a cause.

Rhinitis medicamentosa is most commonly caused by the excessive or prolonged use of topical nasal decongestant drops. These agents should not be used for more than a total of 4 to 5 days at a time. Diagnosis is based on the history, physical examination showing engorged erythematous turbinates, and the lack of the expected decongestant effect on application of a potent nasal decongestant. Cessation of the decongestant spray and substitution of a topical steroid spray will usually allow the condition to ameliorate.

Cleft palate repair in the infant with a compromised nasal airway or associated nasal septal deformity with mucosal turbinate hypertrophy may lead to significant nasal airway obstruction postoperatively. Particularly as soft cleft palate repairs are being closed in many infants between the ages of 3 to 6 months, the subsequent surgical edema at the oropharyngeal level after closure of the cleft will often cause desaturation postoperatively. Management may require temporary placement of a nasopharyngeal airway on the least obstructed side with postoperative monitoring, with oximetry for up to 10 days. Certain children, especially those with Treacher Collins syndrome, are at special risk for postoperative airway compromise. Generally, velopharyngeal incompetence problems are not dealt with in this age group, but similar precautions apply in the older child as to the infant undergoing cleft palate repair. Delayed cleft palate repair with tracheostomy may be necessary for the extreme case. Mechanical trauma secondary to instrumentation, especially insertion of nasogastric tubes or nasotracheal tubes, may cause mucosal edema.

On occasion, overenthusiastic removal of the adenoids or tonsils will cause nasopharyngeal stenosis. This is more common in infants in whom diathermy was applied externally to the adenoid bed, or in whom inflammation was present at the time of the original procedure, or in those children with a predisposition to hypertrophic scar formation. Correction of the stenosis is difficult, with restenosis occurring frequently and requiring multiple procedures.

Trauma

Significant nasal septal deviation may be seen in 1% of neonates, whether delivered vaginally or by cesarean section. Intrauterine forces create nasal molding, which can cause a flattened nasal tip together with nasal septal deformity. A traumatic vaginal delivery, particularly in the occipitoposterior position, can lead to the characteristic deformity of nasal tip deviation, displaced or tilted columella, and asymmetric alae.

In neonates with persistent nasal obstruction, the nasal cavities can be inspected using an otoscope or a plastic septal stent measuring $6 \times 2 \times 100$ mm (the size of a neonatal nasal cavity), which can detect a septal obstruction at 15 to 20 mm from the nares (12). In the majority of infants, the anterior nasal septal deformity will spontaneously correct by the age of 1 month if there is no displacement from the vomerine groove. In the uncommon situation where there is significant external deformity and airway compromise, a closed reduction of the septal deformity can be accomplished using specially devised neonatal septal manipulation forceps. Upward and downward pressure is applied to the nasal bony roof and floor, respectively, prior to the manipulation of the septum to the midline groove (Fig. 14). This follows adequate decongestant and local anesthetic application to the nasal mucosa. Mild septal deformity should be managed conservatively, as the great majority spontaneously correct within the first year of life (13).

Nasal septal injury from direct trauma can cause a septal hematoma with subsequent necrosis of the septal cartilage and growth problems (saddle nose) affecting the cartilaginous portion of the nasal dorsum. This necrosis of the septal cartilage may occur within 48 hours of injury and is best managed by drainage of the hematoma and oral antibiotics to avoid septal abscess formation. Bony nasal injury in other than cases of severe trauma to the face is uncommon.

Infants who place foreign bodies in the nasal cavity generally present with an underlying purulent rhinorrhea and nasal obstruction. Suction and decongestion will allow

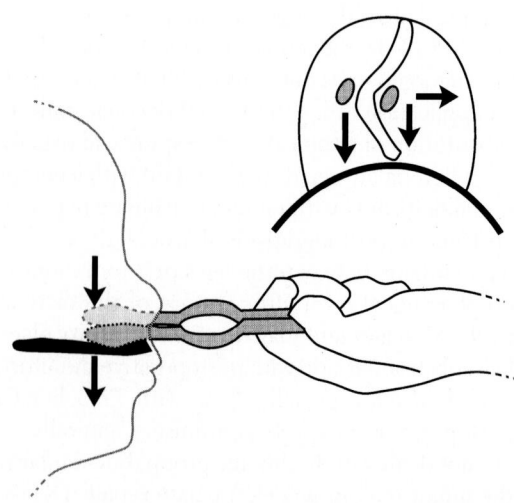

FIGURE 14 Nasal septal manipulation using neonatal nasal forceps. (From Coates HL. Nasal obstruction in the neonate and infant. *Clin Pediatr* 1992; 31:25–29.)

exposure of the foreign body and possible removal using a blunt right-angled hook. Alligator forceps are satisfactory for removal of thin foreign bodies but generally cause a smooth or narrow foreign body to be pushed farther into the nasal cavity (Fig. 15). A successful technique using cotton soaked in a preparation of phenylephrine 0.5% and 5% lignocaine to decongest and anesthetize the anterior nasal cavity will often allow removal of the cotton and the foreign body subsequently, with little resistance from the infant. However, in many cases, previous attempts at removal of the foreign body have caused the infant to be very uncooperative, and controlled removal under a brief general anesthetic is the management of choice. A second foreign body in the other or same nasal cavity should be excluded and in setting of a long-standing foreign body, secondary maxillary sinusitis may coexist and require treatment with local decongestants with antibiotics.

Endocrine

Congenital hypothyroidism may manifest as nasal congestion, as well as the other classic features of the condition. Hormonal replacement therapy will often help reduce the nasal congestion.

Neoplasia

Hemangioma and hemangiolymphangioma of the nose, usually of the nasal vestibule or skin of the external nose, may present with nasal obstruction and are the most common benign neoplasms of the nasal cavity (Fig. 16). Spontaneous resolution occurs in some patients, but occasionally compromise to the airway, hemorrhage, or bony involvement occur and intervention may be necessary. Use of diathermy, cryotherapy, or a carbon dioxide laser may be necessary. Usually, surgical excision is indicated for the noninvoluting cavernous hemangioma. There is no role for radiation therapy of benign disease.

Lymphoma in the infant age group is unusual and is managed by a combination of chemotherapy and radiation therapy. The most common malignant tumor in this age group is a rhabdomyosarcoma, which can present in the nasal cavity or the nasopharynx with obstruction and discharge, and hyponasal speech or secondary middle-ear effusion. The response varies, but usually the prognosis is guarded, especially for lymphoma arising from the nasopharynx.

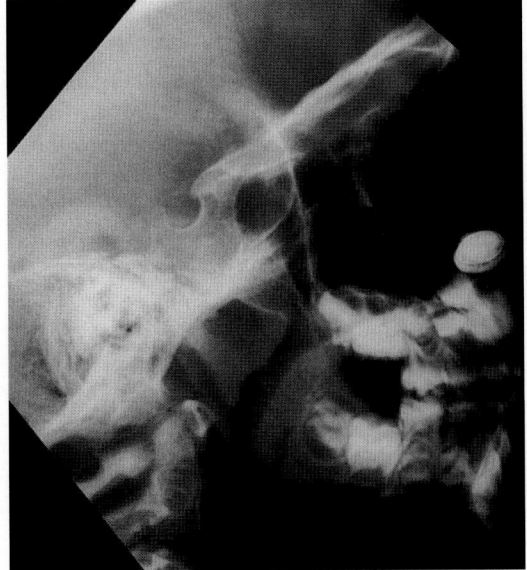

FIGURE 15 Plain radiograph of a radiopaque foreign body in the nasal cavity.

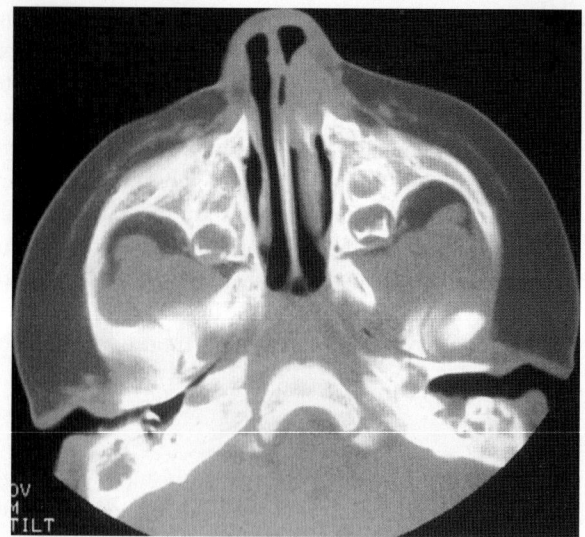

FIGURE 16 Computed tomography of a hemangioma of the left nasal cavity and nares causing significant obstruction.

PEARLS AND PERILS

1. Septal manipulation is useful in the persistent neonatal septal deformity.
2. Never remove "polyps" until computed tomography excludes intracranial extensions.
3. Cromolyn and steroid sprays are useful for reversible mucosal obstruction.

MANAGEMENT OF COMPLICATIONS

Congenital Conditions

Early attempts at choanal atresia repair using blind transnasal surgery led to complications including cerebrospinal fluid leak, meningitis, subluxation of the cervical vertebrae, Gradenigo's syndrome, and brain injury. The introduction of the operating microscope reduced these injuries but exposure and bleeding were still significant problems. The transnasal use of the carbon dioxide laser and subsequently, the Nd:YAG laser enabled more bloodless surgery, and the use of rigid telescopes improved the visualization of the operative area.

Problems with the carbon dioxide laser using the transnasal route include obstruction by the high-arched palate, septal deformity, and turbinate hypertrophy. Care must be taken while operating on infants with multiple congenital anomalies, especially those of the midfacial region, as they may require tracheotomy for airway obstruction (14).

Management of the posterior septal obstruction or turbinate obstruction may require resection or vaporization of portion of the inferior turbinates or posterior septum. Excessive removal of the posterior septum may prejudice normal facial growth. The high-arched palate problem is best managed by rotating the pliable tip of the nose superiorly to allow the laser beam to hit the atresia plate.

A case of fatal gas embolism following contact Nd:YAG laser surgery and the greater risk of thermal injury would indicate that the carbon dioxide laser is a more suitable laser for atresia repair in infancy (15).

The most frequent complication of transnasal repair is restenosis of the choanae, which occurs to some degree in up to 50% of patients. This usually occurs at the lateral and cranial borders of the newly created airway and is associated with excess granulation tissue growth.

The duration of stenting of the airway is controversial. Some authors suggest 6 to 8 weeks of stenting with a silicone stent while others advocate a 2 weeks of stenting with a soft material to reduce further granulation and scarring. Generally, the current practice is to insert a silicone stent (carefully placed to avoid columella damage) in patients with restenosis, and a period of 12 weeks of stenting is advocated.

Although in the neonate and infant the transpalatal approach often offers better visualization of the atresia and posterior septum, there is a higher morbidity, danger of palatal fistulization, and development of crossbite because of removal of the midpalatal suture lesion in more than 50% of the population. The transpalatal approach is not recommended for neonates and infants because of this potential midface complication (1).

Midline nasal masses, principally encephalocele, glioma, and dermoid, must be examined and investigated to rule out intracranial extensions. While the encephalocele is the most likely to have an intracranial extension, the glioma and dermoid can also have a similar communication, albeit rarely. Failure to identify this extension frequently can lead to postoperative fatal meningitis. Early neurosurgical consultation is mandatory if there is clinical radiologic evidence of an intracranial communication, so that a combined intranasal-extranasal approach can be considered.

Rarely, a large basal encephalocele obstructs the entire nasopharynx of a neonate, necessitating either endotracheal intubation or tracheotomy. Similarly, meningitis may be the presenting sign of intranasal encephalocele.

Inflammatory and Traumatic Conditions

Management of allergic rhinitis in infants with nasal sprays, such as cromolyn or steroid nasal sprays, can lead to drying out of the nasal mucosal with secondary bleeding. This bleeding can be prevented in up to 90% of patients by inserting paraffin ointment into the nares prior to using the spray. While cromolyn may safely be used year-round, the author prefers to utilize nasal steroid sprays on a seasonal basis, reducing the dosage to once every second day if possible. Careful counseling of the infant's parents about the dangers of overdosage of topical steroids should help prevent systemic steroid side effects.

Some nonsedating antihistamines interact with erythromycin and may cause a potentially fatal rare cardiac complication. However, with careful use on an intermittent basis, these agents will provide less sedative side effects than conventional antihistamine treatment.

In infants with OSD, the main complication noted is inadequate surgical management that is, removal of the enlarged adenoid only, when there are floppy or significantly enlarged tonsils present. This may lead to the requirement for early reoperation to remove the tonsils because of persistent OSD following adenodectomy. Similarly, the nasal airway should not be forgotten and careful out-fracture of the inferior turbinates may allow an increased nasal airway. As the infant's circulating blood volume is relatively small, extra care with hemostasis during tonsillectomy and adenoidectomy is essential. The author uses a diathermy technique for the tonsillectomy, and following the removal of the adenoid in the conventional manner, suction diathermy is applied to the adenoid bed to secure rapid hemostasis.

Excessive use of decongestant nasal drops can lead to a rebound phenomenon and rhinitis medicamentosa. This complication is generally managed by cessation of the decongestant nasal drops and use of topical steroid nasal drops. Iatrogenic airway obstruction may be caused by repairing a cleft palate or performing pharyngoplasty in an infant with a craniofacial defect such as Treacher Collins syndrome. Tracheostomy may be necessary in these infants, as long-term endotracheal intubation is often not a viable alternative, especially as the airway problem may re-present after extubation.

Long-standing foreign bodies in the nose may be complicated by maxillary sinusitis and there should be a high index of suspicion if symptoms of nasal obstruction or discharge persist after successful removal of the foreign body. Generally, oral broad-spectrum antibiotics taken for 10 days, and topical nasal saline drops, alternating with decongestant drops for 5 days, will be sufficient treatment for this condition.

Neoplastic Conditions

Excessive bleeding from an intranasal hemangioma may require management with diathermy or the laser, or occasionally excision of the lesion. Invasion of bone is a complication requiring definitive surgical excision either directly through the nose or via an alar lifting or lateral rhinotomy approach.

Rhabdomyosarcoma and other malignant tumors of the nasopharynx are generally managed by combination therapy and the complications of chemotherapy and radiation therapy may include nonspecific actions, as well as specific unwanted effects. These may include bone marrow and immune suppression, secondary infection, and retardation of bone growth in the involved area. There is an increased risk of mutagenic effects with a higher incidence of secondary cancers.

PEARLS AND PERILS

1. Deformity of palatal development may follow transpalatal repair of choanal atresia.

2. Contact Nd:YAG laser should not be used for choanal atresia repair.

3. Generally, adenotonsillectomy is more effective than adenoidectomy alone for obstructive sleep disorder.

✳ REFERENCES

1. Pirsig W. *Int J Pediatr Otorhinolaryngol* 1986;11:153–170.
2. Gray LP. *Int J Pediatr Otorhinolaryngol* 1980;2:201–215.
3. Buenting JE, Dalston RM, Drake AF. *Laryngoscope* 1994;104:1439–1445.
4. Carroll JL, Loughlin GM. In: Ferber R, Kryger M, eds. *Principles and practice of sleep medicine in the child.* Philadelphia: WB. Saunders, 1995:163–191.
5. Carroll JL, Loughlin GM. In: Ferber R, Kryger M, eds. *Principles and practice of sleep medicine in the child.* Philadelphia: WB Saunders, 1995:193–216.
6. Brown OE, Pownell P, Manning SC. *Laryngoscope* 1996;106:97–101.
7. Healy GB, McGill T, Jako GT, Strong MS, Vaughan CW. *Am J Otol* 1978;87:658–662.
8. Brown OE, Myer CM, Manning SC. *Laryngoscope* 1989;99:86–91.
9. Hepler KM, Woodson GE, Kearn DB. *Arch Otolaryngol Head Neck Surg* 1995; 121:1423–1425.
10. Hughes GB, Sharpino G, Hunt W, Tucker HM. *Head Neck Surg* 1980;2:222–233.
11. Prescott CAJ. *Arch Dis Child* 1995;72:111–113.
12. Gray LP. *Int J Pediatr Otorhinolaryngol* 1985;8:195–209.
13. Pentz S, Pirsig W, Lenders H. *Int J Pediatr Otorhinolaryngol* 1994;28:183–191.
14. Muntz HR. *Ann Otol Rhinol Laryngol* 1987;96:43–46.
15. Yuan HB, Poon KS, Chan KN, Lee TY, Lin CY. *Int J Pediatr Otorhinolaryngol* 1993;27: 193–199.

H.L. Coates: Department of Otolaryngology, Princess Margaret Hospital for Children, Perth, 6008 Western Australia.

- *Practical Pediatric Otolaryngology*
- edited by Robin T. Cotton and Charles M. Myer, III
- Lippincott-Raven Publishers, Philadelphia © 1999

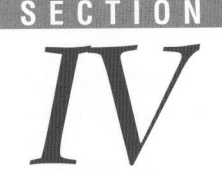
Airway

Section Editor
Robin T. Cotton

Evaluation of the Noisy Infant

Yoram Stern & Robin T. Cotton

Production of a pathologic adventitious respiratory sound may be related to variable sites and causes of airway obstruction. Stridor is characterized by a harsh sound produced by turbulent airflow through a partially obstructed area of the upper airway. Stertor or snoring is a low-pitch inspiratory sound produced by nasal or nasopharyngeal obstruction. Wheezing is a continuous musical or whistling sound produced by turbulent airflow through constricted small airways. The character of the noisy breathing and the respiratory phase in which it appears are determined by the location of the obstruction and the degree of anatomic and physiologic narrowing within the involved airway segment. Therefore, the quality and timing during the respiratory cycle of the pathologic sound can provide clues to its etiology and specific site of anatomic narrowing, as well as help to direct the workup. The supraglottic segment is the most poorly supported in the infant. Physiologic narrowing occurs during inspiration, as the linear movement of air during inhalation causes the supraglottic airway to partially collapse inward. Obstructing lesions within this segment will generally result in high-pitched inspiratory stridor. The glottic and subglottic regions have better cartilaginous support and are rather fixed segments of the infant airway. The lumen through these segments is normally not appreciably altered during the respiratory cycle. With glottic and subglottic lesions, airflow is equally affected during both inspiration and expiration and the stridor is biphasic and of intermediate pitch. Below the thoracic inlet, the intrathoracic trachea and mainstem bronchi undergo circumferential compression and physiologic narrowing during expiration. Obstructing lesions within this segment typically cause expiratory stridor.

Any pathologic respiratory sound in an infant needs immediate attention and should be carefully evaluated. Proper management is possible only after the accurate diagnosis has been established. Therefore, the precise underlying cause must be sought in every patient.

The degree of respiratory distress, including dyspnea, retractions, grunting, apnea, and cyanosis, as well as the degree of feeding difficulties, dictates the urgency of the workup and intervention. When the onset of symptoms is sudden or rapidly progressive and is associated with severe airway obstruction, the first step should be to establish a safe airway. If the respiratory distress is not acute, and there is no evidence of progression, then it is appropriate to proceed with a more thorough history and physical examination.

HISTORY

It is important to assess the urgency of the situation as soon as possible. One should find out whether there have been signs of agitation, blue spells, or apnea and if these are rapidly progressive. The possibility of foreign body aspiration should be addressed. An immediate onset of stridor often accompanied by a choking spell is strongly suggestive of a foreign body.

In the absence of severe respiratory distress, a careful thorough history should be obtained prior to any intervention, since it is one of the most important steps in evaluating noisy breathing in infants.

A history of the nature of the pregnancy and birth should include information or any abnormality in fetal movement or position, as well as any indication of fetal distress, prematurity, difficult or prolonged delivery, birth injury, asphyxia, and evidence of respiratory distress at the time of delivery. Vocal cord paralysis (see Chapter 38), which is the second most common laryngeal anomaly causing stridor in newborns (1), should always be suspected when there is a history of a difficult delivery or evidence of birth injury. Unilateral cord paralysis is more frequent than bilateral cord paralysis and more often involves the left side (2). Other ipsilateral peripheral nerve injuries, including facial nerve palsy, bronchial plexus injury, and diaphragmatic paralysis, are also sometimes seen.

The age at the onset of symptoms is an important factor. Noisy breathing or respiratory distress of immediate onset is most likely secondary to vocal cord paralysis, congenital subglottic stenosis, choanal atresia, or a complete vascular ring, such as a double aortic arch. Intermittent, low-pitched inspiratory stridor that appears within the first 2 weeks of life is typically due to laryngomalacia (see Chapter 39), which is the most common course of stridor in infants (3). Respiratory distress that occurs between 1 and 3 months may be secondary to subglottic hemangioma. Noisy breathing due to infectious lesions, such as croup or bacterial tracheitis, is most likely to appear after the age of 6 months. Recurrent croup should raise the suspicion of anatomic narrowing.

The rate of progression and fluctuation with crying, agitation, and position are also important factors in making the diagnosis. Noisy breathing that worsens with increased airway demands, such as crying, agitation, or feeding, may be secondary to laryngomalacia or subglottic hemangiomas. If the noisy breathing improves during crying, it is most likely secondary to choanal atresia.

The quality (hoarseness) and volume of cry should be addressed. Infants with glottic or subglottic lesions may be hoarse or aphonic, while tracheobronchial obstruction usually does not cause changes in the cry or voice. Infants with unilateral vocal cord paralysis usually have a weak and feeble cry.

Information about the relation of symptoms to feeding and feeding difficulties, such as coughing, choking, regurgitation, or rumination, should be obtained.

A history of previous intubation and surgical interventions should be sought.

Stridor shortly after extubation may be secondary to subglottic edema while distress that starts after 2 to 3 weeks may indicate early subglottic stenosis or vocal cord granuloma.

No history for noisy breathing should be complete without careful, repeated questioning and a high degree of suspicion for the possibilities of foreign body ingestion or aspiration.

PHYSICAL EXAMINATION

The physical examination should begin with careful inspection of the patient. The infant can remain in the parent's arms while the respiratory rate and degree of distress are judged. An increased rate of respiration, nasal flaring, intercostal or supraclavicular retractions, air hunger, or fatigue indicate respiratory distress. Cyanosis is usually a very late sign. If these conditions are present and there is a history of progressive distress, airway stabilization may be required. In a stable child, additional examination can then proceed.

An important part of the examination is auscultation. Listening over the chest should reveal the effectiveness and asymmetry of breath sounds. Sequential listening over the nose, open mouth, and neck should also be performed. Attention should then be directed to the quality and respiratory phase in which the pathologic sounds are present (inspiratory, expiratory, or biphasic).

Next, the nose and oropharynx should be examined. A tongue blade can be used to examine the oropharynx; however, when supraglottitis is suspected, this procedure should be avoided. An appropriate-size feeding tube can be passed through each naris to ensure choanal patency.

The infant should be placed in various positions to determine their effect on the noisy breathing. Noisy breathing caused by laryngomalacia, micrognathia, macroglossia, and innominate artery compression diminishes when the baby lies prone with the neck extended. Respiratory distress due to unilateral vocal cord paralysis may improve when the infant lies on the affected side.

Complete physical examination of the noisy infant should include flexible naso-laryngoscopy. This is a safe procedure when carried out by trained personnel with appropriate precautions, suction and oxygen are available, and the physician is assisted by adequately trained nursing personnel. The examination should always begin with careful bilateral evaluation of the nasal cavities (without application of vasoconstrictors), choanae, and nasopharynx. It is essential to document vocal cord mobility, as well as any abnormalities of the supraglottis. Pooling of secretions in the hypopharynx also should be noted. It is important to distinguish vocal cord paralysis from other causes of vocal cord motion impairment such as cricoarytenoid joint fixation. Fixation of the vocal cord can be ruled out by palpation under general anesthesia during direct laryngoscopy. Direct endoscopy may not be necessary if the diagnosis can be obtained by a combination of radiographic studies and flexible endoscopy. Some authors recommend performing direct laryngoscopy and bronchoscopy in every infant with noisy breathing in order to identify synchronous airway lesions. We believe that it is unnecessary in all patients who have supraglottic or glottic lesions, such as laryngomalacia and vocal cord paralysis, since the incidence of significant synchronous airway lesion below the level of the vocal cords is relatively low and it can usually be detected by high-kilovolt (KV) radiographic studies of the airway (4). However, if the patient shows a progression of symptoms marked by increased noisy breathing, weight loss, feeding difficulties, or cyanotic/apneic episodes, or if the airway x-ray film suggests anatomic narrowing, direct endoscopy is necessary for diagnostic and possibly therapeutic reasons. Esophagoscopy should also be performed when there is a suspicion of esophageal stenosis, esophageal lesions, tracheoesophageal fistula, foreign body, or vascular compression.

ANCILLARY EXAMINATION

After careful history and physical examination, appropriate radiologic evaluation of the airway is indicated for patients without immediate airway distress. Radiographic studies of the airway contribute information as to the location and extent of the obstructive lesion. The airway in children is quite mobile, and if proper technique is not used, misinterpretation is common. The radiographs must be taken during full inspiration with the head in extension. The lateral and anteroposterior soft tissue x-ray (high-KV) films provide the greatest amount of information. The general structure of the larynx can be obtained and the approximate size of the airway column can be ascertained. Normally, the airway appears narrowed between the vocal cords and the subglottic space (Fig. 1). A low-KV view is obtained if a foreign body is suspected, because small bones or other slightly opaque objects can be missed with high-KV radiographs.

Posteroanterior and lateral chest x-ray films complement the neck films. Extrinsic compression of the intrathoracic airway should always be considered as a cause of noisy breathing in infants. It is usually due to aberrant segments of the embryonic aortic arch creating vascular rings or slings, including double aortic arch, aberrant right subclavian artery, anomalous innominate artery, and pulmonary sling. If the plain airway film or the clinical history suggests vascular compression, computed tomography with contrast or magnetic resonance imaging (MRI) with gadolinium should be performed. MRI has proved to be an excellent alternative to angiography for the evaluation of vascular com-

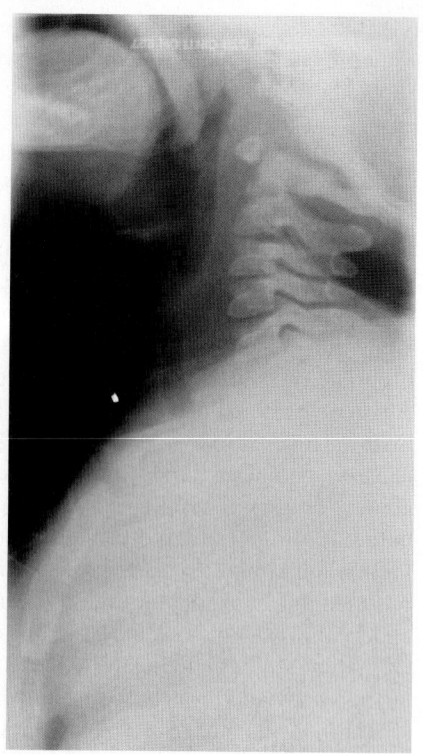

FIGURE 1 Normal lateral radiograph of the upper airway.

pression of the airway (5) (Fig. 2). It is also beneficial in the evaluation of mass lesions in the mediastinum that cause tracheal compression (Fig. 3).

When there is a history of feeding abnormalities or aspiration, a barium esophagram or functional endoscopic swallowing study should be obtained. These studies are helpful in determining the nature of the feeding difficulties and the presence of laryngeal cleft or tracheoesophageal fistula. Indentation on the esophagram can also suggest vascular compression.

Fluoroscopy may be useful to clarify dynamic obstruction or in the evaluation of obstructive sleep apnea, for which it is often combined with polygraphic recording.

FIGURE 2 Coronal MRI. Narrowing of the trachea caused by double aortic arch.

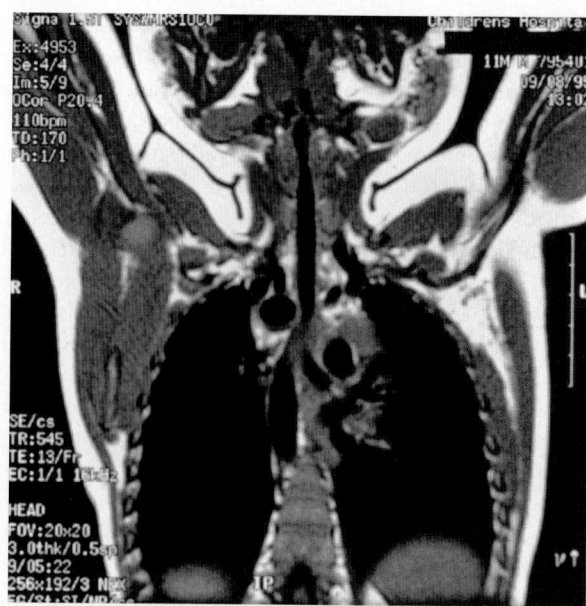

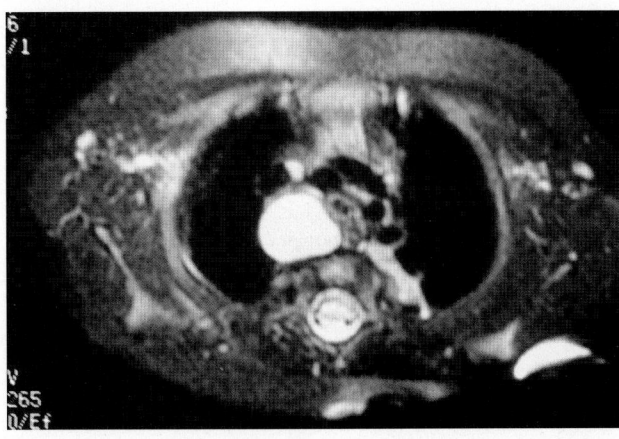

FIGURE 3 Axial MRI. Esophageal duplication cyst compressing the trachea.

Gastroesophageal reflux may exacerbate or cause respiratory tract pathology. Gastric emptying scans, esophageal pH monitoring, and biopsies, either alone or in combination, can be used to evaluate the patient for possible reflux.

Pulmonary function tests, combined with arterial blood gas evaluations, ideally provide useful information in determining the pulmonary status of the patient. Unfortunately, reliable data are difficult to obtain in the pediatric age group. Thus, these tests are not obtained routinely. In patients with lower-airway obstruction and lung parenchymal lesions causing respiratory failure, blood gas and blood pH studies may be required as single or serial examinations to assess the degree of respiratory failure and to assist in the management of respiratory or metabolic acidosis. However, in patients with obstruction of the upper airway, blood gases may remain normal or near normal even with severe obstruction.

TABLE 1: Common Causes of Noisy Breathing in Infants

Supralaryngeal
  Piriform aperture stenosis
  Choanal atresia
  Lacrimal duct cyst
  Nasopharyngeal mass (teratoma, encephalocele)
  Facial skeletal anomalies—micrognathia, glossoptosis
  Macroglossia
  Base of tongue mass (dermoid, lingual thyroid, thyroglossal duct cyst)
  Obstructive adenotonsillar hypertrophy
  Foreign body

Laryngeal
  Laryngomalacia
  Vocal cord paralysis
  Saccular cysts
  Web
  Respiratory papillomas
  Subglottic hemangioma
  Subglottic stenosis
  Laryngeal cleft
  Foreign body

Tracheobronchial
  Tracheomalacia, bronchomalacia
  Vascular anomalies
  Stenosis
  Foreign body
  Tracheoesophageal fistula
  Duplication of trachea or esophagus
  Bronchiolitis
  Bronchitis

TABLE 2: Evaluation of the Noisy Infant

History and Physical Examination

	1. Anteroposterior and lateral neck films (high KV) 2. Anteroposterior and lateral chest films 3. Flexible nasolaryngoscopy	
Normal		**Abnormal**
Stabilization	Progression and/or significant associated symptoms	1. Fluoroscopy 2. Barium swallow 3. Direct laryngoscopy and bronchoscopy 4. Esophagoscopy 5. Echocardiogram/electrocardiogram

Echocardiography and electrocardiography may assist in the diagnosis of cardiovascular lesions that may cause airway obstruction.

Continuous pulse oximetry and apnea and bradycardia monitors provide objective information and can be used at home or during brief hospitalization, while the infant is also observed by professional personnel.

CONCLUSIONS

A wide spectrum of potential causes can produce airway obstruction, most often manifested by noisy breathing (Table 1). All infants with noisy breathing should be evaluated as soon as possible. Careful history, thorough physical examination, and ancillary tests may provide information about the specific site of obstruction and are essential to assess the severity of the airway obstruction and to help the clinician decide whether further intervention is needed. Depending on the clinical picture and suspected lesion, further evaluation of the infant's airway, such as direct laryngoscopy and bronchoscopy, may be required (Table 2).

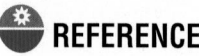 **REFERENCES**

1. Zalzal GH. Stridor and airway compromise. *Pediatr Clin North Am* 1989;36:1389–1402.
2. Cohen ST, Keller KA, Bevins JW, Thompson JW. Laryngeal paralysis in children: a long-term retrospective study. *Ann Otol Rhinol Laryngol* 1982;91:417–423.
3. Friedman EM, Vartola AP, McGill TJI, Healy GB. Chronic pediatric stridor: etiology and outcome. *Laryngoscope* 1990;100:277–280.
4. Mancuro RF, Choi SS, Zalzal GH, Grundfast KM. Laryngomalacia, the search for the second lesion. *Arch Otolaryngol Head Neck Surg* 1996;122:302–306.
5. Myer CM III, Avringer S, Bisset G, Wyatrak B. Magnetic resonance imaging in the diagnosis of innominate artery compression of the trachea. *Arch Otolaryngol Head Neck Surg* 1990;716:314–316.

Y. Stern: Department of Otolaryngology, University of Cincinnati, Children's Hospital Medical Center, Cincinnati Ohio 45229-3039.   •   R.T. Cotton: Department of Otolaryngology, University of Cincinnati, Children's Hospital Medical Center, Cincinnati Ohio 45229-3039.

• *Practical Pediatric Otolaryngology*
• edited by Robin T. Cotton
  and Charles M. Myer, III
• Lippincott-Raven Publishers,
  Philadelphia © 1999

29A

Evaluation of the Pediatric Airway by Rigid Endoscopy

Peter D. Bull

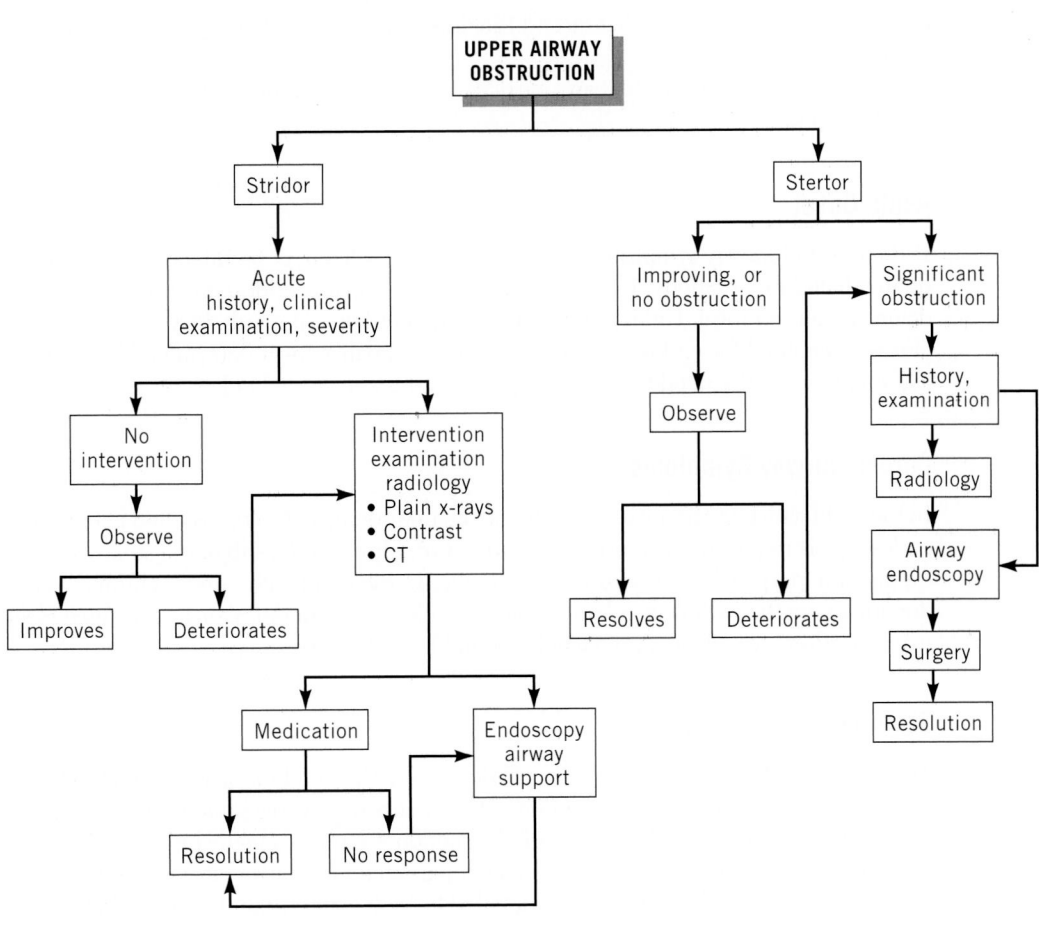

HISTORICAL BACKGROUND

Many attempts to examine the human airway in life had been made until 1854 when the at-once-obvious method of mirror examination was recognized by Manuel Garcia (1). Before this, in March 1828, Babington (2) demonstrated the glottoscope using a single mirror connected to a movable tongue depressor. Liston (3) in 1837 attempted to obtain a better view of the larynx by using a handled dental mirror. Garcia's discovery was communicated to the Royal Society of London in 1855 (4), but it was not until 1858 that

Czermak in Budapest, Hungary started to popularize its clinical use (5). By the early twentieth century, direct examination of the larynx was possible, cocaine having been discovered as a local anesthetic in 1880. Killian in 1912 described suspension laryngoscopy (6). The subsequent development of the operating microscope led to microlaryngoscopy by Kleinsasser. Bronchoscopy had been introduced by Killian in 1897. Instruments with distal lighting were introduced by Jackson and Negus, but it was not until the development of the Hopkins rod telescope and ventilating closed bronchoscopes that rigid bronchoscopy became the safe controlled procedure it is now.

PATIENT ASSESSMENT

Airway endoscopy may be diagnostic, therapeutic, or both. Sometimes the diagnosis is already known, as in laryngeal papillomatosis. Other times, there may be unexplained or undiagnosed disease requiring examination of the airway. It is in the setting of airway obstruction or compromise that most difficulties will occur, and preoperative assessment is vital.

The history is all important and particular attention must be paid to the mode of onset of symptoms.

Acute Onset

If the onset of airway symptoms is acute, the cause is likely to be infective (e.g., croup) or an inhaled foreign body. If the latter is suspected, airway endoscopy is mandatory for diagnosis and removal. Unless the foreign body is radiopaque, radiology cannot be conclusive. The need for endoscopy for acute airway impairment is determined by the clinical findings and the need for airway support, and is considered below.

Chronic Airway Symptoms

In the child with chronic airway symptoms, the underlying pathology is often known, and endoscopy is required for periodic assessment of, for example, subglottic stenosis or for therapeutic purposes, such as bronchial lavage. In the child with a more chronic condition for whom the pathology is known, airway endoscopy is undertaken as a planned elective procedure, usually at a time when the child is as fit as possible.

Severity of Symptoms

The severity of the child's symptoms will determine the need for airway endoscopy and the urgency with which it must be done. This assessment is dynamic in that change in severity is as important as the degree of obstruction. Change can only be assessed by frequent observation and measurement of such parameters as pulse rate, respiratory rate, oxygen saturation, and others that are detailed later. It is important to know whether the situation is deteriorating and urgent intervention is needed or whether it is improving, in which case intervention may do more harm than good. It is vital to intervene early if the clinical condition is getting worse, before crisis becomes disaster.

CLINICAL FEATURES OF AIRWAY OBSTRUCTION

The assessment of the potentially asphyxiating child needs care and experience. It is often undertaken jointly with pediatric and anesthetic colleagues and needs to be a continuing process rather than a single event, that is, a movie, rather than a snapshot.

It is important to record the following:

TABLE 1: Croup Score[a]

	SCORE		
Parameter	*0*	*1*	*2*
Inspiratory breath sounds	Normal	Harsh	Delayed
Stridor	None	Inspiratory	Inspiratory and expiratory
Cough/voice	None	Hoarse cry	Barking
Retraction/flaring	None	Flared nostrils, suprasternal retraction	As for 1, plus intercostal and subcostal retraction
Cyanosis	None	In air	In 40% O_2
Conscious level	Normal	Restless	Obtunded

[a]A score of 7 or more lasting 30 min despite conservative treatment suggests that airway support is required.

1. Oxygen saturation (SpO_2). This is paramount and most easily measured by pulse oximetry, confirmed if necessary by blood gas analysis.
2. Respiratory rate, which is easily charted. Increasing tachypnea is indicative of increasing difficulty. At the same time, respiratory effort must be assessed. Progressive fatigue may result in reduced effort and deterioration in the clinical state.
3. Use of accessory muscles of respiration, which indicates respiratory impairment.
4. Recession. This can be sternal, intercostal, or suprasternal and demonstrates airway obstruction with continuing respiratory effort. It will also decrease with fatigue, but its presence is abnormal.
5. Level of consciousness. An obtunded level of consciousness is a late and serious sign of respiratory insufficiency, and the child needs urgent intervention to support the airway or improve ventilation.

The role of these clinical observations has been formalized into a "croup score." This allocates a score to each parameter (Table 1) and determines when intervention is needed (6). Such intervention nearly always necessitates endotracheal intubation or tracheostomy.

INDICATIONS FOR ENDOSCOPY

Severe stridor will nearly always be associated with significant airway obstruction. Airway support is likely to be necessary and ideally diagnostic laryngoscopy and bronchoscopy should be performed before endotracheal intubation. Once a tube has been passed, the opportunity for diagnosis has been compromised. The degree of cooperation necessary between the endoscopist and anesthetist is total and each must trust the other.

Worsening airway obstruction is another indication for endoscopy. If the overall condition of the child is worsening, it is better to act early. Airway endoscopy will enable a diagnosis to be made and will assist in planning further treatment. Samples for bacteriologic culture can be taken if indicated and definitive treatment of an obstructing lesion can be performed. Early intervention in the setting of worsening stridor may avoid more extreme measures such as endotracheal intubation or tracheostomy. It is essential *not* to allow matters to progress to a degree where urgent airway and cardiovascular support are required.

If to stridor and some measure of airway obstruction are added *poor weight gain* and *difficulty in feeding*, airway endoscopy is advisable to seek a remediable cause. Such circumstances are more likely to be found in chronic conditions such as laryngomalacia.

If *radiology* or *ultrasound scans* suggest an abnormality (e.g., a vascular ring), endoscopy will be necessary to confirm the diagnosis.

If diagnostic uncertainty persists after clinical examination, radiology, and laboratory tests, then careful diagnostic endoscopy will be necessary. This is true for both respiratory compromise and voice abnormality.

PEARLS AND PERILS

1. Endoscopy of the airway is easier at an early stage than late in an asphyxiating child.
2. Discuss the problem case early with pediatric and anesthetic colleagues.
3. If you do not have the necessary facilities (staff and equipment) in your institution, make arrangements for transfer to a specialist unit before matters become critical.

WHY RIGID RATHER THAN FLEXIBLE ENDOSCOPY?

To some extent, flexible and rigid endoscopy are complementary. Fiberoptic examination of the infant larynx is possible in the awake child and gives useful information about cord mobility and laryngeal dynamics. It is only by rigid endoscopy under the controlled conditions of general anesthesia that a magnified leisurely view of the larynx and lower airways can be made. The cords can be viewed with a binocular microscope, affording a stereoscopic view. Only the use of rigid endoscopes allows the lower airways to be inspected safely and in minute detail while at the same time maintaining complete and secure control over ventilation. Flexible bronchoscopes do not allow such control and in a small infant will cause significant if not total airway obstruction. The image quality obtained by rigid telescopes is superior to that obtained by flexible fiberoptic bundles, especially in the smaller sizes, and therefore documentation is clearer (7).

RIGID INSTRUMENTATION

Instrumentation can be considered under three headings: (a) laryngoscopes and bronchoscopes, (b) telescopes, and (c) documentation and teaching.

Laryngoscopes and Bronchoscopes

Laryngoscopes

There is a bewildering array of laryngoscopes available. The author's preference is for those obtainable from Karl Storz GmbH. It is useful to have a small handheld laryngoscope for initial examination, such as the Holinger anterior commissure scope for infants. For more thorough examination of the larynx, instruments designed for suspension are required, and are essential for any endolaryngeal surgery. The Lindholm-Benjamin laryngoscope is available in two sizes, for babies and for toddlers (Fig. 1). For older children, the Lindholm operating laryngoscope and the Benjamin pediatric laryngoscope are well designed and easy to use. Some form of laryngoscope holder will be necessary to support the instrument so as to leave the hands free.

For ease of access both to the operating microscope and to instruments, it is important that the proximal end of the laryngoscope is sufficiently large.

Bronchoscopes

The development of ventilating bronchoscopes has revolutionized bronchoscopy in children and babies and made it a practicable procedure even in the low-birth-weight premature neonate. The features of such an instrument are as follows:

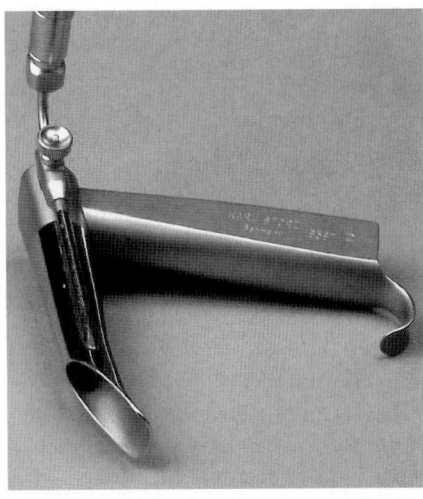

FIGURE 1 Lindholm-Benjamin laryngoscope.

1. A closed gas system allowing connection to an anesthetic circuit, the bronchoscope acting as an endotracheal tube. This will allow either spontaneous respiration or positive-pressure ventilation.
2. A rigid Hopkins rod telescope to allow distal illumination and superb vision down even the smallest-diameter bronchoscope.
3. A side channel for the passage of suction catheters or flexible forceps.

Such bronchoscopes, available from Karl Storz (Fig. 2), can also be used without a telescope, using a glass window to close the system and a swing-away magnifier to aid vision. Used like this, it is a poor second to using a telescope but may sometimes be necessary. The bronchoscope tubes are available in a variety of sizes. Table 2 gives the nominal and actual sizes of the bronchoscopes and indicates the appropriate size for the age of the child (8,9). The small diameter of pediatric bronchoscopes is such that there is a balance to be made between the size of the telescope and the size of the bronchoscope. Below size 4, a telescope of 1.9 mm gives good resolution but is small enough to allow adequate gas exchange and except for the smallest bronchoscope, will also allow the passage of a suction catheter. Larger sizes of bronchoscopes will allow the use of a larger telescope. A review by Marzo and Hotaling (10) clarified the balance between airway resistance and optical resolution. Of great value for the removal of foreign bodies or granulations are the optical forceps. An optical forceps can be introduced through the bron-

FIGURE 2 Storz 3.5 bronchoscope assembled and connected to an anesthetic circuit.

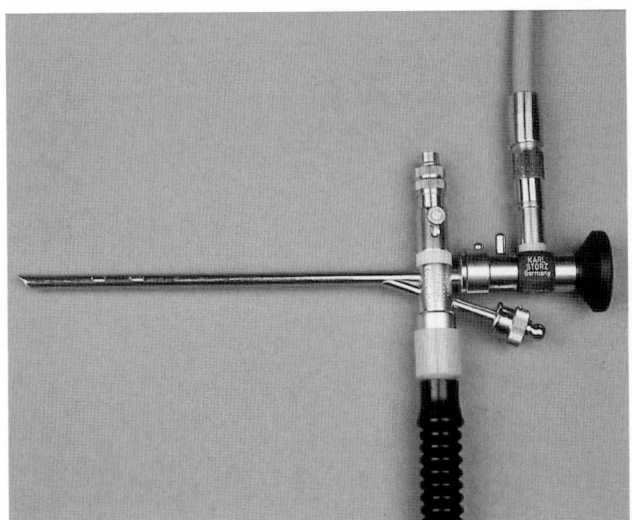

TABLE 2: Bronchoscope Sizes

Nominal Size of Bronchoscope	External Diameter (mm)	Age Range
2.5	4.0	Premature to neonate
3.0	5.0	Neonate to 6 mo
3.5	5.7	6–18 mo
4.0	7.0	18–36 mo
5.0	7.8	3–8 yr
6.0	8.2	>8 yr

choscope tube (through a gas-tight rubber seal) and consists of varying designs of jaws and an axial telescope (Figs. 3 to 5). It is available in different lengths for use with bronchoscopes of different lengths. For pediatric use, the forceps taking a 30-cm telescope with a 20-cm or 26-cm bronchoscope tube is used most often, but also available are forceps using a 36-cm telescope, which can be used in a bronchoscope tube of up to 30 cm long and with a minimum-size 3.5 diameter (external diameter, 5.00 mm).

Telescopes

In 1966 Hopkins introduced the rod lens telescope, allowing a dramatic improvement in resolution and angle of field (Fig. 6). These telescopes now form the basis of all forms of rigid endoscopy and have revolutionized pediatric bronchoscopy by allowing clear vision down a tiny lumen. For the purposes of laryngoscopy, a 4.0 mm × 20 cm 0-degree telescope is ideal (see below) and can be passed through a suspended laryngoscope into the subglottis or trachea. A 30-degree angle of view will allow inspection of the laryngeal sinus and anterior commissure (Figs. 7 to 9).

The size of telescope to be used for bronchoscopy is determined by the size of the bronchoscope. It is often helpful to have a telescope longer than the bronchoscope tube to allow inspection of the more peripheral areas, in addition to the length that matches the tube.

Documentation and Teaching

The development of small high-resolution color television cameras has been of great benefit to the endoscopist. Such a camera can be fitted to the operating microscope or to an endoscopic telescope to allow staff and students to observe the procedure. Video recording is straightforward using an S VHS recorder. Still images can be captured on a

FIGURE 3 Optical forceps and a 26-cm bronchoscope tube.

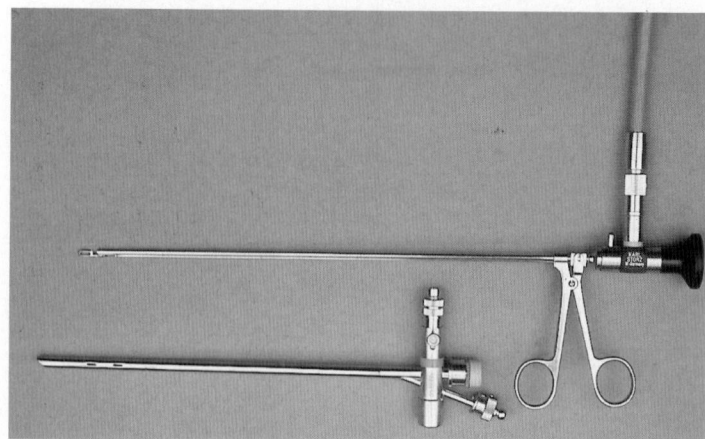

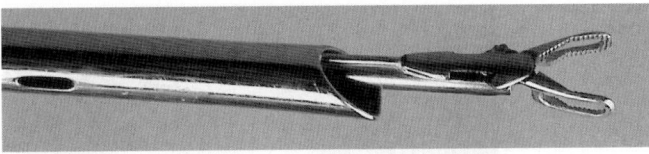

FIGURE 4 Close-up to show jaws of an optical forceps protruding beyond the bronchoscope tube.

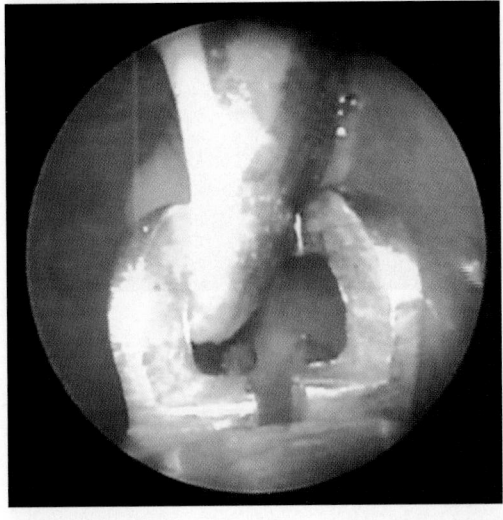

FIGURE 5 A bronchial foreign body (nut husk) being grasped by optical forceps.

still video recorder (Sony Corporation Mavica) in analog form on a magnetic disk. From the camera, the video, or the still video recorder, it is simple to make an immediate color print with a thermal sublimation printer for filing in the patient's record. The image from the magnetic disk can be manipulated to a digital form compatible with computer graphics packages for reproduction or the production of transparencies. The availability of this sort of documentation is invaluable for explanations to patients, for recording operative findings, and for medicolegal purposes. While not yet routine in the United Kingdom, such documentation should be more widely available (Fig. 10).

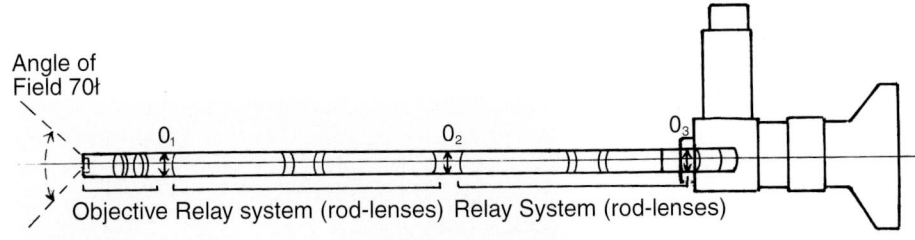

Angle of
Field 70⊦

O_1 O_2 O_3

Objective Relay system (rod-lenses) Relay System (rod-lenses)

FIGURE 6 Diagram to show the inside of a Hopkins rod.

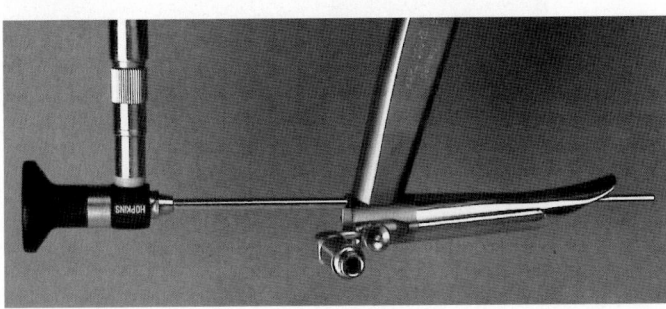

FIGURE 7 Telescope introduced through the laryngoscope.

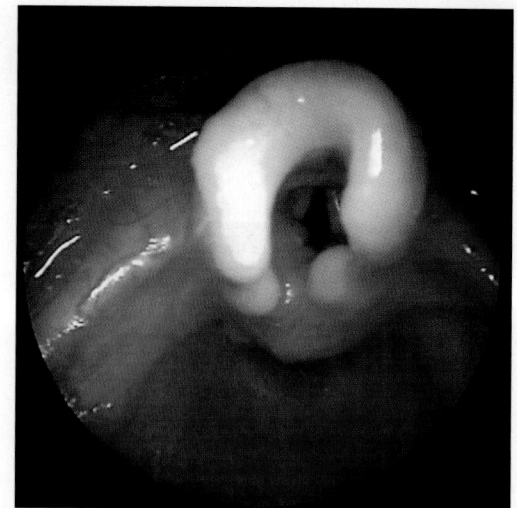

FIGURE 8 A neonatal larynx viewed with a 0-degree telescope.

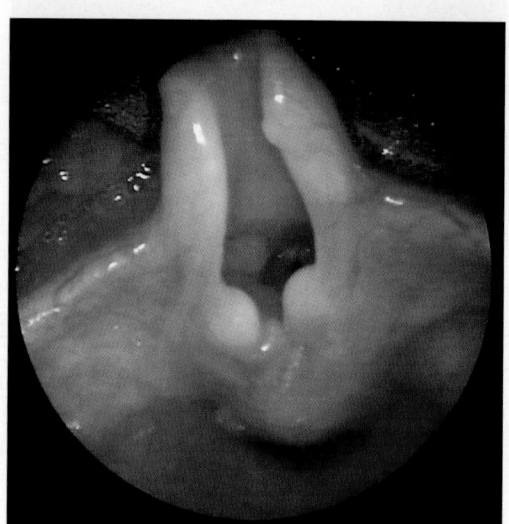

FIGURE 9 The same larynx viewed with a 30-degree telescope.

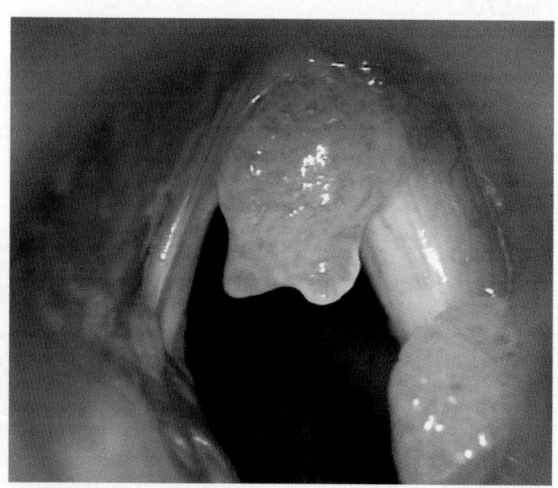

FIGURE 10 Laryngeal papillomas, to illustrate the picture that is filed in the patient's notes.

PEARLS AND PERILS

---

1. Make use of modern technology to make endoscopy as easy and safe as it can be. Do not use outdated equipment.
2. Make sure you are familiar with the instruments and can assemble them easily and confidently. Do not expect the nurse to do it for you if you cannot do it yourself.

ANESTHESIA

In all children, rigid airway endoscopy should be performed under general anesthesia. It is not appropriate for a surgeon to dictate the technique used but the author hopes the following pointers will be unexceptionable.

1. Try to work with the same anesthetist on a regular basis.
2. Never start endoscopy until venous access is secure, even if it means waiting.
3. The additional use of local anesthetic spray to the larynx and trachea improves the operative conditions.
4. A technique avoiding endotracheal intubation is preferable in most instances to allow maximum access to the larynx.
5. If the larynx cannot be visualized by the anesthetist, it will sometimes be accessible to a rigid bronchoscope.
6. Modern practice dictates the use of equipment for monitoring parameters such as continuous pulse rate, SpO_2, end-tidal carbon dioxide level, electrocardiographic data, blood pressure, and ventilatory pressures.
7. If there is upper-airway obstruction, tracheostomy may become necessary as a matter of urgency. Be prepared for such an eventuality.
8. Cooperation and trust between the anesthetist and surgeon should avoid loss of control over the airway.

OPERATIVE TECHNIQUE

Laryngoscopy

In most instances, examination of the larynx should be by telescope or microscope. The child should be positioned on the operating table with some elevation of the shoulders. The head in infants is relatively large and without some neck extension it will be difficult to see the larynx. The laryngoscope is introduced into the right side of the mouth. The left hand rests on the upper jaw and the thumb is used as a fulcrum. Care must be taken not to damage the teeth or the lips. The laryngoscope is advanced along the dorsum of the tongue until it comes to lie in the vallecula. Elevation of the beak of the laryngoscope will then give a good view of the vocal cords, the aryepiglottic folds, the arytenoid cartilages, and often the subglottis. The suspension apparatus is attached to the laryngoscope. Its distal end should rest on a stand attached firmly to the operating table, rather than on the child's chest or abdomen. When the laryngoscope is in place, check that the lips are free and not being damaged by the laryngoscope. At this point, make sure that you are sitting in a comfortable position. If necessary, adjust the operating table. Head-up tilt often gives a better angle of view, particularly with the microscope.

After a brief naked-eye assessment, the larynx can now be inspected with a 4.0-mm Hopkins rod telescope. If a video camera is available, such inspection can be done from the screen, and appropriate recordings made. Some form of antifog solution may need to be applied to the end of the telescope, but saliva from the patient's mouth is sometimes effective. The telescope can be passed through the vocal cords to give a view of the sub-glottis and upper trachea.

If the microscope is to be used for stereoscopic magnified inspection or for endola-ryngeal surgery, it should be fitted with a 400-mm objective lens to provide a suitable working distance. It may be helpful here to note that adult laryngeal instruments are too long for use in children, and instruments with a working length of 18 to 20 cm are pre-ferred.

Once the laryngoscopy is complete, do not withdraw the laryngoscope without con-firming with the anesthetist that you may do so. He or she may be using the instrument to maintain the airway or the anesthetic gas supply to the patient.

Bronchoscopy

Before starting bronchoscopy, make sure the equipment is properly assembled and of ap-propriate size. The light cable must be connected to the telescope and the telescope should be dipped in antifog solution. It is helpful to suck out secretions and residual lo-cal anesthetic solution from the hypopharynx before introduction of the bronchoscope, in order to avoid obscuring the view through the telescope.

The bronchoscope can be introduced in one of several ways. If you are not confident at passing the bronchoscope without delay, it can be helpful to visualize the vocal cords with either a slotted laryngoscope or the anesthetic laryngoscope. The bronchoscope can then be positioned above the cords under direct view. Look through the telescope and rotate the beak of the bronchoscope clockwise so that it slides gently between the cords. Do not push or force it.

An alternative technique if you are not an experienced bronchoscopist is to allow the anesthetist to pass an endotracheal tube. You can then follow the tube to the inlet of the larynx and position the bronchoscope above the cords. Withdrawal of the endotracheal tube will then enable you to pass the bronchoscope between the cords and into the trachea.

If you are more practiced, the bronchoscope can be introduced directly. Remember that until the bronchoscope is in the trachea, you have no control over the ventilation. Hold the bronchoscope in your right hand and support it with the thumb of the left hand, which is resting on the upper jaw (Fig. 11). Slide the instrument down the dorsum of the tongue until the epiglottis is seen. The bronchoscope is next insinuated behind the epiglottis, which is lifted forward. The cords will be visible. Rotate the beak of the bron-choscope clockwise to 45 degrees and slide it gently past the right cord. The scope will then pass into the subglottis. No force should be used. If the bronchoscope will not pass easily, use a smaller size to avoid damaging the subglottis. Once the instrument has been passed, you must confirm its position within the trachea. Identify tracheal rings and the bifurcation. Confirm also that it is possible to ventilate the patient. Only then should you

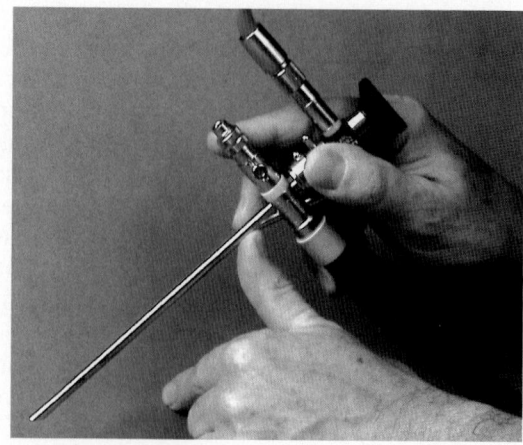

FIGURE 11 Demonstration of holding the bronchoscope for introduction into the pharynx.

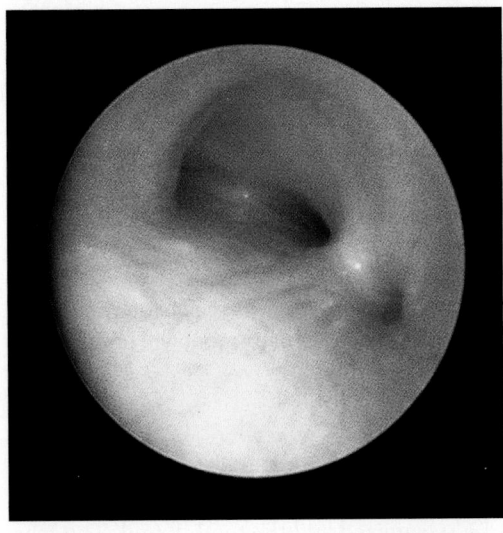

FIGURE 12 The right-upper-lobe bronchus opens directly from the trachea.

proceed to careful examination of the airway and carry out any necessary operative procedures.

The bronchoscope should be passed gently to the carina. By rotating the patient's head to one side or the other, it is then possible to enter each main bronchus in turn. In children, because the structures can be deformed with the bronchoscope, it is usually possible to inspect the opening of the upper-lobe bronchus, particularly on the right. Indeed, the right-upper-lobe bronchus occasionally opens directly onto the trachea above the carina (11) (Fig. 12). If it is not possible to visualize the smaller bronchial divisions, use a telescope longer than the bronchoscope tube. This can be passed beyond the end of the bronchoscope tube with ease. Examination of the airways continues during withdrawal of the bronchoscope. Do not withdraw the instrument from the upper trachea until you have agreed on such a move with your anesthetic colleague. You are handing back control of the airway, and this must be done in a controlled manner.

Once the bronchoscope has been removed, check that there is no injury to the teeth or lips.

PEARLS AND PERILS

1. Be sure that you are completely familiar with all the instruments.
2. Do not start airway endoscopy until venous access has been secured.
3. Airway endoscopy for obstruction should always include examination of the lower airways.
4. Never lose control over this airway.
5. Airway endoscopy is potentially lethal. If you are not sure you can do it safely and have the appropriate equipment, refer to someone who can and does.

COMPLICATIONS OF RIGID AIRWAY ENDOSCOPY

Loss of Control

Loss of control can lead to desaturation, bradycardia, asystole, and hypoxic brain damage. Avoidance depends on familiarity with the procedure, the instruments, and an early recognition that matters are getting out of control. Precipitating factors are as follows:

1. An already compromised airway.
2. Attempted instrumentation at too shallow a level of anesthesia, leading to laryngeal spasm.

3. An underlying cardiac abnormality such as cyanotic heart disease. Positive-pressure ventilation will impede venous return and cardiac filling.
4. A lack of venous access, preventing remedial measures.
5. Unfamiliarity with the instruments.
6. Inexperience on the part of the anesthetist or surgeon.

Injury to the Subglottis

Using too large a bronchoscope will result in damage to the subglottic mucosa, which can lead to postoperative edema and worsening airway obstruction. It may even precipitate the need for endotracheal intubation or tracheostomy. If the instrument will not pass easily, change to a smaller size.

Damage to the Teeth or Gums

Injury to the teeth is more likely to happen during laryngoscopy. Loose primary teeth may be knocked out. Such an event must be recognized and the tooth found. The maxilla in small babies is relatively mobile, and upward displacement of the maxilla may occur during suspension laryngoscopy from pressure by the laryngoscope.

Bleeding

Bleeding from the airway can be severe. Prejudicial factors are as follows:

1. A vascular lesion such as a laryngeal papilloma.
2. Hemangioma. This will not normally bleed on contact but biopsy may produce brisk hemorrhage.
3. Removal of a foreign body. If a foreign body has been present for some time, there may be surrounding granulations that can bleed briskly.

If bleeding occurs, the danger is not blood loss but impairment of gas flow and ventilation from drowning in blood. It is important to leave the bronchoscope in place in order to apply pressure and suction and to protect the other parts of the lungs. The management of airway bleeding is reviewed by Stradling (12).

Pneumothorax

This is more likely to occur with airway obstruction or if positive-pressure ventilation is necessary. Recognition is the key to management with pleural drainage.

Failure to Recognize Abnormalities

Failure to recognize the abnormality present, while not strictly a complication, may necessitate further intervention. Do not embark solo on airway endoscopy unless you are familiar with the abnormalities you may encounter and know how to deal with them.

Hoeve et al (11) reviewed 1,332 rigid laryngobronchoscopies in children and noted a complication rate of 1.9%. They identified the risk factors in 25 cases with complications:

Fallot's tetralogy	4/14	29%
Biopsy/drainage of abscess	5/64	8%
Foreign body extraction	5/75	7%
Tracheal stenosis	2/64	3%
Age <3 months	2/394	0.5%
3 to 12 months	8/361	2.2%
12 to 36 months	8/322	2.5%
>36 months	7/255	2.7%

PEARLS AND PERILS

1. Complications are more likely if some additional intervention is necessary.
2. Early recognition of impending difficulties should avoid the downward spiral into chaos.
3. Try to work regularly with the same anesthetist, so each may trust the other.

REFERENCES

1. Thomson StC. The Garcia centenary and the Jubilee of laryngoscopy. *Laryngoscope* 1905;15:179.
2. Babington BG. Description of the glottiscope. *Lond Med Gaz* 1829;3:555.
3. Liston R. *Practical surgery.* London: J Churchill, 1837:350.
4. Garcia M. Observations on the human voice. *Proc R Soc Lond* 1854–55;7:399–410.
5. Czermak JN. Physiologische Untersuchungen mit Garcias Kehlkopfspiegel. *SBK Akad Wiss Wien* mat-nat CL: 1858;29:557–584.
6. Davis HW, Gartner JC, Galvis AG, et al. Acute upper airway obstruction; croup and epiglottitis. *Pediatr Clin North Am* 1981;28:859.
7. Bush A. Review—neonatal bronchoscopy. *Eur J Pediatr.* 1994;153[Suppl 2]:S27–S29.
8. Benjamin B. *Atlas of paediatric endoscopy.* Oxford: Oxford University Press, 1981.
9. Stankiewicz JA, Holinger LD. Endoscopic sizing: an attempt at uniformity. *Laryngoscopy* 1986;96:997–1001.
10. Marzo SJ, Hotaling AJ. Trade-off between airway resistance and optical resolution in pediatric rigid bronchoscopy. *Ann Otol Rhinol* 1995;104:282–287.
11. Hoeve LJ, Rombout J, Meursing AEE. Complications of rigid laryngobronchoscopy in children. *Int J Pediatr Otorhinolaryngol* 1993;26:47–56.
12. Stradling P. *Diagnostic bronchoscopy,* 4th ed. Edinburgh: Churchill Livingstone, 1981: 120–133.

P.D. Bull: Department of Otolaryngology, Sheffield Children's Hospital, University of Sheffield, Western Bank, Sheffied S10 2TH, United Kingdom.

- *Practical Pediatric Otolaryngology*
- edited by Robin T. Cotton and Charles M. Myer, III
- Lippincott-Raven Publishers, Philadelphia © 1999

29B

Evaluation of the Pediatric Airway by Flexible Endoscopy

Pierre A. Vauthy

Pediatric flexible endoscopy of the airway was initiated in the mid-1970s with the introduction of flexible endoscopes 3.5 mm in diameter. Since that time, newer instruments with suction channels and smaller-diameter bronchoscopes have enabled physicians to visualize the airway of premature infants, infants, and children without the need of general anesthesia and without significantly distorting the anatomy and normal physiology of the upper airway during instrumentation (1–8).

The advantages of fiberoptic airway evaluation are significant when compared to conventional laryngoscopy and rigid bronchoscopy. The procedure may be performed on an outpatient basis and requires little preparation other than making sure the patient has no oral intake 4 to 6 hours prior to the instrumentation. A procedure room is the preferred site for the endoscopy. The room should include: oxygen, suction, pulse oximetry, electrocardiographic and respiratory monitors, a resuscitation cart, and a video system to document the procedure (9).

Personnel requirements include an individual who is trained in monitoring endoscopy patients. The individual should be PALS certified and trained in intravenous (IV) access and conscious sedation. Monitoring of the patient by the endoscopy assistant and with electrical monitors is mandatory to ensure a safe and rapid procedure. The assistant is present to ensure the patient's physiologic status is maintained, as the bronchoscopist may be engrossed by the procedure.

Preparation of the patient for endoscopy is of paramount importance. Psychological preparation of older children results in more comfort and often shorter procedures as well as reduces the dose of sedatives required during the procedure (7).

Infants up to 18 months old can easily tolerate endoscopy utilizing only lidocaine (Xylocaine) jelly in the nose. Endoscopy of these patients has never resulted in laryngospasm. Therefore, they are not routinely premedicated with either atropine or topical anesthesia of the vocal cords (8). Some centers, however, do premedicate patients. The patient is placed on the papoose board with the endoscopy assistant providing oxygen by either mask or nasal cannula. IV sedation has not been required in this age group. The average diagnostic procedure lasts approximately 30 seconds and is videotaped for in-depth evaluations, thus reducing the need to stay in the child's airway for prolonged periods of time. A very informative video can be obtained even with the 2.2-mm bronchoscope. In older children, both psychological preparation and IV sedation are utilized. Nasal lidocaine is used, as in the small children, as well as an aerosolized anesthetic, usually 2% to 4% lidocaine. IV insertion is performed after the site is prepared with Emla, a topical anesthetic that reduces the pain and stress of the procedure. The benzodiazopine midazolam is the mainstay of sedation and the effect can be reversed if necessary. The dose of midazolam is 0.1 per kilogram IV, with a maximum dosage of 3 to 4 mg per procedure. Reversal can be accomplished with flumazenil. Narcotics also have a role and are also reversible. The endoscopist, however, must be highly skilled in both airway management and conscious sedation if he or she is to use these medications.

Postprocedure management in nonsedated children includes examination after the procedure and one-half hour of observation. The patient is then allowed to feed under supervision and, if stable, is discharged following a second one-half hour of observation. Sedated patients are recovered in a postprocedure holding area and are discharged when stable.

SAFETY

The safety of this procedure in this population has been demonstrated in the evaluation of both the upper and the lower airway. There have been 10,000 bronchoscopies performed at the author's center, with zero mortality (8). In the literature, there has been one reported mortality of a patient who underwent bronchial lavage and who was seriously ill (10). If this procedure is performed with close monitoring and performed quickly, with attention to both adequate oxygenation and ventilation of the patient, it is extremely safe in even extremely ill patients (1,6,8,11). Adequate oxygenation of the patient can be accomplished by insufflating oxygen through the suction channel on an intermittent basis throughout the procedure. Morbidity is minimal and usually related to epistaxis, laryngospasm secondary to topical anesthetics, and extremely rare episodes of pneumothorax. There have been four episodes of pneumothorax in over 10,000 bronchoscopies at the author's center. Three were simple pneumothoraces not requiring any intervention, and one was an episode of tension pneumothorax that was treated with closed chest thoracotomy. The latter occurred after vigorous suctioning of an airway filled with thick mucous plugs.

INFANT ENDOSCOPY

The experience at the author's center demonstrates that 58% of fiberoptic bronchoscopies are performed in children less than 1 year old (8) (Table 1). Table 2 lists indications for endoscopy in children under 1 year old. The most common indication, stridor, has many etiologies (Table 3). As can be seen from Table 3, many diagnoses account for this clinical symptom. Of greater importance is the finding that a significant number of patients with stridor have both supraglottic and subglottic pathology. The author's findings corroborate those of Wood and Gonzales and support the need for evaluating the upper and lower airway in stridorous patients (8,12).

Infants as small as 450 g have undergone fiberoptic evaluation with the 2.2-mm Olympus fiberoptic bronchoscope. This instrument allows evaluation of very small infants as well as transtracheal airway evaluation of patients who are intubated with tubes as small as 2.5 mm (2,3,13–15). These small instruments also permit the placement of nasal tracheal tubes in infants with severe deformities of the face, tongue, or mandible (16). Intubation over the fiberoptic bronchoscope is simple and requires insertion of the endotracheal tube over the shaft of the bronchoscope as far proximatively as possible.

TABLE 1: Patient Population

0–1 mo	13%
1–6 mo	27%
6–12 mo	18%
12–24 mo	17%
2–6 yr	12%
8–12 yr	8%
>12 yr	5%

TABLE 2: Indications for Endoscopy

Stridor	48%
Bronchoalveolar lavage	8%
Apnea	7%
Intubation	6%
Foreign body	5%
Atelectasis	4%
Persistent wheezing	4%
Airway trauma	2%
Miscellaneous	1%

This is done to make sure that the mobility of the tip of instrument is not compromised by the endotracheal tube as it is being inserted into the airway (12). The instrument is inserted through the anterior nares. Once the bronchoscope is in the midtrachea, the endotracheal tube is pulled over the instrument and placed into the tracheal lumen. The fiberoptic bronchoscope is then used to confirm the level of the endotracheal tube in the airway as it is pulled out of the patient (17).

In hyperinflation syndromes of a single lung, the fiberoptic bronchoscope not only is useful in evaluating the possible etiology of the pathologic process, but also allows for the placement of the nasal tracheal or oral tracheal tube into the contralateral lung. This allows for the safe deflation of the involved lung in cases of pulmonary interstitial emphysema (18).

PEDIATRIC ENDOSCOPY

Full-term infants up to adolescents tolerate bronchoscopy with the 3.4-mm instruments, which have suction channels that can be utilized for insufflation of oxygen, suction, bronchial brushings, or bronchoalveolar lavage.

ACUTE AIRWAY OBSTRUCTION

Acute airway obstruction in pediatrics is commonly due to viral or bacterial infections of the glottis or subglottic airway. Therefore, the fiberoptic bronchoscope can delineate the level of obstruction and its etiology, and in many instances, it can be used as a therapeutic tool to secure an airway. Membranous tracheitis has become the most frequent diagnosis of airway obstruction in the author's pediatric intensive care unit (1). Affected patients commonly have subglottic edema and the membranes are rarely seen un-

TABLE 3: Stridor Bronchoscopic Findings

Arytenoidal malacia	27
Tracheal pathology	18
Vocal cord paresis/paralysis	11
Subglottic stenosis	10
Membranous tracheitis	9
Subglottic edema	7
No finding	5
Nasal edema or narrowing	12
Both upper- and lower-airway findings	18%

less the trachea is visualized. The patients often respond well to suctioning of the membranes via the bronchoscope. If placement of an airway is necessary, then the endotracheal tube is inserted over the fiberoptic bronchoscope after suctioning has been completed. Intubation for membranous tracheitis without removal of the membranes can be fatal because they can be dislodged distally.

FOREIGN BODY ASPIRATION

Foreign body aspiration is common in children 6 months and older. The fiberoptic bronchoscope can be used to diagnose this problem, especially in patients with a history of acute episodes of aspiration without physical or radiologic findings (12).

The procedure is performed on an outpatient basis and, if a foreign body is found, it is removed by conventional endoscopy. The fiberoptic bronchoscope should not be utilized to remove a foreign body. Persistent wheezing unresponsive to conventional treatment has become an indication for endoscopy, and as with most fiberoptic bronchoscopic procedures, this study can also be performed on an outpatient basis.

BRONCHOALVEOLAR LAVAGE

Bronchoalveolar lavage has become a very useful tool for the diagnosis of infections, gastroesophageal reflux, and the removal of mucous plugs (19–21). The endoscopic procedure is amenable to both inpatient and outpatient settings, and the avoidance of general anesthesia, intubation, and mechanical ventilation reduces the cost and possible complications of these interventions (22).

TRACHEOSTOMY EVALUATIONS

Determining the appropriate time for decannulation of a tracheostomy tube is facilitated by use of the fiberoptic bronchoscope for upper-airway and suprastoma and substoma airway evaluations (4,23). The 2.2-mm fiberoptic bronchoscope is ideally suited for this procedure.

BRONCHOSCOPY IN THE PEDIATRIC INTENSIVE CARE UNIT

The use of the fiberoptic bronchoscope in the pediatric intensive care unit has become a very common procedure for both diagnostic and therapeutic purposes (23–25). The fiberoptic bronchoscope is used to intubate all patients admitted to the author's intensive care unit on both emergent and elective basis. In spontaneously breathing patients, the placement of nasal tracheal tubes by this fashion has resulted in a negligible incidence of subglottic stenosis and accidental extubations. Patients with possible neck injuries or thermal burns are also intubated in this manner. Sedation is given prior to the procedure; however, none of these patients require rapid sequence intubation, which can result in hypoxia if an airway cannot be secured rapidly due to concomitant respiratory paralysis. With the availability of trained endoscopists in emergency rooms and intensive care units, there should be little to no necessity for blind nasal tracheal intubation and its attended complications.

The therapeutic use of the bronchoscope in intubated patients is relegated to the evaluation of upper-airway-structure readiness for extubation in patients with supraglottitis (26). In patients with atelectasis, the bronchoscope is quite useful in either suctioning or lavaging airways that are filled with secretions (27,28). Obtaining specimens for bacteriology is simple, but has many pitfalls owing to contamination that can occur during the passage of the instrument through the airway.

OBSTRUCTIVE SLEEP APNEA

Obstructive sleep apnea is a phenomenon that is seen more and more frequently in children as young as 1 year. The most common findings are enlarged tonsils and adenoids. Often the tonsils are found to fall over the airway when the patient is asleep. Other anatomic and physiologic abnormalities can cause obstructive sleep apnea and are easily diagnosed with the fiberoptic bronchoscope. A positive upper-airway evaluation can make sleep studies of superfluous value.

SUMMARY

The efficacy of fiberoptic bronchoscopy has been documented in multiple publications. The fiberoptic bronchoscope has been a superb diagnostic and therapeutic instrument in the neonatal intensive care unit, the pediatric intensive care unit, and the operating room, as well as at the bedside and in the outpatient setting. In skilled hands, this procedure is safe and has excellent diagnostic yield. In the author's series, 87% fiberoptic evaluations of the airway have been informative (8). The ability to evaluate the upper airway and trachea with the patient awake or lightly sedated provides important information often lost in anesthetized patients. Both children and parents welcome the decreased time spent in the hospital, owing to performing endoscopy on an outpatient basis, as well as the reduced medical costs.

⚙ REFERENCES

1. Vauthy PA, Reddy R. Acute upper airway obstruction in infants and children. Evaluation by fiberoptic bronchoscopy. *Ann Otol Rhinol Laryngol* 1980;89:417–418.
2. Fan LL, Sparks LM, Dulinski JP. Applications of an ultrathin bronchoscope for neonatal and pediatric airway problems. *Chest* 1986;89:673–676.
3. Nusbaum E. Usefulness of miniature flexible fiberoptic bronchoscopy in children. *Chest* 1994;106:1438–1442.
4. Wood RE. Clinical applications of ultrathin flexible bronchoscopes. *Pediatr Pulmonol* 1985;1:244–248.
5. Wood RE. The diagnostic effectiveness of the flexible bronchoscope in children. *Pediatr Pulmonol* 1985;1:188–192.
6. Wood RE. Spelunking the pediatric airway. *Pediatr Clin North Am* 1984;31:785–799.
7. Perez CR, Wood RE. Update on pediatric flexible bronchoscopy. *Pediatr Clin North Am* 1994;41:385–400.
8. Vauthy PA, Snedden SS. Pediatric fiberoptic bronchoscopy without sedation. Abstract presented at the 7th World Congress of Bronchoscopy, Mayo Clinic, October 1992.
9. Riff E, Mitra S, Baker M. Pediatric fiberoptic video bronchoscopy: the use of computer interfacing. *Comput Biol Med* 1993;23:345–347.
10. Wagener JS. Fatality following fiberoptic bronchoscopy in a two year old child. *Pediatr Pulmonol* 1987;3:197–199.
11. Fulkerson WJ. Fiberoptic bronchoscopy. *N Engl J Med* 1984;311:511–515.
12. Wood RE. Pitfalls in the use of the flexible bronchoscope in pediatric patients. *Chest* 1990;97:199–203.
13. Schellhase DE, Graham LM, Fix EJ, Sparks LN, Fan LL. Diagnosis of tracheal injury in mechanically ventilated premature infants by flexible bronchoscopy. *Chest* 1990;98:1219–1224.
14. Wood RE. Clinical applications of ultrathin bronchoscopes. *Pediatr Pulmonol* 1985; 1:255–258.
15. Myers CM III, Thompson RF. Flexible bronchoscopy in the neonatal intensive care unit. *Int J Pediatr Otorhinolaryngol* 1988;15:143–147.
16. Stella JP, Kageler WV, Epker BN. Fiberoptic endotracheal intubation in oral and maxillofacial surgery. *J Oral Maxillofac Surg* 1986;44:923–925.

17. Finer NN, Muzyka D. Flexible endoscopy intubation of the neonate. *Pediatr Pulmonol* 1992;12:48–51.

18. Brooks JG, Bustamante SA, Koops BL. Selective bronchial intubations for the treatment pulmonary interstitial emphysema in newborn infants. *J Pediatr* 1997;91:648–652.

19. Abadco DL, Amaro-Galvez R, Rao M, et al. Experience with flexible fiberoptic bronchoscopy with bronchoalveolar lavage as a diagnostic tool in children with AIDS. *Am J Dis Child* 1992;146:1056–1059.

20. Chan S, Abadco DL, Steiner P. Role of flexible fiberoptic bronchoscopy in the diagnosis of childhood endobronchial tuberculosis. *Pediatr Infect Dis J* 1994;13:506–509.

21. Nusbaum E, Maggi JC, Mathis R. Galant S. Association of lipid laden alveolar macrophages and gastroesophageal reflux in children. *J Pediatr* 1987;110:190–194.

22. Kurland G, Noyes BE, Jaffe R, Atlas AB, Armitage J, Orenstein DM. Bronchoalveolar lavage and transbronchial biopsy in children following heart-lung and lung transplantation. *Chest* 1993;104:1043–1048.

23. Todres ID, Novisk N. Flexible fiberoptic bronchoscopy. *M Sinai J Med* 1995;62:36–39.

24. Olopade CO, Prakash V. Bronchoscopy in the critical care unit. *Mayo Clin Proc* 1989; 64:1255–1263.

25. Fan LL, Sparks L, Fix E. Flexible endoscopy for airway problems in a pediatric intensive care unit. *Chest* 1988;93:556–560.

26. Nusbaum EN. Fiberoptic laryngoscopy as a guide to tracheal extubation in acute epiglottitis. *J Pediatr* 1983;102:269–270.

27. Haenel JB, Moore FA, Moore EE, Read R. Efficacy of intrabronchial air insufflation in acute lobar collapse. *Am J Surg* 1992;164:501–505.

28. Nusbaum EN. Pediatric flexible bronchoscopy and its application in infantile atelectasis. *Clin Pediatr* 1985;24:379–382.

P.A. Vauthy: Department of Pediatrics, Children's Medical Center of Northwest Ohio, Toledo, Ohio 43606.

• *Practical Pediatric Otolaryngology*
• edited by Robin T. Cotton
  and Charles M. Myer, III
• Lippincott-Raven Publishers,
  Philadelphia © 1999

Congenital Anomalies of the Larynx

Robin T. Cotton & Christopher A. J. Prescott

Abnormalities of the airway frequently present with stridor. Stridor is not a diagnosis but rather a symptom, caused by turbulent airflow through a partial obstruction of the airway. Stridor may be inspiratory, expiratory, or biphasic depending on the location of the obstruction in the upper airway. Severe airway obstruction may not be associated with stridor if the rate of airflow past an obstruction is inadequate to generate audible turbulent airflow. Patients with stridor require immediate evaluation, because significant respiratory compromise and death may occur if proper treatment is not initiated in a timely fashion.

Stridor in the majority of infants is due to pathology of the larynx. Less common causes of stridor are tracheal or bronchial lesions. Congenital anomalies of the larynx not only impede the ventilatory function of the larynx, producing stridor, but also impair its ability to protect the lower respiratory tract. Feeding difficulties may result, presenting as frank dysphagia or subtle aspiration. The extent of laryngeal dysfunction is directly proportional to the degree of laryngeal disturbance. Symptoms of congenital laryngeal anomalies frequently present at birth but may be delayed. The common congenital laryngeal anomalies are discussed with regard to their clinical presentation and management.

LARYNGOMALACIA

Laryngomalacia is the most common congenital laryngeal anomaly (1,2). Boys are affected twice as often as girls. It is generally a self-limiting condition, but when severe may produce life-threatening obstructive apnea, cor pulmonale, and failure to thrive (3). It arises from a continued immaturity of the larynx, as if the fetal stage of laryngeal development has persisted. Several anatomic features may be observed. The aryepiglottic folds are short, and often, though not always, the epiglottis is excessively curled, often called an *omega-shaped epiglottis*. The effect of the short aryepiglottic folds is to draw the cuneiform and corniculate cartilages, situated superiorly on the arytenoid cartilage, forward over the laryngeal inlet, in which position it tends to prolapse during inspiration. When supraglottoplasty is planned, it is important to understand that there is more than one obstructing mechanism in laryngomalacia: the prolapsing cuneiform and corniculate cartilages may flop over the airway ("floppers"), the curled epiglottis may indraw ("curlers"), or there may be a combination of both (Fig. 1). Furthermore, the cuneiform, corniculate, and arytenoid cartilages may have a redundant mucosal covering, and the supraglottic laryngeal structures are tethered, practically obstructing the laryngeal inlet (Table 1).

Though laryngomalacia is generally recognized as a cause of stridor and airway obstruction in infants, with growth, laryngomalacia may manifest in different and unex-

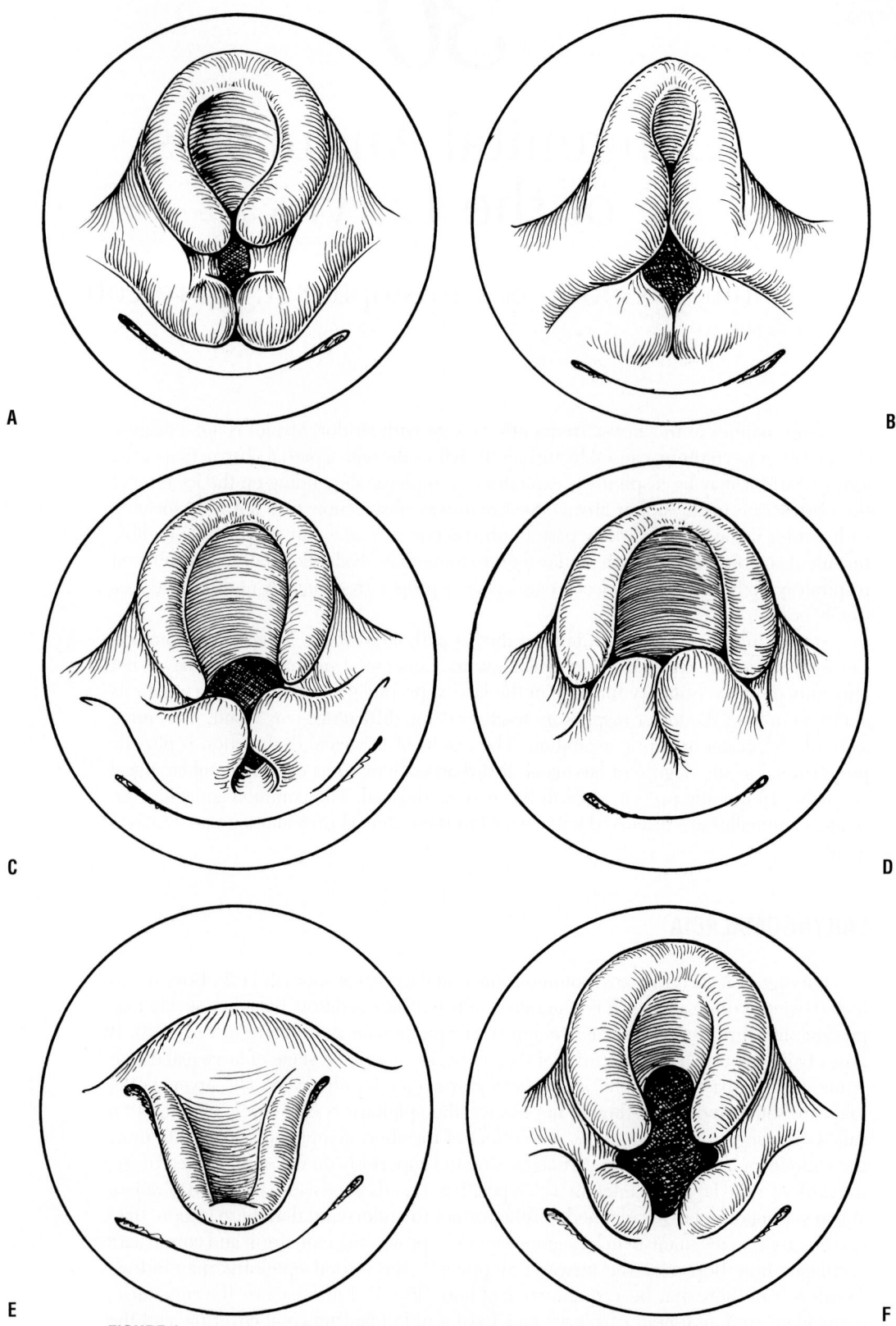

FIGURE 1 Mechanisms of laryngomalacia (after Holinger). **A:** Type I: Inward collapse of aryepiglottic folds. **B:** Type II: Tubular epiglottis. **C:** Type III: Collapse of cuneiform cartilages. **D:** Type III: Collapse of cuneiform cartilages. **E:** Type IV: Epiglottic displacement. **F:** Type V: Short aryepiglottic folds.

TABLE 1: Types of Laryngomalacia

Type I	Inward collapse of the aryepiglottic folds, primarily the cuneiform and corniculate cartilages, which often are enlarged. Obstruction occurs as these cartilages are drawn inward during inspiration. Similar to a one-way valve, they open passively during expiration.
Type II	A long, tubular epiglottis (a pathologic exaggeration of the normal omega shape), which curls on itself and contributes to obstruction during inspiration. This often occurs in association with type I laryngomalacia.
Type III	Anterior, medial collapse of the cuneiform and corniculate cartilages to occlude the laryngeal inlet during inspiration.
Type IV	Posterior inspiratory displacement of the epiglottis against the posterior pharyngeal wall or inferior collapse to the vocal folds.
Type V	Short aryepiglottic folds.

pected ways. Athletes may generate significant inspiratory force to draw the aryepiglottic folds into the endolarynx, causing a subtotal glottic obstruction. This exercise-induced laryngomalacia (4) may be overlooked in children or young adults and be misdiagnosed as asthma, lack of fitness, or functional abnormalities.

 PATIENT ASSESSMENT

Symptoms

Symptoms of laryngomalacia generally present within the first 2 weeks of life. Inspiratory stridor and noisy respiration are noted and can be quite variable, occurring both at rest and when agitated. The circumferential rimming of the supraglottic airway and aryepiglottic folds produces the fluttering quality of the inspiratory noise associated with laryngomalacia. Expiration forces these tissues out of the airway and generally produces no noise. The amount of prolapse depends on the negative inspiratory pressure, and this is increased during more forceable inspiratory efforts. During a quiet inspiratory effort, there may be no significant prolapse, but with increasing inspiratory effort, there is increasing obstruction, which can at times be of such a degree to allow no significant airflow.

The airway noise is frequently related to position. A supine position is classically more aggravating to the condition than a prone position; a reclining position during feeding may also increase the degree of stridor. Neck extension will frequently decrease the intensity of airway noise. Symptoms increase over the first several months. Affected infants will maintain a normal cry without cyanosis, and while dyspnea is rarely experienced, feeding difficulties are not uncommon. The feeding difficulties are related to two mechanisms: First, feeding is a strenuous activity that stresses an already compromised airway; second, gastroesophageal and gastropharyngeal reflux is exacerbated in infants, secondary to the increase in negative intrathoracic pressure generated by inspiratory forces against a partially obstructed supraglottis. While most patients with laryngomalacia have a benign clinical course, some infants develop severe obstruction, pectus excavatum, life-threatening cor pulmonale, obstructive apnea, and failure to thrive. Most often a gradual resolution of symptoms occurs by the age of 18 months.

While several explanations have been proposed for the development of laryngomalacia, none properly explain the distribution of the condition in the population. Most theories incorporate an element of immaturity, either of the cartilaginous elements or of neuromuscular control, to account for the supraglottic structures being drawn into the supraglottic airway. It has been postulated that neurologic immaturity of the brain stem causes inadequate coordination of the laryngeal musculature, resulting in the paradoxical arytenoid movement on inspiration. These theories would predict an increased representation of premature infants and infants with hypotonia. The premature infant does not appear to be at an increased risk for the development of laryngomalacia. The hypotonic infant is difficult to evaluate because hypopharyngeal collapse and glossoptosis seem to exert a much greater effect on the airway than does the laryngomalacia. Histologic studies of the larynx of laryngomalacia patients have failed to demonstrate any significant alterations of the cartilaginous or muscular elements to account for the clinical findings of laryngomalacia. Much work remains to be done to define the factors involved with the development of laryngomalacia.

Diagnosis

Radiographic studies may suggest the diagnosis of laryngomalacia (5). There is frequently medial and inferior displacement of the arytenoids and epiglottis. Because this is a dynamic process, the film must be taken during inspiration and with neck extension to identify the abnormalities. Fluoroscopy is better able to illustrate the dynamic nature of the problem and demonstrate the collapse of the supraglottic structures with inspiration. Hypopharyngeal dilation is also seen on inspiration, accentuating the laryngeal obstruction. Chest radiographs should also be obtained to rule out associated anomalies of the lower respiratory tract, such as innominate artery compression, tracheomalacia, and vascular rings.

The mainstay of diagnosis for laryngomalacia, however, is flexible laryngoscopy. This is best done in an unanesthetized child in an upright position with a 1.9-mm nasopharyngoscope. The scope should be passed through each side of the nose without any preoperative medication, to assess both nasal passages, the nasopharynx, and supraglottic larynx. The anatomic abnormalities outlined above are looked for, and a determination can be made as to the relative obstruction caused by the flopping cuneiform and corniculate cartilages, the curled epiglottis, the short aryepiglottic folds, or the bulky soft tissue of the supraglottis. The vocal cords in laryngomalacia are mobile. With increasing severity of the laryngomalacia, the ability to visualize the vocal cords, however, decreases. In severe laryngomalacia, the vocal cords cannot be seen due to the supraglottic collapse, and very careful examination for a coexisting vocal cord paralysis (unilateral or bilateral) must be undertaken.

TREATMENT RECOMMENDATIONS

The majority of patients with laryngomalacia require no intervention. Continued vigilance on the part of the otolaryngologist is required to ensure adequate feeding abilities, continued growth, and that the child is not developing significant cardiopulmonary complications. In patients with obstructive apnea, failure to thrive, or other complications related to airway compromise, surgical intervention may be required.

In the past, tracheotomy was the preferred surgical procedure for severe laryngomalacia. The area of obstruction was bypassed until the supraglottic pathology spontaneously resolved. Supraglottoplasty (3,6,7) is an alternative method that has proved successful in the correction of the supraglottic obstruction, has avoided the need for tracheotomy, and is now the preferred surgical procedure for the management of severe laryngomalacia. Tracheotomy may be required if there are other obstructing procedures in the airway such as pharyngomalacia (8). Direct laryngoscopy and bronchoscopy must be performed prior to the supraglottoplasty to rule out concomitant pathology contributing to the obstruction of the airway. The precise mechanism of the obstruction is identified by flexible laryngoscopy while the infant is awake and by direct laryngoscopy while the infant is breathing spontaneously under anesthesia. Surgical maneuvers that may be necessary include trimming the lateral edges of the epiglottis, removing a wedge of tissue from restrictive aryepiglottic folds, and excision of redundant mucosa and cartilage in the region of the cuneiform and corniculate cartilages. This may be performed either with sharp dissection using ear instruments or laryngeal microinstruments depending on the age of the infant, or with the carbon dioxide (CO_2) laser (9), with the micropoint manipulator using superpulse on 2- to 3-W power. It is important to be conservative in removing tissue to avoid the serious complication of supraglottic stenosis. Unilateral supraglottoplasty (10) should be considered and the second side operated on only if symptoms do not resolve. Although other methods of surgical relief have been suggested, including suturing the epiglottis to the base of the tongue and hyomandibulopexy, supraglottoplasty is presently the surgical therapy of choice.

MANAGEMENT OF COMPLICATIONS

Complications of supraglottoplasty are unusual; aspiration and supraglottic stenosis may be seen if too much tissue has been removed. It is better to be conservative and perform a unilateral supraglottoplasty, even though this approach occasionally leads to a second procedure. The patients are usually left intubated overnight with extubation the following morning. Antibiotic coverage is maintained for 5 days to prevent supraglottic infection. Perioperative use of antireflux measures (positioning and medications) is recommended to minimize the effect of gastric secretions on raw mucosal surfaces.

VOCAL CORD PARALYSIS

Vocal cord paralysis is the second most common congenital laryngeal anomaly. The paralysis may be unilateral or bilateral. The etiology of congenital vocal cord paralysis is secondary to a neurologic abnormality. In general, bilateral paralysis is secondary to a central nervous system problem, while unilateral paralysis is caused by injury to the peripheral nervous system. The entire course of the recurrent laryngeal nerve must be evaluated in patients with unilateral vocal cord paralysis if the paralysis persists after 2 weeks. A chest x-ray film may demonstrate cardiac or great-vessel anomalies that impinge on the recurrent laryngeal nerve. The left recurrent laryngeal nerve is more prone to injury than the right, owing to the longer course that the nerve takes through the neck and mediastinum. The birth history may elicit a clue as to the etiology of the paralysis. A difficult delivery may result in stretching of the neck, with traction on the recurrent laryngeal nerve that may cause a unilateral paralysis.

Bilateral vocal cord paralysis is usually due to a central disorder. Head ultrasonography or magnetic resonance imaging (MRI) is necessary to diagnose a variety of central nervous system problems such as intracerebral hemorrhage, cerebral agenesis, hydrocephalus, and Arnold-Chiari malformation of the brainstem with herniation. Multiple cranial nerve deficits are common in infants with bilateral vocal cord paralysis. As a result, the incidence of chronic aspiration and dysphagia is increased in these patients. Some cases of vocal cord paralysis will have no identifiable cause. Paralysis of one or both vocal cords occurs occasionally as a complication of surgery for congenital lesions of the cardiovascular system or gastrointestinal tract, despite the best efforts of accomplished surgeons to avoid injury to the recurrent laryngeal nerves. Occasionally, other types of trauma to the nerve can occur either internally (endotracheal tube) or externally (neck surgery). Generalized neurologic disease in infants rarely causes vocal cord paralysis.

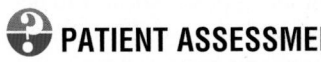 **PATIENT ASSESSMENT**

Symptoms

The symptoms of unilateral vocal cord paralysis may be present at birth or may develop over the first several weeks of life. Unilateral paralysis is often well tolerated by the neonate and delayed diagnosis is not uncommon. Airway obstruction is minimal, and stridor is apparent only with periods of aggravation or stress. A weak or hoarse, breathy cry is commonly present with unilateral paralysis. Feeding difficulties, such as aspiration, may be present but are generally manageable without surgical intervention. Positioning the patient so that the paralyzed vocal cord is inferior during feeding, combined with thickening agents added to the infant's food when necessary, allows adequate nutritional intake in the majority of patients. Positioning the patient with the paralyzed vocal cord inferior will often improve the airway during periods of quiet respiration.

Bilateral vocal cord paralysis presents with acute airway distress. The cry is normal and there is a characteristic high-pitched inspiratory stridor that is present at rest and markedly exacerbated with agitation. Bilateral vocal cord paralysis is poorly tolerated in most neonates and though an artifical airway is not universally necessary (11), emergent intubation is frequently required to stabilize the airway, followed by tracheotomy.

Diagnosis

The diagnosis of vocal cord paralysis is made by flexible laryngoscopy while the infant is awake. Direct laryngoscopy and bronchoscopy are generally reserved for evaluation for bilateral vocal cord paralysis and unresolved unilateral paralysis. Concomitant airway pathology may exist. Awake laryngoscopy is the preferable method of diagnosing vocal cord paralysis, because general anesthesia affects the mobility of the cords. On the emergence from anesthesia, the return of vocal cord function is not symmetric or predictable, so observations of mobility at this time may not be representative of the true picture. Occasionally, the infant's supraglottic airway precludes adequate visualization of the vocal cords with the flexible scope and an awake direct laryngoscopy may be needed.

The differential diagnosis of vocal cord paralysis includes cricoarytenoid joint fixation, posterior glottic web or stenosis, and infiltrative lesions of the vocal cords. For this reason, awake flexible laryngoscopy is supplemented by direct laryngoscopy under general anesthesia. After complete relaxation has been obtained, the arytenoid cartilage is carefully palpated to assess passive mobility and the true vocal cord is palpated for tone and stiffness. The posterior glottis is carefully inspected for any pathology. Complete microlaryngoscopy and bronchoscopy are now performed.

Laryngeal electromyography (12) in infants has been suggested as an adjunct in diagnosis, but in this age group, it is not an established technique for diagnosis. Similarly, ultrasonography (13) has been suggested as an investigation to aid in the follow-up of these patients, but is not widely used.

TREATMENT RECOMMENDATIONS

Unilateral vocal cord paralysis often resolves in the first few weeks of life. Bilateral vocal cord paralysis secondary to neurologic problems often improves when the neurologic problem is treated. Idiopathic vocal cord paralysis may resolve in the first few months of life. If function has not recovered by the age of 2 years, it is unlikely to do so.

Unilateral Paralysis

Most often no therapy is required, because compensation of the opposite vocal cord occurs with time and growth. For this reason, very little laryngeal framework surgery is done in children. On rare occasions, severe aspiration and dysphonia can result from unilateral vocal cord paralysis. While observation and speech therapy are the standard treatment, surgery is appropriate if serious symptoms persist. The choices are vocal cord injection with an absorbable gelatin sponge (Gelfoam) for a temporary effect (14) or laryngeal framework surgery for a more permanent effect.

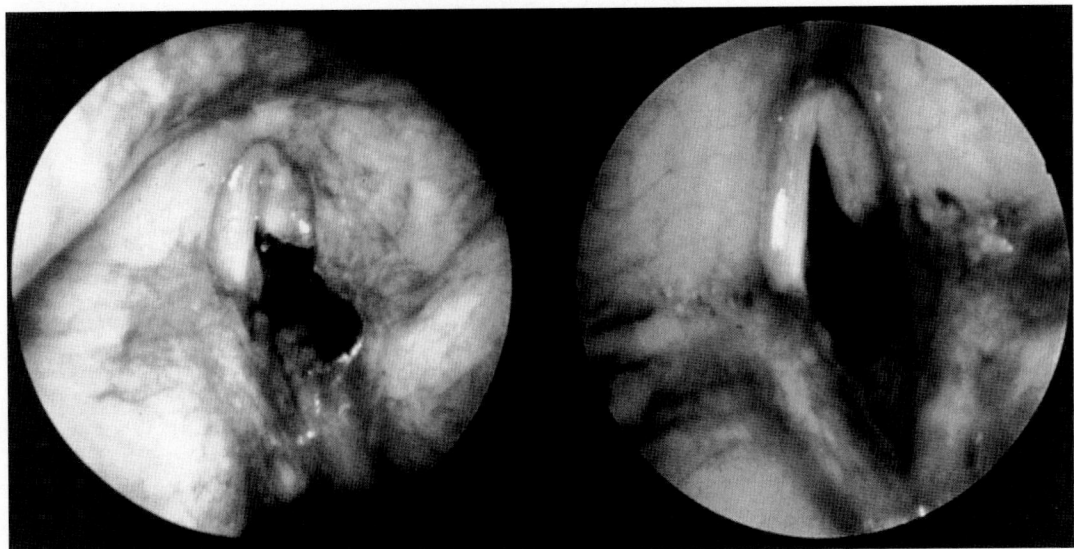

FIGURE 2 Four-year-old with bilateral vocal cord paralysis. **A:** Immediate preoperative. **B:** Six weeks after microlaryngoscopy with posterior cordotomy using carbon dioxide laser.

Bilateral Paralysis

Tracheostomy is generally, though not always, required for idiopathic bilateral vocal cord paralysis. In patients with associated treatable neurologic conditions, a period of intubation for up to 3 months (15) may be considered while the neurologic problem is treated.

Operative management of bilateral vocal cord paralysis is deferred until the age of 2 years. Deferral until adulthood so that the individual can participate in the decision-making process has been suggested. The dilemma facing the surgeon and parents is that any procedure that involves the airway will decrease the quality and volume of the voice. Since these decreases are not dramatic, most people feel this is a worthwhile trade for a lifelong tracheotomy.

A variety of techniques are available for enlarging the glottic airway. Endoscopic techniques include partial or complete arytenoidectomy, but a posterior laser cordotomy is generally sufficient (Fig. 2). The laryngotomy approach with partial arytenoidectomy (16) or arytenoidpexy (17) also produces good results. Expansion surgery with the use of a posterior cartilage graft into the divided cricoid lamina will also create an adequate airway, but the risk of aspiration is greater with this procedure, and should be reserved when other methods fail. Nerve-muscle pedicle reinnervation operations have been disappointing. In the future, electrical pacing with a laryngeal pacemaker may be a realistic alternative.

CONGENITAL SUBGLOTTIC STENOSIS

Congenital subglottic stenosis is the third most common laryngeal anomaly. Congenital subglottic stenosis is divided histopathologically into membranous and cartilaginous types (Table 2). Very often the primary definition of what may be congenital or acquired is somewhat blurred, because children with congenital subglottic stenosis may have a secondary soft tissue stenosis. Subglottic stenosis is present when the lumen of the cricoid region of the airway measures less than 4 mm in a full-term infant, or 3 mm in a premature infant. It is difficult to determine the true incidence of congenital subglottic stenosis, as many patients are intubated in the neonatal period, and therefore by definition would be considered as having an acquired subglottic stenosis.

TABLE 2: Classification of Congenital Subglottic Stenosis

Cartilaginous Stenosis	Soft Tissue Stenosis
Cricoid cartilage deformity	Granulation tissue
Normal shape	Submucosal fibrosis
Small for infant's size	Submucosal gland hypoplasia
Abnormal shape	
Large anterior lamina	
Large posterior lamina	
Generalized thickening	
Elliptical shape	
Submucous cleft	
Other congenital cricoid stenoses	
Trapped first tracheal ring	

The etiology of cartilaginous congenital subglottic stenosis is believed to be failure of the laryngeal lumen to recanalize after it was obliterated during the eighth week of gestation. This mesenchyme condensation within the laryngeal lumen is recanalized beginning during the tenth week of gestation to reestablish the laryngeal lumen. Complete arrest of the process of recanalization will lead to complete laryngeal atresia. Incomplete recanalization will result in various degrees of subglottic stenosis with symptoms ranging from mild to severe. The membranous form of congenital subglottic stenosis is generally circumferential and soft to palpation with an instrument. The mucosa lining the subglottis is thickened secondarily, owing to an increase in the fibrous connective tissue layer of the submucosa. Hyperplasia and dilatation of the mucous glands may also add to the thickness of the obstruction.

The cartilaginous variety of congenital subglottic stenosis is variable in its appearance. Patients with mild stenosis have a normal-shaped subglottic lumen, but the caliber of the lumen is diminished. More commonly, the cricoid cartilage is abnormally shaped, having prominent lateral shelves. This creates a subglottic lumen with an elliptical appearance (Fig. 3).

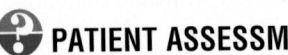 **PATIENT ASSESSMENT**

Symptoms

Children with mild to moderate congenital subglottic stenosis will have no symptoms until the airway is further narrowed by processes such as an upper respiratory tract infection. Recurrent croup may be the only clue to the diagnosis of a congenitally small subglottis. When the subglottic airway is narrowed to the point of generating symptoms, the voice will remain normal, but progressive respiratory difficulty will occur with biphasic stridor, dyspnea, and marked suprasternal and intercostal retractions.

FIGURE 3 Diagram of two forms of subglottic stenosis. **A:** Elliptical cricoid cartilage. **B:** Flattened cricoid cartilage with hyperplasia of submucosal mucous glands.

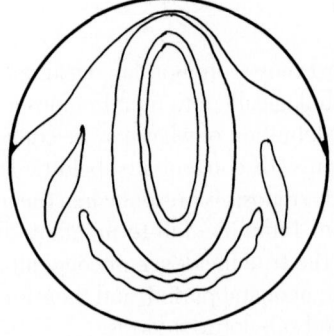

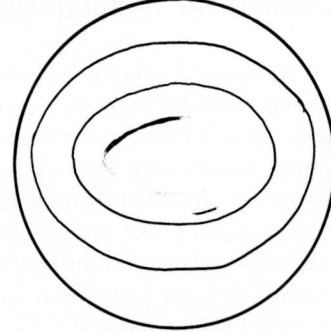

A   B

Diagnosis

Radiographs contribute information as to the location and extent of the subglottic stenosis. High-kilovoltage anteroposterior projections of the neck may demonstrate airway narrowing. A complete physical examination should be performed to rule out any associated anomalies. Flexible laryngoscopy is essential to document vocal cord mobility. The mainstay of diagnosis for subglottic stenosis, however, is rigid endoscopy. Under general anesthesia, the entire laryngotracheobronchial airway can be examined directly. The length of the stenosis, as well as its thickness can be determined. An objective measurement of the residual laryngeal lumen can also be obtained by passing an endotracheal tube of known outside diameter through the stenosis.

Congenital subglottic stenosis may arise as an isolated anomaly or may be associated with other congenital lesions or syndromes. Down syndrome, for example, is well recognized as being associated with a subglottis that is smaller than normal by one-half an endotracheal tube size. Routine intubation for all children must be approached with caution, as a congenitally small larynx can be significantly injured by an inappropriately sized endotracheal tube.

TREATMENT RECOMMENDATIONS

The condition of most patients with congenital subglottic stenosis improves with age. Less than half of the patients with congenital subglottic stenosis will require a tracheotomy for maintenance of their airway. Some patients will require laryngeal reconstruction (18). In general, the reconstructive procedures required for congenital lesions are less radical than those required for the acquired subglottic lesions.

Rational therapy for congenital subglottic stenosis is based on an accurate determination of the histopathology and location of the stenosis. Tracheostomy should be avoided if possible. Dilation has nothing to offer in the management of congenital subglottic stenosis. Use of the CO_2 laser is limited to the management of subglottic cysts, for which decapping with the CO_2 laser followed by short-term intubation is an effective therapy. For cartilaginous stenosis, anterior laryngotracheal decompression (cricoid split), and single-stage laryngotracheal reconstruction with anterior, posterior, or anterior and posterior costal cartilage grafting are effective procedures.

LARYNGEAL AND TRACHEAL CLEFT

The trachea and esophagus share a common lumen during embryogenesis. The tracheoesophageal septum separates these two structures by the thirty-fifth day of gestation. Failure of the interarytenoid tissue or the cricoid cartilage to fuse in the posterior midline will result in a laryngeal cleft. Incomplete formation of the tracheoesophageal septum produces a tracheoesophageal fistula or cleft.

The incidence is less than 0.1% and the majority of cases are sporadic. There is a strong association with other anomalies, most commonly tracheoesophageal fistula. Of special interest is that over 6% of children with tracheoesophageal fistula have a coexisting laryngeal cleft. Of the children who present with tracheoesophageal fistula, the laryngeal cleft goes undetected in three-fourths until persistent aspiration, in spite of successful tracheoesophageal fistula repair, prompts further investigation. Laryngeal or laryngotracheoesophageal cleft is also part of the Pallister-Hall syndrome (autosomal dominant, hypothalamic hamartoblastoma, laryngeal cleft, hypopituitarism, imperforate anus, and polydactyly), as well as G syndrome (dysphagia, hypospadias, hypertelorism, and cleft lip and palate).

The degree of clefting can be relatively minor, involving only a failure of the interarytenoid muscle development, or can extend to the carina and even into the mainstem

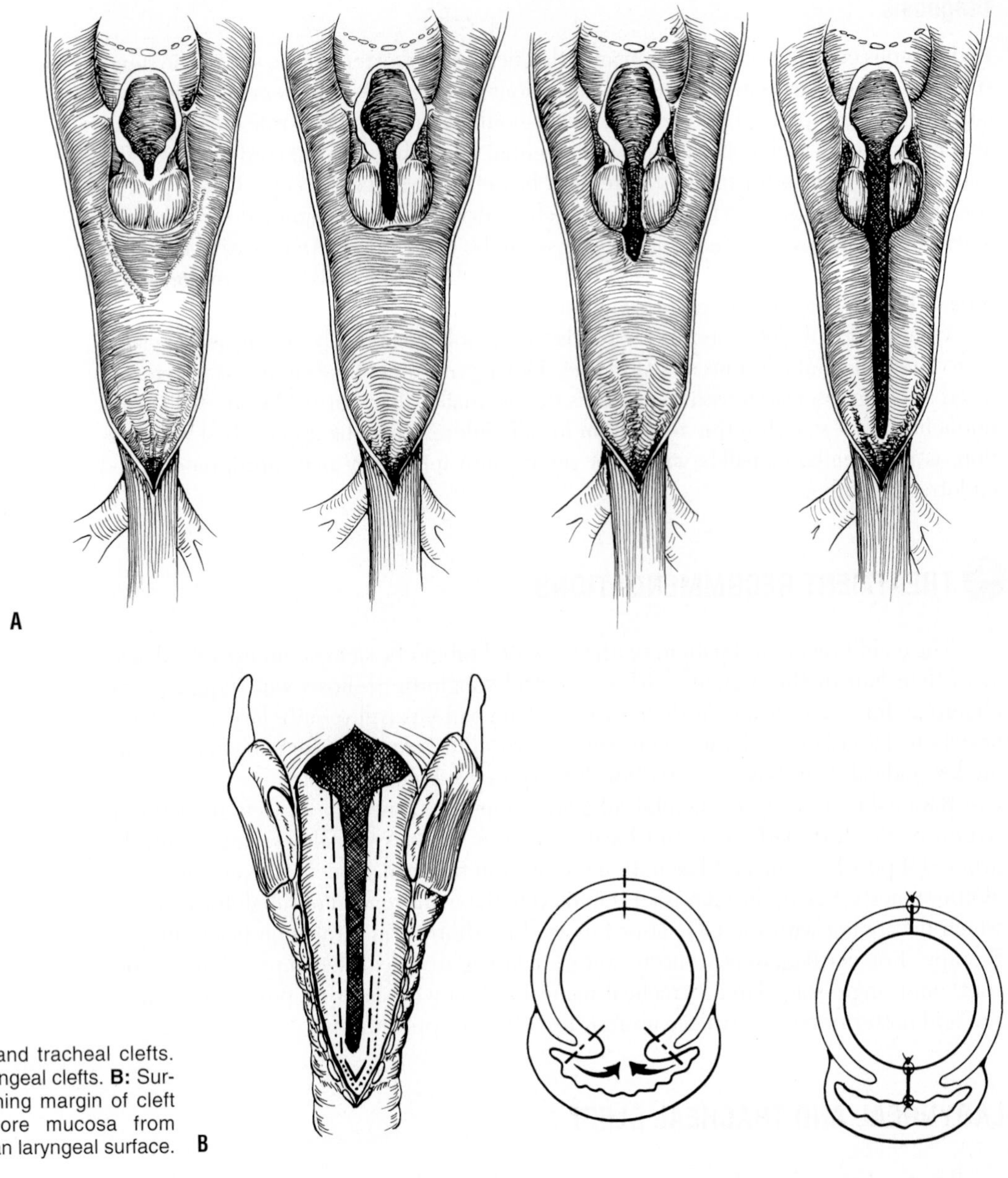

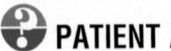

FIGURE 4 Laryngeal and tracheal clefts. **A:** Classification of laryngeal clefts. **B:** Surgical repair by freshening margin of cleft and by removing more mucosa from esophageal surface than laryngeal surface.

bronchi. Multiple classification systems have been used to describe laryngeal clefts. Independent from the numbering system used, it is useful to differentiate the length of the cleft as laryngeal (interarytenoid only, partial cricoid, or complete cricoid), or laryngotracheoesophageal (clefts that extend into the cervical or intrathoracic trachea) (Fig. 4).

🔧 PATIENT ASSESSMENT

Symptoms

Patients with laryngeal clefts present with aspiration and cyanosis during feeding and recurrent pulmonary infections. Increased tracheal secretions with occasional stridor may be noted. Voice abnormalities are present in many patients. Gastroesophageal reflux is a major contributor to the overall pulmonary embarrassment that develops with a laryngeal cleft. The severity of symptoms is related to the extent of the laryngeal cleft.

Diagnosis

Patients suspected of having a laryngeal cleft require radiographic evaluation. Chest radiographs may demonstrate nonspecific infiltrates suggestive of aspiration pneumonia. Contrast esophagrams may show spillover of the barium into the larynx or trachea. Laryngeal clefts may be difficult to visualize radiographically, and frequently multiple studies must be performed prior to demonstrating the defect.

Endoscopy is required to make the definitive diagnosis of a laryngeal cleft. A high index of suspicion is required to identify type I and type II defects. Placement of an anterior commissure scope into the larynx will splay the posterior larynx and demonstrate the inferior extent of the cleft. Great care must be taken to document the relationship of the cleft to the level of the vocal cords. Endoscopy generally underestimates the degree of tracheal clefting, and at the time of surgical repair the cleft is often longer than it appeared to be at the time of endoscopy

 ## TREATMENT RECOMMENDATIONS

Management of patients with a laryngeal cleft begins with protection of the airway from aspiration and maintenance of respiratory support. The longer the tracheoesophageal defect, the more likely a tracheotomy is to be performed. Endotracheal intubation can temporize the situation until the child is medically stable to undergo the procedure. Gastroesophageal reflux is commonly associated with laryngeal cleft and must be managed aggressively. Reverse Trendelenburg positioning and antireflux medications should be implemented. Gastrostomy and Nissen fundoplication must be considered in patients with refractory reflux.

The surgical approach for repair of the laryngotracheoesophageal cleft is dictated by the extent of the defect. Some clefts that are limited to the supraglottic larynx do not require surgical intervention. Treatment methods include evaluation and treatment of gastroesophageal reflux and swallowing therapy. When surgical intervention is required, endoscopic repair may be an option, with open repair reserved for when endoscopic repair fails.

In contrast to the interarytenoid clefts, external surgical repair is required for all laryngeal clefts that extend through the cricoid cartilage. An anterior approach through a laryngofissure is most commonly used. The advantage of this approach is excellent exposure of the entire defect without risk to laryngeal innervation. This should be done preferably without performing a tracheostomy. Intubation for 10 days postoperatively is recommended and tracheotomy is performed only if extubation is not possible at that time. A cleft with increasing length and severe accompanying tracheomalacia increase the need for a tracheostomy. Complete laryngotracheoesophageal clefts that extend to the carina may require a posterolateral approach (19) to allow for a two-layer closure without requiring intraoperative extracorporeal circulation, but can also be considered for repair by an anterior approach.

 ## MANAGEMENT OF COMPLICATIONS

Complications include recurrent laryngeal nerve injury, breakdown of the repair site, excessive granulation tissue formation at the repair site, continued aspiration, and posterior glottic stenosis.

The mortality of infants with laryngeal clefts is usually from associated congenital anomalies, or an excessive delay in making the diagnosis. The mortality associated with intrathoracic laryngotracheoesophageal clefts is high. The incidence of revision surgery also increases with the severity of the cleft. In addition to the length of the cleft, insufficiently treated gastroesophageal reflux may also be associated with a decreased success rate.

SACCULAR CYSTS AND LARYNGOCELES

Congenital saccular cyst of the larynx is an unusual lesion that commonly presents with respiratory obstruction in infants and children (20). This lesion is thought to arise in the saccule of the ventricle of the larynx. It is similar to a laryngocele in that it represents an abnormal dilatation or herniation of the saccule; however, it is distinct from a laryngocele in that there is no opening to the ventricle of the larynx, and it is filled with mucus. Saccular cysts can be classified further into anterior and lateral saccular cysts (Fig. 5). The anterior saccular cyst typically extends medially and posteriorly from the saccule and therefore protrudes into the laryngeal lumen between the true and false vocal cords. The lateral saccular cyst typically extends posterosuperiorly into the false vocal cord and aryepiglottic fold. This is the more common one in infants. The congenital saccular cyst is considered to form as a result of a developmental failure to maintain patency of the orifice between the saccule and the ventricle.

Laryngoceles are defined as a dilatation or herniation of the laryngeal saccule, which is filled with air. This is an uncommon entity, seen predominantly in middle-aged white men, but can be seen, albeit rarely, in the neonatal period (21). The ventricle is the space found between the false and true vocal cords. The saccule is a small blind pouch running superiorly that opens into the anterior one-third of the ventricle of the larynx. As this space runs superiorly, the inner surface of the thyroid cartilage lies laterally and the ventricular band medially. The saccule is surrounded by loose areolar tissue and is lined with pseudostratified columnar epithelium and a mixture of serous and mucous glands in the submucosa.

Laryngoceles are classified into three categories: internal (inferior and within the thyrohyoid membrane), external (above or piercing the thyrohyoid membrane), or mixed (a combination of internal and external components). Clinical significance is interpreted as fulfilling the following criteria: symptomatic, palpable, presenting as an observable le-

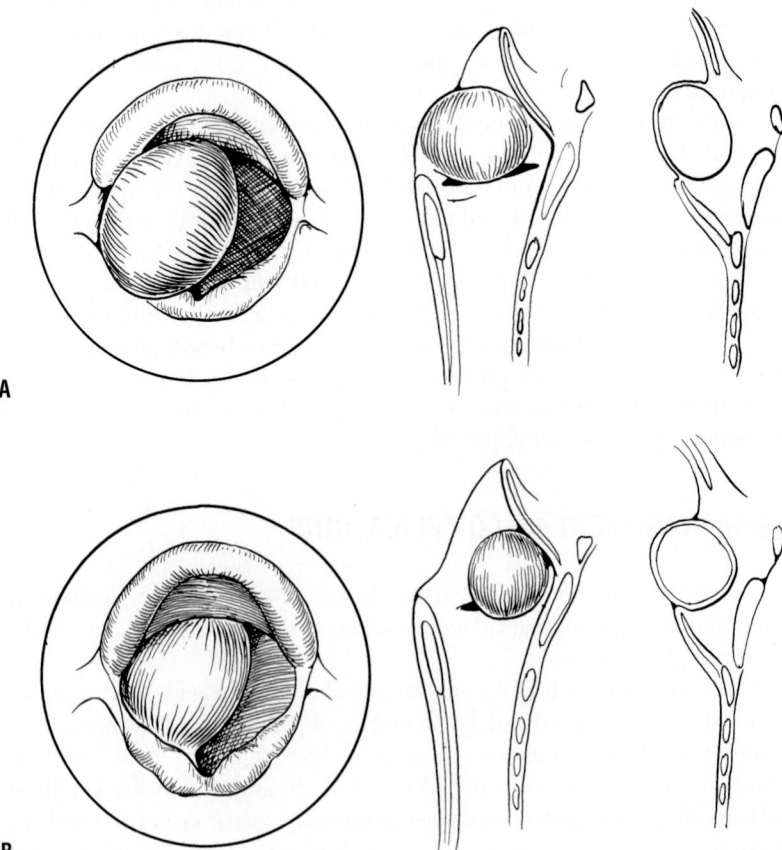

FIGURE 5 Saccular cysts. **A:** Lateral. **B:** Anterior.

sion either by indirect or direct laryngoscopy, and observed surgically or by roentgenogram to extend above the superior margin of the alar of the thyroid cartilage.

As laryngoceles can occasionally be distended with mucus or become infected (laryngopyocele), from a practical point of view a fluid-filled smooth mass distending the aryepiglottic fold may be a saccular cyst or a laryngocele. When filled with fluid, they are considered saccular cysts; if filled with air, they are classified as laryngoceles.

 ## PATIENT ASSESSMENT

Symptoms

Saccular cysts cause respiratory distress most often at birth and are generally diagnosed in the first few days of life. The cry may be muffled, and dysphagia may be encountered. Symptoms of laryngocele are similar though they may present somewhat later; in addition to the above symptoms, which may be worse during crying due to increased distention of air in the laryngocele, an air-containing neck mass may develop.

Diagnosis

The diagnosis of the saccular cyst is suggested by a soft tissue lateral neck radiograph that shows a mucus-filled sac. This can be confirmed easily by fiberoptic laryngoscopy. Both computed tomography and MRI may be helpful in delineating the exact location and the extent of the mass. Direct laryngoscopy and bronchoscopy are performed immediately before surgical repair.

Diagnosis of laryngoceles is based primarily on signs and symptoms in the neonatal age group. Radiography may be helpful in delineating the limits of the laryngocele. Confirmation of diagnosis requires endoscopy, though the findings may be negative in a child with an external laryngocele.

 ## TREATMENT RECOMMENDATIONS

The classic treatment of the lateral saccular cyst has been endoscopic management. Needle aspiration has been suggested as the initial treatment of these cysts but recurrence is the norm because of the difficulty in completely obliterating the cyst by this method. Marsupialization of the roof of the cyst has been advocated; the laser may be employed as an adjunct in marsupialization. Endoscopic excision has been proposed as well. In this method, the cyst is dissected to its base at the orifice of the saccule and then amputated. These methods have frequently required multiple procedures and often a concomitant tracheotomy.

Occasionally, an external laryngofissure approach has been used to remove a recurrent laryngeal cyst (22). This approach provides for adequate exposure with minimal intralaryngeal trauma. The procedure of choice now is a lateral cervical approach extending through the thyrohyoid membrane immediately above the alar of the thyroid cartilage. A portion of the superior alar of the thyroid cartilage may need to be removed (Fig. 6) and short-term intubation employed. This allows for complete excision of the cyst and precludes the need for either a tracheotomy or multiple procedures.

SUBGLOTTIC HEMANGIOMA

Subglottic and tracheal hemangiomas are benign congenital vascular tumors characterized by cellular hyperplasia of endothelial cells, mast cells, fibroblasts, and macrophages. This is in contrast to vascular malformations, which are not neoplastic,

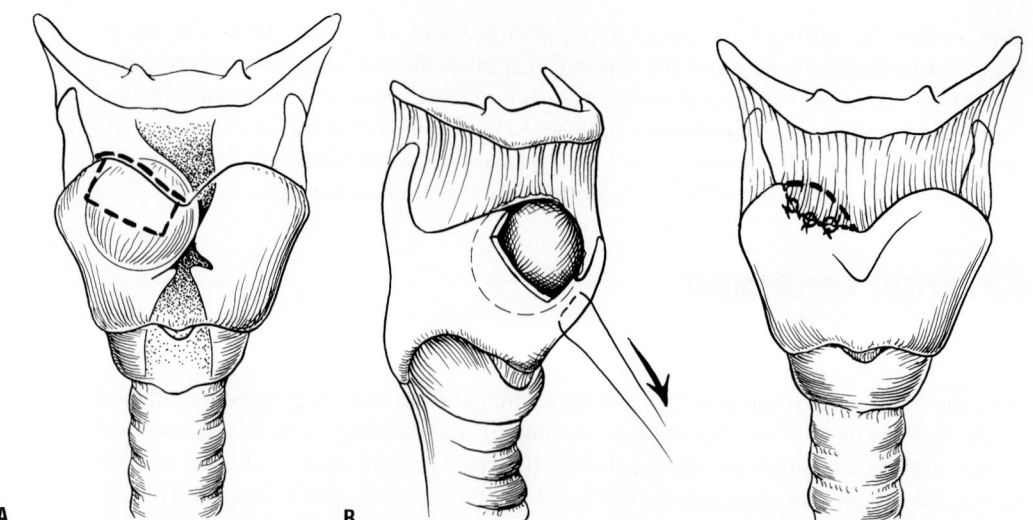

A   **B**   **C**

FIGURE 6 Approach for removal of saccular cysts. **A:** Lateral cervical approach to thyroid ala. **B:** Superior incision of perichondrium of thyroid ala and its preservation. Partial removal of cartilage of thyroid ala to access the cyst. **C:** Closure of perichondrium.

having a normal rate of endothelial turnover, with areas of vascular morphogenesis manifesting as various channel abnormalities (23). Subglottic and tracheal hemangiomas have a rapid growth phase that slows by 12 to 18 months, followed by slow resolution over subsequent months to years. Most patients show complete resolution by 5 years. These hemangiomas are relatively uncommon, with a 2:1 female preponderance.

 ## PATIENT ASSESSMENT

Symptoms

Typically, infants with subglottic or tracheal hemangiomas are asymptomatic for the first few months of life, and become symptomatic by the age of 3 months. Almost all are symptomatic by the age of 6 months. Stridor is initially inspiratory but quickly becomes biphasic with rapid growth of the lesion. The cry may be altered, and the typical infant has a barking cough, hoarseness, and croupy symptoms.

Diagnosis

Asymmetric subglottic narrowing on the anteroposterior neck airway film is almost pathognomonic of a subglottic hemangioma, as this finding is rarely seen with croup, subglottic cysts, subglottic stenosis, or recurrent respiratory papillomas, all of which enter into the differential diagnosis. MRI or computed tomography with contrast medium delineates the limits of the lesion, looking for neck or mediastinal extension. Occasionally, the subglottic lesion is the tip of the iceberg of a much larger lesion.

The diagnosis is made by endoscopic examination under general anesthesia. Diagnosis is usually made without biopsy because of the lesion's typical appearance of a compressible asymmetric submucosal mass, occasionally with a bluish or reddish discoloration and most often found in the posterior lateral subglottic region. Biopsy is generally unnecessary, but if performed, some bleeding may be encountered and can be quickly controlled with compression by an endotracheal tube.

TREATMENT RECOMMENDATIONS

The natural history of subglottic hemangioma is to grow quickly and obstruct the airway, followed by a period of involution to a normal larynx. The decision of what therapeutic measures to take is directed at maintaining the airway while minimizing the potential long-term sequelae of the treatment itself. The goal of therapy should be a normal-looking larynx. Current management options include laser partial excision, open surgical resection, systemic or intralesional steroids, systemic interferon alfa-2a, and tracheotomy. There is no correct therapy, and each case must be individualized.

Bypassing the obstructing lesion with a tracheotomy and waiting for the expected involution will provide for the optimal anatomic result, and is considered by many to be the standard of care by which all other treatment options need to be measured. However, there are significant risks associated with a tracheotomy, such as death from an obstructed or misplaced tracheostomy tube, as well as the delay in speech and language that is routinely encountered when children have a tracheotomy at a young age. Earlier methods of treatment that are no longer used because of the associated morbidity include external-beam radiation, radium and gold implants, and sclerosing agents.

Systemic corticosteroids have been used both in isolation and as adjuvant therapy. Steroids are thought to decrease the size of the hemangioma by blocking estradiol-induced growth or by directly increasing capillary sensitivity to vasoconstrictors. Risks of long-term steroid use include growth retardation and increased susceptibility to infection. These effects may be reduced by using dexamethasone (1 mg per kilogram to a maximum of 15 mg) orally every third or fourth day. Often the growth of the hemangioma can be controlled without the undesirable side effects of steroid use to a degree where other modalities of treatment including tracheotomy are not necessary. If growth continues to produce serious airway obstruction, administration of steroids is helpful in pretreating the hemangioma for 2 weeks prior to CO_2 laser therapy or surgical excision. If tracheotomy becomes necessary, then steroid therapy should be discontinued.

Intralesional injection of corticosteroids with subsequent short-term intubation has also been described to be successful.

The CO_2 laser is one of the treatment cornerstones for subglottic hemangioma and has been used alone or in combination with tracheotomy or steroids. Laser partial excision with or without systemic corticosteroids may avoid a tracheotomy. Use of the laser has been associated with a significant risk of introducing subglottic stenosis, and therefore conservative partial laser excision involving no more than 30% of the circumference of the subglottic larynx is recommended. A maximum of three separate laser treatments at 1-month intervals is advocated. Pretreatment with steroids is recommended for 2 weeks.

Surgical excision of a subglottic hemangioma is being reintroduced as a form of therapy. The decision to utilize an open surgical approach should be reached only after other modalities of therapy are explored with the family. Isolated posterior lateral subglottic hemangiomas that are becoming large enough to obstruct the airway and are not controlled by steroid therapy should be considered for open surgical resection (24,25). This may be performed as a single-stage procedure with a 7- to 10-day period of endotracheal intubation after surgical removal of the hemangioma. Pretreatment with steroids for 2 weeks is recommended.

Interferon alfa-2a therapy has been advocated for life-threatening hemangiomas in infancy and specifically for airway hemangiomas that are corticosteroid resistant and endanger vital structures in the head and neck area. Its use is not indicated for the isolated subglottic hemangioma.

The practice of combining several modalities of therapy increases the probability of avoiding a tracheotomy.

LARYNGEAL WEBS AND ATRESIA

Laryngeal webs and atresias represent failure of recanalization of the larynx during prenatal development. They are uncommon, and most are glottic and have an extension into the subglottic larynx. Congenital webs may rarely occur in the supraglottis.

PATIENT ASSESSMENT

Symptoms

The two major problems of congenital webs of the larynx are airway obstruction and vocal dysfunction. The degree of webbing correlates with the severity of the symptoms. A helpful classification of congenital laryngeal webs (26) is presented in Table 3.

The most consistent evidence of a laryngeal web is vocal dysfunction and may vary from a voice that is aphonic to one that is weak, husky, or breathy. Stridor is the second most common symptom associated with laryngeal webs and again will depend on the degree of obstruction of the web. An extreme form of laryngeal web would be complete failure of recanalization leading to a laryngeal atresia, which would present at birth with maximum respiratory effort, no voice, and rapid death unless an urgent tracheotomy is performed. Less severe forms of web may present with croup at an early age, and this diagnosis should always be entertained in a child with croup-like symptoms before the age of 6 months.

Diagnosis

The diagnosis of a laryngeal web is by a combination of flexible laryngoscopy and direct laryngoscopy under general anesthesia. A well-taken lateral x-ray film of the neck will help to substantiate the degree of cricoid abnormality with subglottic involvement. At direct laryngoscopy, it is important to examine the web very carefully and palpate the web to identify its thickness and extent. Careful examination of the subglottic space is essential to determine subglottic involvement.

TREATMENT RECOMMENDATIONS

Treatment of congenital laryngeal webs is based on the extent of the lesion and the severity of symptoms. A type I web where there are no airway symptoms but only a breathy cry is best initially managed expectantly. Definitive therapy can be delayed until the child is 3 to 4 years old.

Type II glottic webs may be treated by incision along the margin on one vocal fold followed by dilation. Several procedures seem to be necessary to obtain an adequate result. After incision of the web, it is preferable to place a keel either endoscopically or through the thyroid lamina. A young child should have a temporary tracheotomy for 2 weeks while the keel is in position. Because several procedures seem to be necessary, in these cases, serious consideration should be given to perform a laryngotomy with keel insertion, with a temporary tracheotomy.

TABLE 3: Classification of Congenital Laryngeal Webs

Type I	An anterior web involving 35%–50% of the glottis or less. The vocal folds are visible lateral to the thin web. There is little obstruction of the airway, and a breathy cry.
Type II	An anterior web involving 35%–50% of the glottis, which may be thin or moderately thick, with extension into the subglottic larynx. The vocal folds usually are visible within the web and there is little airway obstruction. The voice is husky, weak, and breathy.
Type III	An anterior web involving 50%–75% of the glottis, typically with a thick anterior portion and cartilaginous extension into the subglottic space. These infants have a moderate degree of airway obstruction and a very weak voice.
Type IV	Seventy-five percent to 90% of the glottis is involved by this uniformly thick web, which extends into the subglottic larynx. The individual vocal folds are not identifiable, and may be fused together. The infant is aphonic and airway obstruction is severe, requiring tracheostomy soon after birth. Thickening of the anterior lamina of the cricoid cartilage is always present.

Type III and IV webs generally require a tracheostomy and, again, definitive therapy can be deferred until the patient is 3 to 4 years old, when laryngotomy and insertion of a keel can be carried out. These lesions include a cricoid cartilage deformity, and the techniques of laryngotracheal reconstruction for subglottic stenosis are applicable in this condition. In severe type III and IV webs, an alternative therapy to a tracheotomy is to perform an early single-stage laryngotracheal reconstruction via a midline laryngotomy with submucosal resection of the abnormal cricoid cartilage, preserving sufficient mucosa to cover the interomedial aspect of the vocal cords. An endotracheal tube is then used as an airway stent, as in the cricoid split procedure, and the patient is intubated for approximately 10 days. This prevents the need for a tracheotomy, but there is usually some residual anterior web that can be treated again with laryngotomy and insertion of a keel at about the age of 3 to 4 years. This has the tremendous advantage of avoiding a tracheotomy.

Laryngeal Atresia

Complete laryngeal atresia is incompatible with life, and these infants only survive if emergency tracheotomy is carried out in the delivery room. If the child survives this therapy, then standard laryngotracheal reconstruction techniques are appropriate.

REFERENCES

1. Ferguson CF. *Otolaryngol Clin North Am* 1970;3:185–200.
2. Holinger LD. *Ann Otol Rhinol Laryngol* 1980;89:397–400.
3. Zalzal GH, Anon JB, Cotton RT. *Ann Otol Rhinol Laryngol* 1987;96:72–76.
4. Bent JP, Miller DA, Kim JW, Bauman NM, Wilson JS, Smith RJ. *Ann Otol Rhinol Laryngol* 1996;105:169–175.
5. Tostevin PMJ, deBruyn R, Hosni A, Evans JNG. *J Laryngol Otol* 1995;109:844–848.
6. Hui Y, Gaffney R, Crysdale WS. *Ann Otol Rhinol Laryngol* 1995;104:432–436.
7. Roger G, Denoyelle F, Triglia JM, Garabedian EN. *Laryngoscope* 1995;105:1111–1117.
8. Froehlich P, Seid AB, Denoyelle F, et al. *Int J Pediatr Otorhinolaryngol* 1997;39:9–18.
9. Remacle M, Bodart E, Lawson G, Minet M, Mayne A. *Eur Arch Otorhinolaryngol* 1996;253:401–404.
10. Kelly SM, Gray SD. *Arch Otolaryngol Head Neck Surg* 1995;121:1351–1354.
11. Murty GE, Shinkwin C, Gibbin KP. *J Laryngol Otol* 1994;108:329–331.
12. Gartlan MG, Peterson KL, Luschei ES, Hoffman HT, Smith RJ. *Ann Otol Rhinol Laryngol* 1993;102:695–700.
13. Friedman EM. *Ann Otol Rhinol Laryngol* 1997;106:199–209.
14. Levine BA, Jacobs IN, Wetmore RF, Handler SD. *Arch Otolaryngol Head Neck Surg* 1995;121:116–119.
15. deGaudemar I, Roudaire M, Francois M, Narcy P. *Int J Pediatr Otorhinolaryngol* 1996;34:101–110.
16. Bower CM, Choi SS, Cotton RT. *Ann Otol Rhinol Laryngol* 1994;103:271–278.
17. Triglia JM, Belus JF, Nicollas R. *J Laryngol Otol* 1996;110:1027–1030.
18. Rosenfeld RM, Bluestone CD. *Laryngoscope* 1993;103:286–290.
19. Cotton RT, Schreiber JT. *Ann Otol Rhinol Laryngol* 1981;90:401–405.
20. Holinger LD, Barnes DR, Smid IJ, Holinger PH. *Ann Otol Rhinol Laryngol* 1978;87:675–685.
21. Chu L, Gussack GS, Orr JB, Hood D. *Arch Otolaryngol Head Neck Surg* 1994;20:454–458.
22. Ward RF, Jones J, Arnold JA. *Ann Otol Rhinol Laryngol* 1995;104:707–710.
23. Mulliken JB, Glowacki J. *Plast Reconstr Surg* 1982;69:412.
24. Wiatrak BJ, Reilly JS, Seid AB, Pransky SM, Castillo JV. *Int J Pediatr Otorhinolaryngol* 1996;34:191–206.
25. Phipps CD, Gibson WS, Wood WE. *Int J Pediatr Otorhinolaryngol.* 1997;41:71–79.
26. Cohen SR. *Ann Otol Rhinol Laryngol* Suppl 1985;121:2–16.

R.T. Cotton: Department of Otolaryngology, Children's Hospital Medical Center, Cincinnati, Ohio 45229-4356. • C.A.J. Prescott: Department of Otolaryngology, University of Cape Town, The Red Cross War Memorial Children's Hospital, Rondebosch, Cape Town 7700 South Africa.

• *Practical Pediatric Otolaryngology*
• edited by Robin T. Cotton and Charles M. Myer, III
• Lippincott-Raven Publishers, Philadelphia © 1999

Acquired Anomalies of the Larynx and Trachea

David L. Walner & Robin T. Cotton

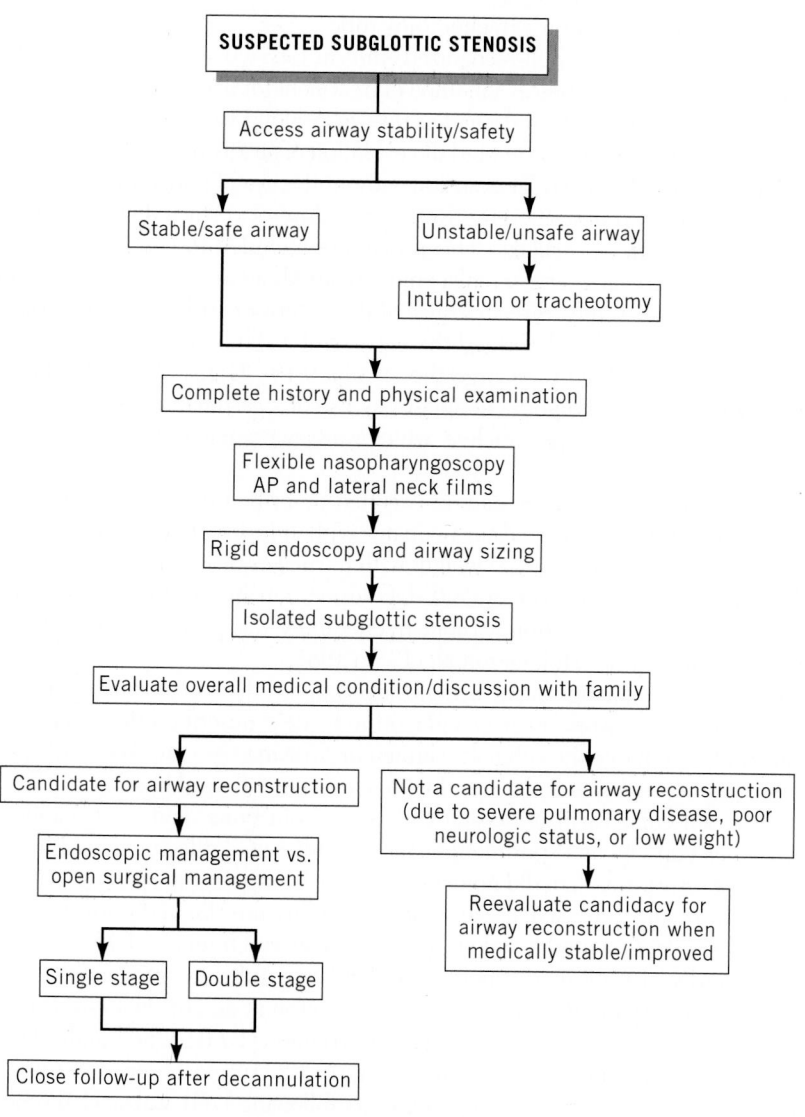

Acquired anomalies of the larynx and trachea must be suspected when children have had any type of therapeutic intervention in their lifetime. This intervention can range from short-term intubation at birth to extensive cardiac surgery later in childhood. The sequelae range from subglottic stenosis (SGS) to vocal fold paralysis. The key point is that a detailed history is essential in the evaluation of any child with a suspected acquired anomaly of the airway.

The majority of this chapter focuses on SGS because it is the most common acquired anomaly of the larynx in children and the most common anomaly requiring tracheotomy in infants younger than 1 year (1,2).

⬛ HISTORICAL BACKGROUND

In the 1930s, Chevalier Jackson (3) commented that children with chronic laryngeal stenosis do not outgrow their problem. In the early twentieth century, acquired subglottic pathology generally had a traumatic or infectious (syphilis, tuberculosis, typhoid, diphtheria) origin (4). These children were often treated with a tracheotomy. Laryngeal stenosis often developed owing to scarring from the infectious process or the high placement of the tracheotomy (5). At this period of time, airway reconstruction had yet to be attempted. Most cases of laryngeal stenosis were treated unsuccessfully with dilatation, leaving children dependent on a tracheotomy tube.

Acquired SGS became a well-recognized entity in 1965 when McDonald and Stocks (6) introduced long-term intubation as a method of treatment for neonates requiring prolonged ventilatory support. The increased incidence of SGS along with estimated tracheostomy mortality rates as high as 24% prompted the evolution of airway reconstruction (7).

Pediatric cricoid framework expansion without the use of grafts was first reported in 1971, when Grahne (8) described the Rethi procedure of vertical division of the posterior lamina of the cricoid cartilage. This procedure included the excision of scar tissue from the posterior cricoid plate, and placement of an Aboulker stent wired to a metal tracheostomy tube, followed by direct closure of the anterior cartilaginous incision. Subsequent reports from Canada described the successful use of anterior and posterior division of the cricoid cartilage to enlarge the airway (9,10). Evans and Todd (11) in 1974 described success with laryngotracheoplasty by use of a castellated incision of the anterior cricoid cartilage and upper trachea, which was sewn open and stented with a rolled Silastic sheet for 6 weeks.

The anterior cricoid split procedure was first described by Cotton and Seid (12) in 1980. The procedure was devised for neonates with anterior glottic or subglottic stenosis who were otherwise of adequate weight with normal or near-normal pulmonary function. The concept was to allow cricoid decompression in an attempt to avoid a tracheotomy. Successful extubation without tracheotomy was performed on 106 (77%) of 138 patients in a study by Holinger et al. (13) in 1987.

Severe pediatric laryngotracheal stenosis prompted the use of cartilage grafts to expand the cricoid framework. Fearon and Cotton in 1972 described the successful use of cartilage grafts to enlarge the subglottic lumen in African green monkeys and in children (7,14). The initial work was done with thyroid cartilage, followed in other studies by septal cartilage, auricular cartilage, costal cartilage, hyoid bone, and sternocleidomastoid myocutaneous flaps. In an experimental study, irradiated cartilage material had a much higher rate of resorption than did nonirradiated fresh autogenous cartilage (15). Survival as well as growth and neovascularization of autogenous anterior and posterior costal cartilage grafts was documented histologically in animals and humans (1,16,17).

The majority of published reports found success utilizing autogenous fresh costal cartilage grafts to expand the subglottic lumen. Cotton et al. (18) in 1989 reviewed 203 children who underwent laryngotracheal reconstruction (LTR). One hundred eighty-six (92%) underwent decannulation after an average of 1.23 surgical procedures per patient. All patients had a minimum follow-up of 2 years following LTR. Zalzal (19) reported on 41 children with moderate and severe SGS. All of these patients underwent anterior and posterior costal cartilage grafting, with a greater than 90% decannulation rate. All of these airways were stented (Aboulker) for an average of 6 weeks.

Four-quadrant cricoid cartilage division in LTR was introduced in 1992 as an option for treating severe acquired SGS (20). It was described as division of the lateral walls of the cricoid cartilage in addition to anterior and posterior cricoid division. This technique was often combined with autogenous cartilage grafts placed anteriorly or posteriorly, or both. The original study involved 29 patients. Twenty-two (76%) of these patients underwent decannulation; 11 of the patients required revision surgery after the four-quadrant split and prior to decannulation.

Single-stage laryngotracheal reconstruction (SS-LTR) has evolved over the past 7 years as an attractive method of short-term stenting. This technique provides stability to the reconstructed airway and allows for removal of the tracheostomy tube and it's associated microbes at the time of surgery. Seid et al. (21) accomplished decannulation in 12 of 13 patients undergoing SS-LTR. The largest series to date involved 107 children; decannulation was achieved in 62 (81%) of 77 patients with a tracheostomy prior to reconstruction and in 26 (87%) of 30 patients not having a tracheostomy prior to reconstruction (22). Postoperative management of SS-LTR patients requires coordination with a well-trained intensive care unit (ICU) staff.

Partial cricotracheal resection (PCTR) with primary anastomosis is the most recent advance in the care of children with severe SGS. Monnier et al. (23) achieved decannulation in 14 (93%) of 15 patients after a single open procedure. Stern et al. (24) recently presented the results of 16 pediatric patients who underwent PCTR. Fifteen (94%) of the patients underwent decannulation; 1 of these 15 required a second open procedure prior to decannulation.

The surgical treatment of SGS continues to evolve. More recently, attention is being drawn toward local factors that may affect wound healing and potentially the surgical outcome (25).

SUBGLOTTIC STENOSIS

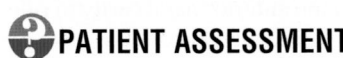

PATIENT ASSESSMENT

Acquired SGS differs from congenital SGS in two ways: (a) It is a complication of medical treatment, and (b) it is generally more severe, leading to greater problems in management. Endotracheal tube intubation is the most common factor responsible for the development of SGS.

History and Physical Examination

When one is called to evaluate these children, it is generally an infant in the neonatal or pediatric ICU with airway distress, having failed multiple extubation attempts. Another scenario may involve a child referred to the office with a tracheostomy already in place, having been given a diagnosis of airway obstruction. Regardless of the presentation, the evaluation must begin with a comprehensive medical and birth history.

- Was the child a product of a term pregnancy?
- If premature, at what week of gestation was the child born?
- What were the child's Apgar scores?
- What was the birth weight?
- Has the child been intubated?
- When and how many times has the child been intubated?
- Have the intubations been difficult or traumatic?
- Has the child tolerated extubation and for how long?
- Has the child ever vocalized?
- Has the child attempted feeding and if so, how was it?
- Does the child aspirate?
- What is the child's pulmonary status (ventilator settings, oxygen requirement)?
- What other medical problems does the child have (neurologic status)?
- If a tracheotomy is present, can the child vocalize around the tube when plugged?

Physical examination should include a complete head and neck examination. The child's overall appearance in terms of failure to thrive versus heartiness is important. If the child is not intubated, is he or she laboring to breathe, retracting, or stridulous? When the child exerts himself or herself, does the breathing pattern change? Conditions such as cleft lip/palate, choanal atresia, retrognathia, and structural facial deformities must be identified. Passing a flexible suction catheter through each naris will ensure nasal patency. Opening, looking, and palpating within the mouth will rule out a cleft palate. Ausculation of the chest will ensure good air movement bilaterally. Ausculation over the anterior part of the neck will reveal restricted air movement at a particular level of the breathing passage.

Radiologic Evaluation

Airway radiographs (anteroposterior and lateral plain films of the neck) can often contribute valuable information. The overall structure of the airway column can be seen, and the length of a stenosis can be estimated. In addition, careful attention can determine if the stenosis begins in the immediate subglottic portion of the airway or further distally involving the upper tracheal rings (just superior to the tracheostomy stoma). Plain films do not always demonstrate a SGS that is actually present. In a recent review at the authors' institution, 15 children who presented with stridor and no tracheostomy tube were found to have SGS on microlaryngoscopy and bronchoscopy. Six of the 15 had a preendoscopy plain film that gave a precise diagnosis of SGS, 6 had films suggestive of the diagnosis of SGS, and 3 had films that either missed the diagnosis or gave a mis-diagnosis (26).

Endoscopic Evaluation

Flexible

All patients with suspected airway pathology should undergo a flexible fiberoptic nasopharyngoscopy while awake. The examination begins in the anterior nasal cavity to rule out a piriform aperture stenosis, and moves posteriorly to rule out a choanal stenosis or atresia. Hypopharyngeal visualization will assess the hypopharyngeal tone. The epiglottis and arytenoid cartilages can be assessed for edema or erythema consistent with reflux esophagitis. In addition, any evidence of laryngomalacia should be noted. Determining the mobility of the true vocal folds is an essential part of this evaluation. Occasionally, a subglottic view is possible with the flexible scope, but in general only the anatomy from the true vocal folds and superior to the folds can be visualized using this method.

The flexible scope allows one to have an idea of what will be found on rigid endoscopy. If all structures appear normal above the vocal folds, then pathology must exist elsewhere within the airway. Accurate evaluation of vocal fold mobility can only be made with a flexible scope while the child is fully awake.

Rigid

Rigid endoscopy remains the mainstay for the diagnosis of SGS and other subglottic or tracheal pathology. Current equipment includes the use of magnified telescopes both for optimal visualization and for teaching purposes (27). It is important to minimize trauma to the airway during endoscopy. This involves meticulous technique and attentiveness of the surgeon, nursing staff, and the anesthesiologist. Having appropriate-size telescopes, bronchoscopes, and endotracheal tubes is essential and necessary.

A full-term infant with a cricoid ring less than 4 mm in diameter has SGS (28). A more practical definition is that a full-term infant should be able to be intubated with a 3-mm (inner diameter) endotracheal tube and still show a leak around the tube at a pressure less than 30 cm H_2O.

Each child's airway must be sized with an endotracheal tube in order to formulate a preoperative plan and to evaluate the response of the airway to a conservative waiting period or airway reconstruction. The use of standard endotracheal tubes allows discussion and comparison with other surgeons and other institutions. The endotracheal tube should be advanced such that the second graduated mark on the endotracheal tube is at the level of the vocal cords. The anesthetic circuit is then connected to the endotracheal tube, and the pressure valve on the anesthetic machine closed. If a tracheotomy tube is present, the tracheostomy tube is removed and a finger placed over the stoma for this portion of the procedure. The surgeon visualizes the subglottis with the endoscope, and the pressure is recorded when a leak around the endotracheal tube is noticed. Pressure should not exceed 40 cm H_2O, to prevent a pneumothorax from occurring. The endotracheal tube that permits a leak at less than 30 cm H_2O pressure is considered the appropriate tube of record.

The original Cotton airway grading system was revised into the Myer-Cotton grading system in order to incorporate endotracheal tube size (Fig. 1) (29). This system classifies SGS into four grades: I—0% to 50% obstruction; II—51% to 70% obstruction (Fig. 2); III—71% to 99% obstruction (Fig. 3); and IV—100% obstruction (Fig. 4).

A careful evaluation must identify the presence of SGS or arytenoid fixation. The position of the each vocal fold should be noted. If a paramedian vocal fold position is present, one must rule out a paralysis. A close look at the interarytenoid tissue should be done to ensure that a laryngeal cleft is not present. If erythema and edema are present on the interarytenoid tissue, one must suspect gastropharyngeal reflux.

Once the stenosis is identified, the length of the stenosis should be measured from its superior to inferior extent. The distance from the undersurface of the true vocal cords to the superior-most aspect of the stenosis should be measured, as should the distance from the inferior-most aspect of the stenosis to the tracheostomy tube (if present). Characteristics of the stenosis such as an elliptical shape, prominent lateral shelves, anterior or posterior predominance, and suprastomal collapse should be noted. Inflammatory changes or granulation tissue present in the airway must be identified.

The trachea and bronchi must be carefully evaluated to rule out malacia, compression, or other abnormalities that will help determine how strong of a candidate the patient is for airway reconstruction.

At the completion of the endoscopy, a quick look at the larynx and subglottis for edema and erythema will give the surgeon a hint as to the reactivity of the airway tissues. Some children have severe subglottic tissue swelling following relatively atraumatic endoscopy. These children are likely going to have the same type of swelling following airway reconstruction, and thus may not be good single-stage candidates.

Gastroesophageal Reflux Evaluation

At this point in time, the verdict is not in on the relationship between gastroesophageal reflux (GER) and SGS. The pH probe has been considered the gold standard for evaluating GER. It must be remembered that in the unusual case of the refluxate being basic in pH, it will not be picked up on the probe, but will be more accurately seen with a nuclear medicine reflux scan.

The authors recently reviewed 74 patients who had known SGS and underwent pH probe testing. This group of patients had a three-fold increase in the incidence of GER as compared to the general pediatric population (30). A high percentage of these children with lower-probe GER had upper-probe (pharyngeal) GER as well.

PEARLS AND PERILS

1. Begin with a complete history including prematurity.
2. Obtain intubation history including when, how often, how difficult, and with what size endotracheal tube.
3. Obtain feeding history including route, texture, progress, and aspiration.
4. Obtain pulmonary history including oxygen requirement and ventilator dependence.
5. Perform physical examination including flexible nasopharyngoscopy.
6. Obtain x-ray films to confirm length of stenosis and rule out other pathology.
7. Perform endoscopy to evaluate larynx, trachea, bronchi, and esophagus.
8. Size the airway by endotracheal tube (Myer-Cotton staging system).
9. Do workup for gastroesophageal reflux.

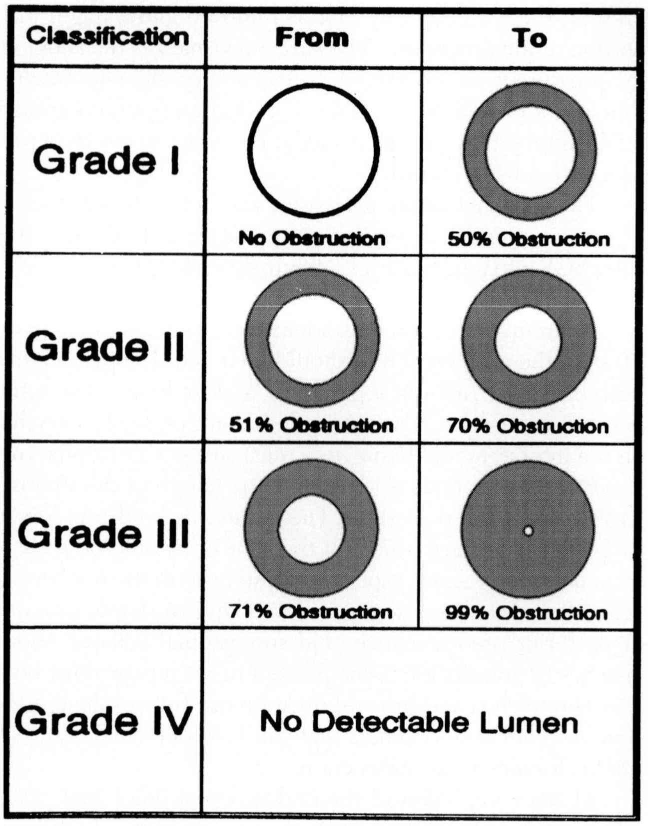

Classification	From	To
Grade I	No Obstruction	50% Obstruction
Grade II	51% Obstruction	70% Obstruction
Grade III	71% Obstruction	99% Obstruction
Grade IV	No Detectable Lumen	

FIGURE 1 Myer-Cotton grading system for subglottic stenosis.

Currently, the authors perform dual pH probe testing in consultation with a pediatric gastroenterologist on all children prior to airway reconstruction. If mild GER is identified, the child is treated medically [cisapride (Propulsid) and ranitidine (Zantac) or Omeprazole (Prilosec)] for 1 month prior to and 12 months following airway surgery. If moderate GER is identified, the child is treated medically and a repeat pH probe test is done prior to surgery. If severe GER is identified, a pediatric surgeon is consulted to consider if a fundoplication is necessary to control the reflux prior to airway surgery.

FIGURE 2 Example of a grade II subglottic stenosis.

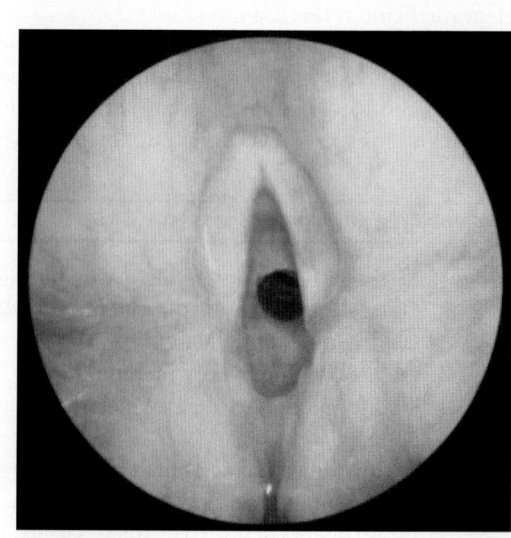

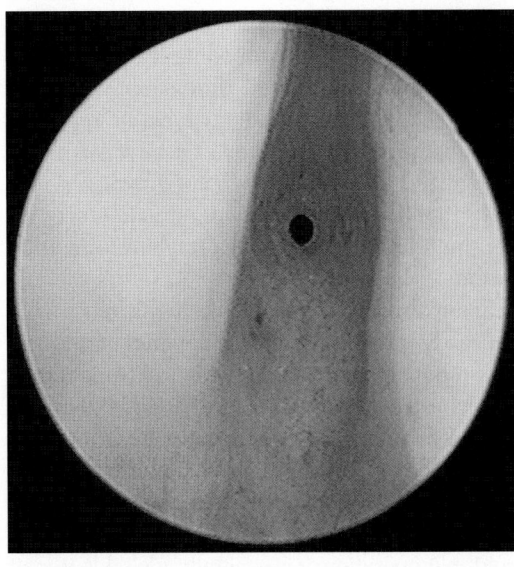

FIGURE 3 Example of a grade III subglottic stenosis.

Preoperative Plan

This should include input from the neonatologist, intensivist, and the child's primary or specialty physicians (pulmonary, cardiology, gastroenterology). The parents must be actively involved in the decision-making process and understand the long-term plan, need for long-term follow-up regardless of the surgical outcome, and potential complications (life-threatening and otherwise) with or without surgical intervention.

For example, a single-stage procedure will generally require ICU admission for a minimum of 1 week and potentially 3 weeks. Often the children will require close airway observation for 1 to 2 weeks after extubation. This requires planning on the part of the family as well as the insurance carrier and ICU staff.

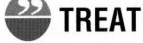 TREATMENT RECOMMENDATIONS

Close Observation

Patients with grade I or mild grade II stenosis can sometimes be observed and not require surgical intervention. These are generally children who do not have tracheostomy

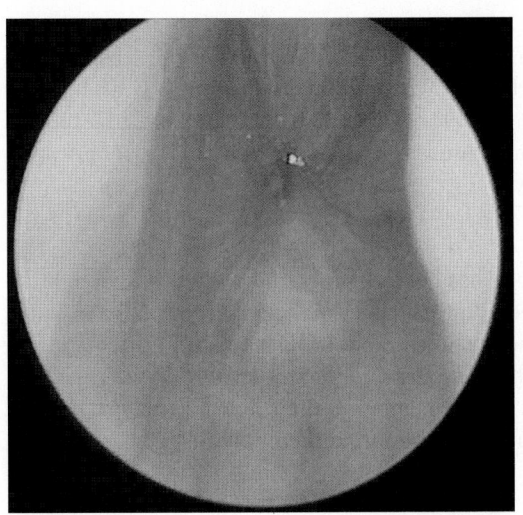

FIGURE 4 Example of a grade IV subglottic stenosis.

tubes, and were intubated for only a short time earlier in life. If these children have only occasional and mild symptoms of stridor without retractions or feeding difficulties and have not required hospitalization for croup or airway-related illness, they may be watched closely. If one chooses to observe these children, endoscopy must be repeated every 3 to 6 months with sizing of the airway, to ensure that the size of the airway is growing along with the child. As soon as it is recognized that the airway is not growing, symptoms of airway problems and hospitalizations for airway distress are imminent. Once this has been identified, airway reconstruction should proceed, before a tracheostomy tube becomes necessary in an emergency situation.

Other scenarios for watchful waiting can involve a larynx that looks highly reactive or edematous. These children are generally already tracheostomy tube dependent and stable and may benefit from waiting a period of months to allow this reactivity to quiet down prior to airway reconstruction. Waiting on reconstructive airway surgery is also advisable if children have pulmonary disease that requires oxygen or frequent hospitalizations due to poor control. Performing airway surgery (single or double stage) on a child with relatively severe pulmonary disease can lead to a less than satisfactory and possibly a devastating postoperative course.

With the exception of the anterior cricoid split operation, it is generally advisable to wait until a child reaches 10 kilograms of body weight prior to performing airway reconstruction.

Tracheotomy

A tracheotomy is usually the most appropriate initial step in safely caring for a child beyond the neonatal period with SGS. It will allow a neonate time to grow and gain weight for future reconstructive surgery. It will allow for a child with bronchopulmonary dysplasia to mature and optimize the pulmonary status prior to reconstructive surgery. The tracheotomy will also allow for an immature stenosis to age and form a more manageable lesion rather than one that is still evolving.

Tracheotomy is not without risk. The morbidity rate for young children with tracheotomy, whose airway is significantly obstructed above the tracheotomy tube is between 6% and 24% (7,18). Language skills are thought to be somewhat delayed in children with a tracheotomy, and in children with complete stenosis vocalization is impossible. For these reasons, early airway reconstruction is attractive and often the safest situation for the child.

Endoscopic

Dilatation

The use of serial dilatations with or without steroid injections for the treatment of SGS has limited application (31). In early SGS, where granulation tissue is present, gentle dilatation may minimize extensive cicatrix formation and maintain some identifiable lumen. Dilatation in the setting of a firm, mature stenosis will not be of any significance in terms of enlarging the subglottic airway.

Laser

Use of the carbon dioxide (CO_2) laser has been described as a treatment option for a circumferential soft SGS (32). The technique involves making incisions in four quadrants within the subglottis with or without micro-trapdoor flaps utilizing the laser, followed by dilatation. It has been the authors' experience that the majority of time, use of the laser to primarily treat SGS results in a worsening of the original problem. Reconstructive surgery following laser use then becomes more difficult because of more severe scar tissue present in the subglottis.

Use of the laser may be appropriate when granulation tissue forms due to early intubation injury. Precise use of the laser in this situation to ablate obstructing subglottic granulation tissue is worthwhile in an attempt to avoid a tracheotomy.

PEARLS AND PERILS
Factors predisposing to failure in treating subglottic stenosis using the CO$_2$ laser

1. Failure of previous endoscopic procedures
2. Significant loss of cartilaginous framework
3. Combined laryngotracheal stenosis
4. Circumferential cicatricial scarring
5. Fibrotic scar tissue in the interarytenoid area of the posterior commissure
6. Abundant scar tissue greater than 1 cm in vertical dimension
7. Severe bacterial infection of trachea following tracheotomy
8. Exposure of perichondrium or cartilage during CO$_2$ laser excision, predisposing to perichondritis and chondritis

---

Open Surgery

Reconstruction of the stenotic airway can be divided into five distinct stages (Table 1) (33). Stage 1 involves complete evaluation of airway (as discussed in the assessment section). Stage 2 involves the expansion of the subglottic lumen with concomitant preservation of function. Stage 3 involves stabilization of the expanded lumen framework, which may involve grafts or stents. Stage 4 is the period required to allow for healing within the reconstructed airway. This period may range from 1 week to 6 months or longer, and likely involves local tissue factors that vary in each individual patient and are not yet well understood. Stage 5 is decannulation, the goal of all reconstructive airway surgery.

There are many approaches to pediatric LTR, and surgeons need to be familiar with a variety of procedures to ensure the best care for their patients. Surgical reconstruction is recommended in mature cases of SGS when conservative efforts to establish a satisfactory airway are inappropriate or have failed. In general, grade III and IV lesions will require open reconstruction. Contraindications to open reconstructive surgery include (a) an absolute contraindication to general anesthesia; (b) conditions in which even if the airway were enlarged sufficiently to allow for decannulation, the patient would still remain tracheotomy tube dependent (a child with chronic severe aspiration); and (c) conditions of severe incompetence of the esophagogastric junction that cannot be controlled medically or surgically.

There are several basic approaches to consider for expanding the larynx, and all approaches yield comparable success when used for the correct indications. For fibrous SGS without significant loss of cartilaginous support, a laryngotracheoplasty with anterior costal cartilage grafting without a stent is successful. If the SGS is combined with severe posterior glottic stenosis or is associated with significant structural damage to the cricoid cartilage, a posterior cricoid split with long-term stenting, a posterior cricoid split with costal cartilage grafting and short-term stenting, or a partial cricotracheal resection would be a treatment options. For stenoses situated in the cricoid and upper trachea with a clear upper resection margin, a partial cricotracheal resection with thyrotracheal anastomosis is recommended.

Meticulous postoperative care and communication with the intensivists caring for the children is essential for all airway surgery.

TABLE 1: Five Stages of Airway Reconstruction

Stage 1: Complete evaluation of the airway
Stage 2: Expansion of the subglottic lumen
Stage 3: Stabilization of the expanded lumen framework
Stage 4: Wound-healing period
Stage 5: Decannulation

Anterior Cricoid Split

The anterior cricoid split is indicated for neonatal acquired SGS in the absence of substantial glottic and tracheal conditions and in the presence of adequate pulmonary reserve. The concept is to avoid tracheotomy in premature children who have failed multiple extubation attempts due to mild anterior subglottic narrowing, and in infants and children who have been extubated but continue to be symptomatic due to a mild narrowing of the subglottis. Interruption of the cricoid ring anteriorly allows the cartilage to spring open and also allows edematous mucosal glands to drain and thus open the airway lumen.

Strict criteria have been established for patient selection (Table 2). If these are not followed, the results following this procedure will be less than satisfying.

The procedure is performed in the operating room after endoscopy has confirmed that other airway pathology does not exist. The patient is intubated with an endotracheal tube and positioned as for a tracheotomy. A horizontal skin incision is made over the region of the cricoid cartilage. The strap muscles are divided in the vertical midline, exposing the lower portion of the thyroid cartilage, the cricoid cartilage, and upper tracheal rings. Stay sutures of 4-0 polypropylene (Prolene) are placed in each side of the cricoid. A Beaver blade is used to make a vertical incision into the airway beginning at the midline of the cricoid cartilage and extending superiorly through the lower half of the thyroid cartilage and inferiorly through the first two tracheal rings (Fig. 5). The skin is loosely approximated around an elastic band drain, which is left in place until after extubation has been attempted. The children are generally left nasally intubated for 7 to 10 days with an endotracheal tube that would be appropriate for their age. Antibiotics are utilized during the intubation period.

These infants generally require sedation while intubated in the ICU, and only if necessary are paralyzing agents utilized. If the endotracheal tube is dislodged in the postoperative period, care must be taken during reintubation that the endotracheal tube does not inadvertently pass out of the airway through the laryngofissure. The stay sutures allow for extra safety for identifying the airway should reintubation be difficult or immediate airway intubation be necessary.

Endoscopy is not performed at extubation. Dexamethasone 1 mg per kilogram daily is administered 12 hours prior to extubation and for 5 days after. Humidification and chest physical therapy are used after extubation. Racemic epinephrine may be used if acute respiratory distress develops. If airway obstruction persists following extubation and time allows, the child should be returned to the operating room for an endoscopy. If granulation tissue is present and can be removed, a tracheotomy may be avoided. However, if the child has clearly failed extubation, a tracheotomy will be necessary. Repeat endoscopy and airway evaluation at a later date will determine what intervention will be necessary to decannulate the child.

Complications of the anterior cricoid split are unusual but can include persisting or severe SGS, wound infection, subcutaneous emphysema, pneumomediastinum, or pneumothorax.

TABLE 2: Criteria for Performing an Anterior Cricoid Split

1. Extubation failure on at least two occasions secondary to subglottic laryngeal pathology
2. Weight greater than 1,500 g
3. Off ventilator support for at least 10 days prior to procedure
4. Supplemental oxygen requirement less than 30%
5. No congestive heart failure for at least 1 mo prior to procedure
6. No acute respiratory tract infection
7. No antihypertensive medication for at least 10 days prior to procedure

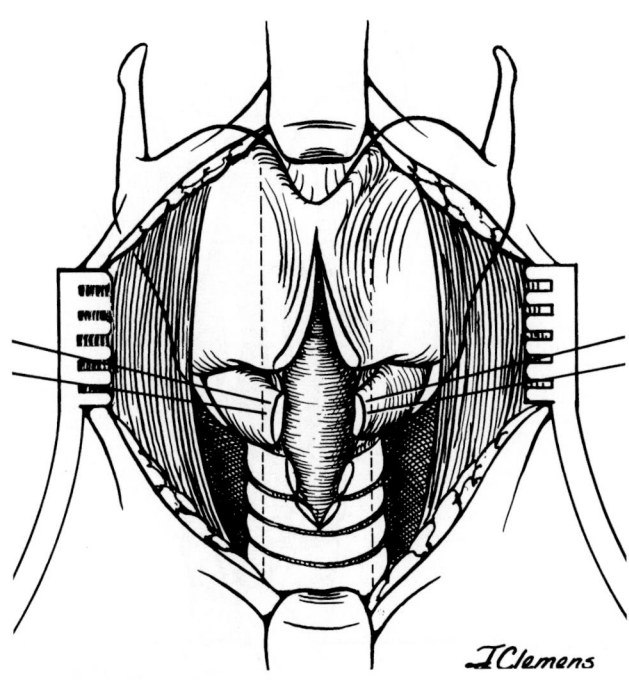

FIGURE 5 Anterior cricoid split. The incision extends from the lower one-half of the thyroid cartilage through the cricoid cartilage and first two tracheal rings.

IClemens

Laryngotracheoplasty Without Cartilage Expansion

This technique performed only in the anterior cricoid was described in the section on anterior cricoid split. For a posterior cricoid split, lateral splits, or the four-quadrant split, the indications and technique differ from those for the anterior split alone. These additional splits are not generally performed in the neonate or infant.

Indications for a posterior split alone include a stenosis that is primarily posterior in location within the subglottis, a stenosis with a glottic component, or glottic obstruction due to vocal fold fixation or a vocal fold located in the paramedian position. Patients for whom splits and no grafts would be considered would include brittle diabetic patients in whom the survival of cartilage graft would be questionable, and older patients who have undergone multiple airway reconstructive procedures with grafts that have failed. Anterior and posterior division of the cricoid is much more commonly used than lateral division. Any patient undergoing posterior or lateral splits without grafting would not be a single-stage candidate, and would require long-term stenting for a minimum of 6 weeks and possibly up to 6 months. The best type of stent to use would be an Aboulker prosthesis secured in position above the tracheotomy tube (above stoma stent). If this is not possible due to stenosis very close or at the tracheotomy stoma, an Aboulker prosthesis wired into a metal tracheotomy tube or a T tube can be utilized.

The larynx may be incised anteriorly in the midline, through the cricoid and thyroid cartilages. The posterior cricoid plate may be divided in the midline. When complete division has been accomplished, the median raphe of the cricopharyngeus muscle and the esophageal constrictors will be exposed (Fig. 6). A blunt hemostat can be used to ensure that the posterior split is complete, by splaying the cut edges of the posterior cricoid plate. An endotracheal tube that would be appropriate for the age of the child can be cut and placed in this portion of the airway, to ensure that the airway has been enlarged to an adequate size.

In rare cases of severe and fibrotic stenosis, a four-quadrant split may be necessary. This will gain maximal expansion of the laryngeal framework. The lateral cuts are made at the 3- and 9-o'clock positions (Fig. 7). The recurrent laryngeal nerves are protected by the outer perichondrium of the cricoid cartilage.

Long-term stenting is generally required if grafts are not utilized.

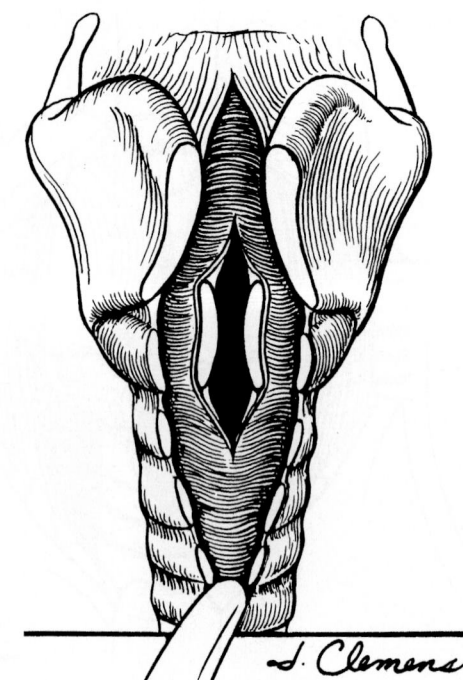

FIGURE 6 Posterior cricoid split. Following creation of a midline laryngofissure, the posterior cricoid plate is divided in the midline to accomplish adequate distraction of the subglottic airway.

FIGURE 7 Four-quadrant split. Lateral cricoid cuts are created at the 3-o'clock and 9-o'clock positions.

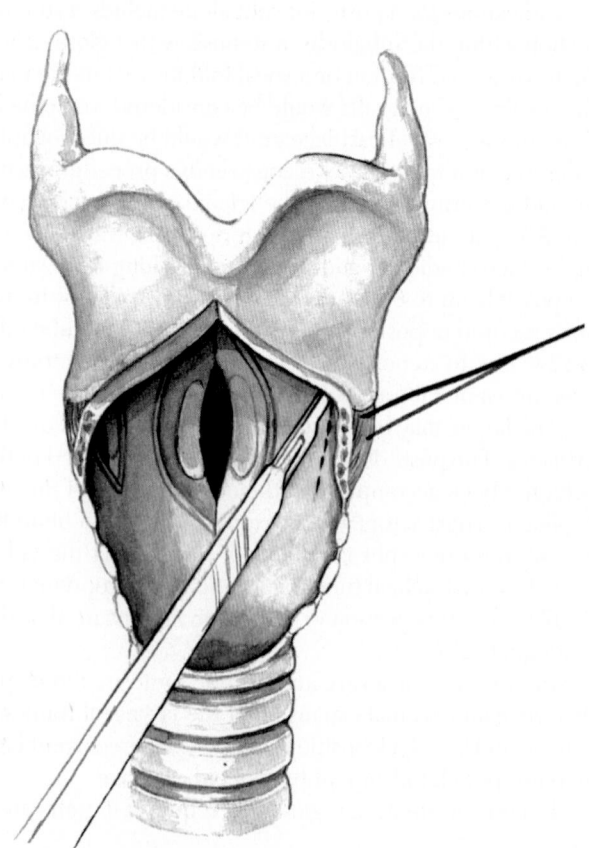

Laryngotracheoplasty with Cartilage Expansion

Expansion and augmentation of the laryngotracheal complex is required when distraction of the laryngotracheal framework must be greater than approximately 3 mm. The material used for expansion can be auricular cartilage, septal cartilage, thyroid cartilage, costal cartilage, or hyoid bone. The authors only use autologous material, harvested at the time of reconstruction. Due to the pliability of auricular cartilage, it is only used in neonates or infants who are candidates for laryngotracheoplasty. For the vast majority of patients, the authors have had great success using costal cartilage, which has excellent rigidity but yet allows for precise trimming and shaping specific for the individual patient's airway.

The technique for harvesting costal cartilage involves a separate sterile field from the neck wound. An incision is made in a horizontal skin crease overlying the right fifth rib to best avoid an unsightly scar. The subcutaneous tissue and underlying musculature are divided to expose the rib from the bony-cartilaginous junction to its sternal attachment. Incisions are made on the superior and inferior aspects of the cartilage through perichondrium. The perichondrium is left attached to the lateral surface of the rib cartilage, and dissected off the medial portion of the rib cartilage. The perichondrium should be left on the deep chest surface to protect against a pneumothorax. The cartilage is incised laterally at the bony-cartilaginous junction and medially at its insertion to the sternum. A 4-cm section of rib cartilage can usually be obtained and is adequate. If additional grafting material is necessary, a second piece of rib cartilage can be harvested from the rib directly superior or inferior to the initial site. Sterile saline solution is placed in the wound and a Valsalva maneuver is performed to ensure that a pneumothorax has not occurred. A Penrose drain is placed in the wound, which is closed in two layers with absorbable suture. This drain is generally removed 24 hours after the procedure.

A neck incision is made at the superior edge of the tracheotomy stoma such that if a single-stage procedure is performed, the stoma and surrounding skin can easily be removed. The strap muscles are divided in the vertical midline, and the cartilaginous airway is exposed. Exposure of the thyroid cartilage and thyroid notch is essential, in order to have a guide to the midline of the airway. The airway is usually entered from the tracheotomy stoma superiorly with a right-angle clamp and Beaver blade. The airway is opened superiorly through the cricoid cartilage and at least the inferior one-half of the thyroid cartilage. If a severe stenosis is present and a posterior graft is to be used, an attempt should be made to avoid a complete laryngofissure. However, it is often necessary to create a complete laryngofissure to allow for adequate visualization of the posterior cricoid plate and room for sewing in a posterior graft. If the laryngofissure is needed, it is of utmost importance to divide directly in the midline at the anterior commissure. If one is unsure of the midline, simultaneous endoscopy can be performed such that the anterior commissure can be divided under direct vision as seen on the monitor. Endotracheal tubes appropriate for the patient's age can be cut and placed in the airway to evaluate the diameter present and what splits or grafts will be necessary to achieve an appropriately sized airway.

When it is decided that the posterior cricoid plate is to be divided, great care must be used to ensure that the incision is in the midline, and at right angles to the plane of the cartilage. A beveled incision prohibits maximal contact between the graft and the cricoid cartilage and predisposes the graft to project or extrude into the lumen. The incision should extend into the interarytenoid area, incising any fibrosis in this region, but not high enough or deep enough to cause an iatrogenic laryngeal cleft. The incision should extend inferiorly 5 to 10 mm into the membranous tracheal wall to allow for adequate distraction and comfortable placement of the graft (see Fig. 6).

The cricoid may be augmented anteriorly, posteriorly, or both. Anterior grafts are considerably larger and thicker than grafts placed posteriorly. The graft is constructed with the perichondrium placed intraluminally, serving as a lattice for epithelialization and thus enhancing survival of the graft. The anterior graft is elliptic in shape. To best preserve acceptable vocal function, the superior edge of the graft should not extend to the level of the anterior commissure. Wide flanges are preserved lateral to the inset por-

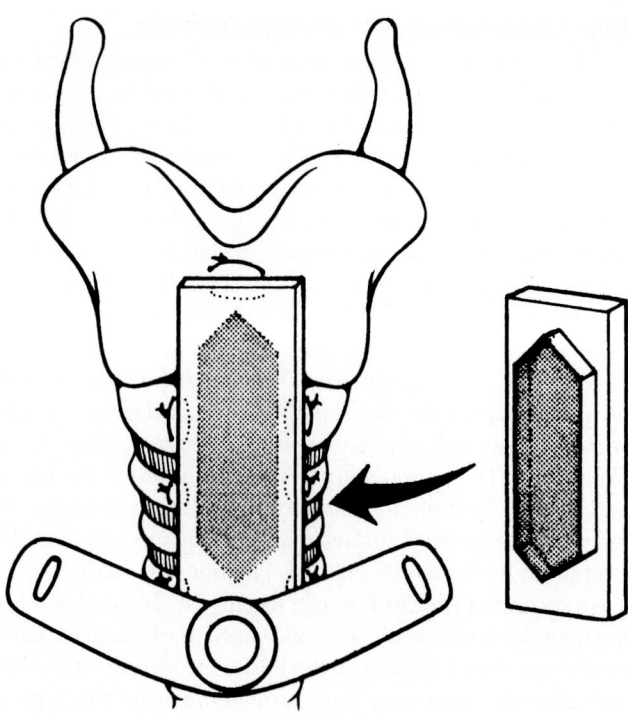

FIGURE 8 Laryngotracheoplasty with anterior costal cartilage grafting.

tion of the graft to prevent prolapse of the graft into the airway. The graft is secured with mattress sutures of 4-0 polypropylene monofilament suture, keeping the sutures extraluminal (Fig. 8). The cartilage must be treated with great care, extra passes with the needle through cartilage increases the likelihood of cartilage necrosis.

Posterior grafts must fit flush between the divided posterior cricoid lamina (Fig. 9). A graft that is excessively thick will compromise swallowing and may lead to aspiration. The graft is carved into an elliptic shape, with 0.05 to 1.00 mm of distraction obtained for

FIGURE 9 Laryngotracheoplasty with posterior costal cartilage grafting. The graft must be flush with the cartilage of the posterior cricoid plate.

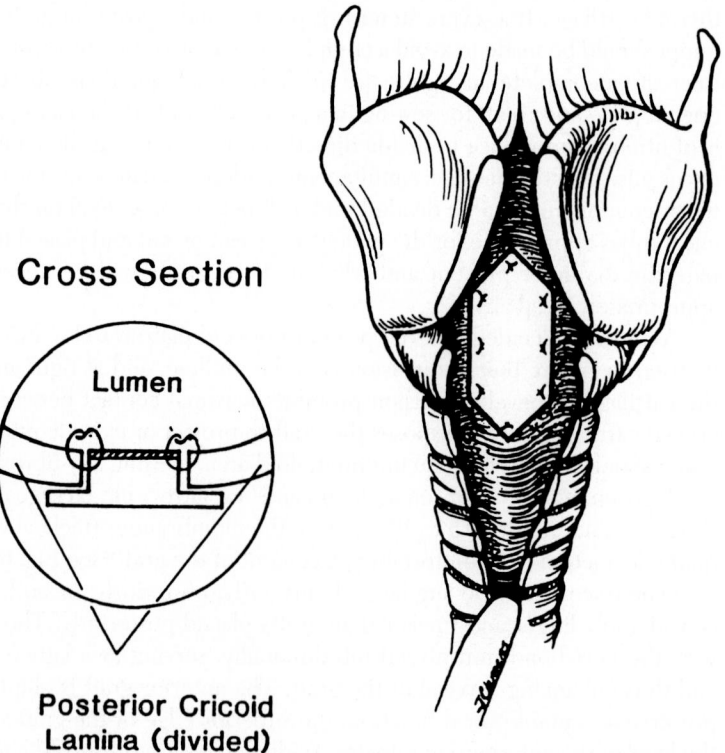

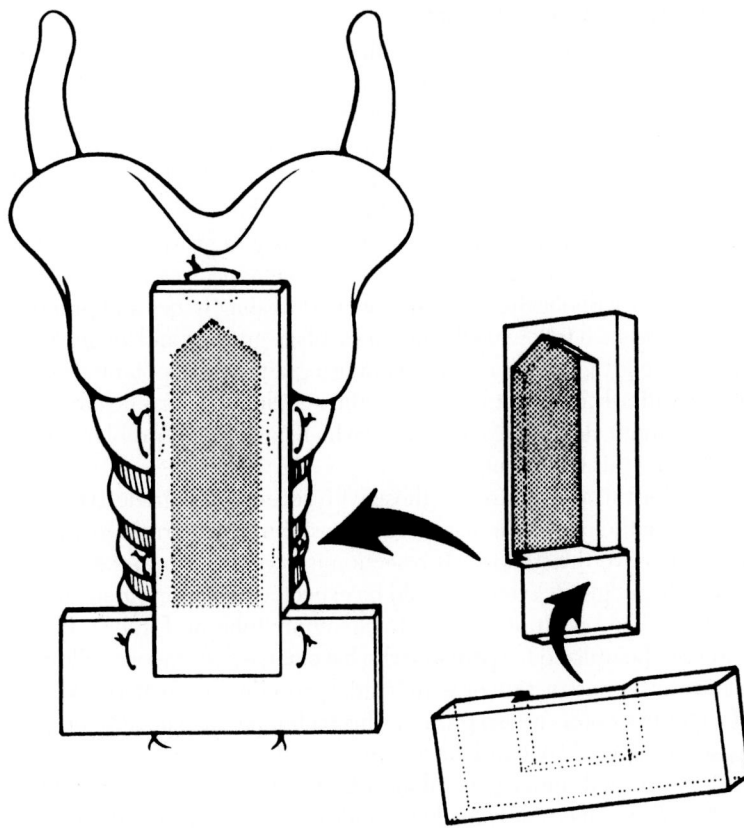

FIGURE 10 Horizontally placed interlocking graft, to add support to the suprastomal framework.

each year of age, up to 1 cm. The graft is sutured into place with 4-0 absorbable suture on a small cutting needle. The knots are buried and remain extraluminal.

In cases of suprastomal collapse, it is sometimes necessary to place cartilage horizontally and create an interlocking notch in its superior surface to receive the conventional anterior graft (Fig. 10).

Based on the severity of the initial stenosis, the surgeon's feeling on the success of the reconstructive procedure, the patient's pulmonary status, and the level of care available at the institution, it is determined whether the procedure is to be single stage or double stage. Single-stage procedures imply that an endotracheal tube is used as a short-term stent. This is usually 7 days for an anterior graft alone and 14 days for a posterior graft alone or an anterior-posterior graft. The vast majority of children can be sedated while intubated without paralysis. This prevents the possible sequelae of paralysis, such as long-term neuromuscular effects and pressure sores.

With severe stenoses, poor pulmonary function, poor intensive care, or an airway that appears or has a history of being highly reactive, a double-stage procedure is advisable. This implies placement of an Aboulker stent secured above the tracheotomy tube, an Aboulker stent wired to a metal trachetomy tube, or placement of a T tube. These stents are secured in place and left in the airway for a period of 6 weeks to 6 months.

Regardless of whether the procedure is single or double stage, the strap muscles are closed over the anterior surface of the graft to allow for revascularization. A Penrose drain is placed underneath the strap muscles and sewn to the skin, to be removed in 48 hours assuming no air leak is present.

A postoperative chest film is ordered to rule out a pneumothorax. Antibiotics are given IV in the operating room and by mouth or nasogastric tube for 1 month following surgery. If reflux is present, antireflux medication is continued for up to 1 year following surgery. Complications can include graft failure or migration, pneumonia, pneumothorax, wound infection or seroma, or subcutaneous emphysema.

Partial Cricotracheal Resection with Anastomosis

Because many of the severe SGSs require multiple reconstructions to achieve decannulation, the concept of a single operation that could remove the diseased segment of the airway and allow decannulation has become attractive. Oftentimes even successful laryngotracheoplasty results in cartilaginous deformities of the airway, or an asymmetric compromised glottis. The advantages of the partial cricotracheal resection with primary tracheal anastomosis are many. Sparing of the glottis, thus allowing for preservation of the normal framework of the larynx and trachea, may improve postoperative voice abilities and laryngeal function. A rounded near-normal-appearing and mucosalized airway follows resection without the associated wound-healing issues and granulation tissue formation that are seen following the use of cartilage grafting and longer-term stenting. Another advantage is the avoidance of obtaining a graft and the potential donor site morbidity. Potential disadvantages to the procedure include recurrent laryngeal nerve paralysis and anastomotic dehiscence, neither of which have been a problem in the authors' experience utilizing this technique.

The best candidates for this procedure are those with severe SGS (grade III or IV) without associated glottic pathology and a margin of at least 4 mm of normal airway beneath the vocal folds and above the stenosis. If resection is necessary up to the level of the true vocal folds, significant glottic edema should be expected and appropriate airway management should be utilized postoperatively (tracheotomy tube or T tube). Partial cricotracheal resection can be utilized for patients who have persisting stenosis following previous attempts at airway reconstruction or as the initial procedure to treat a child with a severe stenosis. If a glottic stenosis is also present, this technique may need to be supplemented with a posterior cricoid split and longer-term stenting.

The procedure is performed under general anesthesia with the neck extended. A horizontal crescent-shaped skin incision is made around the existing tracheotomy tube. The strap muscles are divided in the vertical midline to expose the hyoid bone, thyroid cartilage, cricoid cartilage, and tracheal cartilages above the tracheotomy stoma and at least two rings below the stoma. The soft tissue or scar tissue is sharply dissected off of the thyroid and cricoid cartilages until the cricothyroid joints on each side are identified. The airway is then entered with a Beaver blade in the vertical midline at the level of the cricoid. The incision is carried superiorly to the inferior margin of the thyroid cartilage, unless stenosis is present above this level, at which point a thyrotomy would be necessary (Fig. 11). If the superior extent of the stenosis is unclear, endoscopy can be performed simultaneously such that a precise view of the stenotic segment can be made by watching the monitor. A horizontal cut is made just above the superior extent of the stenosis from anterior to posterior, stopping at the level of the cricothyroid joint (Fig. 12). By staying anterior to the cricothyroid joint, one will avoid injury to the recurrent laryngeal nerves at this level. Lateral cuts are then made anterior to the cricothyroid joints and continued inferiorly through the lateral aspects of the cricoid cartilage, which now exposes the posterior cricoid plate.

Attention is now focused to the inferior aspect of the stenosis, which is generally at the level of the tracheotomy stoma. Stay sutures are placed in the distal, normal tracheal segment. The trachea is then incised just below the inferior aspect of the stenosis through the anterior and lateral portions of the wall. Care is taken to be in a subperichondrial plane during the approach to the lateral aspect of the tracheal wall, to avoid injury to the recurrent laryngeal nerves. At this point, the posterior membranous trachea is incised layer by layer in a horizontal fashion until the party wall is identified between the trachea and esophagus (Fig. 13). If this plane is difficult to delineate, a large bougie placed into the esophagus transorally will allow for definitive identification of the anterior esophageal wall. The lateral and posterior tracheal incisions are then connected, remembering to remain in a subperichondrial plane on the trachea. The stenotic segment of the anterolateral cricoid and upper trachea is then removed, leaving an exposed posterior cricoid plate (Fig. 14). Scar tissue from the inner aspect of the posterior cricoid plate is removed using a small curette or an electrical drill and burr until a thin and flat

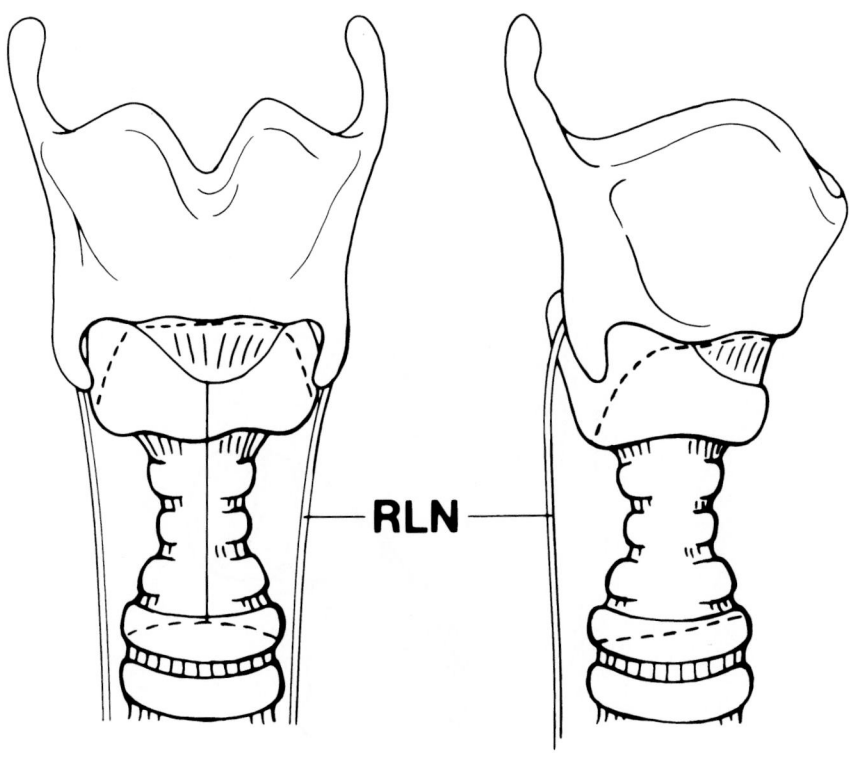

FIGURE 11 Partial cricotracheal resection. Midline vertical incision through the cricoid cartilage and upper stenotic tracheal rings. The ultimate lines of transection are indicated by *dashed lines. RLN,* recurrent laryngeal nerve.

surface is present. No deliberate effort to identify the recurrent laryngeal nerves is made at any stage of the operation, due to significant scarring, especially in reoperations, which renders this dissection difficult and dangerous.

A suprahyoid release is performed to drop the larynx down, and several normal tracheal rings below the anastomosis are released to allow upward mobility of the distal trachea. Interrupted 4-0 polyglactin (Vicryl) sutures are used for the posterior mucosal

FIGURE 12 Partial cricotracheal resection. Incision through the cricoid cartilage anterior to the cricothyroid joints.

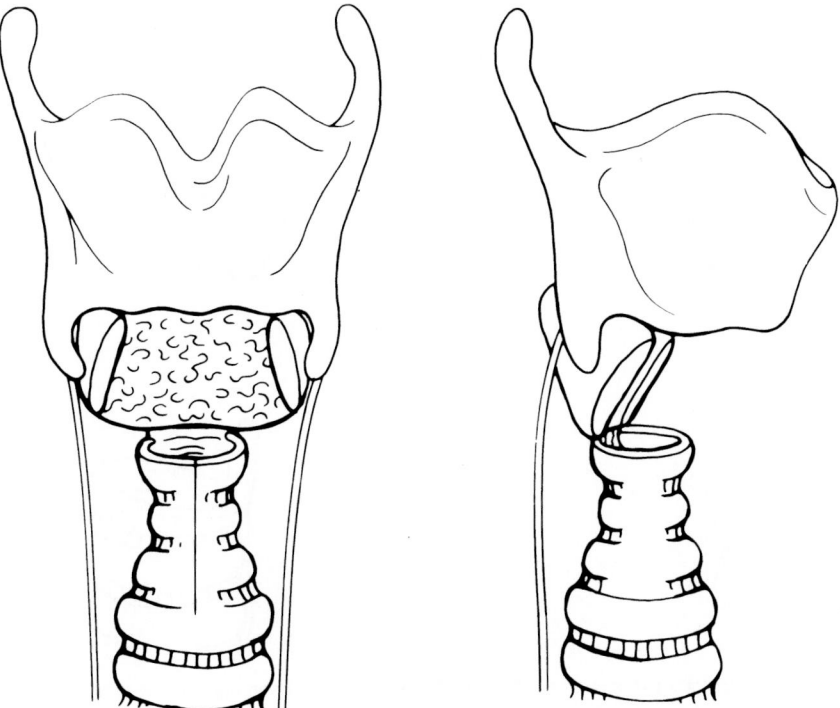

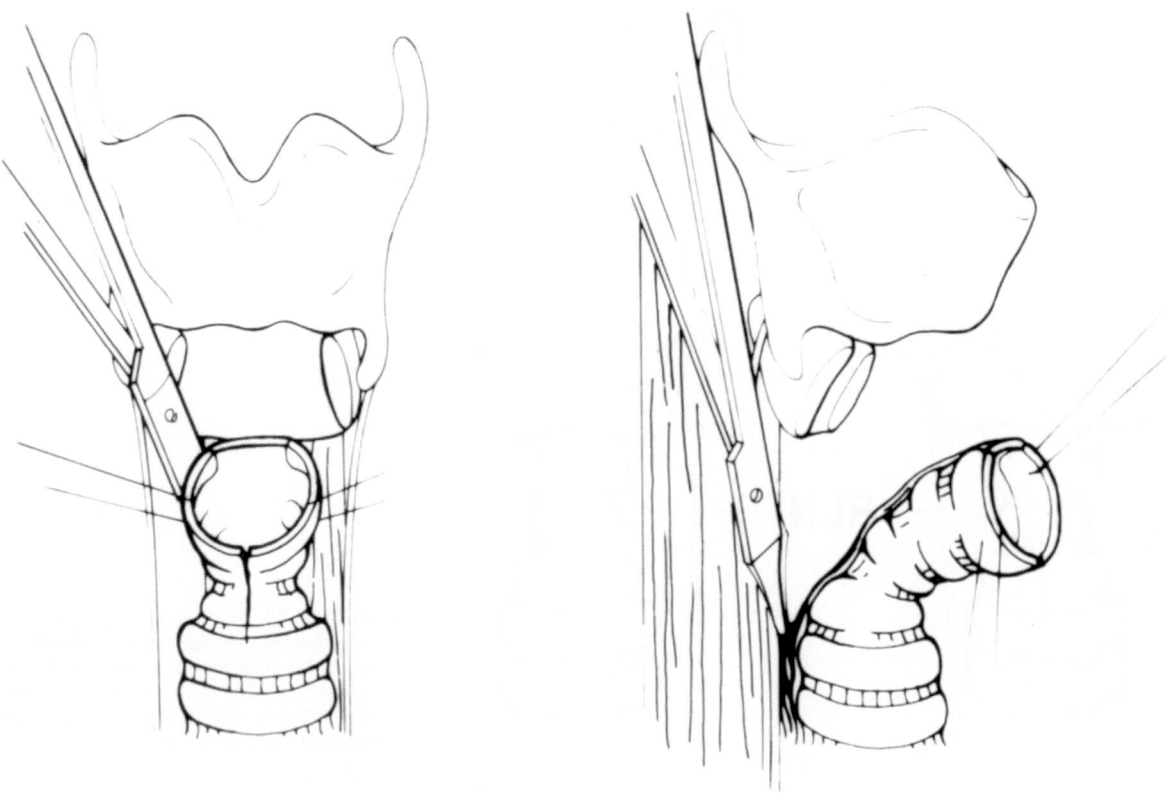

FIGURE 13 Partial cricotracheal resection. Dissection of the upper stenotic trachea away from the esophagus.

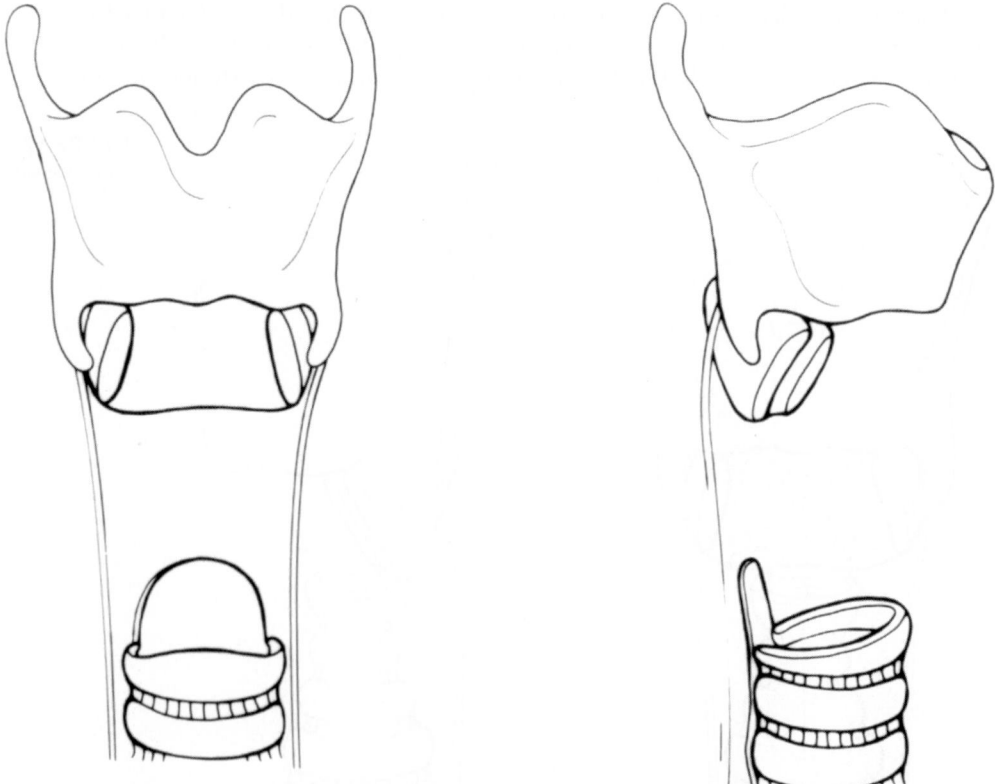

FIGURE 14 Partial cricotracheal resection. The stenotic segment has been resected, leaving the distal trachea with a membranous pedicled flap.

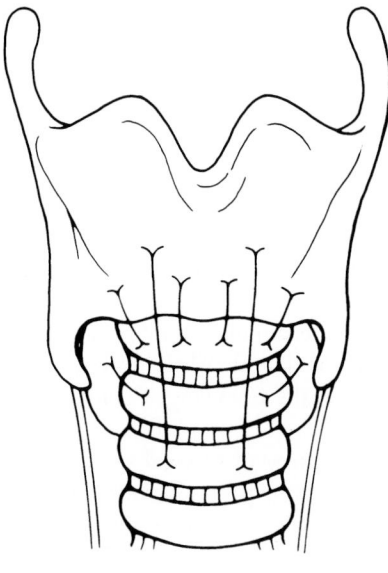 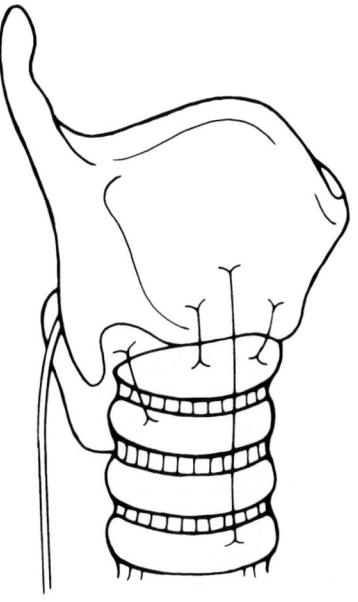

FIGURE 15 Partial cricotracheal resection. Anterior thyrotracheal and lateral cricotracheal anastomosis.

anastomosis. After the sutures are placed, the shoulder roll is removed and the sutures are tied. At this stage, the airway is intubated nasotracheally if a single-stage procedure is to done, or with a T tube if it is decided longer-term intubation is necessary. The anterior and lateral anastomoses are completed by placing 3-0 polypropylene sutures between the thyroid cartilage and the uppermost tracheal ring (Fig. 15). Two or three additional tension-releasing 2-0 polypropylene sutures are placed between the thyroid alae and the tracheal rings below the anastomosis. At the end of the procedure, the neck is maintained in a flexed position and three cutaneous 0 polypropylene sutures are placed from the chin to the chest, to prohibit the child from extending the neck for 1 week postoperatively.

PEARLS AND PERILS

1. Carefully choose candidates.
2. The best candidate is one with a grade III or IV subglottic stenosis without associated glottic pathology and a margin of at least 4 mm of normal airway beneath the vocal folds and above the stenosis.
3. Stay anterior to the cricothyroid joint when resecting cartilage, to avoid injury to the recurrent laryngeal nerves.
4. Stay in a subperichondrial plane when dissecting the lateral tracheal wall to avoid injury to the recurrent laryngeal nerves.
5. Perform a hyoid release to avoid tension at the suture line.
6. Use meticulous technique when creating the anastomosis.
7. Manage the airway appropriately in the immediate postoperative period.
8. Follow the airway closely even after extubation.

In children with minimal glottic involvement and in older children, a single-stage procedure with nasotracheal intubation for a period of 7 to 10 days is appropriate. In children with moderate or severe glottic involvement and in younger children, prolonged glottic edema can be expected, and the airway can be managed with a T tube or tracheotomy tube for a period of 4 to 6 weeks. Placement of small-caliber T tubes in infants and young children should be carefully considered due to the risk of frequent mucous plugging and difficult postoperative care. All children require endoscopy prior to extubation.

Occasionally scar bands will form at the posterolateral aspects of the anastomosis line. These can be managed with dilatation or the CO_2 laser to excise the scar bands. Complications of the procedure include restenosis, aspiration, vocal fold paralysis, dehiscence of the anastomosis, and wound infections.

Postoperative Considerations following Open Airway Procedures

Children who have undergone single-stage procedures must be watched closely, especially in the 2-week period immediately following extubation. Children with tracheotomy tubes in place who are thought to be ready for decannulation must pass an in-hospital minimum 48-hour plugging trial prior to being extubated. All children undergo repeat endoscopy at 4 weeks and 3, 6, 12, and 24 months following reconstructive surgery.

Voice quality following LTR is a very important indicator of surgical success. The majority of patients who had a voice capable of communication preoperatively will have a similar voice postoperatively. It has been estimated that 78% of postoperative larynges have an altered anatomy and as many as 44% have an altered function (34). Continued work in this area in the form of prospective study is essential such that the techniques can continue to evolve and improve.

TRACHEAL STENOSIS

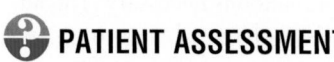 PATIENT ASSESSMENT

Isolated tracheal stenosis in the pediatric age group is not common. Initial evaluation would be identical to that for children with SGS, including a detailed history and physical examination. In a younger child the etiology is more likely to be a problem related to and directly above the tracheotomy tube. In an older child, the etiology is likely to derive from a short-term intubation with too large an endotracheal tube, or a cuffed endotracheal tube that was overinflated.

Regardless of the etiology or age, a careful endoscopy must be performed to ascertain whether the stenosis is anterior, posterior, or circumferential in nature. Sizing of the airway is again imperative to allow for preoperative planning and postoperative comparison. Flexible nasopharyngoscopy should evaluate vocal fold mobility, and a flexible scope passed through the tracheotomy tube will establish if tracheomalacia is at all present.

TREATMENT RECOMMENDATIONS

Endoscopic dilatation is appropriate for tracheal stenoses that are in the acute phase. If the stenosis is progressing or the narrow segment has become a chronic scar, more aggressive treatment will be necessary. The CO_2 laser can be utilized to ablate a single quadrant of the tracheal stenosis, followed by dilatation in attempt to enlarge the airway. This technique works well for short-segment stenoses, limited to one or two rings, and lesions that have an obvious thin lip of scar tissue or are limited to only one quadrant of the trachea. If the lesion has failed to respond to laser therapy, or involves a longer segment, open surgical intervention will be necessary.

Open surgical treatment of tracheal stenosis generally involves a tracheal resection. This is performed via a horizontal cervical incision overlying the third tracheal ring, and incorporating the tracheotomy stoma if one is present. The strap muscles are separated in the vertical midline, and the trachea exposed. Lateral dissection of the trachea should take place in a subperichondrial plane to avoid injury to the recurrent laryngeal nerves. If a tracheotomy is present, the stoma can be utilized as the starting point to opening the trachea in a superior direction in the vertical midline. If a tracheotomy is not present, endoscopy can be performed to precisely identify the stenosis and place a needle into the airway immediately superior and immediately inferior to the stenosis, under direct visualization. Horizontal cuts are made in the interspace immediately superior and immediately inferior to the stenosis. The cuts proceed to the 3- and 6-o'clock positions. Then the posterior membranous tracheal wall is incised horizontally layer by layer until the tissue "party wall" between the trachea and esophagus is identified. The lateral and posterior incisions are then connected with care to hug the trachea in the subperichondrial plane. The stenotic segment is then removed. A suprahyoid release is performed if three or more rings are removed. The posterior anastomosis is created with 3-0 polyglactin suture in an interrupted fashion; then the shoulder roll is removed. The patient is then intubated orally. The anterior and lateral anastomoses are also created with 3-0 polyglactin suture. Tension-releasing sutures are placed from the ring superior to the anastomosis to the ring inferior to the anastomosis with 2-0 polypropylene suture. A drain is placed in the neck, and the wound closed in two layers. A chin to chest suture is placed and left for 1 week. The majority of patients can be extubated in the operating room, and monitored closely in the hospital for 1 week. For smaller children, it may be wise to wait 24 to 48 hours prior to extubation. Follow-up endoscopy is performed to follow the child.

Complications can include restenosis, anastomotic breakdown, pneumomediastinum, and wound infection.

Specific cases of a predominately anterior tracheal stenosis may be best treated by a tracheoplasty and anterior cartilage expansion (similar to the technique described for SGS).

VOCAL FOLD PARALYSIS

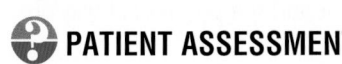 **PATIENT ASSESSMENT**

Acquired vocal fold paralysis in infants and children can have a variety of etiologies. Most commonly these occur secondary to underlying congenital anomalies or secondary to the surgical treatment of such anomalies (35). These conditions include meningomyelocele, Arnold-Chiari malformation, and hydrocephalus. A history of tracheoesophageal fistula repair, surgery for congenital heart defects, previous thyroid surgery, or previous open airway reconstruction can be highly suspected as the etiologic event. As in adults, some children will have paralysis of an undetermined etiology. In newborns with vocal fold paralysis, birth trauma to the recurrent laryngeal nerves has been implicated. The nerves may be unavoidably stretched during delivery, as with a breech presentation.

TREATMENT RECOMMENDATIONS

Unilateral vocal fold paralysis can generally be managed without a tracheotomy. Bilateral vocal fold paralysis can rarely be managed without a tracheotomy, but the majority of times does require a temporary tracheotomy. Operative management of bilateral vocal fold paralysis is usually deferred until the child is 3 to 4 years old. Surgical options include endoscopic laser cordotomy or arytenoidectomy, and open arytenoidectomy or laryngotracheoplasty with posterior cartilage expansion. This subject is discussed in greater detail elsewhere in this text.

VOCAL CORD GRANULOMA

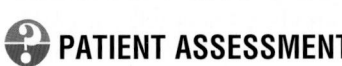 **PATIENT ASSESSMENT**

Response to endotracheal tube intubation usually results in some degree of granuloma formation on the endolaryngeal surface of the true vocal cords. Because the endotracheal tube generally sits in a posterior position, the granulomas are more commonly seen in the posterior half of the glottic inlet. They range in size from barely noticeable, to large completely obstructing lesions. This can be a cause for failed intubation in the infant. The history most often dictates that formal endoscopy be performed to rule out other associated airway pathology.

TREATMENT RECOMMENDATIONS

It is the endotracheal tube that has incited the granuloma formation. By downsizing or removing the endotracheal tube as soon as possible, the granuloma will resolve on its own. Systemic steroids are occasionally used for the days immediately preceding and following extubation. Only rarely in the most severe cases is a tracheotomy necessary to rest the obstructed laryngeal inlet and allow resolution of the granuloma. In this scenario, the tracheotomy tube can be removed as soon as the lesions have allowed for an adequate air passage.

SUBGLOTTIC CYSTS
PATIENT ASSESSMENT

Subglottic cysts are generally the result of short- or long-term intubation due to mucous gland obstruction within the larynx. These can present as long as 5 months following extubation, and must be suspected in children with signs and symptoms of airway obstruction. Symptoms can be very mild or rather significant.

TREATMENT RECOMMENDATIONS

Successful management involves early diagnosis and aggressive endoscopic treatment with laser or cupped forceps excision with mucosal preservation. The bugby (narrow wire-like) cautery, can also be used with the help of a bronchoscope to marsupialize the cyst. Postoperatively the airway can be managed with close observation, or by short-term endotracheal tube intubation if necessary. Repeat endoscopy should be performed 2 to 4 weeks after the initial procedure, to ensure that the cysts have not re-formed. Occasionally, the cysts will recur and reobstruct the airway despite multiple endoscopic attempts. In these cases, an open procedure may be required. This would include creation of a laryngofissure and direct identification of the cyst or cysts present. Micro-trapdoor flaps can then be raised directly over each individual lesion, the cyst and its capsule can be removed, and the flap put back in place. These procedures can generally be done in a single-stage fashion.

SUPRAGLOTTIC STENOSIS
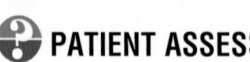 PATIENT ASSESSMENT

Acquired supraglottic narrowing is usually associated with trauma. However, in children with chronic airway obstruction, this condition can also be present following LTR or following tracheotomy (36). Supraglottic stenosis can also develop following an endoscopic surgical attempt to treat laryngomalacia (37). Failure to identify supraglottic stenosis or collapse prior to LTR can lead to difficulty with decannulation following the procedure.

TREATMENT RECOMMENDATIONS

Treatment of supraglottic narrowing is difficult and can be frustrating. Oftentimes, it is best to allow a child to grow rather than intervene and create a more severe stenosis. If the narrowing is due to scarring of the aryepiglottic folds, a modified epiglottoplasty (unilateral or bilateral) can be performed endoscopically with microlaryngeal instruments or the laser, or both. If the problem is primarily due to cuneiform cartilage or excessive arytenoid mucosal prolapse, then endoscopic trimming of these structures can be performed endoscopically. It must be stressed that if any supraglottic work is done, it is done conservatively and often in a staged manner.

REFERENCES

1. Cotton RT. *Laryngoscope* 1991;101[Suppl]:1–34.
2. Tucker GF, Ossoff RH, Newman AN, Holinger LD. *Laryngoscope* 1979;89:866.
3. Jackson C. *Laryngoscope* 1932;2:887–889.
4. Myer CM, Cotton RT. *Ear Nose Throat J* 1995;74:560–564.
5. Jackson C. *Surg Gynecol Obstet* 1921;32:392–398.
6. McDonald IH, Stocks JG. *Br J Anaesth* 1965;37:161–173.
7. Fearon B, Cotton RT. *Can J Otolaryngol* 1972;1:281–289.
8. Grahne B. *Acta Otolaryngol (Stockh)* 1971;72:134–137.
9. Crysdale WS. *J Otolaryngol* 1976;5:479–486.
10. Crysdale WS. *Laryngoscope* 1976;86:1451–1458.
11. Evans JNH, Todd GB. *J Laryngol Otol* 1974;88:589–597.
12. Cotton RT, Seid AB. *Ann Otol Rhinol Laryngol* 1980;89:508–511.
13. Holinger LD, Stankiewicz JA, Livingston GL. *Laryngoscope* 1987;97:19–24.
14. Fearon B, Cinnamond M. *J Otolaryngol* 1976;5:475–478.
15. Hubbell RN, Zalzal GH, Cotton RT. *Int J Pediatr Otorhinolaryngol* 1988;15:67–72.
16. Zalzal GH, Cotton RT, McAdams AJ. *Head Neck Surg* 1986;8:363–374.
17. Pashley NR, Jaskunas JM, Waldstein G. *Laryngoscope* 1984;94:1493–1496.
18. Cotton RT, Gray SD, Miller RP. *Laryngoscope* 1989;99:1111–1116.
19. Zalzal GH. *Arch Otolaryngol Head Neck Surg* 1993;119:82–86.
20. Cotton RT, Mortelliti AJ, Myer CM. *Arch Otolaryngol Head Neck Surg* 1992;118:1023–1027.
21. Seid AB, Pransky SM, Kearns DB. *Arch Otolaryngol Head Neck Surg* 1991;117:408–410.
22. Cotton RT, Myer CM, O'Connor DM, Smith ME. *Laryngoscope* 1995;105:818–821.
23. Monnier P, Savary M, Chapuis G. *Laryngoscope* 1993;103:1273–1283.
24. Stern Y, Gerber ME, Walner DL, Cotton RT. *Ann Otol Rhinol Laryngol* 1997 (*in press*).
25. Walner DL, Heffelfinger SC, Stern Y, Abrams MJ, Miller MA, Cotton RT. 1997 (*submitted*).
26. Walner DL, Ouanounou S, Donnelly LF, Cotton RT. *Ann Otol Rhinol Laryngol* 1997; 106:891–896.
27. Cotton R, Walner D. In: McCafferty G, Coman W, Carroll R, eds. *Proceedings of the XVI World Congress of Otorhinolaryngology Head And Neck Surgery*. Bologna: Monduzzi Editore, 1997:1187–1189.
28. Willging JP, Cotton RT. Subglottic stenosis in the pediatric patient. In: Myer CM, Cotton RT, Shott SR, eds. *The pediatric airway: an interdisciplinary approach*. Philadelphia: JB Lippincott, 1995:111–132.
29. Myer CM, O'Connor DM, Cotton RT. *Ann Otol Rhinol Laryngol* 1994;103:319–323.
30. Walner DL, Stern Y, Gerber ME, Rudolph C, Baldwin CY, Cotton RT. *Arch Otolaryngol Head Neck Surg* May 1998 (*scheduled for printing*).
31. Campbell BH, Dennison BF, Durkin GE, Strigenz MA, Toohill RJ. *Otolaryngol Head Neck Surg* 1986;95:566–573.
32. Shapshay SM, Beamis JF, Hybels RL, Bohigian RK. *Ann Otol Rhinol Laryngol* 1987;96:661–664.
33. Cotton RT, Myer CM, O'Connor DM. *J Pediatr Surg* 1992;27:196–200.
34. MacArthur CJ, Kearns GH, Healy GB. *Arch Otolaryngol Head Neck Surg* 1994;120:641–647.
35. Holinger LD, Holinger PC, Holinger PH. *Ann Otol Rhinol Laryngol* 1976;85:428–436.
36. Walner DL, Holinger LD. *Arch Otolaryngol Head Neck Surg* 1997;123:337–341.
37. Solomons NB, Prescott CAJ. *Int J Pediatr Otolaryngol* 1987;13:31–39.

D.L. Walner: Department of Otolaryngology/Bronchoesophagology, Rush Presbyterian–St. Luke's Medical Center—Chicago, Chicago, Illinois 60612 • R.T. Cotton: Department of Pediatric Otolaryngology, University of Cincinnati, Children's Hospital Medical Center, Cincinnati, Ohio 45229-4356.

• *Practical Pediatric Otolaryngology*
• edited by Robin T. Cotton and Charles M. Myer, III
• Lippincott-Raven Publishers, Philadelphia © 1999

Neoplastic Disorders of the Larynx and Trachea

Gerald B. Healy

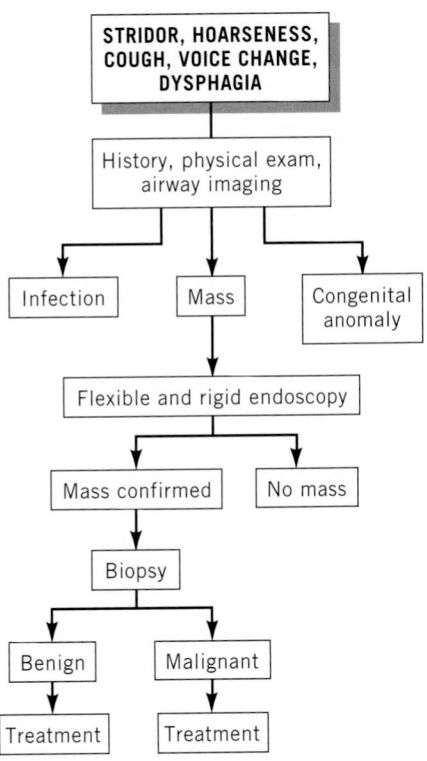

Benign and malignant neoplasms of the larynx and trachea are rare in the pediatric age group. These lesions, however, often present diagnostic and therapeutic dilemmas for the pediatric head and neck surgeon. In a review of 846 patients presenting with laryngeal abnormalities, Holinger and Brown (1) found that only 2% were secondary to tumor. Grillo and Mathisen (2) reviewed 198 tracheal tumors and found that only 6% occurred in patients under 19 years old.

Benign lesions account for approximately 98% of tumors of the pediatric airway, with the most common being squamous papilloma. The next most commonly encountered are those of connective tissue origin such as vascular malformations and neurogenic tumors. Malignant tumors are rare in the pediatric airway and usually are from the sarcoma group. The most commonly encountered lesions are listed in Tables 1 and 2.

TABLE 1: Tumors of the Larynx

Benign	*Malignant*
Epithelial	*Epithelial*
Squamous papilloma	Squamous cell carcinoma
Mixed tumor	Mixed tumor
Adenoma	Adenocarcinoma
Neurogenic	*Neurogenic*
Neurofibroma	Neurofibrosarcoma
Granular cell myoblastoma	
Neurilemoma	*Connective tissue*
	Fibrosarcoma
Connective tissue	Rhabdomyosarcoma
Hemangioma	Chondrosarcoma
Lipoma	Angiosarcoma
Rhabdomyoma	
Chondroma	*Hemotopoietic*
Fibroma	Lymphosarcoma
	Acute leukemia
Miscellaneous	*Miscellaneous*
Lymphangioma	Metastatic tumor

 PATIENT ASSESSMENT

Presentation

Childhood airway neoplasms usually present with signs of upper-airway obstruction. In the newborn and infant, stridor is frequently the first symptom noted. The type and quality of the stridor can often help to more accurately pinpoint the location of the lesion. Inspiratory stridor, associated with a muffled cry and poor feeding, is usually indicative of a pharyngeal or supraglottic obstruction. Aphonia and dysphonia, associated with inspiratory stridor and a mild expiratory component, would most commonly place the lesion at the glottic level. Biphasic stridor, associated with a normal or slightly hoarse cry and reasonably good feeding, suggests that the tumor originates in the subglottic larynx. Expiratory stridor or atypical "wheezing" often represents a tracheal obstruction.

In older children, hoarseness rather than stridor may be the first recognizable symptom of laryngeal pathology. This first symptom can advance to signs and symptoms of upper-airway obstruction if not properly evaluated and treated. Most newborns, infants, and children presenting with these symptoms have inflammatory disorders of the upper respiratory tract. If the symptoms do not improve with appropriate medical therapy,

TABLE 2: Tumors of the Trachea

Benign	*Malignant*
Epithelial	*Epithelial*
Squamous papilloma	Squamous cell carcinoma
Mixed tumor	Mixed tumor
Adenoma	Adenocarcinoma
	Mucoepidermoid carcinoma
Connective tissue	Adenocystic carcinoma
Hemangioma	
Chondroma	*Connective tissue*
Osteoma	Fibrosarcoma
	Chondrosarcoma
	Osteogenic sarcoma
	Leiomyosarcoma
	Myxosarcoma
	Miscellaneous
	Metastatic tumor
	Carcinoid

however, the possibility of a neoplasm must always be considered. In addition, recurrent inflammatory disorders of the larynx may signify an underlying neoplasm that is partially occluding the airway. The diagnostic clue in these cases is the occurrence of infectious symptoms more frequently than one would commonly expect for the age of the child in question. On occasion, diagnosis is delayed because of a misdiagnosis of asthma, recurrent croup, or bronchitis.

Examination

Any child who presents with unexplained or persistent signs of upper-airway obstruction should be fully investigated. In contrast to the adult, it is usually not feasible to examine the infant larynx by indirect laryngoscopy, but the fiberoptic laryngoscope has made it possible to assess lesions of the supraglottic and glottic regions without the need for general anesthesia. This instrument, however, does not allow adequate examination of the subglottic region and trachea. The fiberoptic bronchoscope has been suggested as a means of examining this area, but its introduction into the airway of a small child in an uncontrolled setting can lead to sudden airway obstruction if the airway is already compromised by a partially obstructing lesion.

To define the limits or extension of laryngeal or tracheal lesions, radiographic techniques may be employed. Plain x-ray views of the neck may be valuable in the initial evaluation of stridor in the newborn or infant. This study includes both anteroposterior and lateral projections. Computed tomography (CT) and magnetic resonance imaging (MRI) have found some application in the evaluation of patients suspected of having laryngeal or tracheal neoplasms. CT can demonstrate changes in the laryngeal cartilages that may be indicative of neoplastic invasion whereas MRI can image surrounding soft tissue structures for possible tumor extension. Because of the lack of calcification of the thyroid and cricoid cartilages in patients under 20 years old, CT is limited in its ability to delineate invasive lesions in the pediatric age group. However, MRI is able to give multiplanar views of the airway and further delineate normal from abnormal tissues.

The mainstay in diagnosing laryngeal and tracheal lesions continues to be open tube (rigid) endoscopy. This usually includes direct microlaryngoscopy under general anesthesia in association with bronchoscopy and on occasion esophagoscopy. This allows for evaluation of the entire upper aerodigestive system. The development of fiberoptic instrumentation, in conjunction with the use of the operating microscope and refinements in optical telescopes, now allows the endoscopist to obtain a precise assessment of the lesion and provide the opportunity for appropriate and controlled treatment. Photodocumentation of the pathology seen is helpful both for follow-up and for allowing other physicians participating in the care of the patient to understand the disease process.

TREATMENT RECOMMENDATIONS

Larynx

Benign Laryngeal Lesions

Squamous papilloma is the most common laryngeal tumor of childhood. Strong evidence exists that this lesion is caused by the human papillomavirus (HPV), typically types 6 and 11 (3). Papillomas of childhood, in contrast to the usual solitary adult lesion, tend to occur in clusters and have a relentless propensity for recurrence (Fig. 1). Most commonly, this lesion is located on the true vocal cords but can also occur in the tracheobronchial tree. The frequent clinical pattern of multiple recurrences may be explained by the finding that HPV types 6 and 11 frequently are present in adjacent and clinically normal sites (4). At present, there is no known cure for this disease process. The variety of treatment modalities advocated over the past two and one-half decades for this neoplasm attests to the inadequacy of totally eradicating the disease process. The general

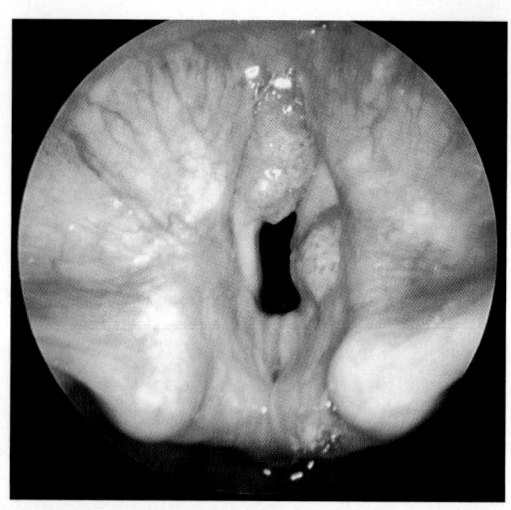

FIGURE 1 Papilloma of the larynx showing glottic involvement.

philosophy of management at present is to control the growth of the papillomas with minimal damage to normal tissues, with the hope that spontaneous regression will take place in time. The mainstay of treatment remains surgical ablation of all visible papillomas, thus maintaining an adequate airway while avoiding damage to normal structures.

Currently, laser therapy is the treatment of choice, with the carbon dioxide (CO_2) and KTP lasers being the most useful. The laser has the ability to ablate or vaporize the papilloma with minimal scarring, bleeding, and edema. This modality has allowed for precise removal without injury to underlying normal structures. Recurrence in the majority of patients necessitates repeated endoscopic procedures performed under general anesthesia to control the disease.

Because recurrent respiratory papillomatosis is a virus-related disorder, *interferon* has been employed in its treatment (5). Interferon is a potent antiviral substance which also possesses antiproliferative properties that inhibit the division of tumor cells grown in culture. The interferon system is a complex defense mechanism involving the release of a substance from cells infected with a particular virus. This substance is then able to confer antiviral resistance on virus-susceptible cells. There are two types of interferon: type 1, which is induced by virus, and type 2, which is induced by antigens. Type 1 interferon is derived from leukocytes (alpha) or fibroblasts (beta), whereas type 2 (immune) is called interferon gamma. At present, interferon alpha has been the most commonly used type for treatment of papilloma. Healy et al. (5) reported a controlled multicenter study on the role of interferon in the treatment of laryngeal papillomatosis. This report suggested that although interferon may be helpful in slowing the disease process, it appears that prolonged use is not curative.

The invasive form of the disease may spread into the pulmonary parenchyma, soft tissues of the neck, or other adjacent areas. Malignant degeneration has also been reported, especially in patients who have undergone radiation therapy in an attempt to control the spread of disease (6).

It appears that the true answer to the control of papillomatosis lies in manipulation of the immune system. Effective methods for such manipulation have yet to be identified.

Subglottic hemangioma is a benign vascular lesion thought to represent a cellular proliferation arising from mesodermal nests of vasoformative tissue. They are not true vascular malformations. The majority of lesions are of the capillary type with vascular spaces surrounded by endothelial cells. These lesions proliferate during the first several weeks of life, with the patient usually presenting with biphasic stridor associated with increasing respiratory distress. Approximately 50% of patients will have an associated cutaneous hemangioma. Endoscopic examination usually reveals a smooth, pink or blue, compressible mass located below the true vocal cords on the posterolateral surface of the subglottic space (Fig. 2).

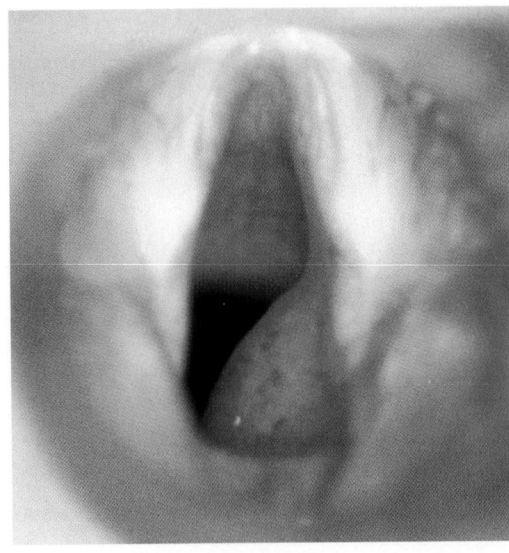

FIGURE 2 Classic subglottic hemangioma in the posterolateral location.

These lesions tend to show spontaneous involution during the first 12 to 18 months of life (7). Some patients, however, develop significant compromise of their airway requiring intervention in the first few months of life. Treatment should be directed at the preservation of normal laryngeal anatomy and function with the avoidance of tracheotomy. Many modalities have been advocated, including radiation therapy, systemic and injectable corticosteroid therapy, and radioactive gold implants (8). These therapies have long-term potential complications and thus, at the present time, laser therapy is a reasonable and safe treatment alternative. Either the CO_2 or the KTP laser appears to be the most appropriate tool for this purpose. A recent report on using open procedures for the correction of this lesion indicated a good outcome (9). However, the endoscopic alternative carries less potential for morbidity and should be considered before opening the cricoid.

In extensive life-threatening hemangiomas, interferon alfa-2a has been shown to be useful. In this situation, interferon acts as an antiangiogenic substance (10).

Tumors of neurogenic origin are rare in the larynx and usually include *neurofibroma, granular cell tumor*, and *neurilemoma*. Laryngeal neurofibroma is frequently a singular lesion but on occasion occurs in association with systemic neurofibromatosis. Lesions are usually supraglottic in location, frequently involving the arytenoids or aryepiglottic folds (Fig. 3).

FIGURE 3 Neurofibroma of the supraglottic larynx.

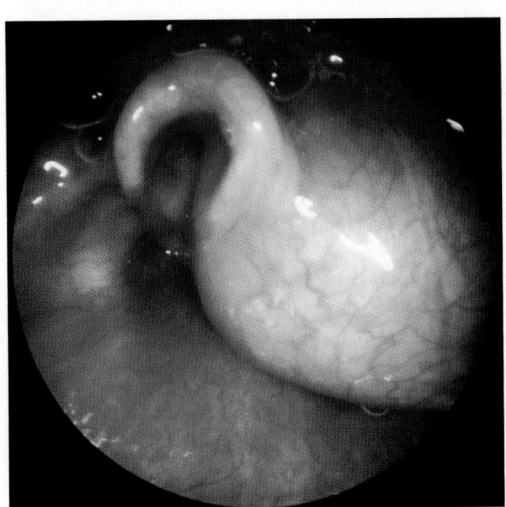

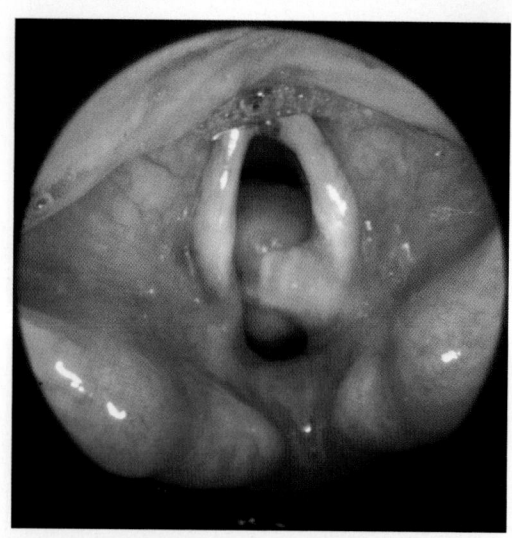

FIGURE 4 Granular cell tumor of the subglottic space.

The goal of therapy should be to keep the airway patent and if possible avoid tracheotomy. This usually involves the careful use of endoscopic resection with the CO_2 or KTP laser.

Granular cell tumor of the larynx occurs much less frequently than neurofibroma, frequently involving the glottic area or subglottic space (Fig. 4). Endoscopic resection is the treatment of choice.

Other rare tumors such as *fibromatosis, rhabdomyoma,* and *fibrous histiocytoma* have been reported (11). Again, endoscopic removal, wherever possible, should be employed. Open surgical excision should be reserved for when the endoscopic approach is not feasible or the tumor has developed significant extension.

Malignant Tumors

Fortunately, malignant tumors of the pediatric larynx remain a rare but challenging entity. The majority of tumors are in the sarcoma group, most commonly *rhabdomyosarcoma* (12). Advances in radiotherapy and chemotherapy treatment modalities have dramatically improved survival over the past 25 years. However, radiation of the pediatric larynx is not without potential complications. Arrest of the growth centers of cartilaginous development, as well as the risk of inducing a second malignant tumor later in life, forces one to reconsider radiation in patients in whom surgical ablation may be possible. Chemotherapeutic agents remain an important defender against distant metastatic spread.

With new treatment modalities, survival rates for patients with head or neck rhabdomyosarcoma have increased dramatically from less than 20% to almost 70% in the last several years (13).

Squamous cell carcinoma of the pediatric larynx is extremely uncommon and treatment is frequently directed along the lines utilized for adult laryngeal carcinoma. The tumor-metastasis-node (TMN) staging system is employed, and patients are treated according to the appropriate staging. Patients with stage I disease may well be candidates for surgical excision of the neoplasm with good tumor margins, thus avoiding the potential hazards of radiation therapy in the young child (14).

Other malignant tumors such as *adenocarcinoma*, tumors of minor salivary gland origin, and varying forms of sarcoma may occur in the larynx (Fig. 5). Treatment must be uniquely designed according to cell type, location of the tumor, and age of the patient.

Trachea

Neoplasms of the trachea in infants and children are rare, and when they do occur, they are usually benign. Patients usually present with signs and symptoms of airway obstruc-

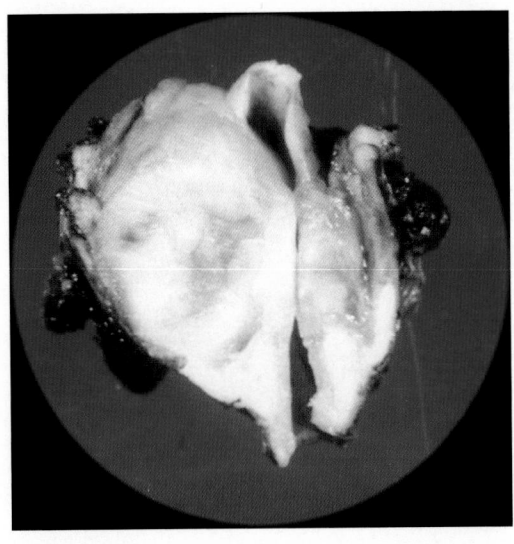

FIGURE 5 Primitive neuroectodermal tumor (PNET) of the larynx in a 1 month old (laryngectomy specimen).

tion including cough, expiratory stridor, recurrent pneumonitis, and occasionally, hemoptysis.

Benign Lesions

Squamous papilloma represents the most commonly seen benign tumor of the trachea in the pediatric population. These patients usually present with simultaneous laryngeal involvement, with tracheal disease frequently representing extension. Many of the patients develop tracheal lesions after tracheotomy, and thus, it has been advised to avoid tracheotomy whenever possible in patients with laryngeal papilloma (15). Unfortunately, in some extensive cases, tracheotomy may be lifesaving and thus cannot be avoided.

Treatment of these lesions involves ablation, usually with laser therapy, although mechanical endoscopic removal or microcautery can be substituted if the laser is not available.

Other less frequently seen benign entities represent either cartilaginous or bony neoplasms emanating from the tracheal cartilages. These usually represent chondromas or osteomas (Fig. 6). Treatment involves endoscopic removal, wherever possible. For tumors that are extremely large, resection with end-to-end anastomosis of the trachea may be necessary.

FIGURE 6 Chondroma of the trachea in a 6-year-old boy.

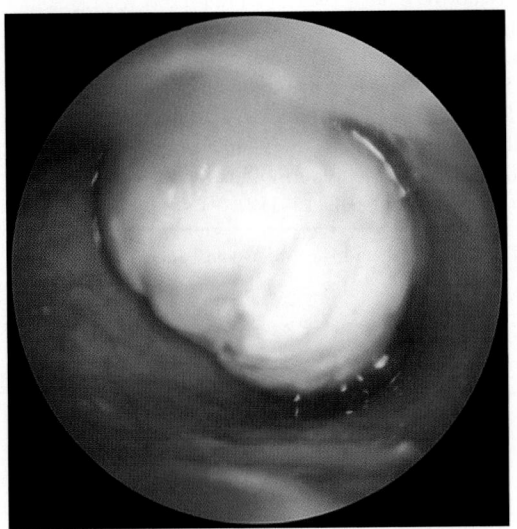

Malignant Lesions

Malignant tumors of the trachea are extremely rare in children, with malignant lesions occurring more frequently in the bronchial system than in the trachea.

Although extremely unusual, *mucoepidermoid carcinoma, adenocystic carcinoma, rhabdomyosarcoma, leiomyosarcoma,* and *myxosarcoma* have been seen (16,17).

Treatment usually involves appropriate application of radiation therapy, chemotherapy, and surgical resection, when feasible. Complete evaluation for local and distant spread must be undertaken as part of the treatment plan.

REFERENCES

1. Holinger P, Brown WT. Congenital webs, cysts, laryngoceles and other anomalies of the larynx. *Ann Otol Rhinol Laryngol* 1967;76:744–752.
2. Grillo HC, Mathisen DJ. Primary tracheal tumors: treatment and results. *Ann Thorac Surg* 1990;49:69–77.
3. Gissman L, Wolnik L, Ikenberg H, et al. Human papillomavirus types 6 and 11 DNA sequences in genital and laryngeal papillomas and in some cervical cancer. *Proc Natl Acad Sci USA* 1983;80:560–563.
4. Pignatari S. Detection of human papilloma-virus infection in diseased and non-diseased sites of the respiratory tract in recurrent respiratory papillomatosis patients by DNA hybridization. *Ann Otol Rhinol Laryngol* 1992;101:408–412.
5. Healy GB, Gelber RD, Trowbridge AL, et al. Treatment of recurrent respiratory papillomatosis with human leukocyte interferon—results of a multicenter randomized clinical trial. *N Engl J Med* 1988;319:401–407.
6. Schnadig VJ, Clark WD, Clegg TJ, et al. Invasive papillomatosis and squamous carcinoma complicating juvenile laryngeal papillomatosis. *Arch Otolaryngol Head Neck Surg* 1986;112:966–971.
7. Healy GB, Fearon B, French R, et al. Treatment of subglottic hemangioma with the carbon dioxide laser. *Laryngoscope* 1980;90:809–813.
8. Ward RF, Healy GB. Neoplasia of the pediatric larynx. In: Fried MP, ed. *The larynx*. St. Louis: Mosby–Year Book, 1996:171–177.
9. Seid AB, Pransky SM, Kearns SB. The open surgical approach to subglottic hemangioma. *Int J Pediatr Otorhinolaryngol* 1991;22:85–90.
10. Ohlms LA, Jones DT, McGill TJ, et al. Interferon alfa-2A and airway hemangiomas. *Ann Otol Rhinol Laryngol* 1994;103:1–8.
11. Ferlito A. Histiocytic tumors of the larynx: a clinicopathological study with review of the literature. *Cancer* 1978;42:611–622.
12. Healy GB. Neoplasms of the pediatric larynx. *Otol Clin North Am* 1984;17:69–74.
13. Healy GB, Upton J, Black PM, et al. The role of surgery in rhabdomyosarcoma of the head and neck in children. *Arch Otolaryngol Head Neck Surg* 1991;117:1185–1188.
14. Ohlms LA, McGill TJ, Healy GB. Malignant laryngeal tumors in children: a 15-year experience with four patients. *Ann Otol Rhinol Laryngol* 1994;103:686–692.
15. Strong MS, Vaughan CW, Cooperband SR, et al. Recurrent respiratory papillomatosis—management with the CO_2 laser. *Ann Otol Rhinol Laryngol* 1976;85:508–516.
16. Gilbert JG. Primary tracheal tumors in the infant and adult. *Arch Otolaryngol* 1953;58:1–5.
17. Watterson KG, Wiseheart JD. Tracheobronchial mucoepidermoid carcinoma in childhood with a ten year follow up. *Eur J Cardiothorac Surg* 1990;4:112–113.

G.B. Healy: Department of Otolaryngology, Children's Hospital, and Harvard Medical School, Boston, Massachusetts 02115.

• *Practical Pediatric Otolaryngology*
• edited by Robin T. Cotton and Charles M. Myer, III
• Lippincott-Raven Publishers, Philadelphia © 1999

Inflammatory Diseases of the Pediatric Airway

Charles M. Myer, III

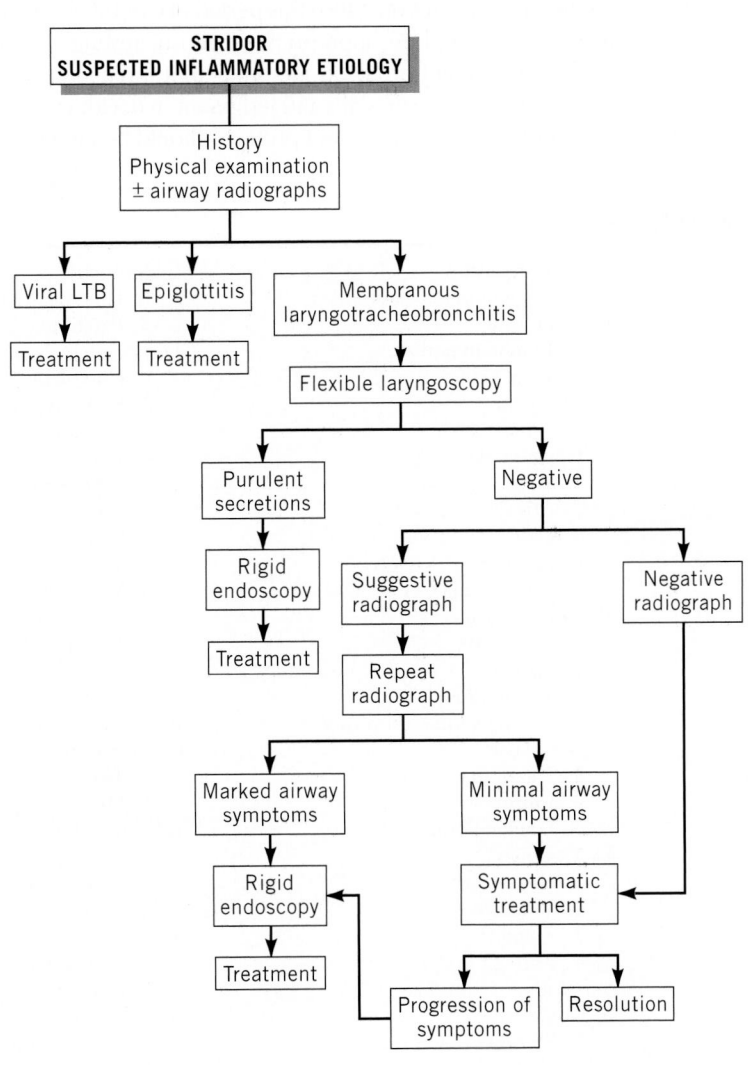

In an overview of inflammatory diseases of the pediatric airway, one is struck by the distinctive features of the major illnesses comprising this broad topic: croup, epiglottitis, and membranous laryngotracheobronchitis. Although each of these processes is marked by respiratory distress, the characteristic presentation of each condition can assist the clinician in the evaluation and management of children with these conditions. This chapter will focus on recognition of the child with inflammatory airway compromise, appropriate radiographic studies that should be obtained, the value of endoscopic evaluation, and the role of intubation or tracheotomy (or both), when aggressive medical therapy fails to prevent progressive airway compromise. A cooperative effort is needed among pediatricians, pediatric intensive care physicians, pediatric anesthesiologists, and pediatric otolaryngologists in the care of these patients.

When a pediatric patient presents with acute onset of respiratory distress, the differential diagnosis generally focuses on the inflammatory conditions enumerated previously. Although other causes of respiratory distress must be excluded (Table 1), analysis of the signs and symptoms of obstruction will allow localization of the site of obstruction (Table 2), thus facilitating disease recognition. Once this period of careful observation by a trained and experienced observer takes place, appropriate diagnostic testing may be undertaken as necessary. Although management protocols are often appropriate as guidelines, the clinician must rely on his or her diagnostic skills and judgment in deciding when an emergency exists and when the diagnostic and treatment protocol should be modified (1–4).

TABLE 1: Differential Diagnosis of Stridor in Children

I. Nose and nasopharynx
   A. Congenital
      1. Choanal atresia
      2. Encephalocele
      3. Dermoid
      4. Glioma
      5. Craniofacial anomaly
      6. Anterior nasal stenosis
   B. Inflammatory
      1. Rhinitis
      2. Obstructive adenoid hypertrophy
      3. Retropharyngeal abscess
II. Oropharynx and hypopharynx
   A. Congenital
      1. Glossoptosis
      2. Lingual thyroid
      3. Dermoid
      4. Vallecular cyst
      5. Cricopharyngeal achalasia
      6. CNS disease/lateral pharyngeal collapse
   B. Inflammatory
      1. Obstructive tonsillar hypertrophy
      2. Retropharyngeal abscess
   C. Neoplastic
      1. Hemangioma
      2. Lymphangioma
   D. Traumatic
III. Supraglottic
   A. Congenital
      1. Laryngomalacia
      2. Laryngocele
      3. Cyst
   B. Inflammatory

      1. Epiglottitis
      2. Angioneurotic edema
   C. Neoplastic
      1. Lymphangioma
      2. Hemangioma
   D. Traumatic
IV. Glottic
   A. Congenital
      1. Web
      2. Atresia
      3. Cleft
      4. Stenosis
      5. CNS/vocal cord paralysis
   B. Inflammatory
      1. Laryngitis
      2. Spasm
      3. Tuberculosis
      4. Gastroesophageal reflux
   C. Neoplastic
      1. Papilloma
      2. Fibroma
      3. Hemangioma
   D. Traumatic
      1. Hematoma
      2. Fracture
      3. Stenosis
      4. Foreign body
V. Subglottic
   A. Congenital
      1. Stenosis
      2. Cyst
   B. Inflammatory
      1. Laryngotracheobronchitis (viral)
      2. Laryngotracheobronchitis (bacterial)

   C. Neoplastic
      1. Hemangioma
      2. Papilloma
   D. Traumatic
      1. Chondritis
      2. Stenosis
      3. Fracture
      4. Foreign body
VI. Tracheobronchial
   A. Congenital
      1. Stenosis
      2. Tracheomalacia
      3. Vascular ring
      4. Tracheoesophageal fistula
      5. Reduplication of trachea or esophagus
      6. Goiter
   B. Inflammatory
   C. Neoplastic
      1. Thyroid
      2. Mediastinal tumors
   D. Traumatic
      1. Stenosis
      2. Foreign body
VII. Pulmonary
   A. Congenital
      1. Hiatus hernia
      2. Diaphragmatic hernia
   B. Inflammatory
      1. Pneumonitis
      2. Toxic
      3. Cystic fibrosis
   C. Neoplastic
   D. Traumatic
   E. Idiopathic

(From ref. 1, with permission.)

TABLE 2: Signs and Symptoms of Airway Obstruction in Children Based on Location of Obstruction

Region	Voice	Stridor	Retractions	Feeding	Mouth	Cough
Oropharyngeal obstruction	Unaffected but may be throaty or full	Inspiratory and coarse; increases during sleep	Sternal and intercostal increasing to total chest when severe	Difficult to impossible with drooling of saliva	Open; jaw held forward	None
Supraglottic laryngeal obstruction	Muffled or throaty	Snoring; inspiratory; fluttering	None until very late	Difficult to impossible	Open; jaw held forward	None
Glottic obstruction	Hoarse or aphonic	Inspiratory early; expiratory as obstruction increases; to and fro with severe obstruction	Xiphoid early and intercostal later; suprasternal and supraclavicular	Normal except with severe airway obstruction	May be closed; nares flared	None
Subglottic obstruction	Hoarse but may be husky or normal	Inspiratory early; expiratory as obstruction increases; to and fro with severe obstruction	Xiphoid early and intercoastal later; suprasternal and supraclavicular	Normal except with severe airway obstruction	May be closed; nares flared	Barking
Tracheobronchial obstruction	Normal	Expiratory and wheezing; becoming to and fro with increasing obstruction	None except with severe obstruction; Xiphoid and sternal	Normal except with severe airway obstruction or when obstruction is due to extrinsic pressure and involves the esophagus	May be closed; nares flared	Brassy

(From ref. 1, with permission.)

CROUP

Acute laryngotracheobronchitis (LTB), or croup, is a viral condition caused primarily by parainfluenza virus types I and II. Other viruses are occasionally implicated, including respiratory syncitial virus (RSV) and influenza virus types A and B. In older children, *Mycoplasma pneumoniae* is commonly found. The age range of affected children is usually between 6 months and 3 years of age, with a peak at age 2 years. The condition is seen primarily in the late fall and early winter, and transmission occurs by direct contact. Although the incubation period is from 2 to 6 days, children infected with parainfluenza type I virus may shed this virus for up to 2 weeks. If a child is hospitalized, strict isolation is appropriate to minimize the possibility of nosocomial spread of infection, especially RSV, since this infection can be devastating in children with congenital heart disease, chronic pulmonary disease, or immunodeficiency (3,5).

Children typically present with a history of an upper respiratory tract infection for approximately 1 to 3 days. This is marked by a low-grade fever, hoarseness, and, typically, a barking cough. A complete blood count is not usually necessary in the evaluation of suspected croup but may be useful in differentiating this condition from epiglottitis or membranous LTB, typically bacterial infections. In fact, croup patients usually have a normal white blood cell count and negative blood cultures.

Although the diagnosis of croup should be suspected clinically, confirmation is generally obtained radiographically. Plain films typically demonstrate hypopharyngeal overdistention, a variable degree of subglottic narrowing with a wider air column noted on expiration in comparison with inspiration, irregular and thickened vocal cords, and a

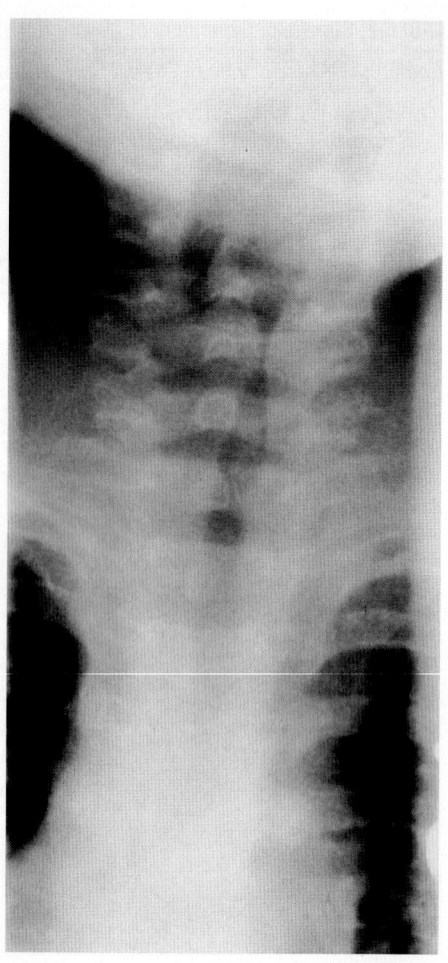

FIGURE 1 Characteristic radiographic features of croup on an anteroposterior view with narrowing of subglottis (steeple sign).

normal configuration of the epiglottis and aryepiglottic folds. These findings on lateral neck radiograph are supplemented with a frontal view demonstrating the classic pencil tip or steeple sign of the subglottic region whereby the normally convex lateral shoulders become convex medially (Fig. 1).

The radiographic features of LTB should be differentiated from those seen in other common subglottic lesions, including subglottic hemangioma and subglottic stenosis. Both of these are static conditions that do not usually demonstrate the changes seen with respiration in croup. In addition, subglottic hemangioma tends to be unilateral, and the radiographs often demonstrate asymmetric narrowing of the subglottis, in contradistinction to the symmetrical narrowing seen with croup and subglottic stenosis (5,6). Although a report from Dawson et al. (7) indicates that a lateral neck radiograph in the evaluation of croup is an inefficient use of diagnostic facilities, this concept appears flawed in children who are evaluated in a hospital setting. In milder cases of LTB, managed in the office, in which the diagnosis is based on clinical symptomatology, radiographic confirmation of pathology is neither necessary nor appropriate. However, in more severe cases, including those that persist or that may constitute a diagnostic dilemma, radiographic confirmation is essential to formulate a treatment plan.

Inflammatory changes may be seen throughout the pediatric airway with LTB. However, symptoms are generally referable to the narrowing found within the subglottis, the narrowest portion of the pediatric airway. There is loosely attached mucosa within the complete ring of the cricoid cartilage, which allows accumulation of submucosal edema and subsequent narrowing of airway diameter. As an example, only 1 mm of edema in an 18-month-old child with an average subglottic diameter of 6.5 mm will decrease the cross-sectional area by approximately 50%, thus leading to the signs and symptoms of airway obstruction enumerated previously (4). It is unclear why some children develop more airway compromise than others and require hospitalization. Although many other underlying airway anomalies, such as chronic lung disease or subglottic/tracheal narrowing, may lead to increased symptomatology, a history of inhalant or food allergies may be seen in those children with a history of severe LTB. Thus, airway reactivity may be related to symptom production (3).

Aside from close observation, the initial form of therapy in most patients with LTB is humidification. At home, parents are often instructed to take a child into the cool night air or into the bathroom with a warm running shower. Improvement is theoretically derived from providing moisture to the inflamed mucosa, preventing drying and crusting. However, little scientific evidence supports this concept, possibly because air is already 100% saturated by the time it reaches the larynx normally (8,9). There is some evidence that croup tents, commonly used in the hospital setting, are detrimental because of their anxiety-provoking qualities, which frequently increase respiratory rate and separate children from their parents. There may be more benefit from parental comforting than from the moisture provided by a shower or croup tent (10). In addition to humidity and comforting, sedation may diminish the work of breathing and allay anxiety. There is always concern about sedating a child in whom respiratory failure may be marked by subtle tiring and lethargy. However, barbituates (pentobarbital 1 to 3 mg per kilogram every 4 to 6 hours) and chloral hydrate (50 to 75 mg per kilogram every 4 to 6 hours) offer predictable sedation and minimal respiratory depression (3).

A second component of therapy that is frequently used is racemic epinephrine inhalation therapy. Racemic epinephrine is an alpha- and beta-agonist containing both levorotatory (L) and dextrorotatory (D) isomers, of which the L form is the active component. Symptomatic relief is provided by vasoconstriction, which reduces subglottic edema, and by beta-2, stimulation, which leads to bronchial smooth muscle relaxation. All patients will improve symptomatically, often within minutes, but there is usually no effect on arterial oxygen saturation (11,12). There appears to be no difference in results whether the medication is delivered by intermittent positive pressure breathing or by nebulization alone, and nebulization is often tolerated better by young children (12–14). Appropriate doses are 0.25 ml of a 2.25% solution in children younger than 6 months of age and 0.5 ml of a similar solution for older children. It can be administered as frequently as necessary, although administration at intervals of less than 30 minutes may herald the need for more aggressive intervention. Because of the possibility of relapse and the fact that the duration of action is less than 2 hours, any child that receives a treatment should be observed for at least 3 hours following medication administration (15). Treatment with racemic epinephrine may not alter the natural history of the disease, but it may postpone or eliminate the need for an artificial airway (12,13). Although side effects are rare, patients with left ventricular outflow obstruction, including tetralogy of Fallot and idiopathic hypertrophic subaortic stenosis, should be treated cautiously with this medication (16).

Steroids

The use and effectiveness of systemic corticosteroids in the management of LTB remains controversial. The rationale of steroid use is solid; steroids exert their effects by decreasing capillary endothelial permeability, thus leading to a decrease in mucosal edema and stabilization of lysosomal membranes, decreasing the inflammatory reaction present. However, their effectiveness remains in question since there have been tremendous variations in research protocols utilizing steroids, including the failure to establish definitive diagnostic criteria for LTB, inconsistency with choice of steroid dose, and lack of consistency in defining the end point in determining improvement (16).

In utilizing systemic corticosteroids, the clinician must remember that it will take at least 3 hours for this medication to produce any substantial physiologic change. Thus, steroid use is beneficial in an anticipatory fashion, whereas racemic epinephrine can provide symptomatic relief on a much more acute basis. Although an initial dose of at least

100 mg of hydrocortisone (or equivalent) is recommended (17,18), dexamethasone sodium phosphate has been used most frequently in evaluating the efficacy of steroids in the management of LTB. Its benefits include an antiinflammatory potency 25 times greater than that of hydrocortisone, as well as a long half-life of 36 to 72 hours. Single-dose therapy of dexamethasone sodium phosphate at 0.6 mg per kilogram appears to decrease the severity of moderate and severe LTB and will decrease the need for racemic epinephrine treatments (19,20). Some recommend repeating this dose on a divided basis daily for 48 to 72 hours. Although the duration of hospital stay does not seem to be altered by steroid use, an adequate initial dose may prevent the necessity for intubation (18,19,21). Similarly, Cruz et al. (22) reported that dexamethasone sodium phosphate (0.6 mg per kilogram) as a single intramuscular injection was effective in the treatment of croup of moderate severity when administered to patients prior to emergency room discharge. No adverse effects have been reported when steroids are used in this manner, but length of hospitalization seems unaffected by steroid use (16,19,20,23–29). As an alternative to oral or parenteral steroids, nebulized budesonide has been utilized. Its efficacy appears to be comparable to that of oral or parenteral glucocorticoids, as opposed to nebulized dexamethasone, which is not effective in reducing hospital admissions or changing clinical outcomes at 24 hours (30).

It is reasonable to consider institution of systemic steroids whenever racemic epinephrine treatments are required, to minimize the risk of intubation and the likelihood of further racemic epinephrine treatments. In some circumstances, one might consider the use of oral corticosteroids on an outpatient basis in less severe cases that do not demand racemic epinephrine therapy and possible admission. However, one must be aware of the lack of clinical trials when treating LTB patients on an outpatient basis with a potent medication such as corticosteroids. Croup is a dynamic process, and patients may worsen in spite of ongoing therapy. Therefore, one must be cautious with recommending this form of treatment in children whose parents are not good observers and not keenly aware of the potential for severe respiratory distress.

Intubation

Placement of an artificial airway is essential when aggressive medical therapy does not prevent progression of airway distress. Although there has been controversy in the past regarding the use of an endotracheal tube or a tracheotomy, initial placement of an endotracheal tube seems appropriate in most children with LTB. There is a reported incidence of subglottic stenosis in less than 3% of children who undergo intubation for croup (20,31,32). Although the development of subglottic stenosis in these children is rare, it may occur secondary to endotracheal tube trauma within the subglottis, the narrowest portion of the pediatric airway. The risk for subglottic stenosis appears to increase with increased trauma to the subglottis, including lack of leak around an endotracheal tube, intubation for greater than 5 days, and a preexisting subglottic stenosis, including children with Down syndrome, who generally have a smaller than normal subglottis. An attempt should be made to utilize an endotracheal tube 0.5 mm smaller than that recommended for a child's age, this being determined from a formula in which one divides the child's age in years by 4 and then adds 4 to this ([age in years divided by 4] + 4) (32). If one is unable to maintain effective ventilation utilizing a smaller than normal endotracheal tube, consideration should be given to endoscopic evaluation and, potentially, a tracheotomy. Whenever possible, the intubation should be done in a controlled fashion; in general, nasotracheal intubation is preferred (32–34). One must keep in mind the possibility of aspiration or postobstructive pulmonary edema in the child who deteriorates rapidly after intubation. Knowledge of this condition will allow for rapid detection and, hopefully, prompt therapy (3).

Once a child is intubated, extubation should not be attempted until the following criteria are met: the child is afebrile, minimal secretions are obtained when the endotracheal tube is suctioned, a leak develops around the endotracheal tube as noted by the child's ability to cough or vocalize, or bubbling can be heard when positive pressure ventilation is given. Even if no leak is present, extubation may be attempted after 5 days of intubation if the child is afebrile and secretions have diminished. Should extubation fail, endoscopic evaluation under anesthesia is appropriate to evaluate the severity of airway pathology. When subglottic stenosis is identified, placement of a tracheotomy would be appropriate (31). If there does not appear to be permanent damage to the subglottis, one might replace the endotracheal tube and make another attempt at extubation several days later. Parenteral corticosteroids may be beneficial prior to any attempt at extubation.

If subglottic stenosis is identified, an anterior cricoid split procedure may be an alternative to tracheotomy. However, should marked inflammatory/infectious changes be noted at endoscopic evaluation, it probably would be advisable to place a tracheotomy initially and allow the inflammation to diminish before attempting surgical reconstruction. If, on the other hand, edema without significant excoriation is noted, a cricoid split may be an acceptable alternative (35).

Endoscopy

Flexible nasopharyngoscopy may play a role in the initial diagnostic evaluation of a patient with the acute onset of stridor. If one is suspicious of croup because of the clinical presentation and radiographic features, flexible endoscopic evaluation of the glottis and subglottis is not necessary. However, when questions arise regarding the diagnosis, flexible endoscopy may be helpful in guiding therapy. If a patient is in severe distress, this evaluation technique is not appropriate, and one should consider formal microlaryngoscopy and bronchoscopy in the operating room instead. During the acute inflammatory process, operative endoscopy should be performed when there is a failure to respond to appropriate and aggressive medical therapy, when a child has failed extubation, in a very young child, or if the diagnosis is in doubt. Endoscopy is performed preferentially utilizing a rigid Hopkins rod telescope only to minimize trauma and to afford an adequate examination of the subglottis. A skilled, experienced endoscopist is needed to avoid iatrogenic complications. In the child who has repeated episodes of croup, endoscopic evaluation of the airway is necessary to eliminate the possibility of subglottic stenosis. One should perform the endoscopy electively about 3 to 4 weeks following the inflammatory event to obtain a true picture of the subglottic airway (4).

SPASMODIC CROUP

Although children with spasmodic croup present like children with viral LTB, i.e., with biphasic stridor and a barking cough, the children are generally afebrile and lack the typical viral prodrome. The pathogenesis is unknown, but an allergic cause has been postulated because of its recurrent nature. Children usually recover within a few hours of onset without treatment (3,4).

MEMBRANOUS LARYNGOTRACHEOBRONCHITIS

A separate condition, but one related to LTB is membranous laryngotracheobronchitis (MLTB), also known as membranous croup. Oftentimes called bacterial tracheitis, this is a misnomer since the diagnosis is based on the clinical appearance of the airway and not on a positive culture result. Like viral LTB, there is a slight male predominance in MLTB, but the age range affected is much broader, with the average age of onset at 5 years. The disease is believed to be due to a bacterial superinfection of a preexisting viral upper respiratory tract infection.

Children with MLTB have a clinical presentation similar to that of viral LTB; they exhibit fever, cough, and stridor but generally have a more toxic appearance. If the patient is not in extremis, radiographic evaluation of the neck and chest is appropriate. When MLTB is present, the radiographs often demonstrate irregular tracheal densities in addition to subglottic narrowing (Fig. 2). If possible, flexible nasopharyngoscopy should be done in an effort to identify purulent secretions within the subglottis and trachea. They often extend into the glottic airway.

Once the diagnosis is suspected, based either on a positive radiographic evaluation, on a positive endoscopic evaluation, or on clinical suspicion, rigid endoscopy in the operating room is essential. One generally finds a markedly inflamed and edematous trachea, with thick, tenacious, adherent secretions (Fig. 3). Careful removal of these secretions is needed and requires the use of suction and foreign body forceps. Cultures are mandatory, and the most commonly recovered organisms are *Staphylococcus aureus* and *Hemophilus influenzae*. Once the diagnosis is made, broad-spectrum antimicrobial therapy should be administered parenterally, always including coverage for the two organisms mentioned previously. An outbreak of bacterial tracheitis in Cincinnati, Ohio, in the winter of 1995 to 1996 demonstrated some changes in the bacterial flora of this condition. The predominant organism in this series of 38 cases associated with an influenza A outbreak was *Moraxella catarrhalis*, but several cases of penecillin-resistant *Streptoccus pneumoniae* were seen, as well as one case of *Pseudomonas aeruginosa* (unpublished data). Endotracheal intubation may be necessary, but this decision should be determined in consultation between the endoscopist and pediatric intensive care unit physician. The secretions generally decrease over 3 to 5 days, and extubation may be attempted at that time if the secretions have decreased and flexible bronchoscopy demonstrates less tra-

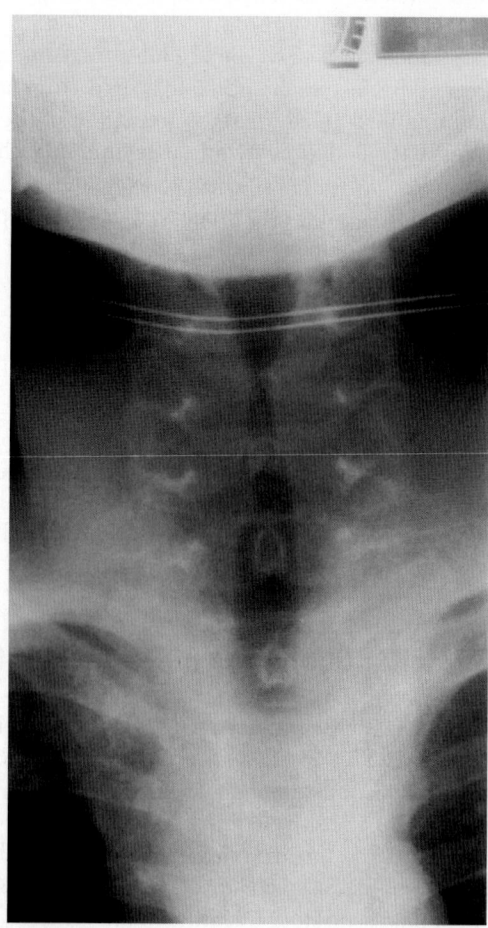

FIGURE 2 Anterior-posterior neck radiograph demonstrating irregular tracheal markings along right lateral wall found in many children with membranous laryngotracheobronchitis (MLTB).

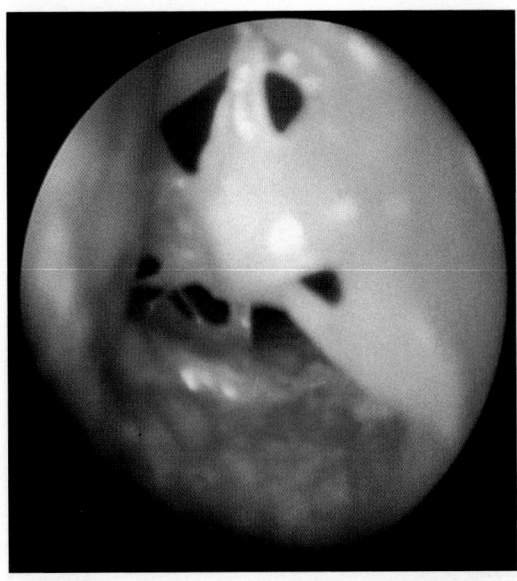

FIGURE 3 MLTB is characterized endoscopically by thick, tenacious secretions within an inflamed edematous airway.

cheobronchial inflammation. There are no standards regarding length of administration of antimicrobial therapy or observation in the hospital, but a conservative posture should be utilized in this potentially life-threatening condition (36–38; see decision tree).

EPIGLOTTITIS

The use of *H. influenzae* type B vaccine has led to a marked decrease in the incidence of epiglottitis (39). However, the potential severity of this condition mandates that the clinician maintain an awareness of its presence and develop a protocol for its treatment. Children with epiglottitis, also known as supraglottitis, present a true airway emergency because of the nature of their disease. Caused primarily by *H. influenzae* type B, it affects children generally between the ages of 3 and 6 years, an older age group than seen with viral LTB (40). It can occur at any time of the year, but it is more common in the winter and spring (41).

In contradistinction to LTB and MLTB, these children generally lack a viral prodrome and often complain of a progressive sore throat. They have a toxic appearance and are generally febrile. Although early in the course of their illness, they may be quite irritable, the patients may become lethargic as airway symptoms progress. Airway distress and pain on swallowing often begin about 4 to 8 hours after the onset of the initial symptoms. The child is generally tachypneic and often sits in the "tripod" position, assuming an upright position with the neck extended and the arms providing support, to maximize the size of the supraglottic airway. As the edematous supraglottic tissues prolapse into the glottis, airway obstruction worsens and severe inspiratory stridor develops. Drooling and a muffled voice are commonly seen (4). If radiographs are obtained, the lateral film will show a thickened epiglottis (thumb sign), thickened epiglottic folds, possible hypopharyngeal distention, and a normal subglottis (Fig. 4) (42).

If one is suspicious of the diagnosis of epiglottis, no radiographic studies are appropriate. Instead, the child should be placed in a setting in which direct visualization of the airway can be accomplished, so that intubation can be performed. Whether this occurs in the operating room, emergency department, or intensive care unit is dependent on the institution and the resources present at any one time. Although some institutions have a protocol that demands the presence of both an anesthesiologist and an otolaryngologist along with bronchoscopic equipment and a tracheotomy set, this is not universal, and one

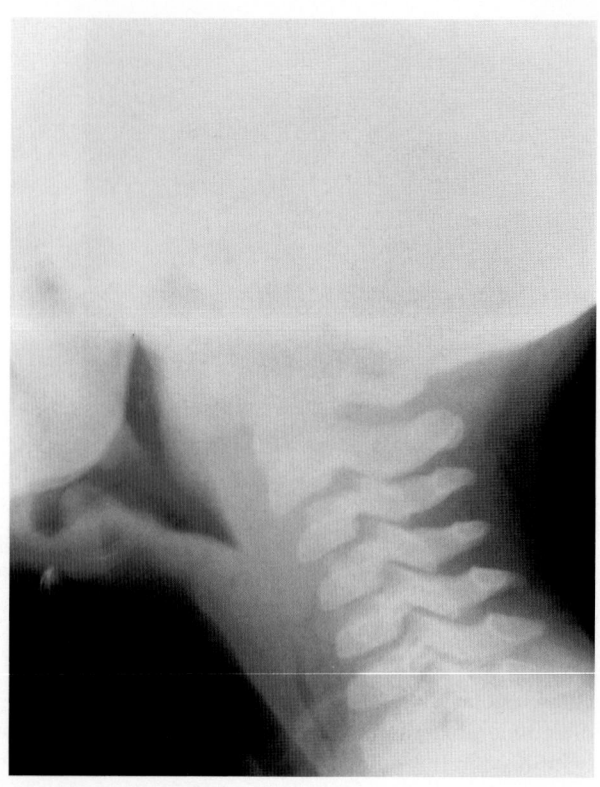

FIGURE 4 Lateral neck radiograph demonstrating the thickened epiglottis and any epiglottic folds typically seen in epiglottitis (supraglottitis).

must establish a protocol that fits one's own institution. The evaluation should be performed with the child breathing spontaneously to optimize care.

An endoscopic evaluation will reveal erythema and edema of all the supraglottic structures, including the arytenoids, aryepiglottic folds, and the epiglottis (Fig. 5). This is consistent with the radiographic findings should they have been obtained prior to intubation. If epiglottitis is not identified, the differential diagnosis of acute supraglottic obstruction should include retropharyngeal abscess or cellulitis, angioneurotic edema of the oral cavity structures, vallecular cysts, epiglottic lymphangioma, or a foreign body of the upper aerodigestive tract.

Following diagnosis, nasotracheal intubation should be attempted. If this is not successful, rigid bronchoscopy should allow the airway to be secured. Should this fail, a tracheotomy may be appropriate. Extubation is usually possible in 48 hours and should be

FIGURE 5 Endoscopic appearance of epiglottitis demonstrates erythema and edema of the epiglottic structures.

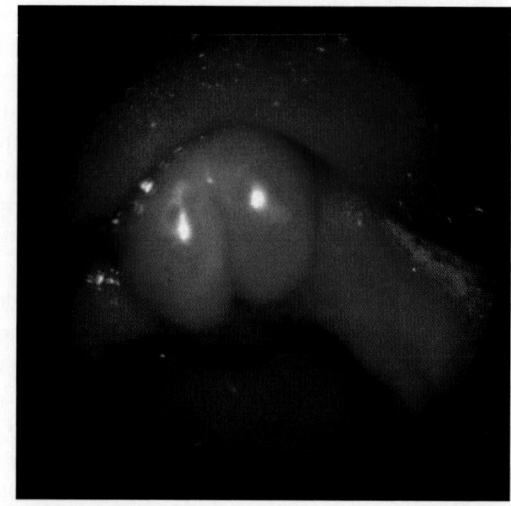

guided by direct visualization of the epiglottis. Normal supraglottic landmarks can be identified with resolution of the edema and erythema (43). Aerobic and anaerobic cultures of the epiglottis should be obtained at the time of endoscopy to permit the choice of an appropriate antimicrobial agent, always initially choosing an agent effective against *H. influenzae* type B. This may include use of a combination of ampicillin and chloramphenicol or third-generation cephalosporins, such as cefotaxime or ceftriaxone. These choices must be made with the knowledge of the emergence of beta-lactamase-producing strains of *H. influenzae*. In some circumstances, rifampin prophylaxis for exposed individuals is appropriate (39).

SUMMARY

An organized approach to the child with respiratory distress secondary to inflammatory changes of the airway is essential. One must be familiar with the clinical radiographic features of LTB, MLTB, and epiglottitis in addition to the treatment alternatives available.

PEARLS AND PERILS

1. Although epiglottitis is rare today, one must obtain cultures for aerobic, fungal, and acid-fast organisms when a suspected case is encountered.
2. When a case of croup seems unusually severe in an older child, one must consider the diagnosis of bacterial tracheitis.
3. Careful evaluation of airway radiographs is essential in inflammatory airway disease because of the possibility of bacterial tracheitis.
4. If intubation is required in the management of inflammatory airway disease, one should have a definite plan regarding timing of endoscopic evaluation and possible tracheotomy.

❋ REFERENCES

1. Myer CM III, Cotton RT. Pediatric airway and laryngeal problems. In: Lee KJ, ed. *Textbook of otolaryngology and head and neck surgery.* New York: *Elsevier,* 1989:658–673.
2. Myer CM III, Cotton RT. Pediatric airway and laryngeal problems. In: Lee KJ, ed. *Textbook of otolaryngology and head and neck surgery.* New York: *Elsevier,* 1995:889–906.
3. Willson DF. Inflammatory diseases of the airway. In: Myer CM III, Cotton RT, Shott SR, eds. *The pediatric airway: an interdisciplinary approach. Philadelphia:* JB Lippincott, 1995:67–99.
4. Cressman WR, Myer CM III. Diagnosis and management of croup and epiglottitis. *Pediatr Clin North Am* 1994;41:265–276.
5. American Academy of Pediatrics. Parainfluenza virus infections. In: Peter G, ed. *1994 Red Book: Report of the Committee on Infectious Diseases,* 23rd ed. Elk Grove Village, IL: American Academy of Pediatrics, 1994:341–342.
6. Swischuk LE. Upper airway, nasal passages, sinuses, and mastoid. In: Swischuk LE ed. *Emergency radiology of the acutely ill or injured child,* 2nd ed. Baltimore: Williams & Wilkins, 1986:133–138.
7. Dawson KP, Steinberg A, Capaldi N. The lateral radiograph of neck in laryngo-tracheo-bronchitis (croup). *J Qual Clin Pract* 1994;14:39–43.
8. Cole P. Some aspects of temperature, moisture and heat relationships in the upper respiratory tract. *J Laryngol Otol* 1953;67:449–556.
9. Cole P. Further observations on conditioning of respiratory air. *J Laryngol Otol* 1953;67:669–681.
10. Henry R. Moist air in the treatment of laryngotracheitis. *Arch Dis Child* 1983;58:577.
11. Newth CJL, Levison H, Bryan AC. The respiratory status of children with croup. *J Pediatr* 1972;81:1068–1073.

12. Taussig LM, Castro O, Beaudry PH, et al. Treatment of laryngotracheobronchitis (croup): use of intermittent positive-pressure breathing and racemic epinephrine. *Am J Dis Child* 1975;129:790–793.

13. Adair JC, Ring WH, Jordan WS, et al. Ten-year experience with IPPB in the treatment of acute laryngotracheobronchitis. *Anesth Analg* 1971;50:649–655.

14. Fogel JM, Berg IJ, Gerber MA, et al. Racemic epinephrine in the treatment of croup: nebulization alone versus nebulization with intermittent positive pressure breathing. *J Pediatr* 1982;101:1028–1031.

15. Ledwith CA, Shea LM, Mauro RD. Safety and efficacy of nebulized racemic epinephrine in conjunction with oral dexamethasone and mist in the outpatient treatment of croup. *Ann Emerg Med* 1995;25:331–337.

16. Hawkins DB. Corticosteroids in the management of laryngotracheobronchitis. *Otolaryngol Head Neck Surg* 1980;88:207–210.

17. Tunnessen WW, Feinstein AR. The steroid-croup controversy: an analytic review of methodologic problems. *J Pediatr* 1980;96:751–756.

18. Davison FW. Inflammatory diseases of the larynx of infants and small children. *Ann Otol Rhinol Laryngol* 1967;76:753–761.

19. Ross JAT. Special problems in acute laryngotracheobronchitis. *Laryngoscope* 1969;79:1218–1226.

20. Postma DS, Jones RO, Pillsbury HC III. Severe hospitalized croup: treatment trends and prognosis. *Laryngoscope* 1984;94:1170–1175.

21. Super DM, Cartelli NA, Brooks LJ, Lembo RM, Kumar ML. A prospective randomized double-blind study to evaluate the effect of dexamethasone in acute laryngotracheitis. *J Pediatr* 1989;115:323–329.

22. Cruz MN, Stewart G, Rosenberg N. Use of dexamethasone in the outpatient management of acute laryngotracheitis. *Pediatrics* 1995;96:220–223.

23. Kairys SW, Olmstead EM, O'Connor GT. Steroid treatment in laryngotracheitis: a meta-analysis of the evidence from randomized trials. *Pediatrics* 1989;83:683–693.

24. Eden AN, Kaufman A, Yu R. Corticosteroids and croup: controlled double-blind study. *JAMA* 1967;200:403–404.

25. James JA. Dexamethasone in croup, a controlled study. *Am J Dis Child* 1969;117:511–516.

26. Koren G, Frand M, Barzilay Z, et al. Corticosteroid treatment of laryngotracheitis vs. spasmodic croup in children. *Am J Dis Child* 1983;137:941–944.

27. Kuusela AL, Vesikari T. A randomized double-blind placebo-controlled trial of dexamethasone and racemic epinephrine in the treatment of croup. *Acta Paedriatr Scand* 1988;77:99–104.

28. Leipzig B, Oski FA, Cummings CW, Stockman JA, Swender P. A prospective randomized study to determine the efficacy of steroids in treatment of croup. *J Pediatr* 1979;94:194–196.

29. Skowron PN, Turner JA, McNaughton GA. The use of corticosteroid (dexamethasone) in the treatment of acute laryngotracheitis. *Can Med Assoc J* 1966;94:528–531.

30. Rowe PC, Klassen TP. Corticosteroids for croup: reconciling town and gown [Editorial]. *Arch Pediatr Adolesc Med* 1996;150:344–346.

31. McEniery J, Gillis J, Kilham H, Benjamin B. Review of intubation in severe laryngotracheobronchitis. *Pediatrics* 1991;87:847–853.

32. Schuller DE, Birck HG. The safety of intubation in croup and epiglottitis: an eight-year follow-up. *Laryngoscope* 1975;85:33–46.

33. Mitchell DP, Thomas RL. Secondary airway support in the management of croup. *J Otolaryngol* 1980;9:419–422.

34. Zulliger JJ, Schuller DE, Beach TP, Garvin JP, Birck HG, Frank JE. Assessment of intubation in croup and epiglottitis. *Ann Otol Rhinol Laryngol* 1982;91:403–406.

35. Cotton RT, Seid AB. Management of the extubation problem in the premature child. Anterior cricoid split as an alternative to tracheotomy. *Ann Otol Rhinol Laryngol* 1980;89:508–511.

36. Gallagher PG, Myer CM. An approach to the diagnosis and treatment of membranous laryngotracheobronchitis in infants and children. *Pediatr Emerg Care* 1991;7:337–342.

37. Seigler RS. Bacterial tracheitis. An unusual radiographic presentation. *Clin Pediatr* 1994;33:374–377.

38. Eckel HE, Widemann B, Damm M, Roth B. Airway endoscopy in the diagnosis and treatment of bacterial tracheitis in children. *Int J Pediatr Otorhinolaryngol* 1993;27:147–157.

39. American Academy of Pediatrics. Parainfluenza virus infections. In: Peter G, ed. *1994 Red Book: Report of the Committee on Infectious Diseases.* 23rd ed. Elk Grove Village, IL: American Academy of Pediatrics, 1994;341–342.

40. Blackstock D, Adderley RJ, Steward DJ. Epiglottitis in young infants. *Anesthesiology* 1987;67:97–100.

41. Lepow ML, Hetherington S. Infections of the lower respiratory tract. In: Bluestone CD, Stool SE, eds. *Pediatric otolaryngology.* 2nd ed. Philadelphia: WB Saunders, 1990:1152–1160.

42. Swischuk LE. Upper airway, nasal passages, sinuses, and mastoid. In: Swischuk LE, ed. *Emergency Radiology of the acutely ill or injured child.* 2nd ed. Baltimore: Williams & Wilkins, 1986:130–133.

43. Gonzalez C, Reilly JS, Kenna MA, Thompson AE. Duration of intubation in children with acute epiglottitis. *Otolaryngol Head Neck Surg* 1986;95:477–481.

C.M. Myer, III: Department of Otolaryngology and Maxillofacial Surgery, University of Cincinnati, and Children's Hospital Medical Center, Cincinnati, Ohio 45229-4356.

• *Practical Pediatric Otolaryngology*
• edited by Robin T. Cotton and Charles M. Myer, III
• Lippincott-Raven Publishers, Philadelphia © 1999

34

Aerodigestive Tract Foreign Bodies

Sharon E. Gibson

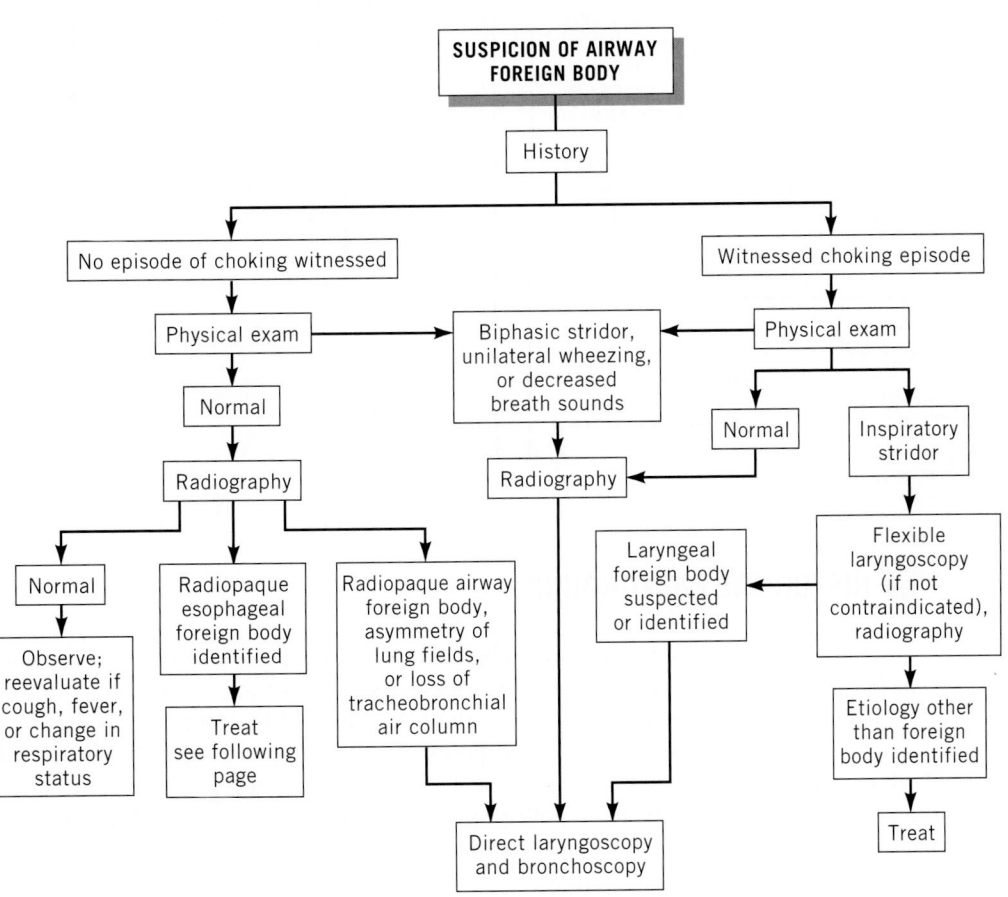

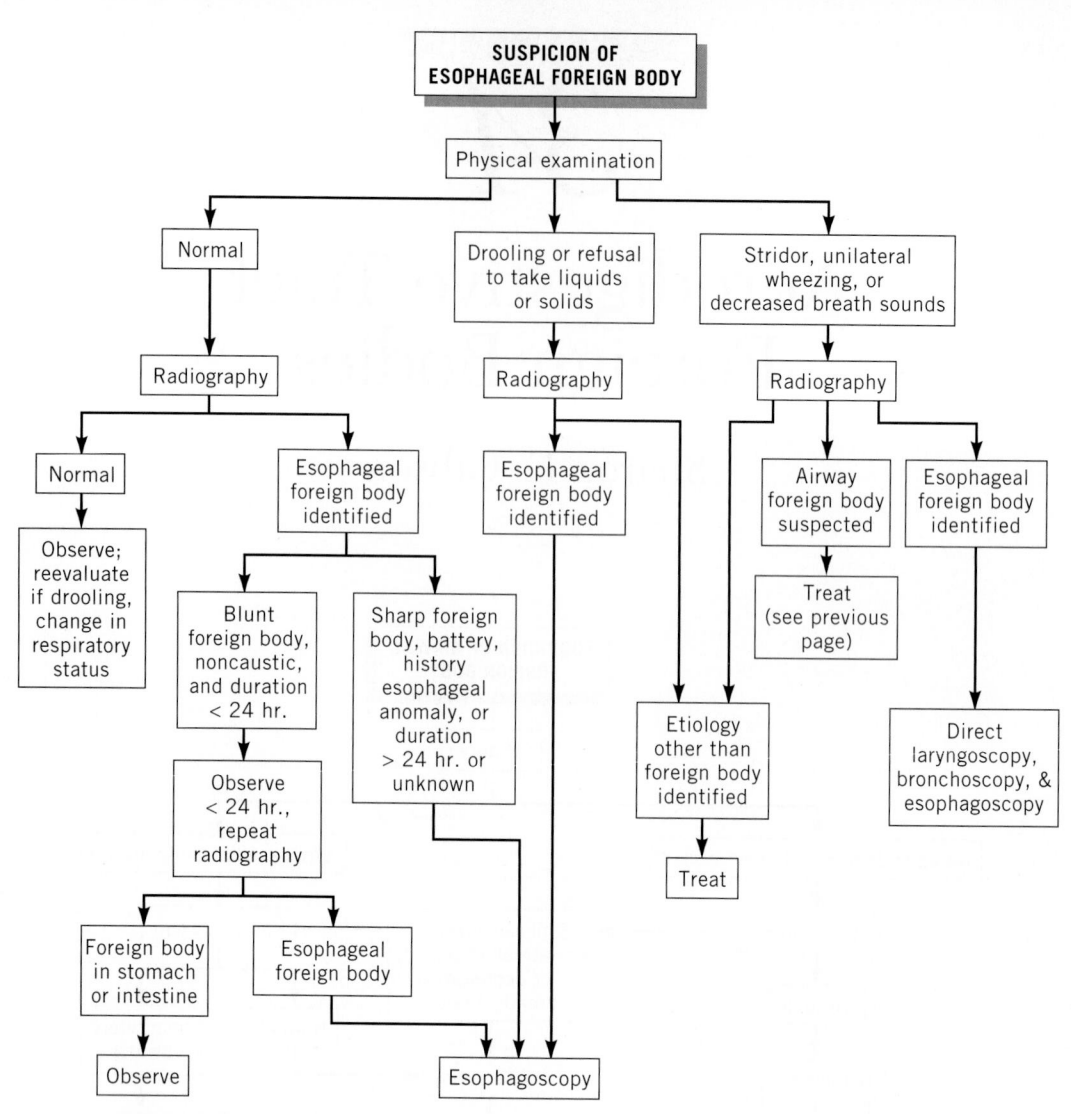

HISTORICAL BACKGROUND

Inhalation and ingestion of foreign bodies are commonplace occurrences in the pediatric population. Children between the ages of 1 and 3 years are the prevailing victims for a number of reasons: toddlers explore their environment by oral tactile means; have sparse dentition, which morselizes food poorly; lack the cognitive ability to distinguish edible objects from inedible; and are prone to distraction and engaging in play while eating. Most foreign objects are expelled spontaneously via protective reflexes, such as coughing or regurgitation, or pass uneventfully through the alimentary canal, yet a significant percentage become impacted within the upper aerodigestive tract. In 1984, the National Safety Council identified foreign body aspiration or ingestion as the fourth leading cause of accidental death in this age group and as the third leading cause for infants under the age of 1 year.

Recent advances in instrumentation and anesthetic technique have led to a lowered complication rate associated with the treatment of upper areodigestive tract foreign bodies. Rod-lens telescopes coupled to esophagoscopes, ventilating bronchoscopes, and grasping forceps provide superior visualization for inspection of the esophagus and tracheobronchial tree and extraction of foreign objects. Continued development of new anesthetic agents and physiologic monitoring devices has resulted in improved safety and expanded options for the delivery of general anesthesia to young children. Despite these improvements in management, the incidence of foreign body ingestion and aspiration remains alarmingly high.

AIRWAY FOREIGN BODIES

 PATIENT ASSESSMENT

History

An accurate history is of tremendous importance in the diagnosis of foreign body aspiration because the remainder of the assessment, the physical examination, and radiographic studies can be deceptively unremarkable after the acute event has lapsed. The characteristic history of an incipient choking or gagging episode, and a subsequent coughing spell, is described by most caretakers if they were present when aspiration occurred (1–3). Serious attention should be paid to such a history witnessed while the child was eating peanuts, seeds, or beans, the primary culprits in foreign body aspiration.

Although most inhaled foreign bodies travel distally into the tracheobronchial tree, laryngeal impaction occasionally occurs. Large or conforming objects (e.g., balloons) are apt to obstruct the glottic inlet and precipitate acute respiratory arrest. These children survive if resuscitated by astute caretakers, paramedics, or emergency physicians and thus are seldom evaluated by the otolaryngologist. Smaller, nonobstructing objects, however, may bypass the supraglottis and lodge in the pyriform sinus, laryngeal ventricle, glottis, or subglottis (Fig. 1). Local inflammation produces complaints of cough, inspiratory stridor, hoarseness, or odynophagia. Because these symptoms mimic the more common infectious maladies of the upper respiratory tract including laryngitis, pharyngitis, and croup, subacute laryngeal foreign bodies may go unrecognized for weeks or longer (4). A witnessed choking episode and the absence of systemic symptoms of infection are important historical clues to the correct diagnosis.

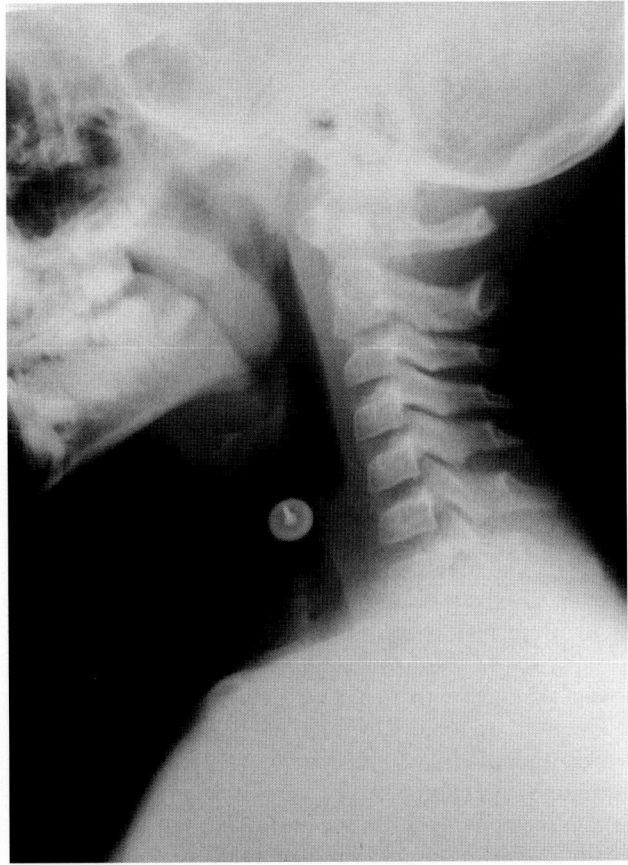

FIGURE 1 Due to its size and shape, this thumbtack was small enough to pass the supraglottic and glottic larynx into the subglottis without causing severe airway obstruction. The resulting symptoms of inspiratory stridor and barky cough can be mistaken for croup.

With rare exceptions, a foreign body that penetrates the larynx and enters the tracheobronchial tree triggers an episode of paroxysmal cough. An asymptomatic lag period often ensues, an interval when the initial mucosal irritation has subsided and the cough reflex has fatigued. This quiescent stage may falsely reassure the parent that the child has effectively cleared the airway. Consequently, only 70% of patients seek treatment within a week following aspiration (5). The first symptoms prompting medical attention may actually represent a complication of foreign body impaction, such as fever and purulent productive cough signaling pneumonia. Chronic cough, recurrent or persistent pneumonia, bronchitis, and atypical asthma are common misdiagnoses (6) assigned to unsuspected airway foreign bodies.

Physical Examination

Physical findings following aspiration are variable and highly dependent on the location and degree of endoluminal obstruction by the foreign body. The child may be quiet and comfortable or may exhibit signs of respiratory distress ranging from mild tachypnea to severe stridor, retractions, and cyanosis. Serial evaluations of respiratory status are advised, since airway edema or foreign body shifting can incite a rapid progression of respiratory distress. Recently aspirated objects are particularly treacherous in this regard.

Findings on physical examination may point to the location of an airway foreign body if it creates significant obstruction to local airflow. Foreign bodies in the larynx or cervical trachea can produce inspiratory or biphasic stridor, and a prolonged wheeze in the expiratory phase is suggestive of intrathoracic tracheal obstruction, although audible stridor is frequently absent with smaller objects in any airway location. Careful auscultation of the chest is the most critical part of the examination. A discrepancy in breath sounds between sides of the chest and unilateral wheezing are the findings of greatest significance, because most aspirated objects impact in the right or left mainstem bronchus (1,2,7). Most signs are subtle, however, and it is important to appreciate that physical examination may be essentially normal. The classic diagnostic triad of unilateral wheeze, cough, and ipsilaterally diminished breath sounds is observed in less than 50% of cases (7), and, in fact, 5% to 40% of patients with an airway foreign body will manifest no obvious signs to suggest the correct diagnosis (1,5). Other findings less frequently observed include hypersonority or dullness on chest percussion, fever, persistent nonproductive or purulent cough, and hemoptysis.

Flexible nasopharyngolaryngoscopy can add valuable diagnostic information when inspiratory stridor is the sole physical finding and a laryngeal or hypopharyngeal foreign body is suspected by history. Laryngomalacia or other nontraumatic etiologies of stridor may be quickly identified and treated accordingly. This examination may precipitate further airway compromise, however, and is contraindicated in small children with severe obstruction, when supraglottitis is suspected, and when airway resuscitative equipment is not immediately available.

Radiography

Plain radiographs remain a helpful adjunct in the assessment of airway foreign bodies. Although most aspirated foreign bodies are nuts, seeds, or plastic items that are radiolucent, posteroanterior and lateral views of the neck and chest may reveal signs of an obliterated bronchial air column or abnormal ventilation of the affected pulmonary parenchyma (Fig. 2). Direct comparison of chest radiographs taken on inspiration and expiration is important. Decreased air entry with atelectasis (inspiratory hypoinflation) or, most commonly, impaired air egress (expiratory hyperinflation) in one lung is characteristic of bronchial foreign body aspiration. Lobar or segmental pulmonary infiltrate from impaired outflow of respiratory secretions usually implies a long-standing impaction of days to weeks. Although radiography is useful for confirmation and localization of foreign body aspiration, up to 25% of bronchial foreign bodies, and over half of

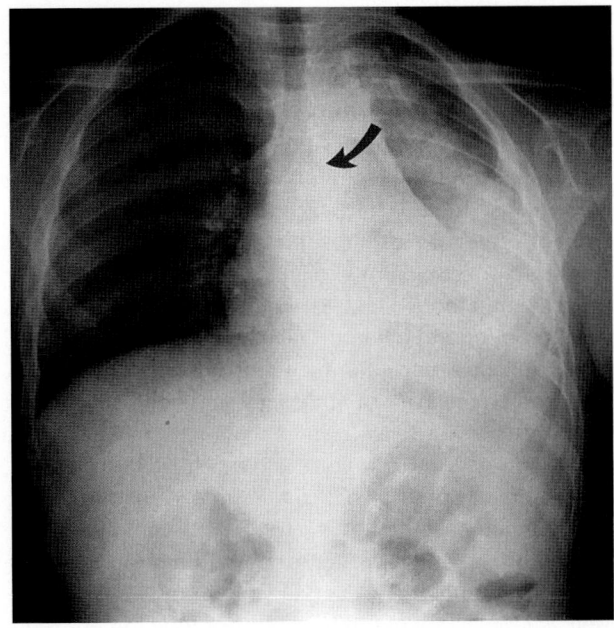

A

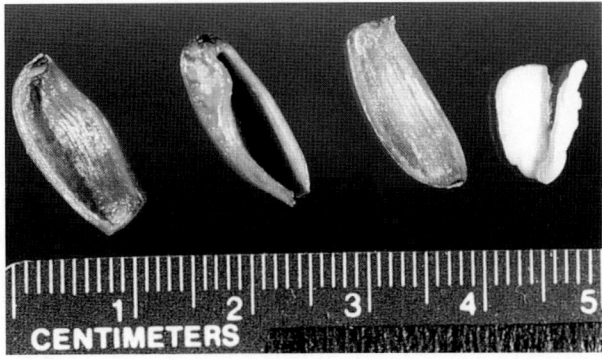

B

FIGURE 2 **A:** Loss of the left bronchial air column (*arrow*), ipsilateral lobar consolidation, and atelectasis demonstrated on this posteroanterior chest radiograph are clues to radiolucent airway foreign bodies. **B:** Upon endoscopy, multiple fragments of a sunflower seed and its shell were found in the left mainstem bronchus.

those within the trachea, yield no abnormalities on plain chest radiograph (5,8). For this reason, foreign body aspiration can never be excluded on the basis of chest x-ray alone. Fluoroscopy has a greater diagnostic sensitivity (2) and may be available and appropriate in some settings. The correct diagnosis is ultimately achieved at the time of the final diagnostic evaluation, the bronchoscopic examination.

PEARLS AND PERILS
Diagnosis of Airway Foreign Bodies

1. A relative lack of symptoms following the choking episode is not unusual with foreign body aspiration and should not be considered evidence against the correct diagnosis.
2. Be highly suspicious of unilateral wheezing and decreased breath sounds. These are the most characteristic physical findings of a bronchial foreign body and must not be mistaken for asthma.
3. Chest radiographs can be normal with a tracheal or bronchial foreign body and can therefore not rule out the diagnosis of aspiration.
4. Subacute laryngeal foreign body impaction is often overlooked because its symptoms mimic more common airway ailments, such as laryngitis and croup.

TREATMENT RECOMMENDATIONS

Preparation and Anesthesia

Once the diagnosis of an aspirated foreign body is entertained, it becomes the responsibility of the endoscopist to confirm its presence and proceed with extraction or to dismiss it from the differential diagnosis. Direct laryngoscopy and bronchoscopy in the pediatric population are most safely and efficiently accomplished by means of a ventilating bronchoscope under general anesthesia. As a rule, endoscopy should be undertaken expeditiously to decrease the hazard of complication (3), particularly in children with laryngeal obstruction or with organic objects, such as beans, which tend to swell when in contact with respiratory secretions and become tightly impacted. A complete mainstem bronchial obstruction, whereby poor alveolar aeration causes shunting of pulmonary perfusion away from the affected lung, is also an inherently dangerous situation. If the foreign body migrates to the contralateral mainstem bronchus, blockage of ventilation to the lung with the only functional alveoli leads to abrupt respiratory decompensation. The urge to rush into operative intervention, however, must be tempered by contingencies of patient status and availability of personnel. When respiratory distress is not apparent or impending, awaiting an adequately empty stomach to reduce the anesthetic risk is indicated, as is judicious postponement of surgery to assemble the endoscopist, anesthesiologist, and operative staff experienced in pediatric airway management (9).

The pediatric airway compromised by a foreign body is a tenuous one, and it harbors the potential for sudden deterioration upon induction of anesthesia or during surgical manipulation. The full complement of endoscopic equipment, including laryngoscopes, ventilating bronchoscopes, foreign body forceps, suction devices, and light cables must be selected, assembled, and ready for use prior to the administration of any anesthetic agent. Rigid bronchoscopes provide direct ventilatory access, excellent visualization, continuous administration of oxygen and anesthetic agent, and a suitable conduit for the introduction and extraction of grasping forceps; they are preferred to flexible fiberoptic instruments for this procedure. One bronchoscope of appropriate dimensions for the child's age and another of a smaller diameter in the event that laryngotracheal edema or stenosis is encountered are chosen. The selection of foreign body grasping forceps is determined by the shape and texture of the object. It is helpful if the parents can furnish a copy of the suspected foreign body if it is extraordinary, both to aid in selection of the best forceps and to practice extraction techniques prior to surgery. Alternate types should be available to accommodate unexpected intraoperative findings.

Continuous monitoring by pulse oximeter, precordial stethoscope, blood pressure cuff, electrocardiogram, and temperature probe must be begun prior to the administration of inhalational anesthetic agents by mask. Maintenance of spontaneous ventilation is preferred and intubation with an endotracheal tube is avoided. During induction, the endoscopist must stand ready to assume control of the airway should ventilation become impaired.

Endoscopy and Foreign Body Removal

Laryngoscopy is routinely performed to provide access for atraumatic bronchoscope insertion, to apply topical anesthetic, which aids in maintaining the appropriate plane of anesthesia for spontaneous respiration, and to examine for hypopharyngeal and laryngeal foreign bodies. Once the bronchoscope has been introduced, the anesthesia circuit is connected to its ventilating port adaptor, allowing oxygen and inhalational agent to be entrained with spontaneous inspiration or positive pressure ventilation to be provided. The bronchoscope is advanced to the point of foreign body impaction when possible. In some instances, the bronchoscope is best positioned with the ventilating ports above the carina to maintain ventilation via the unobstructed contralateral mainstem bronchus.

Extraction of the foreign body requires a delicate touch to avoid incurring further trauma to the respiratory mucosa or pushing the object peripherally out of endoscopic reach. Small objects or fragments may be able to be withdrawn through the bronchoscope while maintaining it in place. More commonly, the forceps with foreign body in tow will not fit through its lumen. The object must be held snugly back against the tip of the bronchoscope and all are removed as a single unit. The anesthesiologist must be forewarned of this maneuver, so that mask ventilation can be immediately provided. If the foreign body becomes disengaged from the forceps while traversing the trachea or larynx, the bronchoscope must be immediately reinserted to push the object back into its previous bronchial location. With an adequate airway reestablished, another controlled attempt at extraction is made. The extraction of sharp objects requires special expertise, employing techniques such as foreign body rotation, bending or sheathing of the point within the bronchoscope to protect the respiratory mucosa during withdrawal (9).

Bronchoscopy should be repeated once the foreign body has been removed. In 5% to 19% of cases (1,3), multiple foreign bodies or fragmented pieces of the original object will be discovered. In addition, direct aspiration of static endobronchial secretions distal to the site of impaction will speed postoperative reexpansion of collapsed alveoli in the affected lung segment.

The vast majority of airway foreign bodies are successfully managed by endoscopic extraction. In the rare case when a very peripheral location or severe chronic inflammatory changes at the site of impaction render endoscopic removal impossible, thoracotomy is warranted.

PEARLS AND PERILS
Removal of Airway Foreign Bodies

1. Laryngoscopy and bronchoscopy should be expedited when an airway foreign body is suspected but should not precede patient preparation and involvement of the appropriately experienced surgical personnel if the child is clinically stable.
2. Ventilating bronchoscopes, with all their accessories, must be assembled and ready for use before any anesthetic agent is given. Only thorough preparation enables the endoscopist to handle airway complications when they arise.
3. Repeat the bronchoscopic examination following foreign body extraction to inspect the tracheobronchial mucosa, to aspirate trapped secretions, and to search for multiple objects or fragments.

Postoperative Management

Chest physiotherapy may be helpful to mobilize retained secretions in the postoperative period, but no other specific interventions are routinely required. Steroids and antibiotics are not customarily prescribed; instead, they are reserved for patients with evidence of complications as outlined below.

MANAGEMENT OF COMPLICATIONS

Complications Related to the Foreign Body

Seldom does the management of complications of foreign body aspiration entail more than removal of the offending object. Foreign body impaction often irritates the adjacent respiratory mucosa, manifesting as mild erythema, edema, tracheitis, bronchitis, or abundant granulation tissue. Beans, nuts, and other organic items are particularly likely to incite a vigorous inflammatory response. A brief course of oral or inhaled corticosteroid has empiric value although controlled efficacy studies are lacking (1).

Stagnant respiratory secretions trapped by the foreign body can give rise to pneumonia, the commonest clinically significant complication, for which systemic antibiotic therapy is indicated. Segmental atelectasis may continue for several days after endoscopy. It may initially be treated expectantly, but the persistence of cough, fever, or consolidation beyond 1 week hint at a retained foreign body (1), and repeat bronchoscopy to search for one is appropriate. Pneumomediastinum and pneumothorax caused by foreign bodies are managed similarly to those arising from other etiologies, simply observed if small and nonrestrictive but with tube thoracostomy performed at the first signs of respiratory or circulatory compromise.

Complications Related to Endoscopy

The most common intraoperative complications are cardiac arrhythmias caused by hypoxia, carbon dioxide retention, or direct pressure during manipulation of the left mainstem bronchus (6). Vigilant intraoperative monitoring is imperative for the early recognition and management of these events to prevent progression to cardiorespiratory arrest. Advancement of an object into an inaccessible distal bronchial segment, traumatic laryngeal edema, maceration of respiratory mucosa, and missed multiple foreign bodies are complications of endoscopic technique avoided chiefly through patience and experience.

ESOPHAGEAL FOREIGN BODIES

 PATIENT ASSESSMENT

History

Parental suspicion that a child has swallowed an inedible object is the most constant historical finding with esophageal foreign bodies (10,11). Symptoms common to foreign body aspiration, such as a choking spell or cough, are prevalent and may raise an initial concern of aspiration rather than ingestion. Older children may be able to describe dysphagia or odynophagia. Young children and infants with esophageal foreign body impaction tend to exhibit subtle or generalized symptoms; a history of fussing, poor appetite, or emesis may be elicited from their parents. For this reason, many unsuspected foreign bodies are initially diagnosed as viral upper respiratory or gastrointestinal illnesses and discovered incidentally on chest radiograph intended to rule out a pulmonary infiltrate (11,12).

Children with a history of a structural or physiologic abnormality of the esophagus are at increased risk of foreign body impaction. A history of acute dysphagia or emesis during a meal should raise the suspicion of food impaction in the child with a known esophageal stricture, dysmotility syndrome, or repaired tracheoesophageal fistula.

Physical Examination

Physical examination may reveal a fussy child who refuses to eat or drink but is commonly unremarkable for any specific findings. Drooling is worrisome and often signifies total obstruction of the esophageal lumen. Large or chronically impacted objects can induce inflammation or erosion of the anterior esophageal wall and thereby compromise the adjacent tracheal airway. Related respiratory symptoms, such as dyspnea and stridor, affect approximately 10% of children with foreign body ingestion (10,12).

Radiography

Unlike foreign bodies of the tracheobronchial tree, esophageal foreign bodies are frequently radiopaque and readily identified on plain chest radiograph (10–12). Coins are by far the most commonly ingested objects. Food products are the second most common, but unlike the vegetable items prone to aspiration, the large pieces of meat, fish, or chicken likely to cause esophageal impaction often contain spicules of bone or cartilage that are radiographically apparent.

The location and orientation of an esophageal coin are characteristic (Fig. 3). The cricopharyngeus muscle at the esophageal inlet forms the narrowest part of the upper digestive tract and is the level at which impactions are most apt to occur. Passage of an object through this sphincter usually portends an uneventful journey through the remainder of the alimentary canal. Esophageal impaction at a lower level is unusual and may be indicative of an unsuspected structural anomaly, such as stricture.

For proper evaluation of an esophageal foreign body, both posteroanterior and lat-

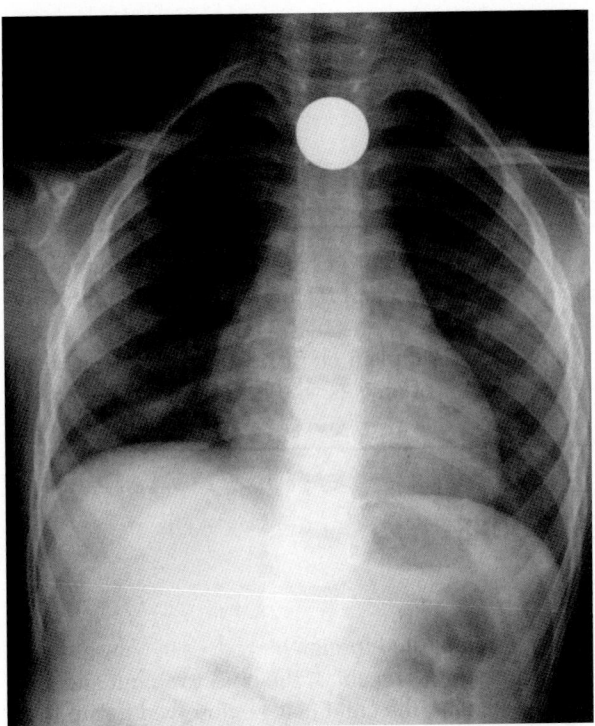
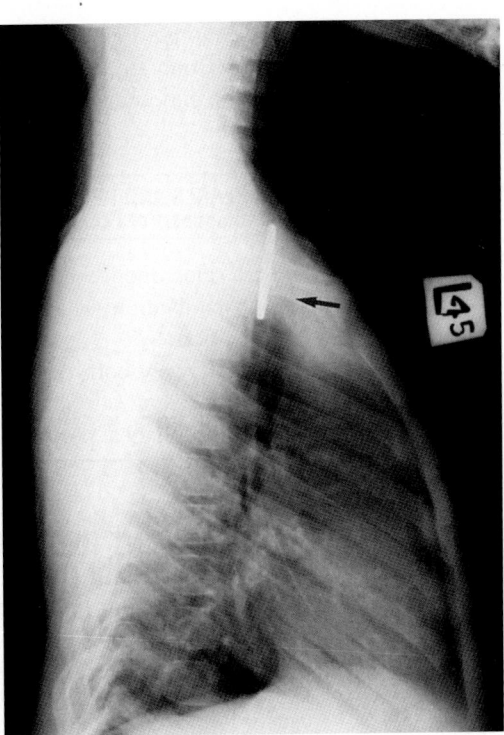

A

B

FIGURE 3 The typical location and orientation of a single esophageal coin as seen on posteroanterior **(A)** and lateral **(B)** radiographic views of the chest. A well-defined tracheal airway (*arrow*) is minimally narrowed anterior to the foreign body.

eral radiographs must be obtained. Details of an object's shape, identification of multiple objects (e.g., multiple coins, which are notorious for "hiding" behind the radiographic shadow of the largest coin), and confirmation of esophageal rather than tracheal location rely on lateral chest radiographs. These views should be studied for evidence of retroesophageal fullness or air suggestive of preoperative perforation when chronically impacted or sharp objects are identified (Fig. 4). Clues to the presence of radiolucent esophageal foreign bodies, which include localized tracheal compression, tracheal deviation, and air within the esophagus, are also best appreciated on lateral films.

In the unusual circumstance that further radiographic evidence of an esophageal foreign body is needed, barium esophagram may outline impaction by a radiolucent object. If the clinical picture is consistent with foreign body ingestion and no medical con-

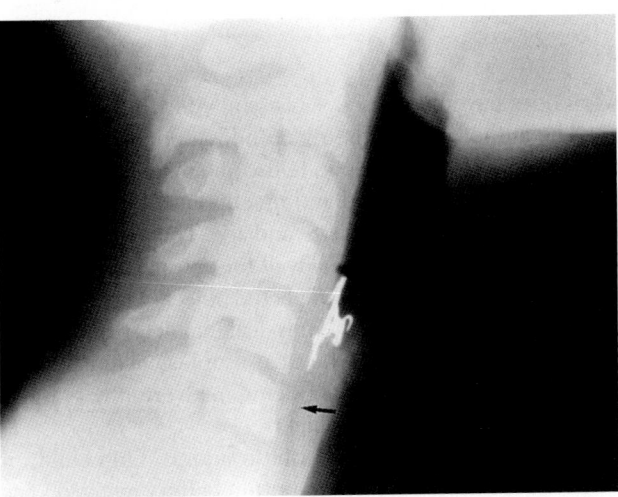

FIGURE 4 With sharp esophageal foreign bodies, lateral neck radiographs should be studied for signs of perforation, such as retroesophageal soft tissue fullness or air, prior to their extraction. In this patient, the air shadow below the foreign body represents air within the esophageal lumen (*arrow*) and is not an indication of perforation.

traindications to general anesthesia are present, awaiting special radiographic studies may serve only to delay intervention. As with foreign bodies elsewhere in the aerodigestive tract, endoscopy is the gold standard for diagnosis.

PEARLS AND PERILS
Diagnosis of Esophageal Foreign Bodies

1. Document whether drooling or airway symptoms are apparent on physical examination. They will influence the timing and technique of surgical intervention.
2. Review both posteroanterior and lateral plain chest radiographs for details of foreign body shape, location, number of objects, and evidence of preoperative esophageal perforation.

 ## TREATMENT RECOMMENDATIONS

When Observation Is Appropriate

Unlike aspirated objects, the presence of an ingested foreign body does not always mandate early surgical intervention. If the ingestion is recent, if the object is blunt and noncaustic, and if respiratory distress is not evident, the child may be observed for up to 24 hours for spontaneous passage of the foreign body. A chest radiograph is repeated, and if advancement past the cricopharyngeus is seen, expectant management is appropriate. Once an object enters the stomach, the risk of subsequent impaction is extremely low, and even most sharp objects can be followed by serial radiographs once they are past the gastroesophageal junction (9).

There are circumstances, however, under which watchful waiting for spontaneous passage of an esophageal foreign body is inappropriate. Any degree of respiratory distress demands foreign body extraction. Total esophageal obstruction leads to pooling and intolerance of oral secretions, carrying with it a risk of aspiration and low likelihood of passage, making it prudent to proceed with extraction. Complication rates also climb with chronically impacted esophageal foreign bodies; those that have remained in the esophagus for more than 24 hours, or for which the duration of impaction is unknown, should not be observed expectantly. Sharp or pointed objects, and corrosives such as button disc batteries, pose a serious risk of esophageal perforation, and their timely removal should not be delayed. Finally, children with known esophageal anomalies are not good candidates for observation, since spontaneous passage is rare (10).

Preparation and Anesthesia

Both rigid and flexible esophagoscopes have been used successfully for the routine extraction of blunt foreign bodies. The author prefers the rigid endoscope, because it accommodates the widest variety of grasping forceps, allows telescopic magnification, and has been proved safe for the treatment of complicated and uncomplicated impactions. The size of the esophagoscope is selected for the child's size and age. The largest safe diameter is selected to hold apart the collapsible esophageal wall for optimal visualization of the lumen and separate the adjacent mucosa from the impacted object. As with airway foreign bodies, grasping forceps are chosen based on the physical characteristics of the object. Special care must be taken with serrated forceps, because esophageal mucosa settled around the foreign body is subject to a greater risk of being inadvertently grasped than the cartilage-supported mucosa of the tracheobronchial tree.

Routine nothing-by-mouth status should be observed prior to surgery. Only children in significant respiratory distress, which is rare, or in whom button battery ingestion has occurred, in which digestive tract mucosal necrosis has been reported within a 4-hour period (13), are exempt from this rule. General anesthesia is induced by inhalation after application of the standard oximetry, temperature, and cardiac monitoring devices. Endotracheal intubation is performed. If respiratory symptoms are apparent, direct laryngoscopy and bronchoscopy, examining specifically for airway narrowing or erosion of the party wall, precede intubation. A muscle relaxant is administered once the airway has been secured.

Endoscopic Evaluation and Removal

The esophagoscope can be introduced directly or following laryngoscopic elevation of the larynx. Use of the laryngoscope provides wide exposure of the hypopharynx and postcricoid space; sometimes the foreign body is visualized with this manuever alone. Frequent suctioning of saliva is necessary to expose the esophageal lumen for safe introduction of the endoscope. The esophagoscope is advanced to the site of impaction, where the esophageal mucosa must be evaluated for signs of preexisting injury or perforation, such as bleeding, edema, purulent or fibrinous exudate, or frank ulceration. After the foreign body is grasped with the appropriate forceps, it is pulled back firmly against the esophagoscope and withdrawn with it. Care must be taken to avoid accidental extubation as the object passes the larynx and hypopharynx. The special techniques as described for the extraction of sharp foreign bodies from the airway apply and are crucial for their safe removal from the esophagus.

Muscle relaxation provided during general anesthesia can allow a loosely impacted object to slip distally as the endoscopist attempts to approximate the esophagoscope to it. If the object traverses the lower esophageal sphincter and enters the stomach, furthering mucosal trauma by extraction back through the esophagus is contraindicated. The two notable exceptions to this rule are open safety pins, which may be advanced into the stomach for version and withdrawal spring first, and needles, which pose a hazard of clinically silent bowel perforation (9).

Esophagoscopy should be repeated following foreign body extraction to ascertain the status of the esophageal wall at the impaction site. Multiple foreign bodies, often of differing composition, are serendipitously identified in 5% of children (11).

Cervical esophagotomy is indicated on the rare occasion that an extraordinarily large, sharp, or chronically impacted foreign body fails all reasonable attempts at endoscopic extraction without inviting esophageal perforation.

PEARLS AND PERILS
Removal of Esophageal Foreign Bodies

1. It is inappropriate to delay extraction of foreign bodies that are sharp, corrosive, or associated with respiratory distress. Those causing total esophageal obstruction or of chronic or unknown duration should also not be observed in hopes of spontaneous passage.
2. Laryngoscopy and bronchoscopy should precede esophagoscopy if airway compromise accompanies an esophageal foreign body.
3. Monitor vital signs closely in the postoperative period for fever, tachycardia, or tachypnea indicative of esophageal perforation. Avoid antipyretic analgesics, which can mask these important signs.

Postoperative Management

Although the rate of complications following extraction of a recently ingested coin is very low, it is prudent to observe all patients, at least briefly, for signs of perforation after removal of an esophageal foreign body. Children should be kept from drinking or eating for a period of 4 to 12 hours while intravenous hydration is maintained, with continued observation as clear liquids are begun and the diet advanced. Vital signs must be checked frequently for tachycardia, tachypnea, and fever, and analgesics that mask these important signals of perforation (e.g., acetaminophen) must be strictly avoided until the child has progressed to an adequate oral intake without event.

Alternate Methods for Esophageal Foreign Body Removal

Balloon catheter extraction of esophageal foreign bodies remains a practice of significant controversy in the surgical literature. Its advocates cite the time and cost savings of avoiding surgery as its prime advantage. By this method, a Foley catheter is introduced orally or nasally and advanced, under fluoroscopic guidance, distal to the impacted object. With the toddler restrained in a head-down position, the balloon is inflated and the catheter withdrawn. Proponents of this procedure have shown it to be effective in up to 90% of cases when limited to blunt foreign bodies, recently ingested, in the otherwise healthy child (14). Failures are then referred for endoscopic extraction under general anesthesia. Because manipulation of the foreign body is blind, preexisting esophageal injury and details of the shape of any coexisting radiolucent foreign bodies cannot be identified. The complications of this method, reported to occur at a rate of 3% to 10%, include emesis, epistaxis, inadvertent balloon placement and inflation within the trachea, laryngospasm, and hypoxia. They underscore the real necessity for resuscitative equipment and personnel skilled in the management of the compromised pediatric airway to be readily available for this procedure. In the author's view, esophagoscopy with a protected airway and the capability to recognize and handle complicated and uncomplicated situations alike represents the safer and more humane method of treatment.

⊕ MANAGEMENT OF COMPLICATIONS

The most feared complication of an impacted esophageal foreign body or its removal is esophageal perforation. Even items as seemingly innocuous as an impacted coin have been reported to penetrate the esophagus and migrate extraluminally with time (15). A localized abscess in the retropharyngeal space can result from perforation at the esophageal inlet or above, presenting with fever, drooling, odynophagia, stiff neck posturing, and potential airway obstruction. Lateral plain radiography or computed tomography of the neck easily demonstrate air or fluid in the retropharyngeal space. Transoral drainage, after appropriate protection of the airway by endotracheal intubation, and parenteral antibiotics are indicated.

Perforation causing retroesophageal abscess or mediastinitis carries a high rate of morbidity and must be treated expediently and aggressively. The onset postoperatively of fever, tachycardia, tachypnea, dyspnea, or odynophagia should prompt the immediate withholding of food, initiation of intravenous fluids, and chest radiography to assess for pneumomediastinum or pneumothorax. If either radiographic finding is present or a worsening clinical status suggests perforation, intravenous antimicrobial therapy and thin barium or Gastrografin esophagram are warranted. The patient should be monitored in an intensive care setting due to the potential for rapid cardiovascular decompensation. Although the cardiothoracic surgeon may elect to observe a very small perforation in the clinically stable patient, mediastinal drainage is required in many cases.

❋ REFERENCES

1. McGuirt WF, Holmes KD, Feehs R, Browne JD. *Laryngoscope* 1988;98:615–618.
2. Wolach B, Raz A, Weinberg J, Mikulski Y, Ari JB, Sadan N. *Int J Pediatr Otorhinolaryngol* 1994;30:1–10.

3. Inglis AF Jr, Wagner DV. *Ann Otol Rhinol Laryngol* 1992;101:61–66.
4. Lima JA. *Laryngoscope* 1989;99:415–420.
5. Mu L, He P, Sun D. *Laryngoscope* 1991;101:657–660.
6. Steen KH, Zimmermann T. *Laryngoscope* 1990;100:525–530.
7. Svedstrom E, Puhakka H, Kero P. *Pediatr Radiol* 1989;19:520–522.
8. Burton EM, Brick WG, Hall JD, Riggs W Jr, Houston CS. *South Med J* 1996;82:195–198.
9. Holinger LD. *Ann Otol Rhinol Laryngol* 1990;99:684–688.
10. Crysdale WS, Sendi KS, Yoo J. *Ann Otol Rhinol Laryngol* 1991;100:320–324.
11. Hawkins DB. *Ann Otol Rhinol Laryngol* 1990;99:935–940.
12. Papsin BC, Friedberg J. *J Otolaryngol* 1994;23:102–108.
13. Kost KM, Shapiro RS. *J Otolaryngol* 1987;16:252–257.
14. Schunk JE, Harrison AM, Corneli HM, Nixon GW. *Pediatrics* 1994;94:709–714.
15. Burton DM, Stith JA. *Int J Pediatr Otorhinolaryngol* 1992;23:187–194.

S. E. Gibson: Department of Otolaryngology, Tufts University Medical School, Boston, Massachusetts, and Department of Surgery, Brown University Medical School, Providence, Rhode Island 02905.

• *Practical Pediatric Otolaryngology*
• edited by Robin T. Cotton and Charles M. Myer, III
• Lippincott-Raven Publishers, Philadelphia © 1999

Tracheotomy in the Pediatric Patient

J. Scott McMurray & Christopher A. J. Prescott

The management of the obstructed pediatric airway is both challenging and rewarding. Because of the small caliber of the infant larynx and trachea, small changes from mucosal edema can rapidly cause dramatic and potentially life-threatening narrowing of the airway. A swift, thorough, and accurate assessment of the acutely asphyxiating child is required of the managing physician. With the relief of the obstruction, through intubation or tracheotomy, the child may then be stabilized. The long-term outcome of the child must be considered, however, as the treatment plan develops.

This chapter will focus on tracheotomy in the pediatric patient. Although it is performed in both children and adults, anatomic and physiologic differences require a separate understanding of this procedure in children. Reviewed in this chapter are the indications, the technique, and the complications unique to pediatric tracheotomy.

INDICATIONS

In theory, intubation may be maintained for prolonged periods without complication, provided that the endotracheal tube causes no mucosal injury. In practice, however, it is difficult to assess whether the endotracheal tube required to provide an adequate airway is injuring the underlying mucosa. Even if mucosal injury can be prevented, the presence of the tube will eventually elicit an inflammatory reaction in the laryngeal mucosa.

Laryngeal injury resulting from intubation has been well described by Benjamin (1). Granulation tissue forming in the localized ulcerated mucosa over the vocal processes can lead to intubation granulomas, healed fibrous nodules, or posterior vocal cord adhesions. Granulation tissue forming in the posterior glottis can cause posterior glottic fibrosis. Ulceration of the subglottis can cause perichondritis, leading to cartilaginous changes and potential subglottic stenosis.

The timing of tracheotomy versus continued intubation remains controversial in the pediatric population (2,3). Consideration of the disadvantages of prolonged intubation helps clarify timing of surgical intervention. The endotracheal tube can cause glottic and subglottic edema and erosion within 72 hours (4,5). Pressure from the endotracheal tube can cause edema, ischemia, and pressure necrosis of the mucosa and cartilage. Although there is no known safe limit for prolonged intubation, it is generally accepted that adult patients requiring intubation for more than 2 weeks have a tracheotomy tube inserted surgically because of the known potential for injury to the larynx and trachea from prolonged intubation (4–6).

In pediatric patients, however, the use of uncuffed endotracheal tubes and recent advances in neonatal care have extended the potential safe period for prolonged intubation. The reported incidence of subglottic stenosis in previously intubated graduates of the Neonatal Intensive Care Unit was as high as 20% in the late 1960s and early 1970s

(7,8). As proper tube size and other supportive measures became more refined in the neonatal intensive care, the reported incidence of subglottic stenosis dropped to 1% to 8% (9–11). The maximum safe time for endotracheal intubation must be determined individually for each child. Since the subglottis is the narrowest portion of the pediatric airway, unlike in the adult, orotracheal or nasotracheal intubation may be more efficient in some infants requiring high-pressure ventilatory support. It is not always practical to insert a tracheotomy tube of sufficient size to overcome the leak generated from high-pressure ventilation. In these cases, it is better to wait until the ventilatory pressures are lower before inserting a tracheotomy.

It can be difficult, however, to find an endotracheal tube small enough to avoid mucosal injury yet large enough to provide adequate pulmonary toilet. Smaller endotracheal tubes are prone to occlusion, requiring frequent replacement. This situation may lead to a cycle of traumatic reintubation and further laryngeal injury. Children at risk of developing permanent laryngeal damage and who may need prolonged pulmonary toilet or ventilation should be considered for tracheotomy.

There are three major indications for long-term tracheotomy in children: airway obstruction, ventilatory support, and pulmonary toilet. Patients requiring tracheotomies for airway obstruction generally received the procedure as very young infants from either congenital or acquired subglottic stenosis. Patients requiring tracheotomy for ventilatory support are a more heterogenous group. Respiratory failure may be associated with prematurity, central nervous system disease, or poor pulmonary reserve. This group has increased in number as medical advances have prolonged the lives of sicker children. Children requiring tracheotomy for pulmonary toilet generally have some degree of aspiration. This is commonly due to dyscoordinated swallowing mechanisms related to neurologic diseases. This group differs from the other two groups in that they have a less immediate dependency on the tracheotomy tube should accidental decannulation occur. They comprise a relatively small patient population.

A child who is a candidate for tracheotomy should have a full endoscopic assessment to diagnose accurately the underlying cause of obstruction if present and to identify any other laryngotracheal disorders that may cause complications. Nasopharyngoscopy gives details about the nasopharyngeal airway, the supraglottis (such as laryngoceles and obstructing papilloma), and the glottis (such as vocal fold motion impairment). Rigid laryngoscopy and bronchoscopy allow for the assessment of arytenoid joint mobility, the subglottis, and the tracheobronchial tree. It is important to rule out concomitant vascular anomalies. Tracheotomy should be avoided, if possible, in patients with vascular anomalies due to the risk of erosion causing a catastrophic fistula.

TECHNIQUE

Obvious anatomic differences between the adult and the pediatric larynx and trachea require a different approach and surgical technique. The infant larynx is higher in the neck and may be shielded by the hyoid bone (Fig. 1). The leading edge of the thyroid cartilage is broad, with an angle of 110°. The cricoid is often the most prominent structure palpable in the extended neck. Palpation to delineate the level of the airway can be difficult. The pediatric trachea also has more lateral mobility than the adult, making it easy to dislodge the trachea out of the surgical field with retraction. All these differences in anatomic characteristics make localization of the pediatric airway more difficult. Care must be taken during exposure of the airway to ensure insertion of the tracheotomy tube at the proper level.

Many techniques have been described. The authors describe here their preferred procedure. The patient is taken to the operating room, with or without an established airway. If the airway has not been secured, an endotracheal tube or bronchoscope is inserted first, if possible. If this is not possible, the airway is initially managed by mask ventilation. An oral airway may facilitate mask ventilation. The laryngeal mask airway has also

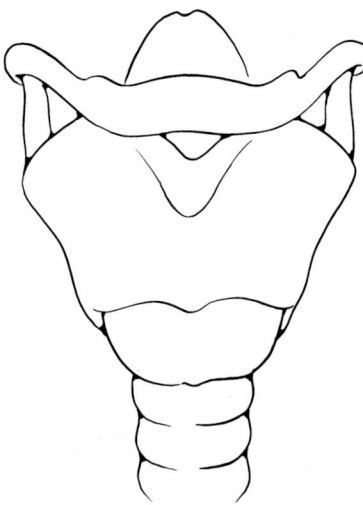

FIGURE 1 Anatomy of pediatric larynx and hyoid bone. Notice that the top of the thyroid cartilage is shielded by the hyoid. The thyrohyoid membrane is more developed in adults and the top of the larynx is easier to palpate. This makes the landmarks in the child different from those in the adult.

been successfully used to manage the airway in children with difficult anatomy such as Pierre Robin sequence. All other indwelling tubes are removed from the aerodigestive tract, so as to avoid mistaking a nasogastric tube in the esophagus for the trachea with an endotracheal tube. A shoulder roll is used to extend the neck, bringing the trachea more anterior and superior. The anesthesiologist sits at the patient's head, holding the bronchoscope or endotracheal tube and the patient's head to provide better extension and exposure (Fig. 2). Local anesthesia 1% lidocaine with epinephrine 1:100,000 is infiltrated into the pretracheal area. Although performed under general anesthesia, this local injection provides better hemostasis and decreases the amount of general anesthetic required.

It is important to ensure that the appropriate instruments are available and ready, including an appropriate array of tracheotomy tubes, before proceeding. The patient is surgically prepped and draped. It is important to give the anesthesiologist immediate access to the airway and neck, however, without sacrificing clean surgical technique. A 2-cm vertical skin incision is made in the midline of the neck, extending to the level of the cricoid cartilage (Fig. 3). Subcutaneous fat is then removed using electrocautery (Fig. 4). This is important to allow for the formation of a matured stoma and prevent anterior dislodgment. It also allows the tracheotomy tube to rest in good position in the trachea, preventing accidental decannulation. The strap muscles are divided in the midline and re-

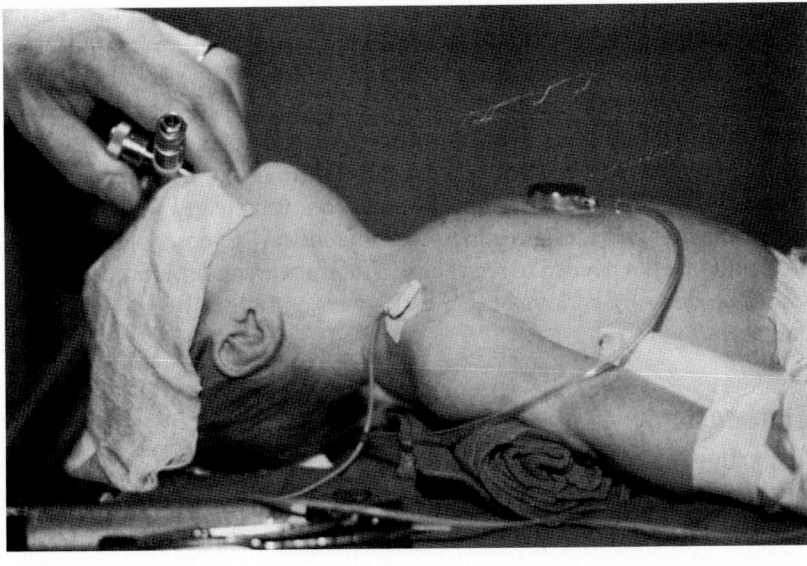

FIGURE 2 The correct position for tracheotomy in the child. Note that the anesthesiologist can stabilize the child's head and assist in extending the neck. (From ref. 21, with permission.)

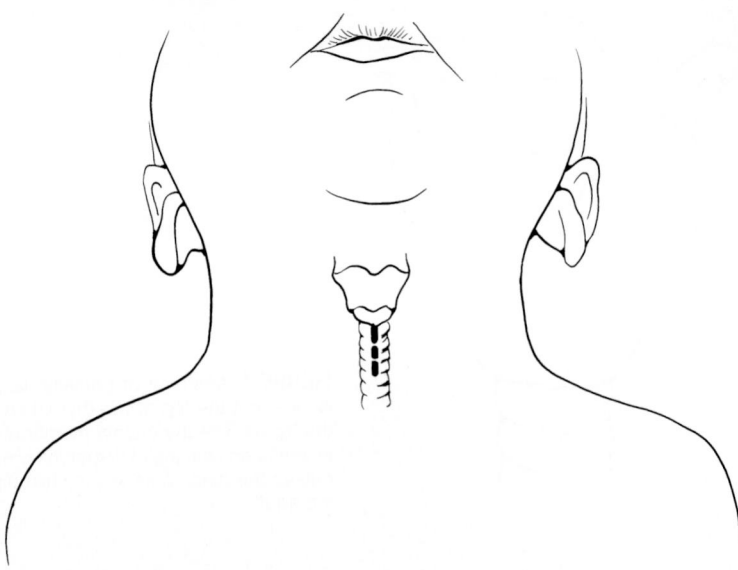

FIGURE 3 The initial incision is made vertically in the pretracheal area. It measures approximately 2 cm long and extends as high as the inferior border of the cricoid.

tracted laterally with small S-shaped retractors. Much of the dissection is performed bluntly with the retractors. The assistant plays an important role in blunt dissection, providing exposure of the trachea with downward and lateral retraction, rather than upward and lateral. This will bring the trachea into view and stabilize it between the retractors. The thyroid gland is divided in the midline with electrocautery. The third and fourth tracheal rings are identified. Vertical 4-0 nonabsorbable sutures are placed through the tracheal cartilage on either side of midline and loosely tied to act as retraction sutures (Fig. 5). These stay sutures will remain taped to the chest, labeled left and right, until the first tracheotomy tube change, as a guide to the tracheal opening should accidental decannulation occur.

The airway is then entered with a scalpel in the midline, creating a tracheostomy appropriately sized for insertion of the tracheotomy tube (Fig. 6). The skin edges are then secured to the tracheal wound with 4-0 chromic gut sutures, fashioning a secure tracheal stoma (Fig. 7). The endotracheal tube or bronchoscope is then withdrawn to the level of the tracheotomy, and an appropriately sized tracheotomy tube is inserted. Ventilation continues until the tracheotomy is in proper position. Once the tracheotomy tube is in

FIGURE 4 Removing subcutaneous fat is important to allow for the development of a well-formed tract. It also allows the tracheotomy tube to sit more naturally in the trachea.

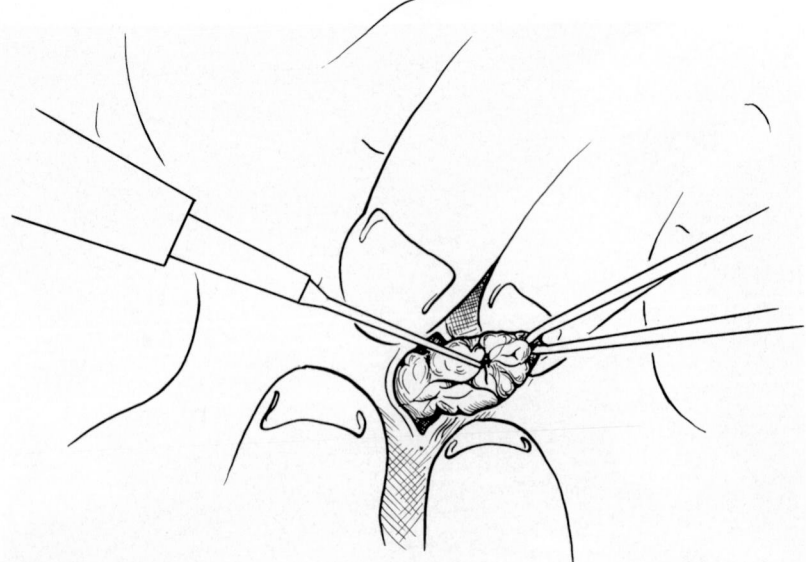

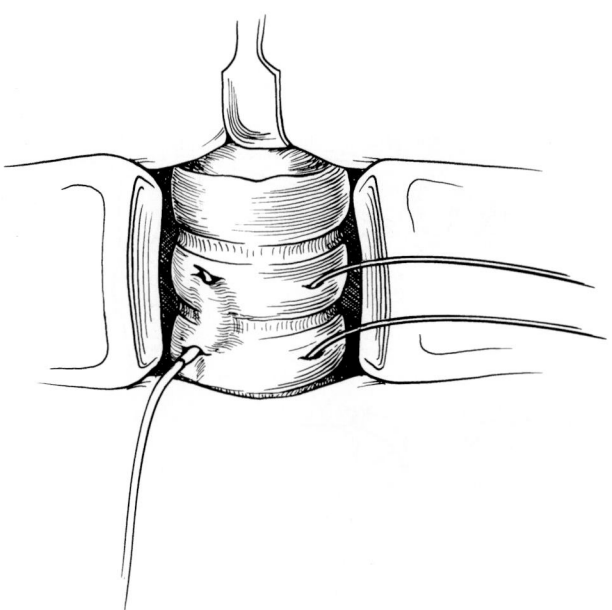

FIGURE 5 Retraction sutures are place vertically around the midline where the trachea will be entered. These are labeled left and right and are taped to the child's chest. They are removed on the fifth postoperative day. In the case of accidental dislodgment, they are used to retract the stoma up to the skin and open. This aids in the proper replacement of the tracheotomy tube.

place, ventilation is then given through the tracheotomy tube. Equal breath sounds and easy ventilation are checked. A flexible suction catheter is also passed through the tracheotomy tube to confirm its position in the tracheal lumen. The position of the distal tip of the tracheotomy tube is confirmed with either flexible or rigid telescopes. It is important to confirm the location of the tip of the tube to prevent encroachment of a long tube on the carina or impingement of a short tube on the posterior tracheal wall. Tracheotomy ties are placed around the patient's neck to secure the tube. They are securely fashioned such that a single finger fits between the skin and the tie (Fig. 8). A chest radiograph is obtained in the immediate perioperative period to identify quickly potential pneumothorax or pneumomediastinum. The tracheotomy ties are changed on the third day. The tracheotomy tube is changed, and the stay sutures are removed on the fifth day.

The appropriate size of the tracheotomy tube depends on the clinical indications for insertion of the tracheotomy and the size of the airway. Generally, the smallest tube that is capable of giving adequate air exchange is chosen. Slightly larger tubes may be required for ventilator-dependent patients. It is possible to estimate the age-appropriate endotracheal tube for orotracheal intubation and then estimate the appropriately sized tracheotomy tube. The formula (age/4 + 4) gives a rough estimate for the age-appropriate endotracheal tube for children above the age of 10 months. Once the age-appropriate endotracheal tube size is calculated, it is easy to convert to the appropriately sized tra-

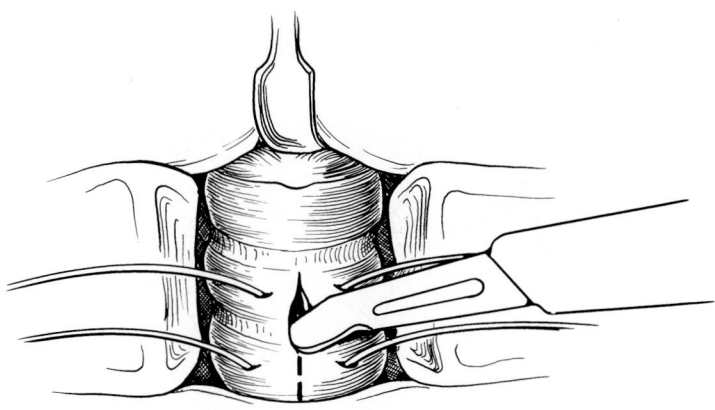

FIGURE 6 A midline tracheotomy incision is made in the trachea. The length of the incision mirrors the outer diameter of the tracheotomy tube.

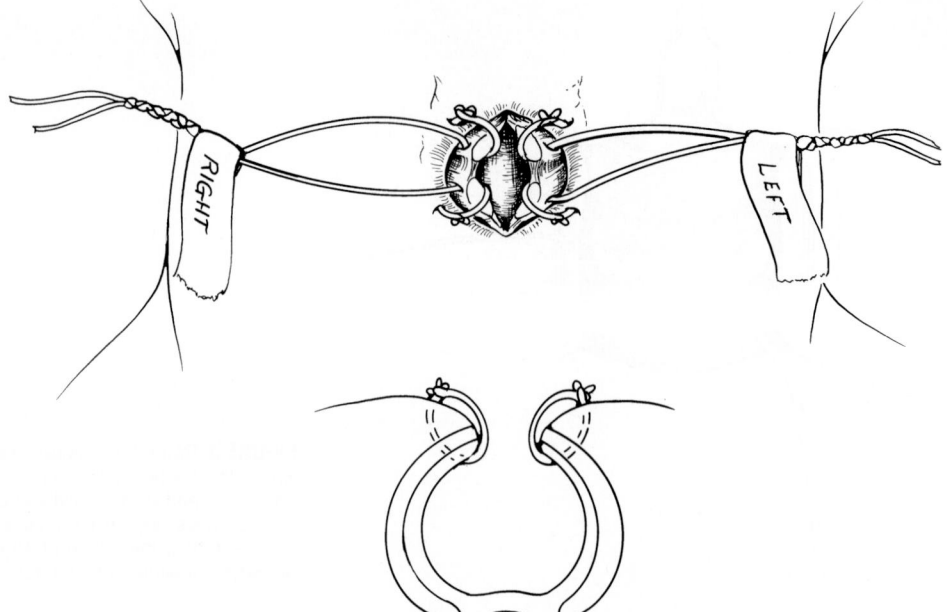

FIGURE 7 The skin edges are secured to the tracheal wall to form a matured stoma. This is important in case of accidental dislodgment. Tacking the skin to the trachea will help to guide the tracheotomy tube through the tracheotomy. This will help prevent the formation of a false passage anterior to the trachea during reinsertion.

cheotomy tube (Table 1). Some tracheotomy tubes are numbered according to the inner diameter, as are most endotracheal tubes. A healthy newborn should accept a 3.5-mm inner diameter tube. A neonate may only accept a 3.0-mm inner diameter tracheotomy tube. The correct size for older children may be estimated with the formula described earlier. More difficult to estimate, however, is the proper length of the tracheotomy tube. Many tracheotomy tubes are manufactured in standard neonatal, pediatric, and pediatric long lengths. Generally, children up to 7 kg may use the neonatal length. Above this weight, the standard pediatric length is generally adequate. Some children with tracheomalacia may need a longer length to stent the airway open with either the standard long tube or a custom length. Again, the only way to determine accurately which length is cor-

FIGURE 8 The tracheotomy ties are secured around the neck. They should allow only one finger between the ties and the skin.

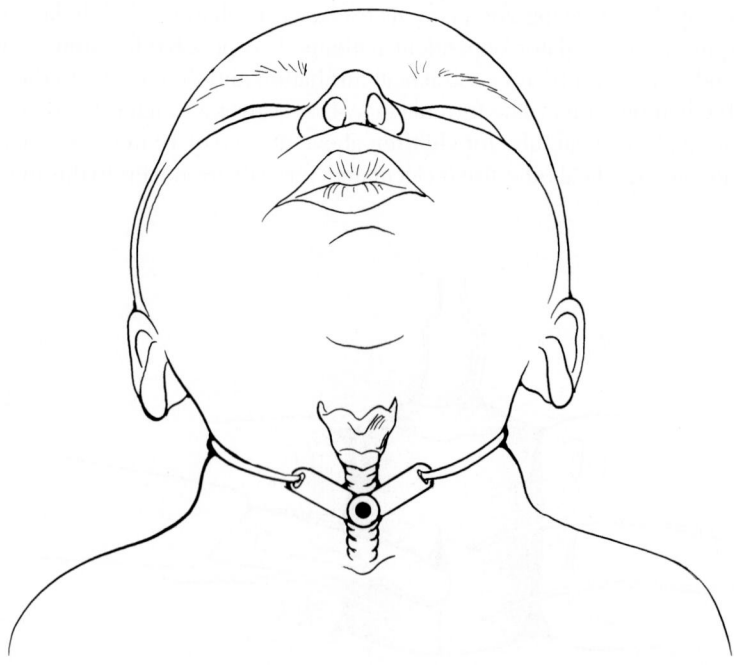

TABLE 1: Size Comparisons of Endotracheal Tubes and Tracheotomy Tubes

Cannula	Inner diameter (mm)	Outer diameter (mm)	Overall length		
			Neonatal (mm)	Pediatric	Pediatric long (mm)
Endotracheal tubes[a]					
2.5	2.5	3.6		12 cm	
3.0	3.0	4.3		14 cm	
3.5	3.5	4.9		16 cm	
4.0	4.0	5.6		18 cm	
4.5	4.5	6.2		20 cm	
5.0	5.0	6.9		22 cm	
5.5	5.5	7.5		25 cm	
6.0	6.0	8.2		26 cm	
Bivona[b]					
2.5	2.5	4.0	30	38 mm	
3.0	3.0	4.7	32	39 mm	
3.5	3.5	5.3	34	40 mm	
4.0	4.0	6.0	36	41 mm	
4.5	4.5	6.7		42 mm	
5.0	5.0	7.3		44 mm	
5.5	5.5	8.0		46 mm	
Franklin[c]					
3.5	3.5	5.0		44 mm	
4.0	4.0	6.0		44 mm	
4.5	4.5	6.7		48 mm	
5.0	5.0	8.0		51 mm	
5.5	5.5	8.5		54 mm	
6.0	6.0	9.3		57 mm	
Portex[d]					
3.0	3.0	5.0		36 mm	
3.5	3.5	5.8		40 mm	
4.0	4.0	6.5		44 mm	
4.5	4.5	7.1		48 mm	
5.0	5.0	7.7		50 mm	
5.5	5.5	8.3		52 mm	
Shiley[e]					
3.0	3.0	4.5	30	39 mm	
3.5	3.5	5.2	32	40 mm	
4.0	4.0	5.9	34	41 mm	
4.5	4.5	6.5	36	42 mm	
5.0	5.0	7.1		44 mm	50
5.5	5.5	7.7		46 mm	52
6.0	6.0	8.3			54
6.5	6.5	9.0			56

[a]Endotracheal tubes are marked with the internal diameter, the outer diameter, and the length.

[b]Bivona Corporation, Gary, IN. Both the inner and outer diameter are marked on the tube.

[c]The Franklin tube of the Great Ormond Street design is manufactured in England and is distributed by Inmed, Norcross GA.

[d]Portex is manufactured by the Simms-Portex Division of Smith Industries, Keene, NH.

[e]Shiley tubes are manufactured by Shiley Laboratories, Irvine, CA. The tube is marked with the outer and inner diameters.

rect is to assess the position of the tip of the tracheotomy tube. This is most easily done with a flexible telescope, but it may also be done with a rigid telescope during bronchoscopy or by chest radiograph.

Some authors have noted that this technique of tracheotomy fashions a more "permanent" stoma, and may result in a persistent tracheocutaneous fistula. Since the major source for mortality in pediatric tracheotomy is accidental decannulation, the added margin of safety created by the matured stoma is justified, particularly during the first few days. Additionally, pediatric tracheotomy is rarely short term (in contrast to adults undergoing certain head and neck cancer operations), and even without the skin sutures, the tract tends to epithelialize permanently over time.

COMPLICATIONS

Complications may be classified as early (perioperative and within the first week) or late. Some complications can occur during both periods, such as accidental decannulation or tube obstruction (Table 2). Some complications are confined to the perioperative period such as pneumomediastinum or pneumothorax. The long-term complications most commonly reported include tracheocutaneous fistula, obstructing distal or suprastomal granuloma, tube obstruction, accidental decannulation, local infection, hemorrhage, long epithelial tract, and tracheoesophageal fistula. In addition, suprastomal tracheomalacia may prevent decannulation.

Unlike adults, children continue to grow, changing the caliber, length, and orientation of the trachea. It is important then to evaluate the airway periodically to ensure that the tracheotomy tube is in the correct position and is the correct size (length and diameter) and that no potential complications are developing. The frequency of interval examination must be tailored to the child. Younger children who are growing more rapidly should be followed more frequently than adolescents.

Early Complications

Pneumomediastinum and Pneumothorax

Although rare, pneumomediastinum and pneumothorax are potentially life-threatening complications that are easily detected through physical examination and chest radiograph. Particularly in infants, the apex of the lung extends into the root of the neck. It is imperative to stay in the midline of the neck to prevent violation of the pleural space.

TABLE 2: Complications of Pediatric Tracheotomy

Early or late
  Accidental decannulation
  Tube obstruction
Early
  Accidental decannulation
  Tube obstruction
  Pneumothorax
  Pneumomediastinum
  Hemorrhage
  Local infection
Late
  Accidental decannulation
  Tube obstruction
  Local infection
  Suprastomal collapse
  Tracheal stenosis
  Tracheocutaneous fistula
  Tracheoesophageal fistula
  Tracheal innominate fistula
  Subglottic stenosis
  Tracheal granuloma
    Distal
    Suprastomal

Equally important is early detection. A small pneumothorax may be conservatively managed expectantly, whereas a larger, progressive, or symptomatic pneumothorax requires chest tube drainage. Avoidance of obstruction of the fresh stoma is important to prevent the development of pneumomediastinum. During forceful coughing, it is not unusual for air to leak around the tracheotomy tube. If a tight dressing is placed on the neck and around the tracheotomy tube before a healed tract can form, the air may dissect into the mediastinum. Pneumomediastinum is treated by enlargement of the neck incision and placement of a drain, allowing a route of escape for the trapped mediastinal air.

Acute Hemorrhage

Acute hemorrhage is generally a problem with technique. It is avoided with meticulous attention to hemostasis during the procedure. Specific attention should be given to the thyroid isthmus, should it need to be divided. If bleeding develops, it may require direct pressure with loose application of hemostatic materials such as Gelfoam (Upjohn, Kalamazoo, MI) or Surgicel (Johnson & Johnson, Arlington, TX) or reexploration to ligate a bleeding vessel. Care should be taking when stomal packing is applied, as it may promote subcutaneous emphysema and pneumomediastinum. Finally, coagulopathy should be considered if bleeding persists.

Accidental Decannulation

Accidental decannulation is a serious complication in the child, especially if the tracheotomy tract is fresh. A false passage anterior to the trachea can easily be formed during emergent reinsertion of the tracheotomy tube. Prevention is the best treatment for this problem. Properly secured tracheotomy ties, a matured tracheal stoma, and stay sutures are the best means to prevent accidental decannulation and to aid in proper replacement of the tracheotomy tube should decannulation occur.

A similar situation can occur in the child with laryngotracheal esophageal cleft. If the cleft extends low enough in the common esophagotracheal wall, the tube may become dislodged from the trachea into the esophagus. This can cause intermittent or complete ventilatory failure. A longer tube may be necessary to position the tip past the end of the cleft. Laryngotracheoesophageal cleft should be kept in mind and its presence disproved when contemplating tracheotomy in the neonate.

Tubal Obstruction

Tube obstruction in the perioperative period can generally be prevented with appropriate tracheotomy care. Frequent suctioning, suctioning with saline, and high humidity will help prevent buildup and plugging of the pediatric single lumen tubes. Meticulous care, observation, and cleaning are imperative in the early perioperative period to prevent diaster. The child with a new tracheotomy tract should be placed in an appropriate setting where the proper level of nursing care can be provided. Constant visual observation is mandatory for the child with a fresh tracheotomy site.

Local Infection

Wound infections occur rarely but may cause significant problems with skin breakdown in the perioperative period. Meticulous tracheotomy tube care and local wound care will help prevent this complication. Occasionally, systemic antibiotics are required for peristomal cellulitis. Local wound care with wet to dry dressing of half-strength Dakin's solution is also helpful for wound breakdown. Some wounds heal more rapidly if a barrier is placed between the tracheotomy tube flanges and the wound dehiscence. In these situations, Duoderm can be applied to help protect the skin from pressure and continued contamination. It is particularly useful in the child with abnormal neck anatomy such as hemangioma or lymphangioma of the neck.

TABLE 3: Long-Term Follow-up in Pediatric Tracheotomy, with Incidence of Selected Late Complications

Author	Year	No.	Airway obstruction	Age range (mo.)	Early complications	Late complications	Tube obstruction	Significant granuloma[a]	Accidental decannulation	Infection	Bleeding	Tracheo-esophageal fistula	Tracheo-malacia	Other	Tracheotomy-related mortality
Gauder et al. (7)	1978	123	63	0–144	30	36	1	5	1	1	0	0	1	27[b]	3
Wetmore et al. (13)	1982	420	164	0–252	n/a	222	23	54	40	18	22	0	12	53[c]	8
Carter and Benjamin (14)	1983	164	126	0–158	n/a	35	3	17	0	7	0	0	4	4	0
Kenna et al. (15)	1987	124	88	0–12	39	47	2	28	0	0	5	1	6	5	3
Crysdale et al. (16)	1988	319	222	0–240	74	101	18	50	5	9	1	10	7	1	3
Gianoli et al. (17)	1990	60	28	0–12	23	33	7	15	2	2	1	0	2	4	1
Zetouni and Manoukian (12)	1993	44	25	0–12	6	6	3	0	2	0	1	0	0	0	2
Totals		1,254	716	0–252	n/a	480	57	169	50	37	30	11	32	94	20

[a]Some authors group suprastomal and distal granuloma together when reporting complications

[b]Includes 15 patients who developed subglottic stenosis, possibly related to underlying conditions or previous intubation.

[c]Includes 42 patients with tracheocutaneous fistula, not considered as a complication in other series.

(Adapted from ref. 22, with permission.)

Late Complications

Many authors have reported their long-term experience in children with tracheotomies (7,12–17) (Table 3, Fig. 9). The most common long-term complications are tracheal granuloma, usually suprastomal, and persistent tracheocutaneous fistula (Fig. 10). Persistent tracheocutaneous fistula is probably underreported, as many authors do not consider it a complication of tracheotomy and do not include it in their series.

Tracheal Granuloma

Distal obstruction of the tracheotomy tube is potentially life threatening. Like many tracheal lesions, this occurs more frequently in the very young patient in whom the margin of safety mirrors the caliber of the airway. The most common cause is granulation, either from trauma at the distal tip of the tracheotomy tube or excessive suctioning. If a vascular anomaly is present, the tip of the tracheotomy tube may rest on the tracheal wall at the level of the vascular anomaly, causing pressure that may induce formation of granulation. It is again stressed that preoperative identification of a vascular anomaly is important and that tracheotomy should be avoided when possible.

The proper position of the tracheotomy tube should be determined by either flexible or rigid endoscope or chest radiographs. The tip of the tube should be well above the carina. Since some tracheotomy tubes come in different standard lengths, it is important to remember to replace the tracheotomy tube with the correct length tube during routine tracheotomy tube changes. It is important that caregivers understand the difference between the neonatal and the pediatric lengths.

Prevention is the best form of treatment for tracheal granulation tissue. Once it has developed, the inciting cause must be removed. A poorly positioned tracheotomy tube should be repositioned away from the site of granulation. Changing the tube length and material may prove helpful. Longer tubes may be inserted past the granulation, but this risks creating granulation tissue more distally. Longer tracheotomy tubes are limited by the carina.

Obstructing granulation tissue may be removed by cup forceps, electrocautery, or laser at bronchoscopy. This may prove difficult in the smaller patient. If the obstruction is minimal, topical steroids may be successful in the reducing the granulation tissue. It is

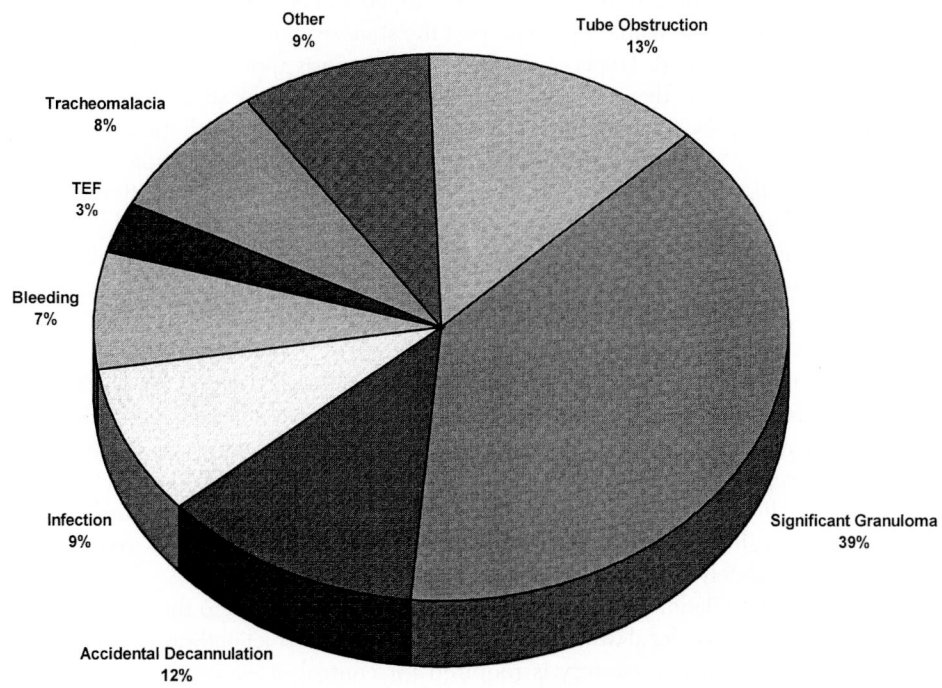

FIGURE 9 Relative proportions of late complications derived from Figure 10. The data are derived from a total of 423 late complications in 1254 patients, excluding 42 patients with persistent tracheocutaneous fistula (since this is not uniformly considered a complication in all the series) and 15 patients with subglottic stenosis (since it cannot be determined that this was actually a complication of the tracheotomy itself). (Adapted from ref. 22, with permission.)

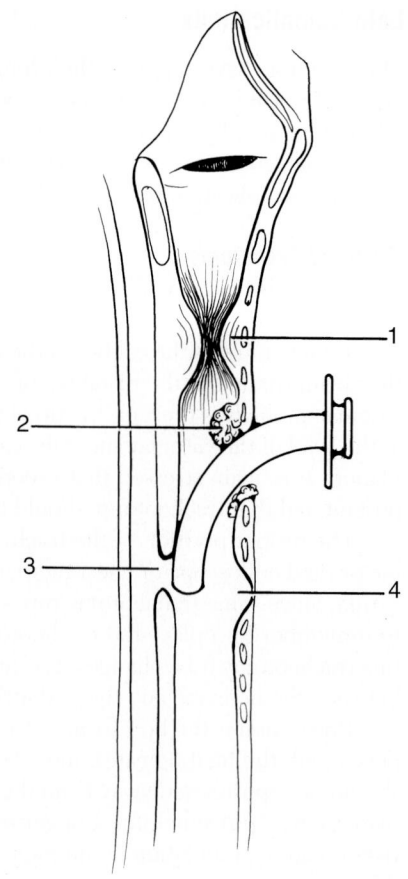

FIGURE 10 Potential late complications from tracheotomy tubes: subglottic stenosis (*1*), suprastomal granuloma (*2*), tracheoesophageal fistula (*3*), and anterior tracheal wall erosion with innominate artery fistula (*4*).

important to treat granulation tissue when present to prevent obstruction or the development of permanent tracheal stenosis.

Tracheal stenosis below the tracheotomy site related to local trauma is even more difficult to manage. Topical steroid preparations are not effective on mature scar. Longer tracheotomy tubes are available to extend past the stenosis, but it becomes problematic as the carina is approached. Tracheotomy-associated stenosis appears to be related to local trauma and not to be the result of interference with growth by surgical intervention in the developing airway. Prevention is the best form of treatment, with meticulous care of the tracheotomy tube and observance of its position. Early identification of stenosis formation may allow for manipulations to be performed before severe stenosis develops. Once tracheal stenosis forms, the inciting factor should be removed, local infection should be treated, and granulomatous diseases should be ruled out. Repeat dilation of the tracheal stenosis may halt its progression. Formal surgical treatment of distal tracheal stenosis is beyond the scope of this chapter, but it generally entails resection with primary anastomosis.

Suprastomal granulomas should be removed if they are obstructing. An obstructing granuloma places the child at increased risk if there is accidental decannulation. The granuloma may be removed at the time of interval bronchoscopy with either optical foreign body forceps or through the tracheotomy with a sphenoid punch (Fig. 11). Bleeding is usually self-limiting. Troublesome bleeding may be controlled with a flexible electrocautery through the bronchoscope. Occasionally, a stomal revision is required to deliver and completely remove giant obstructing granulomas.

Peristomal granulation tissue may also develop at the entrance to the tracheotomy. This usually responses to local wound care and more frequent tracheotomy tube changes. Occasionally, silver nitrate cautery is required for control of exuberant granulation.

Sometimes a formal stomal revision is required to remove granulation tissue and scar that may jeopardize successful tracheotomy tube reinsertion.

Accidental Decannulation

Accidental decannulation can cause tragic results during any period the child is dependent on the tracheotomy. It becomes more frequent as a young child develops the manual dexterity to remove the tracheotomy tube. Constant supervision is required and should be arranged before discharge. At least two caregivers need to be identified and trained before discharge. One of the caregivers must be vigilant at all times, working in shifts. It is important to stress to all the caregivers that tracheotomy ties be secure at all times. No more than one finger should be able to pass under the ties. The caregivers must feel comfortable caring for the tracheotomy tube before discharge from the hospital. This includes competence in changing the tracheotomy tube. A dislodgment plan must be identified and rehearsed with the caregivers so that competency can be demonstrated before discharge. Should the tube become dislodged, frequently the child will be able to breathe comfortably through the open stoma. Calm and controlled reinsertion should follow. Hurried insertion of the tracheotomy tube may cause the development of a false passage, possibly leading to complete airway obstruction.

Subglottic Stenosis

The incidence of subglottic stenosis as a complication related directly to tracheotomy has decreased since Jackson emphasized the dangers of high tracheotomy in 1921. Subglottic stenosis is generally caused by insertion of the tracheotomy too high, close to the cricoid. Factors that may also contribute to the formation of subglottic stenosis include subglottic trauma, generally from endotracheal intubation, and low-grade continued inflammation from local infection originating from the tracheotomy stoma (18). The incidence of this complication can be minimized by meticulous tracheotomy care and placement.

FIGURE 11 Suprastomal granulomas may be removed through the stoma with a sphenoid punch.

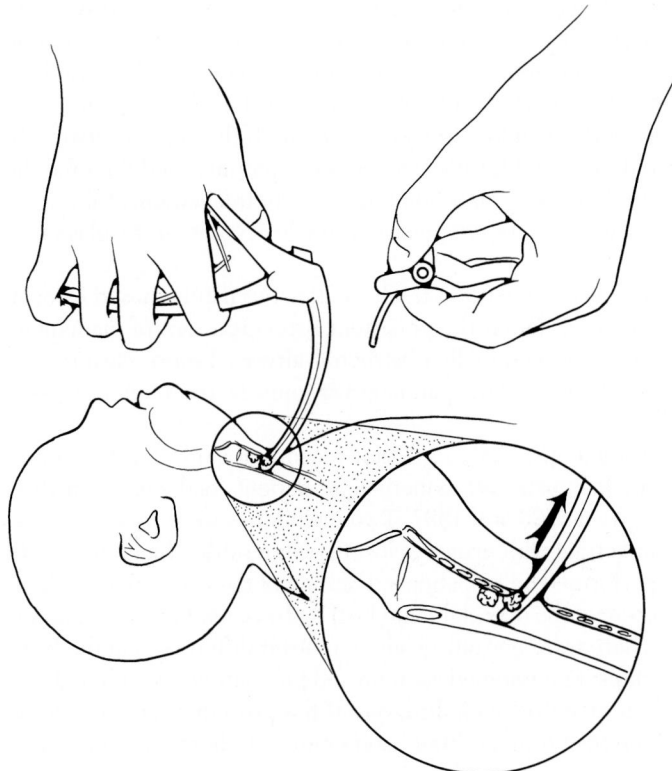

Posttracheotomy stenosis is also associated with emergency surgery in a child with an unsecured airway. Poor technique with poor planning of incisions, rough handling of the trachea, and technical errors account for the development of subglottic stenosis in which a tracheotomy is performed in a hypoxic and unsedated child. Avoidance of subglottic stenosis after tracheotomy can usually be achieved by careful planning, meticulous dissection, insertion of the tube at the correct level, and attention to detail in the postoperative period.

Suprastomal Collapse and Tracheal Stenosis

The incidence of suprastomal collapse increases inversely with the age of the child at the time of tracheotomy insertion. Pressure on the first and second tracheal rings can cause local chondritis and weakening of these tracheal rings. This can cause tracheomalacia in the suprastomal area.

Suprastomal collapse can cause significant obstruction of the airway, making future decannulation impossible without a stomal revision or even tracheoplasty. Relief of the obstruction may require operative intervention. Procedures to relieve the obstruction may be as simple as a revision of the tracheal stoma or as complex as tracheal resection with primary anastomosis.

Prevention of this complication is not always possible. It is more common in young patients who require prolonged tracheotomy (19). Again, insertion of the appropriately sized tube at the correct level in the trachea is the best defense against this potential complication. Removal of cartilage at the time of tracheotomy will further increase the risk of anterior wall collapse and should be avoided.

Persistent Tracheocutaneous Fistula

After the tracheotomy tube has been removed, a persistent tracheocutaneous fistula may develop. The incidence of this occurrence varies from 19% to 42% depending on the series. Some investigators do not consider this a complication and do not report it in their series of tracheotomy complications. The key factor that leads to persistent tracheocutaneous fistula appears to be apposition of the skin to the tracheal mucosa in a nicely formed stoma. The incidence of persistent tracheocutaneous fistula also seems to be inversely proportional to age at tracheotomy and directly proportional to the duration of tracheotomy. The use of tracheotomy for inflammatory disease has decreased recently, decreasing the number of short-term tracheotomies performed. A greater proportion of tracheotomies are performed for airway obstruction. If the chronic airway obstruction is not reconstructed, the need for the tracheotomy continues and the time the child is cannulated increases. A higher proportion of long-term tracheotomy tubes may explain the increase in the relative number of persistent tracheocutaneous fistulas in recent years.

Most important to identify is the persistent tracheocutaneous fistula caused from an airway with a marginal obstruction. Often the persistent fistula is a sign of inadequate reconstruction or persistence of a marginally obstructed airway. Before closure of a tracheocutaneous fistula, the adequacy of the patent airway must be thoroughly assessed to eliminate this possibility.

The closure of tracheocutaneous fistula has been recently reviewed at Children's Hospital Medical Center in Cincinnati (20). Ninety-eight patients had closure of their tracheocutaneous fistula between 1990 and 1997. Two techniques were used. Excision of the tracheocutaneous fistula tract with primary closure over a rubber band drain with short-term intubation was performed on 80 patients. Excision of the fistula tract with insertion of a 3.0-mm tracheotomy tube overnight and healing by secondary intention was performed on 18 patients. There were no statistically significant differences in the long-term outcome of the two groups. Pneumomediastinum and pneumothorax, although not encountered in this series, are potential complications of the procedure and should be identified early. Closure of the tract over a rubber band drain with short-term intubation

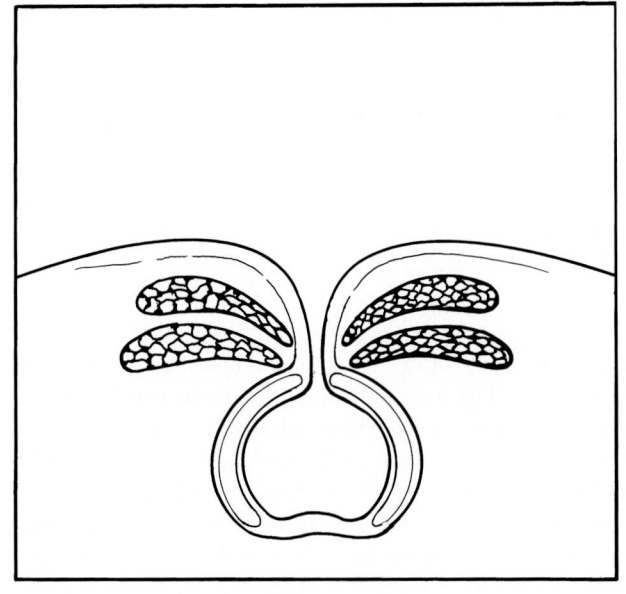

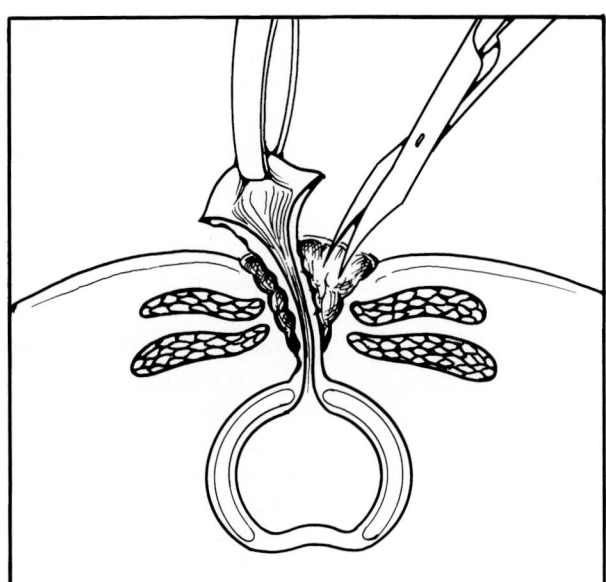

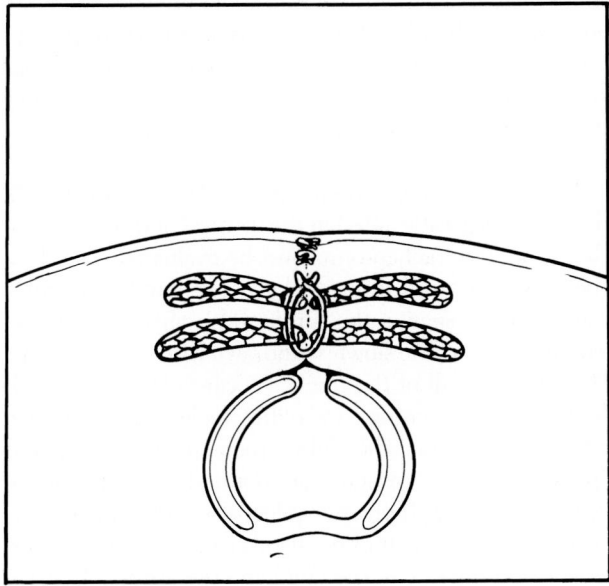

FIGURE 12 Closure of the tracheocutaneous fistula. **A:** The fistula tract is identified, dissected to the trachea, and excised. **B:** The wound is then closed in layers over a rubber band drain. **C:** Short-term intubation is used in the perioperative period. Perioperative pneumothorax and pneumomediastinum must be ruled out.

or allowing the tract to close by secondary intention are two ways to avoid this potential complication. Excision with primary closure (Fig. 12) gives the best cosmetic result and is the procedure of choice according to the authors.

Delayed Tracheoesophageal Fistula

Although rare, erosion of the posterior tracheal wall can cause a fistula to form between the trachea and esophagus. Pressure on the posterior tracheal wall from the distal tip of the tracheotomy tube, as in anterior wall erosion, is the most common cause of this complication. Periodic bronchoscopy will help identify those patients in which the tracheotomy tube is directed posterior and causing granulation. The posterior wall may be in contact with the distal tip of the tracheotomy in patients whose tracheotomy tube is too short or when there is an anatomic abnormality of the trachea such as children with severe scoliosis or kyphosis. This may also occur in a patient on a ventilator with a nasogastric tube. The tissue between the nasogastric tube and the tracheotomy tube may be pinched and undergo pressure necrosis. These patients may begin to have eructation with ventilated breaths as a first sign.

Prevention is the best form of therapy. Symptoms may be nonspecific and can include recurrent pneumonia or coughing with oral feeding. If granulation is present but no fistula, changing the tube length or changing to a softer tube may allow the irritation to subside and prevent fistulization. If fistulization occurs and persists after changing the tracheotomy tube, surgical repair will be needed. Management generally requires an open surgical procedure, with interposition of healthy muscle between the trachea and esophagus.

Tracheal Innominate Fistula

The most dreaded complication of tracheotomy is a tracheal innominate artery fistula. This vessel arises from the aortic arch to cross in front of the trachea and gives rise to the right common carotid and subclavian arteries. Although it generally lies beneath the sternal manubrium, it may occasionally ride high in the neck and should always be identified at the time of tracheotomy. Death from this complication is likely unless it is identified quickly and accurately and corrected promptly. Pressure on the anterior tracheal wall causing erosion is the leading factor of this complication. Cuffed tracheotomy tubes can cause anterior tracheal wall necrosis if the cuff pressure is high. Before the development of softer, more flexible tubes, stiff metal tubes had a higher chance of anterior position and tracheal wall erosion. A high index of suspicion is necessary for prompt identification and successful treatment. Although most bleeding will come from stomal granulation tissue or irritation from deep suctioning, any time blood is reported coming from the tracheotomy tube, the possibility of tracheal innominate fistula must be entertained.

The evaluation requires level-headedness and good judgment. The introduction of the small flexible fiberoptic endoscope has greatly aided in the workup of this complication. Every child who has bleeding from the tracheotomy must be evaluated. The flexible fiberoptic endoscope may be gently inserted through the indwelling tracheotomy tube. Often, areas of suction trauma will be seen at the carina. If no obvious source of bleeding is identified, the tracheotomy tube is then slowly withdrawn with the endoscope situated just distal to the tip. The anterior wall of the trachea is carefully inspected. If bleeding granulation tissue is identified on the anterior wall of the trachea, the presumed diagnosis of a tracheal innominate fistula is made. The child is then taken to the operating room, pediatric thoracic or pediatric general surgeons are notified, and the anterior tracheal wall is explored in a controlled setting. If vigorous bleeding is met, maneuvers to apply direct pressure (until exploration and repair of the fistula can be made) are performed. The maneuver used depends on the size of the child and the airway. A cuffed endotracheal tube or tracheotomy tube positioned such that the balloon may be inflated to tamponade the fistula may help temporize the situation. Sometimes a finger through the stoma is possible, to give direct digital pressure on the bleeding site. This is more often possible in the child with a tracheotomy for chronic ventilation. The tracheotomy is replaced with an orotracheal tube, and a finger may be inserted through the tracheotomy. This would not be possible in the child with a tracheotomy for complete airway obstruction.

Definitive management requires sternotomy and generally involves division of the innominate artery. Fortunately, the risk of cerebral infarction is low in the pediatric population. Repair or replacement of the vessel in a contaminated bed increases the risk of breakdown and rebleeding and is usually avoided. Some authors describe aortography in the workup of potential tracheal innominate artery fistula. This is not recommended. If one's index of suspicion is high enough to desire an arteriogram, it would be unwise to bring a potentially unstable patient to the radiology department. If bleeding is intermittent, the study may be falsely negative. Any patient seriously suspected of impending innominate artery rupture should be explored with a thoracic surgeon available.

HOME CARE

The long-term outcome in children with tracheotomy has improved due mainly to advances in home care. The morbidity and mortality from tracheotomy-related events has dramatically decreased because of advances in this field. Plugging, accidental decannulation, local wound breakdown, mucosal suction trauma, and infections have been addressed by specialists in the field, giving a markedly improved quality of life for the child at home.

Comprehensive home care programs for children with tracheotomies should integrate the skills required to maintain a safe airway while promoting the child's normal development and growth. Individualized training must be given to all caregivers to a level of basic competency. Caregivers should be able to identify proficiently when the child is having an airway-related problem and be able to perform some basic maneuvers to alleviate potential complete obstruction and respiratory arrest. The caregivers should be trained to suction and change the tracheotomy without difficulty. If this cannot be achieved, the child should be placed in a setting where skilled care is available, whether at home with skilled nursing or in a chronic care facility. Optimal procedures for such things as tie securing, humidification, tracheotomy tube changing, and cardiopulmonary resuscitation have been outlined elsewhere by Fitton and Myer (21), and the reader is directed to this reference if further knowledge is desired.

One of the most important jobs of the clinician coordinating home care for a child with a tracheotomy is to ensure that the parents or other caregivers are connected to an appropriate support network, which is available at all times. The surgeon, pediatrician, nurses, speech language pathologist, backup caregivers, and equipment providers should be easily accessible to those primarily responsible for the child's welfare.

Finally, home monitoring is controversial. Mechanical apnea monitors give an alarm with the absence of respiratory effort. They are generally used for central apnea. Cessation of respiratory effort is an extreme late sign of tracheotomy occlusion or dislodgment. Pulse oximetry, on the other hand, is associated with frequent false alarms from failure of the probe to find the pulse or to detachment. It should be stressed that no alarm system is a substitute for adequate training of responsible caregivers. There is a danger that monitoring equipment can give a false sense of security. There is no replacement for constant vigilance of the child with a tracheotomy.

DECANNULATION

Before decannulation is attempted, laryngoscopy and bronchoscopy are performed to evaluate the airway. Decannulation failures are usually caused by the underlying primary airway abnormality that led to the need for the tracheotomy. Suprastomal granulation tissue and suprastomal collapse are the most common sites of obstruction caused by the tracheotomy tube that may need to be addressed before decannulation. Once this pathology has been corrected, progressively smaller tracheotomy tubes are inserted and the patient is observed for 48 hours. The child is watched for signs of respiratory distress. When the smallest tracheotomy tube is tolerated, an inpatient plugging trial is performed. If plugging is tolerated night and day without signs of significant airway obstruction, the tracheotomy tube is removed. An occlusive dressing is applied to the stoma, and the child is closely monitored for 48 hours. If all goes well, the child is discharged and a follow-up laryngoscopy and bronchoscopy is scheduled in 1 month. Formation of significant intraluminal suprastomal granulomas has been identified in decannulated patients at this time. These patients may be asymptomatic, even though they have a significant obstruction by the granuloma. If a large granuloma is identified, attempts at endoscopic removal are tried, and the child remains decannulated.

There is no lower age limit to decannulation. In some smaller infants, however, even the smallest tracheotomy tube occludes most of the airway. In these children, a small fenestration is customized. A plugging trial is then attempted again; if it is successful, decannulation is attempted. Fenestrations are used only in the short term as the open end of the fenestration may predispose to granuloma formation. They can also be difficult to suction as the suction cannula may catch on the fenestration. The suction cannula can also slip through the fenestration during suctioning. The distal tracheotomy tube may not then be cleared of obstructing mucus even though it appears that the suction cannula was inserted completely. To avoid this problem, the tracheotomy tube can be pulled out until the top of the fenestration can be seen. The suction cannula can then be observed passing through the fenestration into the lumen of the tracheotomy tube. Normal suctioning can then be performed. There are alternate methods for decannulation in smaller children who are unable to plug with even the smallest tracheotomy tube because the tube occupies most of the airway. Sometimes a trial of decannulation in a monitored setting under a watchful eye is successful even if capping has not been possible. Stomal revision to remove any suprastomal collapse or granuloma with short-term endotracheal intubation has also been successful in these smaller children.

The patent tracheal stoma generally closes within days to months of decannulation. Water precautions and local wound care are the only restrictions for the open stoma. If the stoma does not close within 6 to 12 months, surgical closure of the persistent tracheocutaneous fistula may be performed, as described earlier in this chapter.

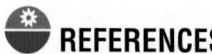

REFERENCES

1. Benjamin B. Prolonged intubation injuries of the larynx: endoscopic diagnosis, classification, and treatment. *Ann Otol Rhinol Laryngol Suppl*, 1993;160:1–15.
2. Senders CW, Muntz HR, Schweiss D. Physician survey on the care of children with tracheotomies. *Am J Otolaryngol* 1991;12:48.
3. Talabere LR. The child with a tracheostomy: a holistic approach to home care. *Top Clin Nurs* 1980;2:27.
4. Whited RE. A prospective study of laryngotracheal sequelae in long-term intubation. *Laryngoscope* 1984;94:367–377.
5. Whited RE. Posterior commissure stenosis post long-term intubation. *Laryngoscope* 1983;93:1314–1318.
6. Dayal VS, Masri WE. Tracheotomy in the intensive care setting. *Laryngoscope* 1986;96:58–60.
7. Gaudet PT, Peerless A, Sasaki CT, et al. Pediatric tracheotomy and associated complications. *Laryngoscope* 1978;88:1633–1641.
8. Fearon B, Ellis D. The management of long term airway problems in infants and children. *Ann Otol Rhinol Laryngol* 1971;80:669–677.
9. Ratner I, Whitfield J. Acquired subglottic stenosis in the very-low-birth-weight infant. *Am J Dis Child* 1983;137:40.
10. Papsidero MJ, Pashley NRT. Acquired stenosis of the upper airway in neonates: an increasing problem. *Ann Otol Rhinol Laryngol* 1980;89:512.
11. Strong RM, Passy V. Endotracheal intubation: complications in neonates. *Arch Otolaryngol* 1977;103:329–335.
12. Zeitouni A, Manoukian J. Tracheotomy in the first year of life. *J Otolaryngol* 1993;22:431–434.
13. Wetmore RF, Handler SD, Potsic WP. Pediatric tracheotomy: experience during the past decade. *Ann Otol Rhinol Laryngol* 1982;91:628–632.
14. Carter P, Benjamin B. Ten year review of pediatric tracheotomy. *Ann Otol Rhinol Laryngol* 1983;92:398–400.
15. Kenna MA, Reilly JS, Stool SE. Tracheotomy in the preterm infant. *Ann Otol Rhinol Laryngol* 1987;96:68–71.
16. Crysdale WS, Feldman RI, Natio K. Tracheotomies: a 10-year experience in 319 children. *Ann Otol Rhinol Laryngol* 1988;97:439–443.

17. Gianoli GJ, Miller RH, Guarisco JL. Tracheotomy in the first year of life. *Ann Otol Rhinol Laryngol* 1990;99:896–901.

18. Sasaki CT, Horiuchi M, Koss N. Tracheostomy-related subglottic stenosis: bacteriologic pathogenesis. *Laryngoscope* 1979;89:857.

19. Benjamin B, Curley JW. Infant tracheotomy-endoscopy and decannulation. *Int J Pediatr Otorhinolaryngol* 1990;20:113.

20. Stern Y, Cosenza M, Walner DL, et al. Management of persistant tracheocutaneous fistula in the pediatric age group. *Laryngoscope*, 1997 (submitted).

21. Fitton CM, Myer CM III. Home care of the child with a tracheotomy. In: Myer CM III, Cotton RT, Shott SR, eds. *The pediatric airway: an interdisciplinary approach.* JB Lippincott, Philadelphia, 1995:171–177.

22. Cotton RT, Rothschild MA, Gerber ME. Airway obstruction managed surgically. In: Stringer MS, Oldhin KT, Mouriquand PDE, Howard ER, eds. *Pediatric surgery and urology: long-term outcomes.* London: WB Saunders, 1998;138–155.

J.S. McMurray: Division of Otolaryngology—Head and Neck Surgery, Department of Pediatrics, University of Wisconsin Clinical Science Center, Madison, Wisconsin 53792-3236. ● C.A.J. Prescott: Department of Otolaryngology, University of Cape Town, Red Cross War Memorial Children's Hospital, Rondebosch, Cape Town, 7700 South Africa.

● *Practical Pediatric Otolaryngology*
● edited by Robin T. Cotton
and Charles M. Myer, III
● Lippincott-Raven Publishers,
Philadelphia © 1999

Caustic Ingestion

Lauren D. Holinger

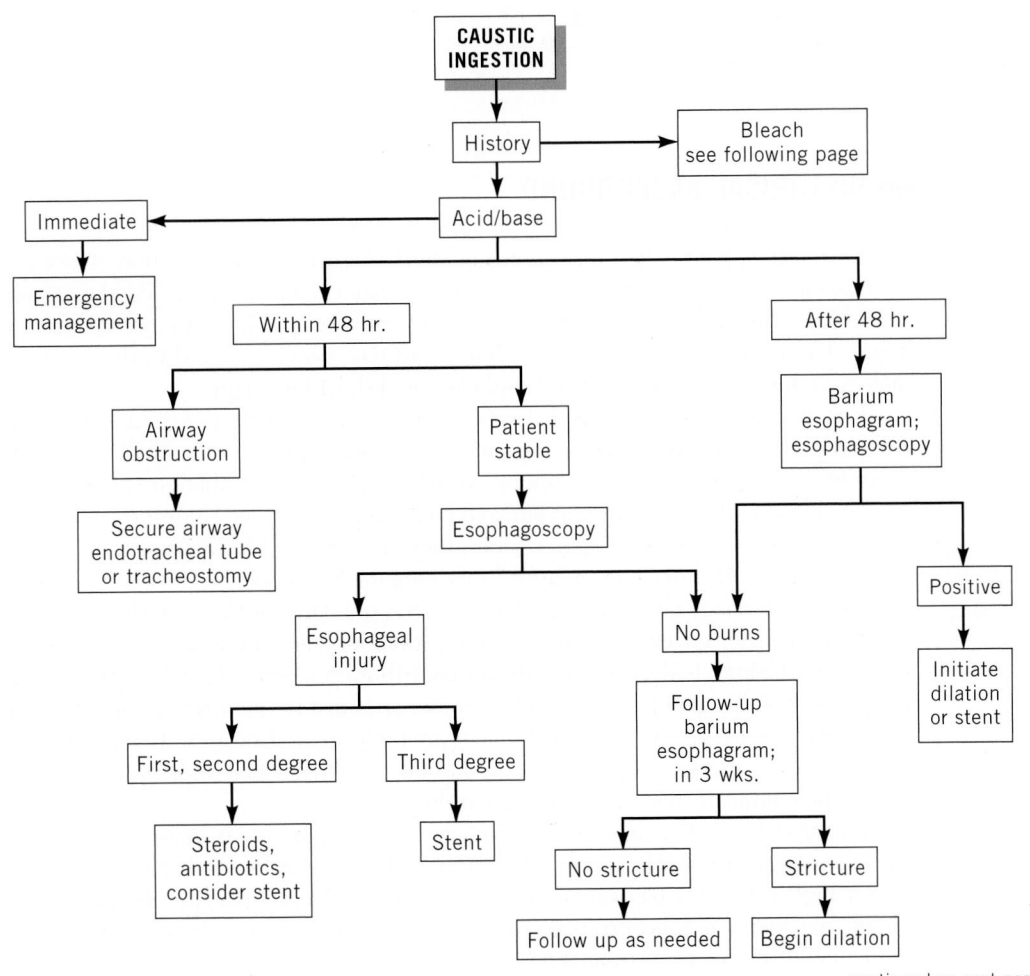

continued on next page

continued

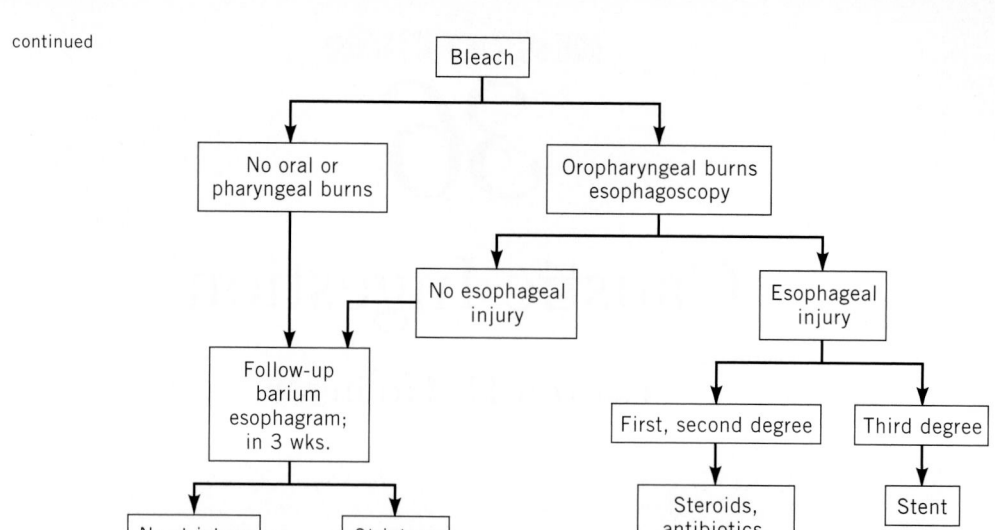

HISTORICAL BACKGROUND

Esophageal, pharyngeal, and laryngeal injury can occur from ingestion of bases (alkalies or caustics), acids, and bleaches. Denture cleaners contain various combinations of these chemicals. Ingestion of substances containing bases produces the most significant injury. These substances include lye (NaOH, KOH), which is found in drain cleaners such as Drano, ammonia (NH_4OH), and electric dishwasher soaps.

Low-phosphate or nonphosphate detergent powders (such as Arm and Hammer) are also part of this group. They are notable because ingestion of a small amount can cause severe upper airway compromise, which may require intubation (1). Symptoms can develop as early as 1 hour or as late as 5 hours after ingestion. Therefore, when these children are seen in the emergency room, they are observed for at least 5 hours. Hair straighteners, "activators," or "relaxers" may contain NaOH or $Ca(OH)_2$ and are especially hazardous since child-proof packaging is not standard for these products (2).

Most ingestions occur at home and in the kitchen. High family stress, both parental and environmental, is the most significant contributing factor. Marital conflict, mental and physical illness, and loss of a family member are most frequently reported. Contrary to what one would expect, an unsafe home is not the primary factor (3). Reporting of suspicious cases of abuse is required by law, and the resulting social intervention may preclude repeat injury to the same child or a sibling.

Fortunately, caustic ingestion is being seen less frequently because of a variety of preventive measures and legislation. The 1971 Federal Hazardous Substance Act and the Poison Prevention Act ban excessively hazardous products, mandate child-proof container caps, and ban concentrations over 10%. Labeling of contents on containers and parental education and awareness has also been a major factor.

PATIENT ASSESSMENT

Evaluation of Extent of Injury

Rational therapy is based on a precise diagnosis. The essence of the evaluation, therefore, is to determine the extent of injury. This begins with a careful history including the type, amount, and brand name of the ingested product. A parent may be sent home to retrieve the container. Any previous home or hospital treatment is documented.

Symptoms of hoarseness, stridor, and dyspnea are noted. Odynophagia, drooling, and refusal of food suggest a more severe injury. Substernal pain, abdominal pain, and rigidity suggest a profound injury and perforation of the esophagus or stomach.

Physical examination of the face, extremities, and chest should not be overlooked in the examiner's enthusiasm to focus on the oral cavity, pharynx, and upper digestive tract. The child is restrained. Good light and suction are made available for examination of the oral cavity and pharynx. The precise location and the extent of any burn or edema are noted. It may be possible to examine the larynx with a mirror or flexible fiberoptic laryngoscope, depending on the age and degree of cooperation of the patient and whether or not the patient has significant symptoms of airway obstruction. In the presence of serious airway obstruction, this part of the examination may be deferred so as not to precipitate an acute severe obstructive episode. Attention is then directed to physical examination of the esophagus and stomach.

For the patient seen within the first 48 hours after ingestion, radiologic examination may include chest radiograph and airway films, particularly if any symptoms of airway obstruction are present. Barium esophagram is of little value acutely in children since it delays the endoscopic evaluation and will not show first- or second-degree injury. If an esophagram is obtained, an atonic, dilated esophagus is an indication of a severe (full-thickness) injury.

Indications for Esophagoscopy

Since the patient's signs and symptoms do not accurately predict the presence or severity of injury, esophagoscopy is carried out in virtually every patient who is suspected of having ingested a caustic substance. It is a more accurate way to evaluate involvement of the esophagus following a caustic ingestion than any other means. Absence of oropharyngeal lesions or pharyngeal symptoms does not exclude esophageal or gastric injury; 8% to 20% of patients without oropharyngeal lesions do have esophageal burns (4). Furthermore, the presence of oropharyngeal lesions does not mean that the esophagus is necessarily involved (5).

Esophagoscopy is contraindicated in the presence of a severe burn with evidence of laryngeal edema and in patients who have been on high doses of steroids. Esophagoscopy is carried out under general endotracheal anesthesia within 24 to 48 hours of ingestion to the upper limit of any full-thickness burn encountered. The oral cavity, pharynx (including pyriform sinuses), and larynx are examined carefully with a laryngoscope. The area of the cricopharyngeus muscle is carefully inspected. A flexible esophagogastroscope is passed to examine the length of the esophagus and the stomach. The type of injury as well as the depth is noted; circumferential burns are more likely to cause strictures than linear injuries.

Bleach ingestion is the one exception to the general rule that "all caustic ingestions get scoped" (6). Bleaches are chlorides (oxidizing agents). Sodium hypochlorite is the most common and is contained in products such as Clorox and Comet. In the United States, bleaches are approximately 5.25% sodium hypochlorite. In the summer months, 6% Clorox (pH 11.4) is distributed because sodium hypochlorite degrades more rapidly in the heat. At these concentrations, bleach produces an ulceration that usually does not result in stricture or residual sequelae. Management of chlorine bleach ingestion includes a careful oropharyngeal examination. If no burns are present, a follow-up esophagram is obtained. When burns are present, esophagoscopy is carried out.

Evaluation for a Patient Presenting more than 48 Hours after Ingestion

Posteroanterior and lateral chest radiograms and barium esophagram are obtained. The patient is hospitalized if there is evidence of an esophageal burn. Dilation is initiated in patients with stenosis. Steroids are not given.

Patients are followed on an ambulatory basis in the absence of any positive findings. A repeat esophagram is carried out in 3 weeks.

PEARLS AND PERILS

1. Management of bleach ingestion varies from standard management of base or acid ingestion.
2. High family stress is the most significant contributing factor.
3. Reporting of suspicious cases of abuse is required by law.
4. Presence or absence of oropharyngeal lesions is not a good predictor of esophageal or gastric injury.
5. Esophagoscopy:
   a. Contraindicated in the presence of severe burn with evidence of laryngeal edema.
   b. Contraindicated if the patient has been on high doses of steroids.
   c. Carried out only to the upper limit of any full-thickness circumferential burn.

 ## TREATMENT RECOMMENDATIONS

Emergency Management

A child who has been observed to have ingested a hazardous substance should drink water or have the mouth thoroughly irrigated by water or milk (a neutral buffer) in large volumes. Fluid intake is limited to no more than 15 ml per kilogram of weight as vomiting may occur with excessive fluid. Gastric lavage and induced vomiting with emetics are contraindicated. Using an acid to neutralize a base (such as administering citrus juices) has been condemned, but recent calculation shows that volume and blood flow will dissipate any heat produced by the exothermic reaction (7).

The child's skin and eyes should be washed with large amounts of cold running water. Garments on which the substance has been spilled are removed immediately. The child is hospitalized for evaluation and management.

Management of Esophageal Injury

If no burns are present in the hypopharynx or esophagus, the patient is discharged and scheduled for an esophagram and reevaluation in 3 weeks. Should there be evidence of stricture at that time, dilation is begun. If first, or second-degree burns are discovered at esophagoscopy, the patient is hospitalized and treated with antibiotics and steroids. Pain and agitation may require analgesics and sedation. Ampicillin, 50 mg per kilogram per day in four doses every 6 hours is administered for 14 days. Antibiotics work by decreasing infection, pyogenic granulation tissue, and scar formation.

Steroids decrease collagen deposition and fibroblasts during healing. Prednisone is given 2 mg per kilogram per day in three doses every 8 hours for days 1 to 6 and then on days 8, 10, and 12. Others use larger doses: methylprednisolone 4 mg per kilogram per day, i.v. for 2 to 4 days; prednisone 5 mg per kilogram per day p.o. tapering to 0.5 mg per kilogram per day for 6 weeks (5). Steroids are thought to be beneficial for moderately severe lye burns but are not indicated for severe lye and acid injury. Gastroesophageal reflux may exacerbate any esophageal injury. Aggressive antireflux therapy is initiated. When third-degree burns are present, the patient is hospitalized, and supportive therapy is initiated. Antibiotics are given. The use of steroids is controversial as it may increase the likelihood of perforation and will mask a perforation should one occur.

Controversy surrounding the use of steroids for treatment of caustic esophageal injury has been exacerbated by a well-written report by Anderson et al. (8). This report of an 18-year clinical study reaffirms the need for endoscopy to document the status of the esophagus following corrosive ingestion. The authors point out that the severity of the initial injury is the most important predictor of stricture formation. Interestingly, they found that 40% (11 of 29) of untreated patients with moderately severe burns developed strictures, whereas only 32% of those treated with steroids developed strictures. Likewise, 24% (7 of 29 patients) in the control group required esophageal replacement, whereas only 13% (4 of 31) treated with steroids required esophageal replacement. However, there were too few cases for these trends to be statistically significant.

The experience of Cardona and Daly (9) suggests that strictures developing in corticosteroid-treated patients may be easier to manage than those that developed in untreated patients. This concept is also supported by the data of Anderson et al. (8) in which esophageal replacement was required by almost twice as many patients in the untreated control group (7 patients) as in the steroid-treated group (4 patients). Again, the trend suggested that steroids indeed are helpful, but the number of patients in this crucial category was too small to be statistically significant.

The equivocal results of the study may also be related to the relatively low dosage of steroids chosen (2 mg per kilogram per day of prednisolone). Hawkins et al. (5) recommended twice the initial dose of Anderson et al. for children. Had Anderson et al. chosen a higher initial dose they might have shown a significant steroid benefit. Unfortunately, the authors conclude (on the basis that their study does not show a steroid benefit) that steroids are not helpful. However, the numbers of patients in the study and the doses of steroids given are inadequate to demonstrate the positive effect of steroids in the treatment of corrosive injuries of the esophagus.

Management of Massive Esophageal Injury

When a massive injury has occurred, as is most common in cases of serious suicide attempt by adults, esophagogastrectomy is considered (10). A nasogastric tube is carefully placed to aspirate the stomach. If stomach contents are alkaline, which does not cease with irrigation, laparotomy may be carried out. Should the stomach be ecchymotic, edematous, or black, esophagogastrectomy is undertaken. If the stomach is intact and the distal esophagus necrotic, only esophagectomy is carried out.

Severe esophageal injuries may be treated with nasogastric intubation for 6 weeks (11). This helps to decrease the likelihood of stricture formation by preventing adherence of the anterior to the posterior esophageal wall while the esophageal mucosa regenerates. Medical grade Silastic tubing can be used in a similar fashion with a feeding tube placed through the lumen. The tubing is anchored superiorly with a Logan bow (12). A Penrose drain fixed distally minimizes reflux.

Severe acid or bleach ingestion can produce similar massive gastric injury, although it is considerably less common than alkaline injury. The protocol for treatment is similar (13). Pyloric stenosis or pernicious anemia may develop as late complications.

PEARLS AND PERILS

1. Esophageal stent placement for 3 to 6 weeks is probably the best treatment for third-degree esophageal injury and severe second-degree injuries.
2. Esophageal lodgement of disc batteries requires immediate endoscopic extraction and treatment of any esophageal injury.

Disc Battery Ingestion

Esophageal lodgment of a disc battery is one of the true urgent foreign body emergencies. Batteries contain NaOH, KOH, and/or mercury. These materials leak around the grommet seal of the battery to produce mucosal damage within 1 hour and involvement of muscular layers within 2 to 4 hours. Perforation may occur within 8 to 12 hours (14). Tracheoesophageal fistula, mediastinitis, death, and esophageal stricture, are all potential complications.

If disc battery ingestion is suspected, an initial radiograph is taken to locate the battery. Continuous pain, especially manifested by crying, is typical with esophageal lodgment. If the battery has passed beyond the esophagus, the patient may be sent home and is observed for fever, pain, and hematochezia. Minor symptoms of vomiting and stool discoloration should not prompt retrieval efforts (15). The parents are instructed to check the stools for the battery. A follow-up radiograph is taken 4 to 7 days after ingestion if the battery has not passed. For a 15-mm (or larger) battery in a child under age 6, a radiograph is obtained 48 hours following observation of the battery in the stomach (15). If the battery remains in the stomach, it is removed endoscopically.

Operative intervention is undertaken at any time if signs or symptoms of bowl perforation develop.

Pill-Induced Esophageal Injury

Esophageal injury occurs when the contents of a pill (capsule or tablet) remain in contact with the esophageal mucosa long enough to produce damage. First reported in 1970, 679 cases due to more than 70 medications in pill form have been reported (16). The incidence is approximately 4 cases per 100,000 population per year (16). Adherent tablets, swallowing the pill without water, or swallowing in the supine position are factors that may cause delay in esophageal transit. Prolonged contact of the pill with the esophageal mucosa then produces the injury.

Several mechanisms may play a role in esophageal injury. Doxycycline, tetracycline, ascorbic acid, and ferrous sulfate produce a pH below 3.0 (in 10 ml of water). Local hyperosmolarity is thought to be the mechanism of injury from potassium chloride tablets. Uptake of the medication by the esophageal mucosa leads to accumulation of toxic concentrations of drugs such as doxycycline, nonsteroidal antiinflammatory agents, and alprenolol. Finally, theophylline and anticholinergic agents may induce gastroesophageal reflux.

Antibiotics and antiviral pills are responsible for 60% of all reported cases, although few injuries seem to occur (10 of 412 cases) (16). Fifty-seven cases of injury have been reported due to antiinflammatory pills, a complication rate of 35%, which represents a more significant problem. Antiinflammatory pills have caused 17 cases of hemorrhage and 4 cases of strictures. Quinidine pills have produced seven cases of esophageal stricture. Six deaths, 4 cases of hemorrhage, and 16 cases of esophageal stricture have been produced by lodgment of potassium chloride pills in the esophagus. The problem is thought to be exacerbated by the relatively mild symptoms associated with KCl tablets: progressive dysphagia with little pain.

Symptoms of pill-induced esophageal injury are typically those of pain, dysphagia, and odynophagia, which cause the patient to seek medical attention. A suspicious history should prompt endoscopic examination of the esophagus to assess the injury and extract the offending pill. Endoscopy is important to differentiate from infection, malignancy, and gastroesophageal reflux disease (16). Typically, discrete, shallow ulcers are observed that may vary from pinpoint to large circumferential ulcers, which may be several centimeters in length. Deep ulceration may lead to mediastinitis, hemorrhage, and death. Esophageal stricture is a long-term complication.

Most injuries heal spontaneously. Prevention is important to avoid repetition of the injury. The typical caustic ingestion protocol is employed based on the severity of the injury. The patient is treated for gastroesophageal reflux to prevent exacerbation of the injury.

🔷 MANAGEMENT OF COMPLICATIONS

Esophageal Stricture

Gentle periodic dilations are carried out using Maloney tapered mercury-filled esophageal bougies. Initially, this may be done on an outpatient basis under general anesthesia. Small, hard strictures may initially require use of Jackson esophageal bougies or hydrostatic dilators under direct vision. When the esophagus has been dilated to a satisfactory caliber, intervals between dilations are increased, and dilations are finally done on a p.r.n. basis without general anesthesia in the office setting. A barium esophagram may be considered from time to time (6 months to 2 years) to follow the progress of the stricture.

The long-term risk of cancer is increased in patients with caustic ingestion who require years of dilations. It should not be assumed that increasing dysphagia is necessarily due to recurrence of the stricture; cancer of the esophagus needs to be ruled out.

More severe strictures and those resistant to dilation require gastrostomy and placement of a string for prograde dilation with Tucker retrograde esophageal dilators. Dilations are most effective when carried out early, before a hard, fibrous, mature cicatricial stenosis has formed. Two or three dilations may be undertaken the first week, one or two the second, and one the third. An attempt is made to double the length of time between subsequent dilations, once an adequate lumen has been attained.

When the esophagus cannot be saved by repeated dilation, esophageal replacement surgery is considered. Use of a segment of isoperistaltic ileum with cecum (17), or transverse or left colon, or a stomach tube are operations commonly considered by pediatric surgeons. Gastric pullup or esophageal replacement with a segment of jejunum are less commonly used in children.

PEARLS AND PERILS

1. A long-term risk of esophageal cancer exists.
2. Bases produce liquefaction necrosis, and esophageal injury may progress during the first few days or weeks following the injury.

✸ REFERENCES

1. Einhorn A, Horton L, Altieri M, et al. Serious respiratory consequences of detergent ingestion in children. *Pediatrics* 1989;84:472–474.
2. Forsen JW, Muntz HR. Hair relaxer ingestion. *Ann Otol Rhinol Laryngol* 1993;102:781–784.
3. Friedman EM. Caustic ingestion and foreign body aspirations: an overlooked form of child abuse. *Ann Otol* 1987;96:709–712.
4. Gaudreault P, Parent M, McGuigan MA, et al. Predictability of esophageal injury from signs and symptoms: a study of caustic ingestion in 378 children. *Pediatrics* 1983;71:767–770.
5. Hawkins DB, Demeter MJ, Barnett TE. Caustic ingestion: controversies in management. A review of 214 cases. *Laryngoscope* 1980;90:98–109.
6. Schild JA. Caustic ingestion in adult patients. *Laryngoscope* 1985;95:1199–1201.
7. Gosselin RE, Smith RP, Hodge HC. *Clinical toxicology of commercial products.* Baltimore: Williams & Wilkins, 1984:245–250.
8. Anderson KD, Rouse TM, Randolph JG. A controlled trial of corticosteroids in children with corrosive injury of the esophagus. *N Engl J Med* 1990;323:637.
9. Cardona JC, Daly JF. Current management of corrosive esophagitis. An evaluation of results in 239 cases. *Ann Otol Rhinol Laryngol* 1971;80:521–527.
10. Ritter FN, Gago O, Kirsh MM, et al. The rationale of emergency esophagogastrectomy in the treatment of liquid caustic burns of the esophagus and stomach. *Ann Otol* 1971;80:513–520.
11. Wijburg FA, Beukers MM, Heymans HS, et al. Treatment of severe esophageal injury. *Ann Otol* 1985;94:337–339.
12. Reyes HM, Hill JL. Modification of the experimental stent technique for esophageal burns. *J Surg Res* 1976;20:65–70.
13. Chong GC, Beahrs OH, Payne WS. Severe acid ingestion. *Mayo Clin Proc* 1979;49:861–868.
14. Maves MD, Carithers JS, Birck HG, et al. Disc battery ingion. *Ann Otol* 1984;93:364–368.
15. Litovitz T, Schmitz B. Ingestion of cylindrical and button batteries: 2382 cases. *Pediatrics* 1992;85:747–772.

16. Pemberton J. Oesophageal obstruction and ulceration caused by oral potassium therapy. *Br Heart J* 1970;32:267–268.
17. Raffensperger JG, Luck SR, Reynolds M, Schwarz D. Intestinal bypass of the esophagus. *J Pediatr Surg* 1996;31:38–41.

L.D. Holinger: Department of Otolaryngology—Head and Neck Surgery, Northwestern University Medical School, and Section of Bronchoesophagology, Children's Memorial Hospital, Chicago, Illinois 60614.

• *Practical Pediatric Otolaryngology*
• edited by Robin T. Cotton
  and Charles M. Myer, III
• Lippincott-Raven Publishers,
  Philadelphia © 1999

37

Feeding Disorders in Children

J. Paul Willging, Claire K. Miller, & Colin D. Rudolph

⬤ HISTORICAL BACKGROUND

The act of feeding a child is a natural and rewarding experience for parents. The infant is comforted by the close contact associated with breast or bottle feeding. The older child interacts with the parent while transitioning to various textures of material. The parent derives a sense of accomplishment by satisfying the child's emotional and nutritional needs from the feeding process. This positive reciprocal interaction reinforces the bonding relationship between the child and the parent. Feeding disorders disrupt this process and cause the parent to develop a sense of inadequacy in the care of the child. In severe cases the child is unable to ingest adequate nutrition for growth and development, further increasing parental frustration (1).

The physical act of swallowing is a complicated process that integrates both structure and function. The process of swallowing is dynamic over time, because of growth and maturational development of the upper aerodigestive tract. The size and position of anatomic structures changes as the child grows, such that the mechanics of swallowing must change to adapt to these alterations. If the child is unable to adapt to changes in structure or neurologic function, the swallow will be ineffective, and problems may arise that could lead to chronic pulmonary disease (from the lack of airway protection during the swallow) or malnutrition.

This chapter discusses the swallowing process as it relates to structure and function in the child. Normal and abnormal swallowing mechanics are outlined, as well as the consequences of these abnormalities. Studies are described to delineate the problems associated with swallowing and to assess the safety of oral feeding. Finally, a brief overview of management approaches to feeding problems is presented.

THE NORMAL FEEDING PROCESS

The Early Swallow

The embryo is seen swallowing as early as 16 weeks of gestation (2). Mouthing patterns persist until about 32 weeks of gestational age, when a disordered pattern of sucking bursts and pauses are observed, being replaced with a stable pattern of rhythmic sucking and swallowing by 36 weeks of gestation. Ingestion of food materials requires coordination of sensory and fine and gross motor skills to move the mouth toward a nipple. The integration of these motor activities and reflexes for feeding represents a complicated challenge to the newborn infant nervous system. Neonates born prior to 36 weeks gestation do not have the neuromuscular development to allow coordination of swallowing with breathing and will require gavage or continuous drip feedings to ensure adequate nutrition.

Neonates beyond 36 weeks of gestation generally have a swallow controlled by bulbar reflexes, with little volitional control of the swallowing process. In term infants, feeding deficits may provide the first indication of an underlying neurologic, pulmonary, or cardiac deficit (3). Infants with tachypnea or borderline respiratory function may have profound difficulties coordinating feeding and breathing. A brief cessation of breathing normally occurs with swallowing, and significant reductions of ventilation may occur, with oxygen desaturations developing during feeding. Cyanosis developing around the time of feeding requires a thorough evaluation (4).

Oral Phase

The anatomy of the oropharynx changes during development, and the motor skills required for developmentally appropriate feeding behavior evolve concurrently (Table 1). The small size and shape of the infant oral cavity is ideal for sucking. The buccal fat pads are large, and they stabilize the lateral and superior walls of the oral cavity. The tongue is relatively large and fills the oral cavity. To suck, the lips close around the breast or nipple, and the tongue seals against the pharynx posteriorly to close the intraoral chamber. The lateral portion of the tongue moves superiorly to contact the palate, creating a central void for accumulation of the bolus. Depression of the tongue and mandible generate a negative pressure of up to 150 mm Hg within the oral cavity.

Liquid accumulation in the oral cavity, between the soft palate and the tongue dorsum, is initiated by compression of the nipple between the tongue and mandible below, and the upper alveolar ridge and palate above. The tongue moves in a peristaltic fashion against the palate to propel the bolus into the pharynx, ending the oral phase of swallowing.

Nipple shape, composition, and hole size determine the rate of milk flow from different nipples. More rapid milk delivery occurs through a nipple with a larger hole. As a consequence of increased flow, the frequency of swallowing will increase, and the time available for respiration will decrease (5). Decreasing nipple hole size increases the work associated with sucking, decreases the frequency of swallowing, and increases available time for respiration. Infants alter their sucking effort to regulate the flow of milk per suck. Inadequate feedback control of flow rates expressed from the nipple can lead to respiratory compromise in infants with neurologic disorders.

As the infant matures, the oral cavity enlarges, the relative size of the tongue decreases, and the buccal fat pads begin to regress. The anatomic relationships no longer exclusively favor sucking by 3 months of age. The child begins to develop tongue movements that allow bolus movement directly from anterior to posterior, with a decrease in tongue extension patterns. By 6 months of age, the infant is able to occlude the lips to remove soft food from a spoon. The bolus is retained in the midline for mastication between the tongue and the palate. Over the next 3 months, mature mastication patterns develop with increased tongue mobility. The tongue lateralizes the bolus for mastication against the alveolar ridges (6).

TABLE 1: Development of Feeding and Oral Motor Skills in Infants

Age (months)	Food type	Oral development
0–4	Breast or bottle feed	Anteroposterior tongue motion
4–6	Pureed foods	Anteroposterior transfer of bolus
6–8	Cup introduced	Emerging chewing patterns
8–12	Ground table foods	Tongue lateralization
12–18	Soft table foods	Munching of food materials
18–24	Meat, fruits, vegetables	Rotary chewing patterns
>24	Table foods	Mature oral motor skills

(Adapted from ref. 24, with permission.)

The oral phase of swallowing requires complex sensory and motor integration. The muscles of the face and mandible function in the oral preparatory phase of swallowing and are innervated by the facial nerve and branches of the mandibular division of the trigeminal nerve. The tongue requires coordinated movement of four intrinsic muscles innervated by the hypoglossal nerve, and four extrinsic muscles innervated by branches from the ansa cervicalis (7). The vagus and glossopharyngeal nerves innervate the muscles of the palate, pharynx, and larynx. Branches from the maxillary division of the trigeminal, facial, glossopharyngeal, and vagus nerves provide sensory inervation. Neural control of the swallowing process is at the level of the brainstem initially, but increasing volitional control is acquired as experience with food materials is accumulated.

Pharyngeal Phase

The pharynx is a common passageway for respiration and alimentation. The pharynx has been divided into the nasopharynx superiorly, hypopharynx inferiorly, and oropharynx between. In the human infant, the larynx is situated high in the neck at the level of cervical vertebrae C-1 to C-3. This enables the epiglottis to pass superior to the free margin of the soft palate, projecting into the nasopharynx. The relatively large size of the arytenoids and epiglottis, as well as their high positions in the oropharynx, functionally separates the respiratory and digestive tracts. Ingested liquids pass over the tongue, divert around the epiglottis into the hypopharynx, and enter the esophageal inlet from the pyriform sinuses (8).

During the first 2 years of life the human larynx remains in this high position in the neck, after which the larynx begins to descend in the neck relative to other cervical structures. By the age of 3 years, the cricoid ring resides adjacent to C-5. The descent of the larynx disengages the epiglottis from the nasopharynx, creating a common area in the oropharynx for the routing of food materials and inspired air (9). This anatomic arrangement is unique to the human and is probably related to the increased vocalization skills achieved by the hominids. As a result of this common chamber accommodating both respiratory and digestive functions, a sophisticated neuromuscular protective mechanism evolved to prevent aspiration (10). Minor anatomic or neuromuscular disorders that are not problematic in an infant have the ability to compromise protective mechanisms when the larynx descends in the neck.

Protection of the respiratory system from contamination is accomplished by a variety of mechanisms. Nonfeeding swallows clear accumulated secretions from the hypopharynx and occur 6 times per minute in the child, decreasing to 6 times per hour in the adult (11). Both mechanoreceptors and chemoreceptors within the larynx and pharyngeal walls mediate reflexive closure of the glottis and cessation of respiration when stimulated. The afferent limb of this reflex is mediated by the superior laryngeal nerve and the pharyngeal plexus of the vagus nerve while the efferent component requires active glottic closure via the recurrent laryngeal branch of the vagus nerve, as well as inhibition respiration. Apnea will be sustained until the noxious stimulus is cleared from the larynx. Hypoxia may result in the neonate due to the lack of respiratory reserve. The cough reflex develops as the infant matures. The cough is expressed after stimulation of the laryngeal receptors, replacing the primary apnea response. Cough may also develop from stimulation of the trachea after an aspiration event. Mucociliary clearance and macrophage activation are also important after aspiration events occur to clear debris from the airway.

Pharyngeal swallows are initiated in an ordered sequential pattern in response to stimulation by food or secretions in the pharynx. Tactile receptors in the pharynx provide sensory stimulation to the medullary swallowing center via the trigeminal, glossopharyngeal, and vagus nerves (12). The medullary swallowing center initiates a swallow by stimulating the nucleus ambiguus and the dorsomedial vagal nucleus. The soft palate closes against the posterior pharyngeal wall to isolate the nasopharynx from the oropharynx as food is propelled posteriorly. The bolus is propelled through the oropharynx by the contraction of the pharyngeal muscles against the tongue located anteriorly. Proprioceptive feedback adjusts the peristaltic activity for different food bolus sizes and consistencies (13). Simultaneous with the initiation of the swallow, respiration is inhibited and the larynx is pulled superiorly and anteriorly. This effectively moves the laryngeal inlet out of the direct path of the bolus. The true and false vocal folds are closed, and the epiglottis retroflexes over the laryngeal inlet with laryngeal elevation to further protect the distal airway. The upper esophageal inlet is pulled open with laryngeal elevation, and the peristaltic contractions of the pharyngeal constrictor muscles propel the bolus into the esophagus (14).

Esophageal Phase

The esophagus is a conduit between the pharynx and the stomach, with muscular sphincters at either end. The upper esophageal sphincter relaxes during swallowing and is actively opened by laryngeal elevation to allow the food bolus to enter the esophagus. Peristaltic contractions propel the bolus down into the stomach. The lower esophageal sphincter relaxes to allow passage of the bolus, after which tonic contraction prevents reflux of gastric contents into the lower esophagus. Propagation of the peristaltic wave is dependent on the intrinsic myenteric plexus and on vagal efferents.

 PATIENT ASSESSMENT

Dysphagia may result from a variety of causes, all of which can be generally grouped into one of three categories: abnormalities of structure, neurologic immaturity or impairment, or abnormal behavior (Tables 2 to 4). It is not uncommon to find a basic defect in one area that has created difficulties in other areas as well (15). A child with an unrecognized laryngeal cleft, for example, will aspirate food materials. If oral feeding continues, oral defensive behaviors may develop because of the noxious stimulation associated with feeding.

Subsequently, the child will fail to develop oral motor skills necessary for proper oral function, which leads to further swallowing dysfunction and increases the risk of aspiration. All of this reinforces the abnormal behaviors associated with feeding, and propagates further feeding problems.

The evaluation of feeding disorders must begin with a complete history and physical examination. The purpose of the history is to identify any potential medical, surgical, developmental, neurologic, or other etiology that could compromise the normal airway protective mechanism or interfere with the swallowing process. The correlation between feeding and symptoms such as gagging, coughing, apnea, or cyanosis should be delineated. The status of the airway before, during, and after feeding should always be explored. Having parents describe a typical feeding session, the types of food materials of-

TABLE 2: Anatomic Causes of Feeding Disorders in Children

Cleft lip/palate
Macroglossia
Ankyloglossia
Pierre Robin sequence
Laryngeal cleft
Tracheoesophageal fistula
Esophageal atresia
Esophageal stricture
Esophageal mass
Vascular ring/sling

(Adapted from ref. 24, with permission.)

TABLE 3: Disorders Affecting Suck-Swallow-Breathe Coordination

Brainstem dysfunction
Choanal atresia
Laryngomalacia
Bronchopulmonary dysplasia
Cardiac disease
Tachypnea

(Adapted from ref. 24, with permission.)

fered to the child, and why they were chosen provides useful information for identification of unconscious modifications in feeding made by the parents in response to the child's reaction to previous feedings. A careful investigation of all medical and surgical interventions sustained by the child, including periods in which no oral nutrition was received, is important. Abnormal oral skills are frequently observed in children who have feeding withheld during critical periods of development, during which a specific feeding stimulus must be experienced to promote subsequent normal development. Beyond this critical period, the particular behavior pattern is difficult to learn (16). Many infants in neonatal intensive care units are prevented from oral feeding due to underlying medical problems. Frequently nonoral stimulation programs cannot be instituted, but unfortunately many of these patients experience recurrent oral stimuli such as oral and nasal suctioning, placement of nasogastric tubes, endotracheal intubations. These negative experiences often result in the child having aversive reactions to anything approaching their face, making feeding difficult. Discriminating between infants who resist feedings because of previous aversive experiences versus those who have current functional problems is a difficult and challenging problem.

The physical examination should be comprehensive. Specific areas of focus should center on the upper aerodigestive tract. Structures related to the oral cavity should be evaluated. The integrity of the lip and palate are important as clefts can have significant impact on swallowing. The relative size and position of the tongue and mandible can influence the swallow and adequacy of the airway during feeding. The status of the craniofacial skeleton may suggest syndromes associated with oral motor difficulties. The absence of a gag reflex may also alert the examiner to other neurologic abnormalities. Examination of the chest should focus on the presence of rales and rhonchi. An abdominal examination should also be performed to rule out associated abnormalities.

All cases of significant feeding dysfunction should have an assessment of laryngeal function. Flexible laryngoscopy allows evaluation of all ages of children, in the office setting without sedation. The procedure can document the mobility of the vocal cords, as

TABLE 4: Disorders Affecting Neuromuscular Coordination of Swallowing

Cerebral palsy
Bulbar atresia
Familial dysautonomia
Tardive dyskinesia
Möbius' syndrome
Myasthenia gravis
Infant botulism
Muscular dystrophies
Oculopharyngeal dystrophy
Polymositis—dermatomyositis
Rheumatoid arthritis
Brainstem tumors
Arnold-Chiari malformation
Myelomeningocele

(Adapted from ref. 24, with permission.)

well as the presence of laryngomalacia or other laryngeal pathology. The general status of the hypopharynx with respect to the amount of retained secretions, tongue position, and sensation can also be ascertained.

Due to the complexity of the behavioral and physiologic components of feeding disorders, the evaluation of an infant or child with a feeding disorder is most readily achieved by a multidisciplinary team approach. Observation of a feeding session by experienced occupational therapists, speech pathologists, psychologists, and nurses provides insight into the underlying feeding problem (17). Positive interactions between the child and parent are noted. The child's responses to offered food materials, including disruptive behaviors, are also noted. These observations highlight primary or secondary behavior problems, which allow future structuring of appropriate behavior treatment interventions.

Attention to the position and posture of the child, as well as the mechanics of feeding skills during the ingestion of various textures, also provides clues regarding any underlying anatomic or physiologic problems. Observations of the ability to handle oral secretions, the pace of feeding, escape of food from the mouth, tongue and jaw movements, number of swallows to clear a bolus, noisy airway sounds after swallowing, coordination of suck and swallow, laryngeal elevation, gagging, coughing, or emesis associated with feedings can indicate a possible underlying neurologic or structural problem. Attention to articulation and voice quality may also provide useful information, as the same structures used for the oropharyngeal phases of feeding are used for speech production. Despite careful observation, however, it is often difficult to ascertain the cause of a feeding disorder or the safety of swallowing using only clinical observations.

Diagnostic Studies

Barium Swallow

Radiographic studies have two separate goals during the evaluation of children with feeding disorders. First, structural abnormalities such as fistulae, vascular rings, strictures, or masses need to be excluded. Second, images of the coordination of movement of a bolus through the oropharynx and esophagus can be studied. The barium esophagram allows anatomic visualization of the esophagus using barium suspensions. Frequently, children with feeding disorders will not ingest an adequate amount of barium for adequate visualization of structures, so a nasogastric feeding tube is passed into the pharynx and barium is instilled to complete the study. Due to the unpleasant nature of this experience, further cooperation of the child is unlikely, and a different session for the evaluation of the functional aspects of swallowing is often required.

Videofluoroscopic Swallowing Study

Functional studies of swallowing are usually best performed by a speech pathologist or occupational therapist in cooperation with a radiologist. Videofluoroscopic swallowing studies are performed on patients with feeding disorders after a careful history is obtained so that the study can be initiated with the child in the best eating position and offered food materials that are most likely to be accepted. Maximizing the likelihood of successful swallows at the beginning of the study ensures that some observations are obtained prior to the patient experiencing discomfort and refusing further efforts at evaluation. Subsequently, other textures are examined and the therapeutic efficacy of modifications in bolus volume, nipple or utensil types, and body posture may all be explored. Videofluoroscopy allows the relatively noninvasive assessment of the oral phase of swallowing as well as determination of consistencies and conditions for safe swallowing. Importantly, there is a large accumulated experience in the interpretation of videofluoroscopic swallow studies, making this test the gold standard method for evaluation of children with swallowing disorders (18). Unfortunately, the exposure to radiation limits the use of fluoroscopy for teaching therapeutic maneuvers and is always a concern when considering repeated examinations over time. In addition, patients must be transported to a facility with expensive fluoroscopy equipment available to perform these studies.

Ultrasound

Ultrasound provides an attractive alternative for the evaluation of the oral phase of swallowing. It allows observation of the coordination of laryngeal elevation during swallows. Unfortunately, ultrasound lacks sensitivity in visualizing pharyngeal motion and for determining whether aspiration has occurred. Therefore it does not provide a reliable method for determining swallowing safety. Ultrasound is useful, however, for studying tongue movements associated with feeding. Bolus creation and manipulation can be documented by ultrasound (19). It may become a useful tool for biofeedback training in compensatory maneuvers because it allows visual feedback regarding tongue and laryngeal movements with no discomfort or risk to the patient. At the present time, ultrasound technology remains a research tool with respect to feeding problems.

Nuclear Medicine Scan

The risk of aspiration occurs not only with feeding, but from the accumulation of oral secretions in the hypopharynx. The radionucleotide thallium injected intravenously will be excreted into the serous secretions of the parotid gland. These radiolabeled secretions can be imaged with a gamma camera. In normal conditions, the image will show all the label in the parotid glands and the stomach. Low levels of the label will be found in the oral cavity, pharynx, and esophagus. In abnormal studies with aspiration, the label will be found distributed throughout the lung fields. This study provides an indication of the volume of oral secretions aspirated over time and can be used to determine the need for surgical intervention to prevent chronic, life-threatening pulmonary disease. Unfortunately, normal data are unavailable in pediatric patients.

Fiberoptic Endoscopic Evaluation of Swallowing

Fiberoptic endoscopic evaluation of swallowing (FEES) is a recently described approach to the evaluation of swallowing performed by passing a flexible laryngoscope into the nasopharynx after anesthetizing the nasal passages (20). In experienced hands this test can be performed in children of all ages. Initially, pharyngeal anatomy and movement of pharyngeal and laryngeal structures can be evaluated during speech. The management of secretions is examined by placing a small amount of green food coloring on the tongue. Accumulation of secretions in the valleculae or pyriform sinus, or aspiration of secretions, may be directly observed. Finally, swallows of varying volumes and textures are administered by mouth, and the coordination of swallowing and efficiency of pharyngeal clearance are assessed. FEES does not provide information regarding the oral phase of swallowing but compares favorably with videofluoroscopy for evaluation of the pharyngeal phase of swallowing. Our preliminary experience with FEES in children indicates similar utility. FEES is particularly valuable for evaluation of swallowing safety in children who refuse to ingest adequate amounts of barium to perform videofluoroscopy. In such cases, studying the anatomy and evaluating the patient's ability to handle the oral secretions provides useful information. In addition, FEES is a useful teaching tool to demonstrate graphically to parents the risk of aspiration when particular food materials are administered to their child.

Endoscopy

Feeding disorders may arise from structural or inflammatory abnormalities of the upper aerodigestive tract. When questions arise with respect to the integrity of the larynx, trachea, esophagus, or stomach, direct visualization of these structures must be obtained. When a child has a history of a single structural abnormality, possible concurrent abnormalities must be considered. When structural deficits are present, such as a persistent tracheoesophageal fistula, laryngeal cleft, vascular ring, etc., the feeding issues will never resolve until the primary problem is addressed. Similarly, children with esophagitis experience pain with feeding and may refuse to eat (21). It is not uncommon for children with structural or inflammatory abnormalities of the airway or esophagus to be misdiagnosed and placed into intensive behavioral modification programs. The index of suspicion must be low when considering whether a child requires endoscopy to rule out structural problems. The risk of general anesthesia is minimal when the procedures are performed at experienced centers with pediatric anesthesiologists, compared with the risks associated with continued aspiration.

Manometry

Manometry is useful for evaluating esophageal peristalsis and more recently has been utilized for evaluating pharyngeal and upper esophageal sphincter function (22). Esophageal manometry is useful for identifying disorders of esophageal motility, such as achalasia. The function of the normal upper esophageal sphincter has been well studied in children. Only isolated cases of primary cricopharyngeal achalasia and abnormalities in the coordination of the upper esophageal sphincter in children with Arnold-Chiari malformations have been reported. The routine role of manometry in the evaluation of pharyngeal swallowing in children requires further investigation.

 TREATMENT RECOMMENDATIONS

The careful evaluation of children with feeding disorders should allow recognition of treatable anatomic or inflammatory lesions. A child may refuse to eat even after an underlying anatomic abnormality has been corrected because of a learned aversion to feeding. Behavior therapy can often overcome this type of "conditioned" food refusal. Unfortunately, many children with feeding disorders have noncorrectable neurologic or anatomic abnormalities that make oral feeding difficult or impossible.

Decisions regarding whether to allow oral feeding depend on balancing the potential risks of aspiration and chronic lung disease with the emotional rewards and convenience of oral feeding. The amount of aspiration that is "safe" depends on the patient's ability to clear the airway with cough and ciliary flow. Society and health professionals often impose a value system on families and patients that stresses the importance of providing nutrition by oral feedings. Some patients cannot obtain adequate nutrition by mouth due to a risk of aspiration. In others, the time required to provide a child with adequate nutrition by mouth consumes the parent's and child's lives, leaving little time for other nurturing activities. Thus, supplying a portion of the patient's nutrition by nasogastric or gastrostomy feedings may be beneficial. Families may need counseling to help them realize that for their child, alternate approaches to providing nutritional support (i.e., gastrostomy feedings) may be better for the child's overall well-being than persisting in efforts to provide nutrition only by mouth. The timing for aggressive behavioral intervention or for the initiation of attempts at oral feeding needs to be decided in the context of the child's overall development and well-being. Because anatomic relationships of the larynx change during development, and disease progression may alter swallowing, episodic reevaluation of the safety or approach to feeding is essential.

Behavior Therapy

Normal preschool children can be induced to change their dietary selections by using a combination of social praise and a program that makes the consumption of preferred foods contingent on eating nonpreferred foods. This type of contingency management has been combined with other therapeutic approaches to treat more serious feeding disorders including food refusal in children with failure to thrive, cerebral palsy, cystic fibrosis, metabolic disorders, and after long-term gastrostomy feedings or other chronic disorders that prevented oral feeding. Treatment strategies utilized include *shaping* by rewarding successive approximations of targeted behaviors, *positive reinforcement* by rewarding a child with praise, access to favored toys, music, clapping, stickers and/or socialization as age appropriate, if they complete a desired behavior, and *ignoring* or inattention when the child engages in inappropriate behaviors. The slow hierarchical advancement of rewarded goals eventually leads to full oral feeding. Successful implementation often requires a structured inpatient management program.

In addition to the immediate goal of achieving oral feeds, it is important to recognize that children with real or perceived feeding disorders are at increased risk of long-term psychosocial problems. Therefore, in cases of nonorganic failure to thrive, a multidisciplinary intervention that includes provisions to ensure access to food, parental training in compensatory approaches to feeding, and efforts to improve family support systems provides the most promise for successful intervention. In children with underlying physiologic disorders, many parents suffer tremendous emotional distress, which also needs to be acknowledged and addressed. Molifying parental feelings of inadequacy and guilt resulting from their previous unsuccessful efforts at feeding is likely to provide therapeutic benefit. Family support services, respite care, and financial assistance programs need to be integrated with the child's chronic care medical needs.

Directed Swallowing Therapy

Combining the clinical history, examination, and videofluoroscopic swallowing study or fiberoptic examination of swallowing allows the therapist to determine the best bolus volume and texture, pace of administration and nipples or utensils for oral feeding. Changes in body and head position may also protect the airway or allow more efficient passage of a food bolus through the oropharynx. For example, tilting the head forward widens the vallecular space, thereby diverting food away from the laryngeal inlet (23).

Even if full oral feeding cannot be achieved, providing some feedings of sterile water may be possible and desirable. This feeding experience will facilitate the possible later introduction of oral feeds and is usually rewarding for the parents. Also, continuing oral stimulation will prevent the development of aversion to oral touch, allowing good dental care. It is essential to remember that the nutritional requirements of every patient must be met by either an oral or alternate route. Similarly, the development of social skills and interactions achieved during mealtimes must be incorporated into the patient's life, despite the lack of oral intake.

Prosthodontics

Prosthodontic approaches to swallowing disorders may be effective in specific cases, particularly when there are major anatomic abnormalities. Use of a palatal prosthesis that increases pharyngeal mechanical stimulation during swallowing has been reported to be effective for treatment of infants with a delayed initiation of the pharyngeal phase of swallowing (23).

✸ REFERENCES

1. Budd KS, McGraw TE, Farbisz R, et al. Psychosocial concomitants of children's feeding disorders. *J Pediatr Psychol* 1992;17:81–94.
2. Pritchard JA. Fetal swallowing and amniotic fluid volume. *Obstet Gynecol* 1966;28:606–610.
3. Hack M, Estabrook MM, Robertson SS. Development of sucking rhythm in preterm infants. *Early Hum Dev* 1985;11:133–140.
4. Selley WG, Ellis RE, Flack FC, Brooks WA. Coordination of sucking, swallowing and breathing in the newborn: its relationship to infant feeding and normal development. *Br J Disord Communi* 1990;25:311–327.
5. Mathew OP. Science of bottle feeding. *J Pediatr* 1991;119:511–519.
6. Stolovitz P, Gisel EG. Circumoral movements in response to three different food textures in children 6 months to 2 years of age. *Dysphagia* 1991;6:17–25.

7. Dodds WJ, Stewart ET, Logemann JA. Physiology and radiology of the normal oral and pharyngeal phases of swallowing [see comments]. *AJR* 1990;154:953–963.

8. Kramer SS. Radiologic examination of the swallowing impaired child. *Dysphagia* 1989;3:117–125.

9. Tuchman DN. Dysfunctional swallowing in the pediatric patient: clinical considerations. *Dysphagia* 1988;2:203–208.

10. Laitman JT, Reidenberg JS. Specializations of the human upper respiratory and upper digestive systems as seen through comparative and developmental anatomy. *Dysphagia* 1993;8:318–325.

11. Thach BT, Menon A. Pulmonary protective mechanisms in human infants. *Am Rev Respir Dis* 1985;131:S55–S58.

12. Kahrilas PJ. Pharyngeal structure and function. *Dysphagia* 1993;8:303–307.

13. Miller AJ. The search for the central swallowing pathway: the quest for clarity. *Dysphagia* 1993;8:185–194.

14. Kidder TM. Esophago/pharyngo/laryngeal interrelationships: airway protection mechanisms. *Dysphagia* 1995;10:228–231.

15. Kramer SS, Eicher PM. The evaluation of pediatric feeding abnormalities. *Dysphagia* 1993;8:215–224.

16. Illingworth RS, Lister JL. The critical or sensitive period, with special reference to certain feeding problems in infants and children. *J Pediatr* 1964;65:839–848.

17. Loughlin GM, Lefton-Greif MA. Dysfunctional swallowing and respiratory disease in children. *Adv Pediatr* 1994;41:135–162.

18. Newman LA, Cleveland RH, Blickman JG, Hillman RE, Jaramillo D. Videofluoroscopic analysis of the infant swallow. *Invest Radiol* 1991;26:870–873.

19. Bosma JF, Hepburn LG, Josell SD, Baker K. Ultrasound demonstration of tongue motions during suckle feeding. *Dev Med Child Neurol* 1990;32:223–229.

20. Langmore SE, Schatz K, Olson N. Endoscopic and videofluoroscopic evaluations of swallowing and aspiration. *Ann Otol Rhinolo & Laryngol* 1991;100:678–681.

21. Dellert SF, Hyams JS, Treem WR, Geertsma MA. Feeding resistance and gastroesophageal reflux in infancy. *J Pediatr Gastroenterol Nutr* 1993;17:66–71.

22. Castell JA, Castell DO. Modern solid state computerized manometry of the pharyngoesophageal segment. *Dysphagia* 1993;8:270–275.

23. Selley WG, Boxall J. A new way to treat sucking and swallowing difficulties in babies. *Lancet* 1986;1:1182–1184.

24. *Rudolph CD. Feeding disorders in infants and children. J Pediatr 1994;125:S116–S124.*

J.P. Willging: Department of Otolaryngology and Maxillofacial Surgery, University of Cincinnati, Children's Hospital Medical Center, Cincinnati, Ohio 45229-4356.   •   C.K. Miller: Department of Speech Pathology, University of Cincinnati, Children's Hospital Medical Center, Cincinnati, Ohio 45229-4356.   •   C.D. Rudolph: Department of Pediatrics, University of Cincinnati, Children's Hospital Medical Center, Cincinnati, Ohio 45229-4356.

• *Practical Pediatric Otolaryngology*
• edited by Robin T. Cotton
  and Charles M. Myer, III
• Lippincott-Raven Publishers,
  Philadelphia © 1999

38

Vocal Cord Paralysis

Robert G. Berkowitz

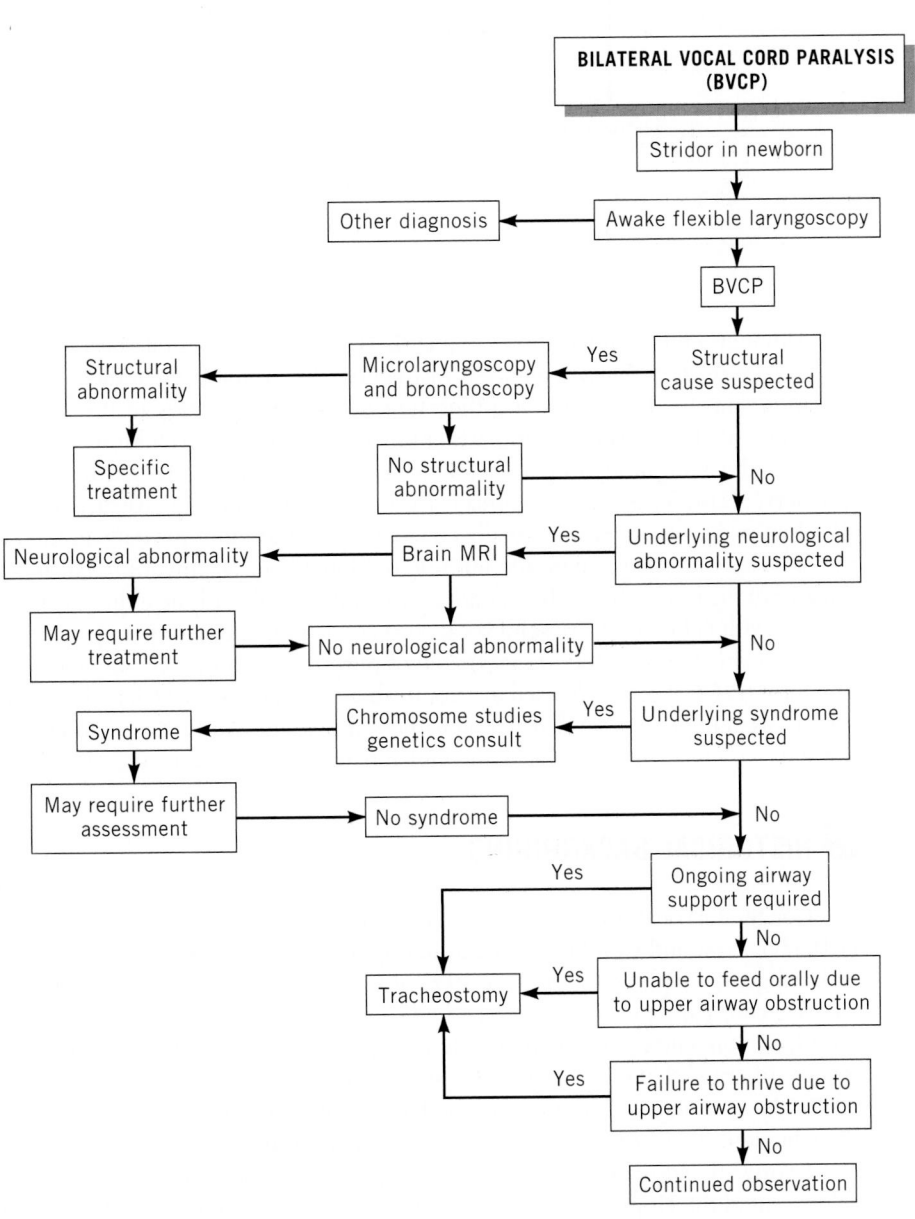

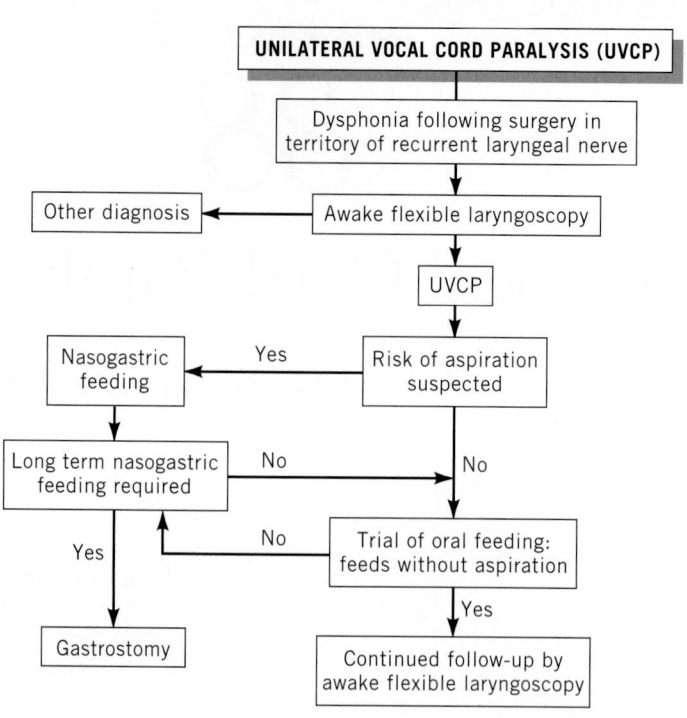

Although unilateral vocal cord paralysis (UVCP) and bilateral vocal cord paralysis (BVCP) are related, they are clinically distinct conditions differing in their etiology, presentation, and treatment, and are therefore discussed separately in this chapter. The management of these two conditions is outlined above. UVCP in children is generally acquired and is seen most commonly following surgical injury to the left recurrent laryngeal nerve. It presents with dysphonia in the absence of significant obstructive symptoms. BVCP in pediatric practice is usually congenital and therefore presents in the newborn period. The condition is typically not one of global paralysis involving all the intrinsic muscles of the larynx, but rather a state in which the vocal cords lie either in an adducted position with failure of purposeful vocal cord abduction (abductor paralysis) or the vocal cords remain abducted and are incapable of purposeful adduction (adductor paralysis). The term BVCP is generally used to refer to abductor paralysis, which is characterized by symptoms of upper airway obstruction without dysphonia. Adductor paralysis is rare and presents with features of laryngeal incompetence (1). It will not be discussed further.

⬮ HISTORICAL BACKGROUND

Congenital vocal cord paralysis was described in association with meningomyelocele in 1932 by New and Childrey (2), and then by Bloch and Lemoine (3) in 1936 in a child with congenital syphilis. Clerf (4) in 1953 reported a series of 19 patients with congenital vocal cord paralysis of whom 13 had other major abnormalities, and in 1964 Platt (5) described congenital vocal cord paralysis occurring on a familial basis. Holinger and Brown (6) noted that congenital BVCP was rarely seen in an otherwise normal infant in 1967. The first major series of pediatric BVCP was reported in 1976 by Holinger et al. (7), who described 149 cases and classified them according to etiology.

Improved endoscopic evaluation and diagnosis have been made possible by the development of the Hopkins rod telescope and the flexible laryngoscope. In particular, the introduction by Silberman et al. (8) in 1976 of a flexible laryngoscope suitable for examination of the upper airway in the awake child has led to increased recognition of disturbances of vocal cord function and other functional abnormalities as being responsible for upper airway symptoms in children.

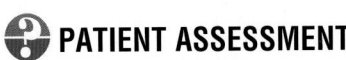 **PATIENT ASSESSMENT**

Bilateral Vocal Cord Paralysis

The key steps in assessment of BVCP are as follows:

1. Make diagnosis of BVCP.
2. Rule out structural cause for limitation of vocal cord abduction.
3. Determine cause of BVCP to predict prognosis both for the child and for recovery of vocal cord abduction.
4. Assess severity and therefore the need for intervention.

Step 1: Make Diagnosis

Clinical Presentation   BVCP is usually congenital and presents with inspiratory stridor, which is often high pitched or "squawking" in nature, associated with respiratory distress (Table 1). Phonation and laryngeal competence are usually normal. Symptoms are present from birth. Endotracheal intubation may be necessary immediately following birth in severe cases.

Occasionally BVCP is acquired and occurs later in the newborn period or at other times during childhood. The degree of paralysis may be complete or incomplete, and therefore the severity of symptoms and extent of impairment of vocal cord abduction observed by awake flexible laryngoscopy may vary.

Awake Flexible Laryngoscopy   The diagnosis of BVCP is suspected clinically and confirmed by flexible laryngoscopy in the awake patient. Awake flexible laryngoscopy in neonates provides the simplest and best assessment of active vocal cord mobility and also rules out structural and other functional causes of upper airway obstruction.

Assessment of vocal cord mobility by awake flexible laryngoscopy may be difficult, however, particularly in cases of partial paralysis or when the neonate cries persistently during the examination. Trans-oral examination may be less distressing than the conventional trans-nasal route and should be performed if excessive crying prevents assessment of vocal cord abduction. Repeat examination or review of the video recording by a colleague may be necessary. Awake flexible laryngoscopy in neonates must always be performed with appropriate monitoring and adequate resuscitation equipment and personnel available.

Step 2: Rule Out Structural Abnormality

Microlaryngoscopy and Bronchoscopy   Bilateral vocal cord immobility may be a consequence of a structural rather than a neurologic abnormality and may be due to

1. Interarytenoid or posterior glottic stenosis, which can develop in neonates following only a relatively brief period of endotracheal intubation.
2. Congenital interarytenoid web, which is rare (9).
3. A nasogastric tube, which may cause inflammation of the posterior cricoarytenoid muscles and lead to temporary paralysis (10).

TABLE 1: Causes of Congenital Bilateral Vocal Cord Paralysis

Structural central nervous system abnormality
Arnold-Chiari malformation
Others, e.g., hydrocephalus unrelated to Arnold-Chiari malformation, hypoplasia of cranial nerve motoneurons, cerebral agenesis
Generalized neuromuscular disorder, e.g., spinal muscular atrophy, congenital myesthenia syndrome, congenital myopathy
Birth hypoxia or head or neck trauma
Idiopathic causes

Microlaryngoscopy and bronchoscopy should be performed when

1. A structural cause for vocal cord immobility is suspected, e.g., history of previous endotracheal intubation or abnormality in the interarytenoid or posterior glottic region observed at awake flexible laryngoscopy.
2. An associated airway abnormality is suspected because the degree of limitation of vocal cord abduction observed is not thought sufficient to explain the child's airway symptoms fully.
3. The diagnosis of BVCP is uncertain; however, the limitations of assessing active vocal cord movement under general anesthetic should be recognized.

Evaluation of the airway under general anesthetic in BVCP is not routinely required.

When performing microlaryngoscopy, in addition to careful examination of the posterior commissure, passive mobility of the arytenoids should be assessed by exerting gentle pressure with a laryngeal sucker.

Laryngeal electromyography cannot be used to differentiate definitively between a structural and neurologic cause of BVCP in neonates because a normal laryngeal electromyogram is also found in idiopathic congenital BVCP (1).

Step 3: Determine Neurologic Cause

Identification of the cause of BVCP is necessary to determine the prognosis for recovery of vocal cord function and also to predict the level of global development and general outcome of the infant. Causes of congenital BVCP are listed in Table 1. Some of these conditions, particularly Arnold-Chiari malformation, may also present later in the neonatal period or in infancy. Acquired BVCP in children has been described following treatment with vincristine (11), with Reye's syndrome (12), and in association with intracranial tumors (13) and raised intracranial pressure (14).

Arnold-Chiari malformation is present in approximately 90% of all infants with meningomyelocele. The hindbrain malformation associated with meningomyelocele has caudal displacement of both the cerebellum and brainstem into the cervical canal and is referred to as the Chiari II anomaly. (The Chiari I anomaly, which is not associated with myelomeningocele, involves caudal displacement of the cerebellum alone.) Although 80% to 90% of infants with Chiari II anomaly will develop hydrocephalus within the first few months of life, only a small minority will have symptoms of brainstem dysfunction, which may include BVCP, central apnea, and dysphagia. Insertion of a ventricular shunt or a posterior fossa decompression may improve these symptoms, but the outcome depends on the degree of preexisting brainstem damage (15).

Children with neuromuscular disorders, which include conditions affecting the anterior horn cells, neuromuscular junction, and muscle, can present with BVCP in addition to weakness and hypotonia. Symptoms of BVCP may not always be present at birth, and, in particular, BVCP in association with spinal muscular atrophy may be progressive.

Birth trauma causing head compression or excessive neck torsion may cause BVCP and should be considered where there is a history of difficult delivery, e.g., rapid labor, large baby, or breech delivery. The degree of BVCP is usually partial and therefore, given the absence of associated severe respiratory distress, the stridor is often attributed to laryngomalacia. Symptoms usually resolve within weeks. Birth hypoxia causing BVCP is associated with global developmental delay.

Idiopathic congenital BVCP is a diagnosis of exclusion and represents a heterogenous group of conditions. The level of resolution available with current magnetic resonance imaging (MRI) scanning techniques is inadequate to identify a specific structural abnormality. Approximately half the cases of idiopathic congenital BVCP occur in otherwise normal neonates; the other half are associated with other significant abnormalities. A variety of chromosomal abnormalities have been described in the latter group. The prognosis is difficult to predict, but recovery may occur in the first year of life, may take a number of years, or may never occur (1). Apart from careful clinical evaluation, the investigations that need to be considered are neuroimaging and chromosome studies.

Neuroimaging and Neurology Consult   As a screening test, cranial ultrasound should be adequate to demonstrate any significant structural central nervous system abnormality. If an underlying neurologic abnormality is suspected, an MRI should be obtained. Specific investigations for a neuromuscular disorder should be performed if hypotonia and muscle weakness are detected.

Chromosome Analysis and Genetics Consult   Chromosome studies and a genetics consult are necessary when BVCP is associated with other significant abnormalities. Although the presence of a chromosomal abnormality does not necessarily preclude spontaneous improvement of BVCP, it may have important prognostic implications for the level of development of the child. A genetics consult is also required if the BVCP is familial, although this is relatively uncommon.

Step 4: Assessment of Severity

The severity of BVCP is determined by

1. Degree of respiratory distress and effort. Loudness of the stridor can be misleading, as soft stridor may be due to poor airflow.
2. Adequacy of ventilation. Continuous monitoring for evidence of oxygen desaturation or bradycardia is necessary. Arterial gases may also be useful to document carbon dioxide retention despite maintenance of normal oxygenation.
3. Ability to feed orally and maintain satisfactory weight gain.

The degree of abductor paralysis documented by awake flexible laryngoscopy alone does not determine the clinical severity of BVCP. Other important factors include the presence of associated airway abnormalities, cardiorespiratory status, and degree of neurodevelopmental impairment of the child.

PEARLS AND PERILS

---

1. Although laryngomalacia is the commonest cause of inspiratory stridor in infants, inspiratory stridor in neonates, especially in association with respiratory distress, is often due to BVCP.
2. Awake flexible laryngoscopy may be the only endoscopic evaluation necessary for the diagnosis of BVCP. Microlaryngoscopy and bronchoscopy only need to be performed when either a structural cause of bilateral vocal cord immobility is suspected or there is a possibility of an additional airway abnormality being present below the level of the vocal cords.
3. A cause is unlikely to be found for BVCP occurring as an isolated abnormality. Extensive investigation in this situation is therefore unnecessary.
4. When BVCP develops after birth in a previously well child, look for evidence of an intracranial tumour or other cause of raised intracranial pressure.

Unilateral Vocal Cord Paralysis

The key steps in assessment of UVCP are as follows:

1. Make diagnosis
2. Rule out arytenoid subluxation
3. Assess severity, particularly with regard to aspiration
4. Consider obtaining prognostic information if thought to be of clinical benefit

Step 1: Make Diagnosis

Clinical Presentation   UVCP is typically acquired following surgery and presents with a weak, breathy cry or voice and poor cough, which develops immediately following surgery. There may also be clinical evidence of aspiration, but stridor is uncommon. The severity and nature of symptoms of UVCP depend on the degree of nerve injury and whether or not there is associated loss of supraglottic sensation due to vagal rather than recurrent laryngeal nerve injury.

In young children, UVCP is usually a consequence of trauma to the left recurrent laryngeal nerve and is classically seen following ligation of a patent ductus arteriosus, other aortic arch procedure, or tracheoesophageal fistula repair. The right recurrent laryngeal nerve can be injured following certain cardiac surgical procedures, particularly right Blalock-Taussig (subclavion to pulmonary artery) shunt, cannulation of the right subclavian vein, and either side can be damaged following thyroid surgery. Injury to the vagus can occur as a result of a skull base surgical approach, cannulation of the great vessels for extracorporeal membrane oxygenation, or following neck trauma. These causes are summarized in Table 2.

UVCP may also be acquired as a result of a variety of conditions responsible for isolated or multiple cranial nerve dysfunction. These include tumors, syringobulbia, granulomatous disease, vasculitis, viral infection, postviral demyelination, or drug toxicity, or it may be idiopathic. UVCP may be present at birth, particularly as a result of birth trauma.

Awake Flexible Laryngoscopy   The paralyzed vocal cord is best visualised at flexible laryngoscopy by passing the laryngoscope through the contralateral nasal airway. Detection of UVCP may be difficult due to the vertical movement of the arytenoids on swallowing or passive movement of the paralyzed vocal cord with changes in air pressure on respiration.

Dysphonia may be due to a "frozen" larynx or poorly mobile vocal cords, which occurs as a temporary consequence of endotracheal intubation, particularly if there has been a long period of intubation. This needs to be differentiated from a postsurgical UVCP.

Step 2: Rule Out Arytenoid Subluxation

Microlaryngoscopy   Arytenoid subluxation or dislocation may occur following traumatic endotracheal intubation or external trauma (16). This diagnosis should be suspected and microlaryngoscopy performed if the symptoms of UVCP develop following endotracheal intubation for a surgical procedure in which the recurrent laryngeal nerve or vagus nerve are not at risk. Laryngeal electromyography and computed tomography scanning also aid in making the diagnosis. Although this diagnosis uncommon, it is important to consider it so that closed reduction of the subluxation can be attempted early while there is still some likelihood of success.

Step 3: Assess Severity

Aspiration   The major criterion for severity of UVCP is the risk of aspiration of oral diet, gastroesophageal reflux material, and rarely saliva. This is particularly a problem following vagal injuries because of the additional sensory loss, and in infants and young children. UVCP is often acquired at a very young age because of its relationship to surgical correction of congenital heart disease and tracheoesophegeal fistula. Young children

TABLE 2: Traumatic Causes of Unilateral Vocal Cord Paralysis

Left recurrent laryngeal nerve
   Ligation of patent ductus arteriosus
   Other aortic arch procedure
   Tracheoesophageal fistula repair
Right recurrent laryngeal nerve
   Insertion of right subclavian venous access line
   Right Blalock-Taussig shunt
Recurrent laryngeal nerve/either side
   Thyroid surgery
Vagus nerve
   Skull base procedure
   Cannulation of the great neck vessels for extracorporeal membrane oxygenation
   Penetrating or blunt neck trauma

with UVCP are particularly prone to aspiration because they have an obligatory liquid diet, an immature swallowing mechanism, and a propensity to gastroesophogeal reflux. In addition, many of these young children have significant cardiorespiratory problems related to their underlying condition that led to their initial surgery; as a consequence, they tolerate aspiration poorly.

Assessment of the risk of aspiration therefore involves an estimation of

1. The degree of glottic closure seen at awake flexible laryngoscopy
2. Factors that may predispose to aspiration, particularly the presence of impaired neurodevelopmental function and gastroesophageal reflux
3. Evaluation of the cardiorespiratory and general health status, which reflects the child's ability to tolerate episodes of aspiration

If it is deemed safe to proceed with oral feeding, this should be initiated slowly and under strict nursing supervision. In addition to coughing or choking with feeding, aspiration must be suspected if there are periods of apnea or bradycardia related to feeding, otherwise unexplained poor lung function or oxygen requirement, or recurrent respiratory infections. Proven gastroesophageal reflux in the presence of any respiratory symptoms is also highly suggestive of aspiration.

Radiologic and nuclear medicine investigations provide information over a limited window of time only and therefore cannot be relied upon to demonstrate laryngeal competence. Ultimately, the diagnosis of aspiration is a clinical one.

Dysphonia　This is best assessed clinically by the impact on the child's ability to communicate. In the young child, a cry that is too soft for the parents to hear poses particular difficulties and some risk. Speech pathology assessment and (in older children) the use of videostroboscopy are of value.

Step 4: Prognosis

Laryngeal Electromyography　The use of laryngeal electromyography to determine whether a neurologic injury is likely to be temporary or permanent is only indicated when surgical intervention is being considered for either aspiration in a young child or dysphonia in an older child. Laryngeal electromyography in a child requires a general anesthetic. The larynx is suspended, and a concentric needle electrode is inserted endoscopically into the thyroarytenoid and posterior cricoarytenoid muscles. Recordings are made while the anesthetic is lightened (1). Great care must be taken in the young child to avoid significant laryngeal trauma by needle insertion as this may lead to laryngeal edema and obstruction.

PEARLS AND PERILS

1. UVCP is usually not associated with stridor. When significant inspiratory stridor or respiratory distress is present, an associated airway abnormality must be sought. The diagnosis may be revised to one of BVCP if there is some degree of paralysis involving the contralateral vocal cord that was not initially detected.
2. UVCP in children is usually acquired following surgery for congenital cardiac disease or tracheoesophageal fistula.
3. A cause for UVCP must always be sought if there is no preceding history of recurrent laryngeal or vagus nerve injury.
4. Make the diagnosis of aspiration clinically. Do not rely on imaging for confirmation.

TREATMENT RECOMMENDATIONS

Bilateral Vocal Cord Paralysis

The neonate with a marginal airway due to BVCP has three hurdles to overcome sequentially to avoid the need for tracheostomy:

1. Maintain adequate respiration and ventilation at rest.
2. Maintain adequate respiration and ventilation while managing oral feeding.
3. Maintain normal weight gain despite the presence of upper airway obstructive symptoms.

Management of BVCP involves providing temporary airway and nutritional support but proceeding with tracheostomy if the airway is inadequate. Occasionally BVCP can be corrected by treatment of the underlying condition, e.g., Arnold-Chiari malformation, interarytenoid/posterior glottic fixation, myesthenia syndrome.

If tracheostomy is required, subsequent enlargement of the glottic lumen can be considered if prognosis for recovery of vocal cord function is considered poor.

Temporary Airway Support

Airway Support   This includes oxygen, nasopharyngeal continuous positive airway pressure to decrease the work of breathing, and short-term endotracheal intubation. Intubation may be associated with a brief period of improvement in symptoms following extubation due to the temporary effect of lateralizing the vocal cords.

Correction of Contributing Factors   Factors such as associated upper airway abnormalities, lower respiratory tract disease, cardiac disease, and gastroesophageal reflux may be contributing to the severity of obstructive symptoms. Reversible factors should be corrected.

Nutritional Support

Nasogastric Tube Feeding   Supplemental gavage feeding or continuous nasogastric tube feeding may be necessary when the neonatal airway is inadequate to cope with the additional demands of feeding. This may need to be continued well beyond the time that airway support is no longer required.

Nutritional Supplements   The adverse effects on growth resulting from increased work of breathing can in part be overcome by close attention to feeding and nutritional requirements.

Charting Weight   The best indicator of an adequate airway despite the persistence of upper airway obstructive symptoms is satisfactory weight gain. Weight should be plotted regularly on a weight percentile chart. A drop in weight across percentiles without a corresponding drop in length despite an adequate calorie intake is indicative of an inadequate airway and suggests that tracheostomy is necessary. Conversely, a child who is thriving is unlikely to have significant upper airway obstruction.

Tracheostomy

Tracheostomy is indicated when BVCP is responsible for significant respiratory distress or effort, inadequate ventilation, or failure to thrive. The tracheostomy rate for BVCP cited in the two largest pediatric series is 48% (7) and 73% (17), but rates as high as 92% have been reported (18). These older studies overestimate the current tracheotomy rate. If tracheostomy is necessary, this should be combined with microlaryngoscopy and bronchoscopy to rule out any other airway abnormality definitively.

Enlargement of the Glottic Lumen

Enlarging the glottic lumen to allow decannulation should be considered if spontaneous resolution of BVCP is considered unlikely. The prognosis for recovery depends on the underlying cause. This may be clear-cut in cases of known neurologic damage, but when no cause is found the prognosis is unknown. The literature suggests that spontaneous resolution of idiopathic BVCP, which represents a significant proportion of cases of congenital BVCP requiring tracheostomy, occurs in about half the cases, but this may take a number of years (1).

Surgical correction should therefore be delayed in idiopathic congenital BVCP until the child is about to attend school to allow spontaneous improvement to occur. If at this time the child remains tracheostomy dependent but there is evidence of some improvement in vocal cord function, surgery should be further delayed. Where there is no prospect of recovery, surgery can be performed earlier. Although some authors recommend surgery within the first year of life (19), 2 to 3 years seems a more appropriate age: the airway is larger and the child is better able to tolerate aspiration that may occur as a complication of surgery.

The surgical options for enlargement of the glottic lumen are listed in Table 3; however, most of the experience with these techniques has been in adults. The most reliable results in children are obtained with external arytenoidectomy via laryngofissure. This approach provides good exposure and a decannulation rate on the order of 80% (20). The procedure is, however, associated with a potential loss of voice quality and a risk of aspiration.

The technique of external arytenoidectomy via laryngofissure involves:

1. Preliminary bronchoscopy. Associated airway abnormalities, particularly tracheostomy-related suprastomal collapse or granuloma, which may preclude successful decannulation, need to be ruled out.
2. Exposure.
   a. Curvilinear skin incision over cricoid cartilage and elevation of subplatysmal flaps.
   b. Strap muscles retracted.
   c. Midline thyrotomy extending through cricoid cartilage and into the first tracheal ring if necessary.
3. Removal of arytenoid.
   a. Mucosa overlying the arytenoid selected for removal is injected with 1% lidocaine hydrochloride with 1:100,000 epinephrine.
   b. Oblique incision over body of arytenoid.
   c. Vocal process freed from thyroarytenoid muscle.
   d. Arytenoid grasped with forceps and division of muscular attachments to aryteroid by sharp dissection.
   e. Cricoarytenoid joint separated and cartilage removed.
   f. Mucosal closure with 5.0 absorbable suture.
4. Lateralization.
   a. Introduction of two 4.0 nonabsorbable lateralization sutures through thyroid ala to posterior vocal cord and back out through thyroid ala.

TABLE 3: Surgical Options for Enlargement of Glottic Lumen

Arytenoidectomy
Endoscopic
External via laryngofissure
Woodman procedure
Arytenoidopexy
Laser cordectomy
Laser ablation of arytenoid process
Cordopexy

b. Lateralization sutures tied under endoscopic vision following closure of thyrotomy.

5. Closure. Closure in layers with wound drain.

A variety of endoscopic procedures have been described. Simple procedures, which can be staged for safety, include laser transverse cordotomy (Fig. 1) and laser ablation of the vocal process. While only increasing the glottic airway by a relatively small amount, these procedures may convert a marginal airway to an adequate one, thereby making decannulation possible.

There is no physiologic basis for employing a nerve–muscle pedicle procedure for treatment of congenital BVCP as this does not overcome the underlying brainstem dysfunction responsible for the BVCP.

PEARLS AND PERILS

---

1. For long-term follow-up of BVCP in a child without a tracheostomy, satisfactory weight gain is the best indicator of an adequate airway.
2. The prognosis for recovery in idiopathic congenital BVCP is uncertain. This must be borne in mind when deciding whether or not to proceed with a glottic enlargement procedure, and on the timing of this surgery.

Unilateral Vocal Cord Paralysis

Traditional methods of treatment of UVCP in adults are not applicable to young children. Aspiration of oral foods associated with UVCP is usually seen in the very young; if they are severe and persistent, gastrostomy is recommended. Dysphonia related to UVCP is not treated surgically. Most cases of UVCP following recurrent laryngeal nerve injury in children resolve spontaneously within weeks to months. Improvement may also occur due to compensatory movement of the normal vocal cord. Long-term problems are uncommon, and treatment is usually not required.

Management of Aspiration

Ingested oral intake, gastroesophageal reflux material, and occasionally saliva may be aspirated. Each of these must be assessed and treated separately. Medialization of a paralyzed vocal cord is usually not an option in young children but could be considered in the management of older children with aspiration (21).

Oral Intake   Feeds should be thickened with corn flour, but if aspiration persists, oral feeding is ceased and the child fed by nasogastric tube. Speech therapy may help oral and pharyngeal function, which improves swallowing and thereby decreases the risk of aspiration. Gastrostomy should be considered if long-term nasogastric tube feeding is required due to persistent laryngeal incompetence and there is evidence of denervation on laryngeal electromyography. Gastrostomy may, however, exacerbate gastroesophageal reflux, and fundoplication in addition may be required. Medialization by vocal cord injection or thyroplasty may be an alternative to gastrostomy in older children.

Gastroesophageal Reflux   UVCP in a child with gastroesophageal reflux is associated with an increased risk of aspiration. Medical treatment of gastroesophageal reflux includes posturing and thickening of feeds and the use of antacids, prokinetic agents (e.g., cisapride), and H2 receptor antagonists (e.g., ranitidine). Fundoplication may be necessary if medical treatment fails.

Saliva   Aspiration of saliva may occasionally be a clinical problem in a child with UVCP despite gastrostomy tube feeding and control of gastroesophegeal reflux. It usually occurs in the presence of an underlying neurologic or neuromuscular disorder and presents with episodes of choking or cyanosis. In the long term, saliva aspiration may lead to chronic lung disease. Treatment initially is with speech therapy (to improve swallowing) and anticholinergic drugs, but if aspiration is severe, tracheostomy may need to be con-

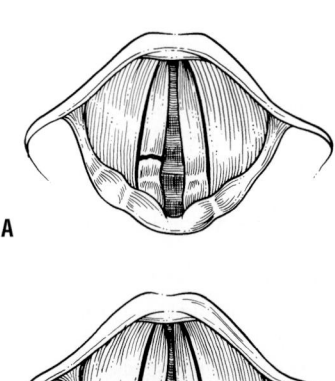

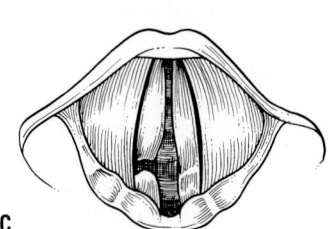

FIGURE 1 Transverse cordotomy **A:** Division of vocal cord immediately anterior to vocal process. **B:** Initial wedge-shaped defect. **C:** Mature rounded defect.

sidered to secure the airway and also provide a means for tracheobronchial toilet. As an alternative to tracheotomy, a procedure to decrease saliva production may be attempted.

Dysphonia

Speech Therapy   In the absence of recovery of UVCP, voice quality may improve with speech therapy and compensatory movement of the normal vocal cord. If the voice is particularly weak, voice amplification with a microphone can be useful.

Surgery   The medialization techniques of vocal cord injection with Teflon and thyroplasty are not appropriate for treatment of dysphonia in very young children with UVCP because of the small size of the airway and the likelihood of causing significant obstruction, the reluctance to implant foreign material in a child, and the loss of medialization with growth of the larynx.

Although there is no ideal procedure in children, fat injection of the vocal cord may be suitable although the benefits appear to be temporary due to resorption of the fat. A reinnervation procedure also appears worthy of consideration, but there has been very little experience with this in the pediatric population.

PEARLS AND PERILS

1. Most cases of UVCP in children acquired following cardiac or tracheoesophageal fistula surgery resolve within weeks to months and do not require treatment.
2. Aspiration in UVCP may involve oral diet, gastroesophageal reflux material, or saliva.

⚙ REFERENCES

1. Berkowitz RG. Laryngeal electromyography findings in idiopathic congenital bilateral vocal cord paralysis. *Ann Otol Rhinol Laryngol* 1996;105:207–212.
2. New GB, Childrey JH. Paralysis of the vocal cords. A study of 217 medical cases. *Arch Otolaryngol* 1932;16:143–159.
3. Bloch A, Lemoine J. Apparition d'une paralysie des dilatateurs chez un nourrisson de 6 mois. *Ann Otolaryngol* 1936;1:427.
4. Clerf LH. Unilateral vocal cord paralysis. *JAMA* 1953;151:900–903.
5. Platt D. Congenital laryngeal abductror paralysis due to nucleus ambiguous dysgenesis in three brothers. *N Engl J Med* 1964;271:593–597.
6. Holinger PH, Brown WT. Congenital webs, cysts, laryngoceles and other anomalies of the larynx. *Ann Otol Rhinol Laryngol* 1967;76:744–752.
7. Holinger LD, Holinger PC, Holinger PH. Etiology of bilateral abductor vocal cord paralysis. A review of 389 cases. *Ann Otol* 1976;85:428–436.
8. Silberman HD, Wilf H, Tucker JA. Flexible fiberoptic nasopharyngolaryngoscope. *Ann Otol* 1976;85:640–645.
9. Benjamin B, Mair EA. Congenital interaryteroid web. *Arch Otolaryngol Head Neck Surg* 1991;117:1118–1122.
10. Sofferman RA, Haische CE, Kirchner JA, Hardin NJ. The nasogastric tube syndrome. *Laryngoscope* 1990;100:962–968.
11. Annino DJ Jr, Mac Arthur CJ, Friedman EM. Vineristine-induced recurrent laryngeal nerve paralysis. *Laryngoscope* 1992;102:1260–1262.
12. Thompson JW, Rosenthal P, Camilon FS Jr. Vocal cord paralysis and superior laryngeal nerve dysfunction in Reye's syndrome. *Arch Otolaryngol Head Neck Surg* 1990;116:46–48.
13. Ross DA, Ward PM. Central vocal cord paralysis and paresis presenting as laryngeal strider in children. *Laryngoscope* 1990;100:10–13.
14. Chaten FC, Lucking SE, Young ES, Mickell JJ. Strider: intracranial pathology causing postextubation vocal cord paralysis. *Pediatrics* 1991;87:39–43.
15. Charney EB, Rorke LB, Sutton LN, Schut L. Management of Chiari II complications in infants with myelomeningocele. *J Pediatr* 1987;111:364–371.
16. Sataloff RT, Bough ID Jr, Spiegel JR. Arytenoid dislocation: diagnosis and treatment. *Laryngoscope* 1994;104:1353–1361.
17. Cohen SR, Geller KA, Birns JW, Thompson JW. Laryngeal paralysis in children. A long-term retrospective study. *Ann Otol Rhinol Laryngol* 1976;85:428–436.
18. Gentile RD, Miller RH, Woodson GE. Vocal and paralysis in children 1 year of age and younger. *Ann Otol Rhinol Laryngol* 1986;95:622–625.
19. Narcy P, Contencin P, Viala P. Surgical treatment for laryngeal paralysis in infants and children. *Laryngoscope* 1990;100:1174–1179.
20. Bower CM, Choi SS, Cotton RT. Aryteroidectomy in children. *Ann Otol Rhinol Laryngol* 1994;103:271–278.
21. Levine BA, Jacobs IN, Wetmore RF, Handler SD. Vocal cord injection in children with unilateral vocal cord paralysis. *Arch Otolaryngol Head Neck Surg* 1995;121:116–119.

R. G. Berkowitz: Department of Otolaryngology, Royal Children's Hospital, Parkville, Victoria 3053, Australia.

• *Practical Pediatric Otolaryngology*
• edited by Robin T. Cotton and Charles M. Myer, III
• Lippincott-Raven Publishers, Philadelphia © 1999

39

Tracheobronchomalacia

David Albert

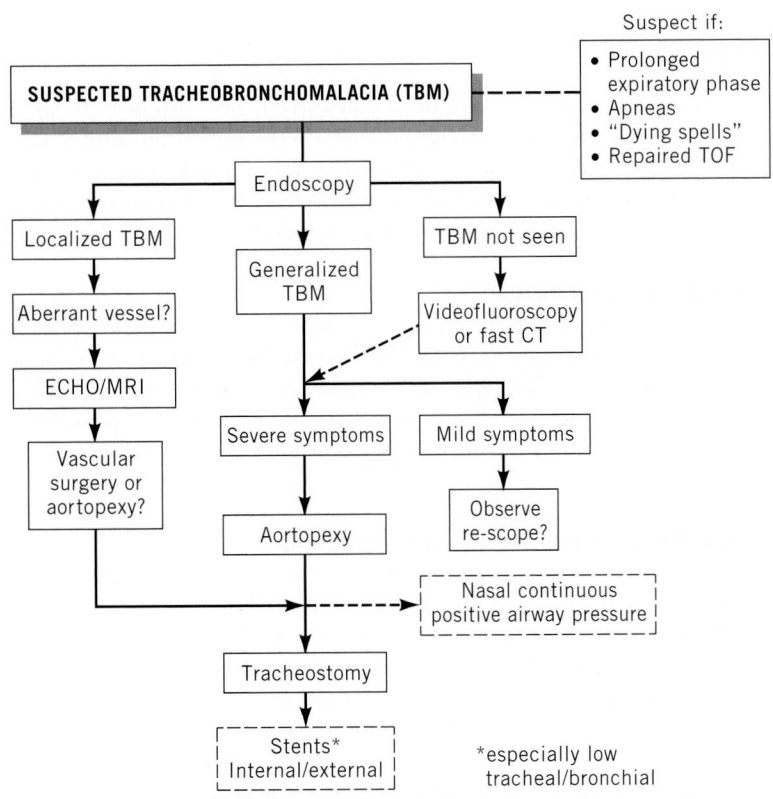

Suspect if:
- Prolonged expiratory phase
- Apneas
- "Dying spells"
- Repaired TOF

SUSPECTED TRACHEOBRONCHOMALACIA (TBM)

Endoscopy

Localized TBM | Generalized TBM | TBM not seen

Aberrant vessel? | Videofluoroscopy or fast CT

ECHO/MRI

Vascular surgery or aortopexy? | Severe symptoms | Mild symptoms

Aortopexy | Observe re-scope?

Nasal continuous positive airway pressure

Tracheostomy

Stents* Internal/external

*especially low tracheal/bronchial

⬤ HISTORICAL BACKGROUND

Mair and Parsons (1) have provided a comprehensive review of the historical aspects of tracheobrochomalacia (TBM), including the 1948 description of pediatric TBM by Gross and Neuman and the endoscopic appearances noted by Holinger et al. in 1952. Of note was the expiratory nature of the collapse and the fact that it could be eliminated by the passage of a bronchoscope. The various treatments developed during the middle of this century (from extended tracheotomy tubes through aortopexy to the more recent use of endobronchial stents) are dealt with separately later in this chapter.

Definition

Tracheomalacia (2) is an abnormal collapse of the trachea that when severe can produce symptoms of airway obstruction. Brochomalacia is the equivalent in the bronchi. The trachea and bronchi of children, and particularly of neonates, are more compliant than in the adult. This compliance can produce a degree of collapse even in normals, particularly for instance if a child coughs during endoscopy because of insufficient topical and general anesthesia. This normal collapse needs to be excluded from any definition of TBM, as does the minor degree of anterior displacement of the trachealis, which unless severe is more often a sign of light anesthesia than of significant malacia. In general, collapse has to be greater than 10% to 20% to be readily appreciated at endoscopy; if the child is well anesthetized at the time, this degree of collapse is usually abnormal although not necessarily clinically symptomatic. To be clinically significant, about 50% obstruction is probably required, less for neonates and more for older children. Different values for collapse are appropriate for other forms of investigation such as radiologic screening (3).

Messineo and Filler (4) describe tracheomalacia as a generalized or localized weakness of the trachea that results in excessive narrowing of the tracheal lumen during expiration or whenever intrathoracic pressure increases.

Classification

Tracheomalacia has classically been categorized into *primary or intrinsic malacia,* in which the collapse is due to an abnormality in the wall of the airway, or *secondary malacia,* which is due to extrinsic compression or other insult causing weakness and collapse. Primary tracheomalacia is seen relatively rarely (5,6), whereas secondary TBM occurs in association with a number of conditions, outlined below.

Tracheoesophageal Fistula

Although a flattened trachea is seen commonly in tracheoesophageal fistula (TEF), significant complications from TBM following fistula repair are relatively rare [1:54 in the series from Spitz (7)]. Spitz also provides a general review of TEF (8). The suggestion that TBM in TEF could arise from pressure of the dilated proximal esophageal remnant is not borne out by the infrequent association of TBM with primary esophageal atresia without TEF (9).

Cardiac Abnormalities and Vascular Anomalies

The anatomic variants of cardiopulmonary circulation that result in extrinsic compression of the trachea and bronchi are illustrated in Fig. 1 (10,11). An aberrant innominate artery compresses the right anterior trachea just above the carina. A double aortic arch surrounds the trachea and main bronchi, producing concentric or triangular-shaped compression at endoscopy. A pulmonary artery sling compresses the right main bronchus, often to the extent that the lumen of the right main bronchus is a thin slit.

Localized Tracheomalacia Associated with a Tracheotomy

Prescott (12) feels that the localized collapse above most long-standing tracheotomies is inevitable and is due to damage to the cartilage. He feels that although some of this may be prevented by careful design of the incision, most is probably secondary to the presence of the tracheotomy tube. Improvements in tube design may offer some hope.

Localized Tracheomalacia Associated with Mediastinal Masses

Even benign masses such as a large cystic hygroma or bronchogenic cyst can produce localized tracheomalacia, perhaps by a pressure effect, or perhaps through localized vascular insufficiency.

Laryngeal Cleft

The association between tracheomalacia and laryngeal cleft (13) presumably stems from the combined embryologic origin with separation of the trachea from the esophagus. Both Larsen's (14) and Hunter's (15) syndromes are associated with TBM, although the embryologic cause is unclear.

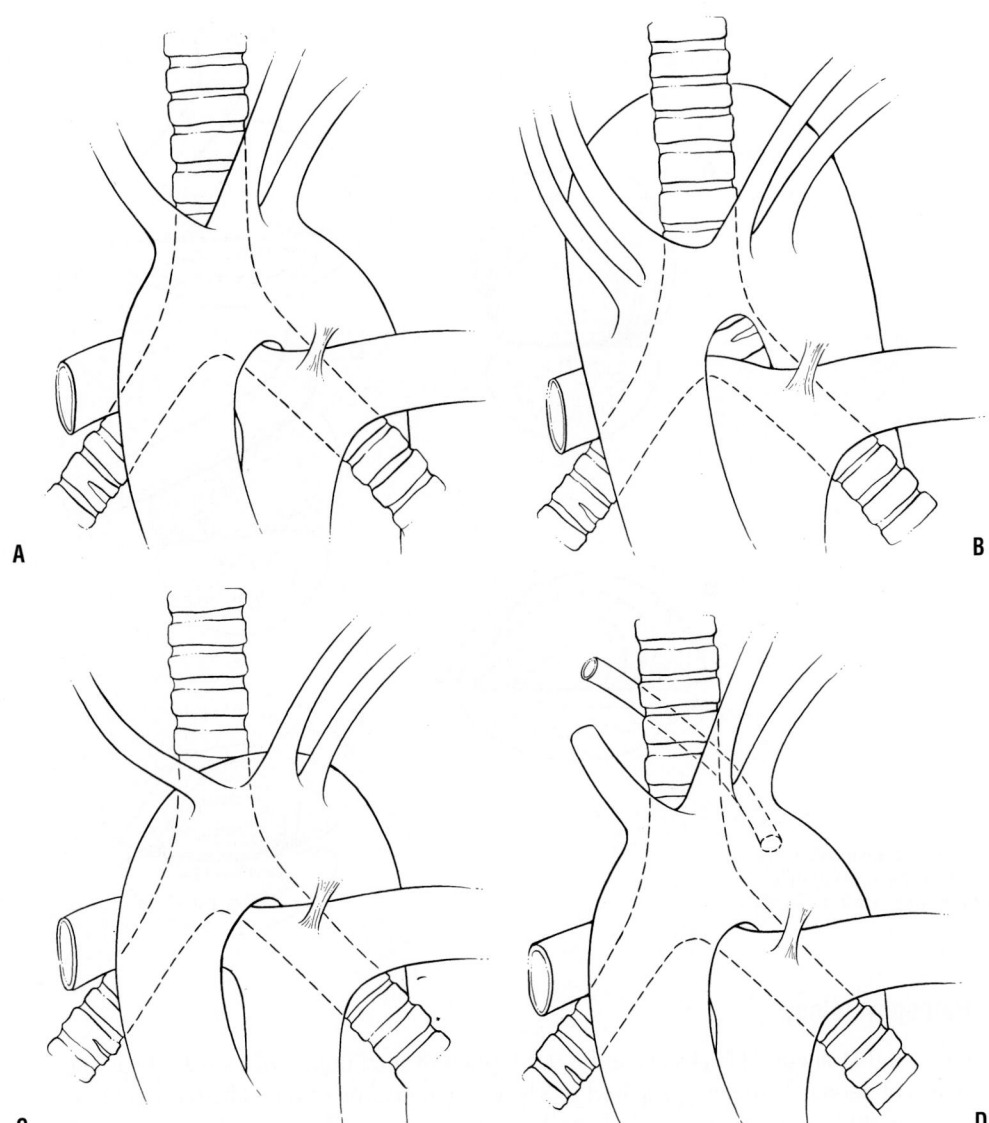

FIGURE 1 Anatomical variants that can lead to tracheobronchial compression (slings and rings). **A:** Normal cardiopulmonary anatomy. **B:** Double aortic arch. **C:** Anomalous innominate artery. **D:** Aberrant subclavian artery.

Major Airways Collapse (a Further Recent Classification)

Based on histopathologic, endoscopic, and clinical findings of the flaccid airway, Mair and Parsons (1) further subdivide secondary tracheomalacia into two types depending on the anatomic ratio of cartilage to muscle and whether external compression is noted. This gives three types of "major airways collapse," a new descriptive term that they hope will define TBM more clearly. Type I (Fig. 2B) is equivalent to primary tracheomalacia and is usually seen with syndromic associations (see below). Type II (Fig. 2C and 3D) is classical secondary malacia occurring from external compression (either congenital, as with abnormal cardiovascular anatomy, or acquired). Type III (Fig. 2E) is acquired TBM either locally as a result of a tracheotomy tube or throughout the tracheobronchial tree as a result of prolonged high-pressure ventilation. Types I and III and most type II forms have widened posterior walls with a cartilage-to-muscle ratio closer to 2:1 than the usual 4:1 or 5:1. So far this new classification does not seem to have been generally accepted.

Mair and Parsons also suggest a staging system analogous to that used for subglottic stenosis (16) with mild describing less than 70% obstruction, moderate 70% to 90% obstruction, and severe greater than 90% obstruction at the end of expiration.

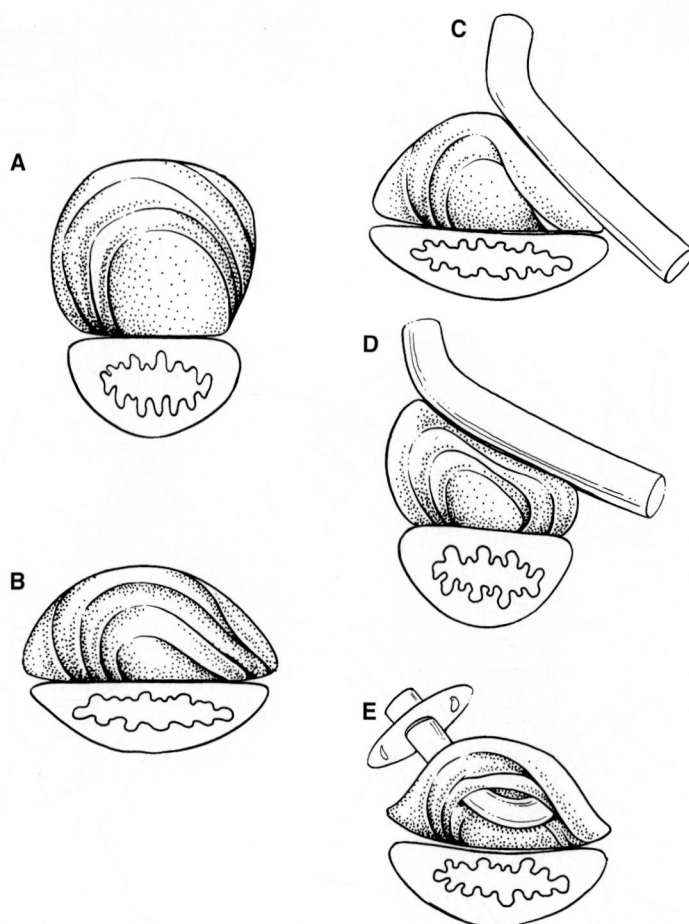

FIGURE 2 Major airway collapse—a new classification by Mair and Parsons (1). **A:** Normal. **B:** Type I, congenital. **C:** Type II, acquired. **D:** Type II (with normal ratio). **E:** Type III, localized.

Pathophysiology

Chen and Holinger (17) give a careful description of the findings of six pathologic specimens of neonatal larynges prepared as whole organ macrosections. The increased muscle-to-cartilage ratio is seen pathologically and endoscopically. Interestingly, one specimen shows thickening of the anterior tracheal ring, i.e., a strengthening rather than a weakening of the cartilaginous part of the trachea.

PATIENT ASSESSMENT

History

The onset of stridor in tracheomalacia is insidious in the weeks following birth and is often episodic, with an unremarkable background stridor and acute exacerbations. It is important to appreciate this variability, as the parents may be describing frightening attacks of severe airway obstruction while the child is sleeping peacefully in the doctor's office. Variability is characteristic of all dynamic conditions including laryngomalacia, although the change from quiet breathing to nearly complete obstruction is much more marked in tracheomalacia. Sometimes the episodes are dramatic, with partial or complete cessation of airflow and cyanosis. Attempts at resuscitation are often carried out by parents and caregivers, giving rise to the term *dying spells*. It difficult to judge in retrospect if these attempts are effective or if most, if not all, episodes of severe tracheomalacia are self-limiting. The attacks are often provoked by severe crying, coughing, and feeding. The stridor in tracheomalacia is typically expiratory, with a few parents being able to differenti-

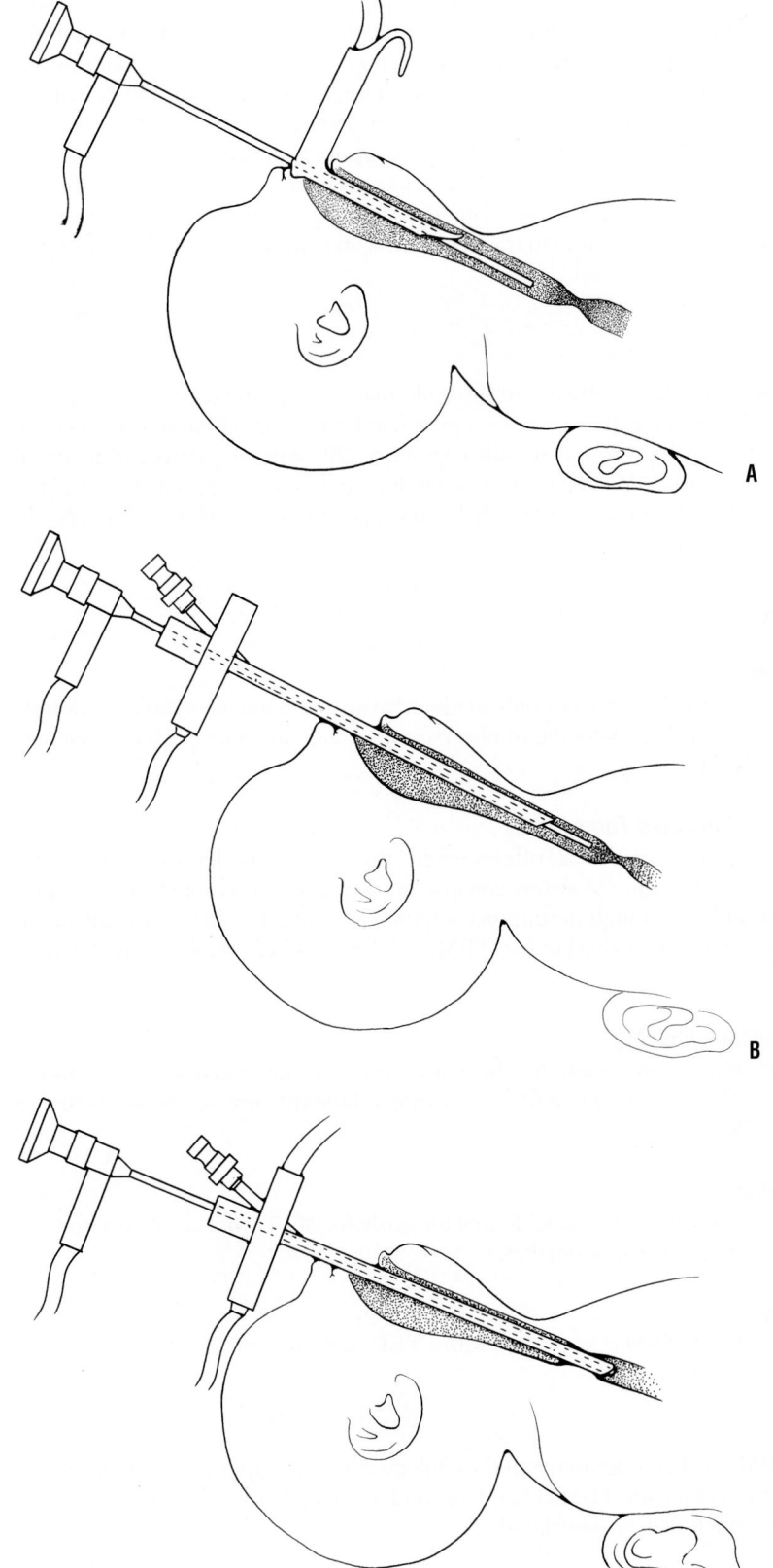

FIGURE 3 Correct and incorrect methods of tracheobronchoscopy to demonstrate tracheobronchomalacia. **A:** Telescope passed through laryngoscope without bronchoscope thus reducing any direct or indirect airway splinting. **B:** Telescope advanced beyond bronchoscope to reduce splinting. **C:** Bronchoscope splinting malacic segment resulting in underdiagnosis of tracheomalacia. (From ref. 1, with permission.)

ate inspiratory from expiratory stridor. Feeding difficulties in neonates with airway obstruction are presumably due to difficulty in coordinating respiration and feeding in the presence of airway compromise. In tracheomalacia there can be increased stridor during feeding but not usually aspiration or choking, which might indicate a vocal cord palsy, a laryngeal cleft, or a tracheocutaneous fistula. Cough (18) can be a sign of tracheomalacia, as can grunting, which may act to provide some positive airway pressure to limit the collapse seen in tracheomalacia. The cough seen in tracheocutaneous fistula may be due to the associated tracheomalacia. Unexplained respiratory distress on the neonatal intensive care unit (5,19) may be due to tracheomalacia and (with the myriad of other possible causes) can often be missed.

Examination

TBM is typically episodic in nature, and the child may seem perfectly well on examination. However, if looked for, there may be a prolonged expiratory phase or even an expiratory wheeze. Stridor if present is usually expiratory (20), with respiratory difficulty at rest only seen in severe TBM. The effect of feeding and crying can, however, be dramatic, with a sudden change from a quietly breathing infant to one who is obviously obstructed and distressed.

Investigations

Barium Swallow

This is a useful investigation not only to identify vascular anomalies such as a double aortic arch but also during screening to observe the change in anteroposterior tracheal dimension seen in TBM.

Ultrafast or Cine-Computed Tomography

These newer modalities (21,22) offer a noninvasive method of determining the site, extent, severity, and dynamics of airway collapse in the trachea and bronchus. Occasionally, without the addition of high-definition computed tomography, they can misdiagnose tracheal stenosis as tracheomalacia (23). TBM is defined radiologically as greater than 50% collapse.

Magnetic Resonance Imaging

This is particularly appropriate for the assessment of vascular anomalies and mediastinal masses but is less sensitive at differentiating a static tracheal narrowing such as a stenosis from TBM (24,25).

Echocardiography

While this has become an invaluable tool for cardiologists it is not always accurate in excluding or defining vascular anomalies.

pH Probe Study

This is important if TBM is associated with a TEF, as there is often associated gastroesophageal reflux (6,26).

Endoscopy

Even if TBM has been demonstrated radiologically, it is important to undertake a full endoscopy to examine the TBM at first hand and to exclude other abnormalities, such as a cleft larynx, which may be associated.

Laryngoscopy Laryngomalacia may be seen, as it is common, but there does not seem to be any association with TBM. Posterior laryngeal cleft needs to be positively excluded by passing a probe between the arytenoids. If the patient has undergone repair of TEF or cardiovascular anomaly it is important to check vocal cord function during laryngoscopy.

Bronchoscopy Bronchoscopy has been considered the gold standard for assessing TBM, but there are many traps for the inexperienced that result both in over- and under-diagnosis. Overdiagnosis can occur with poor anesthesia, resulting in a child coughing as the bronchoscope touches the carina. In infants this can produce collapse in their normally compliant tracheas, mimicking true TBM. This can be avoided by a level of anesthesia sufficiently deep to reduce coughing but still allow spontaneous respiration.

Underdiagnosis occurs with splinting of the airway. Physical splinting from the bronchoscope can be avoided by using a small bronchoscope or advancing a small telescope beyond the tip of the bronchoscope (Fig. 3). Airway splinting due to increased airway pressure can be avoided, again by using a small bronchoscope that has a lower airway resistance and by avoiding the use of positive end-expiratory pressure. Techniques of anesthesia that rely on paralysis and Venturi ventilation will also underdiagnose dynamic conditions such as TBM.

TBM should be carefully recorded as a description for the operative report supplemented by still and video images for later consultation with, for instance, cardiothoracic or general pediatric surgeons. The level and vertical extent as well as the percent of occlusion of the airway are all recorded along with the ratio of muscle to cartilage to help classify the TBM (1).

The common vascular anomalies have sufficiently characteristic findings to aid diagnosis. With an aberrant innominate artery the artery arises from the aorta more posteriorly than normal, compressing the right anterior wall of the trachea as it crosses in front of the trachea from left to right. Endoscopically this oblique flattening of the right anterior wall occurs 1 to 2 cm above the carina. Raising the tip of the bronchoscope can occlude the right radial pulse, best appreciated using pulse oximetry. With a double aortic arch the trachea is encircled by the normal anterior and the aberrant posterior arch, either of which may predominate. The endoscopic finding is of a triangular compression, again just above the carina. In the rare anomaly of pulmonary artery sling, the left pulmonary artery arises from the right pulmonary artery instead of the auricles. It crosses the right main bronchus and then passes behind the trachea to reach the left lung. The endoscopic findings are of a flat lower trachea with a very collapsed right main bronchus. TBM may also be a part of other complex congenital heart defects (27).

PEARLS AND PERILS

1. Suspect TBM in unexplained neonatal respiratory difficulty.
2. Initial endoscopy may be normal either because the airway was supported at the time of endoscopy or there has been progression of the TBM.
3. Entertain a high index of suspicion in repaired TEF.

 TREATMENT RECOMMENDATIONS

Mild Tracheobronchomalacia

Usually no treatment is required for mild TBM as the disease is self-limiting over 1 to 2 years and usually resolves without surgery (28). However, parents need a lot of support and information as well as being taught cardiopulmonary resuscitation if the child has a history of apneas or dying spells. All that may be required with resuscitation is a little positive airway pressure delivered mouth to mouth or with a resuscitation mask and bag. Parents are often told to avoid getting the child upset to prevent attacks relating to crying, although how practical this is with a young child is open to doubt.

Vascular Surgery for Compressing Abnormal Vasculature

If an aberrant innominate artery is causing significant apneas and cyanotic episodes, it can be suspended forward in an innominate arteriopexy. The nondominant (usually anterior) arch in a double aortic arch (29) can be resected, combined if necessary with a vascular suspension procedure. Long-term intubation as a conservative approach has also proved successful (30). With a pulmonary artery sling the left pulmonary artery can be reimplanted anterior to the trachea, but, again, this may need to be combined with tracheopexy (31).

Aortopexy

Aortopexy was initially used in TBM associated with TEF (32,33) but has also been used in TBM without an associated TEF (5,6). Putting a suture through the outer wall of the aorta through a relatively small incision is a significant procedure and should not be undertaken unless there is severe collapse (more than 50%) and symptoms warrant major surgery. The results of lifting the aorta forward are, however, encouraging (22). Pericardial flap aortopexy may prove to be a safer technique (34).

Bronchopexy

Occasionally bronchomalacia can be improved with a suspension procedure (35), although this is less established than aortopexy.

Custom-Made Tracheostomy Tubes

An extended tracheotomy tube (36,37) will effectively support midtracheal tracheomalacia but is less effective for low tracheal and bronchial collapse. A tracheotomy tube reduces airway resistance, making TBM distal to the tube tip worse. However, it is easy to connect a ventilating bag to the tracheotomy tube for resuscitation and increased airway pressure. Longer tubes with a straight cut rather than beveled end can be made to sit just above the carina but at the risk creating a tube tip stenosis at a very difficult site. Recently tubes have been developed to support the carinal area with a bifurcation into two flexible tubes to enter and support the main stem bronchi.

Nasal or Tracheostomy CPAP

Carinal tracheomalacia and severe bronchomalacia can be supported with continuous positive airway pressure (CPAP) (38,39) from a standard home CPAP machine as used in obstructive sleep apnea. The device can be used nasally with a close-fitting mask (with some difficulties of acceptance) or via a tracheotomy tube.

Tracheostomy-Related Collapse

Suprastomal collapse related to tracheotomy can be corrected by a surgical decannulation procedure in which the tracheocutaneous fistula is excised and the stoma formally closed. Sutures are brought laterally to the sternomastoids to support the area of collapse and the patient intubated for 24 to 48 hours (40). If the collapse is particularly severe, a cartilage graft may be required, sometimes placed horizontally between the strap muscles for extra support.

Surgical Alternatives for Severe Disease

External Stents

As open thoracic operations for TBM are traditionally in the domain of cardiothoracic surgeons, early attempts to stiffen the collapsing trachea externally used pericardial patches. Some fibrosed and were successful, and others were as malacic as the original trachea. Marlex and a number of other synthetics have also been tried with sporadically good results.

Internal Stents

Internal stents support the area of collapse well but suffer from migration, extrusion, and localized reactions including granulations and frank infections. Both siliconized plastic and expandable metal stents have been used with success. The expandable metal stents (41–44) are difficult to insert even using an introducer and need to expand at just the right point in the lumen once released. Balloon dilation can be used to increase the lumen further to accommodate future growth (43). The plastic stents are inserted folded or on an introducer and have a variety of external pegs and lips to try to prevent migration.

Segmental Resection

If the TBM is confined to a short segment this can be resected and a primary anastamosis performed (45). Anastamotic stenosis occurs, as it does when segmental resection is employed in short-segment stenosis.

Cartilage Grafting

Rib cartilage grafts can be used to stiffen long-segment tracheal or bronchial malacia with good reepithelialization if the cartilage amounts to 25% or less of the circumference of the airway, but when 30% or more of the circumference is rib graft, epithelialization may be impaired (45).

PEARLS AND PERILS

1. Tracheotomy can make unsupported areas (such as the carina and bronchi) worse by reducing the natural airway pressure.
2. Aortopexy carries a risk of aortic perforation and phrenic nerve palsy but seems to be successful in patients both with and without TEF.
3. Heroic measures such as stenting or resection should be reserved for very severe cases.
4. Severe bronchomalacia can be very difficult to treat even with intubation and/or tracheostomy and CPAP and may therefore be life threatening (46).

MANAGEMENT OF COMPLICATIONS

Sudden Deterioration

The most feared complication of TBM is seen in children whose airway is so collapsed by the effort to exhale that the more they panic the more obstructed they become. These children can change suddenly from being quite well to being obstructed, very quickly progressing to apnea. Sometimes this is in response to crying or coughing and sometimes to feeding. The respiratory arrest may be self-limiting although dramatic, but usually if it is witnessed some form of resuscitation will have been commenced before recovery occurs spontaneously. Some children in hospital have required full cardiopulmonary resuscitation but at home a face mask and CPAP can buy time. Many of the procedures to combat TBM have complications as significant as the disease itself.

Gradual Worsening of Symptoms

Progression of the disease is not uncommon in the first (and second) year of life before the disease improves. Again the parents will have to deal emergently with collapse at home but once in hospital intubation with CPAP may be necessary. In the older child surgical alternatives should be avoided if possible as the disease may be about to "turn the corner." This scenario is particularly depressing for parents if they have been told that their child will grow out of the disease by 18 months.

SUMMARY

Tracheobronchomalacia when mild is common and self-limiting. When it is severe, the child's life is at risk and heroic measures need to be considered but only used if the risk of complication is less than that of the disease itself.

✷ REFERENCES

1. Mair EA, Parsons DS. Pediatric tracheobronchomalacia and major airway collapse. *Ann Otol Rhinol Laryngol* 1992;101:300–309.
2. Filler RM, de Fraga JC. Tracheomalacia. *Semin Thorac Cardiovasc Surg* 1994;6:211–215.
3. Kao SC, Kimura K, Smith WL, Sato Y. Tracheomalacia before and after aortosternopexy: dynamic and quantitative assessment by electron-beam computed tomography with clinical correlation [see comments]. *Pediatr Radiol* 1995;25 [Suppl 1]:S187–193.
4. Messineo A, Filler RM. Tracheomalacia. *Semin Pediatr Surg* 1994;3:253–258.
5. Lassaletta L, Eire PF, Carrero C, Lopez Santamaria M, Borches D, Alvarez F. [Neonatal tracheomalacia. Study of 3 cases treated with aortopexy+] Traqueomalacia neonatal. Estudio de tres casos tratados con aortopexia. *Cir Pediatr* 1993;6:79–83.
6. Malone PS, Kiely EM. Role of aortopexy in the management of primary tracheomalacia and tracheobronchomalacia. *Arch Dis Child* 1990;65:438–440.
7. Spitz L. Gastric transposition for esophageal substitution in children. *J Pediatr Surg* 1992;27:252–257.
8. Spitz L. Esophageal atresia and tracheoesophageal fistula in children. *Curr Opin Pediatr* 1993;5:347–352.
9. Rideout DT, Hayashi AH, Gillis DA, Giacomantonio JM, Lau HY. The absence of clinically significant tracheomalacia in patients having esophageal atresia without tracheoesophageal fistula. *J Pediatr Surg* 1991;26:1303–1305.
10. Rivilla F, Utrilla JG, Alvarez F. Surgical management and follow-up of vascular rings. *Z Kinderchir* 1989;44:199–202.
11. Wiatrak BJ, Myer CM III, Cotton RT. Atypical tracheobronchial vascular compression. *Am J Otolaryngol* 1991;12:347–356.
12. Prescott CA. Peristomal complications of paediatric tracheostomy. *Int J Pediatr Otorhinolaryngol* 1992;23:141–149.
13. Mitchell DB, Koltai P, Matthew D, Bailey CM, Evans JN. Severe tracheobronchomalacia associated with laryngeal cleft. *Int J Pediatr Otorhinolaryngol* 1989;18:181–185.
14. Crowe AV, Kearns DB, Mitchell DB. Tracheal stenosis in Larsen's syndrome. *Arch Otolaryngol Head Neck Surg* 1989;115:626.
15. Morehead JM, Parsons DS. Tracheobronchomalacia in Hunter's syndrome. *Int J Pediatr Otorhinolaryngol* 1993;26:255–261.
16. Cotton RT, Gray SD, Miller RP. Update of the Cincinnati experience in pediatric laryngotracheal reconstruction. *Laryngoscope* 1989;99:1111–1116.
17. Chen JC, Holinger LD. Congenital tracheal anomalies: pathology study using serial macrosections and review of the literature. *Pediatr Pathol* 1994;14:513–537.
18. Wood RE. Localized tracheomalacia or bronchomalacia in children with intractable cough. *J Pediatr* 1990;116:404–406.
19. Duncan S, Eid N. Tracheomalacia and bronchopulmonary dysplasia [see comments]. *Ann Otol Rhinol Laryngol* 1991;100:856–858.
20. Parsons D, Cotton R, Crysdale W. Distal tracheal compression. *Head Neck* 1991;13:251–254.
21. Kao SC, Smith WL, Sato Y, Franken EA Jr, Kimura K, Soper RT. Ultrafast CT of laryngeal and tracheobronchial obstruction in symptomatic postoperative infants with esophageal atresia and tracheoesophageal fistula. *AJR* 1990;154:345–350.

22. Kimura K, Soper RT, Kao SC, Sato Y, Smith WL, Franken EA. Aortosternopexy for tracheomalacia following repair of esophageal atresia: evaluation by cine-CT and technical refinement. *J Pediatr Surg* 1990;25:769–772.

23. Brody AS, Kuhn JP, Seidel FG, Brodsky LS. Airway evaluation in children with use of ultrafast CT: pitfalls and recommendations. *Radiology* 1991;178:181–184.

24. Vogl T, Wilimzig C, Bilaniuk LT, et al. MR imaging in pediatric airway obstruction. *J Comput Assist Tomogr* 1990;14:182–186.

25. Simoneaux SF, Bank ER, Webber JB, Parks WJ. MR imaging of the pediatric airway. *Radiographics* 1995;15:287–298.

26. Guys JM, Triglia JM, Louis C, Panuel M, Carcassonne M. Esophageal atresia, tracheomalacia and arterial compression: role of aortopexy. *Eur J Pediatr Surg* 1991;1:261–265.

27. Davis DA, Tucker JA, Russo P. Management of airway obstruction in patients with congenital heart defects. *Ann Otol Rhinol Laryngol* 1993;102:163–166.

28. Jacobs IN, Wetmore RF, Tom LW, Handler SD, Potsic WP. Tracheobronchomalacia in children. *Arch Otolaryngol Head Neck Surg* 1994;120:154–158.

29. Han MT, Hall DG, Manche A, Rittenhouse EA. Double aortic arch causing tracheoesophageal compression. *Am J Surg* 1993;165:628–631.

30. Reah G, Entress A. Prolonged tracheal intubation in an infant with tracheomalacia secondary to a vascular ring. A useful adjunct to treatment? *Anaesthesia* 1995;50:341–342.

31. Conti VR, Lobe TE. Vascular sling with tracheomalacia: surgical management. *Ann Thorac Surg* 1989;47:310–311.

32. Matute de Cardenas JA, Cuadros Garcia J, Portela Casalod E, Berchi Garcia FJ. [Treatment of tracheomalacia by aortopexy] Tratamiento de la traqueomalacia mediante aortopexia. *An Esp Pediatr* 1992;36:228–231.

33. Corbally MT, Spitz L, Kiely E, Brereton RJ, Drake DP. Aortopexy for tracheomalacia in oesophageal anomalies. *Eur J Pediatr Surg* 1993;3:264–266.

34. Applebaum H, Woolley MM. Pericardial flap aortopexy for tracheomalacia. *J Pediatr Surg* 1990;25:30–31.

35. Kosloske AM. Left mainstem bronchopexy for severe bronchomalacia. *J Pediatr Surg* 1991;26:260–262.

36. Zinman R. Tracheal stenting improves airway mechanics in infants with tracheobronchomalacia. *Pediatr Pulmonol* 1995;19:275–281.

37. Duncan BW, Howell LJ, deLorimier AA, Adzick NS, Harrison MR. Tracheostomy in children with emphasis on home care. *J Pediatr Surg* 1992;27:432–435.

38. Weigle CG. Treatment of an infant with tracheobronchomalacia at home with a lightweight, high-humidity, continuous positive airway pressure system. *Crit Care Med* 1990;18:892–894.

39. Reiterer F, Eber E, Zach MS, Muller W. Management of severe congenital tracheobronchomalacia by continuous positive airway pressure and tidal breathing flow-volume loop analysis. *Pediatr Pulmonol* 1994;17:401–403.

40. Azizkhan RG, Lacey SR, Wood RE. Anterior cricoid suspension and tracheal stomal closure for children with cricoid collapse and peristomal tracheomalacia following tracheostomy. *J Pediatr Surg* 1993;28:169–171.

41. Bugmann P, Rouge JC, Berner M, Friedli B, Le Coultre C. Use of Gianturco Z stents in the treatment of vascular compression of the tracheobronchial tree in childhood. A feasible solution when surgery fails. *Chest* 1994;106:1580–1582.

42. Bousamra M, Tweddell JS, Wells RG, Splaingard ML, Sty JR. Wire stent for tracheomalacia in a five-year-old girl. *Ann Thorac Surg* 1996;61:1239–1240.

43. Mair EA, Parsons DS, Lally KP. Treatment of severe bronchomalacia with expanding endobronchial stents. *Arch Otolaryngol Head Neck Surg* 1990;116:1087–1090.

44. Filler RM, Forte V, Fraga JC, Matute J. The use of expandable metallic airway stents for tracheobronchial obstruction in children. *J Pediatr Surg* 1995;30:1050–1055.

45. deLorimier AA, Harrison MR, Hardy K, Howell LJ, Adzick NS. Tracheobronchial obstructions in infants and children. Experience with 45 cases. *Ann Surg* 1990;212:277–289.

46. Tuma S, Slavik Z, Tax P, Hucin B, Skovranek J. Double aortic arch in d-transposition of the great arteries complicated by tracheobronchomalacia. *Cardiovasc Intervent Radiol* 1995;18:115–117.

D. Albert: Consultant Pediatric Otolaryngologist, Great Ormond Street Hospital for Children, London WC1N 3JH, United Kingdom.

- *Practical Pediatric Otolaryngology*
- edited by Robin T. Cotton and Charles M. Myer, III
- Lippincott-Raven Publishers, Philadelphia © 1999

CHAPTER 40

Recurrent Respiratory Papillomatosis

Craig S. Derkay

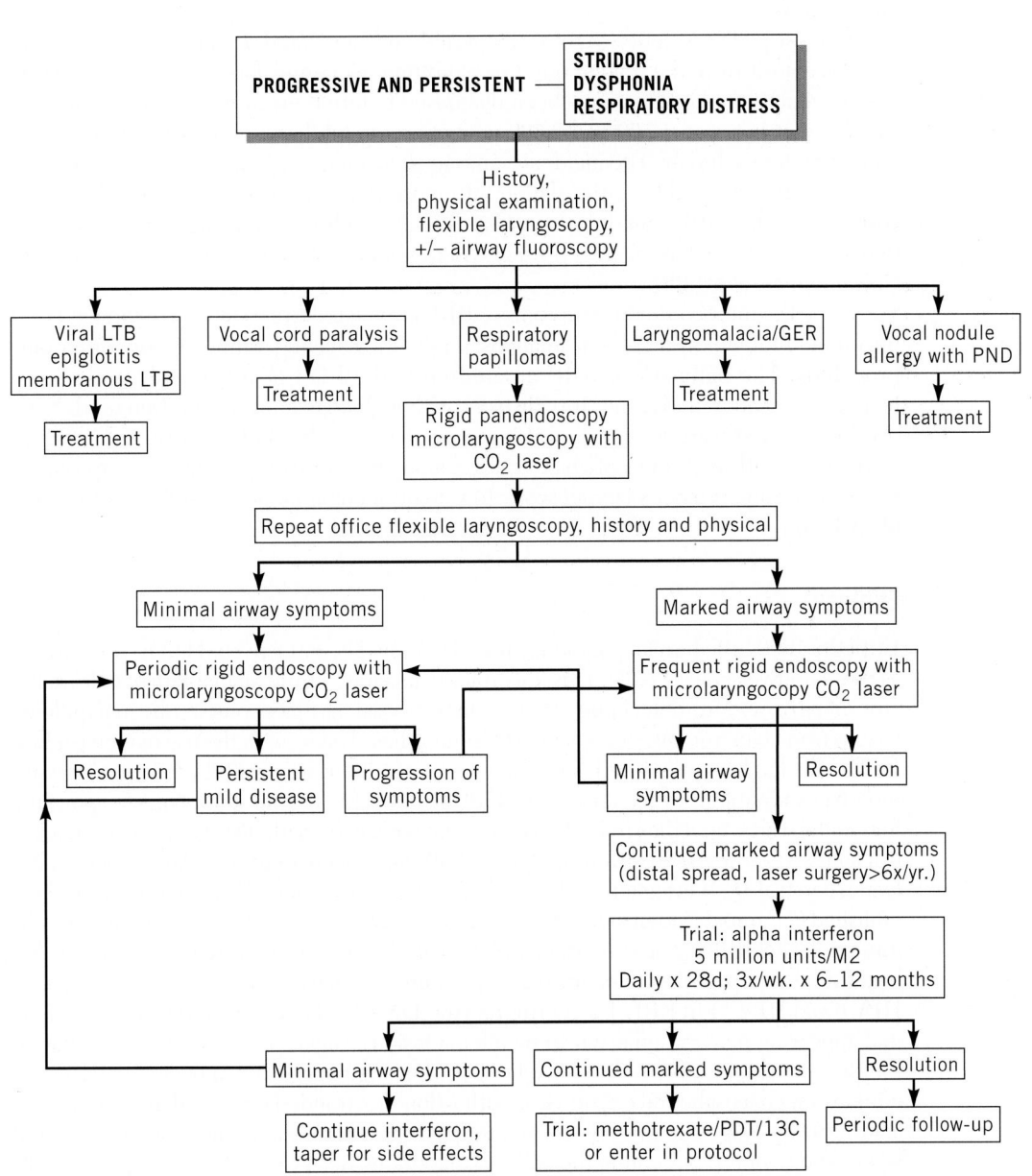

◉ HISTORICAL BACKGROUND

Recurrent respiratory papillomatosis (RRP) is both the most common benign neoplasm of the larynx among children and the second most frequent cause of childhood hoarseness (1). RRP is often difficult to treat because of its tendency to recur and spread throughout the respiratory tract. Although it most often involves the larynx, RRP may involve the entire aerodigestive tract. The course of the disease is variable, with some patients experiencing spontaneous remission and others suffering from aggressive papillomatous growth, requiring multiple surgical procedures over many years. The clinical course is unpredictable, with malignant transformation possible in chronic invasive papillomatosis. RRP may have its clinical onset during either childhood or adulthood. Two distinct forms are generally recognized: a *juvenile* or aggressive form and an *adult* or less aggressive form. The aggressive form, although most prevalent in children, can also occur in adults.

In most pediatric series, RRP is diagnosed between 2 and 3 years of age with a delay in diagnosis from the time of onset of symptoms averaging about 1 year (2). Seventy-five percent of the children have been diagnosed before their fifth birthday (3). It is estimated that between 1,500 and 2,500 new cases of childhood-onset RRP occur in the United States each year. The incidence among children in the United States is estimated at 4.3 per 100,000 children, translating into more than 15,000 surgical procedures at a cost of more than $100 million per year (4). Anecdotal observations suggest that most patients are first-born, have young, primigravid mothers, and come from families of low socioeconomic status (4,5).

Since the most common symptoms of RRP are related to airway obstruction, it is not uncommon for children to be misdiagnosed initially as having asthma, croup, or chronic bronchitis. The hallmark of RRP in children is the triad of relentlessly progressive hoarseness, stridor, and respiratory distress. Although hoarseness in children tends to be overlooked or at least accepted until it reaches a certain level of severity, any infant or young child with symptoms of voice change, along with obstructive airway symptoms or recurrent croup, warrants laryngoscopy to rule out neoplasia, of which RRP is the most likely lesion.

Etiology

Until the 1990s, the human papillomavirus (HPV) had been suspected but not confirmed as the causative agent in RRP. This uncertainty developed from an inability to culture the virus *in vitro,* and from the failure to demonstrate viral particles consistently in papilloma lesions using electron microscopy or HPV antibodies. Today, with the use of viral probes, HPV DNA has been identified in virtually every papilloma lesion studied. The most common types identified in the airway are HPV 6 and HPV 11, the same types responsible for genital warts. Specific viral subtypes may be correlated with disease severity and clinical course (6). Almost 70 different types of HPV have been identified. An association between cervical HPV infection in the mother and the incidence of RRP has been well established (7). Initial evidence for this association was established by electron microscopy, immunocytochemistry, and Southern blot hybridization analysis. Recently, *in situ* hybridization and polymerase chain reaction techniques have confirmed the presence of HPV 6 and HPV 11 in RRP. Furthermore, viral DNA has been detected in areas of "normal appearing mucosa" adjacent to papilloma lesions, suggesting a possible explanation for the recurrence of the disease following thorough surgical removal (8). HPV is a nonenveloped icosahedral capsid virus with a double-stranded circular deoxyribonucleic acid 7,900 bp long. The present understanding is that HPV establishes itself in the basal layer, where viral DNA enters the cell and elaborates RNA to produce viral proteins. In addition to HPV 6 and HPV 11, subtypes 16 and 18 have also been found in RRP lesions. HPV 16 is the most frequently detected HPV in the genital tract. It is only rarely seen in benign aerodigestive tract lesions, whereas it is detected in 5% to 20% of aerodigestive tract squamous carcinomas. In the aerodigestive tract, HPVs frequently cause latent infection, (i.e., viral DNA present in tissue but no evidence of clinical or histologic disease). Brandsma and Abramson (9) reported finding HPV DNA in 4% of random, clinically normal biopsies of the airway. Adult-onset respiratory papillomas could reflect either activation of virus present since birth or an infection acquired in adolescence or adult life.

The universality of HPV in the lower genital tract rivals that of any other sexually transmitted disease in humans. It is estimated that at least 1 million cases of genital papillomas occur per year in the United States (10). These most often manifest as condylomata acuminata involving the cervix, vulva, or other anogenital sites in women or the penis of male sexual partners of affected women. HPV has been noted to be present in the genital tract of as many as 25% of all women of child-bearing age worldwide. Clinically apparent HPV infection has been noted in 1.5% to 5% of pregnant women in the United States (11). As in RRP, HPV 6 and 11 are the most common subtypes identified in cervical condylomata. Ten percent of sexually active men and women with no evidence of disease have been shown to have HPV identified on the penis or cervix by Southern blot hybridization analysis, suggesting the presence of a latent infection (10).

Histology

RRP lesions occur most often at anatomic sites in which ciliated and squamous epithelium are juxtaposed (12). Histologically, RRP appears as pedunculated masses with finger-like projections of nonkeratinized stratified squamous epithelium supported by a core of highly vascularized connective tissue stroma (Fig. 1). The basal layer may be either normal or hyperplastic, and mitotic figures are generally limited to this layer. Cellular differentiation appears to be abnormal, with altered expression and production of keratins. The degree of atypia may be a sign of premalignant tendency, although HPV types and subtypes do not strongly correlate with clinical outcomes (6). The most common sites for RRP are the limen vestibuli, the nasopharyngeal surface of the soft palate, the midzone of the laryngeal surface of the epiglottis, the upper and lower margins of the ventricle, the undersurface of the vocal folds, the carina, and at bronchial spurs (12). In tracheotomized patients, RRP are often encountered at the stoma and in the midthoracic trachea, areas that might be considered iatrogenic squamociliary junctions. Papilloma lesions may be sessile or pedunculated and often occur in irregular exophytic clusters (Fig. 2). Typically, the lesions are pinkish to white in coloration. Iatrogenic implantation of papilloma may be preventible by avoiding injury to nondiseased squamous or ciliated epithelium adjacent to areas of frank papilloma. Ciliated epithelium undergoes squamous metaplasia when exposed to repeated trauma and is replaced with nonciliated epithelium that creates an iatragenic squamociliary junction. It is postulated that an eddying flow of the mucus blanket at squamociliary junctions may concentrate infectious virus particles at these sites.

Epidemiology

RRP may affect people of any age, with the youngest patient identified at 1 day of age and the oldest at 84 years (4). Childhood-onset RRP (arbitrarily defined as patients diagnosed at less than 12 years of age) is most often diagnosed between 2 and 3 years of age. Adult RRP peaks between the ages of 20 and 40 and has a slight male predilection; distribution among boys and girls is approximately equal. Childhood-onset RRP is more common and is more aggressive than its adult counterpart. In a recent survey of practicing otolaryngologists in the United States, half of the adults with RRP had required fewer than five procedures over their lifetime compared with less than 25% of the children. Approximately equal percentages of children and adults (17% children versus 19% adults) had very aggressive RRP (defined as requiring more than 40 lifetime operations), although adults had more years to accumulate these operations (4).

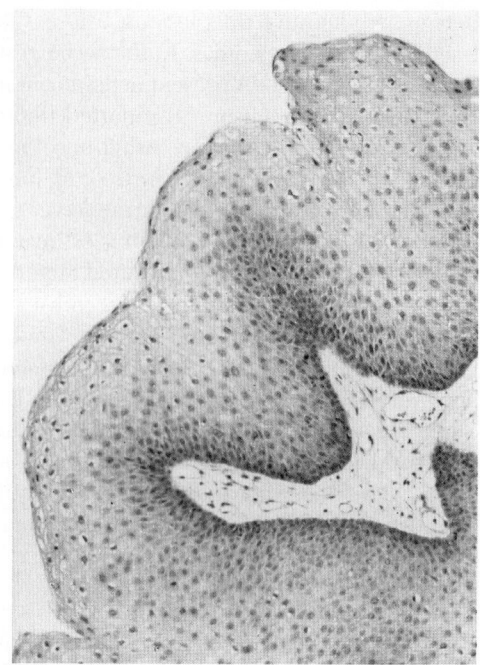

FIGURE 1 Low-power hematoxylin & eosin photomicrograph of respiratory papilloma.

The true incidence and prevalence of RRP are uncertain. In a Danish subpopulation incorporating 50% of the population of that country, the incidence of laryngeal papillomatosis was 3.84 cases per 100,000 (13). The rate among children was 3.62 per 100,000, whereas adult-onset cases occurred at a rate of 3.94 per 100,000. These figures are comparable with those found in a recent U.S. survey, which estimated an incidence in the pediatric population of 4.3 per 100,000 children and 1.8 per 100,000 adults. This translates into roughly 2,300 new pediatric cases per year in the United States (4).

The precise mode of HPV transmission remains unclear. Several studies have convincingly linked childhood-onset RRP to mothers with genital HPV infections, whereas circumstantial evidence suggests that adult disease may be associated with oral–genital contact. Cook et al. (14) first reported an association of juvenile laryngeal papillomatosis with maternal condylomata at the time of delivery. Quick et al. (15) reported that 60% of children with laryngeal papillomatosis were born to mothers who had genital warts at the

FIGURE 2 Endoscopic view of laryngeal papilloma.

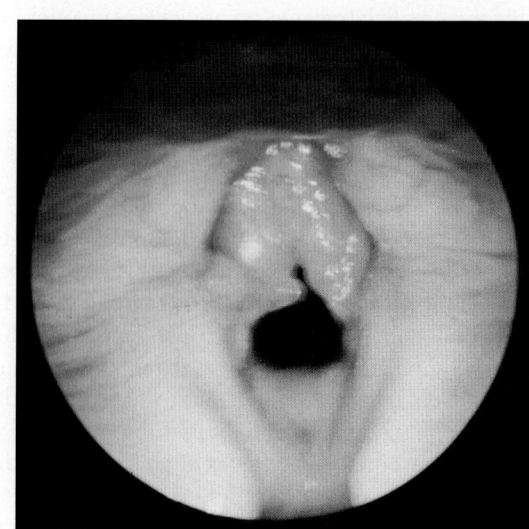

time of delivery. Condylomatas in the male sexual partners were not recorded in any of these studies, and subclinical disease was not detected or investigated.

Retrospective studies and a recent prospective study confirmed that HPV may be passed by vertical transmission from mother to child (11,16). In addition, Kashima et al. (5) found that childhood-onset RRP patients were more likely to be first-born and vaginally delivered than were control patients of similar age. This finding was corroborated by the anecdotal observations in a U.S. survey of otolaryngologists (4). Kashima et al. (5) hypothesized that primigravid mothers are more likely to have a long second stage of labor and that the prolonged exposure to the virus leads to a higher risk of infection in the first-born child. They also suggested that newly acquired genital HPV lesions are more likely to shed virus than long-standing lesions, thus explaining the higher incidence of papilloma disease observed among the offspring of young mothers of low socioeconomic status, the same group that is most likely to acquire sexually transmitted diseases such as HPV. Despite the apparent close association between maternal condylomata and the development of RRP, few children exposed to genital warts at birth actually develop clinical symptoms (17). It is not well understood why RRP develops in so few children whose mothers have condylomata. The most likely method of maternal–fetal HPV transmission is through direct contact in the birth canal (7). This would explain the clinical observation that most children in whom RRPs develop are delivered vaginally to mothers with a history of genital condylomatas. Although HPV could be recovered from the nasopharyngeal secretions of 47% of infants exposed to HPV in the birth canal (18), the number of infants expected to manifest evidence of RRP is only a small fraction of this. Clearly, other factors (patient immunity, timing, length and volume of virus exposure, and local trauma) must be important determinants of development of RRP.

PEARLS AND PERILS

1. RRP, although more frequent in improverished children, crosses socioeconomic lines.
2. Only 50% to 60% of RRP patients will have a maternal/paternal history of HPV.
3. Avoid laying guilt on parents.
4. The vast majority of children will have glottic and/or subglottic disease; if this is not evident on flexible examination, you should still proceed with rigid endoscopy, if the history is suggestive.
5. Although the most common age at presentation is 2 to 3 years, you should still be wary of infants and neonatal intensive care unit graduates presenting in respiratory distress.
6. Some children with RRP will present in acute distress. Be prepared to manage them urgently.

An occasional child with RRP has been delivered by cesarean section. Shah et al. (17) reported that only 1% of 109 childhood-onset RRP cases reviewed gave a history of birth by cesarean section before rupture of uterine membranes. Even though cesarean section would seem to reduce the risk of transmission of the disease, this procedure is associated with a higher morbidity and mortality for the mother and a much higher economic cost than elective vaginal delivery. Shah et al. (17) estimated that the risk of a child contracting the disease from a mother who has an active condylomatous lesion and delivers vaginally is only about 1 in 400. The characteristics that differentiate this one child from the other 399 are elusive. In light of the uncertainty surrounding intrapartum exposure, there is presently insufficient evidence to support delivery by cesarean section in all pregnant women with condylomata (7). Reports of neonatal papillomatosis suggest that, in at least some cases, development of the disease may occur *in utero*. Since cesarean section still does not prevent the development of papilloma disease in all cases, a better understanding of the risk factors associated with RRP is needed before the efficacy of cesarean delivery in preventing papilloma disease can be fully assessed.

Clinical Features

Children with RRP most often present with some degree of dysphonia. Unfortunately, particularly in young children, changes in voice may go unnoticed. Stridor is often the second clinical symptom to develop, beginning as an inspiratory noise and becoming biphasic with progression of the disease. Less commonly, chronic cough, recurrent pneumonia, failure to thrive, dyspnea, dysphagia, and acute life-threatening events may be the presenting symptoms. The duration of symptoms prior to diagnosis varies. Not uncommonly, a mistaken diagnosis of asthma, croup, allergies, vocal nodules, or bronchitis is entertained before a definitive diagnosis is made. When death occurs, it is usually associated with a complication of frequent surgical procedures or caused by respiratory failure due to distal disease progression. RRP presenting in the neonatal period is thought to be a negative prognostic factor with a greater likelihood for mortality and need for tracheotomy. Because of the rarity of RRP and the slowly progressive nature of the disease, some cases may go unrecognized until respiratory distress results from papillomas obstructing the airway. The result is a relatively high need for tracheotomy to be performed in these children. Tracheotomy was necessary at some point in the management of 14% of children reported in two independent series; the frequency of tracheotomy among adults with RRP was estimated at about 6% (4,19). It has been suggested that tracheotomy may activate or spread disease lower in the respiratory tract. Cole et al. (20) reported that tracheal papillomas developed in half of their tracheotomy patients and that, despite attempts to avoid this procedure, 21% of their patients still require a long-term tracheotomy. Prolonged tracheotomy, and the presence of subglottic papilloma at the time of tracheotomy, have been associated with an increased risk of distal tracheal spread. Most authors agree that tracheotomy is a procedure to be avoided unless absolutely necessary. When a tracheotomy is unavoidable, decannulation should be considered as soon as the disease is managed effectively with endoscopic techniques.

Children with bronchopulmonary dysplasia who require prolonged endotracheal intubation may also be at increased risk for development of RRP. Through interruption of the continuous respiratory mucosal surface, an endotracheal tube may have the same role in the mechanical dissemination/implantation of RRP as tracheotomy. Extralaryngeal spread of respiratory papillomas have been identified in approximately 30% of children and in 16% of adults with RRP. The most frequent sites of extralaryngeal spread were, in order of frequency, the oral cavity, trachea, and bronchi (4). A possible link between RRP and immunodeficiency states has also been observed. Both children and adults with the acquired immunodeficiency syndrome or congenital immunodeficiencies or those on immune suppression after organ transplantation have been identified with RRP (4).

Malignant transformation of RRP into squamous cell carcinoma has been documented in several case reports. A total of 26 patients was identified as having progressed to squamous cell carcinoma in the Task Force survey (4). Lindeberg and Elbrond (19) recorded three RRP patients with neoplastic progression. Interestingly, all three had received prior radiotherapy and two were heavy smokers, suggesting that these may be important cofactors for malignant transformation. Lie et al. (21) reported on seven cases of laryngeal carcinomas and one patient with spread of papilloma to the bronchial tree who developed a bronchial carcinoma. The mean time between onset of papilloma and diagnosis of carcinoma was 24 years. In addition to smoking and irradiation, bleomycin was thought to be an important cofactor in Lie et al.'s series (21).

🔊 PATIENT ASSESSMENT

History

Progressive or persistent stridor and dysphonia, with the possible development of respiratory distress, are the most consistent signs and symptoms of RRP in children. In the absence of severe respiratory distress, a careful history should be obtained. Information regarding the time of onset of symptoms, possible airway trauma including a history of previous intubation, and characteristics of the cry are obviously important. Hoarseness, although a common and often benign clinical complaint in young children, always indicates some abnormality of structure or function. Because of the precision of laryngeal mechanics, hoarseness may result from a remarkably small lesion and thus be an early sign in the course of a disease process. On the other hand, if the lesion's origin is remote from the vocal cords, hoarseness may present as a late sign. Although it is histologically the same lesion, a papilloma that produces hoarseness in one patient may produce stridor and obstruction in another, depending on the size and location of the lesion. The quality of the voice change may give only limited clues to its etiology; other characteristics such as age of onset, rate of progression, associated infection, history of trauma or surgery, and the presence of respiratory or cardiac distress may be of much greater significance. A low-pitched, coarse, fluttering voice suggests a subglottic lesion, and a high-pitched, cracking voice, aphonia, or a breathy voice suggests a glottic lesion. Associated high-pitched stridor also suggests a glottic or subglottic lesion. Although stridor that has been present since birth is more often associated with laryngomalacia, subglottic stenosis, vocal cord paralysis, or a vascular ring, it should be realized that neonates can also present with papillomatosis. Associated symptoms such as feeding difficulties, allergic symptoms, vocal abuse, and the presence of hereditary congenital anomalies may help sort RRP from alternative diagnoses including vocal fold nodules, vocal fold paralysis, subglottic cysts, subglottic hemangioma, and subglottic stenosis. In the absence of any history suggesting these lesions, review of the perinatal period may reveal a history of maternal or paternal condylomata.

If the onset of stridor and dysphonia is gradual and progressive over weeks or months, then neoplastic growth compromising the airway must be considered and investigated. Papillomas of the larynx usually do not become symptomatic before 6 months of age. By contrast, subglottic hemangiomas typically appear between 1 and 3 months of age, with 85% present by 6 months. Additionally, 50% of children with subglottic hemangiomas will have an associated skin hemangioma. Certainly not every child with a hoarse voice or cry merits investigation beyond an assessment of the symptom. However, in the presence of hoarseness with respiratory distress, tachypnea, decreased air entry, tachycardia, cyanosis, dysphagia, chronic cough, failure to thrive, recurrent pneumonia, or dysphagia, the larynx must be visualized and a firm diagnosis of the cause of hoarseness made. Any child with slowly progressive hoarseness merits investigation, and the clinician should not wait until total aphonia or airway problems occur. Additionally, the child with rapidly progressive stridor and hoarseness or aphonia in the absence of obvious infectious etiology should raise a high degree of suspicion for an aspirated foreign body warranting urgent intervention.

Physical Examination

Children who present with symptoms consistent with RRP must undergo a thorough and organized physical examination. The child's respiratory rate and degree of distress must first be assessed. The physician should observe the child for tachypnea or the onset of fatigue that may indicate impending respiratory collapse. The child should be observed for flaring of the nasal alae and the use of accessory neck or chest muscles. Increasing cyanosis and air hunger may cause the child to sit with the neck hyperextended in an attempt to improve air flow. If a child is gravely ill, additional examination should not be undertaken outside the operating room, the emergency room, or the intensive care unit, where resuscitation equipment for intubation of the airway, endoscopic evaluation, and possible tracheotomy are readily available. In the stable, well-oxygenated child additional examination can proceed. The most important part of the examination is auscultation with the aid of a stethoscope. The physician should listen over the nose, open mouth, neck, and chest to help localize the probable site of the respiratory obstruction. The author prefers to pull the bell off the stethoscope and listen over these areas with the open tube. The respiratory cycle, which normally is composed of a shorter inspiratory phase and a longer expiratory phase, should then be observed. Stridor of a laryngeal origin is most often musical and may begin as inspiratory but will progress to biphasic with worsening airway narrowing. Infants with stridor should be placed in various positions to determine their effect on the stridor. A child with RRP would not be expected to demonstrate much change in the stridor with position change, in contrast to infants with laryngomalacia, a vascular ring, or a mediastinal mass. Pulse oximetry can add an accurate quantitative analysis of the child's respiratory state. In the stable patient in whom asthma is high on the differential diagnosis, pulmonary function testing combined with arterial blood gas evaluation may also be helpful. Inspiratory and expiratory air flow in relation to lung volume can be assessed by means of a flow–volume loop to assist the physician in localizing obstructions or restrictions of the airway.

Imaging

In the patient without airway distress, appropriate radiologic evaluation of the upper aerodigestive tract may proceed after a careful history and physical examination. Fluoroscopy with the use of barium contrast medium is the radiographic study of choice. This will allow evaluation of both the inspiratory and expiratory phases of respiration. It allows the physician to evaluate the contribution of gastroesophageal reflux or encroachment by an anomaly of the great vessels to the child's airway abnormality as well as to the possible diagnosis of foreign body or airway neoplasm. Computed tomography and magnetic resonance imaging are rarely necessary, although they may be helpful in evaluating the mediastinum for masses or aberrant vessels. I do not find ultrasound or nuclear medicine studies to have any value in diagnosing RRP.

Airway Endoscopy

The preoperative diagnosis of RRP is best made with a flexible fiberoptic nasopharyngoscope. Careful, sequential inspection of the pharynx, hypopharynx, larynx, and subglottis provides the critical information necessary to make the diagnosis of RRP and allows estimation of lumen size, vocal cord mobility, and the urgency of operative intervention. Advances in instrumentation of flexible nasopharyngoscopes have resulted in instruments as small as 1.9 mm in diameter that even allow passage in neonates. Such small-diameter scopes still provide images that can be seen on a video monitor and recorded for later review. Topical decongestion and local anesthesia can be applied by spray, dropper, or pledget. Oxymetazoline is the decongestant of choice because of its lack of cardiac side effects. Either topical ponticaine or lidocaine may be used to enhance patient cooperation, but dosage must be critically monitored in the small infant to avoid cardiotoxicity. The author finds that visualization with the flexible nasopharyngoscope in young children is far superior to that obtained with indirect mirror laryngoscopy. Patient cooperation, however, is required even with good topical anesthesia. In infants, this is not a large issue because they can easily be restrained in a sitting-up position for evaluation in the parent's or nurse's lap. Likewise, most children over 6 or 7 years of age can be "talked into" cooperating for the examination. It is the intermediate age group, between 1 and 6 years of age, who may be the most difficult to examine, taxing the patience and skill of even the most experienced clinicians. Although dynamic evaluation is best appreciated when children are breathing spontaneously, endoscopy in the operating room under anesthesia is warranted in any child suspected to have RRP who cannot be fully examined in the outpatient setting.

 TREATMENT RECOMMENDATIONS

Preoperative Preparation

The gold standard for endoscopic diagnosis of RRP is still operative-direct laryngoscopy. This can be performed with or without general anesthesia in the neonate but requires a general anesthetic for older infants and children. It is ideally performed in the operating room, where resuscitation equipment, small endotracheal tubes, and a tracheotomy set are readily available. Cooperation between the surgeon, anesthesiologist, and operating room staff is imperative in the examination of the upper airway in children. In the child suspected (but not confirmed) to have RRP, consent should be obtained for direct laryngoscopy, bronchoscopy, biopsy, possible use of the CO_2 laser for vaporization, and possible tracheotomy.

Children newly diagnosed with RRP warrant a substantial time commitment on the part of the otolaryngologist and health-care team. Since most RRP patients require frequent office visits, periodic therapies, and endoscopic procedures following the initial diagnosis, it behooves the otolaryngologist to start his/her relationship with the child and its family off on the right foot. The need for continued contact enables the health-care team to get a feel for the child's symptoms and level of distress and the aggressiveness of the disease and provides the family with a frank and open discussion of the disease and its management.

If this is the child's first surgery, the otolaryngologist should discuss all aspects of the surgery, as well as the possibility of laser complications and the need for tracheotomy. Once the child's diagnosis is established, many families benefit from the ability to network with other papilloma patients in their community. This contact is best arranged through the otolaryngologist's practice when feasible. Support groups, such as the Recurrent Respiratory Papilloma Foundation (609-530-1443), can be a tremendous resource to these families for information and stability.

Before the child enters the operating suite, the surgeon, anesthesiologist, and operating room team must select the proper size endotracheal tubes, laryngoscopes, and bronchoscopes and ascertain that all ancillary equipment, including telescopes, light cords, suction tips, and forceps are available and properly functioning. All equipment used for the procedure including the surgical microscope with appropriate size lens, the laser unit, the micromanipulator, filtered suction, and smoke evacuation units should be checked for proper functioning. In our institution, the surgeon personally checks the laser for beam alignment by test firing it prior to the child entering the room.

Laser safety is carefully monitored in our hospital by the laser safety committee. This includes a laser safety officer, a physician for each specialty that uses the laser, nurses from the operating room, a hospital administrator, and a biomedical engineer. All operating room (OR) personnel are required to wear eye protection whenever working around the laser. Specially designed laser masks are required to be worn by OR personnel during the surgery to prevent the inhalation of viral particles liberated during the laser procedure.

Before initiating anesthesia, the surgeon should discuss the pathology with the anesthesiologist. Additionally, the OR staff should be informed of the surgeon's concerns so that appropriate instrumentation is ready. Intraoperative teamwork is enhanced with the use of video monitors during the operation as this allows the entire staff to follow the procedure as it progresses. Dialogue between the surgeon and the anesthesiologist continues throughout the case regarding the current status of ventilation, the amount of bleeding encountered, the motion of the vocal cords, the timing of laser use in conjunction with respiration, and the concentration of oxygen in the anesthesia mix. The ultimate decision about the anesthesia technique should be shared between the anesthesiologist and the surgeon. When utilizing an endotracheal tube, the smallest possible laser-safe endotracheal tube should be used that allows for adequate ventilation. If a cuffed tube is necessary, then the cuff should be filled with saline so that, if it is inadvertently struck by the laser beam, the saline acts as a heat sink and fire extinguisher. Some surgeons prefer to use methylene blue-colorized saline to provide an additional warning in case the cuff is penetrated. The laser-ignited airway explosion is a shocking emergency. Prompt, appropriate management is facilitated if the OR team has previously "rehearsed" and discussed this potential disaster.

PEARLS AND PERILS

---

1. Be prepared in the operating room. Have two of everything and a trach set in the room.
2. Discuss case management with anesthesia and OR staff before the child comes into the OR.
3. Participate in the setup of the laser and other equipment to check on their performance.
4. Establish a team: laser nurse, OR staff, safety program.
5. Avoid unexperienced personnel (CRNA students, junior residents, locum tenem anesthesiologists).
6. Watch depth of penetration of laser and avoid anterior and posterior commissures.
7. Be flexible: develop your skills in the use of the laser bronchoscope, KTP laser, and resectoscope.
8. Send a specimen. Follow children for development of atypia and malignancy. Perform HPV typing.

Operative Procedure

No single modality has consistently been shown to be effective in eradication of RRP. The current standard of care is surgical therapy with a goal of complete removal of papillomas and preservation of normal structures. In patients in whom anterior or posterior commissure disease or highly aggressive papillomas are present, the goal may be subtotal removal with clearing of the airway. Although the CO_2 laser allows for precision of surgery and excellent hemostasis, multiple procedures are often necessary. It is advisable to debulk as much disease as possible while preserving normal morphology and anatomy and preventing the complications of subglottic and glottic stenosis, web formation, and a diminished airway. Frequent interval laser laryngoscopies are recommended in an attempt to avoid tracheotomy and permit the child to develop good phonation with preservation of normal vocal cord anatomy.

The CO_2 laser has been favored over cold instruments in the treatment of RRP involving the larynx, pharynx, upper trachea, and nasal and oral cavities (4). When coupled to an operating microscope, the laser vaporizes the lesions with precision causing minimal bleeding. When used with a no-touch technique, it minimizes damage to the vocal cords and limits scarring. The CO_2 laser has an emission wave length of 10,600 nm and converts light to thermal energy. It provides a controlled destruction of tissues with vaporization of water. It also cauterizes tissue surfaces. The smoke plume contains water vapor and destroyed tissue material. Although the CO_2 laser is the most commonly used laser for RRP in the larynx, the KTP, as well as the Argon laser, could also be used. The newest generation of laser microspot micromanipulator enables the surgeon to utilize a spot size of 250 mm at 400-mm focal length and 160 mm at 250-mm focal length. The 710 Accuspot Sharplan laser is our current choice for managing RRP of the larynx. This unit allows direct visualization of the surgical target with elimination of the parallax problem inherent in earlier models. The author utilizes the Accuspot in the defocused mode to debulk papilloma initially and then focuses the 250 mm spot size to excise papilloma from potentially tricky areas such as near the anterior and/or posterior commissure and along the true vocal cords. I may also combine its use with a subglottiscope for removal of papilloma in the subglottic trachea.

Most children with RRP require repeated laser surgeries with a median of 7 operative procedures in Lindeberg and Elbrond's series (19) and 13 operations in Morgan and Zitsch's series (1). It is helpful when tracking the progression of a child's disease, communicating with other surgeons, and treating patients in a protocol format to have a surgical scoring system to assess severity and clinical course of RRP disease. Kashima (22) devised a relatively simple format that was utilized during the Alpha-n-1-interferon multiinstitutional trial (Table 1). Other scoring systems have been in use at the University of Alabama, Birmingham and the Children's National Medical Center, Washington, DC, and a computerized system is currently being devised at the Centers for Disease Control, Atlanta, Georgia, for eventual application with the national RRP patient registry (23).

Since there is currently no therapeutic regimen that reliably eradicates the HPV, when there is a question about whether papilloma in an area needs to be removed, it is prudent to accept some residual papilloma rather than risk damage to normal tissue and producing excessive scarring. Even with the removal of all clinically evident papilloma, latent virus may remain in adjacent tissue, which may explain the recurrent nature of RRP. Therefore, the aim of therapy in extensive disease should be to reduce the tumor burden, decrease the spread of disease, create a safe and patent airway, improve voice quality, and increase the time interval between surgical procedures. Staged papilloma removal for disease in the anterior commissure is appropriate to prevent the apposition of two raw mucosal surfaces. The surgeon who is not aware of injury to deeper tissue layers with injudicious laser usage may encounter unacceptable scarring and subsequent abnormal vocal fold function. Inappropriate and aggressive use of the laser may also cause injury to nonaffected tissues and create an environment suitable for implantation of viral particles. Use of the CO_2 laser can also result in delayed local tissue damage, which may be related to the total number of laser surgeries and the severity of RRP disease.

After informed consent has been obtained from the appropriate family members, including a discussion regarding potential laser complications and the possibility of tracheotomy, the child is brought into an operating room that has been prepared and in-

TABLE 1: Scoring System for Recurrent Respiratory Papillomatosis

Factor or site	Points
Based on three factors at a variety of sites	
Presence of disease	1
Obstruction of >1/3 of airway lumen	1
Involvement of >1/3 of surface area	1
Sites	Maximum of 27
Epiglottis	
Aryepiglottic folds	
False vocal cords	
Ventricle	
True vocal cords	
Trachea	
Tracheotomy site	
Carina	
Mainstream bronchus	

(From ref. 22, with permission.)

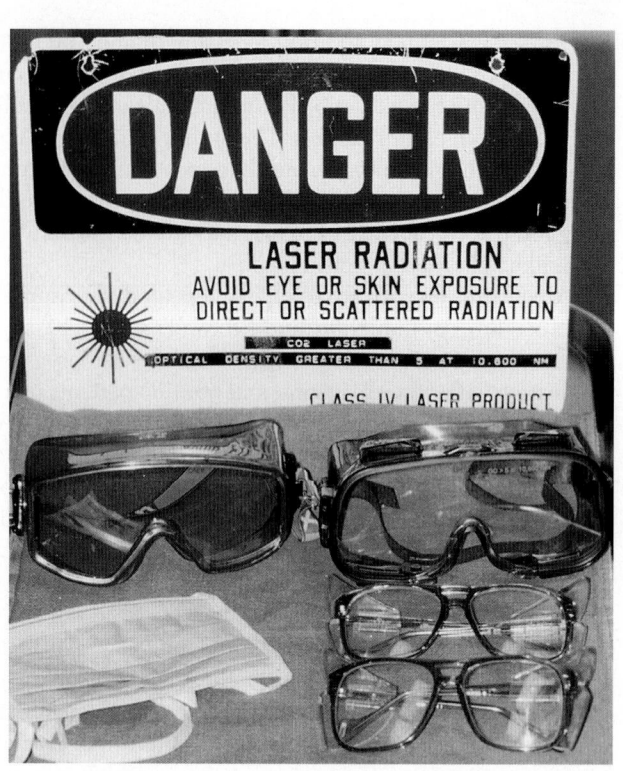

FIGURE 3 Micropore laser filtration masks and protective eyewear utilized by all operating room personnel during RRP surgery.

spected by the surgeon and the laser team. When performing surgery for RRP, it is advisable to have an experienced team of OR nurses familiar with the sequence in which equipment is used and instructed in the proper use of the laser. In our facility we also have a laser safety team and provide yearly updates for the OR staff to ensure everyone's familiarity with the equipment and its potential complications. All our pediatric anesthesiologists are acquainted and comfortable with microlaryngoscopy laser surgery in children. However, in a non-children's hospital or nonacademic setting, if there are but one or two anesthesiologists experienced with these techniques, they should be exclusively utilized, whenever possible. This type of surgery is not well suited to the novice surgeon, anesthesiologist, or OR nurse. It is our practice to insist that the attending anesthesiologist be present with hands-on involvement in all critical portions of the surgical procedure, including induction, securing of the endotracheal tube, positioning of the patient, changing of anesthesia techniques from a laser-safe tube to apnea technique, and extubation.

In our institution the laser team consists of a scrub nurse, a circulating nurse, and a laser nurse. The laser is the responsibility of the laser nurse, which then allows the circulator and scrub nurse to concentrate on their duties. All OR personnel are equipped with micropore laser filtration masks and approved goggles (Fig. 3). The room is set up in advance with a suspension microlaryngoscope (Lindholm), a full set of Parson's laryngoscopes, two appropriately sized ventilating bronchoscopes, and 7200A and 8700A Hopkins Rod telescopes. A microscope with a 400-mm lens is fitted with the AccuSpot 710 micromanipulator (Fig. 4). An assortment of suctions, alligators, cup forceps, and light cords, as well as a pack of neuropathies and topical oxymetazoline drops are also standard. An endoscopy video cart equipped with color TV monitor, VCR, three-chip camera, and xenon light source are also utilized (Fig. 5). Still photography through the endoscope is available as needed. Additionally, a pediatric tracheotomy set is brought into the room, although it is not opened unless specifically requested.

The surgical sequence begins with the mask induction utilizing halothane and the establishment of intravenous access. Cefazolin at 20 mg per kilogram are routinely administered preoperatively. The larynx is exposed utilizing the Parson's laryngoscope attached

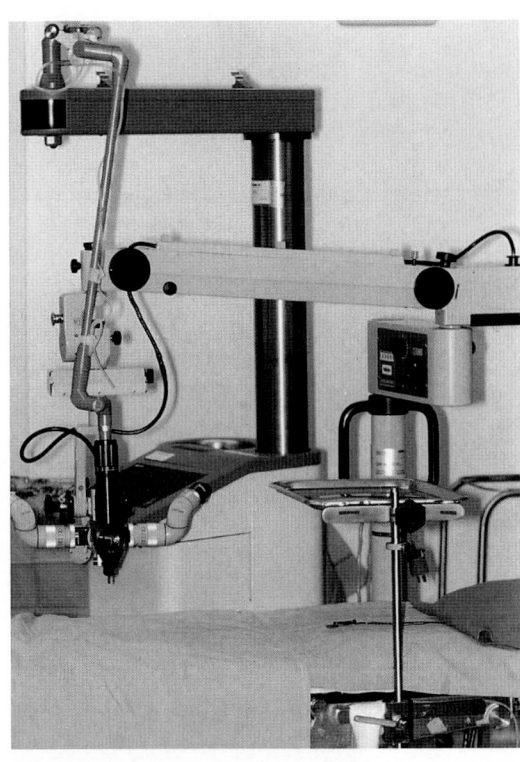

FIGURE 4 Typical microlaryngoscopy setup for RRP surgery.

to 6 L per minute of oxygen flow through its insufflation port, and the vocal folds are then sprayed with 2% lidocaine utilizing a syringe attached to a Cass needle. A diagnostic laryngoscopy is then performed utilizing the 7200A telescope under video control to assess the degree of papilloma disease and its encroachment on the laryngeal airway. Depending on the extent of disease, the child's history, and the interval since the last endoscopy, a full tracheoscopy and bronchoscopy may be performed. Again, depending on the child's level of preoperative and operative distress, the surgeon may choose to perform this maneuver either with the 7200A telescope (if there is a low likelihood of discovering distal disease) or with an appropriate size ventilating bronchoscope (if there is high likelihood of discovering distal disease). Still photography with the 8700A telescope is then performed at this stage, if desirable. If no distal disease is present, then the patient is intubated by the surgeon with a laser safe tube (metal Xomed-Treace) of the smallest caliber that will allow the anesthesiologist adequate ventilation. Once the airway has been secured with the endotracheal tube, the anesthesiologist is given the option to administer muscle relaxants. As an alternative, the child may be maintained on Propofol. It should be stressed that no muscle relaxants are administered until the surgeon has assessed the degree of laryngeal obstruction and ascertained that the airway has been secured. This precaution serves to prevent the situation in which the child has lost his or her respiratory drive, obstructing the airway with papilloma and/or blood or mucus and precipitating hypoxia and a possible laryngospasm.

Once the airway has been secured, the endotracheal tube is taped in place with a single piece of tape (allowing the surgeon easy access for removal of the endotracheal tube in the case of an airway fire) and the child suspended for microlaryngoscopy with the Lindholm microlaryngoscope. The author prefers to suspend the Lindholm to either a Mayo stand attached to the OR table or to a suspension platform fashioned from plexiglass. These two devices allow the microsuspension system to be moved along with the patient and permit angulation of the laryngoscope over a 120° range. The child's eyes are then protected with moist saline-soaked gauze eye pads against any stray laser beam exposure. Lubricant is placed in the eyes and the operative field is draped with moistened

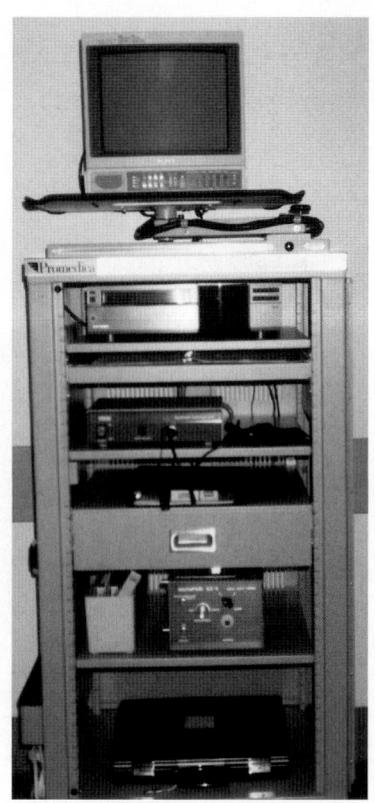

FIGURE 5 Sample video cart setup for RRP surgery.

towels. OR personnel are equipped with ocular protection including side shields, and a sign is posted outside the operating room warning that a laser procedure is occurring. A spare set of safety glasses is left outside the door for operating room personnel who wish to come inside the room while the laser is in operation. Special laser masks with extremely small pores are worn to minimize exposure to the laser plume. A high-volume smoke evacuator is attached to one port of the Lindholm to collect the laser plume. (Fig. 6). A second suction attached to the smoke evacuator is utilized by the surgeon. By this point, the fractional concentration of oxygen in inspired gas (FI,O_2) delivered to the patient should be as close to a room-air mixture as possible. Ideally, the laser is not utilized until the oxygen in the mixture is between 26% and 30%. In selected circumstances, it

FIGURE 6 Smoke-evacuator system utilized for laser RRP surgery.

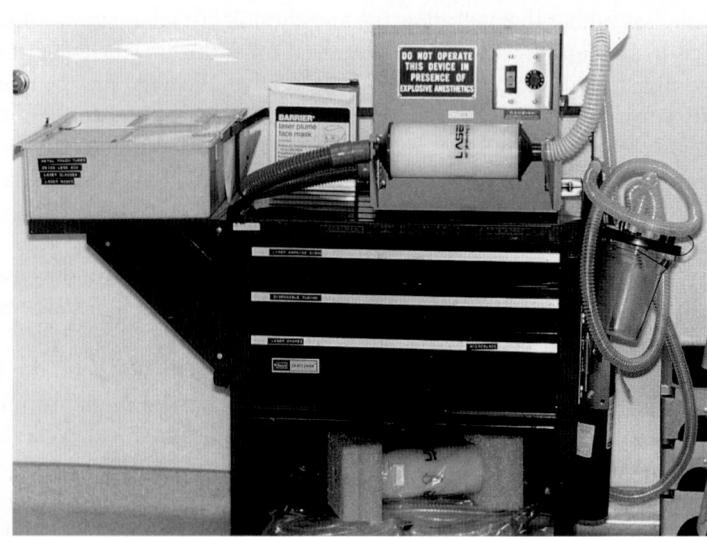

may be warranted to proceed with an FI,O_2 at or below 40%. These precautions are taken to minimize the possibility of a laser-induced endotracheal tube fire.

As an initial procedure, a microcup forceps is utilized for obtaining a biopsy specimen from the bulkiest portion of papilloma. The author utilizes the AccuSpot laser at initial settings of 4 W power, 0.1-second intervals, and repeat mode. Bulky papilloma is handled by defocusing the laser. Moistened neuropathies are placed in the subglottic region to decrease the air leak and to provide a backstop for errant laser shots. These must be kept moist as they too can act as a source of combustion. With the laser refocused, lesions are gradually vaporized to the level of the mucosa, avoiding entry into Reinke's space and the deeper vocalis muscle. The author prefers to use low-power settings to limit thermal injury to the surrounding tissue, although this results in longer operating time. A small-caliber suction device is kept close to the laser impact site to remove the hot steam of vaporization as well as eschar. Neuropathies are soaked in oxymetazoline for removal of eschar and debris as well as hemostasis. The blunt tip of the suction can also be used as a probe and retractor of the false cord or to roll the true cord for exposure of the subglottic region. Care is taken to avoid injuring the anterior commissure, and at least 1 mm of untreated mucosa should be left in this region so that a web does not develop during the healing period (Fig. 7). Similar precautions are taken for the posterior commissure.

The author normally begins the procedure with removal of papillomas in the supraglottic larynx followed by the anterior half of both true vocal cords. If disease has been noted in the posterior half of the glottis or in the subglottic region, then the endotracheal tube obstructs exposure to these areas of the operative field, and an alternative means of anesthesia is sought. The author prefers an apneic technique whereby the endotracheal tube is removed intermittently, and work is performed while the patient's oxygen saturation is monitored. Another alternative would be spontaneous ventilation, although increased circulation of anesthesia gases into the operating room with this technique is an undesirable side effect. Once a decision is made to go apneic, the anesthesiologist increases the FI,O_2 to 100%. The child is extubated although not unsuspended from the microlaryngoscope, the smoke evacuation port of the Lindholm microlaryngoscope is disconnected, and oxygen tubing is connected to this port to a flow of 6 L per minute of O_2. While utilizing an apneic technique, the laser is used for 90- to 120-second intervals initially, and the child is reintubated with a polyvinyl chloride endotracheal tube directly through the microlaryngoscope, utilizing a stylet to stiffen the tube and improve the angulation. The CO_2 and O_2 levels are closely monitored, and the length of "laser-on" time is adjusted appropriately. Typically, the child is reoxygenated for the same period that he or she was apneic before proceeding with the next cycle. At the end of the case, the child is reintubated with a standard endotracheal tube utilizing a Selinger technique to avoid any difficulty in reestablishing the airway on removal of the Lindholm microlaryngoscope. The child is then extubated only when fully awake. High humidity and occasionally racemic epinephrine are administered postoperatively in the recovery room. The patient is then closely monitored for several hours prior to discharge. Often an overnight

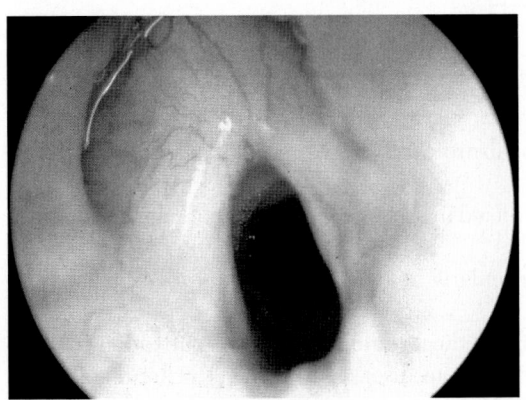

FIGURE 7 Acquired anterior commissure web after multiple procedures for RRP.

stay in a monitored bed unit is necessary. As a general rule, the more extensive the papilloma disease and the more compromised the airway, the more important it is for the child to be monitored postoperatively in an intensive care unit. Additional doses of steroids can be administered at 6-hour intervals if needed, while continuous pulse oximetry is mandatory.

Another anesthetic alternative is the use of jet ventilation for microsurgery of the larynx. Jet ventilation eliminates the potential fire hazard of the endotracheal tube and allows good visualization of the vocal cords. A limitation of this technique is the possibility of transmission of HPV particles into the distal airway. The jet cannula can be placed either above or below the vocal cords, and each has its own particular benefit. The author prefers placement of the cannula proximal to the end of the laryngoscope to decrease the risk of possible pneumothorax or pneumomediastinum. With large laryngeal lesions, narrowed airways, and ball-valve lesions, a high degree of outflow obstruction may develop that could lead to increased intrathoracic pressure and a subsequent pneumothorax. This may also result if there is inadequate muscle relaxation. Jet ventilation also requires constant communication between the operating surgeon and the anesthesiologist. Excessive mucosal drying and damage can occur, as can insufflation of air into the stomach with gastric distention. As mentioned, there is also the potential risk of disseminating papilloma or blood into the tracheobronchial tree.

Postoperative Care

Children with stable papilloma disease requiring fewer than four laser procedures per year, and those with parents that reliably bring them in before showing signs of respiratory distress, can be monitored at home with commercially available infant home intercom-type monitors (Fisher-Price). Those with rapidly reforming papillomas, and those with parents who wait until the child is in distress before seeking medical attention, may require home pulse oximetry with frequent home health visits. Families with RRP patients are encouraged to return to the office or call as often as necessary. The author gives these families carte blanche, explaining to them that their children have a special problem that allows them to speak with the doctors and nurses and to show up unexpectedly at the office whenever they feel their child is in need. The author has yet to experience a family that has abused this privilege; on the contrary, it has enhanced their trust in the health-care team and has avoided urgent and emergent laser procedures.

Children with RRP are followed up regularly in the office, and flexible fiberoptic laryngoscopy in the office is utilized to monitor disease progression. Speech and language therapy is offered early in the course of the disease and is used liberally. Control of other medical factors such as gastroesophageal reflux and asthma are also aggressively pursued. All papilloma families are put in touch with the Recurrent Respiratory Papilloma Foundation support group. Many have found this a tremendous resource for information and support. We have made local arrangements to network papilloma families in our community with good feedback from the participating families.

PEARLS AND PERILS

1. Participation in national/regional protocols are essential to learn more about RRP.
2. A national registry of patients will aid in identification of patients suitable for enrollment in treatment protocols.
3. Family support groups are particularly helpful for parents of recalcitrant RRP patients.
4. Utilize the subspecialists at your medical center to assist you with adjuvant protocols (Hematology/oncology, infectious disease, home health-care teams).

Adjuvant Treatment Modalities

Although surgical management remains the mainstay therapy for RRP, ultimately as many as 10% of patients with the disease will require some form of adjuvant therapy. The most widely adopted criteria for initiating adjuvant therapy are a surgery requirement of more than four procedures per year, distal multisite spread of disease, and/or rapid regrowth of papilloma disease with airway compromise. The most commonly recommended adjuvant therapy is alpha-interferon (4). The exact mechanism by which interferon elicits its response is unknown. It appears to modulate host immune response by increasing production of a protein kinase and endonuclease that inhibits viral protein synthesis. Interferons are a class of proteins manufactured by cells in response to a variety of stimuli including viral infection. The enzymes that are produced block the viral replication of RNA and DNA and alter cell membranes to make them less susceptible to viral penetration. Common interferon side effects fall into two categories: acute reactions (fever and generalized flu-like symptoms, chills, headache, myalgias, and nausea that seem to decrease with prolonged therapy) and chronic reactions (decrease in the growth rate of the child, elevation of liver transaminase levels, leukopenia, spastic diplegia, and febrile seizures). Thrombocytopenia has been reported, as have rashes, dry skin, alopecia, generalized pruritus, and fatigue. Acetaminophen has been found to be effective to relieve the fevers, and interferon injections are best tolerated at bedtime. Interferon produced by recombinant DNA techniques appears to have fewer side effects and better efficacy than blood bank-harvested interferon.

Several large multinstitutional studies regarding interferon have arrived at seemingly conflicting conclusions regarding its efficacy. Healy et al. (24) reported on 123 patients who received 2 million units per square meter of alpha-interferon 3 days per week for 12 months and achieved a significant response that was not sustained at 1-year follow-up. At this dosage, interferon seemed to control disease in the first 3 to 6 months of treatment, but the effectiveness was questionable after 6 months of therapy. Leventhal and Kashima (24) reported on 66 patients who received 5 million units per square meter given initially on a daily basis for 1 month and then 3 times a week for 6 months with sustained or repeated responses in most patients. Twenty-two of the 66 had a complete remission, and 25 of the 66 had partial remission, with a median duration of 550 days. They also found that a response could be reintroduced after a period of nontreatment with interferon. Based on their study, Kashima and Leventhal (25) recommend a 6-month trial of interferon if surgery is required every 2 to 3 months for a year.

Photodynamic therapy (PDT) in the treatment of RRP has been studied extensively at Long Island Jewish Hospital by Abramson, Shikowitz, and Steinberg (26). PDT is based on the transfer of energy to a photosensitive drug. The most common drug utilized is dihematoporphyrin ether (DHE), which has a tendency to concentrate within papillomas more so than in surrounding normal tissue. The ideal photosensitive drug would absorb light and transfer light and energy to triplet oxygen. This then converts it to a highly toxic single oxygen, which is retained in tumor tissue longer than in normal tissue. Patients are typically treated with 2.5 mg per kilogram of i.v. DHE prior to photoactivation with an argon pump dye laser. A small but statistically significant decrease in RRP growth, especially in those patients with the worse disease, was seen with the use of PDT and DHE. The drawback of this therapy is that patients become markedly photosensitive for periods lasting 2 to 8 weeks. A new drug, m-tetra (hydroxyphenyl) chlorine, has shown efficacy in HPV-induced tumors in rabbits with minimal tissue damage, and a clinical trial utilizing this drug is now on-going.

Avidano and Singleton (27) reported on the University of Florida's experience with 34 patients who had severe RRP requiring adjuvant therapy. All 34 were treated with alpha-1-interferon utilizing 5 million units per square meter for 21 to 28 days followed by a maintenance dose 3 times a week for at least 6 months. Interferon was administered by subcutaneous injection, and the drug was held back for severe side effects and then restarted at a lower dosage. Forty-seven percent of patients achieved a complete response, and 35% achieved a partial clinical response. Five of the nonresponders out of the original 34 were subsequently treated with cis-retinoic acid (Accutane). No clinical response was achieved with any of these patients. Three of the 34 patients with minimal response to both interferon and Accutane were subsequently treated with methotrexate. Methotrexate is an antimetabolite used in the treatment of neoplastic diseases. Its mechanism of action is through the inhibition of dihydrofolic acid reductase, blocking synthesis of purine nucleotides and thymidylate, and thus interfering with DNA synthesis. Methotrexate acts best on rapidly proliferating cells and was shown in Avidano and Singleton's (27) series to have some effect in recalcitrant RRP cases. All three patients achieved a significant clinical response, although none had a complete response within 3 to 6 months of initiating methotrexate therapy.

Retinoids, which are analogs of vitamin A, have been evaluated in several small trials with inconsistent results. Bell et al. (28) used 100 mg per square meter per day of oral 13 cisretinoic acid (Accutane) in nine patients without success and with significant toxicity. Alberts et al. (29) experienced more success using a dose of 0.5 to 2 mg per day. Eicher et al. (30) reported success in a single patient with aggressive disease. Transretinoic acid, a similar drug with less potential toxicity, is currently in experimental use at several sites.

Ribavirin is an antiviral drug, used to treat respiratory syncytial virus pneumonia in infants, that has also shown some promise in the treatment of aggressive laryngeal papillomatosis. McGlennen et al. (31) reported on its use in three adults and one infant at a daily dose of 23 mg per kilogram. The authors found a complete response in two of their patients and a partial response in the other two (31). Morrison et al. (32) reported on a single patient with extensive tracheobronchial tree papillomatosis who experienced remarkable regression of this disease on ribavirin without adverse reaction. These authors recommend further evaluation to define the role of ribavirin in the treatment of RRP (32). Ribavirin is currently available only in aerosolized form and costs over $1,000 a day to utilize.

Another antiviral treatment that has received interest in the treatment of RRP is acyclovir. Although the activity of acyclovir is dependent on the presence of virally encoded thymidine kinase, an enzyme that is not known to be encoded by papillomavirus, conflicting clinical results have been obtained in several small series. Theoretically, it would not be expected to have a positive effect. However, it has been postulated that perhaps acyclovir is most effective when there are codisease factors such as a simultaneous infection with herpes simplex virus. Lopez-Agado et al. (33) achieved complete remission in three patients on the drug. Endres et al. (34) observed significant reduction only in patients not previously treated with interferon; patients on interferon developed worsening disease. Morrison and Evans (35) found no response to acyclovir in four patients with aggressive RRP.

Recent interest has focused on chemically pure indole-3-carbinol (I3C), which has been shown to inhibit papilloma formation in mice (36). This compound is found in high concentration in cruciferous vegetables such as cabbage, broccoli, and cauliflower. A small dietary study at Long Island Jewish Hospital showed promise, although there were concerns regarding how much active drug the patients were actually receiving. I3C is now available in pure chemical form, and new trials are ongoing at Long Island Jewish Hospital and the University of Pittsburgh. Preliminary data suggest a linear relationship between the ratio of estrogen metabolism pathways (2-hydroxylation:16 alpha-hydroxylation) and the severity of RRP disease. Ratios of less than 1 are associated with severe disease and those of greater than 3 are associated with mild disease. Efforts are currently under way to expedite Food and Drug Administration approval of I3C as an investigational drug.

It should be stressed that participation in national and regional protocols of adjuvant treatment modalities is essential for the scientific community to learn more about RRP. A national registry of patients with RRP is being formed through the cooperation of the National Institutes of Health and the Centers for Disease Control. This will aid in the identification of patients suitable for enrollment in multinstitutional studies of adjuvant therapies and will better define the risk factors for transmission of HPV and the cofactors that may determine the aggressiveness of RRP.

PEARLS AND PERILS

1. Ounce of prevention: establish a rapport and relationship with families of RRP patients from the outset.
2. Try to avoid the need for laryngotracheoplasty (LTP) and anterior commissure web repairs since these reconstructions may reactivate the disease.
3. Review laser safety yearly with OR staff and your anesthesia team.

Lasers

The CO_2 laser is the mainstay of lasers in otolaryngology. It is the most widely used, well understood, and well studied of the medical lasers and can be used for incision, excision, and vaporization of tissue. It was the first laser to be used clinically in otolaryngology and the first to be used in laryngology. The CO_2 laser is well absorbed by most tissues of the body because of the high water content of soft tissues. Water molecules are excellent absorbers of the CO_2 wave length. This is in contrast to bone and cartilage, which contain minimal water and thus will not absorb CO_2 laser energy. Because the CO_2 wavelength is invisible to the human eye, a helium neon aiming beam is necessary to allow the surgeon to visualize the area of intended application. The advantage of using a CO_2 laser is its superficial extent of injury on tissues and its excellent precision, especially with the microspot micromanipulator. Use of the CO_2 laser results in shallow and predictable tissue penetration with minimal edema. Its hemostatic capability is limited, however, to blood vessels not larger than capillaries (0.5 mm). The CO_2 beam can be focused to create a precise cut and defocused to produce coagulation of small blood vessels. The CO_2 cannot be transmitted through flexible fibers and is delivered through a somewhat awkward articulated mirror system. If used improperly with a large spot size (greater than 0.5 mm), continuous exposure, or high power settings (greater than 10 W) significant mucosal scarring, fibrosis, and poor voice quality can result.

⊕ MANAGEMENT OF COMPLICATIONS

Laser fires can occur in the operating room due to impact of the laser beam on materials such as towels, cloth drapes, or anesthetic tubing. This may be prevented with placing the laser on "standby" when not in use. The most serious complication of laser surgery is an endotracheal tube fire. For combustion to take place, a source of energy (the laser beam), an oxidizable material (the endotracheal tube), and oxygen must all be present. Laser-induced endotracheal tube fires can be avoided by eliminating flammable endotracheal tubes from the procedure, or by utilizing jet ventilation, apneic, or spontaneous anesthesia techniques. If the use of a tube is deemed necessary, then a nonflammable metal endotracheal tube can be utilized. Contrary to previous authors, this author does not recommend the use of red-rubber endotracheal tubes that have been wrapped with aluminum foil by the anesthesiologist. These run too high of a risk of possible flammability if the wrapping is inexact. Whenever possible, a cuffless endotracheal tube is preferred. If a cuff is utilized, it should be protected with wet cottonoids or a metal platform. Studies have shown that the higher the oxygen concentration flowing through the endotracheal tube, the more likely an endotracheal tube fire will occur. Thus the anesthesiologist should ventilate the patient's lungs with the lowest possible oxygen concentration. In an effort to reduce excessive tissue damage, the author recommends utilizing brief intervals of as little as a fraction of a second between laser impacts (repeat instead of continuous mode) to allow dissipation of laser energy and spare the normal tissue. The laser and laryngoscope should be repositioned as frequently as necessary to gain adequate tissue access and visualization. Eschar on tissue that has been lasered should be removed because such tissue absorbs energy and transmits heat to the underlying tissue. Hemorrhage should be controlled with neuropathies soaked in oxymetazoline because blood will absorb laser energy, diminish the laser's effectiveness, and obscure the anatomy. Circumferential lasering should be avoided as this will lead to cicatrix formation and stenosis.

Laser plume should be removed for adequate visualization and because the plume itself may dissipate the CO_2 laser beam. Laser plume has the potential for carrying HPV particles and noxious substances. To date there has been no direct evidence that these particles have caused RRP in the operating surgeon or other OR personnel. However, plume and noxious fumes are irritating to the respiratory tract even if they do not contain infectious particles, and the use of a mechanical smoke evacuator with high-efficiency filters is recommended. Since HPV may be present in a latent state in adjacent tissue, errant lasering should be avoided to prevent reactivation of disease.

Corneal or retinal burns are possible from an acute exposure to the laser beam. This can occur secondary to direct impact of the laser beam on the eye or through indirect reflection off of surgical instruments. The OR should be clearly marked whenever laser surgery is taking place, and all entrances into the room should have additional appropriate eyewear protection located near the door so that OR personnel can use them when entering the room. Patients should have eye protection in the form of gauze eye pads that are taped in place and moistened with saline. The surgeon should wear protective glasses except when using the operating microscope.

A double layer of saline-saturated surgical sponges, towels, or lap pads is used to protect all exposed skin and mucous membranes of the patient outside the immediate surgical field. As previously mentioned, the laser should remain on standby mode whenever it is not in use. Because it is possible for the beam to reflect off the proximal rim of the laryngoscope when performing surgery, the patient's face is completely draped with saline-saturated surgical towels, thereby exposing only the proximal lumen of the laryngoscope.

Finger burns may occur during microlaryngeal surgery if the surgeon does not keep his or her hand out of the line of fire of the laser beam; the surgeon should strive to keep the hand to the extreme side of the operative field.

The anterior commissure of the larynx has to be respected when using the laser. Failure to preserve mucosa on at least one side of the commissure will lead to an acquired glottic web. Subglottic stenosis may occur secondary to laser treatment of circumferential papillomas below the vocal cords. Vocal cord fibrosis may develop following laser surgery in which too much power for too long a period is delivered to the true vocal cord, resulting in partial vaporization of the vocalis muscle. Granulomas can form if the black carbonaceous debris is not removed from the operative site. Prolonged hypoxia and hypercarbia can result when using spontaneous ventilation and apneic techniques of anesthesia; these can be avoided by close monitoring. Jet ventilation techniques can result in pneumothorax if there is significant outlet obstruction. Theoretically, jet ventilation may also result in the distal spread of papilloma disease down the tracheobronchial tree.

Adjuvant therapies using antiviral and antineoplastic drugs can also result in complications. Children placed on these medications are ideally entered into carefully controlled clinical protocols. When this is not possible, the known potential side effects of these medicines need to be monitored. For instance, children placed on alpha-interferon should have liver function studies, a complete blood count, urinalysis, and thyroid function studies obtained at the outset and repeated at least twice a year. It is often appropriate to involve the hematology/oncology or infectious disease subspecialists at your medical center to assist you with managing the potential complications of patients on adjuvant therapy.

The management of RRP that has spread distally in the tracheobronchial tree is both challenging and frustrating. The CO_2 laser can be coupled to a rigid bronchoscope via an universal endoscopic coupler. Custom-designed laser bronchoscopes are now available with the universal endoscopic coupler. Alternatively, the KTP/ND:Yag laser can be utilized through a ventilating bronchoscope. Although the KTP and Yag lasers are more dependent on melanin or pigment for their absorption spectra, they can still be effective in controlling papillomas. The surgeon, however, must be aware that more tissue destruction is possible than with the CO_2 laser. The ND:Yag laser can also be utilized through a flexible fiberoptic bronchoscope. The surgeon should realize that the use of the KTP/Yag laser will require different eye protection for the operating room personnel and the patient. Postoperative atelectasis is common after lasering of tracheal and bronchial papillomas, and aggressive chest physical therapy is needed postoperatively.

The parents of children who are in seeming remission from their papilloma disease and who have developed anterior commissure webbing or subglottic stenosis may request reconstructive surgical therapy for these conditions. Although it may be tempting to embark on this repair, the surgeon must be aware, and the family must be informed, of the possibility of reactivating papilloma disease through the manipulation of this apparently normal tissue. In the author's opinion, whenever possible, laryngotracheal reconstruction and anterior commissure web repairs should be avoided.

Lastly, a comment needs to be made regarding the potential for litigation in RRP patients. This is a frustrating disease because of its often prolonged nature, and there may be guilt on the parent's part regarding vertical transmission from parent to child. The American College of Obstetrics and Gynecology's (37) official statement on HPV disease specifically states that cesarean section is *not* indicated in the prevention of transmission of HPV from mother to child. A comprehensive review of this topic reached the same conclusion (7). Nevertheless, lawsuits have been brought against obstetricians based on a lack of provision of informed consent to parents regarding this disease process. From the otolaryngologist's standpoint, laser surgery for papilloma disease has many potential and even life-threatening complications associated with it. "An ounce of prevention" is the best strategy for avoiding these complications. Additionally, it is wise for the surgeon to establish rapport and a close relationship with the families of their papilloma patients. Informed consent needs to be reviewed with each procedure, and the families need to feel that they have access to the health-care team should their child develop increasing respiratory effort.

Treating children with RRP can be very rewarding as we learn more about HPV. In the future, we look forward to success in reducing the morbidity and mortality of this disease process. The establishment of the national RRP patient registry, as well as coordinated efforts between basic scientists involved in HPV research and clinicians involved in the treatment of RRP, should aid us in this endeavor.

❂ REFERENCES

1. Morgan AH, Zitsch RP. Recurrent respiratory papillomatosis in children: a retrospective study of management and complications. *Ear Nose Throat J* 1986;65:19–28.
2. Mounts P, Shah KV, Kashima H: Viral etiology of juvenile and adult onset squamous papilloma of the larynx. *Proc Natl Acad Sci USA* 1982;79:5425–5429.
3. Cohn AM, Kos JT, Taber LH, Adam E. Recurring laryngeal papilloma. *Am J Otolaryngol* 1981;2:129–5429.
4. Derkay CS. Task force on recurrent respiratory papillomas. *Arch Otolaryngol Head Neck Surg* 1995;121:1386–1391.
5. Kashima HK, Shah F, Lyles A, et al. Factors in juvenile-onset and adult onset recurrent respiratory papillomas. *Laryngoscope* 1992;102:9–13.
6. Mounts P, Kashima H. Association of human papillomavirus subtype and clinical course in respiratory papillomatosis. *Laryngoscope* 1984;94:28–33.
7. Kosko J, Derkay CS. Role of cesarean section in the prevention of recurrent respiratory papillomas: is there one? *Int J Pediatr Otolaryngol* 1996;1:31–38.

8. Rihkaren H, Aaltonen LM, Syranen SM. Human papillomavirus in laryngeal papillomas and in adjacent normal epithelium. *Clin Otolaryngol* 1993;18:470–474.

9. Brandsma JL, Abramson AL. Association of papillomavirus with cancers of the head and neck. *Arch Otolaryngol Head Neck Surg* 1989;115:621–625.

10. Koutsky LA, Wolner-Hanssen P. Genital papillomavirus infection: current knowledge and future prospects. *Obstet Gynecol Clin North Am* 1989;16:541–561.

11. Bennett RS, Powell KR. Human papillomavirus: association between laryngeal papillomas and genital warts. *Pediatr Infect Dis J* 1987;6:229–232.

12. Kashima H, Mounts P, Leventhal B, Hruban RH. Sites of predilection in recurrent respiratory papillomatosis. *Ann Otol Rhinol Laryngol* 1993;102:580–583.

13. Lindeberg H, Elbrond O. Laryngeal papillomas: the epidemiology in a Danish subpopulation 1965–1984. *Clin Otolaryngol* 1991;15:125–131.

14. Cook TA, Brunchswig JP, Butel JS, Cohn AM, Goepfert LL, Rawls WE. Laryngeal papilloma: etiologic and therapeutic considerations. *Ann Otol Rhinol Laryngol* 1973;82:649–655.

15. Quick CA, Kryzek RA, Walt SL, Faras AJ. Relationship between condylomata and laryngeal papillomata: clinical and molecular virological evidence. *Ann Otol Rhinol Laryngeal* 1980;89:467–471.

16. Smith EM, Johnson SR, Pignatari S, Cripe TP, Turek L: Perinatal vertical transmission of human papilloma virus and subsequent development of respiratory tract papillomatosis. *Ann Otol Rhinol Laryngol* 1991;100:479–483.

17. Shah K, Kashima H, Polk BF, Shah F, Aabbey H, Abramson A. Rarity of caesarean delivery in cases of juvenile onset respiratory papillomatosis. *Obstet Gynecol* 1986;68:795–799.

18. Sedlacek TV, Lindeheim S, Elder C, et al. Mechanism for human papillomavirus transmission at birth. *Am J Obstet Gynecol* 1989;161:55–59.

19. Lindeberg H, Elbrond O. Laryngeal papillomas: clinical aspects in a series of 231 patients. *Clin Otolaryngol* 1989;14:333–342.

20. Cole RR, Myer CM, Cotton RT. Tracheotomy in children with recurrent respiratory papillomatosis. *Head Neck* 1989;11:226–230.

21. Lie ES, Engh V, Boysen M, et al. Squamous cell carcinoma of the respiratory tract following laryngeal papillomatosis. *Acta Otolaryngol (Stockh)* 1994;114:209–212.

22. Kashima HK. Scoring system to assess severity and course in recurrent respiratory papillomatosis. In: *Papilloma-viruses: molecular and clinical aspects.* Alan R. Liss, New York, 1985:125–135.

23. Derkay CS, Malis DJ, Zalzal G, Wiatrak BJ, Kashima HK, Koltrera MD. A staging system for assessing severity of disease and response to therapy in recurrent respiratory papillomatosis. *Laryngoscope* 1998 (*in press*).

24. Healy GB, Gelber RD, Trowbridge AL, Grundfast KM, Ruben RJ, Price KN. Treatment of recurrent respiratory papillomatosis with human leukocyte interferon: results of a multicenter randomized clinical trial. *N Engl J Med* 1988;319:401–407.

25. Leventhal BG, Kashima HK, Mounts P, et al. Long-term response of recurrent respiratory papillomatosis to treatment with lymphoblastoid interferon alfa-n1. *N Engl J Med* 19911;325:613–617.

26. Abramson AL, Shikowitz MJ, Mullooly VM, Steinberg BM, Amella CA, Rothstein HR. Clinical effects of photodynamic therapy on recurrent laryngeal papillomas. *Arch Otolaryngol Head Neck Surg* 1992;118:25–29.

27. Avidano MA, Singleton GT. Adjuvant drug strategies in the treatment of recurrent respiratory papillomatosis. *Otolaryngol Head Neck Surg* 1995;112:197–202.

28. Bell R, Hong WK, Itri LM, McDonald G, Strong MS. The use of cis-retinoic acid in recurrent respiratory papillomatosis of the larynx: a randomized pilot study. *Am J Otolarynol* 1988;9:161–164.

29. Alberts DS, Coulthard SW, Meyskens FL. Regression of aggressive laryngeal papillomatosis with 13 cis-retinoic acid (Accutane). *J Biol Respir Med* 1986;5:124–128.

30. Eicher SA, Taylor-Cooley LD, Donovan DT. Isotretinoic therapy for recurrent respiratory papillomatosis. *Arch Otolaryngol Head Neck Surg* 1994;120:405–409.

31. McGlennen RC, Adams GL, Lewis DM, Faras JJ, Ostrow RS. Pilot trial of ribavirin for the treatment of laryngeal papillomatosis. *Head Neck* 1993;15:504–513.

32. Morrison GAJ, Kotecha B, Evans JNG. Ribavirin treatment for juvenile respiratory papillomatosis. *J Laryngol Otol* 1993;107:423–426.

33. Lopez-Aguado D, Perez-Pinero B, Betancor I, Mendez A, Banales EC. Acyclovir in the treatment of laryngeal papillomatosis. *Int J Pediatr Otorhinolaryngol* 1991;21:269–274.

34. Endres DR, Burke D, Bauman NM, Smith RJH. Acyclovir in the treatment of recurrent respiratory papillomatosis: a pilot study. *Ann Otol Rhinol Laryngol* 1994;103:301–305.
35. Morrison GA, Evans JN. Juvenile respiratory papillomatosis: acyclovir reassessed. *Int J Pediatr Otorhinolaryngol* 1993;26:193–197.
36. Newfield L, Goldsmith A, Bradlow HL, Auborn K. Estrogen metabolism and human papillomavirus-induced tumors of the larynx: chemo-prophylaxis with indole-3-carbinol. *Anticancer Res* 1993;13:337–341.
37. Guidelines for perinatal care, 3rd ed. American Academy of Pediatrics/American College of Obstetrics and Gynecology 1990;127–128.

C.S. Derkay: Departments of Otolaryngology and Pediatrics, Eastern Virginia Medical School, Norfolk, Virginia 23507.

- *Practical Pediatric Otolaryngology*
- edited by Robin T. Cotton and Charles M. Myer, III
- Lippincott-Raven Publishers, Philadelphia © 1999

Head and Neck
Section Editor
Charles M. Myer, III

Congenital Malformations of the Head and Neck

Michael J. Cunningham

The vast majority of neck masses in children are benign lesions of inflammatory origin that either spontaneously resolve or respond to appropriate medical therapy. An excisional biopsy for diagnostic or cosmetic purposes becomes necessary in the treatment of persistent or recurrent masses; therapeutic surgical intervention may also be indicated for neck masses that cause aerodigestive tract compromise or present with other worrisome clinical features. The majority of pediatric neck masses requiring surgical therapy prove to be of congenital etiology (1).

Congenital neck masses are likely to be present at birth but some remain unnoticed, even into adulthood, until secondary infection causes acute enlargement (2). Congenital lesions may also initially manifest as an asymptomatic sinus or fistula opening. The anatomic location of the neck mass or sinus/fistula opening on cervical examination may suggest its embryologic origin (Table 1). A midline neck mass, for example, raises suspicion of a thyroid anomaly or cervical dermoid. The most common congenital lesions of the anterior cervical triangle are of branchial origin, although both dermoid cysts and thymic gland anomalies can also occur in this region. Congenital lesions of the posterior cervical triangle are uncommon with the exception of hemangiomas and vascular malformations; these lesions can also involve contiguous neck regions and are discussed in detail in Chapter 56.

Roentgenographic studies can be helpful in the evaluation of neck masses suspected to be of congenital origin. Such studies include ultrasonography, computed tomography (CT), and magnetic resonance imaging (MRI); in specific settings, radioisotope scans or angiographic procedures may supply additional information. Ultrasonography can be used to identify the size, shape, and relationship of the mass to adjacent neck structures; the echogenic pattern of the mass (cystic, solid, or complex) may narrow the list of possible diagnoses (3). Advantages of ultrasonography include relative low cost, absence of ionizing radiation, and ready availability of use even in the uncooperative child. The principal drawback of ultrasonography is the limited image quality. CT and MRI provide much more lucid anatomic detail in multiplanar images (4). MRI provides exquisitely sensitive soft tissue imaging without radiation exposure. However, the soft tissue clarity of MRI is influenced by motion artifact and this dictates the frequent need for sedation, particularly in young children. One particularly important contribution of CT that cannot be replicated by other radiologic techniques is its characterization of potential bone involvement. Etiologic concerns in some circumstances may dictate that both MRI and CT be performed.

The role of additional laboratory studies in the evaluation of suspected congenital anomalies is quite lesion specific. The obtainment of thyroid function studies, for example, may be worthwhile in the evaluation of midline neck masses. A complete blood cell count with differential analysis is appropriate in children presenting with inflammatory neck masses. Fine-needle aspiration (FNA) biopsy of congenital neck masses is not typ-

TABLE 1: Congenital Malformations of the Neck

Midline	Anterocervical	Posterocervical
Thyroglossal duct cyst (ectopic cervical thyroid)	Branchial cyst	Vascular anomalies
Dermoid cyst	Dermoid cyst	Hemangiomas
Laryngocele	Thymopharyngeal duct cyst (ectopic cervical thymus)	Vascular malformations
	Teratoma	
	Vascular anomalies	
	Hemangiomas	
	Vascular malformations	
	Jugular vein phlebectasia	
	Carotid artery aneurysm	

ically recommended; benign cytology and evidence of either acute or chronic inflammation, depending on the clinical presentation, would be the expected findings (5).

MIDLINE NECK MASSES

Thyroid Gland Anomalies

The thyroid gland originates as a diverticulum from the floor of the pharynx, becoming bilobed as it descends in the midline of the neck. During descent the gland remains connected to the floor of the pharynx by a hollow canal, the thyroglossal duct, which eventually involutes. The pharyngeal site of attachment persists as the foramen cecum of the tongue. Arrest in the normal descent of the gland results in ectopic thyroid tissue, whereas persistence of a portion of the embryonic duct is the cause of a thyroglossal duct cyst.

The majority of thyroglossal duct cysts present in children and adolescents as asymptomatic midline neck masses at or below the level of the hyoid bone; however, any relatively midline position from the base of the tongue to the thyroid gland is possible (Fig. 1). Despite the rarity of primary external sinus tracts and a characteristic absence of cyst wall lymphoid tissue, inflammation of thyroglossal duct cysts is common. A variety of both aerobic and anaerobic organisms have been isolated, suggesting a persistent pharyngeal communication, likely via the foramen cecum (2). Recurrent inflammation may result in cyst enlargement, abscess formation, and spontaneous rupture with secondary sinus tract formation (Fig. 2A).

The preoperative radiologic evaluation of patients suspected clinically to have a thyroglossal duct cyst is debated, specifically whether or not a thyroid scan or alternative radiologic study to rule out an ectopic thyroid gland in the clinically euthyroid child is necessary (6). The incidence of ectopic thyroid in a sublingual or thyroglossal location is rare, approximating 1% to 2% (7). Ectopic thyroid tissue usually manifests when the small ectopic gland is unable to keep pace with the increasing metabolic demands of the growing child. Thyroid function tests may be predictive in this situation as levels of endogenous thyroid-stimulating hormone (TSH) should be elevated when a relative deficiency of thyroid hormone production occurs (8). However, a wide range of thyroid function has been documented in children with ectopic thyroid tissue, and the literature contains reports of excised ectopic thyroid tissue clinically and intraoperatively misdiagnosed as thyroglossal duct cyst in patients with normal thyroid function. Ultrasonography is a useful means of assessing midline cervical masses in children. Sonographic documentation of a normal thyroid gland can sometimes be difficult in an actively moving young child, and there is an associated high false-positive rate of the thyroglossal duct cyst itself being interpreted as a solid lesion due to the viscosity of the cyst contents. Consideration should be given to the performance of a thyroid scan in the child in whom thyroid function studies are not definitive and in whom an adequate ultrasound study cannot be performed.

The surgical treatment of thyroglossal duct cysts evolved because of the high rate

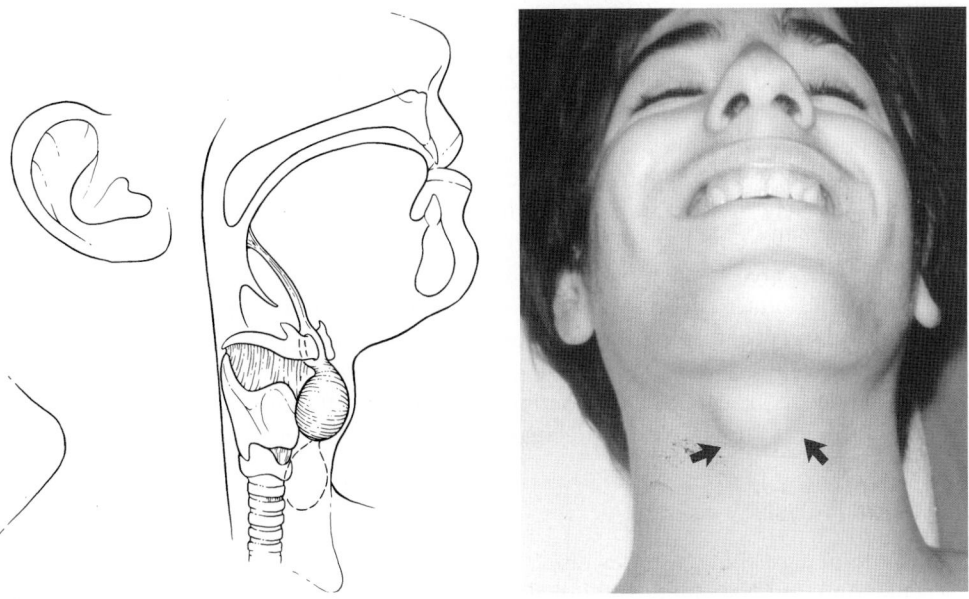

FIGURE 1 A: Diagrammatic representation of thyroglossal duct cyst anterior to the hyoid. **B:** Classic midline cervical thyroglossal duct cyst presentation (*arrowheads*).

of recurrence, approximating 50%, associated with simple cyst excision. In 1893 Schlange (9) proposed removal of the central portion of the hyoid bone in continuity with a thyroglossal duct cyst, reducing the recurrence rate to approximately 20%. In 1920, Sistrunk advocated the additional contiguous removal of a core of tissue through the base of the tongue; he originally recommended excision of the foramen cecum but modified his procedure at a later date to transection in the submucosal plane to avoid entrance into the oropharyngeal cavity (10,11). This form of the Sistrunk procedure remains the treatment of choice for thyroglossal duct cysts today (Fig. 2B). Numerous studies have supported the efficacy of this procedure in terms of markedly decreased recurrence rates ranging from 4% to 6%. Histopathologic studies also lend support to the concept of an en bloc removal of tongue tissue in that many thyroglossal duct specimens demonstrate great anatomic variability with multiple ducts and branching diverticula.

The greatest risk of recurrence is associated with failure to follow the surgical principles of the Sistrunk procedure (12). Rupture of the thyroglossal duct cyst during re-

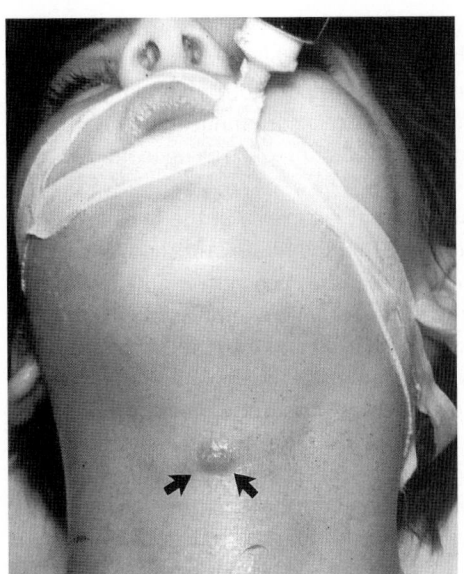

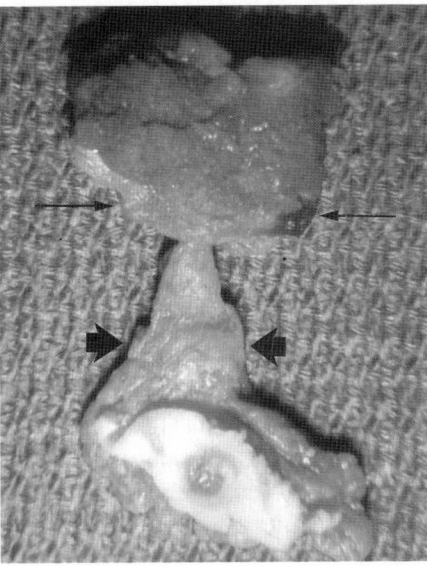

FIGURE 2 A: Secondary sinus tract formation (*arrowheads*) resulting from recurrent thyroglossal duct cyst inflammation. **B:** Complete Sistrunk excision specimen consisting of an ellipse of skin around the pseudofistula, the cyst (*arrowheads*), and a core of tongue tissue in continuity with the central portion of the hyoid bone (*arrows*).

section also increases the likelihood of recurrent disease. Factors that contribute to operative cyst rupture include previous inflammation, prior incision and drainage, and lobulated cysts within close proximity to the skin surface. In such cases, the surgeon should excise the involved or adjacent skin immediately over the cyst in elliptical fashion rather than attempt to preserve an intact skin flap.

Clearly, the best opportunity for curative excision comes at the time of initial presentation. Recurrence rates are much higher in operations performed for recurrent disease. A modification of the Sistrunk procedure incorporating an en bloc anterior dissection is advocated in such patients (13). The dissection begins with a transverse skin incision, including an ellipse of skin around the fistulous tract (if present), and is carried cephalad, removing approximately 3 to 4 cm of strap muscles down to the level of the pretracheal fascia. The central portion of the hyoid bone, or a wider resection of residual hyoid bone, is likewise taken in continuity with a 5- to 10-mm core of tongue tissue. Recurrence rates are significantly decreased after revision surgery using such a technique.

Dermoid Cysts

The term *dermoid cyst* in this discussion refers to those histopathologic cysts lined by epidermis and containing epidermal appendages such as hair follicles and sebaceous glands within the cyst wall. This definition differentiates dermoids from simple epidermal or sebaceous cysts that contain solely ectodermal elements. Cervical dermoid cysts form along lines of embryologic fusion, including the middorsal fusion plane, explaining their potential midline thyroidal and suprasternal presentations.

Dermoid cysts in the midline and paramedian region of the neck are often clinically misdiagnosed as thyroglossal duct cysts. In one study, 11 of 71 midline cysts proved histologically to be dermoid cysts even though they were not recognized preoperatively or intraoperatively to be so; at the time of surgical dissection, 9 of these lesions actually demonstrated attachments to the hyoid bone and 6 had apparent midline tracts (14).

The diagnostic confusion between thyroglossal duct and dermoid cysts is of more than academic interest. The traditional treatment of choice for a thyroglossal duct cyst, as discussed, is the Sistrunk procedure. In contrast, the traditional choice of therapy for a dermoid cyst is simple excision. A recommended approach, based on the clinical similarity of dermoid and thyroglossal duct cysts, is to use the Sistrunk procedure as the uniform treatment for all midline cysts *deep* to the cervical strap musculature.

Laryngoceles

The saccule is a blind pouch that ascends vertically from the laryngeal ventricle between the false cord and the inner surface of the thyroid cartilage. Numerous mucous glands empty into the saccule and provide lubrication for the ipsilateral true vocal cord. If the saccule becomes distended with air and maintains an open communication with the laryngeal lumen, it is termed a *laryngocele*. Secondary infection of a laryngocele results in a laryngopyocele.

Laryngoceles and laryngopyoceles typically present externally in the neck in the region of the thyrohyoid membrane, usually just lateral to the midline. Alternatively or concomitantly, an internal laryngeal mass presentation causing hoarseness and respiratory distress may occur. Whereas laryngoceles are typically soft and compressible, laryngopyoceles are often firm and tender to palpation with both local and systemic signs of inflammation; causative organisms are typically those endogenous to the upper respiratory tract.

Asymptomatic laryngoceles do not absolutely require treatment in children. Symptomatic laryngoceles, including laryngopyoceles, should be excised. An external laryngofissure approach is recommended (15). Care must be taken to avoid damage to the superior laryngeal nerve. In some patients it may be necessary to resect the thyroid ala for adequate exposure. Rarely, a tracheotomy is necessary for airway securement before or at the time of definitive treatment.

ANTEROCERVICAL MASSES

Branchial Cysts, Sinuses, and Fistulas

Many of the symmetrically paired structures of the head and neck arise from the fetal branchial system. This system appears during the fourth week of fetal development as five ridges on the ventrolateral surface of the embryonic head. The ridges are known as *branchial arches* due to their resemblance to the gill arches of fish. Each arch represents a condensation of mesoderm from which cartilage, muscle, and bone will form. The arches are separated from one another by an external cleft of ectodermal origin and an internal pouch of endodermal origin. A thin epithelial plate separates each cleft and pouch.

Branchial system anomalies exist in one of three forms: sinuses, fistulas, or cysts. A sinus tract with either an external or an internal opening is theorized to represent a vestigial cleft or pouch. A complete fistula with both internal and external openings presumably arises from persistence of both cleft and pouch with dissolution of the intervening separation plate. Generally, branchial cleft sinuses with external openings to the skin are associated with the first and second arches. Branchial pouch sinuses with internal openings to the pharynx are associated with the third and fourth arches. The first three branchial clefts and pouches may form complete fistulous tracts joining both pharynx and skin. A cyst is the equivalent of a trapped portion of a cleft or pouch and may occur anywhere along these potential sinus or fistula tracts. The anatomic location of the sinus, fistula, or cyst reflects its presumed branchial cleft or pouch of origin.

The majority of branchial anomalies (65% to 90%) arise from the second branchial system. Next most common are anomalies of the first branchial arch, cleft, or pouch (8% to 25%). Third and fourth branchial system anomalies occur infrequently (2% to 10%) (16,17).

First branchial cleft anomalies can be divided into two separate anatomic types. In a type I first branchial cleft anomaly, the cyst or sinus opening is localized medial, inferior, or posterior to the conchal cartilage and pinna (Fig. 3). If present, the sinus tract parallels the external auditory meatus. In type II first branchial cleft anomalies, the cyst or external opening is localized in the anterior part of the neck, *always superior* to the hyoid bone (Fig. 4). The sinus or fistula tract courses over the angle of the mandible, through the parotid gland, and terminates at or near the bony-cartilaginous junction of the external ear canal. The course of the tract relative to the facial nerve is quite variable. First branchial cleft cysts likewise have a variable relationship to the parotid gland, occurring in both intraparotid and paraparotid locations.

In second branchial cleft anomalies, the external opening, if present, is located along the anterior border of the sternocleidomastoid muscle near the junction of its middle and inferior two-thirds. The internal opening, if present, is located in the tonsillar fossae. Fistula or sinus tracts may course over the hypoglossal and glossopharyngeal nerves and between the carotid vessels. Cysts may occur anywhere along this course, but most commonly they are present in the anterior triangle of the neck *below* the level of the hyoid bone (Fig. 5).

The external opening of a third branchial cleft anomaly, if present, will be found in the same position as those of second cleft derivation; the internal opening, however, is

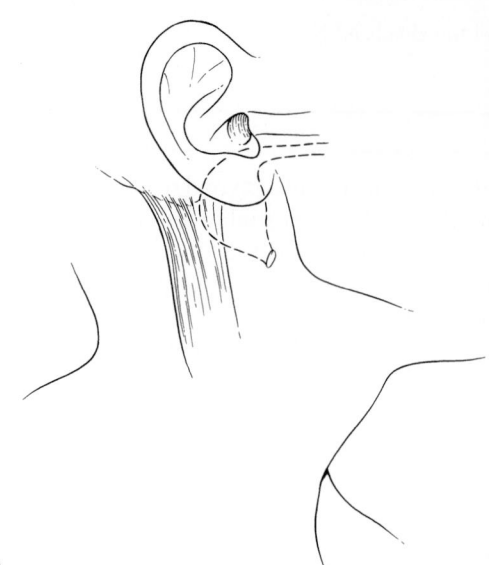

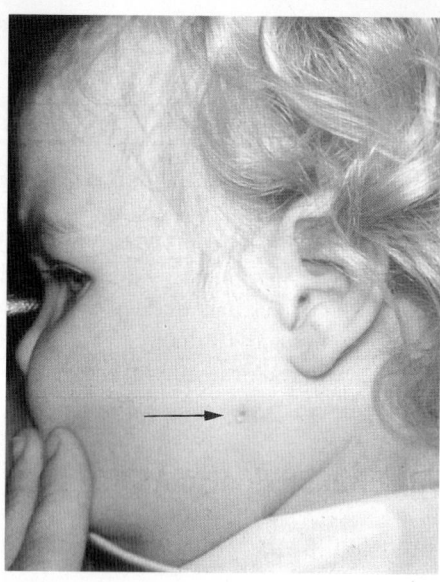

FIGURE 3 **A:** Diagrammatic representation of a type I first branchial anomaly sinus tract and cyst. **B:** Clinical example of an external sinus tract opening (*arrow*).

A

B

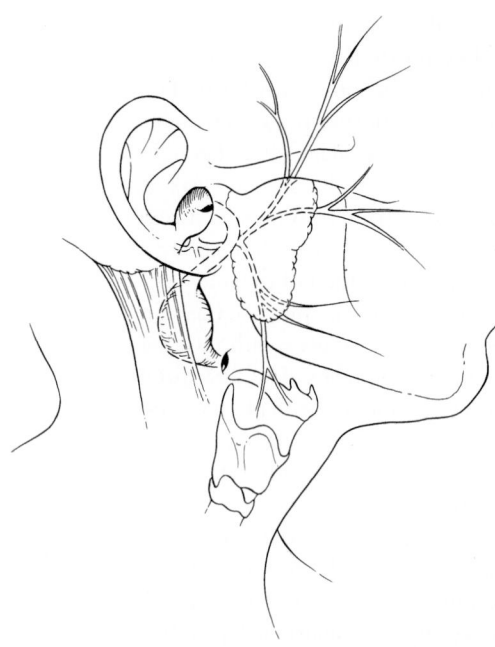

A

FIGURE 4 **A:** Diagrammatic representation of a type II first branchial anomaly fistula tract and cyst. **B:** Clinical example of an external fistula tract opening (*arrow*). **C:** Intraoperative demonstration of a fistula tract (*arrows*) passing beneath the branches of the facial nerve (*arrowheads*) to the cartilaginous external ear canal. The superficial parotidectomy specimen (*P*) and sternocleidomastoid muscle (*S*) are identified.

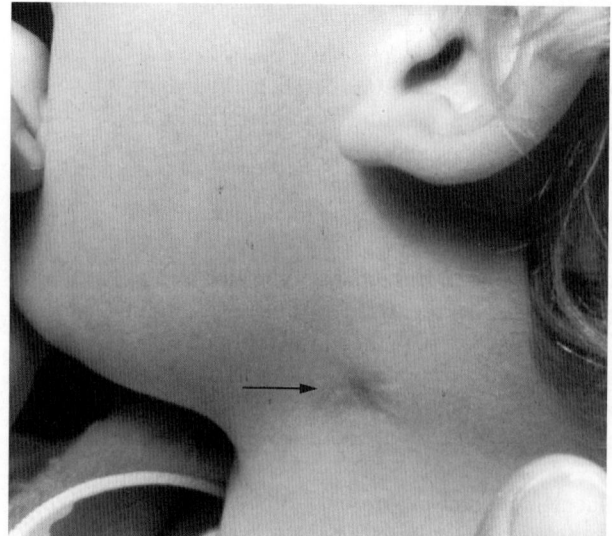

B

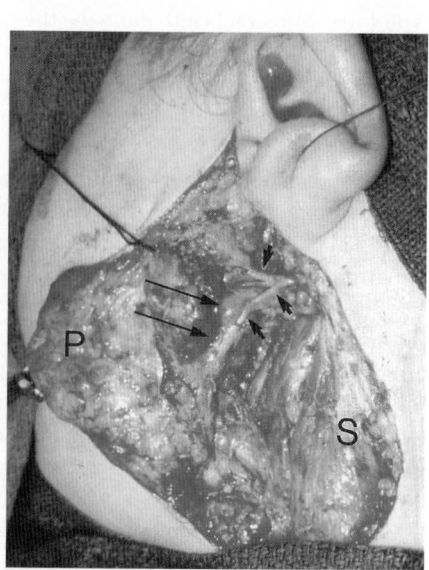

C

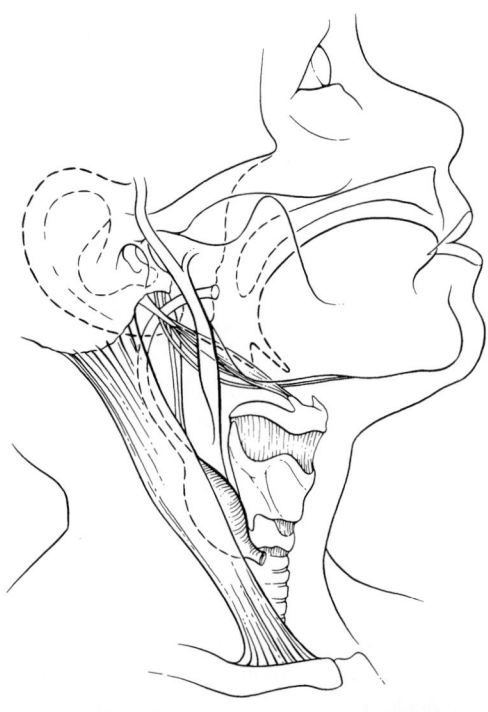

A

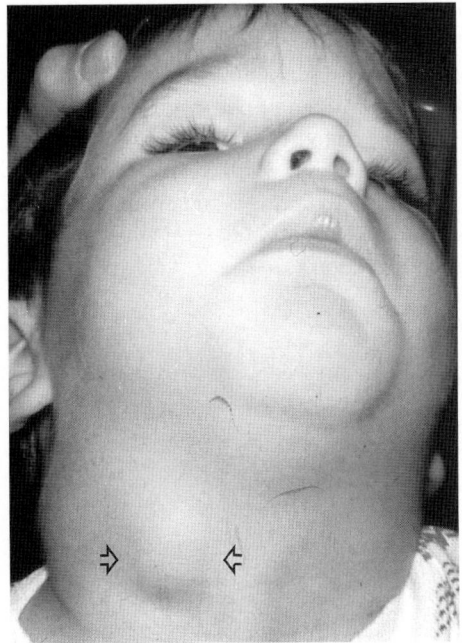

B

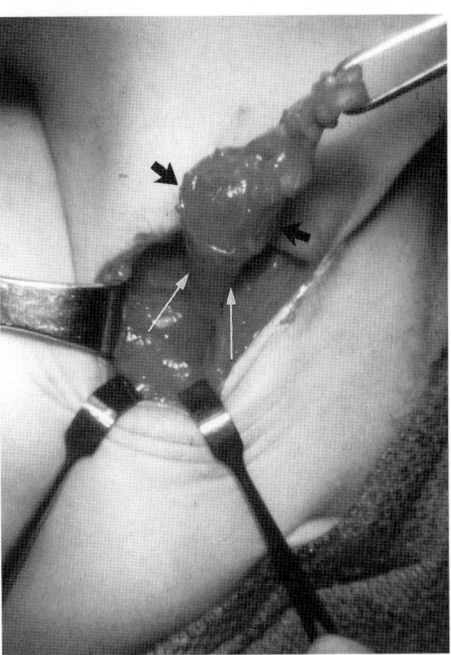

C

FIGURE 5 A: Diagrammatic representation of a second branchial anomaly fistula tract and cyst. **B:** Clinical example of a cyst (*arrowheads*) with no external sinus or fistula tract opening. **C:** Intraoperative demonstration of a cyst (*arrowheads*) and internal sinus tract (*arrows*) terminating in the tonsillar fossa.

located within the piriform sinus. Third cleft fistula or sinus tracts may pierce the thyrohyoid membrane cephalad to the superior laryngeal nerve, cross over the hypoglossal nerve and under the glossopharyngeal nerve, descend behind the internal carotid and along the common carotid artery, and terminate in the anterolateral region of the neck (Fig. 6). Cysts occur anywhere along this course, but most commonly are found in the anteroinferior cervical triangle.

The potential path of a fourth branchial arch derivative must lie between the fourth and sixth arch structures. The internal sinus opening would originate near the apex of the piriform sinus, caudal to the superior laryngeal nerve. The potential tract would descend translaryngeal under the thyroid ala to emerge beneath the inferior constrictor muscle, exiting the larynx near the cricothyroid joint; it would then descend superficial to the re-

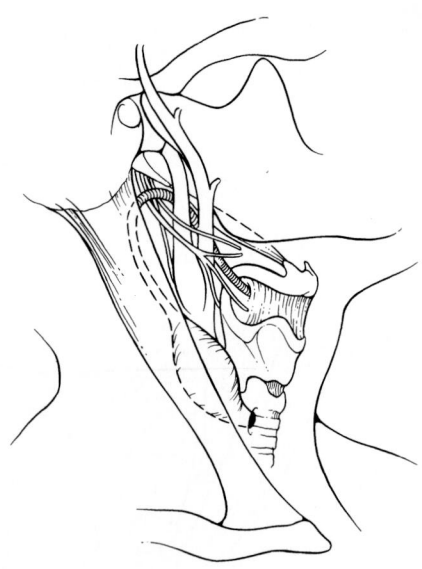

FIGURE 6 Diagrammatic representation of a third branchial anomaly fistula tract and cyst.

current laryngeal nerve in the paratracheal region adjacent to the thyroid gland (Fig. 7). A true fistula of the fourth arch would follow an extremely tortuous course with eventual termination in the anteroinferior region of the neck.

Branchial cysts present in a clinical fashion different from that of sinuses and fistulas. In the absence of infection, branchial cysts typically enlarge gradually and do not become evident until the second or third decade of life. Presentation earlier in childhood is often due to acute, painful enlargement associated with an upper respiratory tract infection (2). Such inflammatory enlargement is attributed to hypertrophy of subepithelial lymphoid tissue characteristically found within branchial cyst walls. Such inflamed cysts may progress to abscess formation with the possibility of rupture and secondary sinus tract formation. Symptomatic branchial cysts in infants are notably rare; when present, aerodigestive tract compromise is a frequent manifestation.

FIGURE 7 Diagrammatic representation of a fourth branchial anomaly sinus tract and cyst.

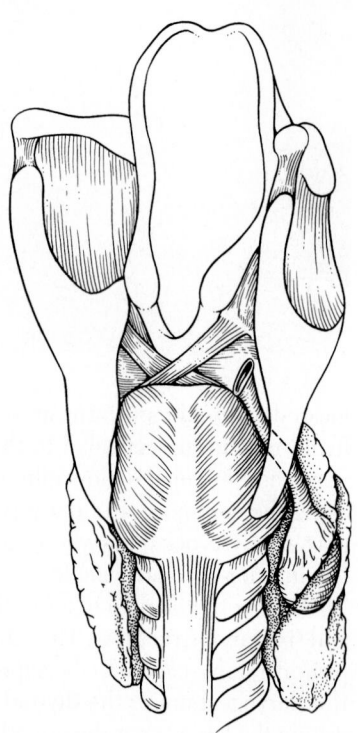

In contrast to branchial cysts, the external opening of a congenital sinus or fistula tract is often detected at birth or soon thereafter during routine physical examination (Fig. 8A); noninfected tracts may secrete a mucus-like material (Fig. 8B). Secondary infection of externally opening sinuses and fistulas frequently occurs. The etiologic organisms in such cases are typically of cutaneous origin, and are most commonly *Staphylococcus aureus* and group A beta-hemolytic streptococci (2). The clinical presentation varies depending on the branchial cleft of origin. For example, infected first branchial cleft anomalies may present with persistent aural discharge in the absence of middle ear disease. If there is a cyst associated with this sinus or fistula tract, the child may present with both a draining ear and a tender lump in the neck. Infected second and third branchial cleft anomalies typically present in similar fashion with an externally draining tract with or without an associated enlarging neck mass.

A less frequent presentation of branchial anomalies is that of a recurrent neck abscess in a child who demonstrates no evidence of an external opening. A vestigial branchial pouch maintaining its internal opening into the tonsillar fossa or, more commonly, piriform sinus is the likely etiology in such cases (18). Third and fourth branchial pouch anomalies have also been recognized as a potential cause of acute suppurative thyroiditis in children. Such children present with fever, paratracheal fullness, and tenderness, typically on the left side. A decrease in radioisotope uptake in the ipsilateral thyroid lobe can be documented on thyroid scans. Operative cultures in these children demonstrate a variety of aerobic and anaerobic organisms consistent with a perithyroidal abscess of pharyngeal origin.

The treatment of children with branchial cleft anomalies begins with a careful and complete physical examination searching for other anomalous systemic findings. Although these lesions typically occur as isolated unilateral or bilateral entities, anomalous branchial system development does occur in both craniofacial and multiorgan syndromes. Branchio-oto-renal syndrome and the DiGeorge sequence are two such examples (Table 2).

Radiographic studies, particularly CT and MRI, can add valuable information in the evaluation of suspected branchial anomalies. Cysts can be defined in terms of location and size (Fig. 9A), and unsuspected sinus tracts may be identified. If an external opening is present, iodinated contrast material can be injected to outline the tract. In the child who presents with a recurrent left lateral neck abscess or suppurative thyroiditis, a barium swallow study may detect an internal sinus opening (Fig. 10); the performance of direct pharyngoscopy is recommended in the absence of such radiologic documentation.

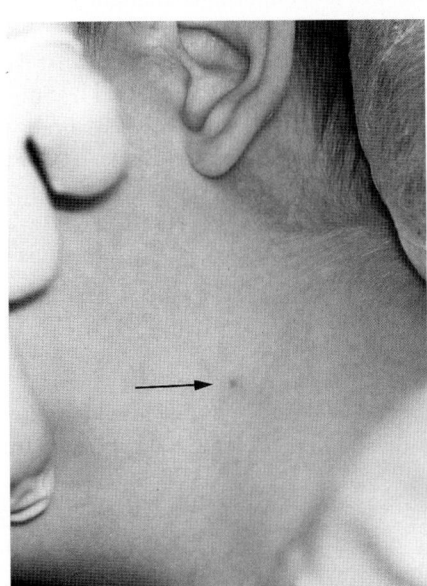 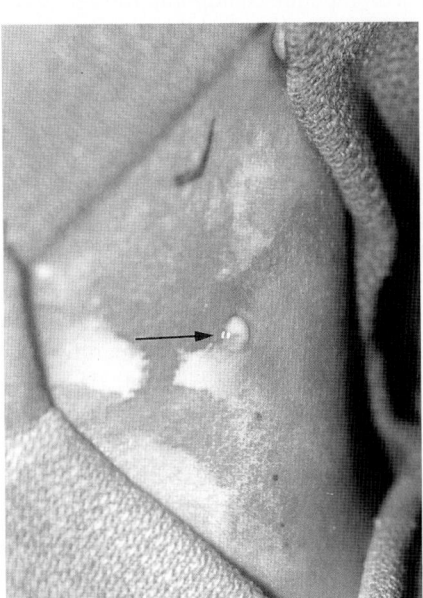

FIGURE 8 A: Second branchial anomaly sinus tract opening (*arrow*). **B:** Neck palpation results in drainage of mucoid material from this site (*arrow*).

A   B

TABLE 2: Representative Branchial Arch Disorders

Branchial Arch Disorder	Cervicofacial Characteristics
Oculo-auriculo-vertebral spectrum (hemifacial microsomia, Goldenhar's syndrome)	Facial asymmetry due to unilateral maxillary, temporal, and malar hypoplasia; wide spectrum of pinna and external ear canal malformation; preauricular cartilaginous tags, pits, and sinus tracts; conductive hearing loss due to external- and middle-ear malformations; aplasia or hypoplasia of the mandibular ramus and condyle; multiple ophthalmologic abnormalities, most commonly epibulbar dermoids
Mandibulofacial dysostosis (Treacher Collins syndrome, Franceschetti-Zwalen-Klein syndrome)	Characteristic narrow facial appearance with downward-sloping palpebral fissures, depressed cheek bones, malformed pinna, receding chin, and large down-turned tongue; cartilaginous ear tags and sinus tracts anywhere between the tragus and angle of the mouth; external- and middle-ear malformations with conductive hearing loss; short neck and malformed mandibular condyles
Branchio-oto-renal (BOR) syndrome	Branchial sinus/fistula tracts with characteristic external cervical opening; usually bilateral, may be unilateral
	Various pinna malformations; narrow or atretic ear canals; cartilaginous preauricular appendages and pits; middle-and/or inner-ear malformations with conductive, sensorineural, or mixed hearing loss
DiGeorge sequence	Complete or partial absence of the thymus gland; if partial, commonly cervical thymic remnants
	Micrognathia; deep-set, low-set, small, posteriorly angulated ears; anteverted nostrils; blunting, clefting, or indentation of the nose; hypertelorism

(From Branchial arch and oro-acral disorders. In: Gorlin RJ, Cohen MM Jr, Levin LS. *Syndromes of the head and neck*, 3rd ed. New York: Oxford University Press, 1990:641–691.)

A complete surgical excision of branchial cysts and sinus/fistula tracts is advocated. A general rule of thumb is to await complete resolution of inflammation in the patient with infection. If possible, incision and drainage procedures should be avoided but may be necessary for acute abscess treatment before definitive resection (Fig. 9B and C). From a therapeutic standpoint, the age of the child is of less importance than the overall clinical presentation. A child of any age with aerodigestive tract compromise requires acute surgical intervention; an otherwise healthy infant with a noninfected sinus/fistula opening can be followed for a few years to allow for a larger operative field and less potential damage to surrounding normal anatomic structures. Any decision to delay surgery must take into account the high incidence of secondary infection of these lesions. Interim infection not only causes acute morbidity but results in postinflammatory fibrosis, increasing the difficulty of excision and the possibility of incomplete resection.

The definitive excision of first branchial cleft anomalies, particularly type II anomalies, requires identification and preservation of the facial nerve (see Fig. 4C) (19). The small caliber of the facial nerve structures and their more superficial position in the very young child increase the risk of operative injury. The insertion of the fistulous tract into the external auditory canal, as well as any previous inflammation and secondary scarring, may further complicate this process. A standard S-shaped parotidectomy incision in the preauricular crease and extending under the mandible is the recommended approach. In older children and adults, the classic landmarks of parotid surgery—the cartilaginous pointer and styloid process—are used to identify the main trunk of the facial nerve. In the young child these landmarks are often absent or poorly developed. The facial nerve in a young child may appear just deep to the parotid fascia as it is separated from the tragal cartilage. If the nerve cannot be readily identified, then it should be sought in the tri-

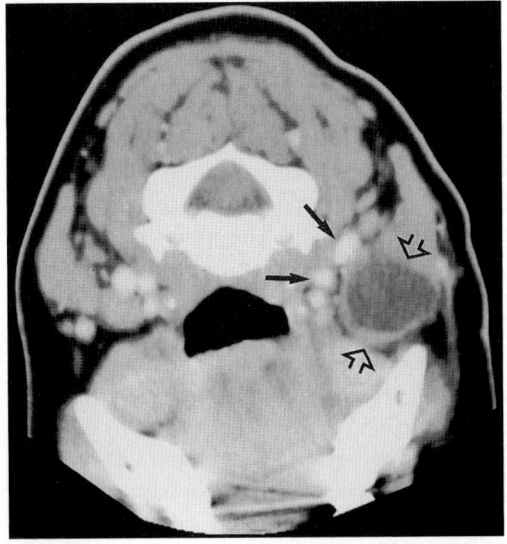

A

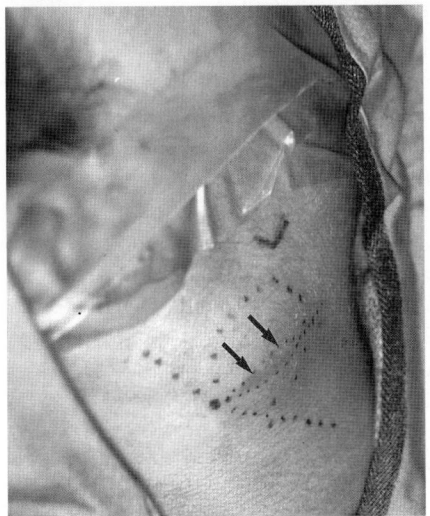

B

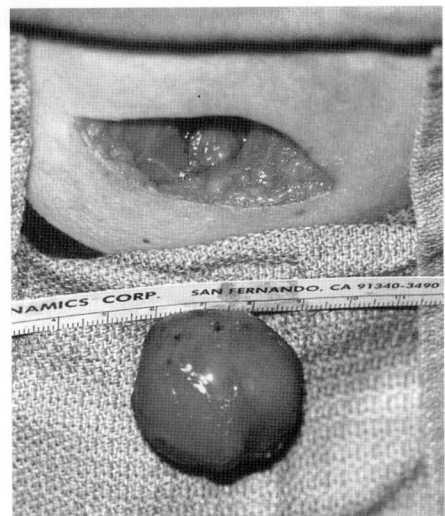

C

FIGURE 9 A: Axial computed tomographic image of a large cystic mass (*open arrowheads*) deep to the sternocleidomastoid muscle abutting the major vessels (*short arrows*) at the level of the oropharynx. **B:** The surgical incision incorporates a previous "incision and drainage" scar (*arrows*); the cyst itself, angle of the mandible, and border of the sternocleidomastoid muscle are also outlined. **C:** Pathologic examination revealed the excised mass to be a branchial cyst.

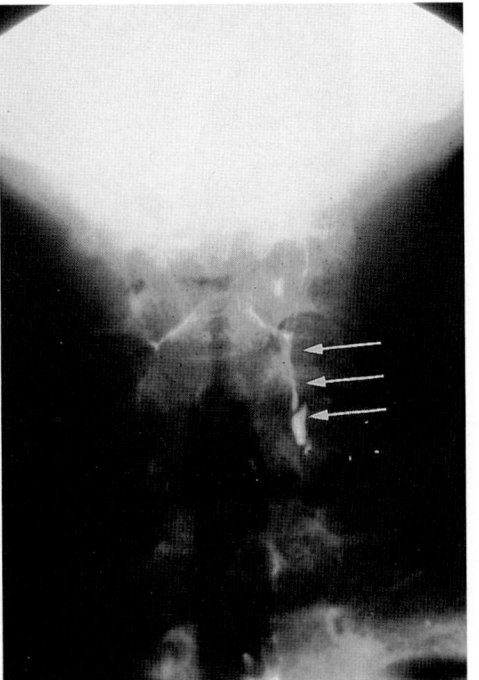

FIGURE 10 Barium swallow fluoroscopy documents a sinus tract (*arrow*) originating from the left piriform sinus in a child who presented with an ipsilateral perithyroidal abscess.

angle formed by the anterior border of the sternocleidomastoid muscle, the posterior border of the digastric muscle, and the cartilage of the ear canal (20). The anterior border of the sternocleidomastoid muscle can be found first in the neck and followed up to this triangle. Once the facial nerve is identified, it is followed into the substance of the parotid gland in standard superficial parotidectomy fashion. The previously dissected tract of the branchial cleft anomaly can then be carefully passed over or under the main branches of the facial nerve as needed (see Fig. 4C). The tract is then followed to its termination in or near the external ear canal; a portion of the cartilaginous canal must often be sacrificed for complete excision. Isolated first branchial cleft cysts in an intraparotid or paraparotid position may clinically masquerade as parotid tumors preoperatively and similarly require a superficial parotidectomy approach.

An elliptical skin incision is recommended around external openings of sinus or fistula tracts in the neck. In the case of a presumed cervical branchial cyst with no external orifice, an incision directly below the inferior margin of the cyst along a neck crease is indicated. Typically the excision of second and third branchial cleft anomalies is carried cephalad until a second, parallel, "stepladder" incision is necessary (Fig. 11). Such stepladder incisions avoid disfiguring vertical scars.

Adequate amounts of connective tissue around the sinus or fistula tract need to be excised to ensure removal of all epithelial remnants. Attempts to enhance the likelihood of complete tract excision have included injections of sterile methylene blue, liquid paraffin, or quick-hardening polymers, and the insertion of esophageal bougies and other blunt probes. A newer approach using a balloon embolectomy catheter has several potential benefits over previously used methods: The catheter is radiopaque for radiographic documentation; it can be secured either externally with a stitch or internally by insufflation of the balloon; and its inherent flexibility and varied diameters allow for intubation of different size tracts (21).

Special mention must be made of those children with recurrent acute neck abscesses who are suspected of having an infected branchial pouch sinus tract. Complete excision of a second branchial pouch anomaly may require a tonsillectomy for internal tract closure. In those children with recurrent suppurative thyroiditis, documentation of a piriform si-

FIGURE 11 Surgical excision of a long fistula tract by means of stepladder incisions. (Photograph courtesy of Eugene Myers, M.D.)

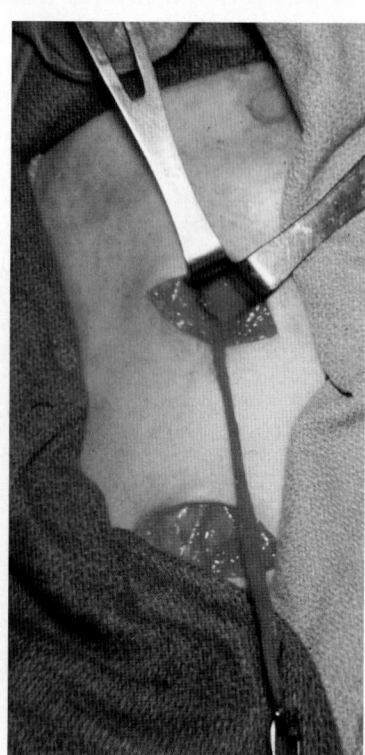

nus internal opening by radiographic or endoscopic means is crucial; the diagnosis should be questioned if careful examination fails to show such a pharyngeal connection. Intubation of the sinus opening with a balloon catheter or blunt instrument may facilitate the external dissection. A standard thyroidectomy collar incision is recommended with exposure of the thyroid gland, larynx, and lateral neck structures. The initial operative findings should allow distinction between the suspected diagnoses of a third or fourth branchial pouch sinus (18,22). As mentioned previously, if the tract pierces the thyrohyoid membrane, a third pouch anomaly would be suspected; identification of a tract in the cricothyroid region would suggest a fourth pouch derivative. Identification and preservation of the recurrent laryngeal nerve is crucial in the latter. A partial or total ipsilateral thyroid lobectomy is often necessary; if possible, the thyroid lobe should be kept attached to the inflammatory mass, and the entire specimen traced cephalad along the carotid sheath toward the piriform sinus. Alternatively, the tract can initially be identified and ligated at the piriform sinus and traced in retrograde fashion toward the thyroid. Retraction of the thyroid alar cartilage anteriorly to facilitate piriform sinus exposure is necessary in completing the excision of fourth branchial pouch anomalies.

Complications of branchial anomaly operations include secondary infection and damage to nearby anatomic structures, most prominently the seventh cranial nerve during first branchial cleft surgery and the recurrent laryngeal nerve during third and especially fourth branchial pouch surgery. Recurrence rates are approximately 3% for patients with no prior infection or surgery, increasing to approximately 20% if there was a previous unsuccessful attempt at removal (16,17). Recurrences are about twice as likely to occur following the excision of branchial sinuses and fistulas compared with isolated branchial cysts. Radiographic evaluation is particularly important in the evaluation of suspected recurrent branchial anomalies, and a functional neck dissection in the patient with recurrent second, third, and fourth branchial cervical remnants is the recommended approach (23).

Thymus Gland Anomalies

The thymus gland principally arises from the third branchial pouch with a possible contribution from the fourth branchial pouch. The thymic primordia arise bilaterally, elongate from the pharynx in a caudal and medial direction, and fuse before descent into the mediastinum. Potential connections to the pharynx remain as hollow epithelial structures termed *thymopharyngeal ducts*. Ectopic solid thymus tissue results from failure of one or both thymic lobes to descend or from sequestration of thymic tissue along the cervical pathways of descent. The thymopharyngeal ducts may also fail to involute with secondary cystic changes in their persistent remnants; the resultant thymopharyngeal duct cyst is also called a *cervical thymic cyst*.

Ectopic solid thymic tissue typically presents as a neck mass during the first decade of life; this reflects the fact that the thymus is of greatest relative size at birth and reaches its greatest absolute size by puberty (24). Thymopharyngeal or cervical thymic cysts similarly present in the pediatric age group as slowly enlarging, painless masses (25). The main entity to be differentiated from a thymopharyngeal or cervical thymic cyst is a branchial cyst of third or fourth pouch origin. These two entities share a clinical predilection for a left paramedian neck location and similar histopathology, differing principally in the presence of thymic tissue within the thymopharyngeal cyst wall. They are apparently both derived from the same vestigial structure and are closely related, if not identical.

The definitive treatment of thymus gland anomalies is surgical excision, utilizing the same principles outlined in the management of branchial cysts (Fig. 12).

Dermoid Cysts

The predilection of dermoid cysts to occur along lines of embryologic fusion includes the junction of the first and second branchial arches, particularly in the submental, sub-

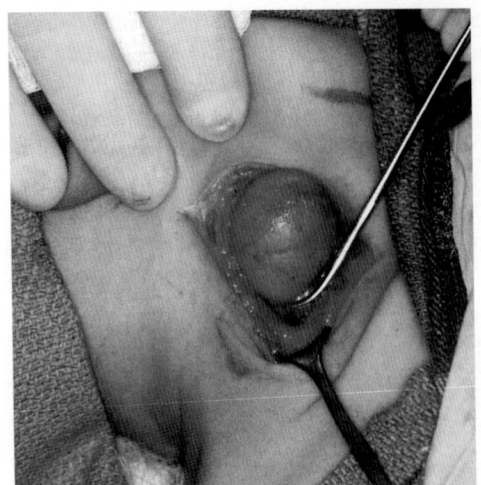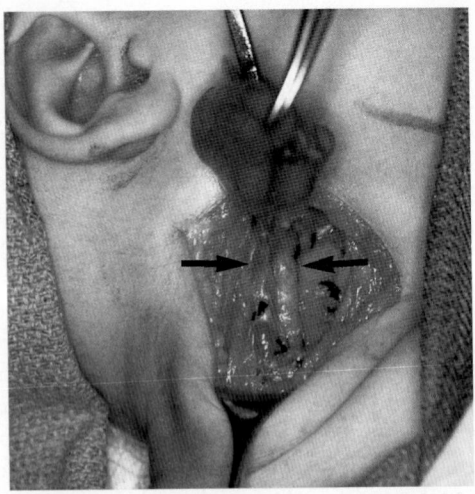

FIGURE 12 A: Intraoperative documentation of an anterocervical solid mass in an infant. **B:** The avascular mass was dissected off the carotid sheath (*arrows*); pathologic examination revealed ectopic thymic tissue. (Photographs courtesy of Michael Williams, M.D.)

mandibular, and thyrohyoid regions. In such locations, preoperative clinical and radiologic differentiation of dermoid cysts from branchial cleft cysts is often not possible. The recommended treatment is similar for both lesions, consisting of complete surgical excision. An incision directly below the inferior margin of the cyst along a neck crease is typically utilized (Fig. 13).

Teratomas

Teratomas are often included under the dermoid lesion category although they differ both clinically and histopathologically. They are rare lesions composed of multiple tissues involving all three germ cell layers (ectoderm, mesoderm, and endoderm) in various degrees of maturity. Teratomas involving the soft tissues of the neck make up about 3% of all childhood teratomas (26). They commonly present at birth as large midline or paramedian lesions causing secondary aerodigestive tract compromise (Fig. 14). There is a 20% to 50% associated incidence of maternal polyhydramnios; the prenatal diagnosis of teratoma is possible in such cases by prenatal ultrasound or MRI.

Children born with massive cervical teratomas often have an immediately compromised airway that requires securement either by endotracheal intubation or by tracheotomy. Extracorporeal membrane oxygenation is extremely valuable in newborn infants in whom airway stabilization is a problem (27).

The radiographic diagnosis of teratoma is suggested by the presence of calcifications on plain films or mixed echogenicity with multiloculated cystic/solid regions on ultrasonography. CT or MRI is particularly useful in demonstrating the anatomic relationship of massive teratomas to surrounding vascular, bony, and visceral structures.

Surgical resection of teratomas is recommended as soon as medically feasible. These lesions tend to be well encapsulated and poorly vascularized, characteristics that enhance the likelihood of total excision. In contrast to adult teratomas, pediatric lesions rarely manifest biologic malignancy.

Vascular Anomalies

The most common congenital vascular anomalies affecting the head and neck region in the pediatric population are hemangiomas and vascular malformations of the venous, lymphatic, capillary, and arteriovenous variety. The presentation and management of these lesions are discussed in detail in Chapter 56. Two vascular anomalies deserve spe-

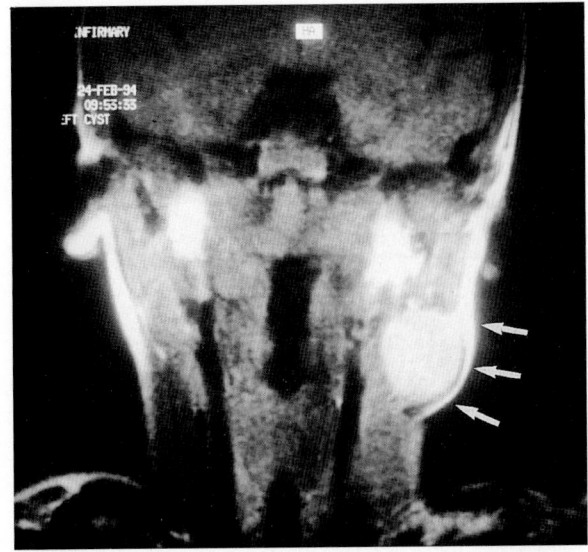

A

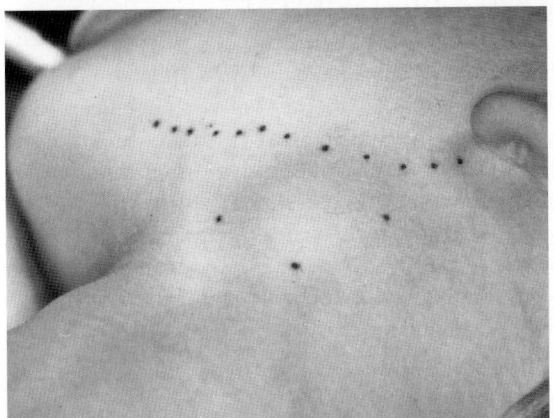

B

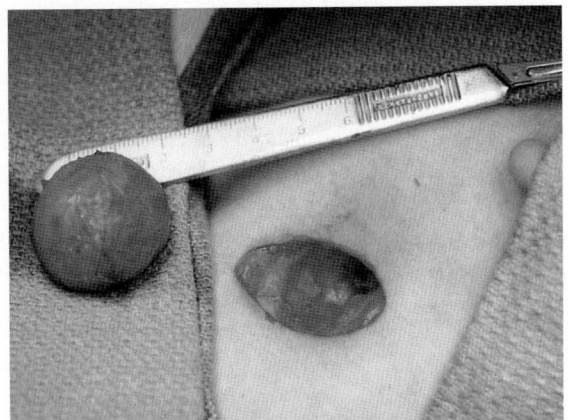

C

FIGURE 13 A: Coronal T$_2$ magnetic resonance imaging scan of a hyperintense, unilocular cystic mass (*arrows*) along the anterior border of the left sternocleidomastoid muscle. **B:** Intraoperative outline of the mass relative to the mandible border. **C:** Pathologic examination revealed the excised mass to be a dermoid cyst.

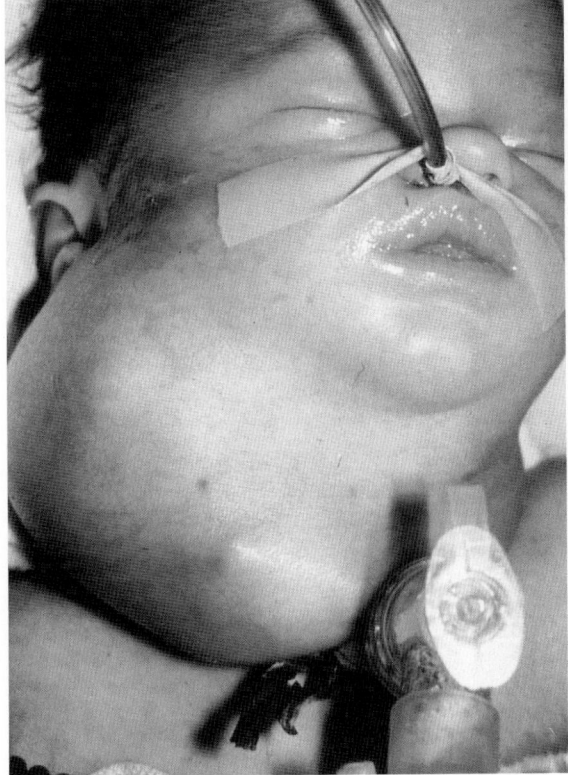

FIGURE 14 Massive right cervical teratoma in an infant requiring emergent neonatal airway support. (Photograph courtesy of Sylvan Stool, M.D.)

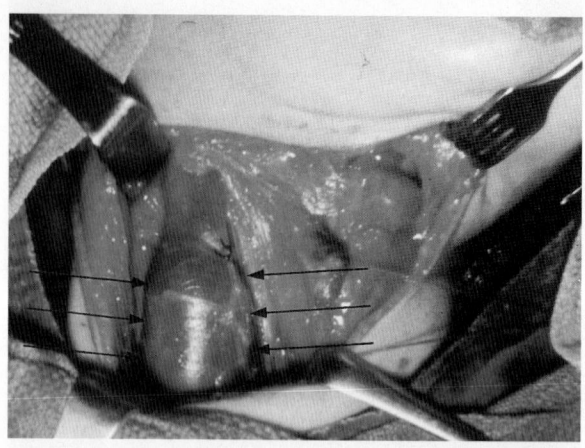

FIGURE 15 Intraoperative documentation of a jugular vein phlebectasia (*arrows*).

cial mention due to their comparative rarity and their capability of masquerading as common cystic pediatric neck masses.

The jugular vein phlebectasia is an isolated saccular or fusiform dilatation of the jugular vein that increases in size with straining, crying, or other Valsalva maneuvers (28). The majority of these venous lesions are noted within the first decade of life as cystic swellings anterior to the border of the sternocleidomastoid muscle. Congenital or mechanical obstruction of the jugular vein in the neck or mediastinum is the suspected etiology. Phlebectasias have historically been diagnosed when surgical exploration has been performed anticipating an alternative etiology (Fig. 15). A suspected diagnosis can be preoperatively established by a variety of radiographic techniques including MRI, CT with intravenous contrast enhancement, or digital subtraction angiography. Confirmed asymptomatic phlebectasias require no treatment.

FIGURE 16 A: Axial computed tomography scan of an enhancing left parapharyngeal space mass (*arrowheads*) in a teenage woman who presented with a several month history of atraumatic swelling in the left side of the neck. **B:** Arteriography revealed the mass to be an aneurysm of the left internal carotid artery just beyond the bifurcation (*arrows*); there is an additional aneurysm dilatation more superiorly at the skull base (*arrowheads*).

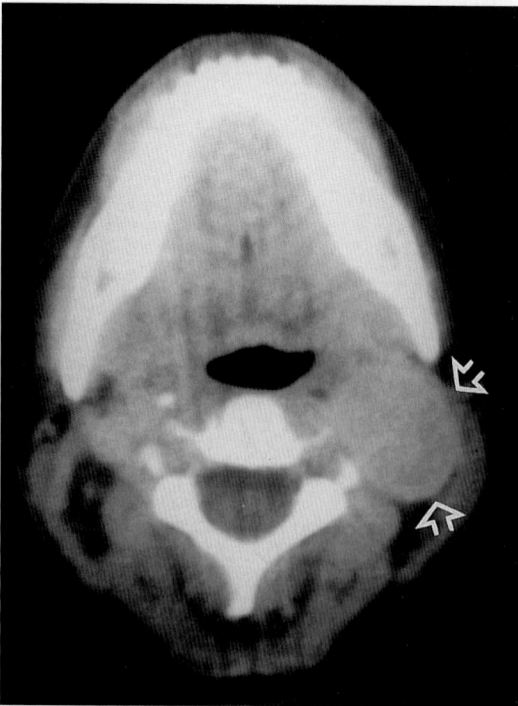

A

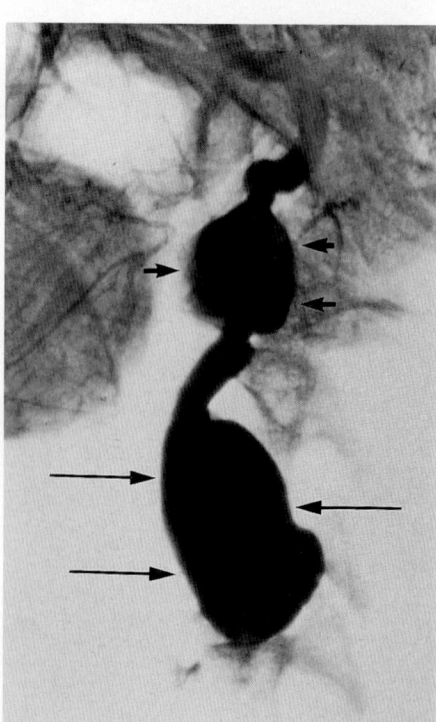

B

An aneurysmal dilatation of the internal or common carotid artery can additionally present as a superior cervical neck mass that characteristically has a pulsatile quality (29). The majority of carotid artery aneurysms occur secondary to predisposing cervical trauma or surgery. Atraumatic arterial wall dissection may occur in patients with angiopathic disorders, and rare idiopathic presentations have also been reported in young adults. Common associated symptoms include unilateral headache and cranial nerve manifestations. The suspected diagnosis can be established by a variety of radiographic techniques, particularly magnetic resonance angiography or arteriography (Fig. 16). Interim anticoagulation is suggested until proximal arterial ligation or definitive surgical repair can be performed.

PEARLS AND PERILS

1. Cysts and external tract openings of first branchial origin always occur superior to the hyoid bone, whereas those of second, third, or fourth branchial origin always present below the level of the hyoid bone.

2. A vestigial pouch maintaining its internal opening into the tonsillar fossa or, more commonly, piriform sinus needs to be sought in the child who presents with recurrent neck abscesses or suppurative thyroiditis.

3. The definitive excision of first branchial cleft anomalies, particularly type II anomalies, requires identification and preservation of the facial nerve.

4. Disfiguring scars following the excision of second and third branchial cleft tracts can be avoided by the use of stepladder incisions.

5. Operative findings during neck exploration best distinguish between the suspected diagnoses of third or fourth branchial pouch anomalies. A tract piercing the thyrohyoid membrane suggests a third pouch anomaly; a tract in the cricothyroid region suggests a fourth pouch derivative.

6. Recurrence rates following the excision of branchial anomalies increase from 3% in patients with no prior infection or surgery to approximately 20% if there was a previous unsuccessful attempt at removal.

7. A preoperative imaging study with vascular enhancement should be performed prior to surgical management of any anterocervical neck mass with a pulsatile quality or significant size increase during a Valsalva maneuver.

REFERENCES

1. Torsiglieri AJ Jr, Tom LWC, Ross AJ III, Wetmore RF, Handler SD, Potsic WP. Pediatric neck masses; guidelines for evaluation. *Int J Pediatr Otorhinolaryngol* 1988;16:199–210.

2. Myers EN, Cunningham MJ. Inflammatory presentations of congenital head and neck masses. *Pediatr Infect Dis J* 1988;7:S162–S168.

3. Friedman AP, Haller JO, Goodman JD, Nager H. Sonographic evaluation of noninflammatory neck masses in children. *Radiology* 1983;147:693–697.

4. Yuh WTC, Sato Y, Loes DJ, et al. Magnetic resonance imaging and computed tomography in pediatric head and neck masses. *Ann Otol Rhinol Laryngol* 1991;100:54–62.

5. Tunkel DE, Baroody FM, Sherman ME. Fine-needle aspiration biopsy of cervicofacial masses in children. *Arch Otolaryngol Head Neck Surg* 1995;121:533–536.

6. Pinczower E, Crockett DM, Atkinson JB, Kun S. Preoperative thyroid scanning in presumed thyroglossal duct cysts. *Arch Otolaryngol Head Neck Surg* 1992;118:985–988.

7. Hawkins DB, Jacobsen BE, Klatt EC. Cysts of the thyroglossal duct. *Laryngoscope* 1982;92:1254–1258.

8. Radkowski D, Arnold J, Healy GB, et al. Thryoglossal duct remnants; preoperative evaluation and management. *Arch Otolaryngol Head Neck Surg* 1991;117:1378–1381.

9. Schlange H. Uber Die Fistula Colli Congenita. *Arch Klin Chir* 1893;46:390–392.

10. Sistrunk WE. The surgical treatment of cysts of the thyroglossal tract. *Ann Surg* 1920;71:121–124.

11. Sistrunk WE. Technique of removal of cysts and sinuses of the thyroglossal duct. *Surg Gynecol Obstet* 1928;46:109–112.

12. Pelausa EO, Forte V. Sistrunk revisited: a 10-year review of revision thyroglossal duct surgery at Toronto's Hospital for Sick Children. *J Otolaryngol* 1989;18:325–333.

13. Mickel RA, Calcaterra TC. Management of recurrent thyroglossal duct cysts. *Arch Otolaryngol* 1983;109:34–36.

14. DeMello DE, Lima JA, Liapis H. Midline cervical cysts in children. *Arch Otolaryngol Head Neck Surg* 1987;113:418–420.

15. Baker HL, Baker SR, McClatchey KD. Manifestations and management of laryngoceles. *Head Neck Surg* 1982;4:450–456.

16. Chandler JR, Mitchell B. Branchial cysts, sinuses and fistulas. *Otolaryngol Clin North Am* 1981;14:175–186.

17. Choi SS, Zalzal GH. Branchial anomalies: a review of 52 cases. *Laryngoscope* 1995;105:909–913.

18. Rosenfeld RM, Biller HF. Fourth branchial pouch sinus: diagnosis and treatment. *Otolaryngol Head Neck Surg* 1991;105:44–50.

19. McCrae RG, Lee KJ, Goertzen E. First branchial cleft anomalies and the facial nerve. *Otolaryngol Head Neck Surg* 1983;91:197–202.

20. Farrior JB, Santini H. Facial nerve identification in children. *Otolaryngol Head Neck Surg* 1985;93:173–176.

21. Feldman JI, Kearns DB, Pransky SM, Seid AB. Catheterization of branchial sinus tracts: a new method. *Int J Pediatr Otorhinolaryngol* 1990;20:1–5.

22. Godin MS, Kerrns DB, Pransky SM, Seid AB, Wilson DB. Fourth branchial pouch sinus: principles of diagnosis and management. *Laryngoscope* 1990;100:174–178.

23. Blackwell KE, Calcaterra TC. Functional neck dissection for treatment of recurrent branchial remnants. *Arch Otolaryngol Head Neck Surg* 1994;120:417–421.

24. Boyd J, Templer J, Havey A, Walls J, Decker J. Persistent thymopharyngeal duct cyst. *Otolaryngol Head Neck Surg* 1993;109:135–139.

25. Nguyen Q, deTar M, Wells W, Crocckett D. Cervical thymic cyst: case reports and review of the literature. *Laryngoscope* 1996;106:247–252.

26. Rothschild MA, Catalano P, Urken M, et al. Evaluation and management of congenital cervical teratoma. *Arch Otolaryngol Head Neck Surg* 1994;120:444–448.

27. Kelly MF, Berenholz L, Rizzo KA, Greco R, Wolfson P, Zwillenberg DA. Approach for oxygenation of the newborn with airway obstruction due to a cervical mass. *Ann Otol Rhinol Laryngol* 1990;99:179–182.

28. Mickelson SA, Spickler E, Roberts K. Management of internal jugular vein phlebectasia. *Otolaryngol Head Neck Surg* 1995;112:473–475.

29. Haynes DS, Schwaber MK, Netterville JL. Internal carotid artery aneurysms presenting as neck masses. *Otolaryngol Head Neck Surg* 1992;107:787–791.

M.J. Cunningham: Department of Otology and Laryngology, Harvard Medical School, and Department of Otolaryngology, Massachusetts Eye and Ear Infirmary, Boston, Massachusetts 02130.

- *Practical Pediatric Otolaryngology*
- edited by Robin T. Cotton and Charles M. Myer, III
- Lippincott-Raven Publishers, Philadelphia © 1999

Neoplastic Disorders: Benign and Malignant

Michael J. Cunningham

The differential diagnosis of a neck mass in a child includes inflammatory lesions, congenital lesions, and both benign and malignant neoplasms. Although comparatively rare, an estimated 5% to 10% of primary malignant tumors in children originate in the head and neck area, and one of every four malignant lesions has eventual manifestations in the head and neck region (1). Any noninflammatory, firm neck mass in a child should be considered of potential neoplastic etiology until proved otherwise.

There are certain historical and clinical findings that increase the suspicion of malignancy. Worrisome historical factors include a family history of childhood cancer, a previous primary neoplasm, a known predisposition to systemic cancer, previous radiation therapy, and exposure to either carcinogenic or immunosuppressive drugs. Clinical findings that suggest the need for urgent biopsy include a history of rapid or progressive growth, fixation of the mass to the skin or deep neck structures, a supraclavicular location, or the occurrence of a firm neck mass in a child with weight loss or prolonged fever in whom a specific diagnosis is uncertain (2). Additional criteria for concern include firm masses of any size in neonates, firm masses greater than or equal to 1 cm in children 6 to 12 months old, or firm masses greater than or equal to 3 cm in diameter in children over 1 year old (3). In the absence of the above findings, observation with serial measurements over several weeks is a reasonable method of discriminating less worrisome underlying pathology such as hyperplastic lymphadenopathy from potential neoplastic disease processes. Subsequent elective biopsy for diagnostic confirmation is recommended if the mass in question increases in size at 2 weeks' follow-up or if the mass in question fails to decrease in size by 4 to 6 weeks' follow-up.

The child suspected of having a cervical neoplasm based on the above historical or clinical features, or both, requires a complete otolaryngologic and systemic examination. The importance of a thorough otolaryngologic examination is underscored by the observation that one of every six children with a malignant neck mass has a primary oronasopharyngeal lesion (4). Otologic, nasal, oral, and neck examinations are easily performed in most children. Flexible fiberoptic nasopharyngoscopes permit direct visualization of the nasopharynx, hypopharynx, and larynx in children of all ages. Direct laryngoscopy and pharyngoscopy under general anesthesia are required for those children who cannot be examined satisfactorily in the outpatient setting. Particular attention during the systemic examination should be directed at the abdomen, axillary, and inguinal areas as the cervical mass may be one manifestation of a generalized neoplastic process involving these additional regions.

The initial workup in evaluating children with potential cervical neoplasms should include a complete blood cell count and chest radiograph. Additional laboratory and roentgenographic studies are performed as indicated. Computed tomography (CT) and magnetic resonance imaging (MRI) are the radiologic studies of choice (5). CT is of value in delineating between cystic and solid lesions, in establishing lesion location relative to other anatomic structures, in determining vascularity when used with contrast infusion, and in allowing documentation of osseous involvement. Advantages of MRI include comparatively greater soft tissue detail, enhanced vascular delineation, multiplanar images, and the absence of radiation exposure. MRI's principal disadvantage is the requirement for sedation in young children, owing to the comparatively prolonged imaging time and the confining nature of the MRI apparatus. In specific clinical circumstances, radioisotope scans and angiographic procedures may supply additional useful information.

Although the physical examination and laboratory evaluation may suggest a diagnosis, biopsy of cervicofacial masses is required for diagnostic confirmation. Biopsy can be performed in either percutaneous or open fashion. The choice between these two techniques is dictated by several factors (6).

Percutaneous fine-needle aspiration (FNA) biopsy is recommended when a preliminary histopathologic diagnosis better selects or eliminates the need for future definitive operative intervention, or when the cervicofacial lesion in question is considered clinically unresectable. In the hands of an experienced cytopathologist, FNA biopsy can distinguish benign from malignant lesions and may also be accurate in predicting specific tumor type (7). Sampling errors do occur, and negative FNA biopsy findings should never be considered definitive when there is clinical suspicion of malignancy. A subsequent open surgical biopsy is necessary in such circumstances.

Open surgical biopsy is additionally advocated in children whose age or level of cooperation would require general anesthesia for the completion of percutaneous biopsy. Open surgical biopsy is also strongly recommended in clinical situations in which surgical excision is the likely definitive treatment of the cervical mass in question, whether benign or malignant. The biopsy incision in such cases should be designed so that it can be incorporated into a formal surgical excision if such proves feasible or necessary.

The obtainment of frozen sections is strongly recommended during open surgical

---

PEARLS AND PERILS

1. Malignancy should be suspected in a child with a *firm* neck mass and any of the associated clinical features:

   History of rapid or progressive growth.
   Fixation to the skin or deep neck structures.
   Supraclavicular location.
   Onset in the neonatal period.
   Size greater than or equal to 3 cm.
   Occurrence in a child with weight loss or prolonged fever in whom a specific diagnosis is undetermined.

2. Consider percutaneous fine-needle aspiration biopsy when:

   A preliminary histopathologic diagnosis better selects, modifies, or eliminates the need for future definitive operative intervention.
   The cervical mass is clinically unresectable.

3. Consider open surgical biopsy when:

   The child's age or level of cooperation dictates general anesthesia for the performance of the biopsy.
   More sufficient quantities of pathologic tissue than obtainable by percutaneous biopsy are required for definitive histopathologic diagnosis (e.g., suspected lymphoma).
   There is clinical suspicion of malignancy despite a negative percutaneous biopsy.
   Excision is the likely definitive treatment of the cervical mass in question.

biopsy, not to necessarily make a definitive intraoperative diagnosis, but to be certain that sufficient pathologic tissue has been obtained from which a future histopathologic diagnosis can be made on the basis of permanent sections. Extensive lesion resection with potential compromise of vital neurovascular structures should not be performed on the basis of frozen section results alone.

Specific clinical situations may additionally dictate preoperative oncology consultation so that arrangements can be made to obtain adjuvant studies such as lumbar puncture or bone marrow biopsy while the child is under anesthesia. Preoperative pathology consultation is also important in suspected lymphoma cases so that fresh tissue preparations can be made for cell culture and lymphoma marker studies.

The definitive treatment of cervical malignancies in the pediatric age group is dictated by the permanent histopathologic diagnosis as well as the extent or stage of the disease. Coordination of treatment often requires the interaction of many pediatric specialists and support services.

BENIGN NEOPLASMS

The most common noninflammatory benign masses that present in the cervical region in children are of congenital origin (8). There are, however, a comparatively smaller number of benign neoplastic and neoplastic-like lesions that can additionally manifest as asymptomatic neck masses. These include pilomatrixomas, lipomas, and peripheral nervous system tumors.

Pilomatrixoma

Pilomatrixomas, also known as Malherbe's calcifying epitheliomas, are solitary, firm, nontender, intradermal or subcutaneous masses histopathologically representative of hamartomas of hair follicle origin. Their firmness reflects a high incidence of calcium deposition and occasional ossification.

Approximately 60% of pilomatrixomas occur in the head and neck, and 40% occur in children under 10 years old (9). They can be of variable size and be clinically confused with lymph nodes, calcified hematomas, and other cervical neoplasms.

They are generally considered benign tumors without malignant potential. Surgical excision is typically curative.

Neural Tumors

Schwannomas and neurofibromas are benign tumors of the peripheral nervous system. The schwannoma is a solitary, often encapsulated, tumor that derives from the Schwann cell of the peripheral nerve sheath. It is estimated that 40% to 50% of all schwannomas arise in the head and neck, with the lateral cervical region being a particularly common site (10). Within the neck, the vagus nerve and sympathetic nerves are most commonly involved. Treatment is complete surgical excision with preservation of the underlying nerve if possible.

Neurofibromas may occur sporadically as solitary tumors, but much more commonly occur as multiple tumors in association with one of two genetic subtypes of systemic neurofibromatosis. Neurofibromas may involve any of the cranial, peripheral, or autonomic nerves. Superficial soft tissue neurofibromas appear as nodular or pedunculated lesions, whereas plexiform neurofibromas occur in deep tissues. Bony abnormalities are a common manifestation of neurofibromas of the head and neck, owing to adjacent bone erosion. Surgical excision is undertaken when the tumor is severely disfiguring or causing functional compromise; complete removal is infrequently achieved.

Lipomas

Lipomas are the most common tumor of mesenchymal origin. Their most frequent head and neck site is in the cervical region where the typical presentation is a slowly enlarging, painless, subcutaneous mass. Deeper lesions may compress the aerodigestive tract with secondary dysphagia or obstructive airway manifestations. Complete surgical excision is the treatment of choice. Two types of lipoma, spindle cell lipoma and pleomorphic lipoma, deserve special mention because of their potential histopathologic confusion with liposarcoma.

Sternocleidomastoid Tumor of Infancy

An additional benign cervical mass unique to the neonatal population is the sternocleidomastoid tumor of infancy (STI). Afflicted infants present with a firm mass within the substance of the sternocleidomastoid muscle at birth or within weeks thereafter. There may be associated torticollis with turning of the infant's head to the opposite side. A history of cervical trauma such as breech delivery or the use of forceps may be obtained, but such lesions also occur in children born by atraumatic vaginal delivery as well as cesarean section (11). The pathologic process appears to involve hemorrhage into the sternocleidomastoid muscle, with a subsequent inflammatory response and eventual fibrosis. Of importance in the evaluation of children with suspected STI is distinguishing this lesion from a malignancy or other congenital anomaly requiring surgical intervention. The radiographic appearance of STI on ultrasonography and CT scans is quite diagnostic. The performance of FNA biopsy, although also informative, is probably unnecessary except when either an uncharacteristic presentation or failure of spontaneous resolution raises the possibility of neoplasm.

STI usually resolves over several weeks to months, with conservative treatment consisting principally of physical therapy; the potential benefit of adjuvant measures such as heat or ultrasound application is uncertain. Those 10% to 20% of children with incomplete resolution can progress to congenital muscular torticollis with the potential for permanent craniofacial asymmetry (12). Therefore, surgical intervention is indicated if STI persists beyond 6 to 8 months; a distal sternocleidomastoid muscle release procedure is recommended.

MALIGNANT NEOPLASMS

Hodgkin's Lymphoma

Hodgkin's disease is a malignancy of the lymphoreticular system that predominantly presents in the cervical region in adolescents and young adults; less than 10% of Hodgkin's disease occurs in children 15 years or younger (13). Boys are afflicted twice as frequently as girls. Enlarged, painless cervical adenopathy, especially in the supraclavicular fossa, is the typical presentation. Associated nonspecific systemic symptoms such as unexplained fever, night sweats, weight loss, weakness, anorexia, and pruritus occur in approximately one-third of patients.

The histopathologic subtype and extent of disease, as determined by the Ann Arbor staging classification system (Table 1), determine treatment. Protocols incorporating multiagent chemotherapy, radiotherapy, or combinations thereof are so effective that the role of otolaryngologic surgery is limited to diagnostic biopsy in most treatment circumstances. More than 90% of all Hodgkin's disease patients, regardless of stage, initially achieve complete remission. Prolonged remission and cure is attained in approximately 90% of patients with early stage I or II disease and in 35% to 60% of those with advanced stage III or IV disease (14).

TABLE 1: Ann Arbor Staging Classification of Hodgkin's Disease

Stage[a]	Definitions
I	Involvement of a single lymph node region, or a single extralymphatic organ or site (IE)
II	Involvement of 2 or more lymph node regions, or localized involvement of an extralymphatic site and 1 or more lymph node regions on same side of the diaphragm (IIE)
III	Involvement of lymph node regions on both sides of the diaphragm, which may be accompanied by involvement of the spleen (IIIS) or an extralymphatic organ or site (IIIE)
IV	Diffuse or disseminated involvement of one or more extralymphatic organs or tissue, with or without associated lymph node involvement

[a]Each stage is subdivided into A and B categories, which indicate the absence or presence, respectively, of documented fever, night sweats, or weight loss (> 10% of body weight in the 6 months before diagnosis).

Non-Hodgkin's Lymphoma

Non-Hodgkin's lymphoma designates a heterogeneous group of solid primary lymphoreticular neoplasms that occur most commonly in the pediatric population between the ages of 2 and 12 years. In contrast to Hodgkin's disease, children with non-Hodgkin's lymphoma more often present with widespread disease, with the head and neck region being one of many involved systemic sites. Asymptomatic lymphadenopathy is the initial presenting manifestation in the majority of patients. Localized extranodal presentations also do occur, with the lymphoid tissue of Waldeyer's ring being commonly involved (15). The early detection of oropharyngeal and nasopharyngeal non-Hodgkin's lymphoma may be difficult because it can mimic common adenotonsillar hypertrophy; tonsillar asymmetry, lymphoid tissue discoloration, or associated systemic symptoms should increase concern of more significant underlying pathology.

Excisional biopsy with pathology consultation for special staining techniques is diagnostically critical. Immunologic typing allows separation of non-Hodgkin's lymphoma into categories of B-cell, T-cell, and true histiocytic origins. The B-cell and T-cell lymphomas are further subdivided based on morphologic appearance and the degree of lymphocytic transformation (Table 2). Resultant classification schemes attempt to group the non-Hodgkin's lymphomas according to their natural histories and responsiveness to therapy.

Chemotherapy is the mainstay of treatment for all non-Hodgkin's lymphomas. Although radiotherapy may apply in some emergency situations, it does not appear to offer

TABLE 2: Subtypes of Non-Hodgkin's Lymphoma: Immunophenotype Classification

Subtype	Growth Pattern	Cell Type	Immunophenotype (%) T Cell	B Cell
Low grade				
Small lymphocyte	Diffuse	Small round cells	99	1
Follicular small cleaved cell	Follicular	Small cleaved cells	100	0
Follicular mixed cell	Follicular	Small cleaved cells and intermediate number of large cells	100	0
Intermediate grade				
Follicular large cell	Follicular	Many large cleaved and noncleaved cells	100	0
Diffuse small cleaved cell	Diffuse	Small cleaved or irregular cells	90	10
Diffuse mixed cell	Diffuse	Mixed small and large cells	60	40
Diffuse large cell	Diffuse	Predominantly large cleaved or noncleaved cells	90	10
High grade				
Immunoblastic	Diffuse	Predominately immunoblasts	80	20
Lymphoblastic	Diffuse	Round or convoluted lymphoblasts	5	95
Small noncleaved cell	Diffuse	Uniform, intermediate-sized round cells	100	0

any therapeutic benefits compared with chemotherapy alone (16). Surgical debulking may be beneficial in selected patients who present with aerodigestive tract compression. Prognosis is associated with stage, and children with leukemic transformation, hematogenous dissemination, and central nervous system involvement do particularly poorly. An overall 76% relapse-free interval of 2 years is reported in children following cessation of initial treatment.

Posttransplantation Lymphoproliferative Disease

Posttransplantation lymphoproliferative disease can present in immunosuppressed pediatric transplant recipients either as a discreet solid tumor or, more commonly, as a diffuse enlargement of lymphoid tissues (17). A grossly distinct tan-brown adenotonsillar discoloration may be observed (18). Airway obstruction may result from hypertrophy of Waldeyer's ring or paratracheal compression. The treatment of such polyclonal B-cell lymphoproliferative disease in transplant recipients is to drastically reduce immunosuppressive therapy; this typically results in prompt and seemingly permanent resolution.

Rhabdomyosarcoma

Rhabdomyosarcoma is the most common soft tissue malignancy in children, accounting for 50% to 70% of all childhood sarcomas (19). Approximately 70% of those children have disease before the age of 12 years, and 43% are younger than 5 years. Rhabdomyosarcoma is four times more common in white children than in any other racial group.

The head and neck region encompasses the most frequent sites of origin, including the orbit, nasopharynx, middle ear–mastoid, and sinonasal cavities. Because of the diversity of potential sites and nonspecific symptomatic presentations, diagnostic delays have historically been common. Direct extension to the skull, brain, or meninges from parameningeal sites is common. Metastatic spread occurs by both lymphatic and hematogenous routes. The incidences of cervical lymph node and distant (lung, bone, bone marrow) metastases with nonorbital rhabdomyosarcoma of the head and neck are 8% and 13%, respectively (20).

The prospectively randomized treatment protocols of the Intergroup Rhabdomyosarcoma Studies have established the superiority of multimodality therapy in the treatment of rhabdomyosarcoma. The clinical staging system utilized is based on the extent of the disease (localized, regional, systemic) and whether or not excision of localized or regional disease, or both, is accomplished (Table 3). Surgery and radiotherapy are

TABLE 3: The Clinical Grouping System of the Intergroup Rhabdomyosarcoma Studies

Group	Definition
I	Localized disease with tumor completely resected and regional nodes not affected
	A. Confined to muscle or organ of origin
	B. Contiguous involvement or infiltration outside the muscle or organ of origin
II	Localized disease with microscopic regional disease, or regional disease with no residual or with microscopic residual disease
	A. Grossly resected tumor with microscopic residual disease (nodes negative)
	B. Regional tumor completely resected (nodes positive or negative)
	C. Regional disease with involved nodes grossly resected but with evidence of microscopic regional disease
III	Incomplete resection or biopsy with gross residual disease
IV	Metastatic disease present at onset

used to control local and regional disease, and chemotherapy is used to control both documented and presumed (micro) metastases. Surgical resection is indicated when removal of the primary tumor imposes no major functional disability on the patient and when resection of the primary tumor will permit the elimination or reduction of radiotherapy dose. A recurring problem is that surgical definitions of disease resectability vary greatly between institutions. Biopsy alone is indicated for orbital rhabdomyosarcoma and for rhabdomyosarcoma in other sites when complete primary tumor removal is not possible. The clinically negative neck requires no treatment beyond chemotherapy and observation. Children with clinically positive lymph nodes benefit from neck dissection with additional radiation therapy if histopathologic findings are confirmatory.

The Intergroup Rhabdomyosarcoma Studies have demonstrated increasingly improved 3-year survival rates. These gains have been most evident in patients with gross residual tumor after surgery but no evidence of distant metastases. Children with tumor in favorable sites, including the orbit and nonparameningeal areas of the head and neck, have an excellent prognosis. The 5-year relapse-free survival rates are 82% to 88% for group I, 68% to 90% for group II, 67% to 79% for group III, and 37% to 40% for group IV patients (21).

Other Soft Tissue Sarcomas

Soft tissue sarcomas other than rhabdomyosarcoma that occur in the head and neck region in children include fibrosarcoma, neurofibrosarcoma, hemangiopericytoma, synovial sarcoma, chondrosarcoma, and extraosseous Ewing's sarcoma (22) (Table 4). These tumors typically present as firm, progressively enlarging masses with additional symptomatology dependent on the specific head and neck location. A multimodality therapeutic approach similar to that employed for rhabdomyosarcoma is generally used for this group of tumors. The prognosis for many of these children depends on achieving local control, and surgical resection with tumor-free margins is advocated for those sarcomatous lesions that are able to be completely excised without creating a severe cosmetic defect or crippling dysfunction. Craniofacial multidisciplinary team approaches employing free flap reconstruction and microvascular techniques have increased the definition of resectability without deformity in many of these patients.

TABLE 4: Clinical Characteristics of the Soft Tissue Sarcomas of the Head and Neck

Tumor Type	Clinical Comments	Management	Prognosis
Fibrosarcoma	Most common sarcoma of the head and neck other than rhabdomyosarcoma	Surgical resection; XRT if residual disease	Excellent if low-grade lesion is resectable
Neurofibrosarcoma	Rare; principally occurs in neurofibromatosis patients	Surgical resection; role of XRT and chemo?	Strongly related to stage at presentation
Hemangiopericytoma	Rare; an infantile variant occurs within first year of life	Surgical resection; role of XRT and chemo?	More favorable in infantile variant
Synovial sarcoma	Rare; parapharyngeal location most common	Multimodality—surgery, XRT, and chemo	Aggressive malignancy; generally poor prognosis
Extraosseous Ewing's sarcoma	Paravertebral predominance in head and neck region	Multimodality—surgery, XRT, and chemo	Relatively good prognosis; stage dependent
Chondrosarcoma	Maxilla more commonly involved than mandible (opposite of osteosarcoma)	Surgical resection; XRT if residual disease	Treatment failure usually due to local recurrence

XRT, radiotherapy; chemo, chemotherapy.

(Adapted from ref. 22.)

TABLE 5: Age Distribution of the More Common Salivary Gland Neoplasms

Tumor Type	Birth to 1 Year	1–10 Years	10–16 Years
Benign mesenchymal			
Hemangioma	++++	++	+
Lymphangioma	++++	++	+
Malignant mesenchymal			
Sarcoma	–	++	++
Benign epithelial			
Pleomorphic adenoma	–	++	+++
Malignant epithelial			
Mucoepidermoid carcinoma	–	++	+++
Acinic cell carcinoma	–	++	+++
Undifferentiated carcinoma	+	++	+
Adenocarcinoma	–	++	++
Adenoid cystic carcinoma	–	+	++

Salivary Gland Malignancies

The most common salivary gland neoplasm in children is the benign pleomorphic adenoma. Malignant salivary gland neoplasms are rare in the pediatric age group. Among those reported, mucoepidermoid carcinomas are most frequent, followed by acinic cell carcinomas, adenocarcinomas, adenoid cystic carcinomas, undifferentiated carcinomas, and sarcomas (23). The characteristic later age at onset of these neoplasms in comparison to the far more common vascular malformations of the salivary glands is illustrated in Table 5. Pediatric salivary neoplasms rarely originate in the submandibular gland; the vast majority involve the parotid gland.

The most common presentation of a salivary gland neoplasm is an asymptomatic firm mass in the periauricular facial region. The reported 50% incidence of firm salivary gland masses being malignant in children poses difficulties in preoperatively distinguishing these malignancies from pleomorphic adenoma as well as from chronic low-grade inflammatory processes such as cat-scratch disease and mycobacterial infections (24). FNA has potential diagnostic benefit in this respect, but the cytologic diagnosis of salivary gland lesions as the basis for management decisions continues to be debated. The preferred diagnostic and often therapeutic procedure is superficial parotidectomy with facial nerve preservation. Rare high-grade malignancies or deep-lobe parotid tumors may require total parotidectomy. Facial nerve sacrifice is performed only when there is clinical and anatomic evidence of malignant neural involvement. Neck dissection is indicated solely in those children with high-grade malignancies or those who have cervical metastases at presentation; adjuvant radiotherapy may also be indicated in such patients.

The survival of children with salivary gland malignancies is chiefly determined by histopathologic findings. Children with low-grade malignancies tend to do well, whereas those with high-grade malignancies do poorly. The prognosis for children with mucoepidermoid and acinic cell carcinomas is particularly good, with 5-year survival rates higher than 90% (25).

Neuroblastoma

Neuroblastoma is a relatively common cancer of early childhood and is the most common malignancy in infants under 1 year old. Ninety percent of these tumors occur in patients younger than 10 years, with birth to 5 years representing the usual age range (26). Primary cervical neuroblastoma typically presents as a firm mass in the lateral part of the neck. The child may additionally manifest heterochromia and an ipsilateral Horner's syndrome. The Horner's syndrome is secondary to cervical sympathetic chain involvement, whereas the heterochromia reflects anomalous neural crest cell derivation. Respiratory distress and feeding difficulties may occur due to direct tracheal and esophageal compression or as a result of entrapment or involvement of cranial nerves IX, X, XI, and XII. Systemic evaluation is necessary to rule out metastatic spread to the head and neck from either the adrenal gland, retroperitoneum, or posterior mediastinum, the more common sites of origin.

The treatment of localized cervical neuroblastoma is surgical excision. Chemotherapy is indicated when complete resection is not possible or systemic disease is documented. Primary neuroblastoma of the head and neck has a better prognosis than that of other sites, attributable to presentation at an earlier stage. Infants younger than 1 year can also generally be cured regardless of extent of disease.

Nasopharyngeal Carcinoma

Nasopharyngeal carcinoma is rare in children. Major institutional reviews reveal an incidence of less than one case per year occurring principally in the adolescent age group, with an increased incidence of nasopharyngeal carcinoma among black teenagers (27). Unilateral otitis media, rhinorrhea, and nasal obstruction are frequent findings. The majority of children with nasopharyngeal carcinoma present with metastatic disease in the neck; the deep superior cervical lymph nodes are most commonly involved. Severe headache or documentation of cranial nerve palsies suggests skull base extension.

Almost all nasopharyngeal carcinoma in young patients is of the undifferentiated (lymphoepithelioma) type. A strong serologic relationship exists between undifferentiated nasopharyngeal carcinoma and Epstein-Barr virus antibody titers, suggesting an infectious etiology. A cause and effect relationship, however, has not been proved. Nasopharyngeal examination and biopsy are required for tissue diagnosis. Histopathologic distinction of undifferentiated nasopharyngeal carcinoma from rhabdomyosarcoma and non-Hodgkin's lymphoma can sometimes be difficult. CT and MRI allow for precise evaluation of primary tumor extension, particularly with respect to the skull base and central nervous system. Systemic evaluation is directed toward ruling out hematogenous metastases, particularly to bone and liver.

Nasopharyngeal carcinoma has traditionally been considered nonresectable, owing to its anatomic location. With present craniofacial surgical techniques, this is no longer categorically true. Undifferentiated nasopharyngeal carcinoma is fortunately a radiosensitive tumor and has historically demonstrated an excellent response to radiotherapy. Such radiotherapy is limited to the primary tumor and regional lymphatic metastases. Adjuvant chemotherapy is required in patients with disseminated systemic disease. The overall 5-year survival rate for children with nasopharyngeal carcinoma approaches 40% (28). Patients with neoplasms confined to the nasopharynx with or without ipsilateral cervical node metastases demonstrate superior survival compared to patients with central nervous system extension or bilateral cervical node metastases.

SUMMARY

The survival of children with cervical malignancies, particularly those with lymphoma and sarcoma, has improved significantly over the past 30 years (29,30) (Table 6). This improvement can be attributed to a number of different factors. These include the identification and incorporation of histologic subtypes with prognostic implication into pathologic staging systems, the establishment of more precise clinical staging systems as a result of advances in radiologic tumor imaging, the development of more effective multimodality treatment protocols, and advances in craniofacial resection and reconstruction techniques applicable to children with neoplasms previously deemed unresectable.

TABLE 6: Overall Survival Trends of Children[a] **for the Five Most Common Malignancies Involving the Head and Neck: Comparative 5-Year Survival Rates (%)**

Tumor Type	1960–1963	1970–1973	1974–1976	1977–1979	1983–1988
Hodgkin's disease	52	90	79	83	88
Non-Hodgkin's lymphoma	18	26	44	56	69
Rhabdomyosarcoma	—	34	53	64	—
Soft tissue sarcomas	—	44	57	67	—
Neuroblastoma	25	40	49	52	55

[a]15 yr or younger.

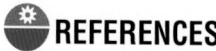

REFERENCES

1. Cunningham MJ, McGuirt WF Jr, Myers EN. Malignant tumors of the head and neck. In: Bluestone CD, Stool SE, Kenna MA, eds. *Pediatric Otolaryngology*. Philadelphia: WB Saunders, 1996:1557–1583.

2. Knight PJ, Reiner CB. Superficial lumps in children: what, when and why? *Pediatrics* 1983;72:147–153.

3. Knight PJ, Mulne AF, Vassy LE. When is lymph node biopsy indicated in children with enlarged peripheral nodes? *Pediatrics* 1982;69:391–396.

4. Jaffe B. Pediatric head and neck tumors; a study of 178 cases. *Laryngoscope* 1973; 83:1644–1651.

5. Yuh WTC, Sato Y, Loes DJ, et al. Magnetic resonance imaging and computed tomography in pediatric head and neck masses. *Ann Otol Rhinol Laryngol* 1991;100:54–62.

6. Cunningham MJ. Tumors of the head and neck. In: Bluestone CD, Stool SE, eds. *Atlas of Pediatric Otolaryngology*. Philadelphia: WB Saunders, 1995:530–570.

7. Mobley DL, Wakely PE Jr, Frable MAS. Fine-needle aspiration biopsy: application to pediatric head and neck masses. *Laryngoscope* 1991;101:469–472.

8. Torsiglieri AJ, Tom LWC, Ross AJ III, Wetmore RF, Handler SD, Potsic WP. Pediatric neck masses: guidelines for evaluation. *Int J Pediatr Otorhinolarngol* 1988;16:199–210.

9. Hawkins DB, Chen WT. Pilomatrixoma of the head and neck in children. *Int J Pediatr Otorhinolaryngol* 1985;8:215–223.

10. Calcaterra TC, Wang MB, Sercarz JA. Unusual tumors. In: Myers EN, Suen JY, eds. *Cancer of the head and neck*. Philadelphia: WB Saunders, 1996:644–669.

11. Thomsen JR, Koltai PJ. Sternomastoid tumor of infancy. *Ann Otol Rhinol Laryngol* 1989;98:955–959.

12. Bredenkamp JK, Hoover LA, Berke GS, Shaw A. Congenital muscular torticollis; a spectrum of disease. *Arch Otolaryngol Head Neck Surg* 1990;116:212–216.

13. Urba WJ, Longo DL. Hodgkin's disease. *N Engl J Med* 1992;326:678–687.

14. DeVita VT Jr, Hubbard SM. Hodgkin's disease. *N Engl J Med* 1993;328:560–565.

15. Weisberger EC, Davidson DD. Unusual presentations of lymphoma of the head and neck in childhood. *Laryngoscope* 1990;100:337–342.

16. Link MP, Donaldson SS, Bernard CW, Shuster JJ, Murphy SB. Results of treatment of childhood localized non-Hodgkin's lymphoma with combination chemotherapy with or without radiotherapy. *N Engl J Med* 1990;322:1169–1174.

17. Sculerati N, Arriaga M. Otolaryngologic management of post-transplant lymphoproliferative disease in children. *Ann Otol Rhinol Laryngol* 1990;99:445–450.

18. Cunningham MJ, Eavey RD. The tan-tonsil sign; a clinical marker of lymphoproliferative disease. *Clin Pediatr* 1992;31:237–240.

19. Wanebo HJ, Koness RJ, MacFarlane JK, et al. Head and neck sarcoma: report of the Head and Neck Sarcoma Registry. *Head Neck* 1991;14:1–7.

20. Lawrence W Jr, Hays DM, Heyn R, et al. Lymphatic metastases with childhood rhabdomyosarcoma: a report from the Intergroup Rhabdomyosarcoma Study. *Cancer* 1987;60:910–915.

21. Crist WM, Jarnsey L, Beltangady MS, et al. Prognosis in children with rhabdomyosarcoma: a report of the Intergroup Rhabdomyosarcoma Studies I and II. *J Clin Oncol* 1990;8:443–452.

22. Miser JS, Pizzo PA. Soft tissue sarcomas in childhood. *Pediatr Clin North Am* 1985;32:779–800.

23. Luna MA, Batsakis JG, El-Naggar AK. Salivary gland tumors in children. *Ann Otol Rhinol Laryngol* 1991;100:869–871.
24. Camacho AE, Goodman ML, Eavey RD. Pathologic correlation of the unknown solid parotid mass in children. *Otolaryngol Head Neck Surg* 1989;101:566–571.
25. Callender DL, Frankenthaler RA, Luna MA, Lee SS, Goepfert H. Salivary gland neoplasms in children. *Arch Otolaryngol Head Neck Surg* 1992;118:472–476.
26. Jaffe N, Cassady R, Petersen R. Heterochromia and Horner's syndrome associated with cervical and mediastinal neuroblastoma. *J Pediatr* 1975;87:75–77.
27. Roper HP, Essex-Kater A, Marsden HB, Dixon PF. Nasopharyngeal carcinoma in children. *Pediatr Hematol Oncol* 1986;3:143–152.
28. Pao WJ, Hustu HO, Douglass EC. Pediatric nasopharyngeal carcinoma: long term follow-up of 29 patients. *Int J Radiat Oncol Biol Phys* 1989;17:299–305.
29. Silverberg E, Lubera J. Cancer statistics, 1987. *Cancer J Clin* 1987;37:2.
30. Boring CC, Squires TS, Tong T. Cancer statistics, 1993. *Cancer J Clin* 1993;43:7.

M.J. Cunningham: Department of Otology and Laryngology, Harvard Medical School, and Department of Otolaryngology, Massachusetts Eye and Ear Infirmary, Boston, Massachusetts 02130.

• *Practical Pediatric Otolaryngology*
• edited by Robin T. Cotton and Charles M. Myer, III
• Lippincott-Raven Publishers, Philadelphia © 1999

Salivary Disease in Children

Sally R. Shott

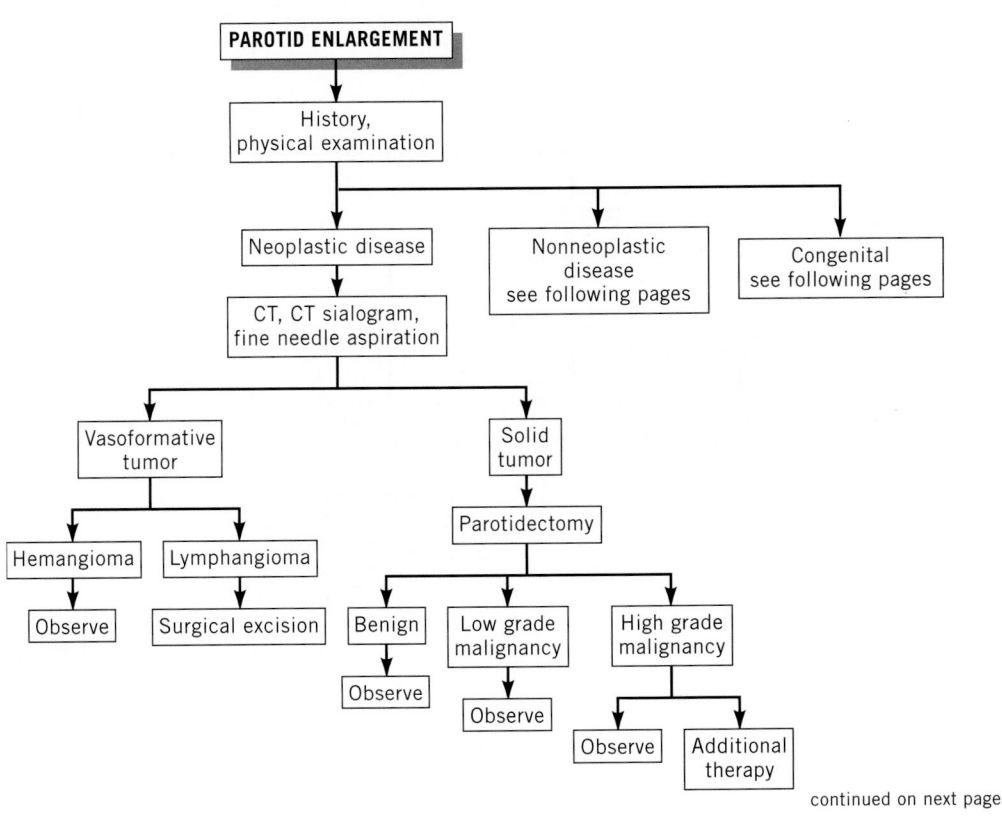

continued on next page

continued

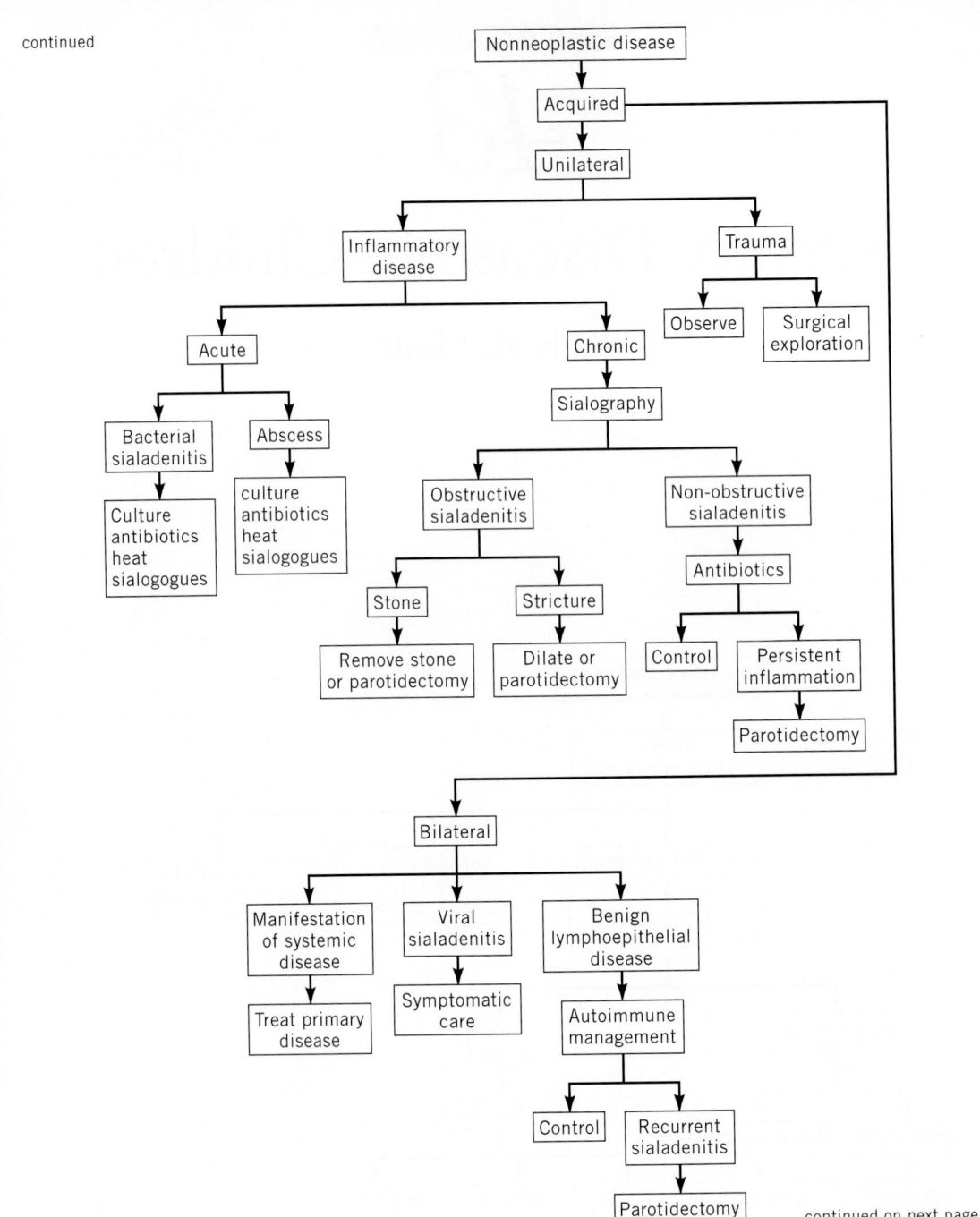

continued on next page

continued

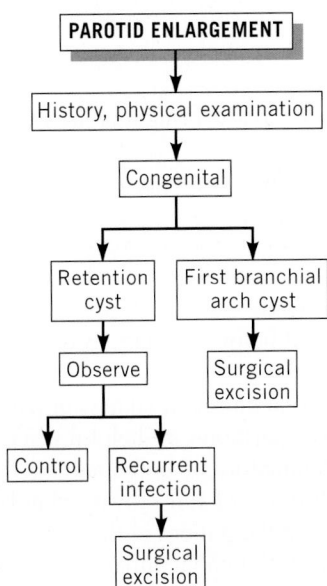

 ## HISTORICAL BACKGROUND

The major salivary glands include the parotid and submandibular glands. These two sets of glands produce almost 90% of the 500 mL of saliva that is produced daily. Salivary disease and salivary gland neoplasms, both benign and malignant, do not occur very often in children. In general, both the pediatric and the adult population are affected by the same disease processes but the frequency of each disease varies between the two groups. However, there are a few disorders unique to the pediatric age group. These include neonatal sialoadenitis, vascular or vasoformative tumors such as hemangiomas and lymphangiomas, congenital anomalies involving the salivary glands, and sialorrhea. Recurrent inflammatory disorders of the salivary glands are more likely to occur in children than in adults.

Salivary disease is divided into neoplastic and nonneoplastic disorders, as seen in the decision tree. Although inflammatory diseases are more common, a firm nontender mass in a salivary gland has a much higher chance of being malignant in the pediatric population than in adults. The goal of the initial assessment of the patient is to determine which pathway is most likely.

PATIENT ASSESSMENT

History and Clinical Assessment

When a child presents with a salivary gland abnormality, a full history and physical examination are in order. Regardless of the specific salivary gland involved, certain baseline historical and clinical characteristics of the abnormality need to be established:

Is there a history of trauma to the area?
Is there a cheek-chewing habit?
Has there been any swelling or involvement of the other salivary glands, especially the opposite-side gland?

A history of any type of systemic diseases, especially immunologic, should also be sought. Medications and possible infectious disease exposure should be reviewed. Ask specific questions about the clinical presentation of the area of concern:
- How long has the involved area been a problem?
- Is the area painful or nonpainful?

- Did the area of concern arise overnight or has there been a gradual onset of the problem?
- Is there any change in the area when the patient eats—does the gland hurt more or get bigger during eating?
- What happens if the patient cries or strains?
- Has the character of the area changed—did it used to be soft, but now it is firm, or has the opposite occurred?
- Has this ever happened before—did the problem spontaneously resolve or was specific treatment needed?
- Has there been any facial muscle weakness or paralysis?

The answers to these questions are helpful while evaluating the patient and determining whether an inflammatory or potentially malignant process is present. For instance, inflammatory diseases of the salivary glands tend to be painful and present acutely. Increased pain or enlargement of the gland with eating suggests a lesion that is obstructing salivary flow. With benign, inflammatory lesions, the pain may take hours to slowly resolve. With discrete neoplasms, the pain and swelling resolve more quickly. A progressively enlarging, nonpainful mass suggests neoplasm. Facial nerve involvement is highly suggestive of a malignant process and one should consider facial nerve involvement equal to malignancy until proved otherwise.

Physical Examination

The physical examination of the involved area should include a bimanual examination. This involves simultaneous intraoral and extraoral palpation. From the examination, the physician should be able to answer the following questions: Is the lesion tender? Is the overlying skin erythematous? Is the lesion discrete or diffuse? Is it fixed or mobile? Is it firm, soft, or cystic? Are there multiple lesions within the gland?

Because of the dense fascia overlying the parotid gland and because lesions can be in the deep lobe of the gland, abnormalities that present within the parotid may be quite subtle. The bimanual examination increases the sensitivity of the physical examination and is an essential tool in these situations. Even subtle irregularities within the parotid gland should be taken seriously.

Examine the area of the salivary ducts for trauma. Trauma from either dental appliances or cheek biting can cause inflammation with secondary infection or scar tissue formation, with resultant obstruction of salivary outflow from the duct.

Check salivary secretions at all ducts. It is best to wipe the area of the duct dry and then while observing the duct puncta, palpate the gland, applying pressure from a posterior to anterior direction, essentially milking the duct. Normal saliva should be clear fluid. If purulent fluid is expressed, a culture should be done. If there is no salivary flow, obstruction of the duct is possible.

Document the appearance of the duct. An inflamed ductal punctum with clear saliva suggests a viral infection.

Evaluate and make a notation of the patient's facial function.

Diagnostic Tests

Adjunctive tests that may provide further information as to the etiology of the salivary gland disorder include laboratory evaluation of the saliva, radiologic tests including plain x-ray films, sialography, ultrasonography, computed tomography (CT), and magnetic resonance imaging (MRI), and fine-needle aspiration biopsies.

Plain x-ray films have limited use but can potentially identify an obstructing stone or calculi within the gland. They can also be used to evaluate adjacent structures and can delineate dystrophic calcifications.

Sialography has limited use in the pediatric population because it requires significant patient cooperation. This type of study is also contraindicated in the setting of an acute inflammation. In addition, most of the information supplied by this test can be obtained by use of ultrasound and CT scans.

Ultrasonography is noninvasive, requires no radiation exposure, can be easily repeated, and is inexpensive. Ultrasonography can help to differentiate a solid mass in the gland from a cystic lesion. It can delineate dilated ducts in the case of duct obstruction. Sialectasis has a characteristic appearance, with ultrasound showing small punctate echogenic densities throughout the gland (1). Ultrasonography can also help to clarify whether the mass in question is within or outside the body of the gland.

Despite all of the advantages of the ultrasound evaluation, the resolution of the images is still somewhat primitive. Although CT exposes the patient to ionizing radiation, this type of imaging more distinctly defines the lesion and clearly differentiates an intrinsic from an extrinsic mass. Contrast can demonstrate the vascularity of the lesion and will show ring enhancement at the border of an abscess.

MRI requires no use of ionizing radiation but may require sedation of the child. This study is also useful in demonstrating the facial nerve within the parotid gland (1).

Radionucleotide studies of glands have limited use in children, but can be helpful in the rare case of congenital agenesis of the parotid submandibular gland where no gland is visualized.

Though helpful, these radiologic studies provide only indirect information about the disease process in question and because any lesion in a salivary gland has a higher chance of being malignant, tissue diagnosis is usually ultimately needed. Because of the risk of tumor seeding, incisional biopsy is contraindicated. Fine-needle aspiration cytology (FNAC), however, can help establish a diagnosis and differentiate a benign from a malignant lesion. The sensitivity of identifying a neoplasm as malignant is approximately 90% while the specificity of a malignant diagnosis is 95% to 100% (2,3). FNAC can help establish whether a lesion is inflammatory and can provide tissue for culture purposes. The diagnosis of a malignant lesion is helpful for preoperative surgical planning and allows the surgeon to appropriately educate the patient's family about the possible surgical consequences (i.e., facial nerve sacrifice). Unfortunately, cooperation is not always possible in pediatric patients. In addition, the success of this procedure is highly dependent on the experience of the pathologist.

PEARLS AND PERILS

1. Rapid enlargement of a salivary mass suggests a malignant process.
2. Slow enlargement suggests a benign disease of the salivary gland.
3. The dense fascia covering the parotid gland can make accurate palpation difficult. If suspicious, perform further diagnostic tests.
4. Facial nerve weakness suggests a malignant lesion.
5. A solid lesion is more likely to be malignant in a child than in an adult.

DIFFERENTIAL DIAGNOSIS AND TREATMENT RECOMMENDATIONS

Salivary disease in children can be divided into three main categories: congenital, nonneoplastic diseases, and neoplastic diseases.

Congenital Absence or Malformation of the Salivary Glands

Congenital absence of the salivary glands is rare. Less than 15 cases are reported in the literature (4,5). Frequent presenting symptoms include excessive dry mouth and dental caries because of the loss of the protective mechanism of saliva. Agenesis can affect all of the major salivary glands or be only partial in nature. The latter is probably missed clinically because saliva is made by the uninvolved glands. Parotid gland agenesis can be associated with first branchial arch anomalies and hemifacial microsomia. Lacrimal dysfunction is frequently also present.

Diagnosis is made by first technetium 99m pertechnetate radionucleotide scanning and then either CT or MRI. The nuclear scan will establish if there is a functioning gland but the latter studies are needed to truly define whether tissue is present or not.

Congenital anomalies of the gland ducts can also occur. Duplication anomalies as well as imperforate ducts have been reported (6). Dilation of the duct and ranula formation will occur if imperforate submandibular ducts are not appropriately treated. Simple marsupialization and ductoplasty are usually adequate (6). MRI study will delineate duplicated ducts. Treatment includes excision of the accessory duct with preservation of the primary duct.

Abnormal parotid duct fistulas opening onto the face have also been reported (7). The external fistula can originate from the parotid duct or from auxiliary parotid gland tissue.

Congenital Cysts

Congenital cysts of the salivary glands occur most frequently in the parotid glands (8). Congenital cysts of the salivary glands include dermoid cysts, first branchial cleft cysts, first branchial pouch cysts, and retention cysts. The dermoid cyst will present as a firm, rounded mass within the body of the parotid gland. The mass can be nontender, but if it becomes infected, it will be painful. If the mass is located near the duct, ductal compression and secondary parotitis can occur. Elements of all three germinal layers will be present. Total excision by subtotal parotidectomy is necessary to prevent recurrence.

First branchial cleft cysts will also present as a painless mass in the parotid gland. Work (9) classified first branchial cleft cysts into two distinct types, each with a different embryogenesis and different clinical behavior. Type I first branchial cleft cysts are duplication anomalies of the external auditory canal. They commonly present as a sinus tract or cystic mass in the preauricular area, the conchal bowl area, or the postauricular sulcus. Infection and abscess formation are common. They can course superficial to, deep to, or through the branches of the facial nerve. Complete surgical excision, with facial nerve identification and preservation, is needed.

Type II first branchial cysts are due to duplication anomaly of the external canal and a rudimentary pinna. These cysts are composed of ectodermal elements (hair follicles, squamous epithelium sebaceous glands) and mesodermal elements (cartilage). Type II cysts frequently present in the neck and also easily become infected. They can extend into the external ear canal or into the middle-ear space. Similar to type I cysts, their tract can course superficial to, deep to, or in between the branches of the facial nerve. Surgical excision should be done only after infection has resolved, and complete removal requires exposure and dissection of the facial nerve.

First branchial pouch anomalies present occasionally in the retromandibular area of the parotid gland. Complete excision with special attention to the cyst's relationship to the facial nerve is needed.

Retention cysts of the salivary glands most commonly affect the minor salivary glands. They can occur on the palate or tongue and appear as thin-walled bluish, mucus-filled lesions. Surgical excision is the treatment of choice.

Retention cysts of the parotid gland can be congenital or acquired and are due to obstruction of the duct within the parotid body, most frequently the lobular portion. Observation is advised unless there are repeated episodes of infection, in which case excision by means of parotidectomy with facial nerve preservation is needed.

It is also possible to have congenital ectopic rests of salivary tissue that can manifest as draining sinuses in the area of the neck, mandible, or cervical lymph nodes (10).

TABLE 1: Nonneoplastic Disease

Viral sialoadenitis
    Viral parotitis—mumps
        Coxsackie A virus
        Echovirus
Acute suppurative sialoadenitis
Parotitis of infancy
Chronic sialoadenitis
    Recurrent parotitis of childhood
    Strictures
Sialolithiasis
Granulomatous lesions
Diffuse parotid swelling
Trauma
Systemic disorders
    Endocrine and metabolic disorders
    Cystic fibrosis
    Drug reactions and allergies

Nonneoplastic Disease

Nonneoplastic diseases of the salivary glands can be categorized into viral, bacterial, and granulomatous etiologies. In addition, some salivary diseases are secondary to either systemic diseases or secondary inflammatory diseases (Table 1).

Viral Diseases

Mumps Mumps sialoadenitis is the most common of all salivary gland inflammatory diseases. However, with the availability of a vaccination, it is now uncommonly seen in the United States. Classically, children 4 to 5 years old are affected. Fever, malaise, headache, and painful swelling of the parotoid glands are present. Seventy percent have bilateral involvement. Classically, Stensen's duct is swollen and erythematous but clear saliva is expressed. The submandibular glands can also be affected. Serum antibodies to the mumps S and V antigens, with a titer higher than 1:192, indicate recent infection. The patient achieves immunity with infection.

    Treatment of mumps is largely supportive. However, because the potential sequelae from mumps can be quite severe, and because this is so rarely seen today, it is important to keep this in the differential diagnosis. Local salivary gland sequelae include parotid gland sialectasia with recurrent and chronic suppuration. More distant and potentially more severe sequelae include sensorineural hearing loss, usually unilateral; diabetes secondary to pancreatic fibrosis; sterility secondary to orchitis; and meningoencephalitis.

    Other viral etiologies of parotitis include Coxsackie A virus, Echovirus, and the virus of lymphocytic choriomeningitis. Positive diagnosis requires either viral isolation or acute and convalescent serology. Treatment is supportive.

Bacterial Diseases

    Bacterial infections of the parotid glands can be divided into acute and chronic diseases. Acute disease includes acute suppurative sialoadenitis and acute suppurative parotitis of infancy. Chronic diseases include acute recurrent sialoadenitis, specifically, recurrent parotitis of childhood, and local duct obstruction from a stricture. Sialolithiasis can cause either acute or chronic infections and is examined separately.

Acute Suppurative Sialoadenitis Acute suppurative sialoadenitis is characterized by sudden painful swelling of the salivary glands and overlying tissues with fever and leukocytosis. Bimanual palpation will reveal a firm, indurated, and tender gland. Milking the gland will express purulent fluid from the duct orifice. Predisposing etiologic factors include dehydration, calculi, and duct stricture. Trauma, particularly chewing on the buccal mucosa near the parotid duct, can cause inflammation and blockage of the duct and result in an acute infection. Dental appliances, especially braces and appliances used for maxillary expansion, are other important etiologic factors in children. Surgical parotitis, secondary to dehydration in the immediate postoperative period as well as debilitation, confinement to bed, and electrolyte imbalance, has been estimated to occur in 1 in 1,000 postoperative patients, with bilateral presentation in 20% (8).

Staphylococcus aureus and *Streptococcus viridans* are the most common organisms in acute parotitis. *Streptococcus pneumoniae* and *Escherichia coli* have also been reported (11). In addition, Brook et al (11) cultured anaerobic bacteria in 50% of the patients they evaluated with acute suppurative parotitis.

Treatment of acute suppurative parotitis includes systemic antimicrobial therapy using a penicillinase-resistent antistaphylococcal agent, local heat and massage, fluids, and sialagogues such as lemon juice or sour candy to stimulate salivary production and flow.

If progressive induration and fever occur in spite of appropriate antibiotic management, an abscess formation may be present and surgical drainage must be considered. An abscess of the submandibular gland responds well to incision and drainage, with subsequent excision of the gland following resolution of the acute infection. Abscess formation within the parotid gland can be more difficult to diagnose because of the insulating nature of the parotid fascia. If edema and induration progress despite appropriate antibiotic therapy, incision of the parotid abscess should be considered. After elevation of a skin flap superficial to the parotid fascia, a hemostat is introduced into the parotid gland and spread in the direction of the branches of the facial nerve.

Acute Suppurative Parotitis of Infancy   Acute suppurative parotitis of infancy is a unique process to newborns. Forty percent of those affected are premature infants. It is more common in the parotid gland than the submandibular gland. The higher mucus content from the submandibular gland conveys a relative immunity from infection by the bacterial effect of the mucus (12). *S. aureus* is the most common organism, with streptococci, *E. coli*, *Pseudomonas aeruginosa*, and *Branhamella catarrhalis* also cultured. Treatment includes hydration and antimicrobial therapy. Resolution is usually within 1 week and recurrence is uncommon.

Chronic Inflammatory Disease

Recurrent parotitis of childhood is uncommon but next to mumps it is the most common inflammatory salivary disease in the pediatric population (13). Characterized by recurrent acute or subacute swelling of the parotid gland, it is frequently accompanied with symptoms of fever and malaise. The inflammation is usually unilateral and between episodes the child is free of symptoms. Numerous studies suggested that the symptoms resolve with puberty but persistent disease also occurs (13,14). The incidence is higher in the male than the female population. Infections occur every few months, lasting several days to 2 weeks.

Diagnosis is usually made by the clinical examination, the clinical behavior of repeated short-lived episodes of parotitis responding to antimicrobials, and tests ruling out any type of stone or mass causing the recurrent infections. Because it has been suggested that recurrent parotitis of childhood may be the first manifestation of Sjögren's syndrome, this disease should be considered (14).

Ultrasonography may be helpful in establishing a diagnosis. Small hypoechoic areas in the superficial lobes of one or both of the parotid glands were seen in the study by Nozaki et al. (15). These areas were round and 2 to 4 mm in diameter. Unfortunately, these small hypoechoic areas can also be seen with other inflammatory parotitides including mumps and Sjögren's syndrome. However, it was suggested that because ultra-sonography is such a convenient procedure, particularly in children, it should be used as a first-line investigational test (15).

Etiologic factors that have been suggested include congenital malformation of the parotid ducts, hereditary etiologies, primary or secondary infection, allergy, and immunologic factors. Encson et al. (13) noted a high relationship between clinical symptoms and possible sialectasis on sialograms. Because the disease process was common in small children, even infants, they believed that congenital sialectases may be one of the important factors in the pathogenesis of recurrent parotitis, as this led to a predisposition for bacterial colonization (13). Others (14) suggested a repeated ascending ductal infection with accumulation of cells, mucus, and pus forming a mucous plug.

Between periods of parotid swelling, clinical recovery occurs and normal clear saliva flow is established. Therapy should be conservative in view of the "burnout" that seems to occur with puberty. Dilation of the parotid ducts may be useful to break up any mucous plugs blocking the ducts (14). Antimicrobial therapy with each acute inflammatory episode is important to guard against further scarring and sialectasis. Massage, warm heat, and sialagogues may also be helpful. Steroid therapy has been suggested, but although parotid swelling may be decreased on a short-term basis, the incidence of recurrence is unchanged. In more severe situations where episodes are frequent, painful, and progressive, surgery may need to be considered. Parotid duct ligation with resultant gland atrophy has been somewhat successful (14).

Sialolithiasis

Sialolithiasis or salivary calculi occur more frequently in the submandibular gland (90%) than in the parotid gland. The sublingual gland and minor salivary glands are rarely affected. Several factors account for this higher incidence in the submandibular gland. The more alkaline pH of its secretions and higher viscosity with higher mucin content as well as higher calcium concentration predispose to calculi formation. In addition, the submandibular duct runs a long narrow course against gravity, so stasis of secretions can occur more easily (16).

Salivary calculi are made up predominantly of calcium phosphate in the form of hydroxyapatite (17). Infection produces a change in the mucoid element of the saliva that favors deposition of calcium (18). Stone formation does not appear to be related to serum calcium and phosphate levels but increased levels of serum uric acid have been linked to uric acid stone formation in gout (19,20). Interestingly, despite the increased viscosity of salivary secretions, children with cystic fibrosis do not have an increased incidence of salivary gland stones (20). Other etiologic factors suggested include fungal infections as well as bacterial infections (17). Repetitive biting around the duct orifices can lead to ductal obstruction and salivary stasis.

Sialolithiasis occurs infrequently in children. The average age at presentation is usually around 10 years. Boys seem to be affected more frequently than girls, with an approximate 3:1 ratio. Intermittent pain and swelling, particularly related to eating, are a frequent presentation. With eating and increased saliva production, pain and swelling occur against an obstructed duct. Between meals, the swelling and discomfort may decrease or resolve. Symptoms can range from mild discomfort to localized cellulitis, malaise, fever, and obvious purulent drainage from the involved duct. Sialolithiasis is frequently missed diagnosis, with approximately 65% of patients with chronic sialoadenitis finally diagnosed with salivary stones (18).

Diagnosis can frequently be made by bimanual palpation. It is best to palpate from a posterior to anterior location, milking the duct. Plain x-ray films will delineate a radiopaque calculus in the submandibular gland in 80% to 90% of the cases (17,20,21). A dental occlusal x-ray study will show stones in the anterior two-thirds of the duct. A distal oblique x-ray film is needed to show stones involving the posterior third of the duct (22).

Because 10% to 20% of submandibular calculi and the majority of calculi in the parotid duct are nonpaque, other diagnostic studies may be needed. In addition to its near 100% diagnostic effectiveness, sialography allows better determination of the location of the stone in relation to the gland's parenchyma. This can assist with surgical planning. It also gives information about the functional abilities of the gland and may help diagnose a rupture of the duct by the stone with surrounding parenchymal involvement or even abscess formation (21). Sialography, however, is contraindicated in the setting of an acute infection. In addition, most children are unwilling participants in sialography. Therefore, axial CT of the floor of the mouth or cheek, which can also identify calculi within the gland or ductal system, may be the diagnostic test of choice if a stone is not seen on plain films or if more detailed information is desired (16).

If caught early and if there is no history of recurrent infections, spontaneous extrusion of the calculus may be possible with aggressive sialagogues to stimulate salivary flow (16). If the stone can be palpated in the proximal aspect of Stensen's or Warthin's duct, the stone might be removed by probing and dilation of the duct and actually milking the stone out. A palpable calculus not able to be milked out of the duct can be removed by local incision into the submandibular duct. After a stay suture is placed around the duct distal to the palpable stone so the stone will not slip back into the gland, an incision is made into the duct over the stone and the stone is removed. A similar approach can be used for a stone in the parotid duct, but injury to the buccal branch of the facial nerve is possible. In addition, there is a higher incidence of postoperative stricture and narrowing of the parotid duct with this approach, and repair and stenting of the duct should be done once the stone is removed (20). Although it is possible to remove the stone under local anesthesia in adults, general anesthesia is usually required in children. If the stone is in the parenchyma of the gland, gland excision is needed.

Complications of salivary gland calculi include ductal stenosis, erosion of the stone through the ductal wall with formation of an abscess, prolonged ductal obstruction leading to chronic sialoadenitis, and parenchymal gland destruction (23). Occasionally despite stone removal, chronic sialoadenitis persists after removal of the calculi. This suggests that irreversible scarring within the gland and ductal structures has occurred and gland removal is then suggested (24).

Granulomatous Sialoadenitis

Granulomatous disease of the salivary gland more frequently occurs in the parotid gland than in the submandibular gland (25). There can be diffuse glandular involvement or localized interparotid or periparotid lymph node enlargement. The lesions are usually painless and slowly progressive in size, with minimal to no surrounding inflammatory reaction. Salivary secretions are usually normal (20). As these findings are also quite characteristic of a neoplastic disorder, diagnosis through biopsy is usually needed. Granulomatous diseases involving the parotid include tuberculosis caused by *Mycobacterium tuberculosis* or atypical *Mycobacterium* species, cat-scratch disease, actinomycosis, sarcoidosis, brucellosis, and histoplasmosis (25,26).

In the diagnosis of tuberculosis involvement of the parotid gland, acid-fast staining or culture of the saliva may be used to confirm the presence of *M. tuberculosis*, but frequently no growth occurs (25). Skin tests can be quite helpful in evaluating the diagnosis in this situation. Biopsy and culture of the tissue are important in determining whether further systemic antituberculosis treatment is necessary.

Forty percent of patients with sarcoidosis present initially with parotid swelling (27). The parotid swelling is constant and pain is minimal. Facial palsy may occur. Pulmonary disease is seen in approximately 90% of the patients, with perihilar adenopathy seen on chest x-ray films.

Because granulomatous disease can mimic neoplasm, tissue diagnosis or diagnosis by positive cultures is necessary. Fine-needle aspiration biopsy and cytology can be used for both of these studies (27).

Trauma

Dental appliances or chronic cheek chewing can cause localized trauma to the major salivary ducts. Chronic irritation and inflammation of the punctum can lead to stricture formation and resultant infection, both chronic and acute. Direct acute trauma to the salivary gland can occur with any type of facial trauma. Evaluation and treatment of an injury to the parotid gland must include an evaluation of facial nerve function and parotid duct integrity. Any laceration through the parotid fascia and posterior to a vertical line along the lateral canthus of the eye requires facial nerve exploration if there are any signs of facial nerve weakness. With any laceration anterior to this line, nerve branches most likely will reinnervate satisfactorily (20).

It is advised that exploration of the facial nerves be done within 72 hours of the injury so that electrical stimulation of the distal nerve segment is still possible (20). Epineural repair using 6-0 to 8-0 ophthalmic nylon suture is performed. A cable graft should be considered if there is any tension whatsoever.

If a laceration courses through the masseter muscle, evaluation of the parotid duct's integrity is necessary. Pooling of saliva in the wound suggests that the duct has been violated. Treatment options include duct ligation, ductal rerouting with a new intraoral opening, or ductal repair suturing the severed ends over polyethylene tubing. The tubing, acting as a stent, should remain in place at least 10 days (20). Failure to repair a severed duct can lead to an interstitial inflammatory process with sinus tract formation, recurrent infection, and abscess formation as well as obstructive cysts (20).

Systemic Disorders—Diffuse Parotid Swelling

Diffuse bilateral salivary gland enlargement can be seen with generalized endocrine and metabolic dysfunctions such as obesity, starvation, diabetes, alcoholism, malnutrition, chronic pancreatitis, uremia, thyroid disease, autoimmune diseases, abnormalities of the pituitary-adrenal axis, and cystic fibrosis (1,20,26). The enlargement may be due to infiltration of the gland by fatty tissue in the case of diabetics and grossly obese people, or may be a functional hypertrophy in patients who consume a carbohydrate diet exclusively (1). It can also be the result of an autoimmune process as in Sjögren's disease. The submandibular gland is enlarged in more than 90% of patients with cystic fibrosis. Therefore, a sweat chloride test should be considered in any young child who presents with diffuse salivary gland enlargement with no obvious etiology or infection (20).

Agents that can cause an asymptomatic salivary gland enlargement include thiourea, methimazole, isoproterenol, phenylbutazone, phenothiazine, thiocyanate, iodine compounds, and heavy metals such as lead and copper (20,26). The reaction to iodine products may have a delayed onset, 2 to 3 days after oral ingestion or injection, and can last almost a week (26).

Allergy may also play a part in occasional episodes of bilateral painless parotid swelling. Allergies to certain foods such as strawberries and seafood may cause a sudden, short-lived episode of parotid swelling. Other signs of allergy such as hives and bronchospasm are seen with the parotid swelling. Though the exact mechanism is not clear, it is postulated that a rapid increase in the viscosity of the saliva may be responsible (1). Diagnosis can be established using provocative testing, cytologic examination of the saliva looking for eosinophils, and a differential white blood cell count showing a high eosinophil count and normal white blood cell count.

Acquired Cysts

As discussed in the section on congenital lesions of the salivary glands, the parotid gland can be affected by retention cysts, both congenital and acquired due to obstruction of the duct within the parotid body. Acquired parotid retention cysts can develop from obstruction of the parotid duct caused by either recurrent infection, ductal strictures, neoplasm, calculi, or direct trauma to the parotid duct. Secretions made by the cyst's lining lead to progressive growth. Unless secondarily infected, the cyst contents resemble clear saliva. Parotidectomy with facial nerve preservation is recommended after treatment of any secondary infection (20).

Polycystic disease of the parotid gland has also been described. Characterized by replacement of the lobular portion of the parotid gland by multiple epithelial-lined cysts, this disease is thought to arise from the intercalated ducts and may be due to a developmental abnormality of the intercalated duct cysts (28).

A ranula is a retention cyst originally from the sublingual gland, one of the minor salivary glands. Ranulas are believed to develop secondary to either degeneration of the sublingual gland or ductal obstruction. Trauma with mucous extravasation into the surrounding soft tissue can also lead to ranula formation. The simple ranula presents as a bluish, slowly growing, nontender mass in the floor of the mouth. Simple ranulas are usually localized to one side of the mouth, although they can occasionally cross the midline (29). A plunging ranula represents extravasation of the mucin through or around the mylohyoid muscle into the soft tissues of the neck. Some plunging ranulas are believed to be secondary to incomplete removal of simple ranulas where the sublingual gland was not removed (29). These tend to be larger in size, secondary to mucous extravasation with secondary inflammation. Plunging ranulas frequently present with not only a cervical mass but also an intraoral mass. They can also extend posteriorly as far as the skull base, and inferiorly to the superclavicular region and the superior mediastinum (29).

Treatment of simple ranulas includes marsupialization of the cyst or sublingual gland excision, or both. A combination of both procedures is suggested to best eliminate the risk of recurrence. With plunging ranulas, a combined cervical and intraoral approach is advocated, with special attention to preserving vital structures. Failure to remove only the cervical mass and not the sublingual gland can lead to recurrence.

Sialorrhea

Excessive production of saliva is not a common entity seen in children. However, sialorrhea or excessive drooling and an inability to handle salivary production is seen. Most patients with sialorrhea have an underlying neurologic dysfunction such as cerebral palsy, mental retardation, or head injury. Other factors that may contribute include a patient's head position and sitting posture, concentrating ability, tongue size and control, and dental malformations. Only occasionally are otherwise normal children unable to handle their oral secretions. The defect is not due to an overproduction of saliva but rather is a defect in the oral or voluntary phase of swallowing. This defect leads to overflowing of the secretions that build up in the anterior portion of the mouth. In children with cerebral palsy there is a dysfunction in motor activity of the oral cavity, and initiation of swallowing is less frequent as well as less coordinated and inefficient.

Sialorrhea can also be due to chronic nasal obstruction. Therefore, evaluation should also rule out adenotonsillar hypertrophy, or nasal obstruction due to turbinate enlargement, nasal septal deformity, or rhinorrhea. Both medical and surgical treatments should first address these potential problems prior to any consideration of decreasing the amount of saliva produced.

Therapy is oriented to oral stimulation and swallowing therapy and then surgical intervention when this fails. Medical management with anticholinergic drugs cannot be considered for this chronic problem, because of the side effects of the medication. Radiation therapy, known to decrease saliva production, is contraindicated because of the risk of malignant transformation.

Surgical management with bilateral submandibular gland excision and bilateral parotid duct ligation is the current treatment of choice. Lesser procedures, such as duct rerouting and denervation procedures, have only short-term success (30,31). Removal of the submandibular gland removes the major source of saliva production in the resting state. Ligation of the parotid duct leads to atrophy of the parotid gland and eliminates the major source of saliva produced by stimulation by food ingestion. The remaining minor salivary glands account for 10% of all saliva produced and provide adequate lubrication of the oral cavity without an increased incidence seen in dental caries or problems with xerostomia (30).

Although sialorrhea may first appear to be treated for only cosmetic reasons, closer examination illustrates the serious medical and psychosocial consequences associated with this condition. Sialorrhea may be associated with difficulty in speech clarity, inability to eat a normal diet, an increase in oral and perioral infections, and dehydration (31). Sialorrhea can be the factor holding back a special needs child from being accepted into a mainstream environment.

Neoplasms

Salivary gland neoplasms (Table 2) are uncommon in children, with less than 5% of the salivary gland tumors occurring in patients under 16 years old (20). The histologic types of tumors encountered in the pediatric and adult populations are not different but the frequencies of each type are different between the two populations. Children are more likely to have tumors of vascular origin, with adults having an increased incidence of solid tumors. However, a solid salivary mass in a child has a much higher likelihood of being malignant than is a solid tumor in an adult.

Neoplasms of the parotid gland can be divided into benign, including the vascular tumors, and malignant tumors. The latter is further divided into low-grade and high-grade malignancies.

Benign Neoplasms

Hemangiomas account for 50% of the neoplasms in the pediatric population (32). Girls are more commonly affected. The hemangiomas present either at birth or in the first few months of life. The tumor is usually contained within the intracapsular portion of the gland but can extend into the overlying subcutaneous tissue and skin. Capillary, cavernous, mixed, and hypertrophic hemangioma types have been described. Although the ductal structures are unaffected, the parenchyma of the gland is replaced by vaso-

TABLE 2: Neoplastic Disease

Vascular origin
   Hemangioma
   Lymphangioma
Benign
   Pleomorphic adenoma
   Warthin's tumor
   Oncocytoma
   Adenomas
   Neurofibroma
Low-grade malignancies
   Mucoepidermoid
   Acinic cell carcinoma
High-grade malignancies
   Mucoepidermoid
   Squamous cell carcinoma
   Adenoid cystic
   Adenocarcinoma
   Carcinoma ex pleomorphic adenoma
   Undifferentiated
Other
   Mesenchymal sarcomas
   Rhabdomyosarcoma
   Malignant epithelial tumors
   Neuroblastoma
   Lymphoma

formative elements. Clinically, the mass is soft and compressible. It enlarges and becomes tense with crying or straining. The facial nerve is not affected.

Treatment of salivary gland hemangiomas is conservative and sometimes controversial. Because of the cosmetic deformity, the families of the patient frequently ask for or even demand early surgery. Although an exact time course is difficult to predict, the majority of these lesions will undergo spontaneous resolution over several years and treatment should be conservative. Situations where surgical excision is indicated include excessive rapid growth of the mass, functional impairment, infection, hemorrhage, and ulceration (33).

The differential diagnosis to be considered in these lesions includes infected cystic lesions, lymphangiomas, and neurofibromas. The absence of typical findings of pain and erythema can usually eliminate an infective source. MRI can be helpful in confirming the diagnosis (34). Other options include the use of radiolabeled red blood cell pool imaging with technetium 99m. The specificity for hemangioma is reported to be near 100% if both hypoperfusion in the early phase and increased activity in the delayed imaging are present (32). This would be a reasonable option as a diagnostic tool, particularly in a child who could not tolerate the sedation needed for an MRI. Ultrasonography is helpful in differentiating a vascular lesion from a cystic or solid lesion but cannot show the true extent of the lesion or give a firm diagnosis (34).

A lymphangioma or cystic hygroma is the second most common benign neoplasm of the salivary gland. Derived from an abnormality in the development of the lymphatic system, lymphangiomas usually present as a diffuse mass involving not only the parotid but also surrounding structures of the head and neck. Isolated occurrence within the parotid gland, though rare, can occur (35). Similar to hemangiomas, lymphangiomas are soft and can progressively enlarge. Transillumination is frequently possible. In contrast to the hemangiomas, lymphangiomas of the salivary gland do not replace the normal glandular parenchyma, but rather islands of normal salivary tissue are next to thin-walled lymph-containing vessels (36). The three histologic patterns, simple or capillary, cavernous, and cystic, can coexist in the same lesion (33).

Similar to hemangiomas, the majority of lymphangiomas are present at birth, with approximately 50% to 60% of tumors presenting before age 1 and 90% presenting prior to the end of the second year of life (33).

Although the usual clinical behavior is of slow enlargement, rapid enlargement can occur with trauma, upper respiratory tract infections, or hemorrhage into the cyst (35). This acute type of enlargement can be associated with upper-airway compression, particularly if the lymphangioma involves the surrounding neck structures. Facial weakness, most likely from compression of the facial nerve, has also been reported (35).

Definitive diagnosis of a lymphangioma can best be established by either CT or MRI studies. Ultrasonography may confirm a cystic-type lesion but these former more detailed studies delineate the true extension of the mass.

Unlike hemangiomas, lymphangiomas do not resolve spontaneously. Surgical excision is the treatment of choice. Aspiration of the lesion is not recommended because of the risk of infection and hemorrhage into the cyst (37). Sclerosing agents, radiotherapy, and electromagnetic treatment have been used without significant success and have the potential for serious complications (37). The timing of surgery is somewhat controversial. If the lesion is associated with any type of airway obstruction, prompt excision is advocated. This is more common with lymphangiomas of the sublingual glands, submandibular glands, or the minor salivary glands. Because of concerns of infection resulting in inflammation and fibrosis around the facial nerves in the case of a lymphangioma of the parotid gland, excision should not be delayed beyond the age of a few years. Gross residual disease can potentially lead to regrowth and recurrence rate of lymphangiomas is approximately 10% to 15% within the first year (36,37). Recurrence is uncommon if all gross tumor is removed. Small amounts of residual tissue may atrophy or fibrose.

The benign salivary tumors include the mixed or pleomorphic adenoma, Warthin's tumor, oncocytoma, and adenoma. Of these, the pleomorphic adenoma is the most common in the pediatric population and represents the most common solid tumor mass seen in children. Frequently presenting as a small, approximately 1-cm, slow-growing, firm discrete nodule with good mobility, this lesion presents in an older age group than do the vascular tumors. The incidence is higher in the female than the male population. Although it appears to be quite discrete, the capsule is actually quite thin with an irregular surface and microscopic projections of tumor coming through the capsule. Multicentric satellites are also possible. Neoplasms frequently present during the adolescent years.

CT and MRI are helpful in delineating the extent of the tumor and in surgical planning. Simple incisional biopsies are not suggested because of the risk of seeding the surrounding tissue with tumor. In the past, simple enucleation of an apparently well-circumscribed mass was done but this was wrought with frequent recurrences. With the minimal biopsy procedure of a superficial parotidectomy with facial nerve preservation or submandibular gland excision now advocated, recurrences are rare. However, because this is a slow-growing tumor, recurrences can occur quite late after the original surgery and a long-term follow-up policy is advocated. Tumors involving the deep lobe have a higher chance of recurrence (38).

Pleomorphic adenoma of the minor salivary glands, though rare, has been reported (39). A lesion of the hard palate may mimic a torus palatinus, as the lesion is usually smooth, nontender, and not fixed to the overlying mucosa, and ulceration is rare. Again, CT and MRI are helpful in delineating the extent of the lesion and in regards to the hard palate, clarifying if there is any bone involvement. Surgical excision with removal of at least the periosteum is suggested for palatal lesions (39).

Other benign neoplasms that occur in the parotid gland include neurofibromas, basal cell adenomas, and cystadenomas. These all, however, are quite rare.

Malignant Tumors

In their review of salivary gland neoplasms, Schuller and McCabe (36) found an incidence of 57.5% malignancy in a solid firm mass within the salivary glands of children. This is in contrast to adults, in whom only 25% of salivary gland neoplasms are malignant (33). Therefore, these lesions should be taken quite seriously and not ignored.

In general, malignancies of the salivary glands occur in later childhood whereas the vasoformative lesions occur in early childhood. However, high-grade malignancies tend to occur in the younger child than do the low-grade or benign lesions (36).

Malignant tumors sometimes have warning signs. Any facial nerve involvement is highly suggestive of a malignant process. Involvement of the lingual, hypoglossal, or marginal mandibular nerve points to a malignancy involving the submandibular gland. Local pain is also highly suggestive, especially if the pain seems out of proportion to the surrounding inflammatory reaction. Rapid growth or fixation suggests a high-grade malignancy. Location also may contribute to the prognosis (40,41).

Diagnosis is established with the help of CT and MRI for evaluation of the location and extent of the mass in question, but true diagnosis must be histologically confirmed. Incision biopsy is never indicated because of the risk of seeding of the tumor. Although FNAC can be helpful, this is not always an option in the pediatric population. Because of the high risk of malignancy with essentially every salivary gland mass, surgical planning should include the potential for aggressive resection. Parents should be aware of this prior to surgery on their child.

Primary malignant tumors of the salivary glands are quite rare in children. Salivary gland malignancies represent only 3% to 8% of the tumors that can occur in the head and neck region in children, which are themselves quite rare (40,42,43). Similar to the benign tumors, the parotid gland is involved more frequently than the submandibular gland. Shikhani and Johns (41) found that not only were malignancies more common in the parotid gland but also masses that occurred in the parotid gland had a higher chance of being malignant when compared to a similar firm mass in the submandibular and sublingual glands.

Rasp and Permanetter (40) reviewed nine reported series of salivary gland tumors in children. Mucoepidermoid carcinomas were the most common tumors, at 51.7%. This was followed by acinic cell carcinoma (16.8%) and undifferentiated carcinoma (8.7%). Adenocarcinoma (8.1%) and adenoid cystic carcinomas (7.6%) were also seen. The very rare tumors included squamous cell carcinoma, rhabdomyosarcoma, and other sarcomas including neurosarcomas, fibrosarcomas, and osteosarcomas, as well as neuroblastomas and malignant lymphomas.

Most of the information available in terms of behavior of these tumors is sketchy at best, except for the mucoepidermoid tumors, because the overall numbers and series sizes are so small. Mucoepidermoid carcinoma is derived from the intralobular salivary ducts. This tumor has been subclassified into low and high grades and it is believed that its behavior correlates closely with the histologic morphology. With the mucoepidermoid tumors, despite a move from enucleation to parotidectomy as the treatment of choice, the relapse rate has only improved from 50% for the lesser procedure to 30% for the more aggressive surgery (41). Lymph node metastasis can occur in up to 20%, with an overall 5-year survival rate of 90% for patients treated with both aggressive surgery and postoperative radiation.

Similar to the behavior seen in adults, an acinic cell carcinoma may have an excellent 5-year control rate but is characterized by late recurrences after 20 to 25 years. The prognoses for adenocarcinomas and adenoid cystic carcinomas is significantly worse. Adenocarcinoma, when diagnosed in early childhood, can have a high malignant potential. This form of neoplasm may require a more radical resection or adjunctive treatment, or both (43).

Treatment of malignancies of the parotid gland requires superficial parotidectomy for low-grade malignancies and total parotidectomy with facial nerve preservation for high-grade malignancies. For the submandibular gland, total gland removal is indicated.

There is an overall higher rate of local recurrence and cervical lymph node metastasis in children compared to adults with the same type of tumor (42,43). Radical neck dissection, however, is only indicated in the presence of clinically evident cervical lymph nodes (41,43) and perhaps should be considered for poorly differentiated and high-grade carcinomas (33).

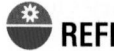 **REFERENCES**

1. Seibert RW. Diseases of the salivary glands. In: Bluestone CD, Stool SE, eds. *Pediatric Otolaryngology.* Philadelphia: WB Saunders, 1990:948–960.
2. Derias NW, Path MRC, Chong WH, O'Connor FF. Fine needle aspiration cytology of a head and neck swelling in a child: a non-invasive approach to diagnosis. *J Laryngol Otol* 1992;106:755–757.
3. Smith Frable MA, Frable WJ. Fine-needle aspiration biopsy of salivary glands. *Laryngoscope* 1991;101:245–249.
4. Myers MA, Youngberg RA, Bauman JM. Congenital absence of the major salivary glands and impaired lacrimal secretion in a child; case report. *J Am Dent Assoc* 1994;125:210–212.
5. O'Malley AM, Macleod RI, Welbury RR. Congenital aplasia of major salivary glands in a 4 year-old child. *Int J Paediatr Dent* 1993;3:141–144.
6. Pownell PH, Brown OE, Pransky SM, Manning SC. Congenital abnormalities of the submandibular duct. *Int J Pediatr Otorhinolaryngol* 1992;24:161–169.
7. Kun Z, Li-Min W, Dao-Yi Q. Congenital extraoral fistula from an auxiliary parotid duct. *J Oral Maxillofac Surg* 1992;50:752–753.
8. Travis LW, Hecht DW. Acute and chronic inflammatory disease of the salivary glands: diagnosis and management. *Otolaryngol Clin North Am* 1977;10:329–338.
9. Work WP. Cysts and congenital lesions of the parotid glands. *Otolaryngol Clin North Am* 1977;10:339–343.
10. Morgan DW, Pearman K, Raafat F, Oates J, Campbell J. Salivary disease in childhood. *Ear Nose Throat J* 1989;68:155–159.

11. Brook I, Frazier EH, Thompson OH. Aerobic and anaerobic microbiology of acute suppurative parotitis. *Laryngoscope* 1991;101:170–172.

12. Myer CM, Holmes DK, Cotton RT. Salivary gland disease in children. In: Granick MS, ed. *Salivary gland disorders.* Baltimore: Williams & Wilkins, 1992:241–249.

13. Encson S, Zetterlund B, Ohman J. Recurrent parotitis and sialectasis in childhood—clinical, radiologic, immunologic, bacteriologic and histologic study. *Ann Otol Rhinol Laryngol* 1991;100:527–535.

14. Mandel L, Kaynar A. Recurrent parotitis in children. *NY State Dent J* 1995;61:22–25.

15. Nozaki H, Harasawa A, Hara H, Kohro A, Shigeta A. Ultrasonographic features of recurrent parotitis in childhood. *Pediatr Radiol* 1994;24:98–100.

16. Bodner L, Fliss DM. Parotid and submandibular calculi in children. *Int J Pediatr Otorhinolaryngol* 1995;31:35–42.

17. Lustman J, Shteyer A. Salivary calculi—ultrastructured morphology and bacterial etiology. *J Dent Res* 1981;60:1387–1395.

18. Levy DM, ReMine WH, Devine KD. Salivary gland calculi. *JAMA* 1962;181:1115–1119.

19. Hiraide F, Nomura Y. The fine surface structure and composition of salivary calculi. *Laryngoscope* 1980;90:152–158.

20. Myer CM, Cotton RT. Salivary gland disease in children: a review. Part 1: acquired non-neoplastic disease. *Clin Pediatr* 1986;25:314–322.

21. Blatt IM. Studies in sialolithiasis. III. Pathogenesis, diagnosis and treatment. *South Med J* 1964;57:723–729.

22. Bodner L, Azaz B. Submandibular sialolithiasis in children. *J Oral Maxillofac Surg* 1982;40:551–554.

23. Ballenger JJ, Yeh S. Sialadenolithiasis. In: English GM, ed. *Otolaryngology.* Philadelphia: JB Lippincott, 1994;3(62):1–9.

24. Isaccson G, Lundquist P. Salivary calculi as an aetiological factor in chronic sialadenitis of the submandibular gland. *Clin Otolaryngol* 1982;7:231–236.

25. Smith RJH. Non-neoplastic salivary gland diseases. In: English GM, ed. *Otolaryngology.* Philadelphia: JB Lippincott, 1994;3(61):1–29.

26. Wurster CF. Non-neoplastic salivary gland disorders. In: Gates GA, ed. *Current therapy in otolaryngology head and neck surgery.* St. Louis: Mosby–Year Book 1994:238–243.

27. Wakely PE, Silverman JF, Holbrook CT, Fairman RP, Daeschner CW, Joshi VV. Fine needle aspiration biopsy cytology as an adjunct in the diagnosis of childhood sarcoidosis. *Pediatr Pulmonol* 1992;13:117–120.

28. Smyth AG, Ward-Booth RP, High AS. Polycystic disease of the parotid glands: two familial cases. *Br J Oral Maxillofac Surg* 1993;31:38–40.

29. Tavill MA, Poje CP, Wetmore RF, Faros H. Plunging ranulas in children. *Ann Otol Rhinol Laryngol* 1995;104:405–408.

30. Myer CM. Sialorrhea. *Pediatr Clin North Am* 1989;36:1495–1500.

31. Shott SR, Myer CM, Cotton RT. Surgical management of sialorrhea. *Otolaryngol Head Neck Surg* 1989;101:47–50.

32. Liu KKW, Lam WWM. Parotid hemangioma in infancy: diagnosis with technetium 99m-labeled red blood cell pool imaging. *Otolaryngol Head Neck Surg* 1995;112:780–781.

33. Myer CM, Cotton RT. Salivary gland disease in children: a review. Part 2: congenital lesions and neoplastic disease. *Clin Pediatr* 1986;27:353–357.

34. Huchzermeyer P, Birchall MA, Kendall B, Bailey CM. Parotid haemangiomas in childhood: a case for MRI. *J Laryngol Otol* 1994;108:892–895.

35. Tsui SC, Huang JL. Parotid lymphangioma. A case report. *Int J Pediatr Otorhinolaryngol* 1996;34:273–278.

36. Schuller DE, McCabe BF. Salivary neoplasms in children. *Otolaryngol Clin North Am* 1977;10:399–412.

37. Emery PJ, Bailey CM, Evans JNG. Cystic hygroma of the head and neck. *J Laryngol Otol* 1984;998:613–619.

38. Phillips PP, Olsen KD. Recurrent pleomorphic adenoma of the parotid gland: report of 126 cases and a review of the literature. *Ann Otol Rhinol Laryngol* 1995;104:100–104.

39. Noghreyan A, Gatot A, Moar E, Fliss DM. Palatal pleomorphic adenoma in a child. *J Laryngol Otol* 1995;109:343–345.

40. Rasp G, Permanetter W. Malignant salivary gland tumors: squamous cell carcinoma of the submandibular gland in a child. *Am J Otolaryngol* 1992;13:109–112.

41. Shikhani AH, Johns ME. Tumors of the major salivary glands in children. *Head Neck* 1988;10:257–263.
42. Rush BF, Chambers RG, Ravitch MM. Cancer of the head and neck in children. *Surgery* 1963;53:270–284.
43. Ogata H, Ebihara S, Mukai K. Salivary neoplasms in children. *Jpn J Clin Oncol* 1994; 24:88–93.

S.R. Shott: Department of Otolaryngology and Maxillofacial Surgery, University of Cincinnati, and Children's Hospital Medical Center, Cincinnati, Ohio 45229–3039.

• *Practical Pediatric Otolaryngology*
• edited by Robin T. Cotton
  and Charles M. Myer, III
• Lippincott-Raven Publishers,
  Philadelphia © 1999

Deep Neck Infections: Recognition, Evaluation, Therapy

Andrew J. Hotaling

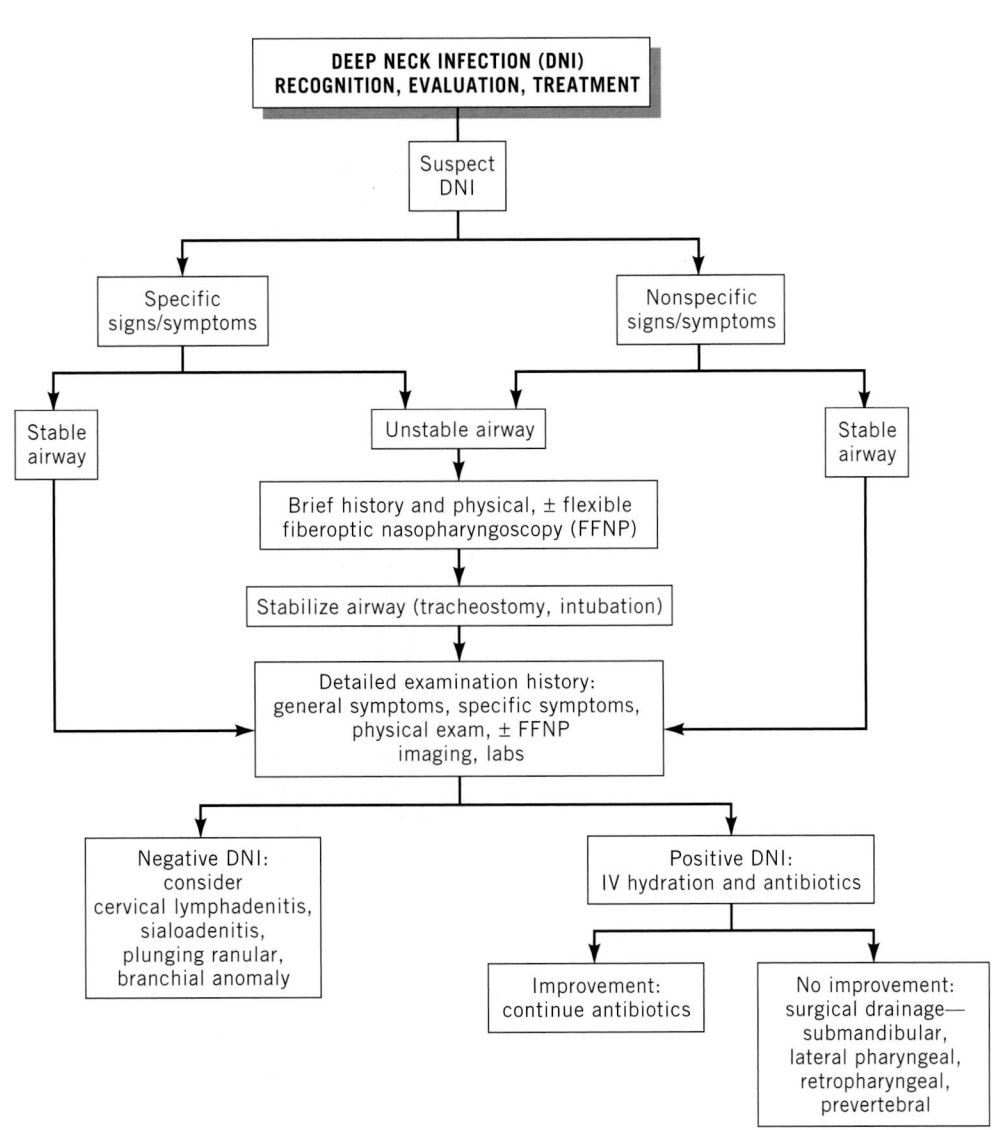

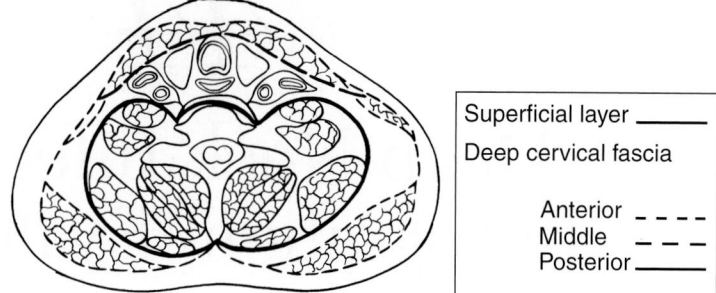

FIGURE 1 Axial section of the neck through the level of the T-1 vertebra. (From ref. 1, with permission.)

OVERVIEW AND ANATOMY

This chapter reviews the recognition, evaluation, and treatment of deep neck infections (DNIs). Because the anatomy of the fascial spaces in the neck is complex and has been complicated by multiple synonyms, the beginning section introduces the terminology chosen for use in this chapter. The terminology is followed by a detailed review of the anatomy, the key element to understanding and treating DNIs. A generalized discussion of the signs, symptoms, and workup of DNIs follows. The chapter concludes with a review of specific DNIs.

Terminology

There are three major fascial layers of the head and neck: the superficial fascial layer, the deep fascial layer, and the visceral layer (Figs. 1 and 2). The superficial fascia is defined as the subcutaneous tissue of the head and neck enclosing the voluntary muscles of facial

FIGURE 2 Sagittal section demonstrating the anterior, middle, and posterior layers of the deep cervical fascia. (From ref. 1, with permission.)

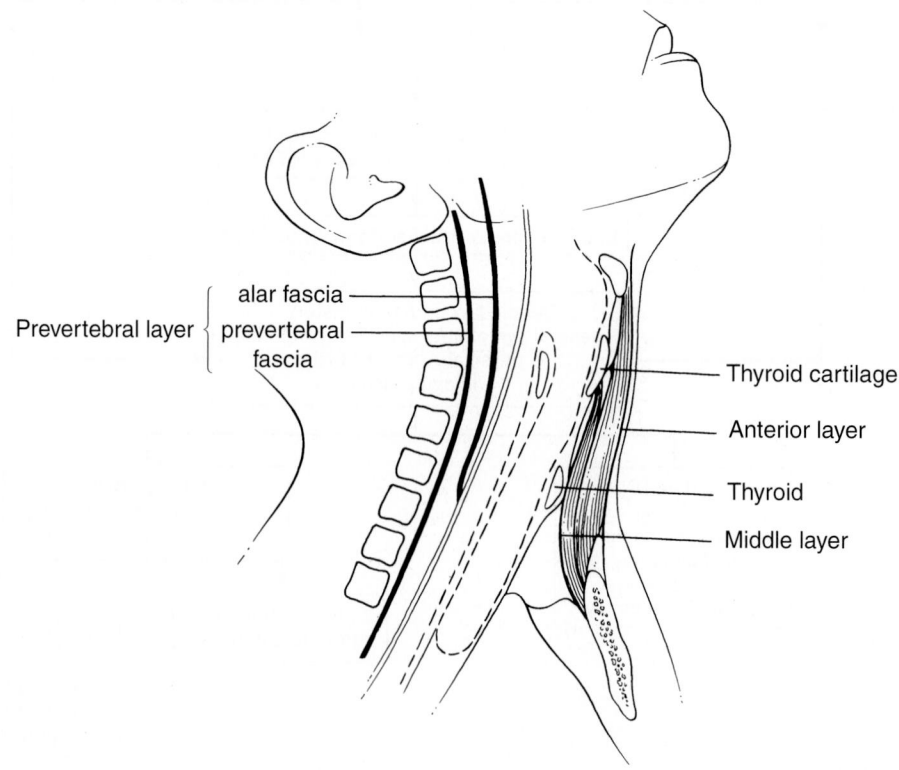

TABLE 1: Cervical Fascia Layers and Synonyms[a]

A. Superficial cervical fascia
B. Deep cervical fascia
   1. Anterior layer—*Superficial investing*
   2. Middle layer—*Pretracheal*
   3. Posterior layer—*Deep*
     a. Alar layer
     b. Prevertebral layer
C. Visceral fascia—*Buccopharyngeal*

[a]Regular type indicates terminology used in this review; *italics indicates synonyms.*

(Adapted from ref. 1, with permission.)

expression and the platysma muscle. The deep fascial layer is subdivided further into three layers: anterior, middle, and posterior. The posterior layer again subdivides into alar and prevertebral layers. The visceral fascia surrounds the esophagus, trachea, and thyroid gland. Table 1 lists the fascia as they are discussed in this review and provides synonyms for the fascial terminology employed in this chapter (1).

From these layers, spaces are formed, divided by the hyoid bone into suprahyoid and infrahyoid. Table 2 lists the spaces as they are encountered, moving from superficial to deep in this review, and synonyms for these spaces. In the suprahyoid region, the anterior layer of the deep fascia divides to form the following spaces: body of mandible, submaxillary gland, masticator, and parotid. Moving from superficial to deep, the peripharyngeal spaces represent the second layer of fascial spaces. These spaces include lateral pharyngeal space, retropharyngeal space, and submandibular space. These three spaces all lie deep to the anterior layer of the deep cervical fascia. Completing the list of suprahyoid spaces are the danger space and the prevertebral space. The danger space is formed by the separation of the alar and prevertebral layers and allows access into the mediastinum. Posterior to the danger space is the prevertebral space. Three of these spaces communicate from the suprahyoid to the infrahyoid level: retropharyngeal, danger, and prevertebral.

TABLE 2: Fascial Spaces and Synonyms[a]

  I. Spaces created by splitting the anterior layer of deep cervical fascia
    A. Above level of hyoid bone
      1. Space of body of mandible
      2. Space of submaxillary gland
      3. Space of parotid gland
      4. Masticator space—*masseteric, mandibulopterygoid, temporal pouch*
    B. Spaces deep to anterior layer of deep cervical fascia
      1. Retropharyngeal space—*retrovisceral space, retroesophageal visceral compartment (posterior)*
      2. Lateral pharyngeal space—*parapharyngeal, peripharyngeal, pharyngomaxillary, pterygopharyngeal, pterygomandibular, pharyngomasticatory*
        a. Anterior—*prestyloid*
        b. Posterior—*poststyloid*
      3. Submandibular space
        a. Sublingual—*floor of mouth*
        b. Submylohyoid—*submaxillary, submandibular*
    C. Other spaces
      1. Danger space
      2. Prevertebral space—*paravertebral space*
      3. Carotid sheath
      4. Pretracheal space—*visceral compartment (anterior)*
      5. Peritonsillar space

[a]Regular type indicates terminology used in review; *italics indicates synonyms.*

(Adapted from ref. 1, with permission.)

The pretracheal space begins below the hyoid and consists of connective tissue surrounding the trachea, lying anterior to the esophagus. (Note: Some authors describe a visceral compartment, not a space, consisting of anterior and posterior subcompartments, corresponding to the pretracheal and retropharyngeal spaces, respectively.) These spaces communicate around the esophagus and thyroid gland between the inferior thyroid artery and the superior border of the thyroid cartilage. The space of the carotid sheath also continues above and below the hyoid as it follows the carotid artery.

Cervical Fascia

The superficial fascia creates no fascial spaces, owing to its tight inherence to the underlying muscle and bone. As stated already, the superficial fascia is defined as the subcutaneous tissue of the head and neck enclosing the muscles of facial expression in the head and the platysma muscle in the neck.

The deep cervical fascia is divided into three layers. The most superficial is the anterior layer, which originates from the vertebral spinous processes and ligamentum nuchae, the fibers that descend vertically from vertebral spinous processes. The anterior layer of the deep cervical fascia encircles the entire neck and splits to enclose the trapezius, omohyoid, and sternocleidomastoid muscles (2). The strap muscles lie medial to the anterior layer, which attaches to the hyoid and extends from the hyoid superiorly to the mandible where it splits to enclose the inner and outer tables of the mandible. From the outer table of the mandible, the anterior layer continues superiorly to the zygoma and temporalis muscle. Superior to the mandible, it splits to encompass the parotid gland and the masseter and internal pterygoid muscles. Between the hyoid and the mandible, it forms the floor of the submandibular space.

Beginning at the lateral border of the strap muscles, the middle layer of the deep cervical fascia originates from the anterior layer, traveling posterior to the strap muscles and anterior to the trachea and thyroid. Its superior extent is the hyoid bone. Inferiorly, it joins the fibrous pericardium (see Fig. 2).

The posterior layer of the deep fascia, like the anterior layer, originates from the vertebral spinous processes and encircles the neck. Superiorly, it extends to the base of skull, lying deep to the trapezius muscle and enclosing the vertebral muscles. From the transverse processes of the vertebrae, the posterior layer splits to form two separate layers: the anterior alar fascia and the posterior prevertebral fascia. The prevertebral fascia covers the longus colli muscle.

The third major fascia layer is the visceral fascia, described as the connective tissue surrounding the esophagus, thyroid gland, and trachea. (Note: The visceral fascia is a separate entity from the visceral compartment.) Above the level of the hyoid, some authors define the visceral fascia as the buccopharyngeal fascia. No spaces are formed as this fascial layer is tightly adherent to underlying structures.

Fascial Spaces

The various fascial layers combine to form spaces. These are listed in order of their presentation from superficial to deep. Table 2 lists the spaces as they are identified in this chapter, and common synonyms (1). Table 3 lists the contents of the spaces (1). Again, no spaces are formed by the superficial layer, which is the subcutaneous tissue of the head and neck tightly adherent to the facial and platysma muscles. The splitting of the anterior layer of the deep cervical fascia around the inner and outer tables of the mandible forms the space of the body of the mandible. In reality, it is a potential space as no soft tissue lies within this space, limited anteriorly by the attachment of the anterior belly of the digastric muscle to the mandible and posteriorly by the internal pterygoid muscle.

Similarly, the parotid space and the space of the submaxillary gland are formed by

TABLE 3: Major Contents of Cervical Spaces

Space	Contents
A. Splitting of anterior layer	
1. Space of parotid gland	Parotid gland, facial nerve, lymph nodes
2. Space of submaxillary gland	Submaxillary gland, lymph nodes
3. Masticator space	Muscles (temporalis, masseter, internal pterygoid)
	Internal maxillary artery, mandibular nerve
4. Space of body of mandible	Potential space
B. Peripharyngeal spaces	
1. Retropharyngeal space	Loose connective tissue, lymph nodes
2. Lateral pharyngeal space	
a. Anterior	Connective tissue, lymph nodes
b. Posterior	Cranial nerves IX, X, XII; cervical sympathetics, carotid sheath
3. Submandibular space	
a. Sublingual	Sublingual gland, lingual nerve and artery, genioglossus, and geniohyoid muscles, submandibular duct
b. Submylohyoid	Digastric muscle
C. Other	
1. Danger space	Loose connective tissue
2. Prevertebral space	Longus colli muscle
3. Carotid sheath	Internal jugular vein, carotid artery, cranial nerve X
4. Pretracheal space	Connective tissue
5. Peritonsillar space	Faucial tonsils

(Adapted from ref. 1, with permission.)

splitting the anterior layer. These spaces contain their respective glands and associated nodes. The glands are tightly adherent to their surrounding fascial layers. To be discussed in more detail later, the lateral pharyngeal space lies deep to the parotid space and may become involved if infection spreads medially from the deep lobe of the parotid.

The masticator space encloses the ramus of the mandible, the masseter, internal pterygoid, and lower portion of the temporalis muscles and is formed by splitting of the anterior layer. Most of the branches of the mandibular nerve and the internal maxillary artery are contained within this space.

Moving medially, the next series of spaces are peripharyngeal, forming a ring around the pharynx. The peripharyngeal spaces include the retropharyngeal, lateral pharyngeal, and submandibular spaces, all lying deep to the anterior layer of the deep fascia. These three spaces are in communication with each other via the muscles and vessels passing through them.

The retropharyngeal space extends from the base of skull to the bifurcation of the trachea and lies behind the pharynx and esophagus. Two chains of lymph nodes lie on either side of a midline raphe, formed by attachment of the superior constrictor muscle to the alar layer of the deep cervical fascia.

The lateral pharyngeal space also extends from the base of the skull and is contiguous with the retropharyngeal space. This space is described as conical in shape, with its base the petrous portion of the temporal bone. The apex is the hyoid bone. Medially it extends to the lateral pharyngeal wall, and laterally is bounded by the mandible, parotid gland, and internal pterygoid muscles. It is divided into anterior and posterior compartments by the styloid process and associated musculature. The anterior compartment is composed primarily of fat and connective tissue. The posterior compartment contains cranial nerves IX, X, and XII, the internal jugular vein and common carotid artery, and the cervical sympathetic chain.

The most anterior of the peripharyngeal spaces is the submandibular space, bounded superiorly by the lingual mucosa and inferiorly by the anterior layer of the deep fascia. This space is divided into two portions by the mylohyoid muscle. These are the sublingual and submaxillary subcompartments that communicate posteriorly at the posterior border of the mylohyoid muscle. The sublingual portion contains the submandibular duct, lingual nerve, and the hypoglossal nerve. The anterior belly of the digastric muscle is contained in the submaxillary portion.

Several other spaces need to be defined. The danger space exists between the alar and prevertebral fascia, extending from the base of the skull to the diaphragm. It is a space that potentially can be involved with infection extending anteriorly from the prevertebral space or posteriorly from the retropharyngeal space. It provides another avenue for infection to spread to the mediastinum.

The most anterior of the fascial spaces below the hyoid bone is the pretracheal space; others include the retropharyngeal, danger, and prevertebral spaces. The pretracheal space is defined anteriorly by the middle layer of the *deep* fascia and posteriorly by the esophagus. Superiorly, it extends to the hyoid bone; inferiorly, to the level of the fourth thoracic vertebra along the arch of the aorta.

Finally, the carotid sheath forms a potential space for infection to spread. The carotid sheath encloses the carotid artery, internal jugular vein, and cranial nerve X. It is formed by contributions from all three parts of the deep cervical fascia. Anteromedially, it is formed by the anterior layer, deep to the sternocleidomastoid muscle, and posteriorly by the lamina from the anterior layer prior to dividing to form the middle layer. The cervical sympathetic chain lies posteromedial to the carotid sheath but superficial to the posterior fascial layer. The carotid sheath has been referred to as "Lincoln's highway" of the neck by Mosher (3), as it traverses the posterior compartment of the lateral pharyngeal space and descends into the mediastinum.

PEARLS AND PERILS

1. Carotid sheath known as "Lincoln's highway" is a potential pathway from the lateral pharyngeal space into the mediastinum.
2. Frequent bacteria in deep neck infections include aerobic streptococcus and nonstreptococcal anaerobes.

MICROBIOLOGY

Currently, aerobic streptococcal species and nonstreptococcal anaerobes are the bacteria causing the majority of DNIs. These bacteria are present in normal oral flora and become virulent when normal mucosal barriers are broken.

The *Streptococcus* species are divided into the hemolytic and nonhemolytic strains. Hemolytic strains are predominately group A species. The nonhemolytic strains are classified as alpha and gamma species, with further subclassification of the alpha species into group D or nongroup D subspecies. In odontogenic infections, the most common streptococcal species is alpha nonhemolytic streptococcus. Contrastingly, hemolytic group A strains are more commonly isolated from pharyngeal infections.

The most commonly isolated anaerobes include *Peptostreptococcus, Fusobacterium,* and *Bacteroides* (4). In a retrospective review of neck abscesses, streptococcal isolates were most frequent. Thirty-two streptococcal species were isolated from 36 patients with positive cultures, most commonly, alpha nongroup D strains and group A beta-hemolytic strains (5). Among the anaerobes, *Bacteroides* and *Peptostreptococcus* organisms were most common. Recently, there has been an increase in isolation of the anaerobe *Eikenella corrodens,* which is frequently resistant to clindamycin (6).

Gram-negative rods are rarely isolated in DNIs but may be found in immunocompromised, debilitated, elderly, and diabetic patients (4).

PATIENT ASSESSMENT AND
TREATMENT RECOMMENDATIONS

To successfully manage DNIs, the initial critical factor is evaluation of the airway and, if necessary, control of an unstable airway. Signs and symptoms can be divided into two groups: general and specific. Generalized symptoms include fever, chills, loss of appetite, and malaise.

PEARLS AND PERILS

1. Key to DNI management: Evaluation of airway: if unstable, control.
2. Posterior pharyngeal wall swelling: Symmetric—prevertebral, asymmetrical—retropharyngeal.
3. Any sign of bleeding from the head or neck indicates possible carotid artery involvement.
4. If airway is threatened, secure via intubation or tracheotomy.

Specific symptoms include odynophagia, dysphagia, sore throat, neck stiffness, torticollis, neck pain, trismus, and voice changes. Specific signs include neck swelling, fullness in the floor of the mouth, drooling, and bulging of the pharyngeal wall. Classically, prevertebral infections cause symmetric bulging of the posterior pharyngeal wall, contrasted with unilateral swelling for retropharyngeal space infections due to the midline raphe previously described for the retropharyngeal space, preventing involvement of the contralateral side.

Airway signs include dyspnea, stridor, shortness of breath, and a "hot potato" voice. When these signs are present, immediate steps to evaluate and, if indicated, secure the airway are required to avoid airway obstruction and respiratory arrest.

Any bleeding in the head and neck may be a sentinel bleed, ranging from ecchymosis of the skin to frank blood from the ear, nose, or mouth. Such bleeding may represent a mycotic process of the carotid artery with a potentially lethal outcome.

The evaluation of a patient with a suspected deep neck abscess (Fig. 3) should proceed in an orderly fashion, beginning with a brief history and physical examination to assess the potential threat to the airway. If the airway is threatened, immediate steps are required to stabilize the airway, usually by endotracheal intubation or tracheotomy.

If there is no immediate threat to the airway or if the airway has been secured, a comprehensive history and physical examination is initiated. The physical examination should include a complete head and neck evaluation, paying specific attention to the airway and intraoral examination. Specific areas to evaluate include the floor of the mouth, the oropharynx, and the pharyngeal walls. Difficult to see on an intraoral examination and more easily visualized on flexible fiberoptic nasopharyngoscopy (FFNP) is bulging posterior to the palatopharyngeal fold or the posterior tonsillar pillar, where such bulging may indicate a lateral pharyngeal space infection. Based on the findings of the history and physical examination, relevant radiographic studies can be requested.

PEARLS AND PERILS

Keys to successful management of DNI:
1. Evaluation, and if necessary, control of airway.
2. Intravenous antibiotics.
3. Empiric antibiotic choice: high-dose penicillin or third-generation cephalosporin.
4. Surgical drainage, if required.

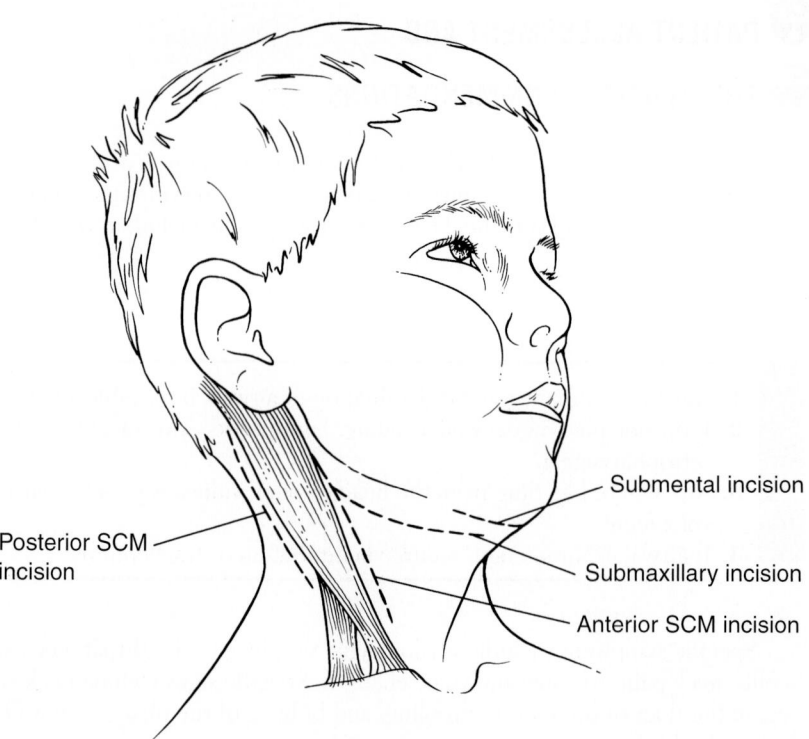

Submental incision

Posterior SCM
incision

Submaxillary incision

Anterior SCM incision

FIGURE 3 External approaches to the deep
neck spaces. (From ref. 1, with permission.)

When surgical drainage is performed, any purulent material obtained via aspiration
or incision and drainage should be cultured aerobically and anaerobically to guide subsequent antibiotic therapy. A Gram stain of the material may aid in initial antibiotic selection. When the abscess cavity is opened, a biopsy on a portion of the wall can be performed to help exclude the possibility of an abscess secondary to tumor.

As an initial antibiotic choice, high-dose penicillin is reasonable, as are third-generation cephalosporins. The use of clindamycin as a single agent is not recommended (7).

Radiology

Multiple imaging techniques are available. The simplest is a lateral cervical neck film, applicable when there is suspected retropharyngeal or prevertebral space involvement
(Fig. 4). It is critical that these films be obtained during inspiration, as the bulging of the
posterior pharyngeal wall can be interpreted falsely if the film is taken during expiration.
Interpretation of lateral cervical films is based on measuring the distance between the
anterior aspect of the vertebral column to the air column of the posterior pharyngeal
wall. In both children and adults, the normal distance may be as wide as 7 mm at C-2. At
C-6, the distance may extend to 14 mm in children and 22 mm in adults. A significant
false-negative rate has been reported for these films, and other imaging modalities may
be indicated (2,4).

PEARLS AND PERILS

1. High false-positive rate if lateral film taken in expiration.

Ultrasonography has not been useful in the evaluation of DNIs. Contrastingly, computed tomography (CT) provides excellent imaging to confirm the presence of the abscess and the surrounding anatomy (Fig. 5).

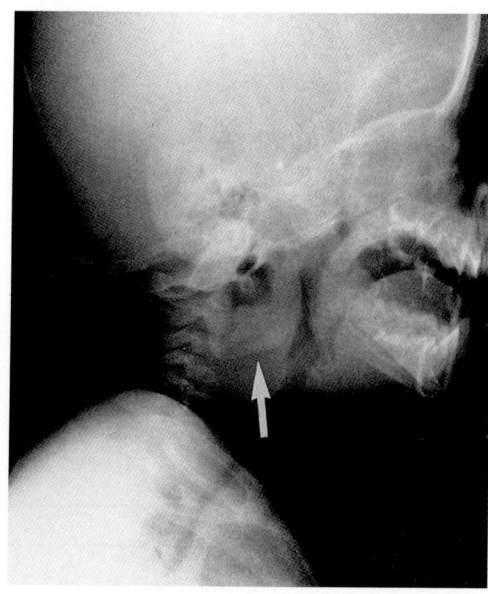

FIGURE 4 Lateral neck film demonstrating increased soft tissue column representing a retropharyngeal space abscess in a 4-year-old patient. The *arrow* shows the increased soft tissue width. (From ref. 1, with permission.)

Magnetic resonance imaging (MRI) can also provide accurate information about the anatomic detail. However, MRI has the disadvantage of frequently requiring transportation of patients away from the acute hospital complex and, consequently, away from personnel needed for rapid intervention to stabilize the airway. The transport thus presents a potential hazard to patients as their condition may deteriorate rapidly in an environment where they cannot be treated expeditiously. CT is generally preferred because it is more readily available, is less expensive, and can effectively localize abscesses in the head and neck. It should be emphasized that no imaging should be performed in an acute situation where there is the potential of respiratory complications from DNIs.

The chest x-ray study remains useful to help assess for complications from DNIs including mediastinal extension, lung abscess, pyopneumothorax, and aspiration. If mediastinal involvement is documented, aggressive management of the patient should be anticipated.

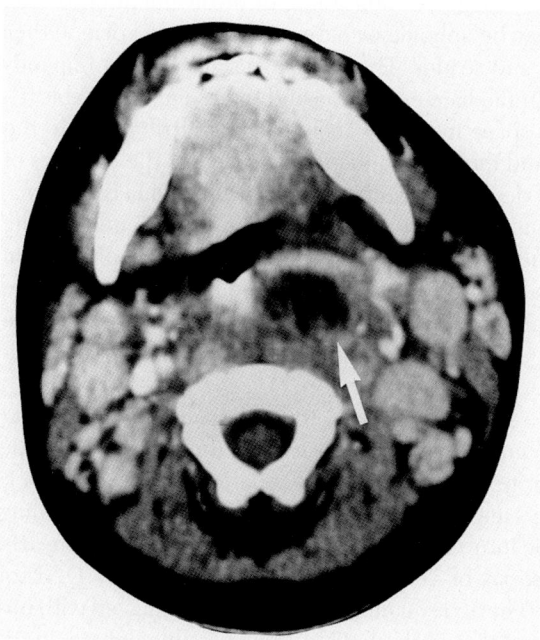

FIGURE 5 Computed tomography scan demonstrating a retropharyngeal space abscess in a 4-year-old patient. Note that the abscess is off midline. The *arrow* denotes the abscess capsule. (From ref. 1, with permission.)

SPECIFIC SPACE INFECTIONS

Submandibular Space

Submandibular space infections are the most common DNIs. Submandibular space infections can involve either or both of the subcompartments: the sublingual or the submylohyoid. Frequently, both are involved in a submandibular space infection as they communicate at the posterior border of the mylohyoid muscle. The prototypic infection in this space is Ludwig's angina; by definition, this infection requires that both subcompartments be involved. The usual source of submandibular space infection is odontogenic, occurring in 70% to 85% of cases. Other etiologies include disruption of the mucosal layer by a laceration or mandibular fracture and by tumor, sialadenitis, and lymphadenitis. Alpha-hemolytic streptococcus is most commonly isolated from this space.

PEARLS AND PERILS

1. Usual source of submandibular space infection: odontogenic.
2. Tongue displacement in submaxillary DNIs may significantly impair the airway.
3. Empiric antibiotic of choice: high-dose intravenous penicillin.
4. Tracheotomy remains the gold standard to control the airway.

The patients are typically 20 to 40 years old and otherwise healthy. Sixty percent are men. They present with pain in the oral cavity, anterior-neck stiffness, sialorrhea, and dysphagia. The presentation of submandibular space infection is provided in Table 4 and is contrasted with those signs presenting with other DNIs. External swelling is limited, due to the strength of the anterior layer of the deep fascia that forms the inferior aspect of the submandibular space. However, the distensible tissue in the floor of the mouth can be easily elevated, precipitating anterior or posterior tongue displacement.

On physical examination, the tongue is enlarged, edematous, and anteriorly displaced. The floor of the mouth is usually swollen, indurated, and erythematous. The suprahyoid area of the neck is tender with woody induration. Fluctuance is rarely present. Trismus is atypical and, if present, suggests extension to or involvement of the lateral pharyngeal space. The patient may be aphonic or have a "hot potato" voice. Other signs include fever, chills, tachypnea, and stridor. The latter two signs suggest impending airway obstruction, necessitating immediate evaluation and treatment (see Table 4).

Complications of submandibular space infections include those attributable to the infection occurring within the space and those when the infection leaves the confines of the space. The most common cause of death in patients with Ludwig's angina is asphyxia, secondary to upper-airway obstruction, commonly due to posterior displacement of the tongue. Extension beyond the submandibular space occurs through the buccopharyngeal gap, the point at which the styloglossus muscle exits the submandibular space between the middle and superior constrictor muscles. This gap serves as a pathway for infection to enter the lateral pharyngeal space. Other complications include tongue necrosis, aspiration pneumonia, and lung abscess.

As with all DNIs there are three primary components in treating submandibular space DNI. These include evaluation and possible stabilization of the airway, antibiotic therapy, and surgical intervention. Protection of the airway is paramount as asphyxia is the primary cause of death in Ludwig's angina. Airway management is varied, including observation, oral intubation, fiberoptic intubation, cricothyrotomy, and tracheotomy (8).

Patterson et al (8) described a series of 20 patients with submandibular DNI, of whom only 7 required airway control. The 13 remaining patients were managed with observation. However, it must be stressed that such observation is possible only in an in-

TABLE 4: Clinical Features of Deep Neck Infections

Space	Pain	Trismus	Swelling	Complications Dysphagia	Dyspnea	Other
Submandibular	Present	Minimal	Floor of mouth	Present	Present	Asphyxias, tongue necrosis, aspiration pneumonia, lung abscess
Lateral pharyngeal						
Anterior	Severe	Prominent	Anterior oropharynx	Present	Occasional	—
Posterior	Minimal	Minimal	Posterior oropharynx behind posterior pharyngeal pillar	Present	Severe	Carotid artery erosion, internal jugular thrombosis, lateral and cavernous sinus thrombosis
Retropharyngeal	Present	Minimal	Posterior pharynx, off midline	Present	Present	Mediastinitis, pyopneumothorax, bronchial erosion
Prevertebral	Present	None	Posterior pharynx, midline	Present	Occasional	—

(From ref. 1, with permission.)

tensive care unit when the progression of infection does not require surgical drainage and control of the airway can be achieved quickly if the infection rapidly progresses.

High-dose intravenous penicillin is the drug of choice until culture results are available. Additional anaerobic coverage can be obtained with metronidazole or clindamycin. In those patients who fail to respond to appropriate antibiotic therapy or who have rapid progression threatening the airway, surgical intervention is required. Drainage can be intraoral or by external incision. Intraoral drainage is indicated only when the submandibular space infection is limited to the sublingual compartment and is uncomplicated. In all other cases, an external approach is recommended.

The external submental incision is illustrated in Figure 3. This incision is made only after airway control has been achieved. The gold standard for airway control remains tracheotomy. The usual landmarks on the mandible for the incision are frequently obscured. An incision starts four fingerbreadths (about 8 cm) below the auricle at the anterior border of the sternocleidomastoid muscle. The submaxillary incision follows a line parallel to the body of the mandible to preserve the marginal mandibular nerve. The incision continues to the midportion of the contralateral submandibular gland. The anterior fascia is transected and the mylohyoid is entered in the midline using blunt dissection, being careful not to penetrate the oral mucosa from below as an orocutaneous fistula could result. Drains are placed through the mylohyoid, and the incision is loosely closed. Wet-to-dry dressings are applied postoperatively. Typically, surgically decompressing the abscess and treating with intravenous antibiotics will achieve resolution within 10 days.

Lateral Pharyngeal Space

There are various etiologies for infection in the lateral pharyngeal space, including penetrating trauma and extension of infection from another area. Extension can occur laterally from a peritonsillar abscess, posteriorly from a submandibular space infection, and from the masticator space, the most common source of extension. Of note, a peritonsillar abscess occurs medial to the lateral pharyngeal space, separated from this area by the superior constrictor muscle. Only with lateral extension does a peritonsillar abscess extend into the lateral pharyngeal space.

As noted earlier, the lateral pharyngeal space has anterior and posterior compartments, each with different contents. The presentation in each subcompartment depends on the contents of the compartment. With contents of fat, connective tissue, lymph nodes, and muscle, the typical anterior-compartment infection presents with pain, trismus, and dysphagia. Systemic signs including fever and chills may also be present. Typically, there is an antecedent pharyngitis or tonsillitis within the preceding 10 days. Classically, four signs are described for an anterior-compartment infection: trismus, medial bulging of the pharyngeal wall, swelling at the angle of the mandible, and systemic toxicity. Fluctuance is frequently encountered although abscesses may occur.

PEARLS AND PERILS

1. *Lateral pharyngeal DNI.* Anterior compartment: symptomatic. Posterior compartment: "asymptomatic."
2. Signs of impending bleed: shock, prolonged course, Horner's syndrome, hemorrhaging, hematoma, neuropathies of cranial nerves IX to XII, and persistent peritonsillar swelling.
3. Lateral DNI empiric antibiotic choice: penicillin and metronidazole or clindamycin.
4. Surgical drainage of lateral DNI: if vascular/mediastinal complication unlikely, use submaxillary approach; if vascular/mediastinal complication likely, use anterior sternocleidomastoid approach.

Infection of the posterior compartment of the lateral pharyngeal space is often more difficult to detect. Trismus is usually absent as there are no muscles within the compartment to be affected. On intraoral examination, the posterior presentation is difficult to visualize. While systemic signs of fever and toxicity are present, infections of the space are often described as fevers of unknown origin. If swelling is present in the lateral pharyngeal wall, it is usually posterior to the palatopharyngeal arch and thus difficult to see on intraoral examination. The use of FFNP aids in the detection of this subtle sign.

Vascular complications may occur from infectious processes involving the carotid sheath. Most commonly, suppurative internal jugular vein thrombosis is seen (9). With antibiotic therapy, the preantibiotic mortality has been reduced significantly. With adequate surgical drainage of the lateral pharyngeal space and intravenous antibiotics, suppuration of the internal jugular vein can be managed without ligation of the vein if the patient is otherwise stable (10). Internal jugular vein thrombosis can precipitate bacteremia, septic pulmonary emboli, metastatic abscess formation, and thrombosis of the lateral and cavernous sinuses (11).

The most severe complication is erosion of the carotid artery. While the use of antibiotics has significantly lowered the mortality of internal jugular vein thrombosis, carotid arterial erosion still carries a 20% to 40% mortality rate. Some patients with this complication will die of acute exsanguination, but the majority asphyxiate. In order of frequency of involvement, the internal carotid artery is most frequently affected, then the external carotid artery, followed by the common carotid (12). An impending bleed may be signaled by various signs, including the onset of shock; a protracted clinical course; an ipsilateral Horner's syndrome (ptosis, meiosis, and anhydrosis); recurrent small hemorrhaging from the ear, nose, or mouth; hematoma in nearby tissues; unexplained neuropathies of cranial nerves IX to XII; and peritonsillar swelling after the abscess has resolved (see Table 4) (12).

The therapy is, again, control of the airway, antibiotics, and surgical drainage. In contradistinction to the submandibular DNI, in lateral pharyngeal DNI, the airway is less difficult to control. If tracheotomy is required, the midline landmarks are more easily identified than in a submandibular space infection. As anaerobes are found more frequently in lateral pharyngeal space infections, the addition of metronidazole or clindamycin to high-dose penicillin is advocated.

The method of surgical drainage of the lateral pharyngeal space varies, depending on the clinical situation. In the initial cellulitic phase, drainage is discouraged as it will not hasten resolution. Intraoral drainage is avoided as the carotid sheath may be difficult to control. In patients in whom vascular complications or mediastinal spread are unlikely, the submaxillary (Batson) approach is useful (see Fig. 3). Beginning three to four fingerbreadths (6–8 cm) below the auricle, an incision is made along the anterior border of the sternocleidomastoid muscle and is then carried horizontally to the midportion of the submandibular gland. After the anterior fascia is divided, a band of fascia connecting the parotid and submandibular glands is usually identified. Blunt dissection through this fascia under the angle of the mandible is performed in a mediosuperior direction to drain the lateral pharyngeal space. A Penrose drain is placed, and the incision is loosely reapproximated.

If there is concern about the integrity of the carotid artery, an anterior sternocleidomastoid (Mosher) approach (see Fig. 3) is employed. This incision begins at the same point as the submaxillary incision but continues along the anterior border of the sternocleidomastoid muscle. Of note, the head is left in the midline so that the sternocleidomastoid muscle does not cover the carotid sheath. After the carotid sheath is identified and opened, the common carotid artery is isolated with a vessel loop. Then, a submaxillary incision is made at the superior aspect of the vertical incision (see Fig. 3), extending horizontally to the anterior submandibular gland. The submandibular gland is elevated from inferior to anterior. The lateral space can then be entered and drained. If there is concern about the integrity of the carotid artery, the vessel loop can be left around the artery as a precaution while the infection resolves (2).

Retropharyngeal Space

The retropharyngeal lymphatic chains laying on either side of the midline raphe usually involute by age 5. Thus, infections in the retropharyngeal space are rare after this age due to suppurative lymphadenitis. The retropharyngeal space also can be infected by penetrating trauma, blunt trauma, instrumentation such as esophagoscopy, intubation, or passage of nasogastric tube, or from an extension of infection from other spaces. Most commonly, an extension can occur from the lateral pharyngeal space posteriorly to the retropharyngeal space or from anterior spread from the prevertebral space.

The diagnosis of a retropharyngeal space infection is difficult to make, especially in children in the early phase. Superior swelling may be not detected or may be mistaken for adenoidal inflammation or hypertrophy. Many children do not complain of a sore throat but may refuse to eat. If trismus is present, the possibility of extension to the lateral pharyngeal space should be considered, as this is an unusual finding in a process confined to the retropharyngeal space. There may be modest constitutional symptoms, including a low-grade fever. A "hot potato" voice can develop if swelling presents in the supraglottic region of the retropharynx. If the swelling occurs below the palate, a mass may be seen on the posterior pharyngeal wall on one side of the midline (see Fig. 5). Cervical adenopathy and nuchal rigidity may also occur. Significant respiratory distress is unusual if mediastinal extension does not occur (see Table 4). The review by Gianoli et al (13) suggests that trauma is an increasingly frequent cause of retropharyngeal space infection, which they noted occurred in an older population than previously reported.

As the retropharynx has communication with the anterior and posterior compartments of the superior mediastinum, extension to this region should be considered. The anterior mediastinum can be reached by extension via the pretracheal space. The posterior mediastinum can be accessed to the level of the tracheal bifurcation through the retropharyngeal space. Thus, complications of retropharyngeal space infection include pyopneumothorax, mediastinitis, purulent pericarditis, and bronchial erosion. If the abscess ruptures, it can precipitate aspiration, empyema, or pneumonia.

The mortality rate remains very high, approaching 50%, in patients developing mediastinitis (14). Sepsis is the usual cause of death. The mediastinum can be drained effectively via a cervical route early in the process; however, if the infection is advanced, thoracotomy is mandatory.

Transoral drainage and intravenous antibiotics will resolve most uncomplicated retropharyngeal infections, as the vascular sheath is not at risk. If the lateral space is involved, an external approach is required. For transoral drainage, the patient is positioned as for adenoidectomy. The initial localization of the abscess should be performed with needle aspiration to rule out the presence of blood and to confirm the presence of purulent material. If blood is encountered, the external approach should be performed. When pus is encountered, the cavity can be incised vertically and opened widely using blunt dissection.

PEARLS AND PERILS

---

1. Retropharyngeal DNI approach: transoral with initial needle aspiration.
2. If pus is found, continue transorally.
3. If blood is found, use the external approach for vascular control.

When an external approach is required, the incision is made along the anterior sternocleidomastoid muscle (see Fig. 3). This incision is made from the level of the hyoid to the cricoid. If there is inferior dissection, the neck incision can be extended to the clavicle. Adequate transcervical drainage usually can be obtained to the level of the fourth thoracic vertebra. The anterior border of the sternocleidomastoid muscle is identified and lateralized. The carotid sheath is identified and medialized. Following the prevertebral fascia with medial retraction of the larynx, trachea, and thyroid, the abscess cavity is opened and drained.

Prevertebral Space Infection

Classically, infection of this space is attributed to tuberculosis involving a vertebral body, known as Pott's abscess. Other etiologies include trauma, surgery, anterior extension of osteomyelitis, and posterior extension from a retropharyngeal space infection.

The presentation of a prevertebral space infection is nonspecific (see Table 4). Many patients have only minimal complaints such as neck or shoulder pain. Other symptoms include dysphagia and less commonly, respiratory compromise.

On physical examination, a midline bulge of the posterior pharynx may be visible. Complications include extension into the danger or retropharyngeal space, with the complications discussed previously. As well, neurologic sequelae can ensue following destruction of vertebral bodies, precipitating subluxation or epidural compression. The antibiotic therapy is directed toward *Staphylococcus aureus*, the usual organism. If the infection is refractory to the usual antibiotics, treatment for *Mycobacterium* infection should be considered.

If respiratory compromise is feared, the airway must be secured, with tracheotomy remaining the gold standard. Surgical drainage is dependent on the location of the infection. Prevertebral space infections from C-1 to C-3 can be approached transorally in a manner similar to the retropharyngeal abscess drainage. The limiting factor may be the ability to achieve adequate removal of bone. Externally, two approaches are used: an incision anterior to the sternocleidomastoid muscle or an incision posterior to the sternocleidomastoid muscle (see Fig. 3). The dissection proceeds to the prevertebral fascia, permitting drainage through the prevertebral and alar fascia.

CONCLUSIONS

With knowledge of the anatomy of the fascial planes and spaces, DNIs can be evaluated in a systematic manner. Initially, the airway must be evaluated, and if threatened, secured with intubation or tracheostomy. The history, physical examination, and imaging will usually determine if DNI is present. Initial management is performed with intravenous antibiotics. If there is no improvement or if there is deterioration, surgical drainage of the involved space or spaces is indicated.

ACKNOWLEDGMENT

Thanks to my secretary, Susan Whelton, for her assistance in the lengthy preparation of this chapter.

REFERENCES

1. Marra S, Hotaling AJ. *Am J Ootolayngol* 1996;17:287–298.
2. Brown DF, Richstmeier WJ. *Infections of the deep fascial spaces of the head and neck.* Continuing education program, American Academy of Otolaryngology—Head and Neck Surgery Foundation, Washington, DC, 1987.
3. Mosher HP. *Trans Am Acad Ophthalmol Otolayngol* 1929;34:19–36.
4. Blomquist IK, Bayer AS. *Infect Dis Clin North Am* 1988;2:737–764.
5. Tom MB, Rice DH. *Laryngoscope* 1988;98:877–880.
6. Tami TA, Parker GS. *Arch Otolaryngol* 1984;110:752–754.
7. Beck AL. Ann Otol Rhinol Laryngol 1952;61:515v532.
8. Patterson HC, Kelly JH Stroone M. *Laryngoscope* 1982;92:370–377.
9. Yau PC, Norante JD. *Arch Otolaryngol* 1980;106:507–508.
10. Lemierre A. *Lancet* 1936;2:701–703.
11. Salinger S, Pearlman SJ. *Arch Otolayngol* 1933;18:464–509.
12. Blum DJ, McCaffrey TV. *Otolaryngol Head Neck Surg* 1983;91(2):114–118.
13. Gianoli GJ.Espinola TE, Guarisco, JL, et al. *Otolaryngol Head Neck Surg* 1993;105:92–100.
14. Estera AS, Landay MJ, Grisham JM, et al. *Surg Gynecol Obstet* 1983;157:545–552.

A.J. Hotaling: Departments of Otolaryngology—Head and Neck Surgery and Pediatrics, Loyola University Medical Center, Maywood, Illinois 60153–3304.

- *Practical Pediatric Otolaryngology*
- edited by Robin T. Cotton and Charles M. Myer, III
- Lippincott-Raven Publishers, Philadelphia © 1999

Section Editor
Peter J. Koltai

Craniofacial Skeletal Trauma in Childhood

Peter J. Koltai

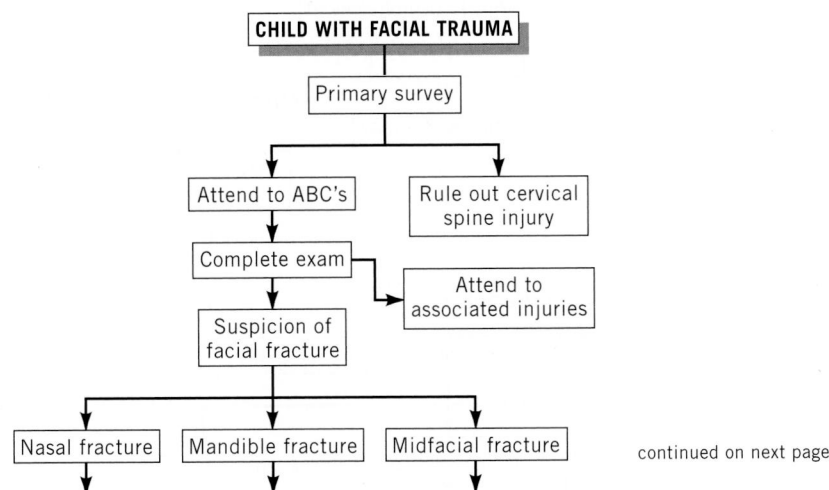

continued on next page

continued

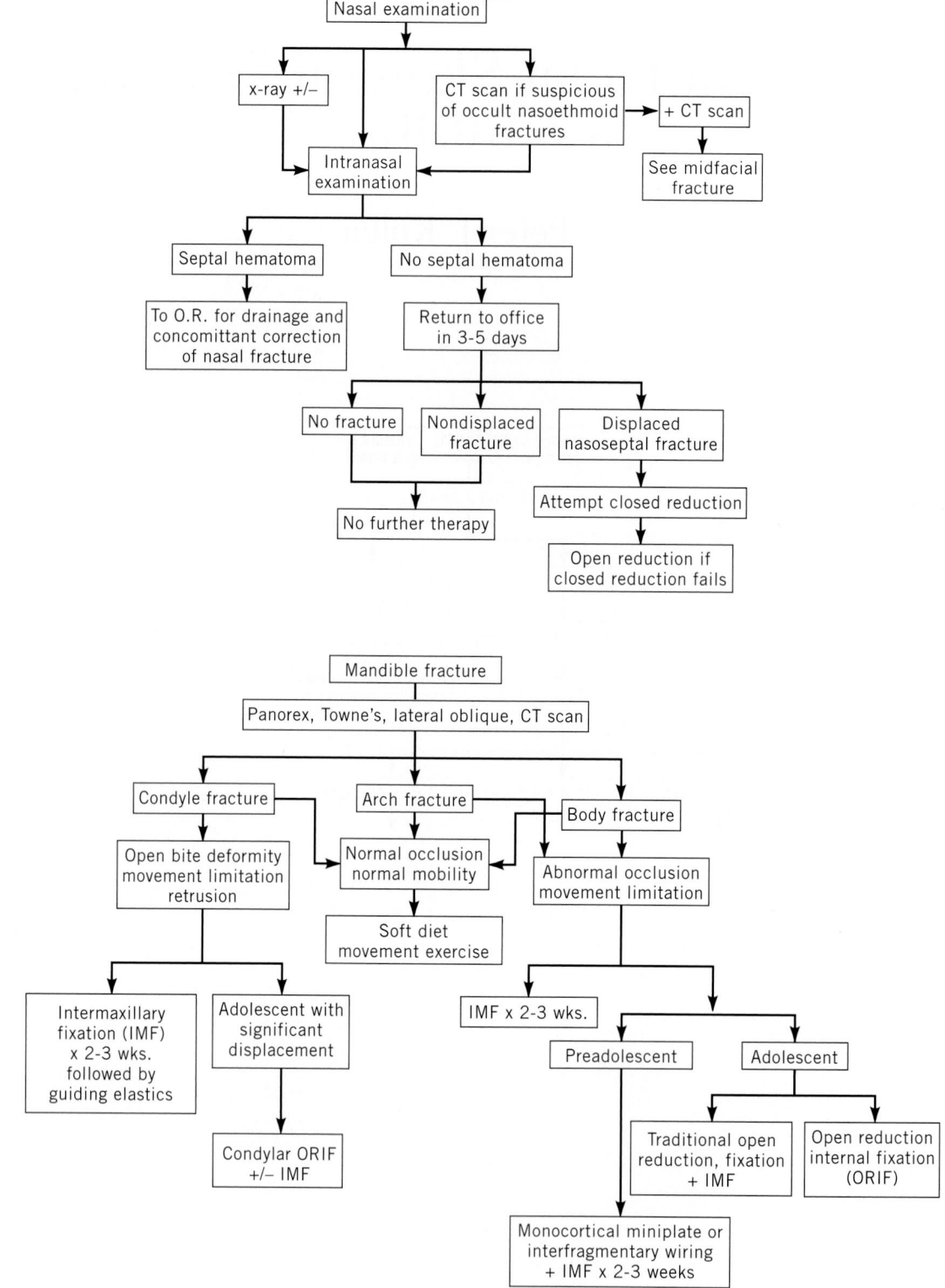

continued on next page

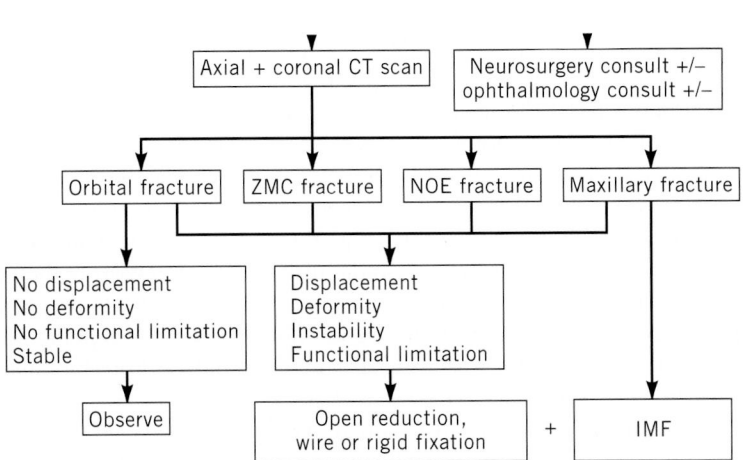

OVERVIEW

The leading cause of death among children is trauma; nearly 15,000 children die each year, 100,000 are permanently disabled, and $15 billion is spent on this epidemic of childhood injuries. Despite this appallingly high incidence of pediatric injuries, serious facial fractures in children are relatively rare. When they occur, correct treatment requires an understanding that there are differences between the facial skeleton of a child and that of an adult, and that the reconstructive techniques used in appropriate management must be modified to account for the potential of deformity as a consequence of change in facial growth resulting from the trauma.

Over the past 15 years the use of rigid fixation via camouflaged extended exposures has become a practical reality for adult maxillofacial trauma victims; however, its utility in children is not as obvious (1–5). Unresolved questions remain about the effects of metal plates and screws on the growing face, and there is concern that wide soft tissue exposure may alter the growth of bone (6). The paradox in the treatment of severe pediatric facial fractures is that reconstructing the normal three-dimensional proportions, a goal that offers the best prospect for normal facial appearance, function, and development, is best accomplished by techniques that may adversely effect growth. While this dilemma cannot be completely resolved, a rational approach to treatment that yields satisfactory results can be formulated from a careful reading of the experimental and clinical literature. This chapter presents an overview of the author's experience in the elective use of both traditional and contemporary techniques in the management of pediatric facial trauma.

VITAL STATISTICS

Pediatric facial fractures accounted for 9% of all maxillofacial injuries at the author's Institution over a 5-year period (6). However, the incidence has been reported to be as low as 1.5% and as high as 15%. Under the age of 5, children have an even lower risk, somewhere around 1% (6–16). The author has not seen much variation among the different age groups, but has found that adolescents are more likely to have severe injuries that require more complex reconstruction. Pediatric facial fractures are fairly consistent among boys and girls, and this may reflect the high frequency of motor vehicle passenger accidents, a mechanism of injury that tends to be gender neutral (8).

Nasal fractures are probably the most common facial fracture in children; however, because these are often treated in an office setting, exact statistics about their frequency are difficult to come by (9). Mandible fractures are the most common facial injuries that require hospitalization and account for one-third to one-half of facial injuries (6). The condyle tends to be the most vulnerable part of the child's mandible and accounts for more than half of all mandible fractures (12–14). This is especially true for younger children in that there is an increased incidence of symphyseal, body, and ramus fractures in adolescents. Tooth avulsions and dentoalveolar fractures are often treated in a dental setting and as a result it is difficult to gauge their frequency. Mid and upper facial injuries in children are rare, and their sporadic distribution emphasizes their uniqueness and highlights the limited experience one surgeon may have with these more complicated injuries. Orbital fractures reportedly account for 20% to 25% of pediatric fractures; zygomaticomalar complex fractures, for 10% to 15%; and Le Fort–type maxillary fractures, for 5% to 10% (6–11).

Pediatric facial fractures have a high incidence of associated injury. In the author's series, 30% of children with facial fractures sustained associated neurocranial and orthopedic injuries (6). Intracerebral trauma, often associated with a concurrent skull fracture, is particularly problematic and the incidence has been reported as high as 60%, especially among younger children (8). Such a high incidence emphasizes the necessity of a complete and systematic assessment of the child with facial trauma and may complicate timing of the reconstruction, in that bone healing may begin before the child is medically ready for surgical correction.

The developmentally specific anatomy of the child's face, and the type of force that results in injury, are the two main considerations in understanding the etiology of pediatric facial fractures. Living in protected environments, children have a reduced risk of major injuries. The forces children are subject to during child's play are not generally sufficient to cause serious damage; nevertheless, by sheer numbers childhood play is the most frequent cause of pediatric facial fractures. On the other hand, the primary etiology of serious pediatric facial fractures is motor vehicle accidents.

An appreciation of facial development is also helpful in understanding the differences between pediatric and adult facial fractures. This fact is highlighted by a recent study of 40 children with orbital fractures (16). Orbital roof fractures were significantly more likely to occur among younger children, were associated with a high incidence of neurocranial injury, and rarely required surgical reconstruction. Lower orbital fractures occurred generally after the age of 7, were not usually associated with cranial injuries, and frequently required surgical reconstruction. The age distribution of roof fractures, a type of skull fracture, was thought to reflect the greater craniofacial ratio of the young child, the vulnerability of the large cranium to trauma, and the lack of pneumatization of the frontal sinus. On the other hand, the age distribution of lower orbital fractures, which are types of facial fractures, was interpreted to reflect the growth and development of an area of the face that unfolds from beneath the overhanging cranium and becomes more vulnerable to trauma. The pneumatization of the paranasal sinuses appeared to determine paths along which the impacting force was dissipated, resulting in the pattern of orbital fractures that was observed.

There are other characteristics that render the face of a young child less prone toward facial injuries. These include the thick layers of muscle and fat that cover a more elastic softer bone, buttressed by unerupted teeth and unweakened by the development of the paranasal sinuses. A greater proportion of cancellous bone and thinner cortical plates accounts for the higher incidence of greenstick fractures in children.

PATIENT ASSESSMENT

In the initial assessment of a child with facial fractures, the basic principles of trauma management should be followed. An immediate evaluation needs to be made of the airway, breathing, and circulation; the ABCs. The type and severity of the injury will define the options available for managing the airway. Where the injury is limited to the maxillofacial skeleton, careful posturing of the child is usually adequate. Gentle suctioning of the oral cavity to remove secretions, blood, or sometimes loose teeth and bone fragments is a simple additional measure. A midline traction suture may be needed to prevent retrodisplacement of the tongue, which is seen with some types of mandible fractures.

Orotracheal intubation should be performed when positioning is inadequate to maintain the airway, or when there is concomitant neurologic injury, significant bleeding, or airway obstruction associated with fracture. Radiologic evaluation of the cervical region of the spine is mandatory, and manipulation of the neck during orotracheal intubation should be avoided unless cervical spine injury has been ruled out.

Cricothyrotomy or crash tracheotomy is almost never warranted; however, a controlled tracheotomy in the operating room is often necessary for severe panfacial fractures or when there are fractures with associated injuries. Severe hemorrhage associated with the facial injury is a double threat resulting in hypovolemic shock as well as risk to the airway. The airway can be secured by intubation and volume expansion will require intravenous administration of crystalloid solution. On occasion, transfusion with type-specific red blood cells may be necessary.

An orderly head and neck examination must be made after the primary survey has been completed and the ABCs have been attended to. This includes neurologic evaluation, examination of the neck and cervical region of the spine, and inspection of the eyes, ears, nose, and oral cavity. Ophthalmologic assessment is necessary to rule out intraocular trauma, evaluate ocular motility, and check pupillary reflexes. Otologic examination will reveal anterior canal wall injuries from condylar fractures. Anterior rhinoscopy will reveal potential septal injuries, septal hematoma, and even cerebrospinal fluid (CSF) rhinorrhea.

The face is examined visually and manually. Edema, ecchymosis, periorbital swelling, facial asymmetry, trismus, and malocclusion are all highly indicative of underlying fractures. Areas of tenderness and crepitations are highlighted by manual examination. Midfacial mobility is assessed by grasping the upper incisors and rocking the premaxilla, while the head is being held steady by the opposite hand. The maxillary buttresses are palpated intraorally for irregularities, and the gingivolabial sulcus can be inspected for the presence of ecchymosis. The temporomandibular joints are palpated intraorally and examined externally by placing fingers in the external auditory canal. Fractures of the mandibular arch will also be revealed by intraoral digital examination.

Computed Tomography (CT) greatly facilitates the imaging of facial fractures in both adults and children (1,9). Axial CT is useful for orbital and maxillary fractures. Much useful information can be obtained from coronal projections; however, these can be difficult to obtain in an injured or uncooperative child. With complex fractures, both projections will be necessary to precisely define the full extent of the fractures. Three-dimensional reconstructions are a useful adjunct to two-dimensional CT for surgical planning (17). Axial CT scans can also be helpful with mandible fractures; however, the most useful x-ray study is the panoramic view, which demonstrates the entire jaw. This study requires a cooperative patient, which is not always possible with a child, and alternative views may be required for documentation of the injuries. A Towne's view, which is an anteroposterior projection, is specific for the condyle, while the lateral oblique projection is useful for the ramus, angle, and body. X-ray films of nasal fractures are inevitably obtained in the emergency department when there is a question of injury. The author generally has found these of little utility, and prefers digital palpation and visual inspection as the primary diagnostic tool. It is, however, worth noting that significant nasal fractures, which result in flattening of the nasal dorsum, warrant proper imaging with CT to rule out an occult nasoethmoid injury.

⬤ TREATMENT RECOMMENDATIONS

Rigid Fixation and Facial Growth

The characteristics that distinguish a child's face from that of an adult result from the combined process of growth and remodeling. Adult deformities as a consequence of childhood trauma are due to the alteration of proportional growth attributable to the injury; however, they are not inevitable. A review of the many reports that tried to determine the consequence of early fractures on growth of the face is beyond the scope of this chapter (18–21). Nevertheless, several basic insights are readily understood. Injuries that adversely affect the future growth of the face typically occur at specific, vulnerable locations such as the multiple suture sites of the midface, the nasal septum, and the head of the condyle. Posttraumatic development is also affected by functional factors such as the constant motion of the mandible, which results in a dynamic adaptation of the bone and soft tissues and thus the mandible is less vulnerable to traumatic deformity than is the midface.

The use of rigid plate fixation is controversial for younger children because its use may have negative impact on facial growth. The concern is that transient skeletal stabilization will result in permanent growth retardation. Numerous animal studies showed that miniplate fixation across the suture lines results in significant growth reduction across the plated sutures and adjacent bones (22). It is difficult to draw any firm conclusions from these animal studies about the use of plate and screw fixation following trauma in young children, except that it should be done with caution and reserved for fractures where the original features are difficult to restore by other means. The alternative of no correction is unacceptable because the soft tissue will shrink and contract to mirror the abnormal skeletal infrastructure, and interfragmentary wiring can yield an unstable reconstruction and still result in growth retardation. Based on the information available in the literature, as well as the author's own experience, there is currently no good alternative to rigid fixation for certain complex fractures. In view of the questions about the potential for growth restrictions from the implants, consideration for removal is valid, but must be weighted against the additional injury to the facial soft tissues required by their removal. The prospect of restorable plates and screws is fortunate and may placate much concern.

Surgical Approaches

Most pediatric facial fractures, such as zygomatic arch fractures, nasal fractures, and even condylar fractures, can be easily treated by manual manipulation or with limited open techniques. However, when there is need for extensive reconstruction due to severe injuries, hidden extended incisions for complete exposure are most useful (3, 23). The upper third of the face, including the zygoma, orbital rims, and the nasoethmoid region, can be exposed through a coronal incision. The infraorbital rim and floor can be exposed by a subciliary or transconjunctival incision. The anterior buttresses of the maxilla can be exposed by an upper gingivolabial sulcus incision. This incision can be extended into a midfacial degloving to reach the nasoethmoid area. The mandibular arch can be exposed through a lower gingivolabial sulcus incision, although comminuted mandible fractures, as well as angle and ramus fractures, are probably best exposed through an external approach.

The coronal incision begins with the preauricular crease above the tragus and traverses across the cranium to the opposite side, camouflaged in the hairline (Fig. 1). The incision should be made with a scalpel to prevent hair loss, while the bleeding is controlled with Raney clips. The incision is made to the depth of the calvarial periosteum and temporal fascia and the flap is elevated superficially to the periosteum and fascia until approximately 2 cm above the supraorbital rims (Fig. 2). At this point the periosteum is incised and the dissection carried forward between the periosteum and the bone. The

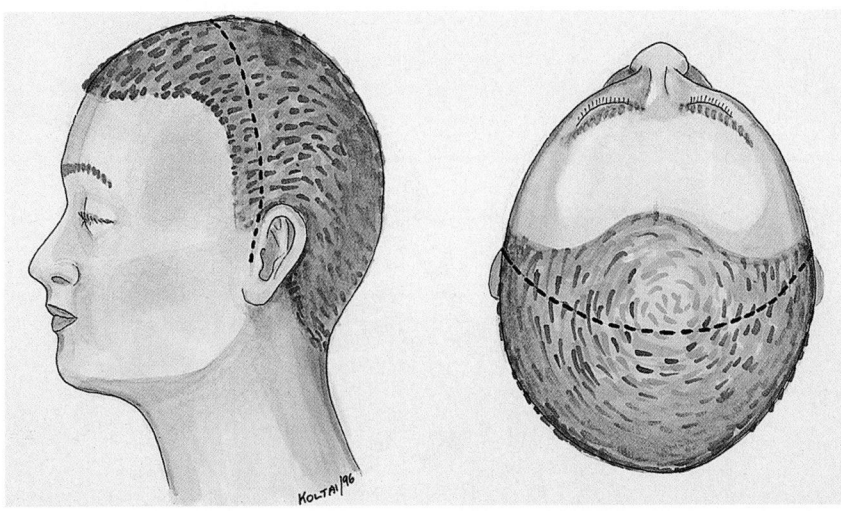

FIGURE 1 The incision line for bicoronal exposure. It begins in the preauricular crease above the tragus and enters the hairline above the attachment of the auricular helix, where it can be stepped posteriorly. The line traverses the cranium, and is kept 4 to 6 cm behind the hairline.

temporal fascia is incised laterally above the temporal fat pad, and the elevation is continued between the fascia and the fat pad in order to protect the frontal branch of the facial nerve (Fig. 3). Dissecting in the subperiosteal plane, the entire superior part of the orbit, the zygomatic arches, and the medial canthal ligaments can be accessed (Fig. 4).

A subciliary or transconjunctival incision will facilitate exposure of the lower half of the orbit. The subciliary incision is made approximately 1 mm below the lashes of the lower eyelid through the skin and the orbicular muscle to the orbital septum. The dissection then follows the orbital septum down to the orbital rim where the periosteum is incised and the floor exposed, yielding excellent access to the medial part of the orbit, as well as to the floor and lateral orbital wall.

The transconjunctival incision has similar utility; however, when it is done in conjunction with a lateral canthotomy, it provides greater exposure of the lateral orbital rim (Fig. 5). Several variations of the transconjunctival dissection exist; however, the author prefers the approach posterior to the orbital septum. While this results in exposure of the orbital fat, the approach is more rapid and is less likely to cause problems with the eyelid postoperatively (Figs. 6 and 7).

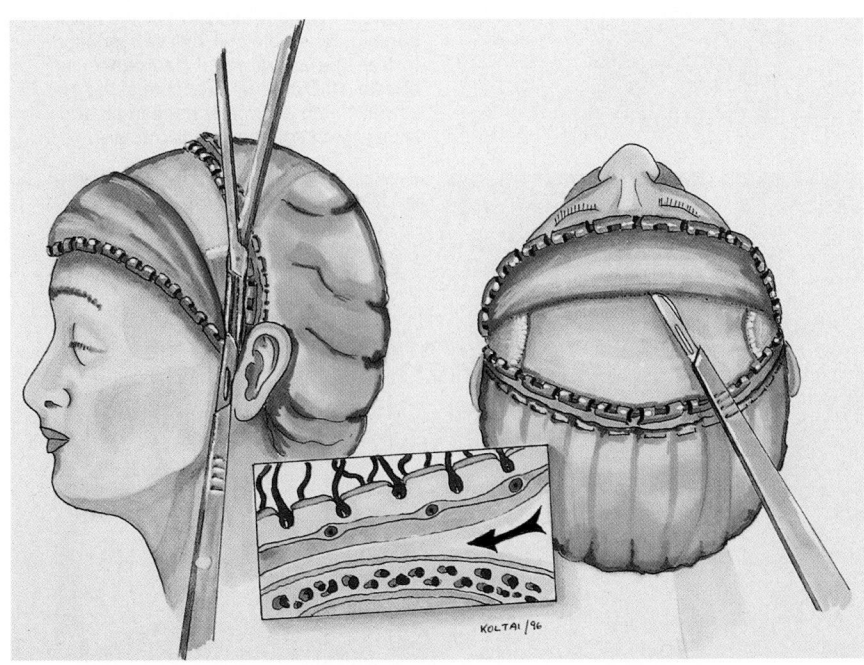

FIGURE 2 The incision is made to the depth of the calvarial periosteum across the cranium, and to the depth of the temporal fascia laterally. The flap is elevated with a knife or by blunt finger dissection in the subgaleal plane (**inset**). Over the temporal muscle blunt dissection with a hemostat or scissors is utilized between the fascia and the scalp. The scalp is then incised over the instrument to prevent penetration of the temporal fascia, which will result in bleeding.

FIGURE 3 The subgaleal elevation ends 2 cm above the supraorbital rim, where the calvarial periosteum is incised and the dissection is carried forward between the periosteum and the bone. Laterally, the temporal fat pad can be seen under the temporal fascia, which at this point is incised, and the dissection is bluntly carried forward between the fascia and the fat pad. This deeper dissection protects the frontal branch of the facial nerve, which lies superficially in the layer continuous with the temporoparietal fascia (**inset**).

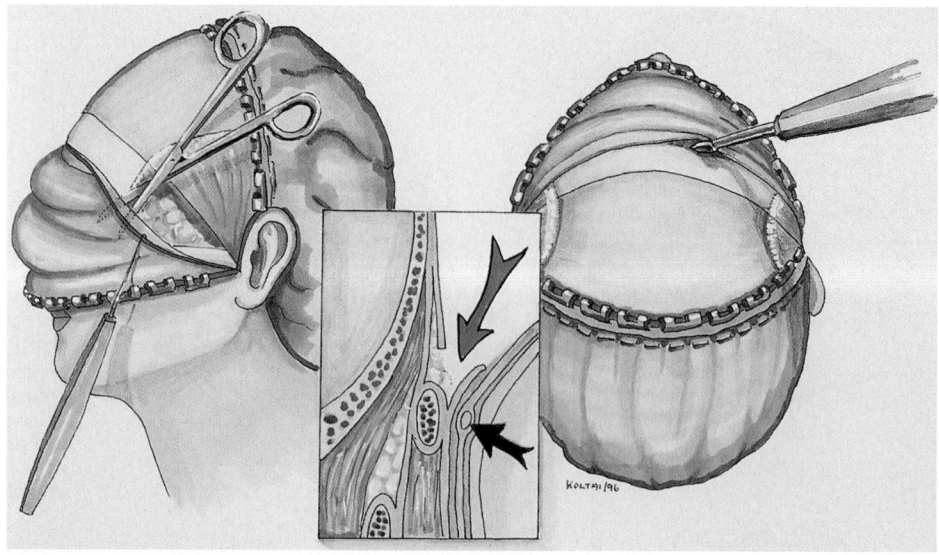

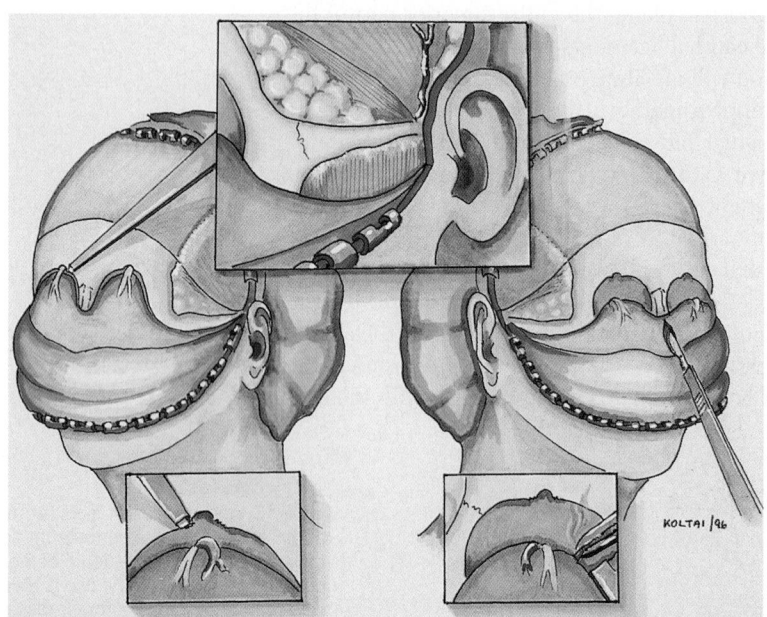

FIGURE 4 A: The incision through the temporal fascia begins at the root of the zygomatic arch. The superior surface of the zygoma and the malar bone is exposed by sharp dissection of the periosteum (**upper inset**). The supraorbital neurovascular bundle is released from its foramen by chiseling away the bone on either side of its inferior aspect (**left inset**). The medial region of the orbit is exposed with blunt elevation and the anterior ethmoidal neurovascular bundle, if still intact, is divided after bipolar cauterization (**right inset**). A relaxing incision of the periosteum over the nasal dorsum allows for greater exposure of the lower dorsum. **B:** An otologic drill can be used to free the supraorbital neurovascular bundle. **C:** Bicoronal exposure of the zygomatic arch and malar bone in an adolescent with right Le Fort III fracture.

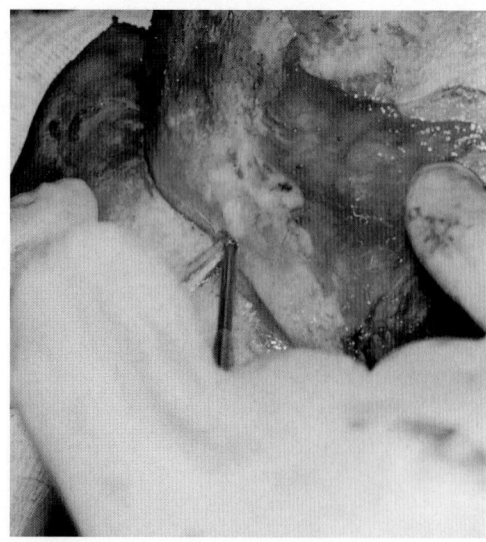

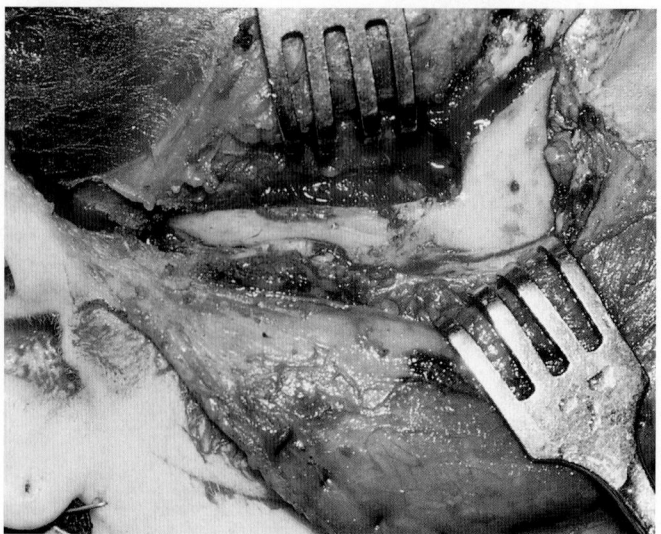

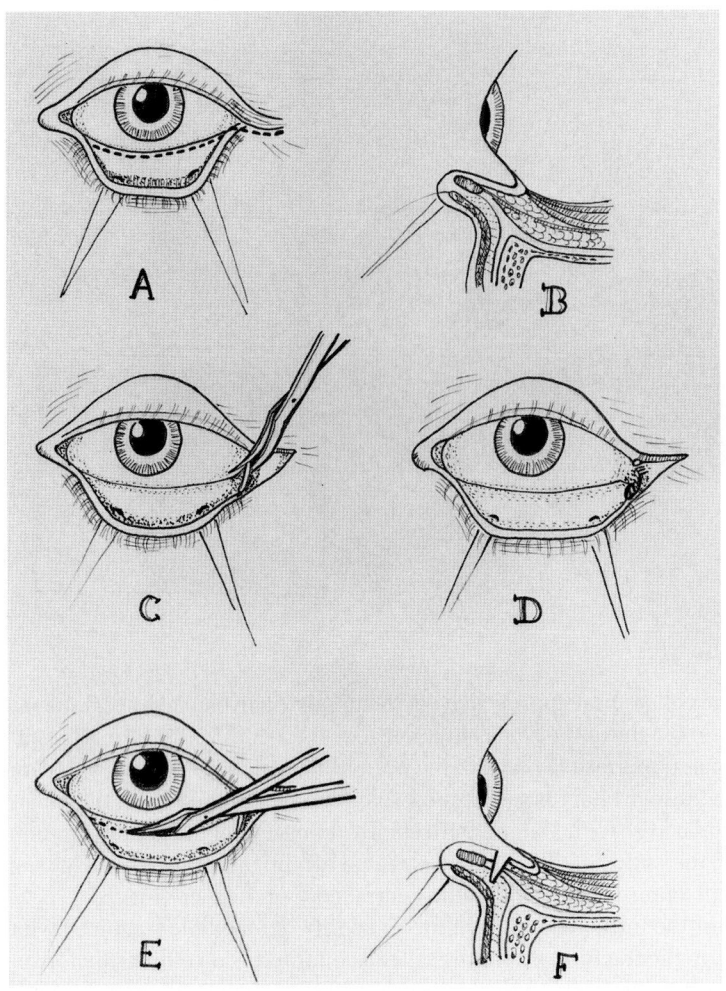

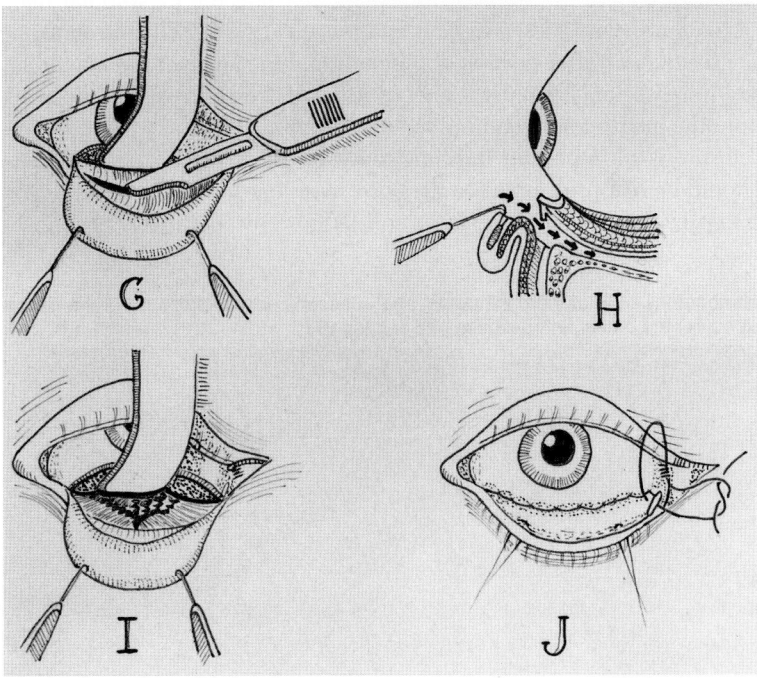

FIGURE 5 **A–F:** The transconjunctival incision begins with traction sutures in the lower lid. Scissors are used to make the lateral cantholysis (see Fig. 6). Through the lateral canthopexy, scissors are introduced in the subconjunctival plane and blunt dissection is carried out inferior to the tarsal plate, and medially to but not past the lacrimal punctum. The conjunctiva is then incised below the tarsal plate (**E**). Two routes are now possible. By incision of the orbital septum, the dissection can be made preseptally, just behind the orbicular muscle (**F**). The dissection can also be carried out behind the orbital septum, anterior to the postseptal fat pad. **G–J:** The periosteum on the orbital rim is exposed and incised, allowing access to the floor. The closure involves a continuous running 6-0 chromic suture of the conjunctiva. The canthopexy is repaired with 5-0 Polydioxanone (PDS) or Polyglactin (Vicryl) suture (From Koltai PJ. The management of facial fractures in the pediatric age group. *Adv Otolaryngol Head Neck Surg*, 1996;10:1375–1379, with permission.)

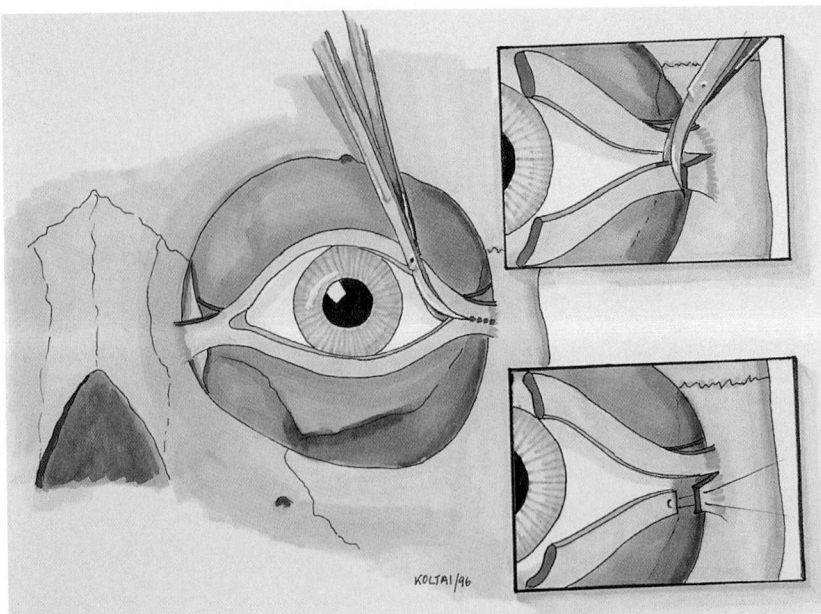

FIGURE 6 Detail of the lateral canthopexy. The lateral canthal tendon is divided horizontally into an inferior and superior limb with scissors. The inferior limb is then released with a vertical scissor cut (**upper inset**). The cut inferior limb of the lateral canthal tendon is closed with a 5-0 PDS or Vicryl suture. Some surgeons do not reanastomose the tendon and rely on it to heal on its own.

The body of the maxilla is best approached via the upper gingivolabial buccal sulcus, with the incision a little bit above the sulcus in order to leave a cuff for closure. The soft tissues are elevated in a subperiosteal plane to the infraorbital rim and zygoma, with care taken not to injure the infraorbital nerve. The masseter can be stripped from the malar prominence to give full access to the lateral buttress. By doing a circumferential incision in the nasal vestibule, the entire midface can be elevated off the underlying bone, giving total exposure from the outer facial frame to the central core of the face (Fig. 8).

The author prefers the intraoral approach for a majority of mandible fractures, with the incision centered on the fracture, extending several centimeters on either side for access. A 3-mm cuff of soft tissue is left on the labial side of the gingivolabial sulcus for later closure. The elevation is done in the subperiosteal plane down to the mandibular margin. It is important to identify and preserve the inferior alveolar nerve. The intraoral approach can be done for the posterior portion of the body and the angle of the mandible; however, this will require working though the cheek, utilizing sleeves to protect the overlying soft tissue from the instruments required for rigid fixation (Fig. 9).

Appropriate closure is an important finishing touch to craniofacial exposures (24). The periosteum should be reapproximated to the corresponding section of the underlying bone in order to prevent sagging of the facial soft tissues postoperatively. An exam-

FIGURE 7 Clinical photographs of a lateral canthopexy and transconjunctival exposure of the orbital floor (**A**). After full exposure, the orbital rim has been microplated (**B**).

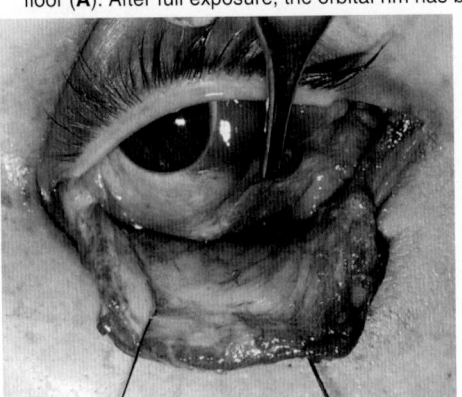

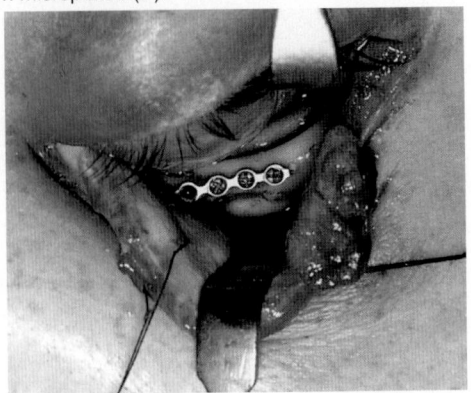

A   B

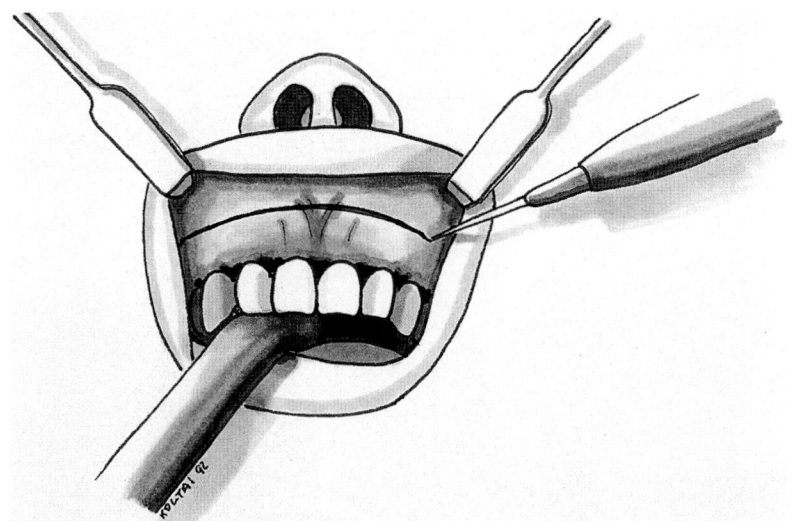

A

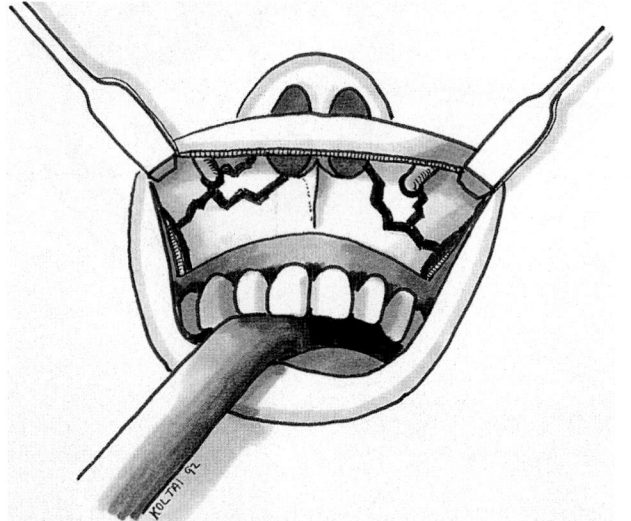

B

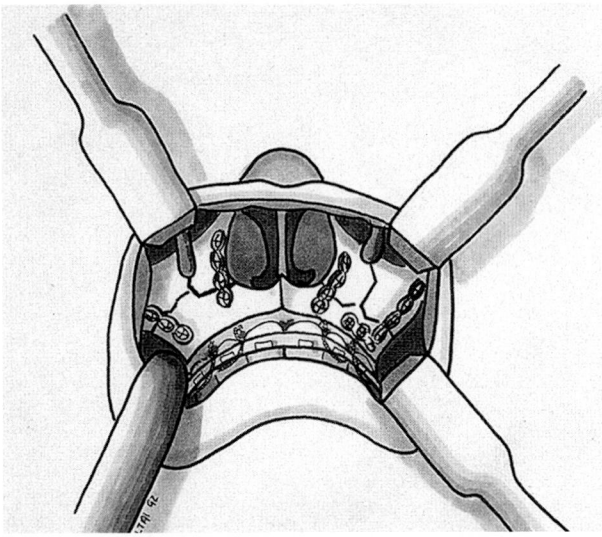

C

FIGURE 8 **A:** The gingivolabial sulcus incision is made with a cautery, with a 3 mm cuff of tissue on the labial side left for closure. **B:** The fractures of the anterior and lateral buttresses have been exposed. In a child, the infraorbital nerve is low, since the vertical growth of the maxilla is incomplete. **C:** The buttresses have been reduced and plated. (From Koltai PJ. The management of facial fractures in the pediatric age group. *Adv Otolaryngol Head Neck Surg*, 1996;10:, with permission.)

ple of this would be the resuspension of the anterior face from the infraorbital rims, and the suturing of the temporal fascia to the periosteum of the zygomatic arch.

Nasal Fractures

A child's nasal architecture differs significantly from that of an adult. Soft compliant cartilage is the primary projecting tissue of a child's nose, and this will easily bend from the force of a blow; thus the energy is dissipated across the soft tissues of the face and the maxillary buttresses. This results in edema over the central portion of the midface with loss of anatomic specificity. The tip cartilages usually do not sustain permanent injury except perhaps for dislocations from the bony framework. On the other hand, the more rigid septum, which is surrounded by bone and has a tight perichondrial cover, is more likely to be fractured.

Septal trauma takes several forms. The septal perichondrium can detach from the cartilage when it is deformed during injury, with bleeding from the internal lining of the perichondrium resulting in a septal hematoma. The septum can also be avulsed from its bony attachments to the vomer, the perpendicular plate of the ethmoid, and the maxillary crest, resulting in immediate nasal obstruction and possibly long-term hypertrophic growth disturbances (25,26). The caudal border of the septum is prone toward stellate

FIGURE 9 A: Gingivolabial sulcus incision for the intraoral approach to parasymphyseal fractures of the mandible. **B:** Intraoral exposure of the fracture. **C:** Wire osteosynthesis of the fracture. (From Koltai PJ. The management of facial fractures in the pediatric age group. *Adv Otolaryngol Head Neck Surg* 1996;10: 135, with permission.)

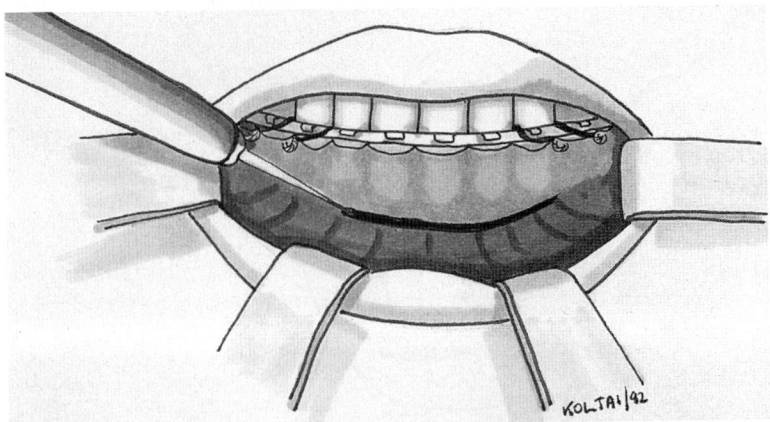

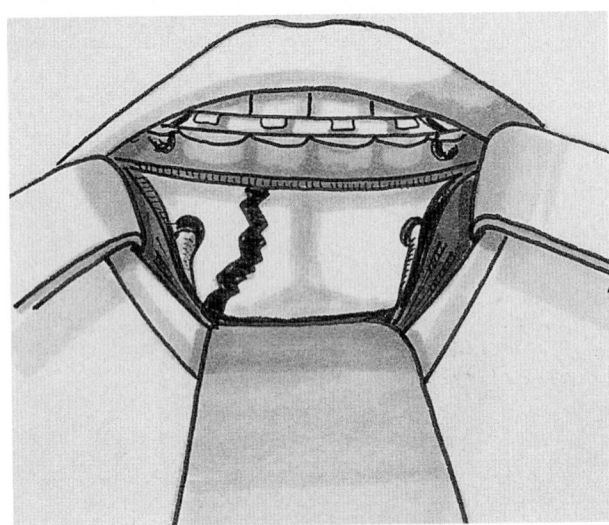

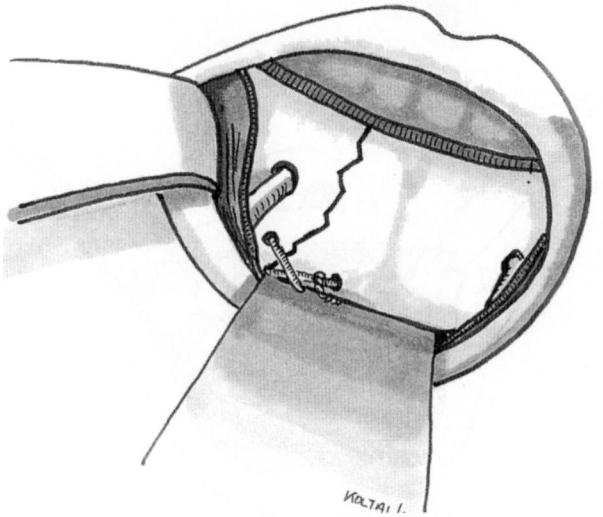

and vertical fractures of the cartilage, resulting in nasal obstruction, as well as delayed growth disturbances with twisting deformities.

The nasal bones of the very young children are not frequently broken because of their minimal projection; however, when they occur, these typically are greenstick-type injuries. Midline injuries can result in open book–type fractures resulting in a central depression and lateral flaring of the nasal bones. Occult orbital and nasoethmoid fractures should always be suspected when there appears to be significant nasal injuries.

The initial examination of a child with a nasal fracture may be of limited value because of the edema that tends to occur over the entire midface. It is difficult to differentiate between soft tissue swelling only and a modestly displaced fracture. Several days are required for the swelling to go down before one can appreciate the full extent of the deformity. Yet the initial evaluation is important with regard to the presence of septal injury, especially septal hematoma. It is the child who has difficulty breathing through the nose after injury who should arouse the greatest suspicion of septal hematoma, observed as a purple bulge usually confined to one side of the nose. The hematoma is generally compressible with cotton pledget; however, it will not vasoconstrict with oxymetazoline or phenylephrine (Neo-Synephrine).

In young children the treatment of a septal hematoma will require a general anesthetic. The hematoma should be evacuated through an ipsilateral hemitransfixion incision and the rest of the septum should be examined for other fractures. The septal leaflets can be reapproximated to the cartilage utilizing a through-and-through mattress 4-0 chromic suture on a mini-Keith needle. Silastic splints will further support the septum and are held in place with a through-and-through nylon suture. The author generally also packs the nose with an antibiotic-impregnated gauze for 2 to 3 days while the child is maintained on broad-spectrum antibiotics. While the child is under anesthesia for treatment of the septum, the rest of the nose needs to be evaluated as well.

In most cases there is no septal hematoma and the child is asked to be brought back 3 to 4 days after the injury, so that a more accurate assessment of the nose can be made. Demonstrable bony or septal fractures resulting in an external deformity or a fixed obstruction require definitive management. Closed reduction is generally adequate for most bony fractures, and is performed with intranasal instrumentation and bimanual external manipulation. Open reduction may be necessary if there are significant dislocations or if the injury is older than 2 weeks. Occasionally with greenstick fractures, a completion osteotomy may be necessary to properly reduce the fragments. If the fragments are unstable and the reduction cannot be maintained, intranasal packing is used to support the repair. Externally the reconstruction is supported with a cast of thermoplastic (Aquaplast) applied over Steri-Strips.

It has been the author's experience that the septum is more difficult to reconstruct, especially by closed techniques, and subperichondrial exposure of the broken cartilages may be necessary to properly realign the fragments. Resection should be avoided in view of the potential consequence of growth retardation at this critical site.

PEARLS AND PERILS

1. Septal hematoma will not vasoconstrict with oxymetazoline (Afrin).
2. Reexamine in 3 to 4 days for accurate assessment of deformity.
3. Immediate nasal obstruction suggests septal hematoma.
4. Use mattress suture to reapproximate septal leaflets.
5. Closed reduction should be within 10 days of fracture.
6. Greenstick fractures can be hard to reduce and may need completion osteotomies.
7. Do not overread nasal bone x-ray films.
8. Do not overlook occult nasoethmoid fracture.
9. When in doubt, obtain computed tomography scans.
10. Do not resect displaced septal cartilage—open, realign, and splint with Silastic.

Mandible Fractures

The management of pediatric mandible fractures differs significantly from that of adults due to developing dentition and the future growth of the mandible. Prior to the age of 2, the deciduous teeth are incompletely erupted, and it is difficult to achieve adequate immobilization. However, the imperfect alignment achieved with an acrylic splint will usually be compensated for by later growth. Between the ages of 2 and 5 the primary teeth have firm roots that can be utilized for cap splints and arch bars. Reabsorption of the deciduous roots between the ages of 6 and 12 years will require arch bars to have additional support from suspension wires from the piriform aperture and around the mandible. The permanent teeth, generally in place after the age of 13 years, are excellent supports for the fixation of arch bars. The condyle is the most common site of mandible fractures in children, and there are three anatomic variants. Intracapsular crush fractures of the condylar head are the least common and pose the greatest threat to normal function of the mandible. High condylar fractures through the neck above the sigmoid notch are also uncommon, but are not associated with a bad prognosis. The third type, which is the most common, is a low subcondylar fracture often of a greenstick variety (Fig. 10). Numerous clinical and experimental reports advocated a conservative approach to the management

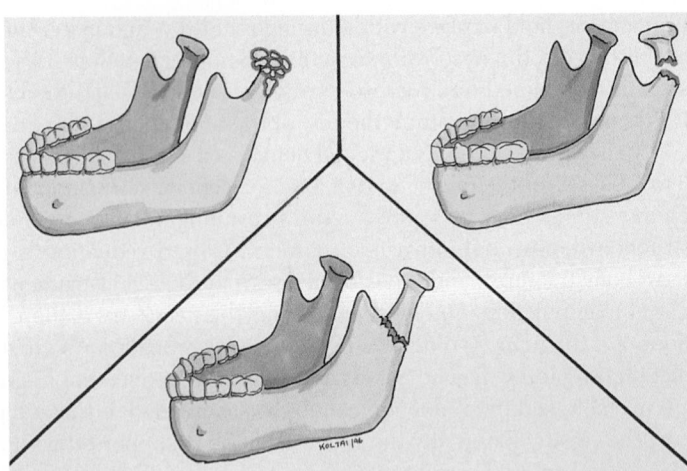

FIGURE 10 Three types of condylar fractures in children: crush injuries of the condylar head, high condylar fractures of the neck, and low subcondylar fractures.

of most condylar fractures in children (6,9,12–15). The primary decision in management is generally not whether to open the fracture, but whether the child needs immobilization.

Unilateral and occasional bilateral condylar fractures will present with normal occlusion and normal jaw mobility. A soft diet and movement exercises are all that are usually necessary for these types of injuries (Fig. 11). On the other hand, if there are movement limitations along with an open bite deformity and retrusion of the mandible, then immobilization for 2 to 3 weeks with intermaxillary fixation, followed by the use of guiding elastics, yields excellent results. The author generally considers an open reduction of a condylar fracture only in adolescents who have sustained substantial loss of vertical height of the mandible or have significant dislocation of the condylar head.

FIGURE 11 **A:** High condylar fracture in a 5-year-old child. Note the comminution of the condylar neck. **B:** Same child 6 months later. Treatment consisted of a soft diet and symptomatic analgesia. Note remodeling of the condyle into a normal anatomic position.

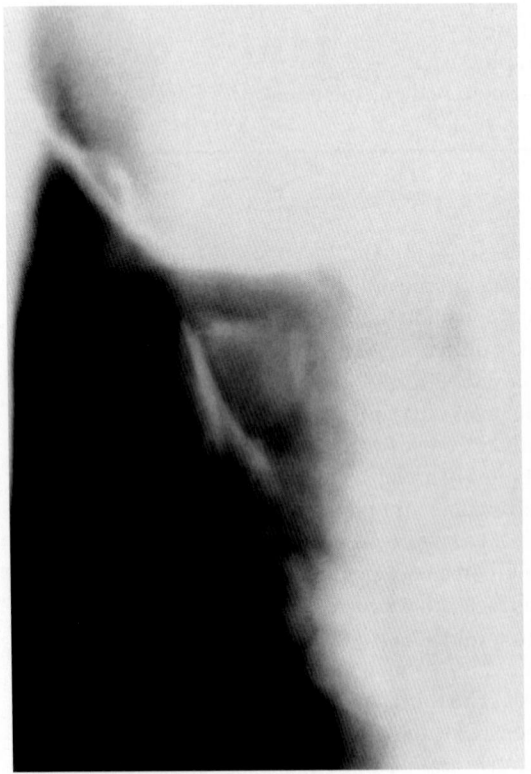

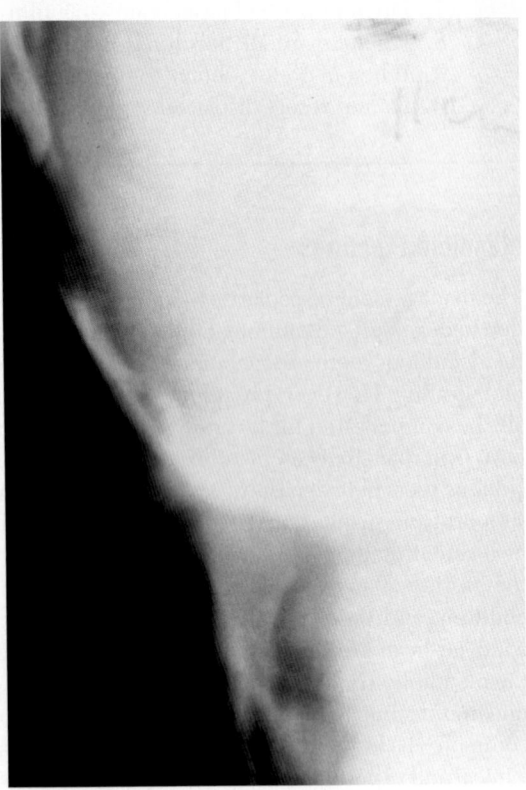

A

B

For fractures of the mandibular arch in children, treatment can range from simple observation to open reduction with rigid fixation. Symphyseal or parasymphyseal fractures with minimal to moderate displacement can often be realigned and immobilized with interdental wiring, arch bars, or cap splints. In very young children an acrylic splint stabilized by circummandibular wires is highly effective (Fig. 12). While conservative management will suffice in a majority of arch and body fractures, some complex injuries will require open reduction with internal fixation to achieve adequate bone-to-bone reapproximation of the fragments. Interfragmentary wiring or monocortical miniplate fixation in conjunction with intermaxillary fixation can achieve this goal. It is imperative to recognize that both techniques risk injury to the developing tooth buds; therefore,

FIGURE 12 A: Towne's view of a 3-year-old girl with a right parasymphyseal fracture. **B:** Clinical photographs of the same child. **C:** Acrylic splint fabricated on a plaster cast made from the mandibular impression in the same child. The plaster cast was refractured, to establish the occlusion with a plaster cast made from an impression on the maxillary teeth. After correct alignment of the mandibular cast was obtained, the acrylic splint was fabricated. **D:** The acrylic splint held in place on the mandibular teeth with circummandibular wires.

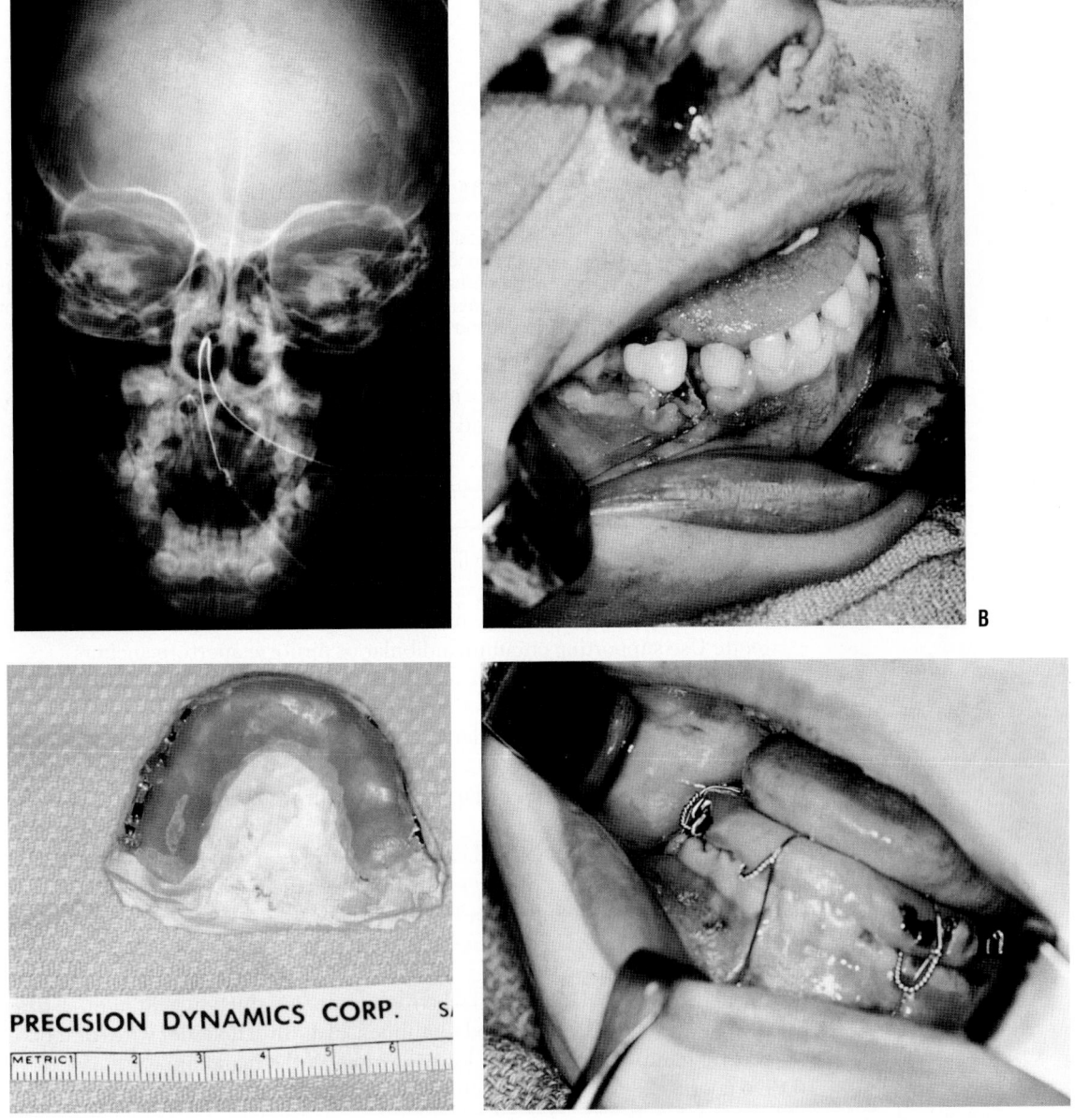

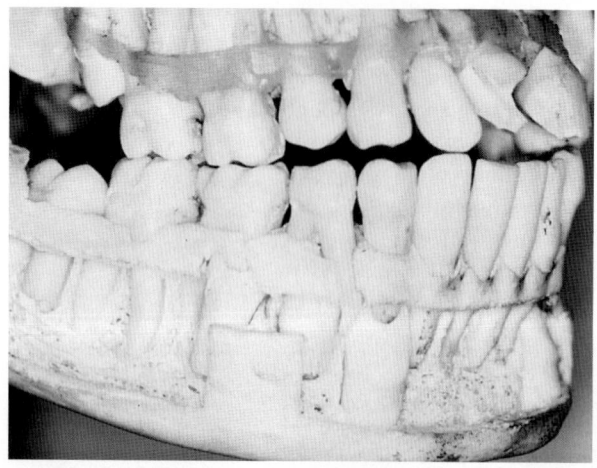

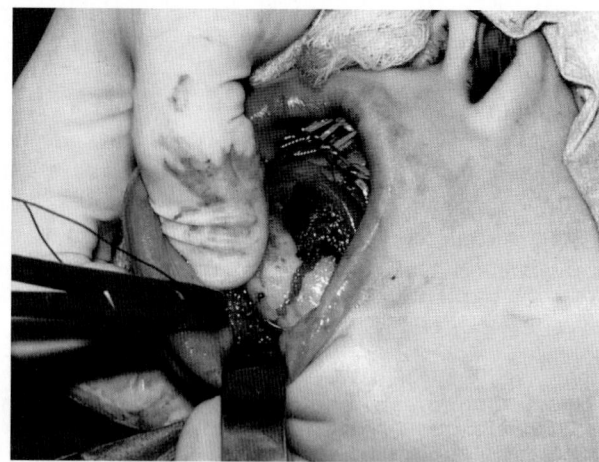

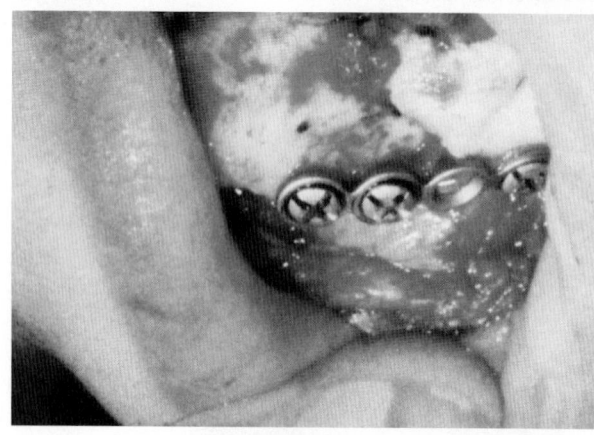

FIGURE 13 **A:** Proximity of the unerupted teeth to the lower border of the mandible. **B:** Transoral wire osteosynthesis in a 10-year-old child with a parasymphyseal mandible fracture. **C:** Transoral monocortical miniplate osteosynthesis in a 6-year-old child with a parasymphyseal mandible fracture. For the patients in B and C, great care was taken with drill hole placement to prevent injury to the developing toothbuds.

great care is required with drill hole placement (Fig. 13). In adolescents with permanent dentition, the principles of bicortical rigid fixation are applicable.

PEARLS AND PERILS

1. In young children, use an acrylic splint on the lower teeth, fixed with circummandibular wires, to correctly align the fracture fragments.
2. Between ages 6 and 12 is the most difficult time to anchor arch bars to only teeth. Use supporting circummandibular or piriform aperture anchors.
3. After 13 years, treat like an adult but check panoramic x-ray views for unerupted teeth.
4. Wait 3 to 5 days before considering intermaxillary fixation (IMF) for condylar fractures.
5. Crush fractures of the condylar head need early continued mobilization and ongoing physiotherapy.
6. Get an avulsed tooth replaced within an hour. Keep it in milk in the interim.
7. Do not leave condylar fractures in IMF longer than 3 weeks. Treat asymmetric movement with guiding elastics.
8. Do not open condylar fractures except in rare instances of severe displacement in adolescents.
9. In children under 13 years old who require open reduction with internal fixation, be aware of the unerupted toothbuds. Place drill holes for wires or monocortical miniplates in the very lower margins of the mandible.
10. Do not take dentoalveolar fractures out of IMF too early.

Dentoalveolar fractures are not the serious dental emergency in children with primary teeth as they are in adults. Nevertheless, it is sometimes difficult to be certain about whether a tooth is a primary or a secondary one, and since the survival of the tooth depends on reimplantation within an hour of injury, reimplantation should always be attempted. The incisors and canines are the most common site of injury, as a result of their prominence. The avulsed tooth should be cleansed in saline solution and replaced in the socket. If the child is unable to cooperate, then the tooth can be kept in saline solution or a bowl of milk until reimplantation and stabilization can be achieved. It has been the author's experience that dentoalveolar fractures with avulsion of the surrounding bone result in difficult malocclusions and will often require prolonged immobilization.

Midfacial Fractures

The midface, which includes the orbit and the nasoethmoid region, is aesthetically prominent and injuries can leave children with significant deformities. The extent of these injuries is determined by the magnitude of the impacting force, and consequently they can range from simple fractures of the orbital floor to highly comminuted injuries with complete loss of the architectural supports of the face. Thus, the surgical management needs to be tailored to the severity of the injury and can vary from observation to extensive craniofacial reconstruction. The orbit is a key component of all of these fractures, and accurate management requires a complete assessment of both the functional and structural changes by physical and radiologic examination. Ophthalmologic evaluation is essential for measurement of visual acuity. The position of the globe must be assessed for exophthalmos, enophthalmos, and vertical dystopia. This is often made difficult by concomitant periorbital edema, ecchymosis, and subconjunctival hemorrhages seen with major facial injuries. Voluntary range of motion and force duction tests are used to assess ocular mobility. Intraocular pressure is measured. Infraorbital and supraorbital nerve integrity is tested. Traumatic hypertelorism is assessed by measurement of the intercanthal distance. The rims are palpated for discontinuities and an attempt is made to identify the medial canthal ligaments.

Zygomaticomalar Complex Fractures

Fractures of the zygomaticomalar complex (ZMC) are generally not seen before the age of 5 as they usually parallel the pneumatization of the maxillary sinus. Fractures of the malar bone prior to this age do occur, but tend not to involve the orbital floor. ZMC fractures can be classified according to the patterns of the fractures seen on CT scan (27). Low-impact injuries result in separation of the frontozygomatic suture, infraorbital rim disruption with extension along the zygomaticomaxillary suture, "greenstick" fracture of the zygomatic arch, and cracks along the orbital floor and lateral orbital wall. Varying degrees of comminution of the buttresses, orbital wall, and infraorbital rim generally indicate a more forceful impact. The most severe injuries present with a high degree of comminution and can often be associated with more extensive maxillary fractures. A strong indication of an unstable fracture is lateral displacement of the malar fragment on CT scans and this indicates that a more extensive reconstruction will be required.

Bone displacement is usually an indication for surgical correction of ZMC fractures, and this requires adequate exposure of the fractured buttresses, a process called *triangulation* since it involves control of three key sites; the frontozygomatic suture, the infraorbital rim, and the zygomaticomalar buttress. Subciliary and brow incisions or a transconjunctival incision with lateral canthotomy in conjunction with an upper buccal sulcus incision will yield full exposure. However, in noncomminuted fractures the reduction of the infraorbital rim fracture and the frontozygomatic fracture can often be controlled by external palpation, while the malar fragment is manipulated into position via the gingivolabial sulcus exposure of the zygomaticomalar buttress. A hemicoronal approach may be necessary for high-energy injuries that require reconstruction of the zygomatic arch. Most injuries can be reconstructed utilizing one-point fixation of the zygo-maticomalar buttress. Comminuted fractures may require additional open reconstruction of the infraorbital rim and frontozygomatic suture. Sagging of the orbital contents into the maxillary sinus can be supported with Gelfilm if the defect is small, or with calvarial bone graft if the defect is large. The zygomatic arch can be repositioned by the standard Gillies approach through the brow or through a lateral canthotomy.

PEARLS AND PERILS

1. Under age 5, zygomaticomalar complex (ZMC) fractures do not tend to involve the orbital floor, but are confined to the malar bone and arch.
2. Lateral displacement indicates an unstable fracture.
3. With displaced fractures, one- or two-point visualization may be inadequate for correct realignment.
4. Do not forget about the orbital floor and potential for enophthalmos.

Nasoethmoid Fractures

Nasoethmoid fractures are defined by dislocation at the nasofrontal suture, the nasal bones, medial orbital rim, and inferior orbital rim. This describes a four-sided fracture that yields a core called the *central fragment* (27). The severity of the fracture and the difficulty of the reconstruction are determined by the extent of comminution of the central fragment (Fig. 14). This can be determined from a CT scan, which is invaluable for an accurate diagnosis. Axial views demonstrate the retrodisplacement of the central fragment and the coronal view identifies the disruptions of the orbital walls. Traumatic hypertelorism should be suspected, and is evaluated by defining the integrity of the medial canthal ligaments. This is best accomplished under anesthesia at the time of surgical correction with a hemostat inserted into the nose up toward the medial orbital rim. Mobility of the underlying fragments suggests that the bone with its canthal attachment has been displaced and will need to be repositioned and stabilized with transnasal wiring (Fig. 15). The easiest mistake in children is to set the intercanthal distance too wide, since intraorbital growth is nearly complete by the age of 8 years. Nasoethmoid fractures are usually treated by open reduction and internal fixation. It is generally better to overtreat these injuries since the secondary deformities from undertreatment are extremely difficult to correct (28). Favorable existing lacerations can be utilized for access to the fracture; however, in most cases coronal exposure provides the best opportunity for an adequate reconstruction. In order to get the coronal flap down low enough on the nasal bridge, the globe has to be mobilized along the orbital roof. This allows access to the medial canthal tendon, which is usually attached to a sizable bony fragment. If the

FIGURE 14 Classification of nasoethmoid fractures. Type 1 fractures have a solid central fragment. Type 2 fractures have a superficially comminuted central fragment with fragmentation of the nasomaxillary buttress. Type 3 fractures have a deeply comminuted central fragment with fragmentation of the bone to which the medial canthal tendons attach.

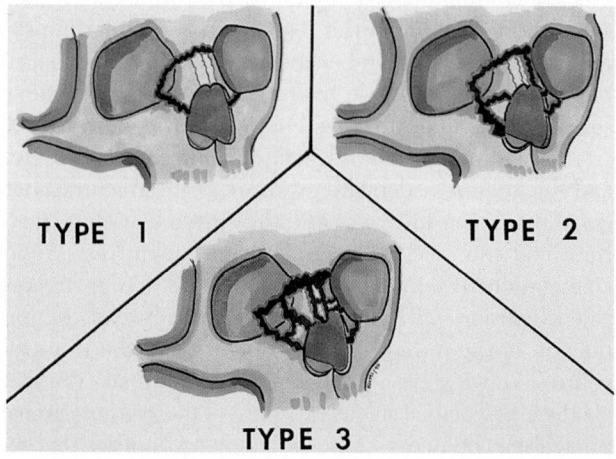

TYPE 1   TYPE 2

TYPE 3

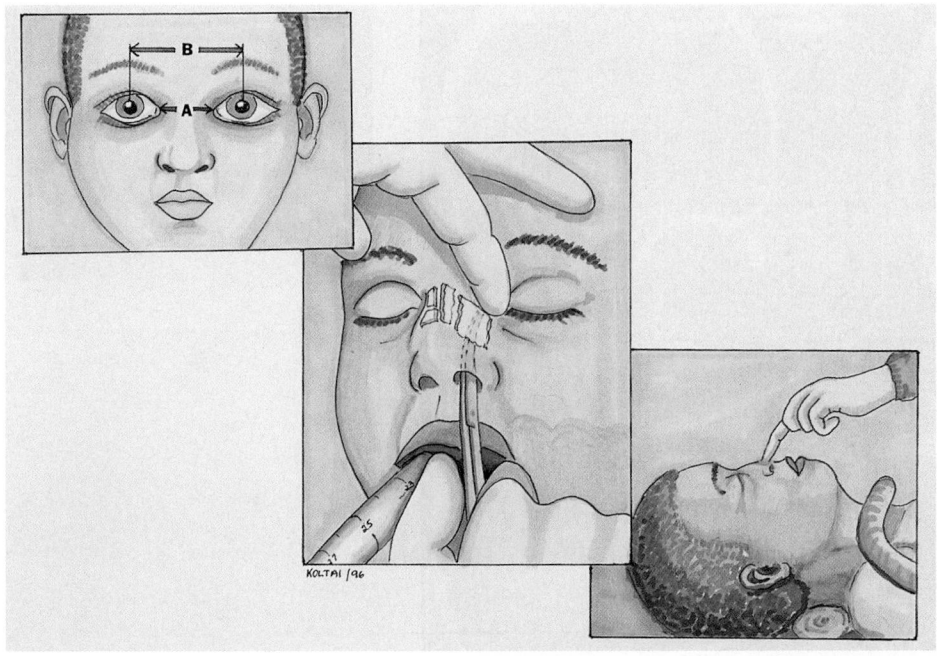

FIGURE 15 Physical findings in children with nasoethmoid fractures. Intercanthal and interpupillary measurements must be taken (**left frame**). The medial canthal integrity is tested while the child is anesthetized, utilizing the bimanual examination (**central frame**). Digital palpation of the nasal dorsum resulting in collapse suggests the need for a cantilever bone graft (**right frame**).

canthal tendon has been inadvertently stripped from its bony attachment, it has to be identified for later reconstruction. Once the tendon has been accounted for, the nasomaxillary buttress and the medial orbital rims are reduced and reconstructed with microplates (Fig. 16). Medial wall bone grafting may be necessary to separate the orbital contents from the ethmoidal sinus. Medial canthal reconstruction is the next and perhaps most important step in the repair. A drill hole is placed in the anterior lacrimal crest above the insertion of the anterior limb of the tendon. A second hole is made in the posterior crest just behind the insertion of the posterior limbs. Contralateral holes are similarly placed and a 28-gauge stainless-steel wire is passed transnasally between the two

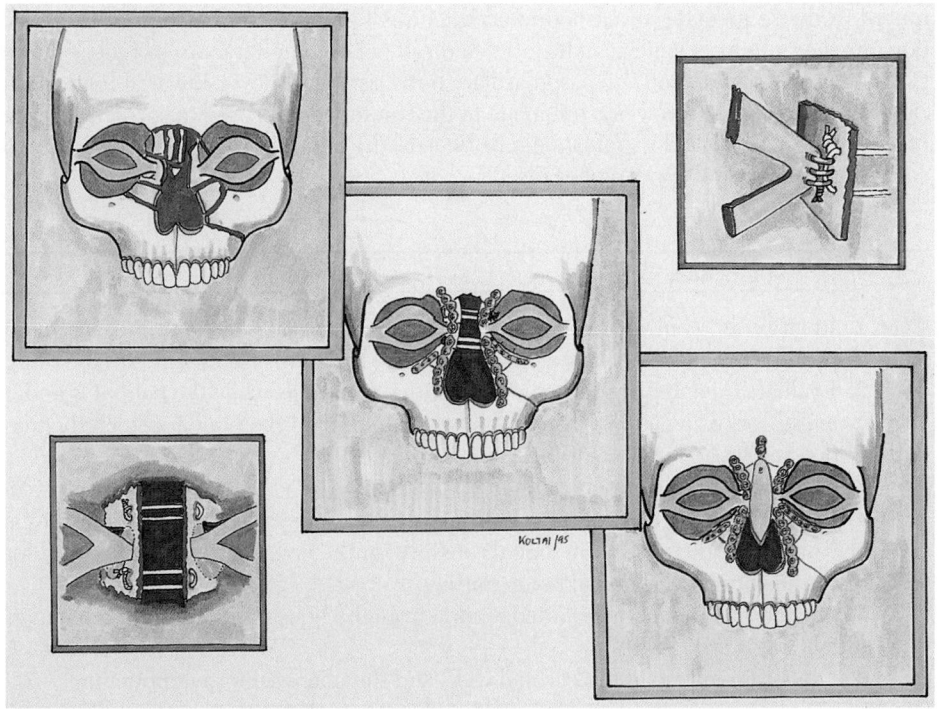

FIGURE 16 Sequencing of comminuted nasoethmoid fractures begins with reconstruction of the nasomaxillary buttress (**central frame**). Transnasal wiring is performed next. If possible, wires are placed above and below the tendons and each is oriented anterior/posteriorly (**left lower frame**). If the tendon is avulsed from the underlying bone, then the tendon should be sewn to the transnasal wire with permanent (4-0 polypropylene) suture. Incorporating the tendon with the transnasal wire runs the risk of shredding the tendon (**right upper frame**). After the nasomaxillary buttress and medial canthal reconstruction, a cantilever cranial bone graft is used for the reconstruction of the nasal dorsum (**right lower frame**).

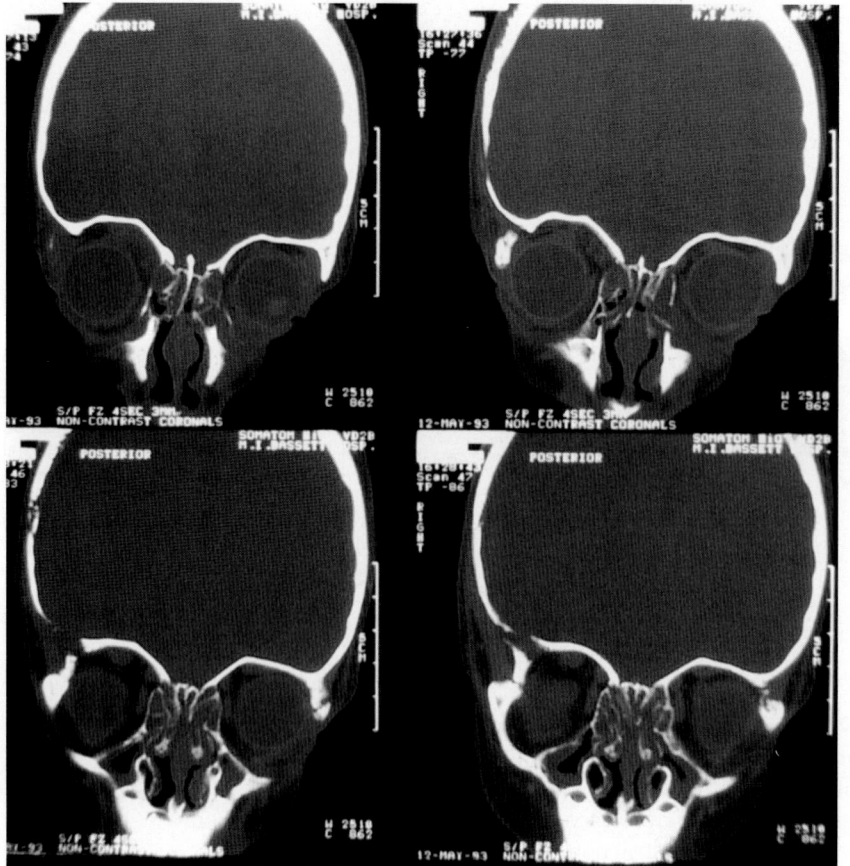

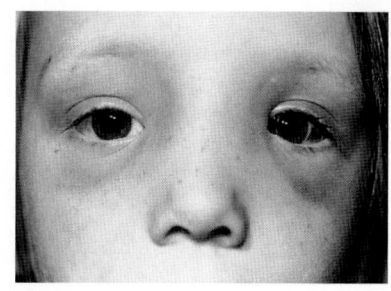

FIGURE 17 A: Coronal computed tomography scan of a 2-year-old child with a deeply comminuted nasoethmoid fracture. Note the associated skull fractures. **B:** Clinical photograph of the same child showing marked widening of the intercanthal distance, with rounding of the left medial canthal area.

fragments and tightened in an effort to overcorrect the deformity. A final step may be required in the sequencing of nasoethmoid fractures for the reconstruction of the nasal dorsum, the support of which can be lost as a result of combined fractures of the septum, the nasofrontal suture, and the nasomaxillary buttress. A cantilever calvarial bone graft, rigidly fixed with a lag screw or a miniplate to the frontal bone, is used to correct this type of deformity. The tip of the graft should be deep to the upper border of the lower lateral cartilages for a natural appearance (Fig. 17).

PEARLS AND PERILS

1. Identify the central fragment—recognize its comminution and the degree of posterior displacement into the ethmoids or lateral displacement into the orbit.
2. Evaluate the integrity of the medial canthal ligaments while the patient is under anesthesia using an intranasal hemostat. Mobility of the bone to which the tendon is attached indicates a need for canthopexy.
3. Overcorrect the canthopexy.
4. Evaluate the integrity of the nasal support while the patient is under anesthesia. Collapse of the nose from digital pressure on the dorsum suggests the need for cantilever calvarial dorsal bone grafting.
5. Do not strip the medial canthal tendon from the bone fragment to which it is attached.
6. Do not forget the medial orbital walls and the potential for enophthalmos.

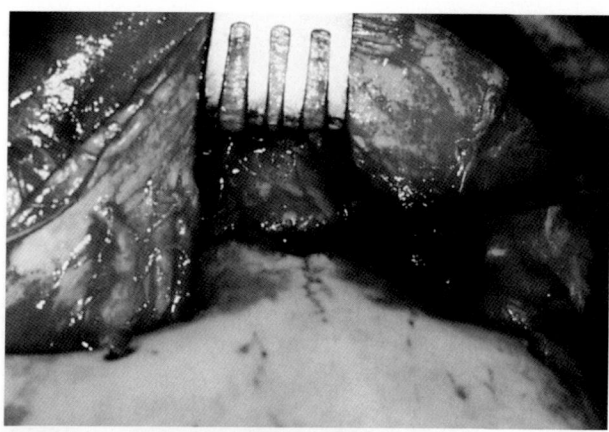

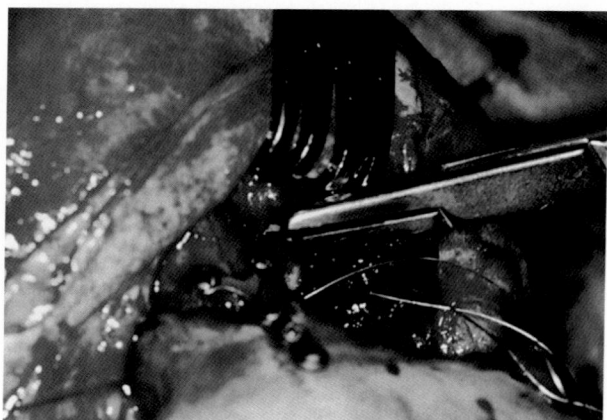

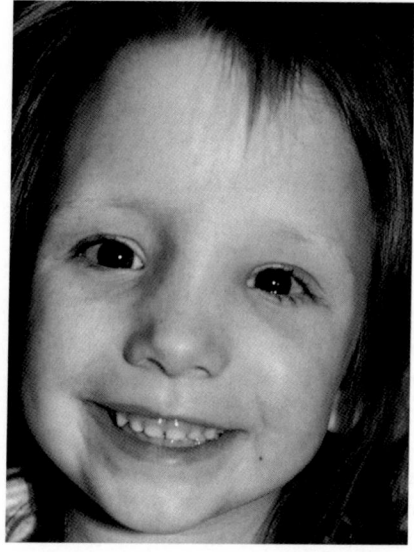

FIGURE 17 *Continued.* **C:** Reosteotomy of the broken fragments was required since the reconstruction was delayed for 3 weeks secondary to associated neurocranial injuries. **D:** After reconstruction of the central fragment with Y-miniplate osteosynthesis at the nasofrontal separation, transnasal wiring is performed. **E:** Six-month postoperative view.

Orbital Fractures

Orbital floor fractures are determined by the pneumatization of the maxillary sinus, and thus are rarely seen before the ages of 5 to 6 years. Yet in older children they are the most common isolated type of orbital fracture. As previously noted, they can be seen in conjunction with ZMC or maxillary fractures; however, they are often isolated injuries. Several configurations occur, depending on the forces involved. "Trapdoor" fractures are when the blow out is hinged on one surface with the orbital contents herniated into the maxillary sinus and trapped by fragments of bone. A "saucer"-type fracture occurs when there is a depression of the floor into the maxillary sinus with an increase in orbital volume resulting in enophthalmos. Linear floor fractures typically extend into the inferior orbital rim, while severe injuries result in the total loss of globe support by disruption of the floor. Clinically, orbital floor fractures share common physical findings with other types of facial injuries. It is common to see immediate periorbital ecchymoses, edema, and subconjunctival hemorrhage. Diplopia can be a consequence of muscle entrapment, muscle contusion, or cranial nerve damage. More severe injuries result in greater degrees of loss of globe support and enophthalmos. While rarely permanent, infraorbital hypoesthesia is a common early sign with most types of orbital floor fractures. As noted with most orbital injuries, globe damage is uncommon. Coronal CT best demonstrates floor defects, while axial CT is useful for the evaluation of changes in orbital volume (Fig. 18). It is essential that the patient have an ophthalmologic evaluation. Forced duction

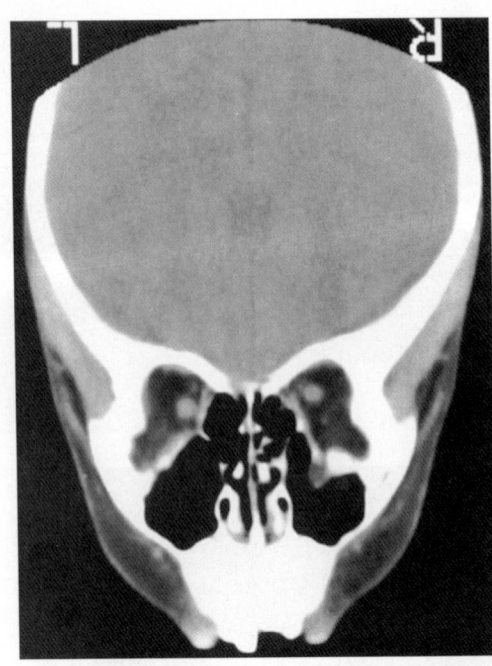

FIGURE 18 Coronal computed tomography scan of a "trapdoor" orbital floor fracture in a 6-year-old child. Note entrapment of the inferior rectus muscle.

testing is important to differentiate entrapment from muscle contusion or cranial nerve damage.

The management of orbital floor fractures has been unnecessarily controversial. There is little disagreement of the necessity of orbital floor exploration in conjunction with repair of concurrent maxillary injuries. Large orbital floor injuries are routinely explored, as are fractures that show muscle entrapment on CT scans. It is probably best to observe children with less severe injuries for 7 to 10 days. If at the end of that period the child continues to have enophthalmos, extraocular muscle restriction, or pain on movement, then exploration is appropriate. In about half the children, the symptoms resolve during the 7- to 10-day waiting period, and surgical intervention is not required.

FIGURE 19 Calvarial bone graft for reconstruction of the orbital floor.

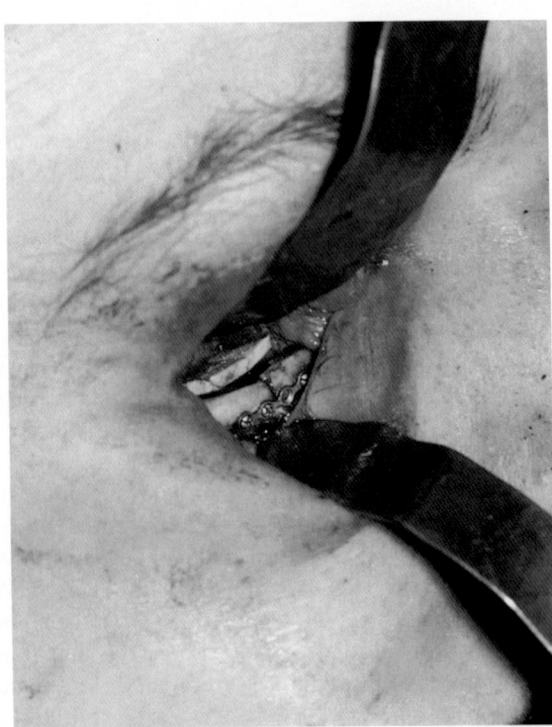

The author's approach to isolated orbital fractures has been primarily through the transconjunctival technique, although the subciliary approach can also be used. Herniated soft tissue is carefully pushed back into the orbit and the bony fragments are elevated into position. It is rarely necessary to remove any of them. For small defects or areas of weakness, an implant of saline-soaked Gelfilm is usually adequate for children. For the reconstruction of larger pediatric defects, the author prefers calvarial bone grafts to rigid alloplastic materials (Fig. 19). Harvesting calvarial bone grafts in children may require full-thickness removal, with splitting and replacement of the outer table (Fig. 20). The key step of a successful reconstruction depends on the accurate clinical estimation and restoration of the bony volume of the orbit.

PEARLS AND PERILS

1. With extensive fractures, early surgery is appropriate. With more limited isolated injuries, waiting 7 to 10 days may prevent an unnecessary exploration.
2. Transconjunctival, postseptal approach to the floor yields the least postoperative lid problems. Be prepared to deal with orbital fat.
3. Gelfilm works well for small floor defects.
4. Orbital emphysema indicates a medial wall fracture.
5. Use an external ethmoidectomy approach to the medial wall.
6. Most orbital roof fractures do not require reconstruction. Observe for 7 to 10 days for persistent exophthalmos and vertical dystopia.
7. Late-developing periorbital hematoma suggests an orbital roof fracture.
8. Greenstick fractures of the supraorbital rim are very hard to reduce. Use an otologic drill to eliminate step-off deformity.
9. Do not try to harvest calvarial bone graft in one step by trying to remove the outer table. Get a neurosurgeon to harvest a full-thickness section of parietal bone and then split it on the back table. Use the inner table and replace the outer table.
10. Do not approach the floor via the maxillary sinus.
11. Do not overlook apex injuries when there is a lateral wall fracture.
12. Do not overlook developing frontal sinus after the ages of 6 to 7 years. Injury to the nasofrontal duct may result in mucocele several years later.

FIGURE 20 A: In children younger than 12, the author prefers removing a full-thickness quarter section of the calvarium, which is then split into the outer and inner layers. The inner layer is used for the reconstruction, while the outer layer is replaced back into the harvest site on the calvarium. **B:** In older children the calvarial bone graft can be harvested with an otologic drill, which is used to make a trough on the outer cortex, outlining the harvest site. The graft is then removed with either a right-angle saw or a chisel and mallet.

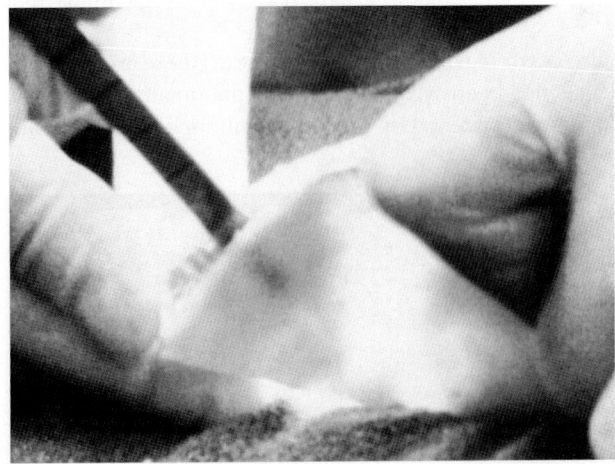
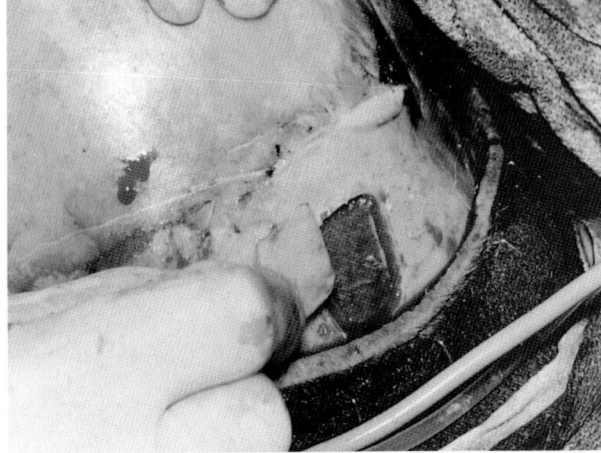

A   B

Orbital Wall Fractures

Isolated lateral and medial orbital wall fractures are very uncommon. Medial wall fractures are typically associated with nasoethmoid injuries. Isolated fractures of the lamina papyracea tend to occur as a result of trauma to the nose and medial rim of the eye, or of the globe itself. CT scans will generally reveal orbital emphysema as well as medial displacement of the lamina papyracea. Isolated injuries often resolve on their own; however, if there is a persistent enophthalmos or entrapment of the medial rectus in the ethmoidal sinus, then surgical reconstruction is required. This is accomplished through an external ethmoidectomy approach, which yields an excellent exposure of the medial orbital wall with minimal postoperative scarring. The orbital contents can be reduced from the ethmoidal sinus, and calvarial bone graft replacement of the lamina papyracea can then be performed.

Lateral wall fractures are typically seen with ZMC or Le Fort III fractures and the orbital repair is part of the overall reconstruction (Fig. 21). The lateral rim can be reduced with microplates with exposure through the brow, lateral canthotomy, or coronal flap. Severe lateral wall fractures that result in enophthalmos from an increased orbital volume may require postbulbar bone grafts. Sphenoid wing injuries impinging on the orbital apex can be accessed through a hemicoronal incision with detachment and retraction of the temporal muscle.

Orbital Roof Fractures

With the availability of direct coronal CT evaluation of children with facial injuries, orbital roof fractures have been more commonly observed (16–29). These are frequently seen in conjunction with head injuries, and suspicion should be raised by the presence of a late-developing periorbital hematoma. Proptosis and dystopia can be delayed findings.

Since the orbital roof is a part of the cranial cavity, concomitant intracranial injury is present in a substantial portion of patients. While permanent morbidity is an ever-present concern, usually as a consequence of neurologic damage, the globe and the orbital soft tissues rarely sustain permanent damage. Three types of fractures are generally seen: nondisplaced fractures; blow-out fractures, which are displaced into the anterior cranial fossa; and blow-in fractures, which result in reduced orbital volume. Most children do not require repair of roof fractures; however, there have been rare cases of blow-in fractures causing permanent exophthalmos, vertical dystopia, and even orbital encephalocele. As a consequence, the author generally observes these children for a 7- to 10-day period and if the exophthalmos and vertical dystopia have failed to resolve, then reconstruction is undertaken via a basicranial approach or via a combined neurosurgical maxillofacial approach with intracranial exposure of the orbital roof (80). Severe disruption of the roof will require a split calvarial bone graft, fixed rigidly with microplates, for definitive repair. The timing of repair may be complicated by the neurologic injury that the child has sustained.

Supraorbital rim fractures also occur in young children; however, these are not common because the frontal bone has not been weakened by the pneumatization of the frontal sinus (Fig. 22). When fractures occur, they are commonly in association with

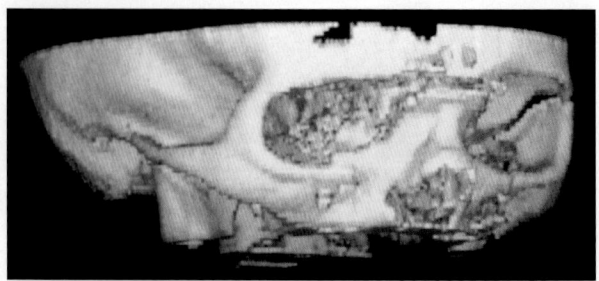

FIGURE 21 Three-dimensional computed tomography scan of an adolescent with a right Le Fort II and left Le Fort III fracture. Note the wide separation of the left lateral orbital wall.

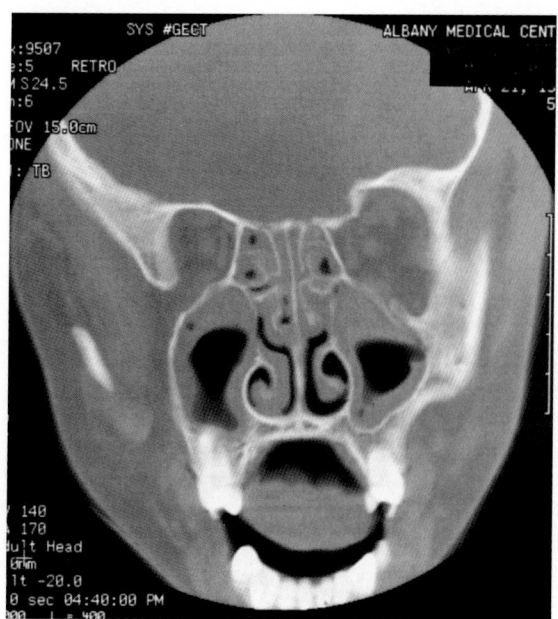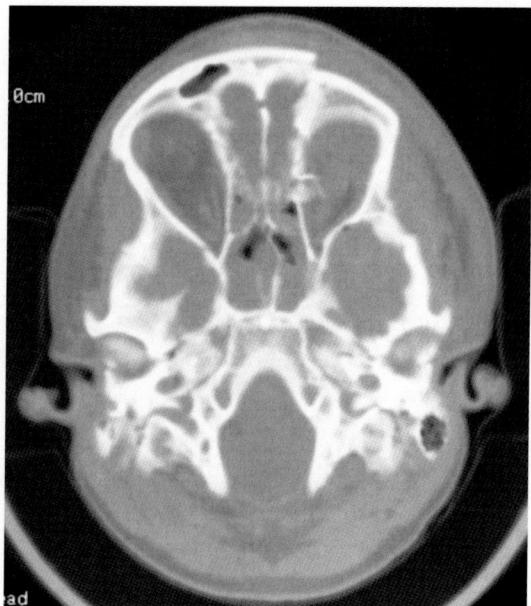

FIGURE 22 A,B: Coronal and axial computed tomography scans of a 12-year-old with a supraorbital rim and "blow-in" orbital roof fracture.

frontal skull fractures and orbital roof fractures. It is rarely necessary to repair orbital rim fractures unless the dislocation will leave a permanent step-off deformity in the brow. It has been the author's experience that isolated rim fractures are typically "greenstick" in nature, and are difficult to reduce. Recontouring of the displaced edges with an otologic drill can camouflage step-off deformities. Repair can be a concomitant part of the neurosurgical procedure and can be approached either through an extension of the overlying laceration or by coronal craniofacial exposure. When the need for exposure is limited, a brow incision may be sufficient.

In older children who have had pneumatization of the frontal sinuses, supraorbital rim injuries may be evaluated for frontal sinus fractures and these are treated similarly to those in adults. The anterior wall can be reconstructed with wire or microplates. Posterior-wall fractures require basicranial exploration, evaluation of the dura, assessment of the nasofrontal ducts, and reconstruction of the bony walls. Obliteration is only required when the supraorbital fractures involve the nasofrontal duct. When this occurs, the author strips the sinus of its mucosa, burrs the walls with an otologic drill, closes the nasofrontal duct with muscle and bone, and obliterates the sinus with abdominal fat.

Maxillary Fractures

As with adults, fractures of the maxilla in children are classified using the Le Fort system. Le Fort I fractures separate the palate from the maxilla, extending through the floor of the nose, maxillary sinus, and pterygoid plates. Le Fort II fractures result in separation of the midface from the cranium, extending through the pterygoid plates, anterior maxillary walls, medial orbital walls, and the nasofrontal suture. Le Fort III fractures separate the entire face from the cranium, extending through the zygomatic arch, frontozygomatic sutures, lateral orbital walls, medial orbital walls, nasofrontal suture, septum, and pterygoid plates. It is important to understand that this is an anatomic classification and that these types of maxillary fractures are as unique as a ZMC fracture or a nasoethmoid fracture. Hence, the classification does not adequately describe the severity of the injury, and is inadequate as a communication tool for surgical planning. The author has utilized a functional classification for maxillary fractures, and found it useful in predicting the difficulty of the reconstruction (6). Type I fractures are minimally displaced and

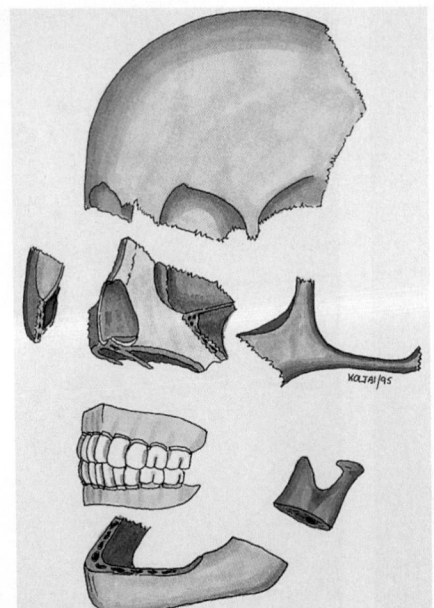 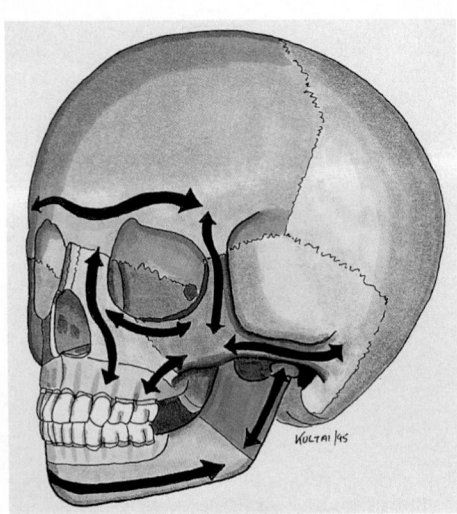

FIGURE 23 A: An exploded view of a child's facial skeleton into component units. **B:** With severe complex fractures, the component units are reconstructed individually and then connected to each other and to the cranium via their associated buttresses. (From Koltai PJ, Rabkin D. Management of facial trauma in children. *Pediatr Clin North Am* 1996;43(6): 1272, with permission.)

A

B

generally not comminuted. With these types of injuries the major buttresses are "greenstick" and the fragments are close to their original anatomic location and orientation. Type II fractures are moderately displaced with some areas of comminution. With these injuries the buttresses are clearly recognizable, and the fragments are robust enough to readily accept plate and screw fixation. Type III fractures are severely displaced with multiple comminutions of the major architectural supports, resulting in highly unstable injuries that require extensive three-dimensional stabilization utilizing bone grafts and screws and plates for reconstruction of the shattered buttresses. These are rare pediatric injuries, and clinically present with severe facial edema, periorbital ecchymoses, and malocclusion. Associated neurocranial injuries are common, as a force large enough to cause maxillary fractures is of a magnitude that is transmitted to the cranial cavity. Appropriate radiologic assessment is the key to complete diagnosis and axial and coronal CT scans are indispensable for assessing the severity and degree of bony displacement, as well as in the development of an appropriate operative plan.

Contemporary care of the multiply injured child requires coordination among a team of physicians including the pediatric intensivist, ophthalmologist, neurologist, neu-

FIGURE 24 Traditionally, sequencing begins with reconstruction of the occlusion and the mandible, which then serves as a template for the upper face.

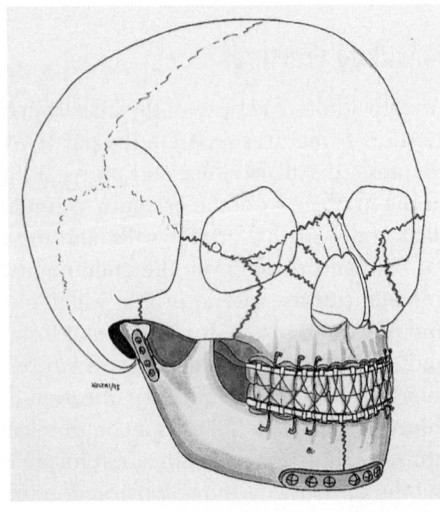

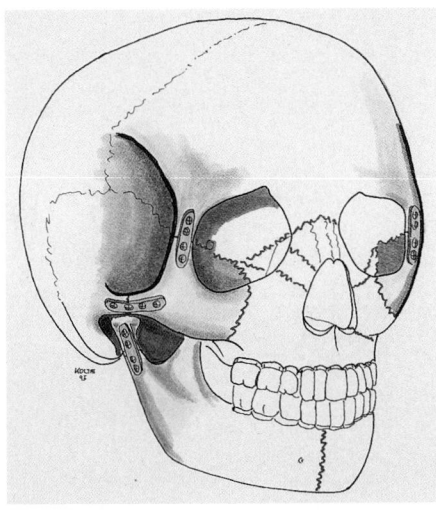

FIGURE 25 The outer facial frame is reconstructed with emphasis on the zygomatic arch in order to narrow and reproject the face.

rosurgeon, anesthesiologist, and the maxillofacial reconstructive surgeon. Medical contraindications may preempt early operative intervention; however, significantly displaced fractures should be reduced within 10 days of the injury because rapid interfragmentary healing makes later correction very difficult. As with all facial injuries, the goals of therapy are to restore facial symmetry, accurate occlusion, and normal architectural support (Fig. 23B). When there is minimal or no displacement, surgical correction is not required; however, alterations of form and function necessitate surgical intervention. The sequencing of surgical repair of severe maxillary fractures, especially panfacial fractures, is an important consideration in the reconstructive effort. Traditionally, complex reconstruction began with the reestablishment of the occlusion. This was followed by correction of mandible fractures, which formed the foundation on which the upper face was reconstructed (Fig. 24). Over the last 20 years differing strategies about sequencing have evolved (4). One strategy is to begin the reconstruction with the external frame of the face, including the frontal bar, zygomatic arches, and orbital rims (Fig. 25). This approach emphasizes the importance of the zygomatic arch in the control of the facial width and its reciprocal, facial projection (Fig. 26). On occasion the author has followed an al-

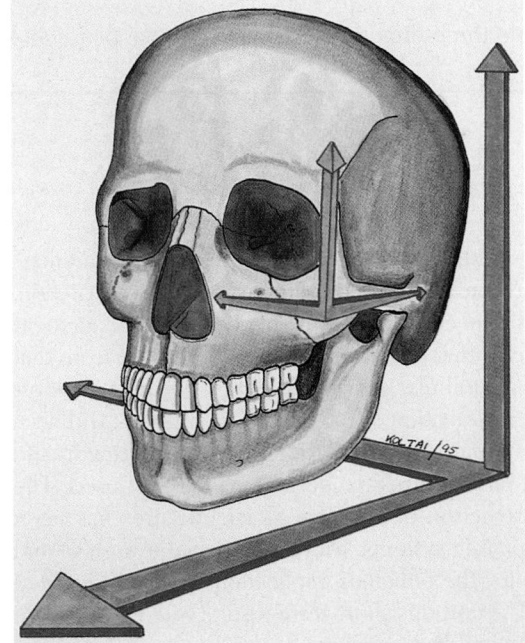

FIGURE 26 Correct reconstruction of the zygomatic arch can be the key to maintaining the projection and narrowing the width of the face, which are reciprocal measures of each other.

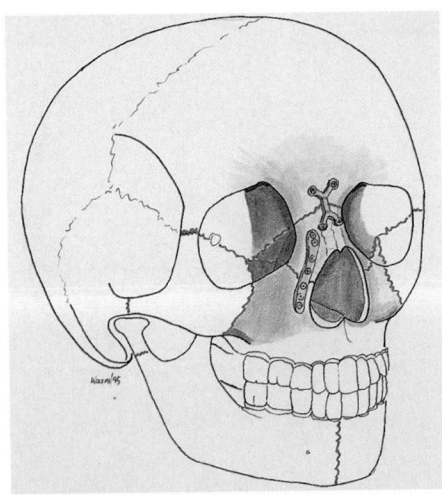

FIGURE 27 Reconstruction begins with the central core of the face using the anterior skull base as the template, with the goal of improving the accuracy of the repair of the aesthetically most significant component of the face.

ternative strategy in children with complex maxillary fractures, based on the recognition that the nasoethmoid area is the most prominent aesthetic unit of the face and is often the most difficult to reconstruct. If there are concomitant mandible fractures, the author begins surgical repair by establishing the occlusion and reducing the mandible. Upper facial reconstruction starts with the nasoethmoid region, followed by positioning of the orbits and the outer facial frame to the central core (Fig. 27).

PEARLS AND PERILS

1. These are complicated fractures. Sequencing of reconstruction should begin with IMF followed by reestablishment of the central core of the face. An alternative is to start with the outer facial frame.
2. Get adequate craniofacial exposure.
3. Look for the introduction of absorbable plates.
4. Delays longer than 10 days make reduction of fractures very difficult. May need to refracture with osteotomies.
5. Wiring does not provide a stable three-dimensional reconstruction; plates and screws can.

CONCLUSION

In today's busy and mobile culture, children occasionally sustain serious craniomaxillofacial injuries that require careful and considerate three-dimensional reconstruction. Facial growth is the fourth dimension that needs to be appreciated in the management of pediatric facial fractures and is the factor that differentiates their treatment from that of adult facial fractures. Anticipation of mandibular growth simplifies repair, since most injuries can be treated conservatively by observation or intermaxillary fixation. Midfacial injuries, on the other hand, appear to be more sensitive to alterations of growth, and when bones are displaced significantly, more aggressive management is required. The technique of three-dimensional reconstruction of complex facial fractures has been greatly facilitated with the use of rigid plating systems, wide craniofacial exposure, and bone grafting. There is sound rationale for the judicious application of these advanced techniques in severe pediatric injuries. The author's short-term results with their use are excellent, and their long-term value looks highly promising.

ACKNOWLEDGMENTS

Sincere appreciation is expressed to Loretta Lynne Crowe for the preparation of this manuscript.

REFERENCES

1. Manson PN, Markowitz BL, Mirvis S, Dunham CM, Yaremchuk MJ. Toward CT based facial fracture treatment. *Plast Reconstr Surg* 1990;85:202–214.
2. Gruss JS, Mackinnon SE. Complex maxillary fractures: the role of buttress stabilization and immediate bone grafting. *Plast Reconstr Surg* 1986;78:9–22.
3. Shumrick KA, Kersten RC, Kulwin DR, Sinha PK, Smith TL. Extended access/internal approaches for the management of facial trauma. *Arch Otolaryngol Head Neck Surg* 1992;118:1105–1112.
4. Kelly KS, Manson PN, VanderKolk CA, et al. Sequencing Le Fort fracture treatment (organization of treatment for a panfacial fracture). *J Craniofac Surg* 1990;1:168–178.
5. Manson PN, Crawley WA, Yaremchuk JF, Rochman GM, Hoopes JE, French JH. Midface fractures: advantages of immediate extended open reduction and bone grafting. *Plast Reconstr Surg* 1985;76:1–10.
6. Koltai PJ, Rabkin D, Hoehn J. Rigid fixation of facial fractures in children. *J Craniomaxillofac Trauma* 1995;1(2):32–42.
7. Gussack GS, Lutterman A, Rodgers K, Powell RW, Ramenofsky ML. Pediatric maxillofacial trauma: unique features in diagnosis and treatment. *Laryngoscopy* 1987;97:925–930.
8. McGraw BL, Close RR. Pediatric maxillofacial trauma. *Arch Otolaryngol Head Neck Surg* 1990;116:41–45.
9. Kaban LB. Diagnosis and treatment of fractures of the facial bones in children 1943–1993. *J Oral Maxillofac Surg* 1993;51:722–729.
10. Tanaka N, Uchide N, Suzuki K, et al. Maxillofacial fractures in children. *J Craniomaxillofac surg* 1993;21:289–293.
11. Posnick JC, Wells M, Pron GE. Pediatric facial fractures: evolving patterns of treatment. *J Oral Maxillofac Surg* 1993;51:836–844.
12. Hardt N, Gottsauner A. The treatment of mandibular fractures in children. *J Craniomaxillofac Surg* 1993;21:214–219.
13. Thoren H, Iizuka T, Hallikainen D, Lindquist C. Different patterns of mandibular fractures in children. An analysis of 220 fractures in 157 patients. *J Craniomaxillofac Surg* 1992;20:292–296.
14. Norholt S, Krishnan V, Pedersen S, Jensen I. Pediatric condylar fractures; a long term follow-up study of 55 patients. *J Oral Maxillofac Surg* 1993;51:1302–1310.
15. Siegel MB, Wetmore RF, Postic WP, Handler SD, Tom LWC. Mandibular fractures in the pediatric patient. *Arch Otolaryngol Head Neck Surg* 1991;117:533–536.
16. Koltai PJ, Amjad I, Meyer D, Feustel PJ. Orbital fractures in children. *Arch Otolaryngol Head Neck Surg* 1995;121:1375–1379.
17. Koltai PJ, Wood GW. Three-dimensional CT reconstruction for the evaluation and surgical planning of facial fractures. *Otolaryngol Head Neck Surg* 1986;95:10–15.
18. Grymer LF, Gutierrez C, Stoksted P. Nasal fractures in children: influence on the development of the nose. *J Laryngol Otol* 1985;99:735–737.
19. Grymer LF, Gutierrez C, Stoksted P. The importance of nasal fractures during differential growth periods of the nose. *J Laryngol Otol* 1985;99:741–744.
20. Osterhout DK, Veargervic K. Maxillary hypoplasia secondary to midfacial trauma in childhood. *Plast Reconstr Surg* 1987;80:L491–499.
21. Precious DS, Delaire J, Hoffman CD. The effects of nasomaxillary injury on future facial growth. *Oral Surg* 1988;66:525–530.
22. Laurenzo JF, Canady JW, Zimmerman B, Smith RJH. Craniofacial growth in rabbits: effects of midfacial surgical trauma and rigid plate fixation. *Arch Otolaryngol Head Neck Surg* 1995;121:556–561.
23. Manson PN, Crawley WA, Yaremchuk MJ, Rochman GM, Hoopes JR, French JH. Midfacial fractures: advantages of immediate extended open reduction and bone grafting. *Plast Reconstr Surg* 1985;76:1–10.

24. Phillips JG, Cruss JS, Wells MD, Chollet A. Periosteal suspension of the lower eyelid and cheek following subciliary exposure of facial fractures. *Plast Reconstr Surg* 1991;88:145–148.

25. Pirsig W, Lehmann I. The influence of trauma on the growing septal cartilage. *Rhinology* 1975;13:39–44.

26. Pirsig W. Morphologic aspects of the injured nasal septum in children. *Rhinology* 1979;17:65–71.

27. Paskert JP, Manson PN, Iliff NT. Nasoethmoidal and orbital fractures. *Clin Plast Surg* 1988;15:209–223.

28. Ellis E. Sequencing treatment for naso-orbito-ethmoid fractures. *J Oral Maxillofac Surg* 1993;51:543–558.

29. Messinger A, Radkowski MA, Greenwald MJ, Pensler JM. Orbital roof fractures in the pediatric population. *Plast Reconstr Surg* 1989;84:213–216.

30. Denny AD, Rosenberg MW, Larsen DL. Immediate reconstruction of complex cranio orbital fractures in children. *J Craniofac Surg* 1993;4:8–20.

P.J. Koltai: Section of Pediatric Otolaryngology, Cleveland Clinic Foundation, Cleveland, Ohio 44195-4939.

• *Practical Pediatric Otolaryngology*
• edited by Robin T. Cotton
   and Charles M. Myer, III
• Lippincott-Raven Publishers,
   Philadelphia © 1999

46

Blunt and Penetrating Neck Trauma in Children

Éréa-Noël Garabédian & Denis Ayache

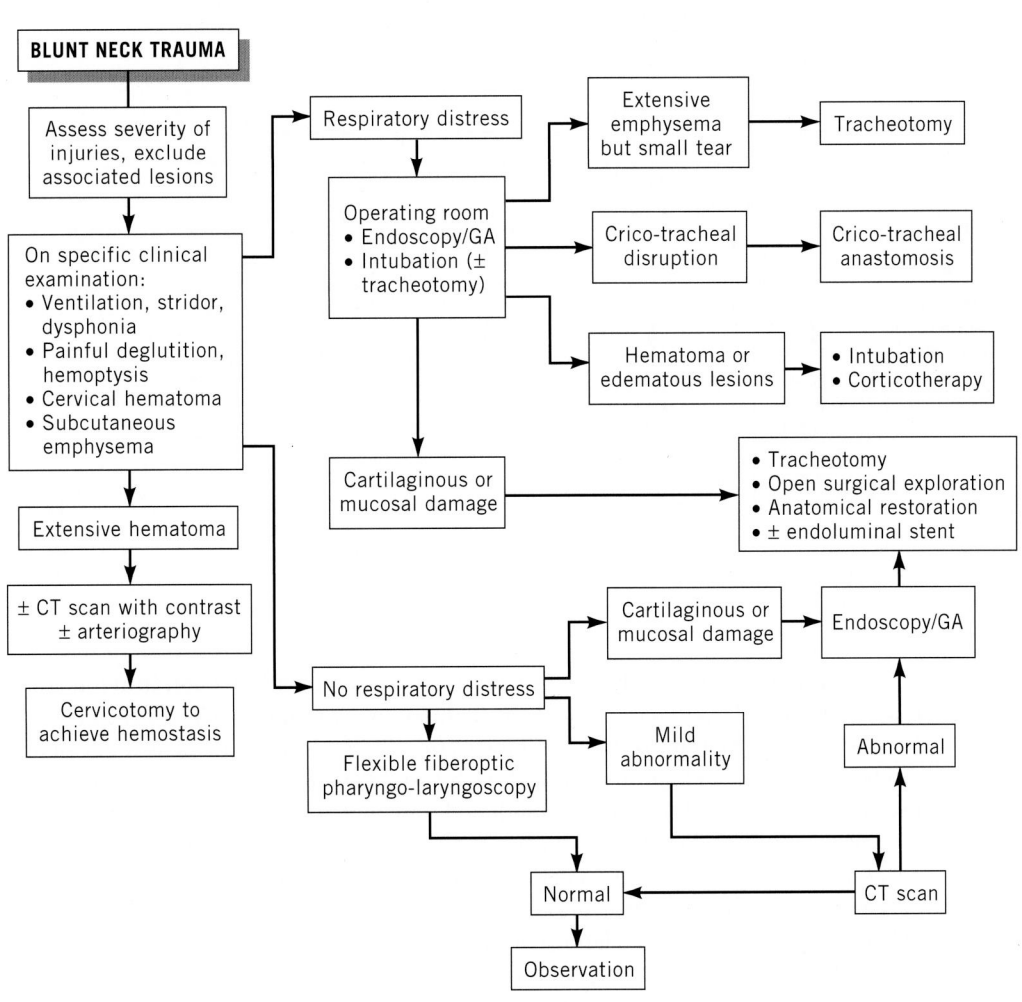

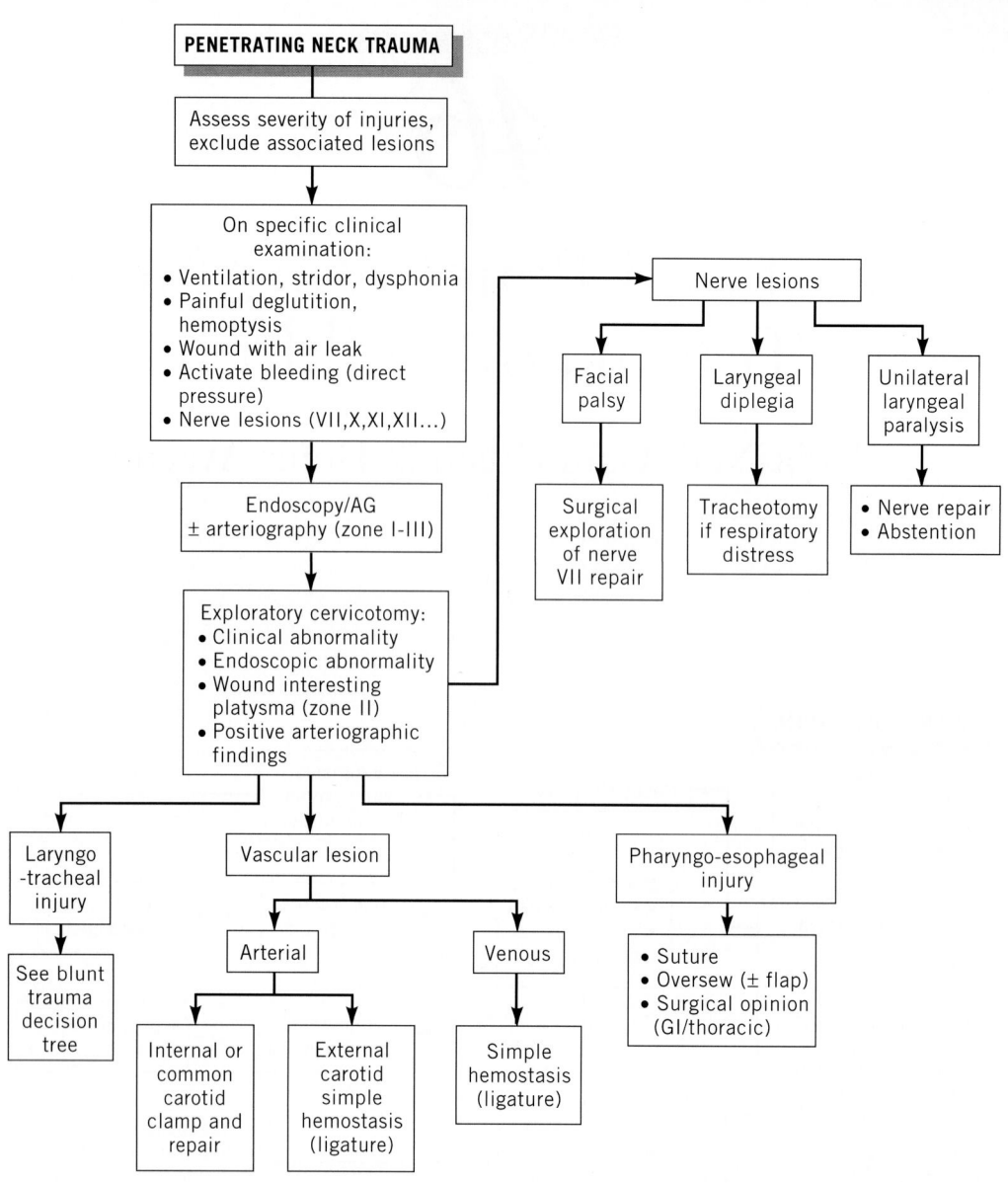

PENETRATING NECK TRAUMA

Assess severity of injuries, exclude associated lesions

On specific clinical examination:
- Ventilation, stridor, dysphonia
- Painful deglutition, hemoptysis
- Wound with air leak
- Activate bleeding (direct pressure)
- Nerve lesions (VII,X,XI,XII...)

Nerve lesions

Facial palsy → Surgical exploration of nerve VII repair

Laryngeal diplegia → Tracheotomy if respiratory distress

Unilateral laryngeal paralysis →
- Nerve repair
- Abstention

Endoscopy/AG ± arteriography (zone I-III)

Exploratory cervicotomy:
- Clinical abnormality
- Endoscopic abnormality
- Wound interesting platysma (zone II)
- Positive arteriographic findings

Laryngo-tracheal injury → See blunt trauma decision tree

Vascular lesion

Arterial
- Internal or common carotid clamp and repair
- External carotid simple hemostasis (ligature)

Venous → Simple hemostasis (ligature)

Pharyngo-esophageal injury →
- Suture
- Oversew (± flap)
- Surgical opinion (GI/thoracic)

Neck trauma is relatively rare in children. Compared with the literature on adults, few publications have been devoted to childhood neck trauma (1–8). In the report by Ford et al. (5), neck trauma (blunt or penetrating) represented 0.5% of all admissions to the trauma unit of a children's hospital. Head and neck injuries accounted for approximately 1% to 2% of admissions for childhood trauma in a study by Cooper et al. (1) and for 1.9% in a study by Hall et al. (6). In a study, Lee (9) demonstrated that severe laryngeal fractures mainly occurred in patients over 61 years old, probably due to calcification of the cartilages; however, they also occurred in patients less than 20 years old, presumably from the thinness of the laryngeal cartilages. Despite the relatively protected position of the pediatric larynx, the child with neck trauma may develop respiratory distress more quickly than the adult because of the relatively small size of the pediatric airway and the propensity for soft tissue edema of the pediatric larynx.

As in adults, there is a clear male predominance to neck trauma in children.

Accidents account for the majority of cases. Blunt neck trauma in children is largely associated with bicycle accidents from falling onto the handlebar or clothesline injuries.

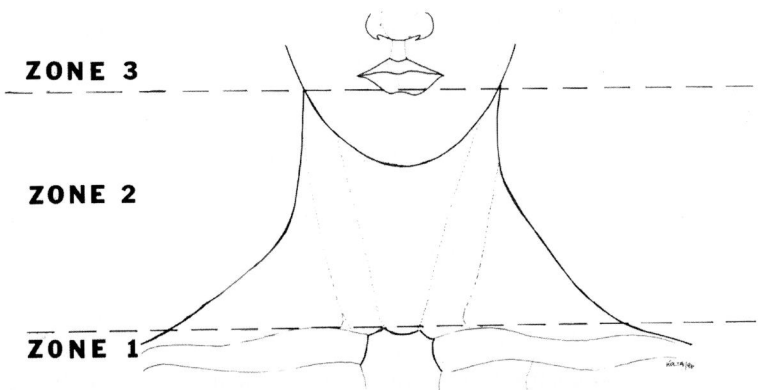

FIGURE 1 The three zones of injury in penetrating neck trauma.

Penetrating neck trauma is usually from accidental falls onto a sharp object, animal bites, stab wounds, and missile wounds.

The low frequency of pediatric neck trauma can be attributed to certain anatomic characteristics of children (2,3,5). The neck is shorter, the larynx is higher, and the whole is protected by the arch of the mandible. The laryngotracheal cartilages are more elastic and there is greater mobility of the laryngotracheal axis, which tends to decrease the risk of fracture.

The neck region is anatomically divided into three zones (10–12). This classification is particularly relevant for the management of penetrating neck trauma (Fig. 1):

- Zone I: The lower neck region is situated below the sternal notch. Many vessels such as the aorta, subclavian artery, innominate artery, carotid artery, vertebral artery, and jugular veins are at risk of injury by traumatic lesions affecting zone I.
- Zone II: The middle neck region stretches from the sternal notch to the angle of the mandible. The major vessels that traverse this region are the jugular veins, common carotid artery, and the proximal parts of the internal carotid artery and of the external carotid artery and its branches.
- Zone III: The upper neck region extends from the angle of the mandible to the base of the skull. This region also has many vessels at risk including the external carotid artery and some of its branches (internal maxillary, facial, ascending pharyngeal, middle meningeal, lingual), the jugular veins, and the vertebral plexus.

 PATIENT ASSESSMENT

General Measures

Initial Assessment of Life-threatening Injuries

At the scene of the accident or in the emergency department, the severity of the trauma must be assessed rapidly and if necessary, the patient is resuscitated prior to investigating and instituting specific treatment of the neck injury. In such situations, the child's ventilatory status usually dictates the immediate management. Thus, it is necessary to recognize obstructive injury of the pharyngolaryngotracheal axis by symptoms of stridor, suprasternal or intercostal retraction, and inspiratory hypoventilation. Respiratory distress can also be an indication of cardiopulmonary injury, which must also be excluded. When respiratory distress is present due to obstruction, the child should be taken to the operating room for endoscopy and airway control. Indications for intubation or tracheotomy are discussed later.

In the child with hemorrhagic neck wounds, bleeding can usually be controlled by direct compression (12). If this proves to be unsuccessful, the patient should be operated on immediately to achieve surgical hemostasis. Blind clamping must be avoided as it reduces the chances of vascular repair and may lead to neural lesions (10).

In comatose patients or those at risk of aspiration, protection of the lower airway should be ensured by endotracheal intubation or tracheostomy (10).

Medical History

The circumstances of the trauma should be ascertained by questioning the child or witnesses to the event. Important information to be collected includes the time and circumstances of the event, evolution of the symptoms, and the mechanism of the trauma, which can be especially helpful in predicting the possible tract of the penetrating object in neck wounds.

Associated Injuries

Associated injuries must systematically be searched for in patients with isolated neck trauma as well as in those with multiple trauma. In view of the anatomic proximity, the presence of ophthalmologic, neurologic, or thoracic lesions, must be excluded. With major blunt or penetrating trauma, where the vertebral column might be affected, the head and the neck must be immobilized in a neutral position, until cervical spine radiographs have ruled out a vertebral fracture or dislocation (2). If airway control is necessary in a case of proved or suspected cervical spine trauma, extreme care must be taken to avoid neck hyperextension during intubation, and fiberoptically controlled intubation should be considered.

Blunt Neck Trauma

Clinical Examination in the Emergency Room

In a child with blunt neck trauma the physical examination should assess the presence of respiratory distress. Signs include hypopnea with retractions and stridor, which may be biphasic. Complaints of dysphonia, dysphagia, and hemoptysis indicate laryngopharyngeal injury. Other important indications of significant injury include cervical pain, cervical ecchymosis, and hematoma formation. Digital palpation will reveal changes in the contour of the laryngeal cartilages, with loss of the thyroid prominence and possibly subcutaneous emphysema.

The clinical picture can be extremely misleading, with little or no initial symptomatology but with a risk of subsequent deterioration. Most authors emphasized that mortality and morbidity are directly associated with a delay in diagnosis (3,5,6).

Fiberoptic laryngeal examination plays a central role in assessing the patient and in determining the course of treatment (4,13,14). This technique is simple and safe and allows the site and the type of trauma as well as airway patency to be ascertained. The examiner needs to assess vocal cord and arytenoid mobility, as well as morphologic changes such as edema, ecchymosis, hematoma, mucosal ulcerations, exposed cartilage, epiglottic disruption, avulsed true cord, and arytenoid dislocation.

Even in the absence of respiratory distress, fiberoptic endoscopy should be performed in the emergency room, as this will provide guidance for the further management of the patient. If the fiberoptic endoscopy findings are normal, patients need to be admitted for observation for 24 to 48 hours, owing to the risk of secondary deterioration.

If minor lesions such as laryngeal edema, hematoma, or minor ulcerations are present, or if the symptomatology is not severe and the patient is stable, then an emergency computed tomographic (CT) scan of the neck ought to be obtained. If the findings are normal, patients are admitted for supervision and symptomatic treatment.

If on the other hand fiberoptic examination reveals severe mucosal or cartilaginous damage, or if CT scans show potentially unstable laryngotracheal lesions, laryngotracheobronchial and esophageal endoscopy must be performed under general anesthesia in the operating room. Pharyngoesophageal examination should be performed with a rigid endoscope to look for the rare pharyngeal or esophageal laceration. The results of endoscopy will provide guidance for therapeutic management.

When there is respiratory distress at presentation, the patient must be immediately transferred to the operating room, to perform endoscopy in the safest conditions possible under general anesthesia. If possible, this should be preceded by fiberoptic endoscopy to assess laryngeal function. Control of the airway must be secured by intubation or tracheotomy before other aspects of the patient's management can be considered.

If the patient's condition required intubation or tracheotomy at the scene of the accident, a CT scan of the neck should be carried out on arrival to the emergency department. If CT confirms a diagnosis of a comminuted laryngeal fracture or cricotracheal separation, then an immediate tracheotomy (if the patient is intubated) with open surgical exploration is indicated. Under these circumstances extubation for the purpose of diagnostic endoscopy, even in the operation room, could prove to be dangerous. Blunt neck trauma associated with an extensive cervical hematoma is a rare finding and demands urgent treatment. Bleeding may be due to damage to the carotid vessels caused by a fragment of fractured thyroid cartilage or by a rupture of the thyroid gland. If the condition of the patient permits, a four-vessel arteriography or a contrasted CT scan should be considered but should not delay surgical intervention to achieve hemostasis.

Ancillary Diagnostic Studies

Following the physical examination, additional diagnostic studies can be performed, depending on the clinical context and given that surgical intervention is not urgently needed (7,13,14).

Cervical spine radiographs (anterior view, lateral) allow the detection of vertebral fractures or dislocation, but may also reveal subcutaneous emphysema, displacement of the trachea, or narrowing of the airway. This investigation ought to be routinely done if the condition of the patient permits.

Chest x-ray films (anteroposterior, lateral) must also be obtained very early on, depending on the patient's condition, in order to detect a pneumomediastinum or mediastinal shift, pneumothorax, or hemothorax.

CT of the neck permits excellent views of the laryngotracheal skeleton and the endolaryngeal and perilaryngeal soft tissues (Fig. 2). It is recommended for patients with mild clinical symptomatology or minimal, fiberscopic abnormalities. However, it is not likely to modify the therapeutic management of patients with severe laryngeal lesions that require immediate surgical exploration or, on the contrary, of patients with no clinical symptoms or fiberscopic findings.

Laryngotracheobronchial and pharyngoesophageal endoscopy under general anesthesia (if possible, preceded by laryngeal fiberoptic endoscopy to assess the mobility of the vocal cords) allows a complete assessment of the injuries, although the interpretation of the findings may prove to be difficult. The endoscopic examination must be performed with care, preferably with the aid of telescopic magnification. It is indicated when there is subcutaneous emphysema, respiratory distress, evidence of mucosal or cartilaginous damage on fiberoptic endoscopy, or significant laryngotracheal injury identified on a CT

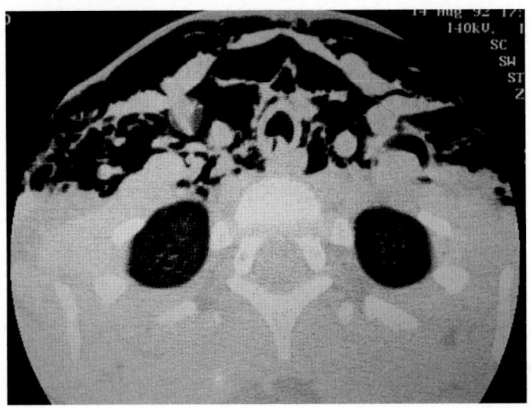

FIGURE 2 Computed tomography of the neck demonstrating air in the subcutaneous and deep spaces, as well as posterior tracheal laceration. (From the collection of J. M. Triglia, M.D.)

scan. Pharyngeal or esophageal lacerations or wounds, laryngeal edema, submucosal hematoma, mucosal ulceration, exposed cartilage, epiglottic disruption, vocal cord disruption, arytenoid dislocation, comminuted laryngeal fracture, cricotracheal separation, and tracheal wounds (in particular, posterior laceration) can be identified during endoscopy.

Arteriography does not play an important role in blunt neck trauma, except in rare cases of extensive cervical hematoma.

Penetrating Neck Trauma

Clinical Examination in the Emergency Room

In the child with penetrating neck trauma, the following manifestations must be looked for immediately; damage to the laryngotracheal axis, respiratory distress, stridor, dysphonia, hemoptysis, subcutaneous emphysema, and wounds with an associated air leak (1,6,10,12,15). If there is respiratory distress, the priority is the reestablishment of the patency of the airway.

Pharyngoesophageal damage must be ruled out even though a patient might sometimes present with minimal signs at first, such as painful swallowing, dysphagia, hemoptysis, and subcutaneous emphysema (16).

If there is external bleeding (10,12,17), the clinical signs of hypovolemic shock are an indication of the extent of the hemorrhage. The venous or arterial (pulsatile) nature of the blood loss should be ascertained. Bleeding from a penetrating neck wound should initially be controlled by digital compression while awaiting transfer to the operating room for exploratory cervicotomy (blind clamping must be avoided). In addition, one should exclude occult internal hemorrhage by examining for the signs of blood loss or the presence of a cervical or pharyngeal hematoma, which could potentially deteriorate into pharyngeal obstruction and thereby cause respiratory distress. Finally, it should be pointed out that a lesion of the common or internal carotid artery may have consequences in the central nervous system, which need to be recognized preoperatively.

Physical examination of the patient should take into account the possibility of lesions affecting the major neural structures exiting the skull base including cranial nerves VII, X, and XI, the recurrent laryngeal nerves, the brachial plexus, and the phrenic nerve.

Examination of the cervical injury must be extremely detailed. The nature of the wound, its location (zone I, II, or III), the tract of the penetrating object, the presence of external bleeding and foreign bodies, and the vitality of the soft tissues must be assessed. Traditionally, the plane of the platysma muscle is used to differentiate between superficial and deep injuries. The debate between the advocates of exploratory cervicotomy in all patients with injury penetrating the platysma and advocates of selective surgical exploration only in symptomatic patients is discussed in "Treatment Recommendations." However, one must be wary of being complacent when dealing with puncture wounds, since the size of the entrance wound may not correspond to the depth or breadth of the neck lesion.

If the patient's ventilatory and hemodynamic status is stable, nasopharyngeal fiberoptic endoscopy should be performed in the emergency room in order to identify pharyngolaryngeal lesions and to evaluate vocal cord mobility. However, if the patient is unstable, an exploratory cervicotomy preceded by endoscopic examination is required.

Ancillary Diagnostic Studies

Following the physical examination, additional diagnostic studies can be performed, depending on the clinical context (10,11,12,17).

Cervical spine radiographs (anterior, lateral) allow visualization of cervical spine lesions, especially in cases of ballistic trauma or of lesions near the vertebrae. They can also be helpful in identifying displacement of the trachea and subcutaneous emphysema.

They are not required routinely, as in blunt trauma, but the context of the trauma and the clinical state of the patient should dictate their definitive need.

Chest x-ray films (anteroposterior, lateral) ought to be obtained very early on, in order to detect associated thoracomediastinal lesions, if the condition of the patient allows.

A barium esophagography is employed in patients with suspected esophageal injury, which is identified by extravasation of the contrast material. It allows confirmation of the diagnosis and localization of the level of the lesion. Nevertheless, esophageal injury cannot be ruled out by a normal-appearing esophagram.

Rigid panendoscopy with telescopic magnification must be performed when laryngotracheal or pharyngoesophageal injury is clinically suspected. This should be preceded by fiberoptic endoscopy if possible. It must also routinely be employed before any exploratory cervicotomy of a neck injury, regardless of the indication for the cervical exploration. Pharyngeal and esophageal wounds or lacerations and laryngotracheal lesions such as vocal cord transection or disruption, false vocal cord injuries, epiglottic disruption or injury, arytenoid dislocation, cricotracheal separation, tracheal injury, mucosal ulceration, submucosal hematoma, and exposed cartilage must be excluded.

Four-vessel arteriography is indicated in patients with extensive hematoma of the lower neck, and injuries to zones I and III of the neck.

PEARLS AND PERILS

1. Undetected associated lesions must be systematically searched for by physical examination, because of the anatomic proximity of the face, the base of the skull, the cervical spine, and the thorax. Suspicion of associated injuries demands appropriate imaging techniques.
2. All patients with blunt trauma, even those with few or no symptoms, must remain under medical supervision for 24 to 48 hours due to the risk of delayed deterioration.
3. The size of the entrance wound of the neck injury may not correspond to the depth and breadth of the wound. A small puncture wound may be associated with major vascular or visceral lesions.

 ## TREATMENT RECOMMENDATIONS

The following is based on the authors' preferences.

Therapeutic Indications

Role of Medical Treatment (1,4,10,13,14)

The initial management, of a child with blunt or penetrating neck trauma should follow the basic principles of trauma resuscitation.

The airway is secured if there is respiratory distress, by intubation or tracheotomy. Cervical hemorrhage is controlled with homolateral neck compression. Venous access is obtained with a large-bore cannula and blood loss is replaced with colloid solutions or packed red blood cells, or both. When evaluating blood loss in children, it is important to take into account the child's age and weight. The intravenous line is usually situated in the upper limb. However, in patients presenting with a lower neck wound, it is preferable to have intravenous access located in the lower limb, because of the risk of lesions to the subclavian or innominate vessels. These measures must be carried out prior to arteriography or surgical exploration.

In patients with blunt or penetrating neck trauma that might involve the spinal column, the head and neck are immobilized in a neutral position, until radiologic investigations of the cervical region of the spine have been performed.

The authors recommend the systematic use of antibiotics in all patients with penetrating neck trauma and in patients with blunt neck trauma associated with laryngotracheal or pharyngoesophageal wounds. When there are obvious infectious complications (mediastinitis, parapharyngeal abscess), the authors use broad-spectrum antibiotics (covering *Streptococcus, Staphylococcus,* gram-negative, and anaerobic organisms), which are changed as dictated by culture results. In the absence of obvious infection, the authors prescribe an 8-day course of prophylactic antibiotics (usually amoxicillin–clavulanic acid). Antitetanus vaccination must be ascertained, just as for other types of penetrating injuries. Antirabies treatment should be considered after animal bites.

The administration of corticosteroids locally (aerosol therapy) or systemically is mainly employed in patients with edematous or inflammatory laryngotracheal lesions. In patients with edematous or inflammatory laryngeal lesions or in the presence of laryngeal hematoma with no respiratory distress (which therefore does not require the reestablishment of the airway), the authors combine local and systemic corticosteroid therapy at a dose equivalent to 1 mg of prednisone per kilogram per day for 5 days, and then progressively decrease and stop the therapy over 5 days. If intubation or stenting has been required during the treatment of a laryngotracheal lesion, the authors give corticosteroids to cover the extubation or the removal of the stent. They also use corticosteroids if the postoperative course is complicated by the development of inflammatory granulation tissue.

Criteria for Surgical Intervention in Penetrating Trauma

There is a great deal of controversy regarding the management of a deep neck wound penetrating the platysma muscle. There is agreement that surgical exploration is indicated when the symptomatology is suggestive of a vascular, visceral, or airway lesion.

However, when a patient with a cervical wound does not present any symptoms, management differs among authors. Some advocate systematic surgical exploration of all deep wounds while others employ selective surgical exploration based on the results of ancillary diagnostic studies, and a few suggest observation only of asymptomatic patients. The arguments in favor of systematic surgical exploration are the low rate of morbidity and mortality associated with this procedure and the fear of occult lesions (10). The arguments in favor of selective exploration are the high rate of negative explorations (36% to 63%) and the safety and efficacy of this approach (15,18).

The authors' management of asymptomatic patients is based on the site of the injury. They systematically explore all deep wounds situated in zone II. Indeed, a surgical approach to lesions in this region does not represent a major operative risk and is not technically difficult. After endoscopy, surgical exploration is performed via the orifice of the wound, which sometimes has to be enlarged, and follows the entire length of the penetrations tract. If an injury is found and cannot be repaired via the original wound, a new more appropriate incision should be made.

The authors selectively explore neck wounds involving zone I depending on the results of arteriography and endoscopy. Finally, they selectively explore neck wounds involving zone III depending on the results of arteriography.

Criteria for Surgical Intervention in Blunt Trauma

Vascular and pharyngoesophageal lesions are relatively rare in patients with blunt neck trauma. The diagnosis is based on the clinical examination and endoscopy and radiologic investigations.

The criteria for operating on patients with laryngotracheal trauma are complicated (13,14). It is beyond the scope of this chapter to give an exhaustive list of all laryngotracheal lesions that may be encountered, but indications for open neck exploration should include displaced fractures of thyroid or cricoid cartilages, cricotracheal separation, disruption of the vocal cords (in particular at the level of the anterior commissure), epiglottic disruption, extensive endolaryngeal mucosal lesions, and large tracheal wounds.

Intervention should be performed early, ideally within 12 to 24 hours of the injury and after having secured a stable airway.

Patients who do not require airway management or surgical intervention are hospitalized and followed with daily fiberoptic examination (4,13,19).

Treatment Principles for Specific Lesions

Management of Laryngotracheal Lesions

Restoration of Airway Patency   Securing the airway is essential in patients with respiratory distress and laryngotracheal lesions necessitating surgical intervention. While most authors (13,20) recommend performing tracheostomy with local anesthesia for adults, this is not possible in children.

The authors prefer an initial endotracheal intubation with an undersized endotracheal tube, which can be replaced by an elective tracheotomy if required. Apart from extreme emergencies where field intubation is required, intubation should ideally be performed in the operating room during endoscopy under general anesthesia. The use of a rigid bronchoscope is helpful if a standard endotracheal tube proves to be difficult to place or in trauma cases where there is a risk of sudden deterioration. An example of this would be a cricotracheal separation for which the rigid bronchoscope can ensure the child's ventilation while a tracheostomy is performed. The decision to perform a tracheostomy is dependent on the ventilatory status of the patient and the results of endoscopy.

The authors have found that tracheostomy is essential when there is trauma to the larynx and the trachea that requires open surgical intervention, especially if stenting might be needed later postoperatively. In certain cases where there is extensive and compressive subcutaneous emphysema due to a small tear of the air passages, especially a posterior tracheal tear, and where surgical repair is not essential, a tracheostomy may also be the treatment of choice as it establishes patency of the airway and allows evacuation of the leaked subcutaneous air. However, if respiratory distress is caused by purely inflammatory or edematous laryngeal lesions or by submucosal hematomas, the authors avoid tracheostomy and prefer endotracheal intubation for 2 to 4 days combined with a course of corticosteroids.

General Principles of the Surgical Management of Laryngotracheal Trauma   In view of the range of lesions that can be encountered, the authors present certain general principles that can be adapted to each situation (12,13,20,21,22).

Several types of skin incisions can be employed two of which are shown in Figure 3. The first is a horizontal incision with a slight concavity superiorly between the thyroid

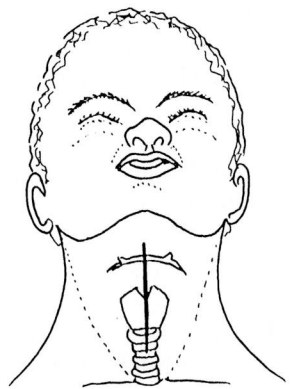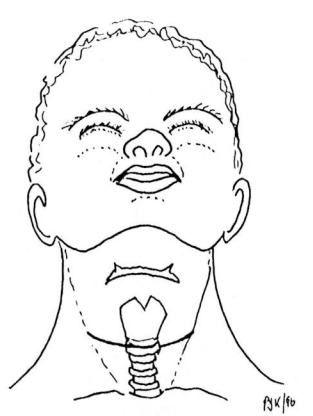

FIGURE 3 Incisions utilized for the exploration of laryngotracheal trauma.

notch and the cricoid cartilage. The other is a vertical midline incision from the hyoid bone to the inferior border of the cricoid. If possible, the authors try to keep a band of skin between the cervical incision and the tracheotomy. Occasionally, the laryngotracheal axis can be reached via the wound itself in cases of penetrating trauma.

The endolarynx sometimes can be approached through a thyroid cartilage fracture, especially in cases of paramedian fracture. If there is no preexisting fracture, the best approach is provided by a midline thyrotomy.

The goal of operative repair of the lesions is restoration of the normal anatomy. Mucosal lesions must be carefully sutured, avoiding any tension, with absorbable sutures (4-0 or 5-0). Where there has been a loss of tissue, the damage should be repaired using local mucosal flaps from the epiglottis, the false vocal cords, and the aryepiglottiic folds, or mucosal grafts from the hypopharynx or buccal cavity.

The restoration of the cartilaginous skeleton must also be extremely thorough, with great attention paid to the external perichondrium. This is best do with absorbable perichondrial sutures or transcartilaginous steel sutures.

The use of internal stenting is a matter of debate but must sometimes be considered. Many different stents are available, including the Aboulker stent, the Montgomery stent, a finger of surgical glove filled with foam sponge, and a Silastic Swiss roll. The authors have primarily used the Silastic Swiss roll fixated by translaryngeal sutures, as described by Evans for laryngotracheal reconstruction.

Unstable comminuted cartilage fractures and major mucosal damage are indications for stenting. Based on the authors' experience with the surgical treatment of childhood laryngotracheal stenosis and a review of the literature (13,23), the duration of stenting should be 2 to 4 weeks.

Special Cases (20,21,22) Trauma to the thyroid notch of the thyroid cartilage is frequently associated with a disruption of the stalk of the epiglottis and of the vocal cords. The stalk of the epiglottis must be secured to the thyrohyoid membrane or by transcartilaginous sutures to the thyroid cartilage. If the epiglottic stalk cannot be properly stabilized, it is resected and the proximal epiglottis is fixed to the hyoid bone. Similarly, the vocal cords must be stretched and fixed either to the external perichondrium, to cartilage, or to prelaryngeal muscles.

Cricotracheal separation, when complete, is frequently associated with transection of the recurrent laryngeal nerves. The emergency treatment consists of cricotracheal reanastomosis, starting with the posterior wall. Exploration for the recurrent nerves often proves to be difficult and may be of questionable value since reanastomosis is not known to restore laryngeal function. Nevertheless, if the transected ends of recurrent laryngeal nerve are found, primary end-to-end neurorrhaphy can be attempted.

Comminuted fracture of the anterior arch of the cricoid is associated with risk of chondronecrosis and secondary subglottic stenosis. If the arch cannot be restore then it should be excised and a thyrotracheal anastomosis performed. When arytenoid dislocation occurs as an isolated lesion, an initial endoscopic repair is possible. If this is unsuccessful or if there are associated lesions, the repositioning must be performed by a translaryngeal approach with mucosal oversewing of denuded areas and arytenoidopexy.

Management of Vascular Injuries

Vascular injuries are seen in 40% of patients with penetrating neck trauma and represent one of the main causes of mortality (12). After diagnostic evaluation suggests a vascular wound, surgical intervention must be urgently performed.

The surgical approach will depend on the site of the wound and the results of arteriography (12,17).

Adequate access to zone I (Fig. 4) is usually gained by an oblique incision just above and parallel to the clavicle. Resection of the medial half of the clavicle can enhance visualization. If exposure is still inadequate, access to the right subclavian or innominate vessels can be achieved by a median sternotomy. Access to the left subclavian artery requires

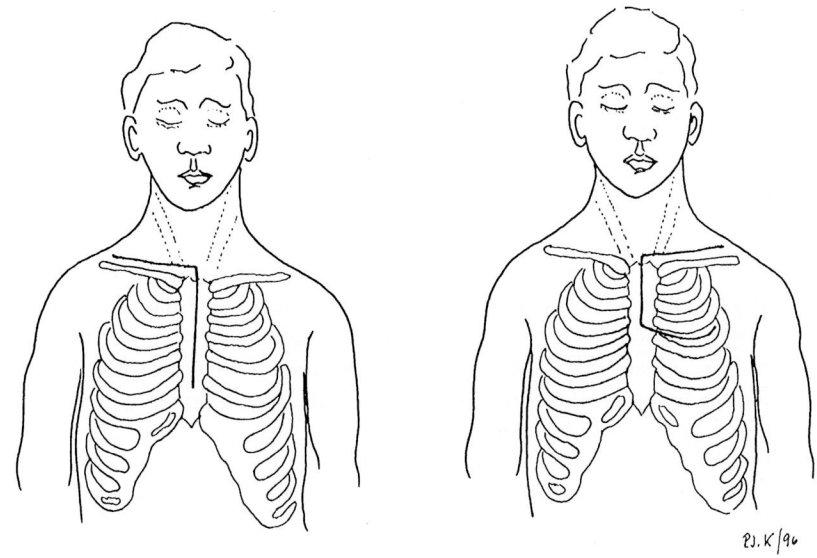

A   B

FIGURE 4 Primary neck incision for injury involving zone I of the neck with potential thoracic extensions. **A:** For right subclavian or innominate injuries. **B:** For left subclavian injuries.

anterolateral thoracotomy through the third or fourth intercostal space. The two transverse cervical and thoracic incisions can be connected by a superior median sternotomy, thereby resulting in a "book" thoracotomy. Exposure of zone II (Fig. 5) is usually performed by a standard incision made along the anterior border of the sternocleidomastoid muscle or through the wound itself. Injuries involving zone III (see Fig. 5) are particularly difficult to manage surgically because of the problems in gaining access to the skull base. Parotidectomy can provide partial access and further exposure can be achieved by mandibular subluxation or lateral mandibulotomy. In situations of surgically uncontrolled hemorrhage or when vascular lesions are inaccessible to surgical intervention as revealed by arteriography, embolization should be considered (11).

Depending on the lesions, surgical hemostasis can be achieved by a variety of techniques, including lateral suturing, primary end-to-end suturing, vein grafting, synthetic bypass material grafting, or ligation. Overall, conservation and reestablishment of blood flow should be employed in patients with common carotid artery and internal carotid

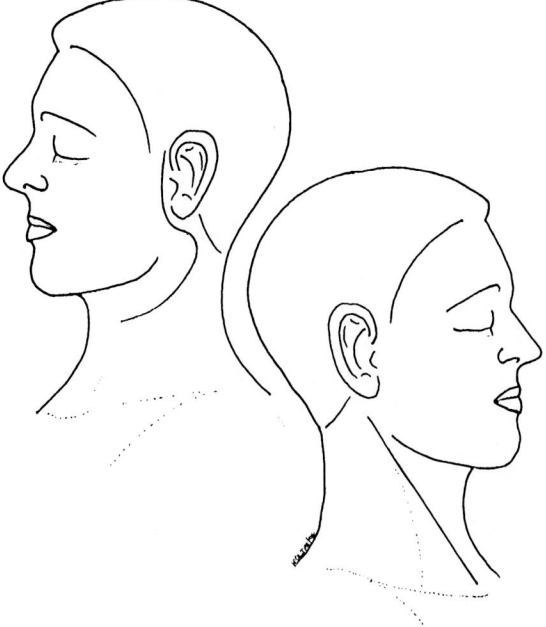

FIGURE 5 **A:** Incision utilized for exploration of penetrating neck trauma involving zone III. **B:** Incision utilized for exploration of penetrating neck trauma involving zone II.

artery lesions. Ligation is safe for the external carotid system, the vertebral artery, and the internal jugular vein.

Management of Pharyngoesophageal Lesions (12,21,22)

Most puncture wounds of the pharynx or esophagus can be medically treated. A nasogastric tube is inserted, the patient is kept off of oral intake, and intravenous antibiotic therapy is instituted.

With major disruptions, surgical repair must be carried out as soon as possible. A nasogastric tube should be inserted prior to surgery in order to facilitate visualization of the digestive tract. Surgical repair involves closure of the mucosal layer with inverting sutures and closure of the muscular layer with absorbable sutures. When there is excessive loss of pharyngeal mucosa and primary repair is not possible, than a draining pharyngotomy is required. This will heal on its own in time.

If combined tracheal and esophageal injuries are present, the interposition of a strap muscle flap between the trachea and the esophagus is performed to prevent a tracheoesophageal fistula.

Management of Nerve Injuries

Peripheral nerve injuries may occur with penetrating neck trauma. Immediate primary repair offers the best chance of restoring a severed nerve. Unfortunately, surgical repair is not always possible due to the difficulty of visualizing the proximal and distal nerve ends in a traumatic surgical field. Despite the fact that the consequences of neglecting nerve lesions are variable and that the results of surgical repair are unpredictable, the authors nevertheless believe that it is important to attempt to reanastomose the facial nerve, the recurrent laryngeal nerves, and the phrenic nerve.

The authors use microsurgical techniques with the aid of an operating microscope. The nerves are sutured without tension with nonabsorbable 9-0 monofilament sutures. If necessary, a free nerve graft is used between the cut segments. Adequate access to lesions of the facial nerve can be obtained via a superficial parotidectomy.

The correct treatment of recurrent nerve injuries is a subject of great controversy. Many techniques have been proposed, including neurorrhaphy, free nerve grafting, use of a neuromuscular pedicle, and selective anastomosis, but consistent outcomes remain elusive. Nevertheless, when the local conditions are favorable, the authors utilize a simple neurorrhaphy, with free nerve graft when necessary.

Management of Other Injuries (23)

Submandibular gland lesions may result in hemorrhage or a leak of saliva, and should be treated with submandibular gland excision.

Parotid gland injuries result in devitalized tissue, hemorrhage, and facial nerve injury. After facial nerve exploration, the devitalized tissue is debrided and hemostasis is obtained. When the parotid duct has been severed, primary end-to-end anastomosis and stent insertion (silicone tube or Teflon catheter) for 2 weeks should be attempted. If the degree of trauma precludes repair, a parotidectomy should be considered.

The thyroid gland is a highly vascular structure and injuries are associated with brisk hemorrhage. Although it is desirable to preserve the parenchyma of the thyroid while at the same time achieving hemostasis, sometimes it is impossible to control the bleeding without a hemithyroidectomy or a subtotal thyroidectomy. Under these circumstances, the basic principles of thyroid surgery should be followed including the location of the recurrent laryngeal nerves and the parathyroid glands and the postoperative monitoring of thyroid function and serum calcium.

Thoracic duct lesions need to be excluded if there is trauma to the lower region of the left side of the neck. Such lesions may manifest themselves by the presence of an effusion of lymph in the wound. Identification of the duct may be difficult; however, ligation is the proper treatment.

MANAGEMENT OF COMPLICATIONS

Laryngotracheal Stenosis

External trauma to the larynx and to the trachea is a known cause of acquired laryngotracheal stenosis. Several prognostic factors that predispose children to the development of stenosis have been identified (14,19,23). These include blunt trauma, major trauma with mucosal or cartilaginous damage, the need for a stent, laryngeal immobility, delayed treatment, and postoperative infection. Such stenoses are often complex and will require laryngotracheoplasty for decannulation.

The risk of developing laryngotracheal stenosis can be minimized by early intervention, meticulous repair of mucosal and cartilaginous lesions, endolaryngeal stenting of cohort duration, perioperative antibiotics, and regular endoscopic surveillance with excision of granulation tissues. The role of gastroesophageal reflux in the pathogenesis of laryngotracheal stenosis is a matter of great debate. The authors recommend antireflux treatment systematically during the postoperative period.

Phonatory Sequelae of Laryngeal Trauma

The prognostic factors cited above with respect to stenosis are also predictive of poor phonatory outcomes (19,23). Recent publications (24,25) showed that minimally displaced fractures of the thyroid cartilage can lead to poor voice quality, indicating the vulnerability of voice to laryngeal trauma. Applying the principles previously outlined is the best way to optimize the postinjury voice; however, results tend to be very unpredictable and secondary therapeutic interventions are of limited value.

Vascular Complications

Vascular trauma, especially if undiagnosed, can be complicated by the development of arterial aneurysms, with an associated risk of rupture, infection, or thrombosis or the development of arteriovenous fistulas, with a risk of cardiac decompensation. In view of these late risks, the authors believe that all penetrating neck trauma, even if asymptomatic, must be evaluated with arteriography for lesions to zones I and III, and cervicotomy for wounds involving zone II.

CONCLUSIONS

Neck trauma is rare in children but can be life-threatening and can lead to long-term ventilatory, phonatory, and neurologic sequelae. The management of such patients must take into account the possible involvement of all the anatomic structures in the region of the neck. Even with apparently minor trauma, a rational structured approach as outlined is necessary and will allow a reduction in the morbidity and mortality associated with these types of injuries.

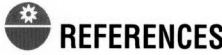
REFERENCES

1. Cooper A, Barlow B, Niemirska M, Gandhi R. *J Pediatr Surg* 1987;22:24–27.
2. Lusk RP. *Clin Pediatr* 1986;25:445–447.
3. Myer CM III, Orobello P, Cotton RT, Bratcher GO. *Laryngoscope* 1987;97:1043–1048.
4. Gold SM, Gerber ME, Shott SR, Myer CM III. *Arch Otolaryngol Head Neck Surg* 1997;123:83–87.
5. Ford HR, Gardner MJ, Lynch JM. *J Pediatr Surg* 1995;30:331–335.
6. Hall JR, Reyes HM, Meller JL. *J Trauma* 1991;31:1614–1617.
7. Humar A, Pitters C. *Pediatr Emerg Care* 1991;7:291–293.
8. Martin WS, Gussack GS. *Laryngoscope* 1990;100:1288–1291.
9. Lee SY. *Ann Otol Rhinol Laryngol* 1992;101:270–274.
10. Saletta JD, Lowe RJ, Lim LT, Thornton J, Delk S, Moss GS. *J Trauma* 1976;16:579–587.
11. Sclafani SJA, Panetta T, Goldstein AS, et al. *J Trauma* 1985;25:871–879.
12. Miller RH, Duplechain JK. *Otol Clin North Am* 1991;24:15–29.
13. Schaefer SD. *Arch Otolaryngol Head Neck Surg* 1991;117:35–39.
14. Gussack GS, Jurkovich GJ, Luterman A. *Laryngoscope* 1986;96:660–665.
15. Jurkovich GJ, Zingarelli W, Wallace J, Curreri PW. *J Trauma* 1985;25:819–822.
16. Weigelt JA, Thal ER, Snyder WH, Fry RE, Meier DE, Kilman WJ. *Am J Surg* 1987;154:619–622.
17. Livingstone AS. *Otol Clin North Am* 1983;16:671–678.
18. Ayuyao AM, Kaledzi YL, Parsa MH, Freeman HP. *Ann Surg* 1985;202:563–567.
19. Cohn AM, Larson DL. *Arch Otolaryngol* 1976;102:166–170.
20. Fabre A, Menard M, Lacau St. Guily J, Brasnu D, Laccourreye H. Editions Techniques—*Encycl Med Chir* (Paris, France). Oto-rhino-laryngologie, 1987.
21. Guerrier Y. *Traité de technique chirurgicale ORL et cervico-faciale.* Paris: Masson, 1988.
22. Buffe P, Poncet JL, Verdalle P. Editions Techniques—*Encycl Med Chir* (Paris, France). Techniques chirurgicales—Tête et cou, 1993.
23. Leopold DA. *Arch Otolaryngol* 1983;109:106–111.
24. Hirano M, Kurita S, Terasawa R. *Arch Otolaryngol* 1985;111:59–61.
25. Stanley RB, Cooper DS, Florman SH. *Ann Otol Rhinol Laryngol* 1987;96:493–496.

E-N. Garabédian and D. Ayache. Department of Pediatric Ear, Nose, and Throat, Children's Hospital Armand-Trousseau, 75012 Paris, France.

- *Practical Pediatric Otolaryngology*
- edited by Robin T. Cotton and Charles M. Myer, III
- Lippincott-Raven Publishers, Philadelphia © 1999

47

Pediatric Facial
Soft Tissue Trauma

Kevin A. Shumrick

OVERVIEW

Children are subjected to a wide variety of facial soft tissue trauma due to their relative incoordination, low height (compared to the adult world), and lack of sophistication with regard to their external environment. In fact, it must be the rare child who makes it to adolescence without the need for management of some sort of facial injury. Fortunately, most of these injuries are not a serious threat to the physical health of the child; nonetheless, facial injuries may have significant psychological sequelae. For instance, just the process of having a facial wound sutured in an emergency room setting may be extremely traumatic for a child, leaving life-long negative feelings regarding hospitals and physicians. Additionally, facial wounds that fail to achieve optimal results (with scarring or deformity) have the potential to set the stage for self-image and self-confidence problems that may alter the individual's adult personality and have a significant impact on the course of the child's life. It is the purpose of this chapter to provide an overview of pediatric facial soft tissue injuries and effective methods for not only managing the physical damage, but also minimizing the psychic trauma.

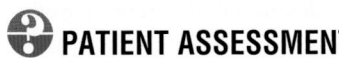 PATIENT ASSESSMENT

Clinical History

An accurate clinical history regarding the cause of pediatric facial trauma is invaluable for completely and accurately assessing a wound and, most importantly, planning appropriate treatment. Unfortunately, many pediatric facial injuries are not witnessed and the traumatic event must be reconstructed retrospectively. As such, it is common that much valuable information is lost regarding the wounding agent, degree of contamination, and other associated injuries. Additionally, the clinician treating pediatric facial trauma must always keep in mind the possibility that the facial injuries were not accidental, but intentionally inflicted, and it is every physician's responsibility to investigate any unusual or suspicious injuries to a child. Particular attention should be given to cases in which the child is too young to have been in the traumatic situation (such as an infant who cannot walk falling against a table) or multiple injuries on both sides of the head when there was only one traumatic event reported (such as multiple facial bruises and contusions when the child supposedly only fell once).

Historical issues of concern include the following:

What was the mechanism of injury?
Was the patient mobile, restrained, or stationary?
Was the impacting object mobile or stationary?

Was the injury the result of blunt or penetrating trauma? Both?

Can you estimate the degree of energy transfer—high versus low?

Were there coincident fatalities?

Are there associated thermal or chemical injuries?

Assessment of Soft Tissue Injuries

There are a number of possible types of soft tissue facial injuries, including contusions and avulsions, but the most common soft tissue injuries, particularly in children, are lacerations. Lacerations may range from simple, superficial wounds, easily repaired, to injuries that penetrate to involve deeper structures including muscles, nerves, and ducts. Major lacerations, improperly treated, can leave dysfunctional and deforming sequelae. The single most important factor in managing any injury is proper initial evaluation and assessment in order that relevant concerns are identified and a comprehensive treatment plan formulated.

It should also be mentioned that chart documentation is an integral part of modern-day medical care, for both medical follow-up and medicolegal concerns. The following specifics of soft tissue injury should be noted and documented:

1. Laceration shape. Is the wound a straight laceration with clean margins? If so, it can probably be closed primarily with an acceptable result. Is the wound stellate with multiple trifurcations? It should be noted whether the wound margins are very irregular or have adjacent devitalized tissue, as this may have implications for treatment and outcome. While a simple clean laceration may be repaired primarily, a complicated wound with devitalized tissue may require resources not available in the emergency room.
2. Surrounding soft tissue injury—associated contusion. Contusions often result in a very irregular disruption of the skin with surrounding devitalized tissue. These wounds should be documented and managed conservatively. The parents (and sometimes the child) should be informed that these injuries often result in depressed scars that may benefit from scar revision when mature.
3. Loss of soft tissue coverage or lining. Fortunately actual loss of soft tissue is uncommon, but when it occurs, it has significant implications for wound management and eventual outcome. These injuries should be carefully documented and the parents informed accordingly.
4. Injury to structural margins or borders. Soft tissue injuries involving the eyelid, nasal alar rims, auricular helical rims, and the oral stoma must be examined carefully and noted. Full-thickness injuries involving these structures have significant cosmetic and functional implications. The specifics of repairing these structures are discussed later in this chapter.
5. Penetrating soft tissue injuries. Penetrating wounds are dangerous because while the exterior entrance point may seem relatively benign, the possibility of deeper structures being involved must be considered and a thorough physical examination should be performed to rule out the possibility of injury to a significant structure such as a branch of the facial nerve, parotid duct, or the lacrimal apparatus. Timely identification of such an injury is important because delay in repairing these structures can significantly decrease the chances of a successful outcome.

Special Considerations

While most pediatric soft tissue trauma is superficial and involves only the skin and subcutaneous tissue, children may also sustain more severe injuries that are usually associated with adults. Because these injuries may be subtle, and the child is unable to voice symptoms, if the treating physician is not alert to their possibility recognition of these injuries may be delayed and the final outcome compromised.

Facial Nerve

The status of the facial nerve and all its branches should be noted and recorded on the initial evaluation of all facial trauma patients. It is not uncommon for a facial nerve deficit to be noted in a delayed fashion. The question then arises as to whether the deficit occurred immediately (implying a severance of the nerve requiring repair or decompression), or on a delayed basis secondary to tissue edema (implying a contusion of the nerve, which will recover spontaneously). Additionally, during the repair of a facial laceration using local anesthesia, it may be noted that there is a facial nerve deficit. If the functional status of the nerve has not been documented at the initial assessment, there will be uncertainty as to the cause of the palsy and whether it is the result of the initial injury, anesthesia induced (transient), or iatrogenic (during the repair). It is important to establish early on if there has been a transection of the nerve or one of its branches, because an early and accurate repair maximizes the chances of functional regeneration. Note also the fact that the distal portion of the nerve can be stimulated for up to 72 hours following injury, which greatly facilitates accurate identification of the distal end of the nerve for coaptation and repair.

Parotid Duct

Injury to the parotid (or Stensen's) duct should always be considered with any deep cheek laceration or penetrating injury. While an injury or transection of the duct is relatively uncommon, the morbidity of an unrecognized and unrepaired ductal injury is high and can be avoided with timely surgical intervention. The parotid duct exits the parotid gland at approximately the posterior border of the masseter muscle and then travels across the lateral border of the masseter. At the anterior border of the masseter the duct turns medially and enters the oral cavity just lateral to the second upper molar. It should be remembered that the facial nerve lies just lateral to the duct and there is almost always an associated injury to a buccal branch of the facial nerve with any parotid duct injury (Fig. 1). The most common sign of a ductal injury is saliva draining from the wound. The most direct way to confirm a ductal injury is to cannulate the duct intraorally with a lacrimal probe and use the probe to check the integrity of the duct in the depths of the wound. If a laceration or transection is discovered, it should be repaired with fine nylon suture (8-0 or 9-0) using magnification. Some authors advocate leaving a Silastic stent in place for 7 to 10 days after repair (see Fig. 1). If a ductal injury is unrecognized, the patient will return with a sialocele that is often infected. Repair of the duct after formation of a sialocele or fistula is very difficult because of the maceration and friability of the tissues. If a Stensen's duct laceration is diagnosed on a delayed basis and repair is not possible or fails, then conservative therapy is instituted, with anticholinergics to decrease saliva output and pressure dressings with the hope that the gland will atrophy or the ductal injury will seal itself. If the fistula persists, a superficial parotidectomy may be required.

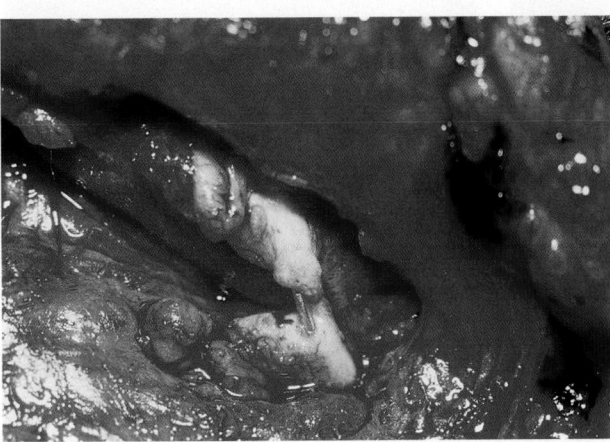

FIGURE 1 Laceration of Stensen's duct with a Silastic tube connecting proximal and distal lumens. Additionally, note the severed buccal branch of the facial nerve lying lateral and superior to the duct. Both the nerve and the duct were repaired with 8-0 nylon.

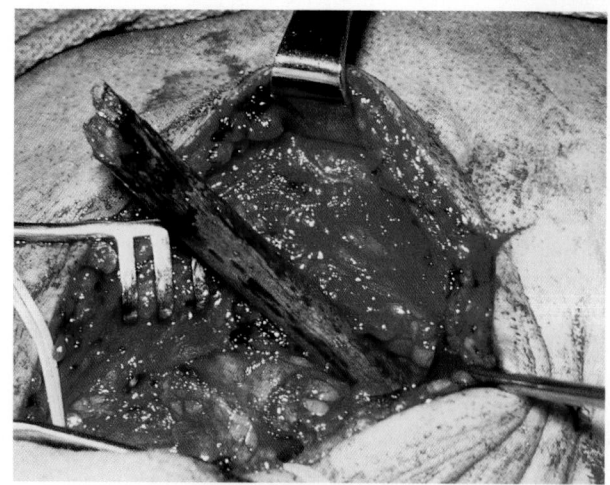
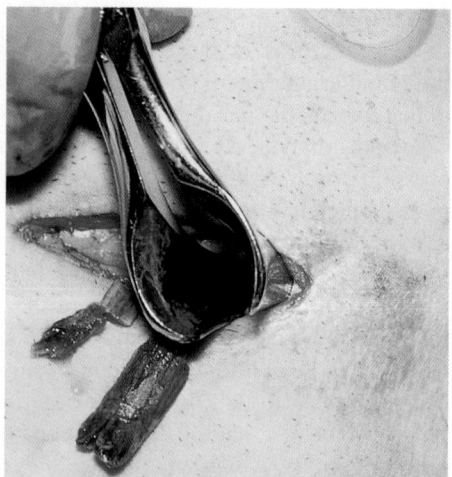

FIGURE 2 **A:** Penetrating wound with tree branch at the time of primary treatment. **B:** Several weeks later the wound began to fester and reexploration revealed retained pieces of wood. This highlights the fact that the physician should always be vigilant of possible retained foreign bodies in penetrating wounds, especially wooden objects.

Lacrimal Apparatus

There should be a high index of suspicion for injury to the lacrimal drainage apparatus with any laceration involving the medial portion of the upper or lower eyelid in the region of the medial canthus laceration. The major sequela of a lacrimal canalicular laceration is epiphora, but this may not be obvious in the acute setting due to associated pain and edema. If there is a question of a canalicular laceration or lacrimal duct laceration, the lacrimal punctum and duct should be cannulated with lacrimal probes and the laceration examined to see if they appear in the wound. If a laceration is identified, it should be repaired over Silastic stents under magnification with fine (8-0) sutures.

Retained Foreign Body

The treating physician should always consider the possibility of a retained foreign body in penetrating injuries involving glass or wood or resulting from striking the ground (Fig. 2). Special mention should be made of the phenomenon of "debris tattooing" resulting from particulate matter being embedded in the dermis and not appropriately removed (Fig. 3). Typically this occurs as a result of abrasions sustained from falling and sliding along the ground or pavement. The epidermis is denuded and dirt, stones, and

FIGURE 3 **A:** Periocular debris tattooing from a blast injury. **B:** Debris tattooing due to abrasion from pavement. In both cases the wound has healed and removal of dermal debris is now extremely difficult.

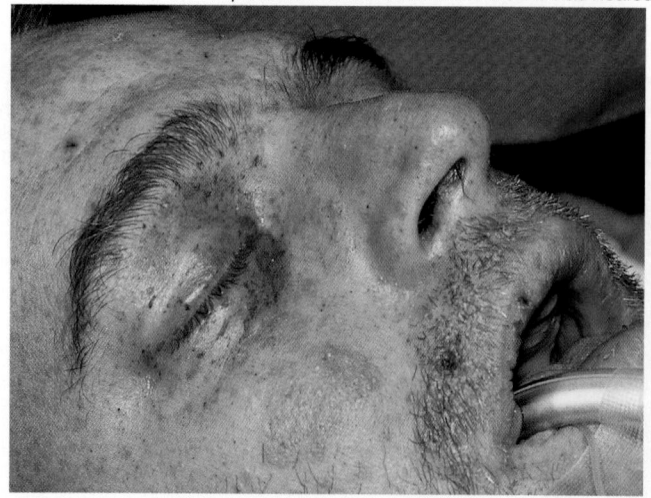
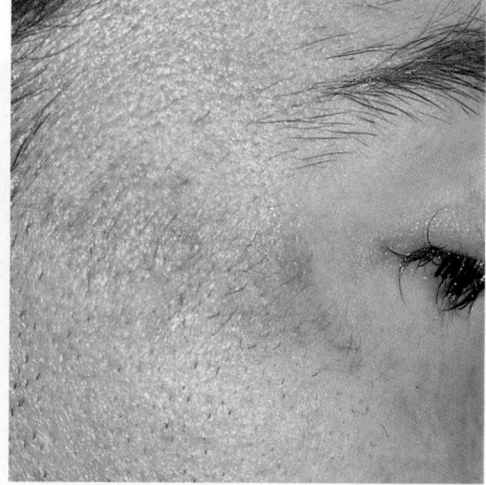

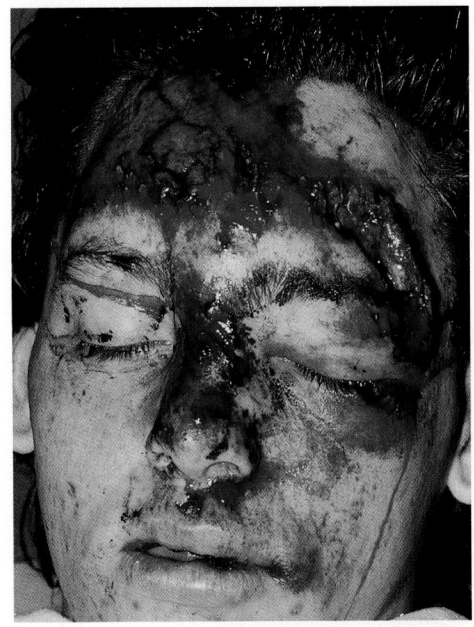

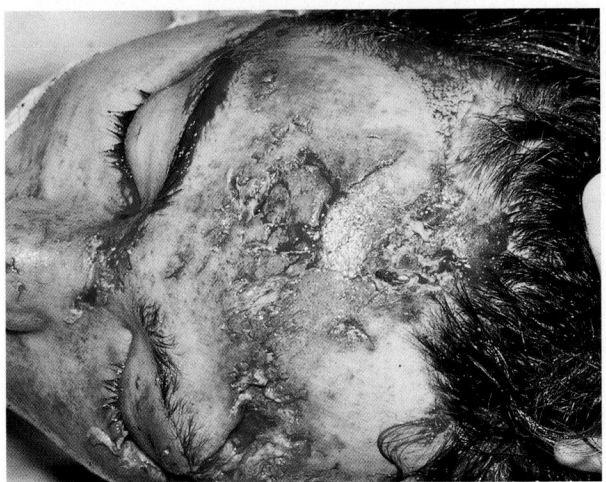

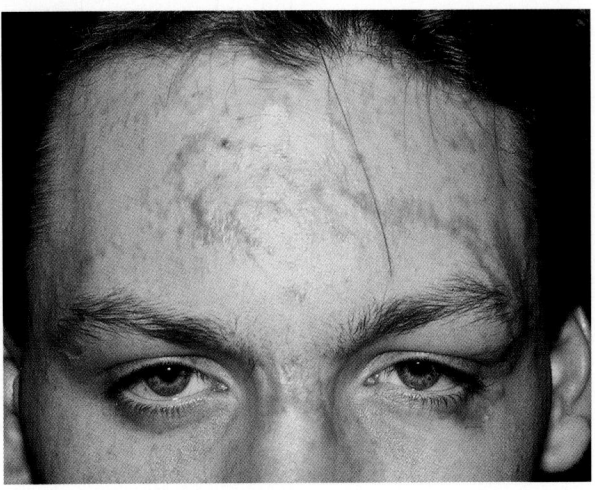

FIGURE 4 A: Facial abrasions sustained from a motorcycle accident with large amounts of debris ground into the wound. **B:** Patient in the operating room after irrigation and acute dermabrasion. **C:** Three-month postoperative result showing some residual scar redness but no debris tattooing.

other debris implanted in the dermis. The epidermis will then resurface the wound and the retained material will be visible externally. Once the epidermis has sealed the wound, it is virtually impossible to remove the visible debris short of full-thickness excision of the affected area (late dermabrasion has been disappointing, laser vaporization may eventually prove useful). Therefore, it is important to identify wounds with the potential for debris tattooing because the optimum time to treat this condition is at the time of injury when the epidermis is still open and the foreign material can be removed by scrubbing, irrigation, or dermabrasion (Fig. 4). It should be noted that it is extremely difficult to achieve adequate local anesthesia for debridement of large areas of abraded tissue and this is probably best performed in the operating room with general anesthesia.

TREATMENT RECOMMENDATIONS

Repair of Soft Tissue Injuries

After injuries to associated deep structures are ruled out, attention may be turned to repair of the superficial soft tissue injury. As noted, the treating physician should always take the time to meticulously remove all foreign bodies from the wound. If the wound appears grossly contaminated, it should be irrigated with copious quantities of saline solution under mild pressure. With regard to debridement of tissue in acute wounds, it is generally accepted that conservative removal of only obviously devitalized tissue should be performed. The specific method of repair or treatment depends primarily on the wound morphology and etiology, and those other relevant factors noted during the wound evaluation.

In what follows, technical pointers are emphasized for the repair of a clean, simple laceration. Additional guidelines are provided regarding management of wound-complicating factors and those cosmetically challenging injuries involving margins and borders.

For repair of a straightforward uncomplicated laceration, the aim should be to provide an anatomically accurate, secure repair. This is best accomplished with complete anesthesia, fine instruments, excellent lighting, and comfortable working conditions for the surgeon. Often these conditions are not met in the usual emergency room setting and the surgeon has a duty to the patient to ensure that the proper conditions and resources are available before beginning a repair. This may mean taking the patient to the operating room, and utilizing general anesthesia, particularly if the patient is uncooperative.

Instruments and Suture Material

Before beginning a discussion of the technical aspects of facial wound repair, it seems appropriate to take a moment to consider instrumentation for facial wound repair. Often, the physician suturing a child in the emergency room is faced with the prospect of using rather crude instruments that do not lend themselves to atraumatic soft tissue handling and optimal soft tissue repair. While maximum soft tissue coadaption may be of little consequence on the hand or trunk, scars on the face are of significant cosmetic, social, and psychological importance, and every effort should be made to minimize the visibility of a facial scar. Toward this end of minimizing facial scarring, an accurate primary repair is the first step. To achieve an accurate repair, the surgeon requires instruments commensurate with the fine work that must be accomplished. The two most important instruments involved in fine suturing are a fine pair of tissue forceps and a fine needle holder. Unfortunately, these are the two instruments most lacking in emergency room suture packs. Typically, the emergency room provides a thick pair of Addison toothed forceps and a long-handled thick-jawed needle holder. These bulky instruments really are inadequate to achieve fine soft tissue work and every effort should be made to upgrade the available instruments, even going so far as to have plastic instruments brought from the operating room. Many facial plastic surgeons own a few key instruments and bring them to the emergency room for facial repairs (Fig. 5).

The next issue to consider is that of suture material. As with instrumentation, the results achieved are often indirectly related to the caliber of the suture material employed (the finer the suture, the better the results). The author rarely uses anything larger than a 6-0 suture on the face (particularly in pediatric patients) and never larger than 5-0. The only time the author would use a 5-0 suture on a pediatric patient would be in the scalp and on a visible soft tissue surface. For absorbable subcutaneous sutures, the author uses 6-0 polyglycolic acid and tries to use as few buried sutures as possible. For the skin sutures, the ideal suture would be a 7-0 monofilament suture. The 7-0 suture, while somewhat fine, provides the best soft tissue approximation. However, the author usually only uses 7-0 permanent suture on patients who may be cooperative for suture removal. Perhaps, the only thing more frustrating than performing a suture repair on an uncooperative child is trying to remove sutures from an uncooperative child. Meticulous hard-fought closures can be destroyed because of a child struggling against suture removal. Therefore, for children who may be uncooperative for suture removal, the author employs a 6-0 fast-absorbing gut suture that is made by Ethicon. This suture is different from the commonly available "mild-chromic" suture, which often persists longer than needed and has needles that are not ideal. This fast-absorbing gut suture has a needle

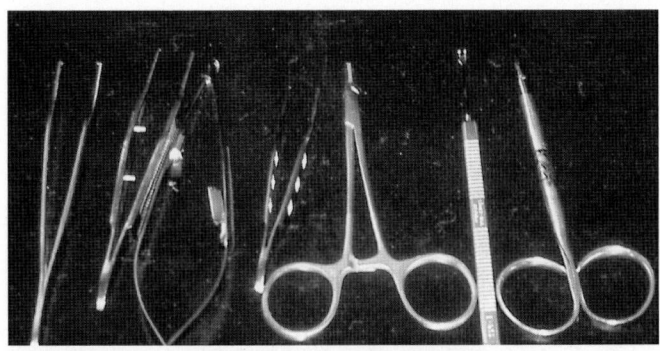

FIGURE 5 Basic set of soft tissue instruments with fine pickups, needle holder, scissors, and skin hooks.

conducive for soft tissue repair and the suture will usually be gone from the wound in 3 to 5 days. The rapid dissolution of this suture prevents the cross-hatching seen with sutures that are left in place longer than a 3 to 5 days and does so without the need for the trauma of suture removal.

Anesthesia for Pediatric Facial Lacerations

Without a doubt the single most important determinant of a positive experience for both the patient and the physician during the management of a pediatric facial laceration is obtaining adequate anesthesia with minimal trauma. In the past, the most commonly employed method of obtaining anesthesia for laceration repair was to infiltrate local anesthetic via a needle stick. Anesthetic infiltration had two negative psychological effects. First, the child's perception of a needle being stuck into an open wound was enough to generate extreme anxiety and would heighten any negative stimuli subsequently encountered. Second, infiltration of the local anesthetic, as expected by the child, is painful from the hydrostatic and chemical properties of the anesthetic. The combination of heightened expectation followed by painful stimuli is often enough to put a child "over the edge" and the child then becomes completely uncooperative with any subsequent endeavors, even if adequate anesthesia has been obtained. This hysterical response then requires placement of restraints, which further aggravates the child, and the following repair is an ordeal for all involved. If the physician is able to achieve anesthesia of the wound without inflicting any additional anxiety or pain, the suture repair is usually simplicity itself. Toward this end TAC anesthesia has been developed, and effectively used, in the management of facial lacerations (1,2).

TAC anesthesia is a topically applied combination of tetracaine (0.5%), adrenaline (1:2,000), and cocaine (11.8%). This solution is applied topically into a facial wound and it usually obviates the need for injected anesthetics. The primary advantage of TAC anesthesia is that the child is never hurt. It has been the author's experience that if the physician can avoid hurting the child initially, wounds in even small infants can be sutured without requiring restraints such as the papoose board.

Technique of TAC Anesthesia

The application of TAC anesthesia is simplicity itself. The wound can be briefly cleaned, but no attempt should be made to perform a complete scrubbing as this may be interpreted by the child as being painful. It is necessary to remove from the wound any clot that may be present so that the solution has a chance to diffuse into the surrounding tissue. At the author's institution the TAC solution comes in 3-mL vials. The simplest way to apply TAC solution is to place it in a medicine cup and use sterile cotton-tipped applicators to absorb the solution and then place the applicators directly into the wound (Fig. 6). The applicators should be placed fully into the wound and should be completely saturated with the TAC solution (Fig. 7). An accepted rule of thumb for utilizing TAC is that 1 mL of TAC per centimeter length of wound should be used. Up to 10 mL for a to-

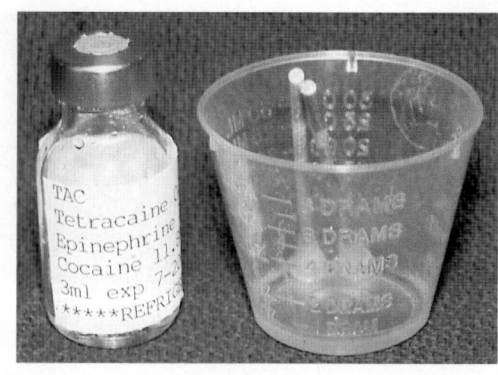

FIGURE 6 A 3-mL vial of tetracaine-adrenaline-cocaine (TAC), with a cotton-tipped applicator soaking. Cotton dental rolls may also be used.

tal wound length of 10 cm can be safely applied. However, the author believes this is much more than is generally required and has never had to use more than 1 to 2 mL of the solution, even for wounds of considerable length. Once the applicator is in the wound, it is generally changed every 4 to 5 minutes to make sure that there is a maximal concentration of the TAC solution within the wound. It generally takes 7 to 12 minutes for the TAC solution to become effective. However, the duration to achieve anesthetic effect can vary and perhaps the most reliable sign that the solution is working is to look for a ring of blanching around the wound margin, which indicates that the solution has moved out into the surrounding tissues and has now become effective. Once this blanching has occurred, the physician can be assured that the anesthetic effect has taken effect and can begin the repair.

A variant of TAC has been described using lidocaine instead of cocaine (referred to as LAT) with concentrations of 4% lidocaine, 1:2,000 adrenaline, and 11.8% tetracaine (3). Ernst et al (3) reported that LAT seemed to have better control of pain than did TAC and that the cost per dose for LAT was $3 versus $35 for TAC. Given the fact that there should be little chance for systemic toxicity with LAT and the low potential for abuse, LAT may well become the topical anesthesia solution of choice.

Indications and Contraindications of TAC Anesthesia

The author has used TAC anesthesia on lacerations involving the entire face, and head and neck region. However, there are several areas where TAC is probably con-

FIGURE 7 Lip laceration in a 3-year-old anesthetized with tetracaine-adrenaline-cocaine (TAC). Note how calm the patient is because he has not been hurt. Note also that TAC does not distort the vermilion border as an injectable anesthetic would. In general, it is not recommended that TAC be used on mucous membranes, due to increased absorption and possible toxicity, but in this case it was thought that the mucosal extent was minimal.

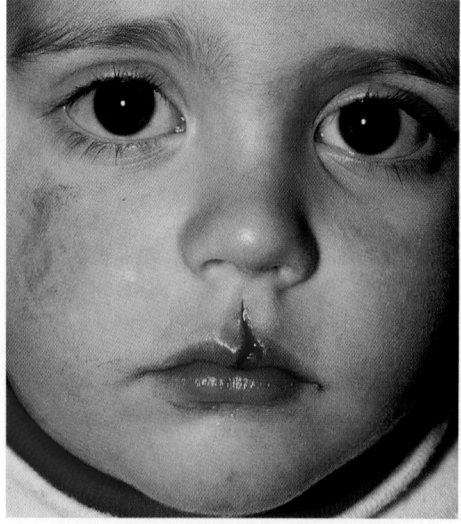

A

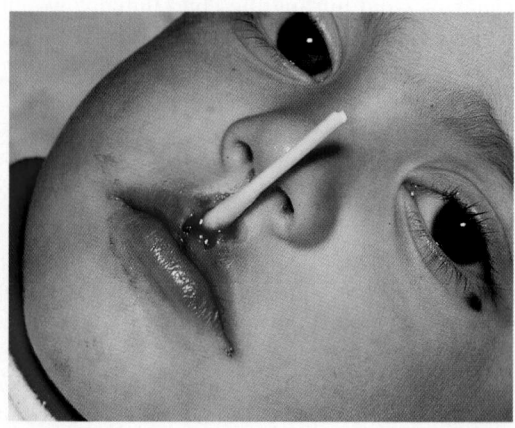

B

traindicated. Because TAC does contain cocaine, one of the major concerns regarding its use would be about systemic absorption of cocaine sufficient to cause toxic symptoms. The fact that TAC is mixed with a vasoconstrictor lessens the possibility of a systemic dose due to the intense local vasoconstriction. However, all the instances of toxic symptoms occurred when TAC was used around mucosal membranes. The proposed explanation for this increased toxicity of TAC when used on mucous membranes is that owing to the high blood flow in mucosal membranes, enough of the cocaine is picked up to cause systemic symptoms. Therefore, it is generally recommended that TAC anesthesia not be used on significant mucosal lacerations of the lips or nose. Additionally, because of its vasoconstrictive effect, concern has been expressed over using it on end-arterial situations such as the tip of the nose or ear, or when pedicled flaps of tissue are encountered.

An additional note should be made of the fact that TAC administration will cause a positive result on a urine or blood test for cocaine (4). While this would only rarely be of concern in children, it could cause significant difficulty in adults undergoing routine drug testing.

Minimizing Pain with Injectable Anesthetics

In the author's experience, TAC anesthesia has been extremely effective and a large number of pediatric patients have been managed with it as the only anesthesia. However, there are situations where it is believed inadvisable to use TAC anesthesia, such as for lip lacerations extending well onto the mucosa, lacerations in which a flap has been raised, or where the vascularity of the lacerated area is in question. Additionally, TAC may not be available in all emergency rooms, particularly smaller community hospitals where limited numbers of pediatric patients are treated. In these situations the physician may need to resort to the standard injectable anesthetic. It is well known that the injection of a local anesthetic is painful, but what is not generally appreciated is that most of the pain associated with local anesthetic injection is not from the injection procedure itself, but from the chemical properties of the anesthetic. Specifically, the pH of most commercially available anesthetics is about 4.0. It is this acidic pH that causes most of the stinging encountered with local anesthetic injection. If the anesthetic solution is buffered so that the pH is brought up to the physiologic range, then the pain of the local injection is considerably diminished. Neutralization of the anesthetic solution can be achieved by mixing sodium bicarbonate with the local anesthetic solution. Generally, 1 mL of 8.4% sodium bicarbonate is mixed with 9 mL of 1% lidocaine with 1:100,000 epinephrine, which will raise the pH to approximately 7.0. Sodium bicarbonate solution is available in multiple-use bottles or may be obtained from the pharmacy in single-use viles used for injection on emergency resuscitation carts (Fig. 8). The cost of a sodium bicarbonate vile

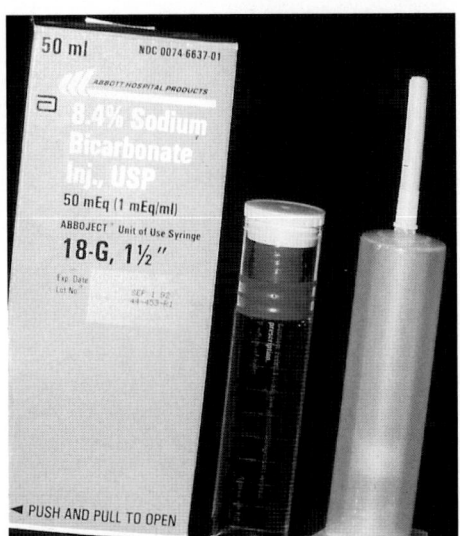

FIGURE 8 Commonly available vials of 8.4% sodium bicarbonate that can be used for buffering local anesthetics. One milliliter of sodium bicarbonate is mixed with 9 mL of 1% lidocaine with 1:100,000 epinephrine to achieve a pH of approximately 7.0.

is approximately $2. If one does not need 10 mL for injection, a proportional solution can be made up, such as using 0.5 mL of sodium bicarbonate with 4.5 mL of local anesthetic. Using this buffered anesthetic solution with a very fine needle (27 or 30 gauge) can significantly diminish, and often eliminate, the pain of local anesthetic injection. If done properly with concealment of the needle, very slow injection technique, and some form of distraction, it is often possible to administer the anesthesia with little or no discomfort noticed by the patient.

It should be mentioned that with the use of buffered local anesthetic solution, the duration of effective anesthesia is definitely lessened. However, it has been this author's experience that the treating physician can expect at least 30 to 45 minutes of substantial anesthetic effect, which should be sufficient for most pediatric lacerations.

While the vascular supply of the facial skin is probably the best of the entire body, necessitating the addition of a vasoconstrictor to the lidocaine, there may be situations where the use of a vasoconstrictor is inappropriate. In particular, vasoconstrictors should probably be avoided in situations where there is clearly a limited pedicle-type blood supply. Examples of this type of limited blood supply would include the tip of the nose or ear or an avulsion-type injury where a pedicled flap of skin has been raised. In these types of injuries consideration should be given to using plain anesthetic without epinephrine or performing the repair under regional or general anesthesia.

Management Issues with Complicated Wounds

Contusions

Blunt trauma often presents with an associated stellate laceration resulting from the skin being caught between the striking object externally and the facial skeleton internally (Fig. 9). In these situations the skin is actually ripped rather than cut and this gives rise to widespread surrounding tissue disruption. These wounds often do poorly from an aesthetic standpoint, even with the most meticulous repair. The scars are irregular, often widen, and tend to become depressed. Initial treatment should be directed at obtaining as accurate a repair as possible. As a general rule, extensive debridement should not be performed at the time of primary repair because of the difficulty in assessing what tissue will be important for the final outcome. When the wound has fully matured (a minimum of 6 months and ideally a year), a scar revision may be considered.

FIGURE 9 A: Significant soft tissue contusion with stellate lacerations. **B:** One-year result. No tissue was debrided. Instead, meticulous attention was paid to accurate soft tissue realignment with a fine suture (7-0).

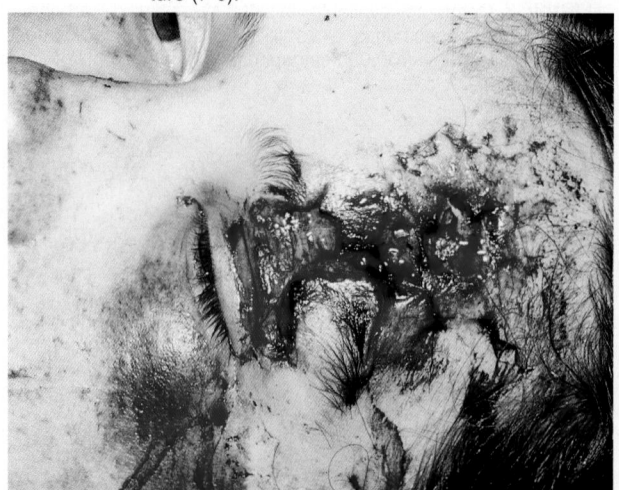
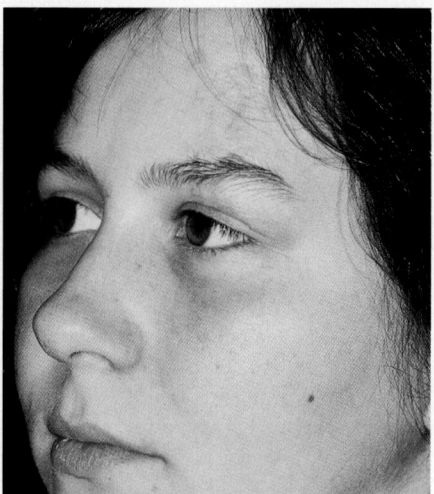

A

B

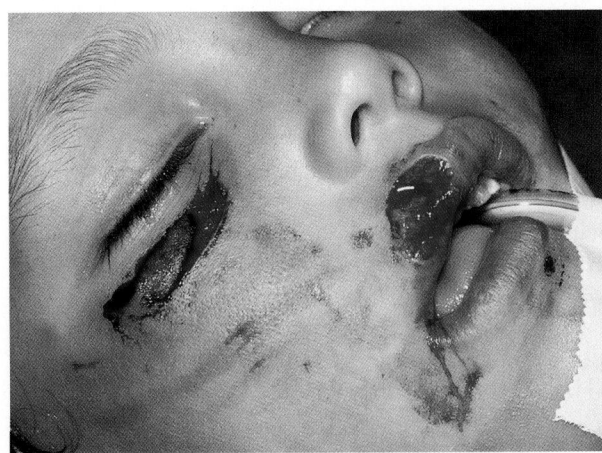

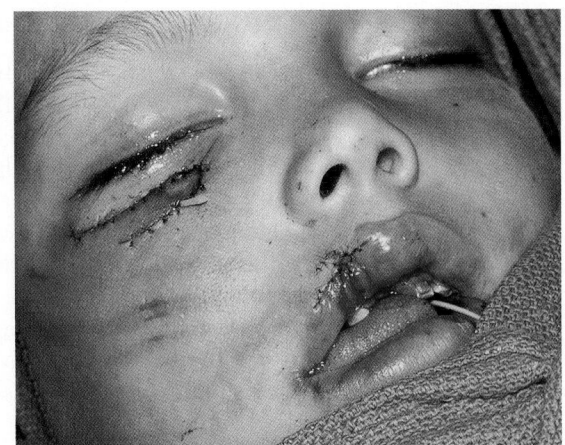

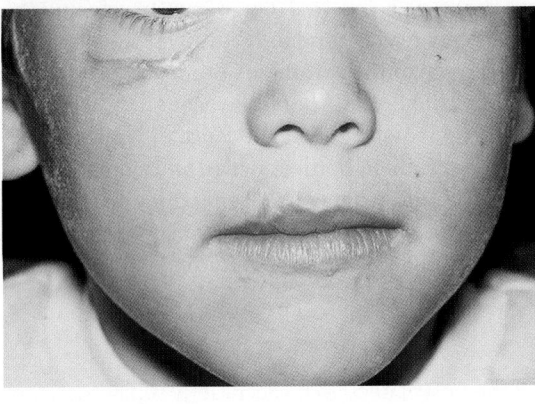

FIGURE 10 A: Avulsion of a portion of the upper lip secondary to a dog bite. **B:** Because the defect was only of moderate size, soft tissue undermining and primary closure was performed. **C:** One-year follow-up with acceptable lip scar. Note that a portion of the avulsed cheek skin flap died, resulting in a hypertrophic scar.

Avulsions

Actual loss of soft tissue represents one of the most difficult wound management situations. If the soft tissue is available, it is not unreasonable to try and reattach it as a full-thickness graft. Some authors feel hyperbaric oxygen may facilitate the survival of these grafts. Adjunctive treatment might include some form of anticoagulation or platelet inhibition. If it is a large portion of tissue with identifiable blood vessels, such as a scalp or ear, then a microvascular reattachment may be considered. If the reattached portion survives long enough to develop venous stasis, surgical leeches can used, with some success, to provide temporary venous decompression until the peripheral circulation reestablishes itself. If the avulsed tissue is not available, then the surgeon must manage the wound in its absence. If the defect is not too wide, an attempt at primary closure with undermining can be considered (Fig. 10). However if there is going to be excessive tension on the wound that distorts anatomic landmarks (i.e., lip, eyebrow, etc.), then it is probably best to allow the wound to granulate and heal by secondary intention, with a revision when the wound is stable. No matter how tempting, there is almost no situation (except perhaps with massive tissue loss) where split- or full-thickness skin grafting is indicated. Placement of a skin graft where soft tissue has been avulsed or lost stops the wound contraction of secondary healing (which can be very helpful in closing a wound) and almost always provides a poor tissue match. This is particularly true where full-thickness skin and subcutaneous tissue has been lost. Where there has been loss of skin and subcutaneous tissue, placement of a split- or full-thickness skin graft not only will result in a poor tissue match but also will leave a very noticeable contour deformity. It is usually best to allow these wounds to stabilize and plan a local or regional flap repair with facial skin that matches the skin surrounding the wound.

Lacerations Involving a Margin or Border

Special consideration should be given to any laceration that extends through an anatomic margin or border because of the aesthetic and functional importance of these junctional structures. From an aesthetic consideration, the eye is attracted to discrepancies in facial lines and contours and a misaligned margin or border will be readily noticed. Technically these structures are somewhat more demanding to repair because they have an external and internal surface, both of which may be involved with the laceration. If an optimal repair is to be performed, all three layers (internal, middle, and external) must be completely and accurately realigned. In particular, if the internal-surface laceration is not repaired, the wound contraction associated with secondary wound healing may cause distortion of the external surface or margin of the lacerated structure. The sites that merit particular attention are discussed below:

Vermilion Border of the Lip

This smooth line of transition between the pale, external, cutaneous lip skin and the red mucosa is a critical facial landmark and any malalignment, by even as little as a millimeter, will be quite noticeable. With any lip repair the vermilion border should be a primary focus of attention and the continuity of the border should be accurately realigned first, to ensure that repair of the rest of the lip structures will not cause distortion of the vermilion border (Figs. 11 and 12). With the vermilion border aligned and stabilized, the rest of the lip layers (inner mucosa, muscular, and cutaneous) are repaired in the standard fashion. Generally, the inner mucosa is closed loosely with 4-0 plain gut sutures; the muscular layer, with 6-0 polyglycolic acid; and the external skin and mucosa, with a fine monofilament.

Nostril Margin

Lacerations involving the margin of the nostril need to be accurately repaired, to ensure that unsightly notching does not occur. Additionally, it must be remembered that in the medial portion of the nostril and superior columella, the lower lateral cartilages are quite close to the margin and relatively superficial. If a coincident laceration of the lower lateral cartilage is not recognized and repaired, there is a high likelihood that the nose will shift and twist as the forces of healing put stress on the ipsilateral side of the nose and the ends of the lower lateral cartilage slip over one another (Fig. 13). If the inner mucosa is not repaired, the contraction resulting from secondary wound healing may cause superior retraction of the nostril margin. Because the nose has such a high aesthetic importance, and secondary repair of the complications discussed herein is so difficult, lac-

FIGURE 11 A: Left upper-lip laceration from a dog bite. After tetracaine-adrenaline-cocaine (TAC) anesthesia, the repair was carried out painlessly for the patient and without distorting the vermilion border. **B:** Six-month result after a multilayered repair focusing on accurate realignment of the vermilion border.

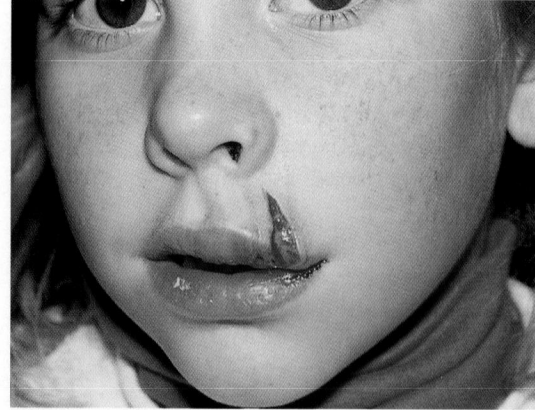
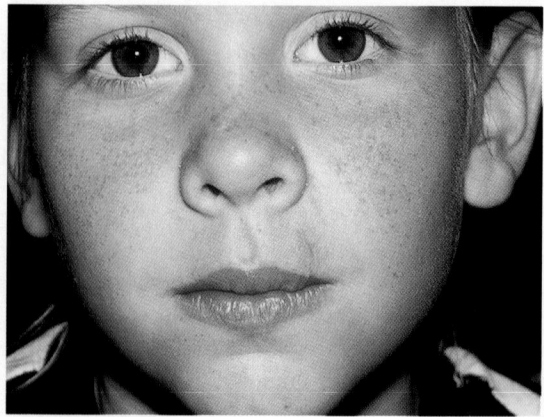

A   B

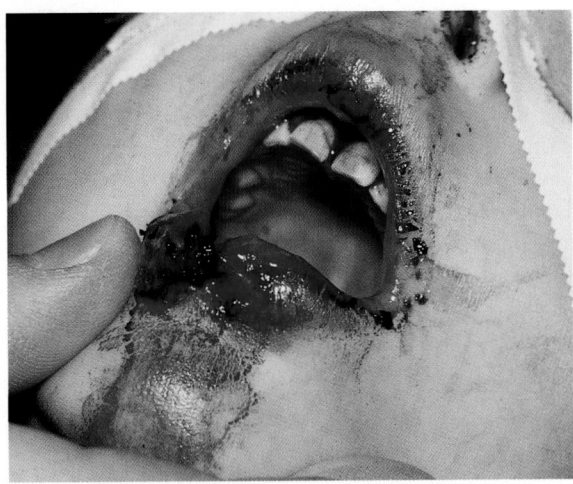
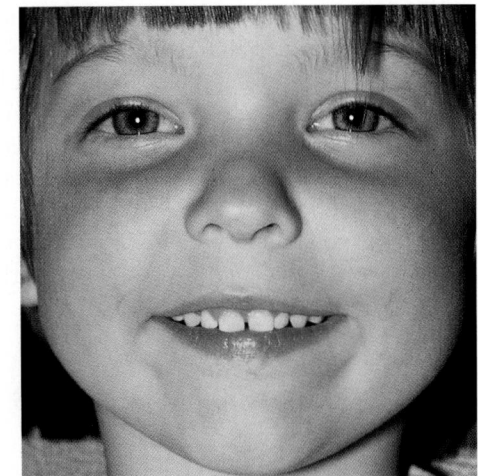

FIGURE 12 A: Severe lip laceration and contusion requiring debridement and then a multilayered repair in the operating room. **B:** One-year postrepair result. Note that the vermilion border has been accurately realigned.

erations of the nostril margin are often best repaired in the operating room. The principal of a three-layer closure is followed with the exception that a laceration of the lower lateral cartilage is identified and repaired with 5-0 or 6-0 clear monofilament nylon in order to impart some permanent strength to the wound.

Auricular Helical Rim

Lacerations of the helical-rim which traverse skin and cartilage require a three-layer repair with accurate reapproximation of the auricular cartilage, as in the nose, in order to avoid notching. Again, the perichondrium of the cartilage is reapproximated with 5-0 or 6-0 clear nylon and the skin with 6-0 nylon.

Eyelids

Management of eyelid lacerations could well take up an entire chapter on its own, but a few brief remarks are in order. While laceration of the globe is a primary concern (this should be ruled out with appropriate ophthalmologic consultation and examination), there are several structures that may be involved with eyelid trauma that must also be considered. With upper-eyelid lacerations, the surgeon should also consider the possibility of injury to the levator palpebrae, which could cause ptosis of the upper lid if not repaired. The lacrimal gland may be involved with lacerations of the lateral portion of the

FIGURE 13 A: Initially benign-appearing laceration of the left nostril margin. **B:** However, further investigation showed a full-thickness injury with a laceration of the lower lateral cartilage. A three-layer closure with repair of the cartilage was performed in the operating room.

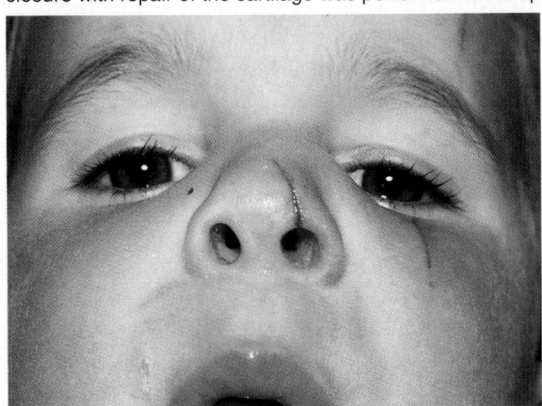
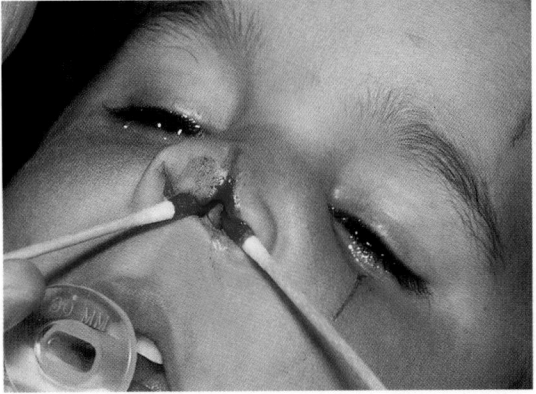

upper lid and may be mistaken for orbital fat. There are reports of the lacrimal gland being excised under the mistaken assumption that orbital fat was being debrided. In the lower eyelid the possibility of a laceration to the lacrimal system should always be considered with any medial lid laceration. In both the upper and lower eyelids, special concern should be given to lacerations that involve the lid margin. As with lacerations that involve margins elsewhere on the face, unsightly notching may occur if the edges are improperly repaired. Briefly, repair of a lid-margin laceration involves a three-layer closure with a fine, 6-0 or 7-0 plain gut suture on the conjunctival side (to avoid irritation of the scleral conjunctiva), a fine absorbable suture in the tarsal plate, and a fine monofilament on the external surface.

PEDIATRIC FACIAL BURNS

General Comments

A separate category of pediatric soft tissue facial injuries is that of burns. While the term *burn* implies a thermal injury, burns can also be caused by cold or freezing, electric current, chemicals, or ionizing radiation. Regardless of the exact etiologic agent, the common histologic picture of a burn is that of widespread cell death in the affected tissue. Typically, this extends from the skin surface medially for a variable depth. In fact, burns are classified on the basis of the depth of extension of cell death into the soft tissue. First-degree burns are defined as a superficial injury involving just the epidermis and resulting in pain and redness but little significant tissue damage, and they heal without scarring. Second-degree burns extend into the dermis for a variable distance. The identifying features of a second-degree burn are pain (often severe) and blistering. Second-degree burns will reepithelialize spontaneously and generally have limited scarring (unless deep into the dermis). It should be mentioned that a deep second-degree burn may be converted to a full-thickness injury by improper wound management or infection. Third-degree burns extend through (or nearly through) the full thickness of the dermis and destroy all the adnexal structures, which are the source of epithelial regeneration, blood vessels, and nerve endings. Severe third-degree burns can extend through the dermis into the subcutaneous tissue, even involving bone. Clinical evaluation of third-degree burns is deceptive as to the severity of this type of injury. By definition, in a third-degree burn, blood vessels and nerves are destroyed so there is no bleeding, inflammation, blistering, or pain in the area of full-thickness injury, although there may be pain in surrounding areas with just partial-thickness injury. Pricking a third-degree burn with a needle elicits no bleeding or pain. The initial relatively benign appearance of a third-degree burn belies the serious nature of this injury. Because the full thickness of the dermis has been lost, there is no possibility of regeneration or reepithelialization of this portion of skin. A third-degree burn of the skin will result in an eschar that will eventually slough or require debridement, leaving a full-thickness wound that on its own can only heal by secondary wound contraction (with severe hypertrophic scarring). Additional methods of closing third-degree burns are skin grafting and resurfacing with some form of flap. With regard to flap choice it should be noted that while there are a wide variety of flaps available to fill the wound, generally only local or regional flaps, using facial skin, give acceptable aesthetic results. Due to the limited availability of facial skin flaps in patients with generalized burns, local flaps are usually only available in patients with limited or localized burns.

Acute Management

The major concern with the acute management of facial burns relates to making sure that systemic life-threatening issues are addressed. The facial burns themselves are not definitively treated for 10 to 14 days. Third-degree burns of any size are a serious injury and may be fatal with as little as 20% of the body surface burned. Formerly, the major cause of death in burn patients was "burn shock" due to massive extravascular fluid shifts. With modern-day physiologic monitoring and improved replacement fluids, mortality from burns has been steadily dropping over the last several decades. An in-depth discussion of the intricacies of burn fluid resuscitation is beyond the scope of this chapter.

Definitive Management

A generally accepted treatment principle for facial burns is that the sooner burns of the face and neck are sealed by either spontaneous reepithelialization or skin graft, the better the ultimate cosmetic and functional outcome will be. Complete closure of the wound should be accomplished by the third or fourth week following the injury. If a burn spontaneously heals within 10 to 14 days, there will usually be little scarring and good-quality skin. However, if healing has not taken place by then, the chance of unsatisfactory hypertrophic scarring increases dramatically. Therefore, at approximately 10 days the wound is assessed with regard to its ability to heal spontaneously. If it is determined that there will be a significant delay in healing, the burn eschar is tangentially excised until viable tissue is reached and then skin grafting is performed. While awaiting eschar excision and grafting, a major source of potential morbidity lies with colonization and superinfection of the eschar itself. In the past a major cause of burn sepsis was the heavily infected eschar having direct access to the bloodstream via the adjacent viable tissues. Topical antimicrobial agents have significantly reduced the dangers of eschar superinfection and the most commonly used preparation is silver sulfadiazine applied twice a day.

When planning skin grafts to the face, it is important to keep Gonzalez-Ulloa's unit theory of facial reconstruction in mind and replace entire facial units (i.e., perioral region, cheek, forehead, or nose) rather than just portions of a unit (5,6). Failure to follow the unit concept of facial reconstruction will result in a patchwork appearance with diminished aesthetic results. As a general rule, the thicker the skin graft, the closer to normal the final result will be. However, full-thickness skin grafts create more donor site morbidity; therefore, split-thickness grafts at 0.015- to 0.035-inch thickness are the most common alternative. Postgrafting care is directed at avoiding scar contracture through vigorous physical therapy, splints, and pressure garments.

Special Considerations

Eyelids

With thermal injuries to the periorbital region, it is rare to have a direct injury to the eye, but there may be severe long-term ocular sequelae. The major concern in patients with eyelid burns is maintenance of adequate corneal covering. Corneal exposure typically does not occur until the initial periorbital swelling subsides and scar contracture begins to occur. Treatment consists of early eschar removal and skin grafting (thick split-thickness grafts for the upper lids and full-thickness grafts for the lower lids) with meticulous attention to corneal lubrication with ointment and appropriate ophthalmologic consultation. Tarsorrhaphy, once routinely recommended, is now reserved for very difficult cases with a high chance of corneal ulceration (7).

Ears

Due to their exposed position and thin skin, ears are often severely injured in any major facial burn. Ninety percent of all burns of the face involve the ears (8,9). Conservatism is the best course of therapy in the acute care of the burned ear. Previously, a major source of morbidity in burned ears was progressive chondritis due to infection of the exposed cartilage, which led to the admonition of early radical debridement and closure of all ear burns regardless of size. With the addition of topical antimicrobials, the complication of progressive chondritis has virtually disappeared. The presently recommended treatment is liberal use of silver sulfadiazine, continuous conservative debridement, and grafting when a suitable recipient bed is available. Definitive reconstruction is then carried out secondarily.

Oral Commissure Burns

A characteristic pediatric burn is of the oral commissure from an electric current. These injuries occur most commonly in children 2 to 3 years old. Typically oral commissure burns result from the child biting an electric cord, with an arc of electric energy at the oral commissure where the cord was in contact with the lip. Because this injury results from the electric current passing through the tissue, rather than heat applied to the skin surface, the initial injury may seem limited, but progressive necrosis unfortunately becomes evident over the next 36 to 48 hours. Owing to the difficulty in distinguishing viable from nonviable tissue, early debridement and primary closure are generally not recommended. Instead, it is advocated that the wound be treated conservatively with topical antibiotics and progressive gentle debridement. Earlier literature attached considerable importance to the possible complication of delayed hemorrhage from the labial artery when the eschar separates, but several large recent series had a zero incidence of this complication (10,11). Management of the resultant oral commissure deformity is somewhat controversial. For some time, oral splints were routinely advocated, but Donelan (10) and Canady et al (11) both questioned whether splints truly have much benefit, and thought they may actually do some harm. Presently, the consensus appears to be to treat the wounds conservatively until the scar matures and softens, and then perform the definitive repair with one of a variety of commissureplasties.

REFERENCES

1. Anderson AB, Colecchi C, Baronoski R, DeWitt TG. Local anesthesia in pediatric patients: topical TAC versus lidocaine. *Ann Emerg Med* 1990;19:519–522.
2. White WB, Iserson KV, Criss E. Topical anesthesia for laceration repair: tetracaine versus TAC (tetracaine, adrenaline, and cocaine). *Am J Emerg Med* 1986;4:319–322.
3. Ernst AA, Marvez-Valls E, Nick TG, Weiss SJ. LAT (lidocaine-adrenaline-tetracaine) versus TAC (tetracaine-adrenaline-cocaine) for topical anesthesia in face and scalp lacerations. *Am J Emerg Med* 1995;13:151–154.
4. Altieri M, Bogema S, Schwartz RH. TAC topical anesthesia produces positive urine tests for cocaine. *Ann Emerg Med* 1990;19:577–579.
5. Gonzalez-Ulloa M, Castillo A, Stevens E, Fuertes GA, Leonelli F, Ubaldo F. Preliminary study of the total restoration of the facial skin. *Plast Reconstr Surg* 1954;151–161.
6. Gonzalez-Ulloa M. A quantium method for the appreciation of the morphology of the face. *Plast Reconstr Surg* 1964;34:241–246.
7. Constable JD. Thermal injuries of the head and neck. In: Stark RB, ed. *Plastic surgery of the head and neck,* 1st ed. Vol. 1. New York: Churchill Livingstone, 1987:275–281.
8. Hammond JS, Ward CG. Burns of the head and neck. *Otolaryngol Clin North Am* 1983;16:679–695.
9. Dowling JA, Foley FD. Chondritis in the burned ear. *Plast Reconstr Surg* 1968;42:115–122.
10. Donelan MB. Reconstruction of electrical burns of the oral commissure with a ventral tongue flap. *Plast Reconstr Surg* 1990;95:1155–1163.
11. Canady JW, Thompson SA, Bardach J. Oral commissure burns in children. *Plast Reconstr Surg* 1995;97:738–744.

K.A. Shumrick: Department of Otolaryngology, Division of Facial Plastic Surgery and Maxillofacial Trauma, University of Cincinnati Medical Center, Cincinnati, Ohio 45267–0528.

- *Practical Pediatric Otolaryngology*
- edited by Robin T. Cotton and Charles M. Myer, III
- Lippincott-Raven Publishers, Philadelphia © 1999

Unilateral Cleft Lip

Craig W. Senders & Jonathan M. Sykes

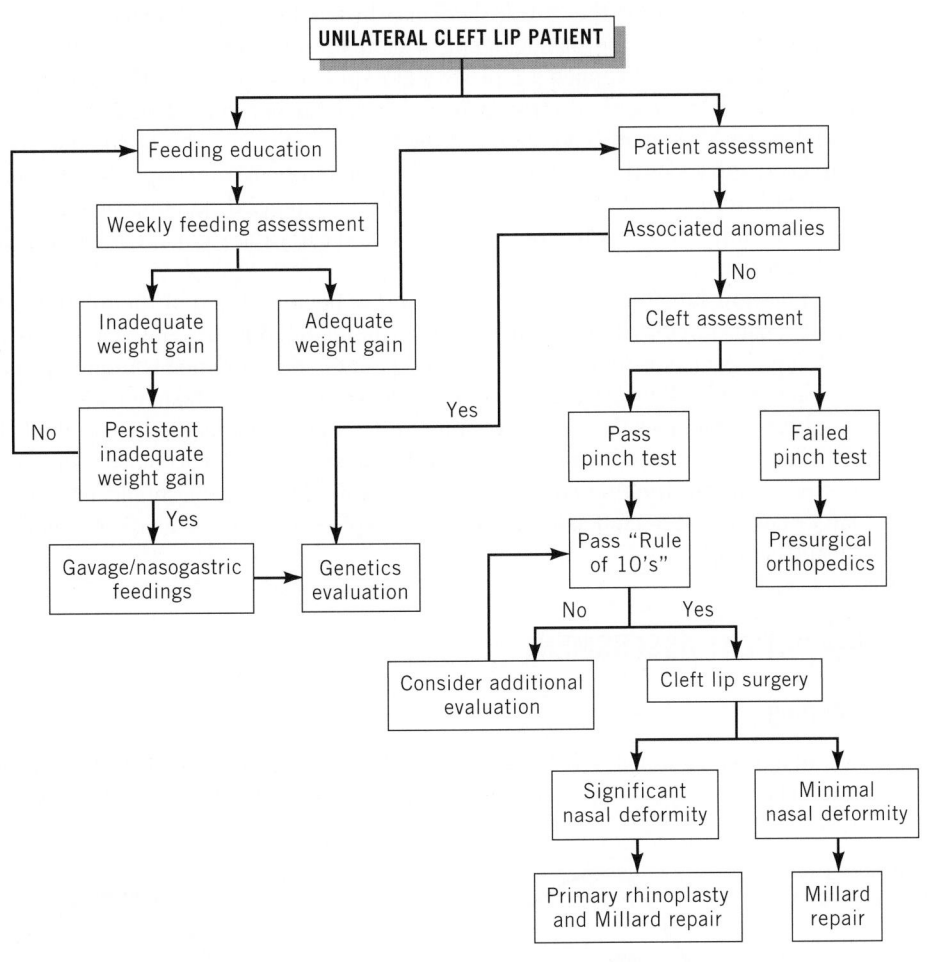

🌑 HISTORICAL BACKGROUND

The earliest records of cleft lip surgery date back to 300 AD during the Tien dynasty in China (1,2). In this primitive technique, the cleft lip edges were simply cut and sutured together. In 1564, Ambrose Pare utilized a similar straight line closure, which was reinforced with a needle passed through both lip segments and a figure-of-eight wraparound thread (2). Even though at its best this technique would leave a residual whistle deformity; it continued to be advocated by J.A. Pancoast in the mid-1800s (3) (Fig. 1).

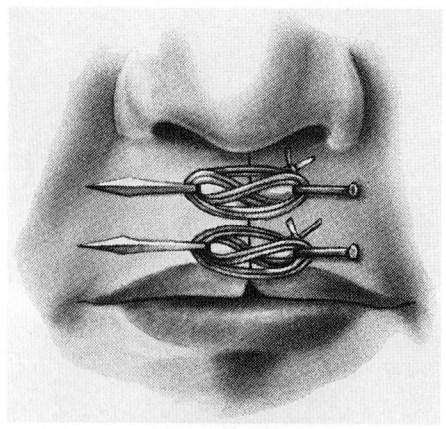

FIGURE 1 The cleft lip repair was reapproximated using a needle and a figure-of-eight wraparound thread between the mid-1500s and mid-1800s. (From ref. 2, with permission.)

Efforts at avoiding the whistle deformity by lengthening the lip have resulted in significant advances in the management of cleft lip deformity in this century. In 1952, Charles Tennison (4) applied a Z-plasty technique to add length to the cleft lip. In 1959, Peter Randall (5) described a triangular repair that further refined the Z-plasty technique and defined mathematically the size of the triangles (Fig. 2). This technique gave excellent lip length and is the preferred method of a minority of surgeons today. The main disadvantage is that most of the scars do not fall in the relaxed skin tension lines of the lip. Consequently, most repairs are easily visible and carry the stigmata of a triangular geometric scar.

For most surgeons, the triangular repair has been replaced by the rotation-advancement repair developed by Ralph Millard in the mid-1950s (6). This is a "cut as you go" technique. A higher degree of surgical judgment and experience is required to achieve excellent results. Because the incisions are closer to the relaxed skin tension lines and the resulting scar mimics the philtral column, the aesthetic results can be excellent (Fig. 3).

The inexperienced surgeon is warned against a tendency to narrow the nostril excessively with the rotation-advancement technique. The surgeon should aim for a slightly larger nostril on the cleft side by using "active placement of the alar base" with the surgical technique.

PATIENT ASSESSMENT

Feeding

All infants with a unilateral cleft lip have some compromise in feeding that requires additional time and often specialized techniques to overcome. Approximately two-thirds of

FIGURE 2 The triangular repair as described by Peter Randall. (From ref. 1, with permission.)

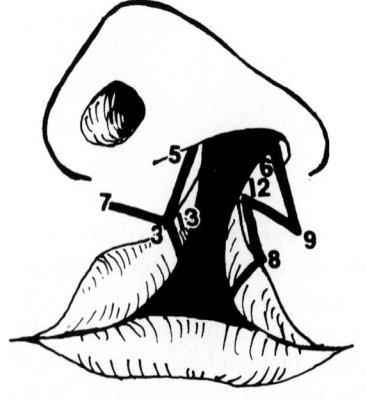
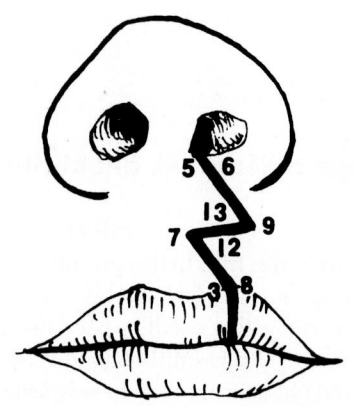

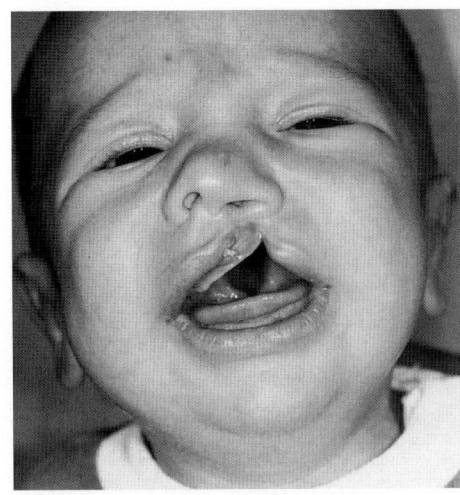

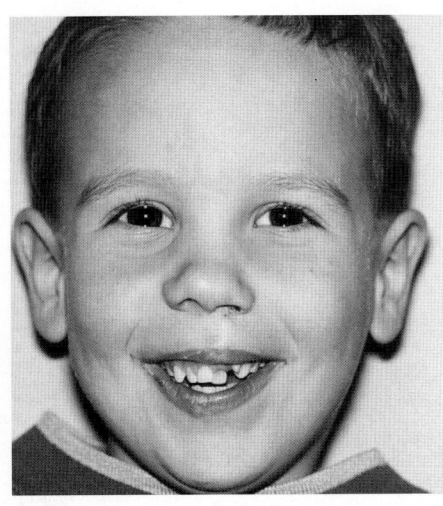

FIGURE 3 Millard repair. **A:** Preoperative view. **B:** Two years after operation.

the children with a cleft lip will also have a cleft palate, which leads to increased problems with feeding. Children with an associated cleft palate require specialized cleft feeding techniques, and breast feeding is not recommended. In the one-third of patients with a cleft lip deformity alone, breast feeding is typically successful.

The lack of separation between the oral and nasal cavities in a cleft palate results in a decreased suck. The remainder of the child's swallowing mechanism should be entirely normal. Therefore, our specialized feeding techniques are aimed at making it easier for the infant to receive milk or formula despite the inefficient suck. This can be achieved by the following measures:

1. Enlarging the openings in the nipple, thereby requiring less suck to extrude formula or milk.
2. Using a longer nipple, which bypasses and/or occludes a portion of the cleft palate.
3. Utilizing a squeeze bottle, such as the Mead Johnson Cleft Palate Nurser. With a squeeze bottle, the parents can squeeze the bottle in coordination with the infant's suck. With practice, parents become very adept at this coordinated technique. It is rare in our institution not to be able to achieve adequate nutritional intake in a child with an isolated cleft of the lip and palate.

All children with a cleft palate should be seen weekly until consistent weight gain is demonstrated. These visits can be made with the infant's pediatrician or surgeon. Joint responsibility between the surgeon and the pediatrician is optimal, as these early visits allow the family to bond with the surgeon, and they can improve the referral relationship between the pediatrician and the surgeon.

The infant is expected to have a 10% weight loss in the first week of life (Table 1). Thereafter, the infant should gain 20 to 30 g per day. An infant requires approximately 50 calories per pound per day (115 calories per kilogram per day) (7). Breast milk and normal formula contain 20 calories per ounce. Therefore, an infant should take approximately 2.5 ounces per pound per day (6 ounces per kilogram per day). Weight gain of less than 15 g a day will require admission to the hospital for extensive feeding instruction or nasogastric feeding.

TABLE 1: Expected Weight Changes

Time	Weight
1st week	Lose up to 10% of birth weight
2nd week	Regain birth weight
3 months	Double birth weight
12 months	Triple birth weight

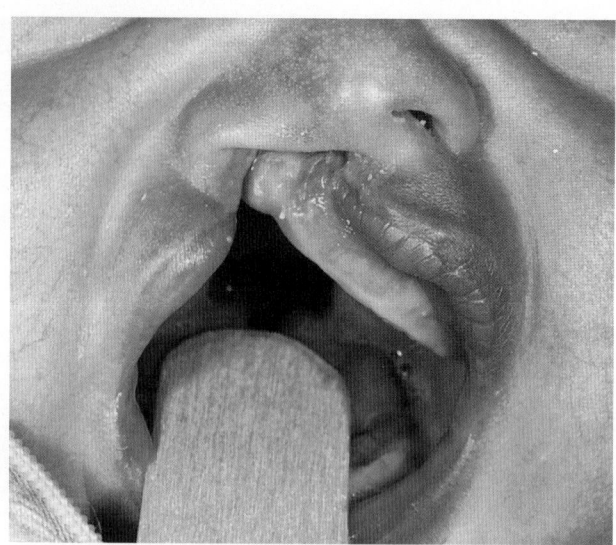

FIGURE 4 The cleft nasal deformity involves all layers of the nose, including external skin, cartilage, soft tissue, and mucosa, as well as skeletal support. The inappropriate insertion of the orbicularis oris muscle pulls the caudal septum and columella to the non-cleft side and further deforms the ala laterally.

Cleft Assessment

The unilateral cleft lip is always associated with a nasal deformity. The extent of the nasal deformity is related to the degree of cleft lip deformity and whether there is a Simonartz band. A Simonartz band is an epithelial bridge across the sill of the nose in a child with an otherwise complete cleft lip and palate. The cleft nasal deformity is the combined result of the deformation inherent in the cleft lip and the abnormal muscle tension created from the inappropriate insertion of the orbicularis oris muscle (8,9). The abnormalities involve all layers of the nose including external skin, mucosa, cartilaginous and soft tissue, and skeletal support (Fig. 4).

The extent of lip deformity varies with the severity of the cleft lip, from an incom-

FIGURE 5 The orbicularis oris muscle inappropriately inserts into the alar base and the columella. The superior labial artery inserts near the base of the nose on the both sides of the cleft. (From ref. 9, with permission.)

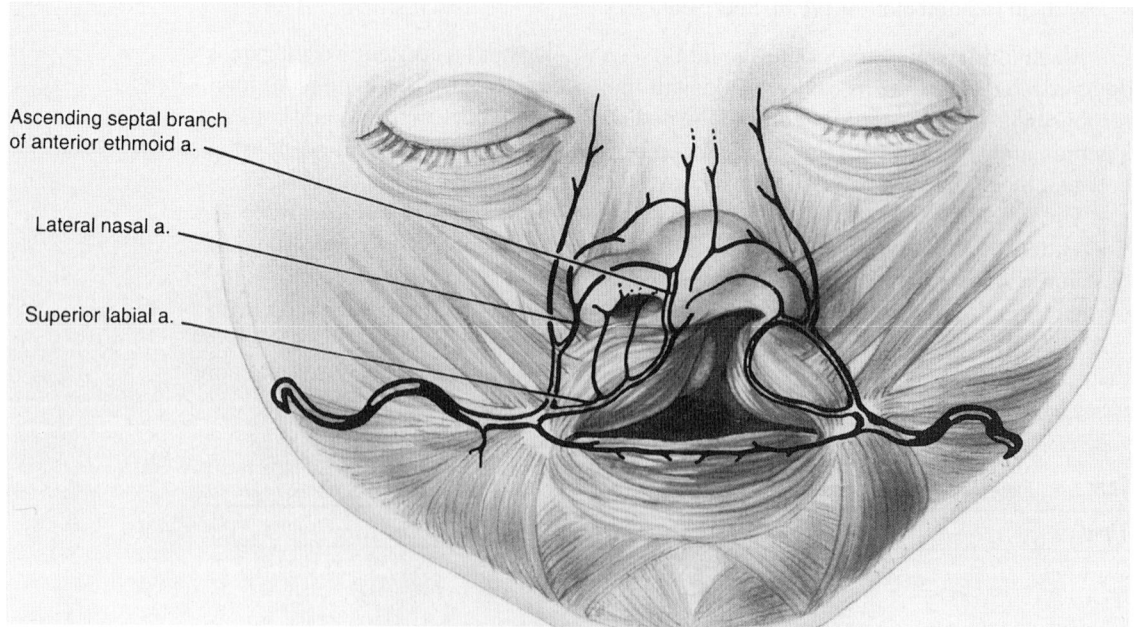

Ascending septal branch of anterior ethmoid a.

Lateral nasal a.

Superior labial a.

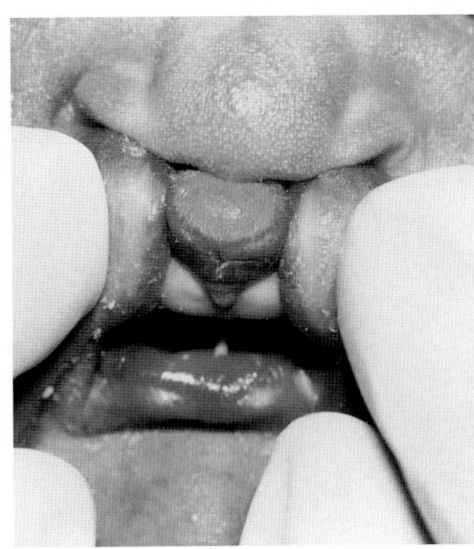

FIGURE 6 The pinch test can be utilized to determine whether presurgical orthopedics or a lip adhesion is necessary prior to lip repair.

plete cleft involving the vermilion only to a complete cleft of the lip extending into the palate. As a result of the cleft, the orbicularis oris muscle inappropriately inserts laterally into the ala and medially into the columella of the nose (Fig. 5). The pull from these aberrant insertions increases the cleft nasal deformity. This is evidenced by the caudal deflection of the septum and columella to the noncleft side (10) (Fig. 4). The arterial supply mimics the course of the muscular abnormalities and follows the edges of the cleft to the base of the nose.

Most surgeons follow the "rule of tens" to determine eligibility for cleft lip repair: a hemoglobin greater than 10, weight greater than 10 pounds, and age greater than 10 weeks. All children who do not meet these criteria and those who have an unusual facies or other abnormalities should be seen by a geneticist, as there are now over 300 syndromes associated with clefts (11). Six percent of patients with a cleft also have cardiac abnormalities and should have a careful cardiac examine by a pediatrician prior to cleft lip repair.

The "pinch test" is used to evaluate whether a cleft will be easily closed by primary repair or would benefit from presurgical orthopedics and/or a lip adhesion (Fig. 6). The surgeon grasps the lip on both sides of the cleft and determines the ease with which the cleft edges approximate. Some experience is required to interpret this test. Nevertheless, if the cleft edges will not approximate at all, some sort of presurgical orthopedics and/or a lip adhesion is required prior to lip repair.

PEARLS AND PERILS

1. The surgeon should assume responsibility for feeding education and for following the patient for weight gain.
2. Expect the infant to lose up to 10% of its body weight in the first week and regain its birth weight by the second week. Thereafter, the infant should gain a minimum of 20 g per day for the first 3 months.
3. Use the "pinch test" to evaluate whether a cleft can be closed easily or will require presurgical orthopedics.
4. Operate when the "rule of tens" is met (hemoglobulin 10, weight 10 pounds, age 10 weeks).

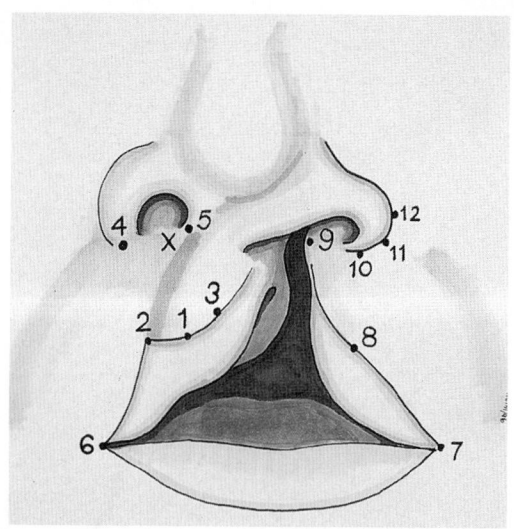

FIGURE 7 Basic reference points of the Millard advancement rotation advancement repair.

💬 TREATMENT RECOMMENDATIONS

Rotation Advancement Cleft Lip Repair (Millard Repair)

Markings

The markings for the rotation advancement technique are complex and require time. The surgeon should make the surgical markings carefully and not feel rushed. The numbered points indicated in Figure 7 are the same as those described by Dr. Ralph Millard (2). This is out of respect for the man who developed this technique and to make it easier for surgeons to compare variations in the technique. The reference points are summarized in Table 2 (12).

The first point to identify is the low point of the cupid's bow. This marks the center point of the lip. Because of the deviation of the columella to the noncleft side (NCS), it is sometimes necessary to place a small amount of traction on the lip to identify this point. The maxillary frenulum can also help identify the midline. Point 2 is the high point of the cupid's bow on the NCS. If this point is ill defined, one should avoid making it too lateral by keeping the distance from point 1 to point 2 less than 3.0 mm (this can be increased in older children). Point 3 is important and represents the calculated peak of the cupid's bow on the medial segment of the cleft side (CS). The distance from 1 to 2 should equal that from 1 to 3 (Fig. 8). Point 4 marks the base of the ala on the NCS. Point 5 represents

TABLE 2: Reference Points for Rotation Advancement

Point	Definition
1	Low point of cupid's bow
2	Peak of cupid's bow, non-cleft side (NCS)
3	Medial peak of cupid's bow, cleft side (CS)
4	Alar base (NCS)
5	Columellar base
X	Backcut point
6	Commissure (NCS)
7	Commissure (CS)
8	Lateral peak of Cupid's bow (CS)
9	Medial tip of advancement flap
10	Midpoint of alar base
11	Lateral alar base
12	Maximum extent of alar incision

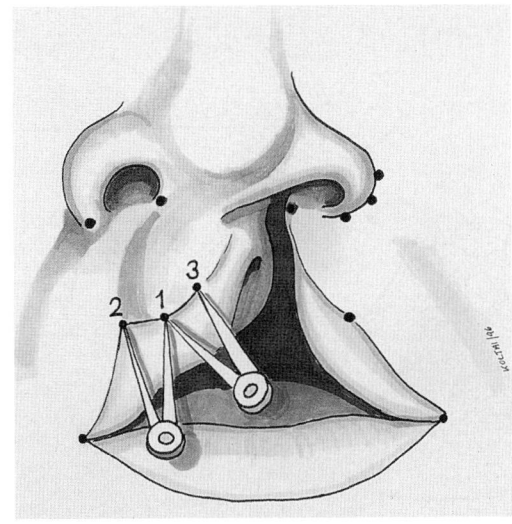

FIGURE 8 Point 3 is calculated by measuring the distance from point 1 to point 2 and marking a similar distance on the opposite side of point 1.

the superior extent of the rotation incision at the base of the columella. This point is located closer to the noncleft nostril than the cleft nostril, but never closer than two-thirds of this distance. Point X represents the backcut for the rotation advancement flap as performed from point 5 at a 45° angle for a distance of 1 to 2 mm. The incision from point 5 to point X is frequently utilized when additional rotation is needed to give adequate length to the lip.

The commissures are represented by point 6 on the NCS and point 7 on the CS. Point 8 represents the high point of the cupid's bow on the lateral segment of the CS (Fig. 9). Point 8 can be located by measuring the distance from point 2 to point 6 and finding a similar distance on the CS. This point should never be more medial than the point at which the white roll of the vermilion cutaneous junction disappears.

Point 9 represents the medial tip of the advancement flap. The distance from point 8 to point 9 should equal the distance from point 3 to point 5 to point X (Fig. 10).

Point 10 represents the midpoint of the alar base on the CS. Point 11 is located in the alar facial crease at the junction of the nasal labial crease. Point 12 represents the furthest lateral extension of the advancement incision that may be necessary during the repair.

After marking these points, the height of the lip on the NCS and CS should be compared. The distance from point 8 to point 10 should almost equal the distance from point 2 to point 4 (Fig. 11). If the distance from point 8 to point 10 is short, one must keep in

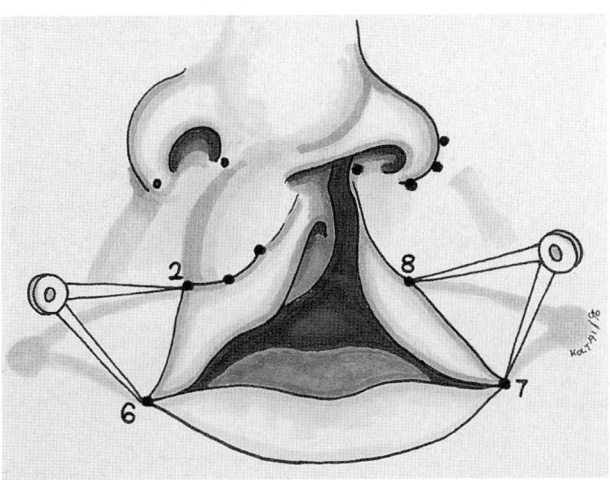

FIGURE 9 The peak of the cupid's bow (point 8) can be determined on the non-cleft side by measuring a similar distance on the non-cleft side.

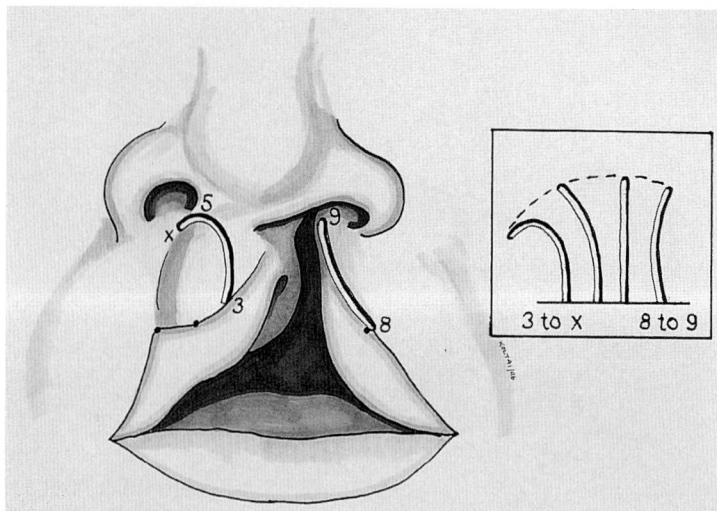

FIGURE 10 The distance from point 3 to point 5 to X should equal the distance from point 8 to point 9. A wire can be used to ensure that these two lengths are equal.

mind that with advancement of the lateral lip segment, point 10 will move closer to point 11. If the difference between the distance from point 8 to point 10 is still over 1 mm shorter than the distance from point 2 to point 4, the surgeon needs to consider moving point 8 more laterally. Alternatively, the surgeon could abandon the rotation advancement repair and perform a triangular repair.

After the reference points are marked, the incision lines are drawn. The rotation incision from point 3 to point 5 should be a gentle curve with an effort to maintain a healthy sized c-flap (Fig. 12 and Table 3). The lateral extent of the c-flap is defined by the mucosal cutaneous junction and extends into the sill of the nose. Every effort is made to preserve tissue for the c-flap, particularly as it extends into the sill of the nose (Fig. 13).

The incision for the advancement flap (B-flap) follows the cutaneous mucosal junction between points 8 and 9 and extends into the sill of the nose. As this incision extends into the nose, tissue is preserved on the alar flap (D-flap) for closure of the floor of the nose. Once this incision reaches the pyriform aperture, it turns anterior to the inferior turbinate (Fig. 13).

Both the rotation and advancement mucosal incisions should be started by making a vertical incision in the vermilion (relative to the lip) that extends approximately the thickness of the lip. These mucosal markings should parallel the cutaneous mucosal markings

FIGURE 11 The distance from the base of the ala to the height of the cupid's bow should be similar on both the cleft and non-cleft sides.

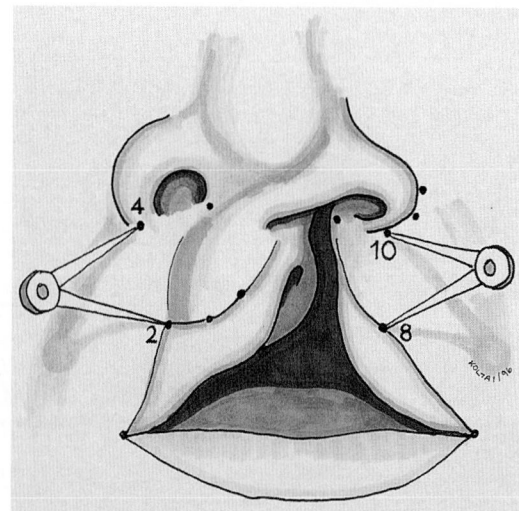

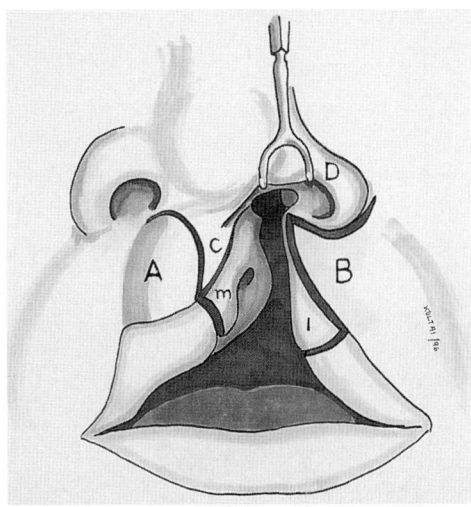

FIGURE 12 The incisions from the Millard repair are outlined. *A*, rotation flap; *B*, advancement flap; *c*, columella flap; *D*, alar flap; *m*, medial mucosal flap; *l*, lateral mucosal flap.

to leave an m-flap or l-flap that is hinged on the alveolar mucosa. From this point, the incision of both the rotation and the advancement flap extends in the gingival buccal sulcus. On the rotation flap, it is important the incision include all of the frenulum, as cleft patients often have a very low attachment of the frenulum between the two central incisors. Leaving redundant tissue in this area results in unsightly cosmetic problems (Fig. 13).

Prior to making incisions, point 3 and point 8 are tattooed using a 27-gauge needle. A small amount of infiltration of lidocaine with epinephrine (1% lidocaine, 1:100,000 epinephrine) is used to vasoconstrict the superior labial artery laterally near the commissure, the columella, the entire tip of the nose, and the base of the nose on both the CS and the NCS, as well as the buccal alveolar mucosal incision points.

Development of the Advancement Flap

A #11 blade is used to make the right angle cut from point 8 through the vermilion. Following this, a #15C blade is used to make all the cuts in the cutaneous skin, and a #15 blade is used to make all mucosal cuts. The lateral mucosal flap (l-flap) is elevated, leaving the muscle attached to the B-flap.

Lip Release   It is necessary to release the lip from both the nose and the face of the maxilla. Therefore, the incision between point 8 and point 11 is connected to the mucosal incision in the buccal alveolar sulcus. Every effort is made to take all the inappropriately inserted fibers of the orbiculus oris muscle with the advancement flap. Scissors are utilized to release the lip from the face of the maxilla. Care is taken not to injure the inferior orbital nerve (Fig. 14).

TABLE 3: Flaps

Letter	Name
Full thickness flaps	
A	Rotation
B	Advancement
D	Alar
Skin or mucosa flaps	
c	Columellar skin
m	Medial mucosal
l	Lateral mucosal

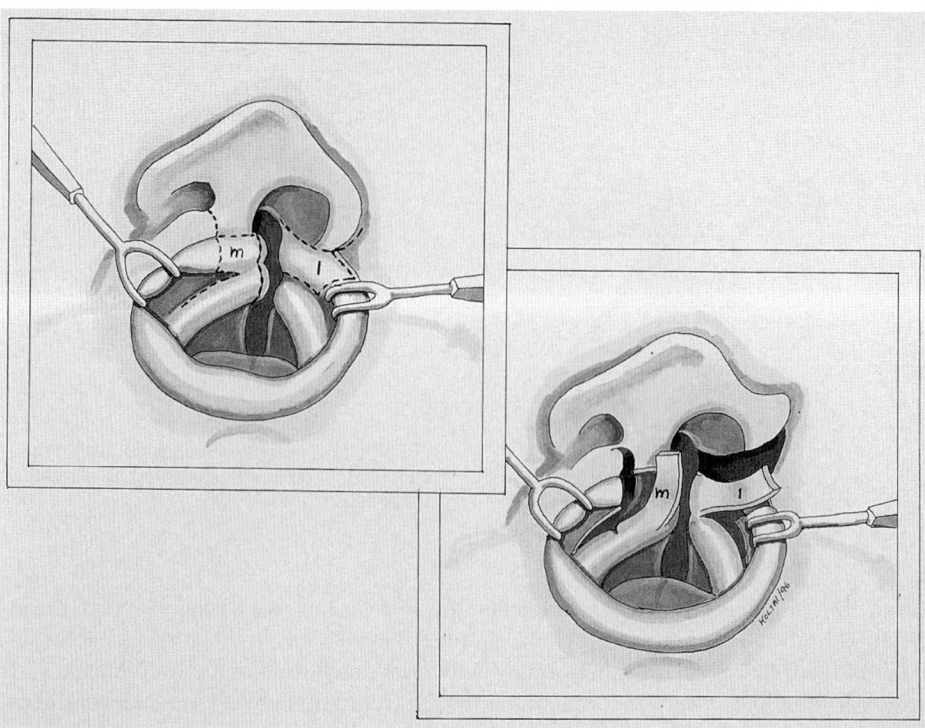

FIGURE 13 The internasal and mucosal incisions are outlined.

Alotomy (Nasal Release)   An alotomy is now performed to release the lateral portion of the ala completely from the pyriform aperture (Fig. 15). At the completion of the alotomy and lip release, both the ala and the lip should be completely free of each other and their movements independent.

Undermining   Generally, the skin is undermined approximately 2 mm from the underlying muscle. The vermilion mucosa should be undermined from the muscle by approximately 3 mm. The remainder of the mucosa generally does not require undermining.

FIGURE 14 The lip release requires dissection off the face of the maxilla. Care is taken not to injure the infraorbital nerve. The shaded areas represent areas undermined on both the cleft and non-cleft side.

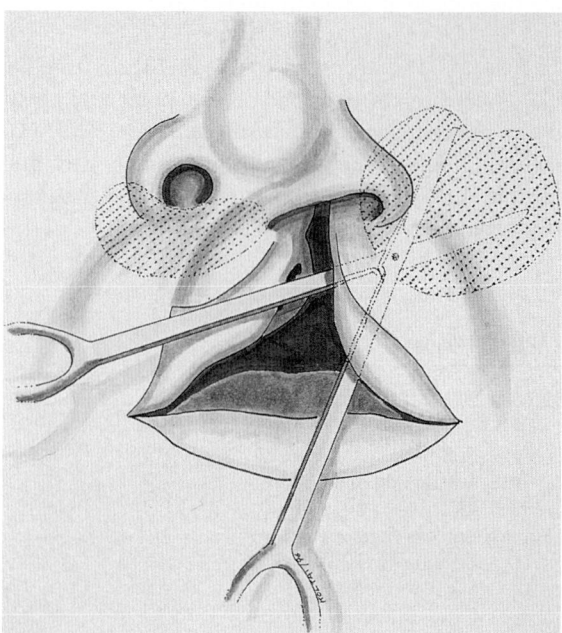

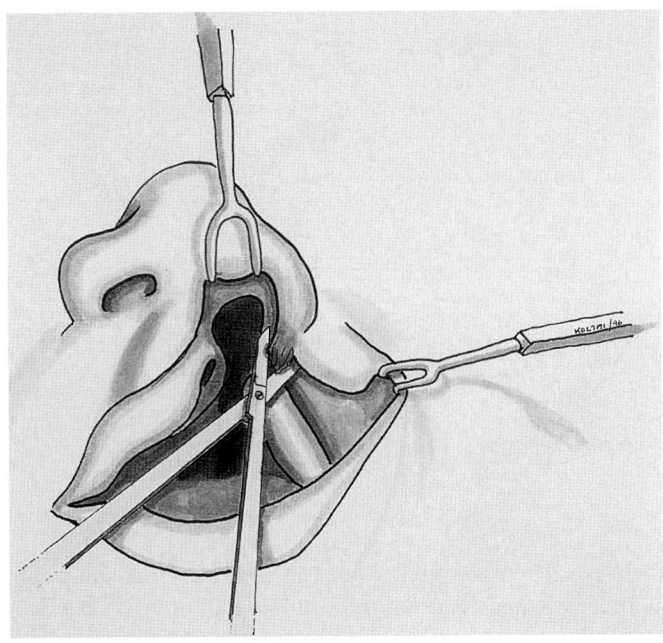

FIGURE 15 The lateral nasal release is accomplished by an alatomy and complete freeing of the lateral ala from the pyriform aperture.

Development of the Rotation Flap

Incisions   A #11 blade is used to make the right-angle cut from point 3 through the vermilion. A #15C blade is used to make the cutaneous incisions.

The m-flap and c-flap are both elevated without underlying muscle. Generally, the m-flap is elevated first, followed by the c-flap. In the floor of the nose, the c-flap is elevated off the septum to give adequate tissue for closure of the floor of the nose.

Lip Release   Using a #15 blade or scissors, the external rotation incision and the buccal sulcus incision are connected. Every effort is made to retain all the inappropriately inserted orbicularis oris muscular fibers with the rotation flap. This includes dissection of the depressor nasi muscle from the columella. The extent of muscle dissection from the base of the nose is greater than the extent of the cutaneous and mucosal incisions.

Backcut   With a hook at point 3, a #11 blade is used to make a backcut in the skin only. [The muscles should have been previously dissected from this area (Fig. 16).] It is im-

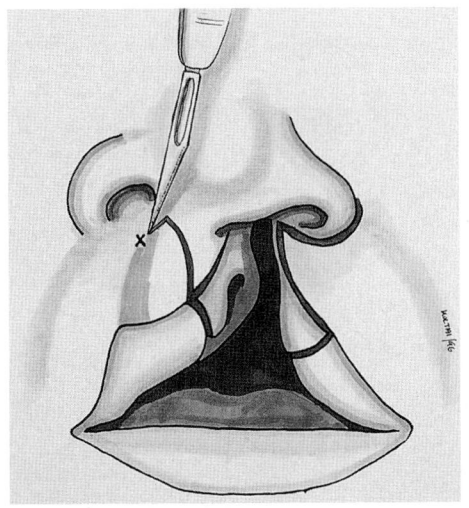

FIGURE 16 With a skin hook providing inferior traction, a backcut is made to allow the cleft side of the cupid's bow to be even with the non-cleft side of the cupid's bow.

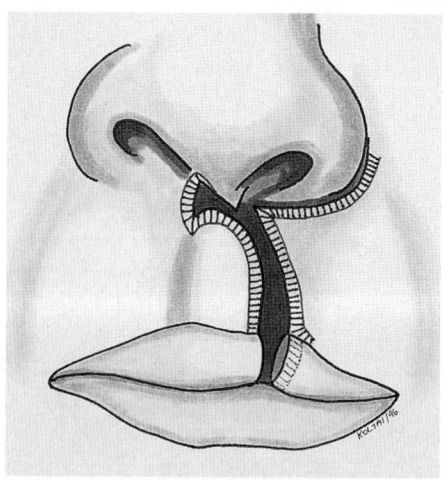

FIGURE 17 The cutaneous undermining is indicated by shading. More undermining is necessary near the vermilion.

portant to allow enough of a backcut to allow point 3 to easily reach a horizontal plane with point 2. Failure to achieve an adequate backcut will result in a short lip on the CS.

Undermining The skin is undermined approximately 2 mm from all incisions including the internasal incisions (Fig. 17). In the area of the columella, 1 mm is adequate. At the vermilion, approximately 3 mm is necessary. Generally, additional mucosal undermining is not required.

Closure Test With skin hooks at point 3 and point 8, the cupid's bow is approximated. If there is adequate lip release, point 9 of the advancement flap should easily reach to point X of the rotation flap (Fig. 18). If the advancement flap is too short for the amount of rotation necessary to give adequate length to the lip, it becomes evident at this time. If this is evident, there are two "cut as you go" techniques to resolve this situation. If there is a large c-flap that will not be necessary for closure of the floor of the nose, it can be used to close the superiormost portion of the rotation defect. Alternatively, point 8 can be extended further laterally to give an increased length to the advancement segment (Fig. 19). This comes at a cost, as the lateral portion of the lip on the CS will be smaller than on the NLS. However, generally discrepancies up to 3 mm are aesthetically well tolerated.

FIGURE 18 A closure test can demonstrate whether additional lip release is required and can allow the surgeon to determine whether the advancement height is adequate to close the rotation defect.

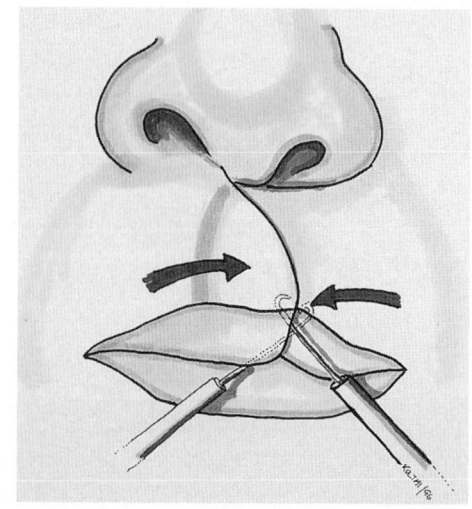

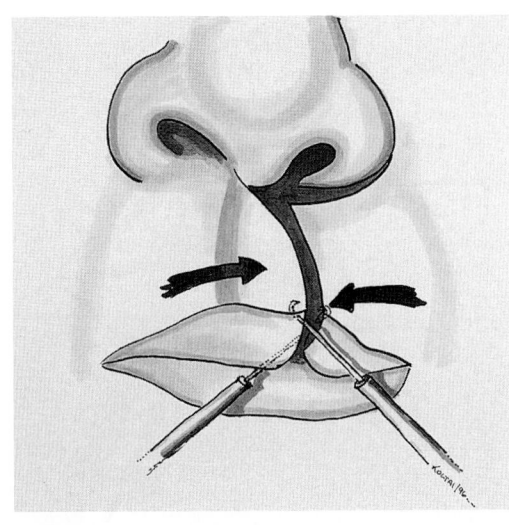

FIGURE 19 When the advancement flap is too short, point 8 can be extended laterally to give increased height. Alternatively, the c-flap can be closed on itself to close a portion of the rotational flap defect.

Primary Rhinoplasty

Using scissors through the existing incisions, the lower lateral cartilage on the CS is freed from the overlying nasal skin (13,14). This can be approached laterally and, if necessary, medially (Figs. 20 and 21). Early in our experience, the authors used both approaches to free this area, but increasingly, the lateral approach alone has been found to be adequate. The area of undermining generally extends over the entire tip of the nose, including inferior and medial portions of the upper lateral cartilage on the CS, as well as the medial portion of the upper lateral cartilage and lower lateral cartilage on the NCS. No attempt is made to separate the mucosa from the cartilage, as the authors have seen significant nasal stenosis when excessive scar contracture occurs.

Closure

Nose   A deep suture of 4-0 or 5-0 polydioxanone (PDS; Ethicon) is used to reposition the columella in the midline. The floor of the nose is then closed with 4-0 or 5-0 chromic suture. Closure of the floor of the nose by necessity affects the final resting position of the ala. The nostril on the CS should be ½ to 1 mm larger than on the NCS. Under no circumstance should it be smaller. Additionally, closure of the floor of the nose affects the vertical height of the ala in relation to the opposite ala. Symmetry at this junction of the procedure will have a significant affect on long-term aesthetic nasal results.

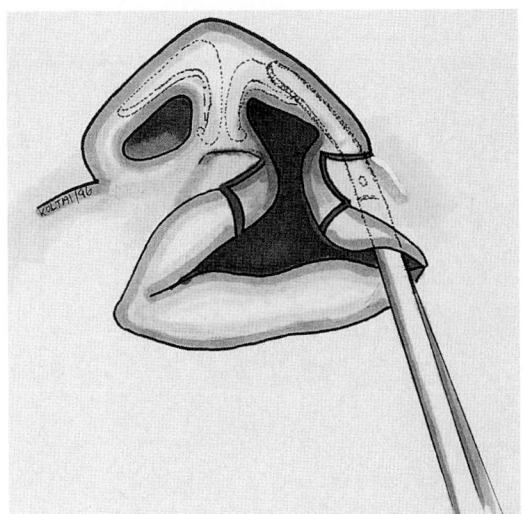

FIGURE 20 The primary rhinoplasty can be accomplished without additional incisions. The lower lateral cartilage is separated from the overlying skin.

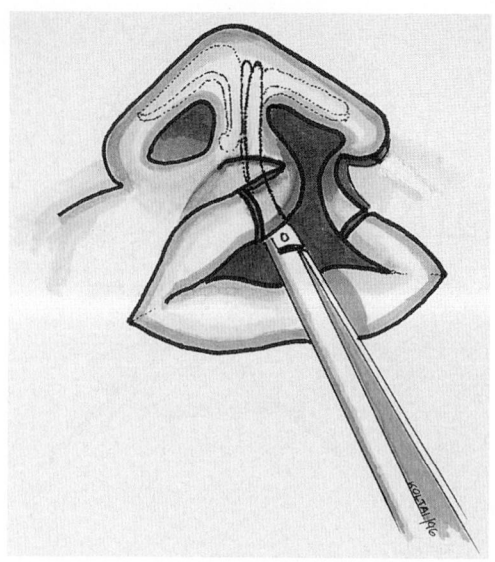

FIGURE 21 Sometimes it is necessary to dissect both medially and laterally to free the lower lateral cartilage completely.

Mucosa   The mucosa must be closed prior to the approximation of the lip muscle (Fig. 22). The m-flap can be used to enhance the frenoplasty. Care should be taken not to make the lip too full on the NCS with the use of too much m-flap tissue. If this tissue is not needed, it should be discarded. The l-flap can be used to reinforce the floor of the nose closure, particularly in the area of the alveolus. Heroic efforts to close the floor of the nose in this area are not warranted, and often the l-flap is discarded. The buccal alveolar sulcus is loosely closed (Fig. 23). The closure of the mucosa has a significant affect on the fullness of the vermilion on both the CS and the NCS. Any discrepancies with mucosa should be made up distantly from the vermilion cutaneous junction. The last few mucosal and vermilion sutures are placed after skin closure.

FIGURE 22 Mucosal closure demonstrating a use for both the m-flap and the l-flap. Often these flaps are discarded.

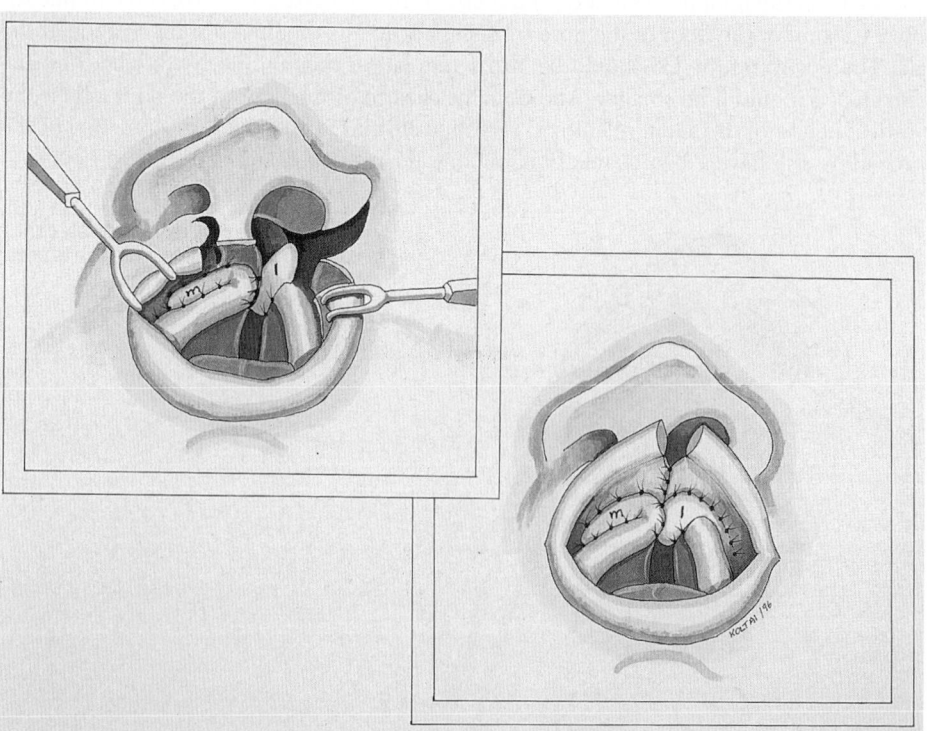

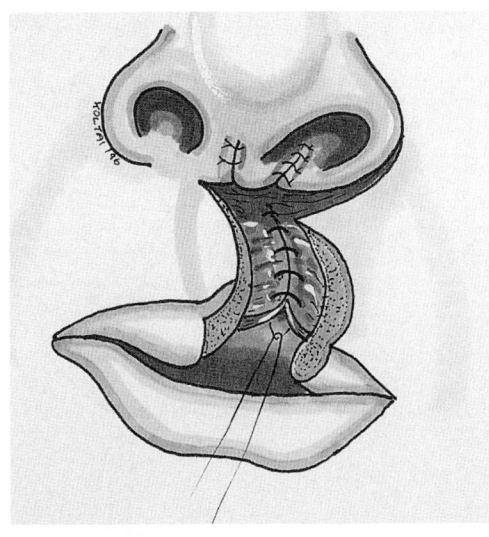

FIGURE 23 The muscle is closed by bites of absorbable suture. Adequate closure inferiorly will prevent a whistle deformity.

Muscle Often a temporary nylon suture is placed at the vermilion cutaneous junction to ensure alignment and to provide inferior traction while the muscle is approximated. It generally requires four or five stitches of 4-0 PDS suture to approximate the muscle (Fig. 24). Superiorly, every effort is made to realign the inappropriately directed orbicularis oris muscle fibers with the opposite side. After the temporary nylon suture is removed, extra care is taken to ensure a slight overapproximation of the muscle fibers inferiorly. This prevents a whistle deformity in this area.

Skin Two or three intradermal 5-0 PDS sutures take the tension off the skin closure. Most of the skin is closed with 6-0 Fast Absorbing Gut (Ethicon). The use of two or three 6-0 nylon sutures is acceptable in key locations. However, removal of nonabsorbable sutures in a young infant can be problematic, and overuse is cautioned against.

Active Placement of Alar Base Because of the movement of the advancement flap medially, the ala on the CS often appears small and elevated in relation to the opposite

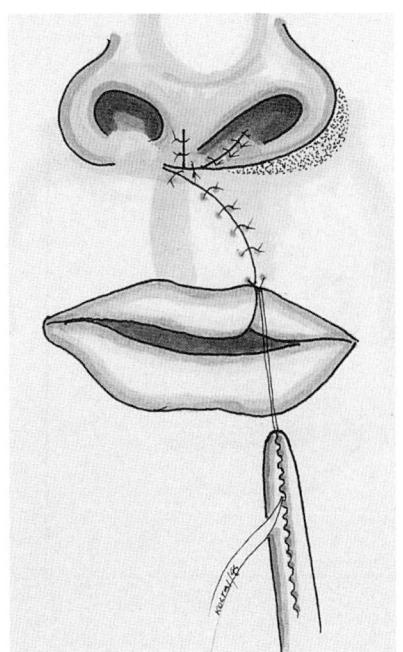

FIGURE 24 Active placement of the alar base often requires excision of skin (*shaded area*) to allow a symmetric nostril to be created.

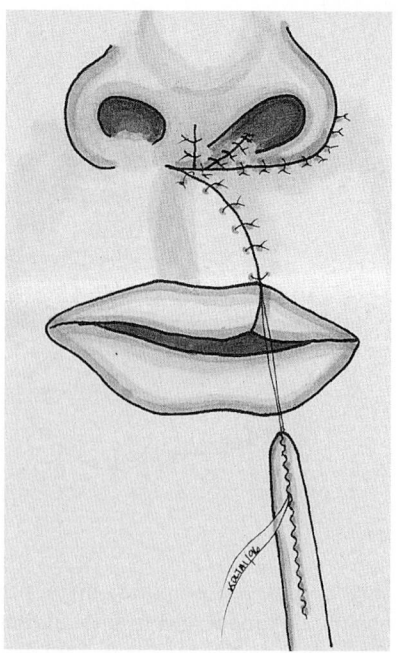

FIGURE 25 After excision of the skin, the nostril is symmetric or slightly larger on the cleft side.

side. If the surgeon had a balanced ala prior to the lip closure, then the simple excision of skin to allow proper placement of the ala will achieve an excellent result (Figs. 25 and 26).

White Roll Flap   The use of a white roll flap is optional, but it can help prevent a widening of the scar at the high point of the cupid's bow and the false appearance of a short lip (pseudo-elevation of the cupid's bow). The white roll flap involves making a 1½-mm triangle that contains cutaneous skin and vermilion from the lateral lip segment. This tri-

FIGURE 26 A white roll flap can be used at the vermilion cutaneous junction to give better definition to the white roll.

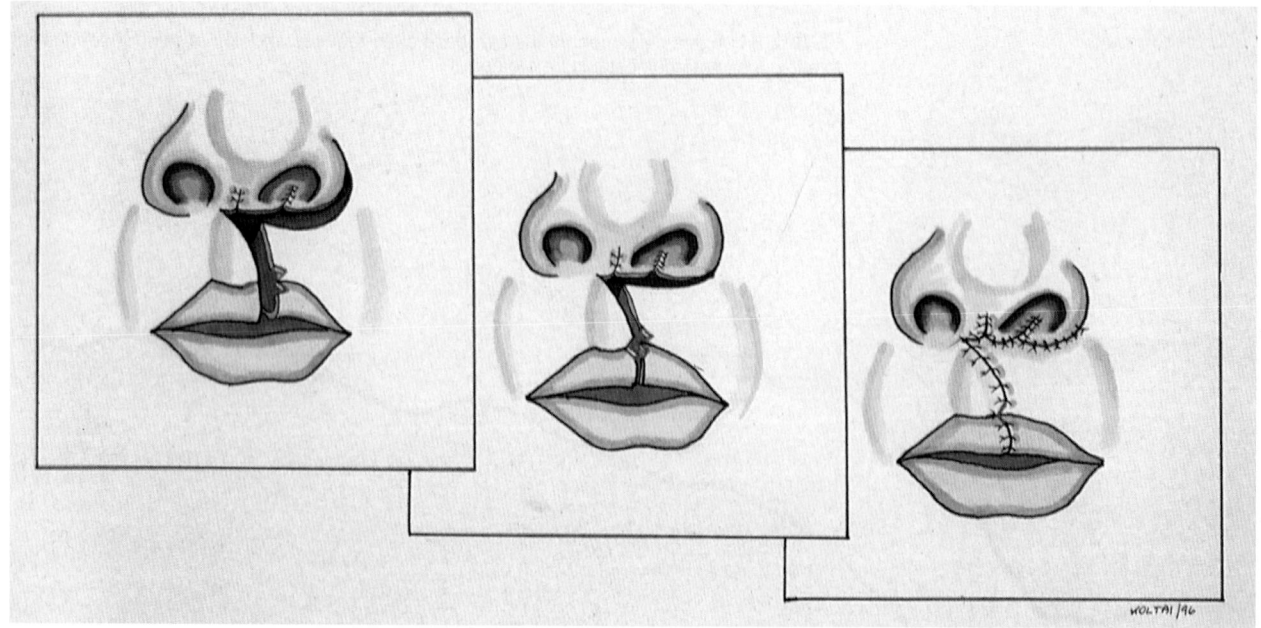

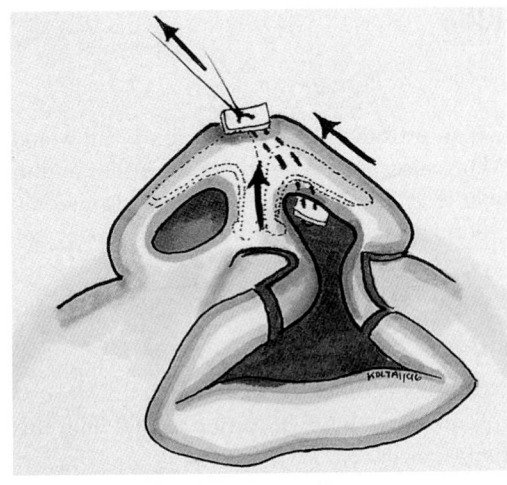

FIGURE 27 Bolsters using Teflon pledgets are utilized to reposition the dome of the lower lateral cartilage superiorly and medially. This decreases hooding and gives a more symmetric nasal tip appearance.

angle is inserted into a similarly shaped cut at the vermilion cutaneous junction on the rotation side of the lip (Fig. 26). A small portion of skin and mucosa is excised from the advancement flap; occasionally, a small piece of mucosa needs to be excised from the rotation flap to allow this to sit appropriately.

Vermilion   The vermilion is closed with 5-0 chromic suture. Often there is redundancy of tissue, which requires excision to avoid fullness of this area. Some surgeons perform a Z-plasty routinely to avoid a whistle deformity. This is not necessary if the orbicularis oris muscle has been properly approximated along the inferior border.

Tip Rhinoplasty   As the dome of the lower lateral cartilage on the CS is generally displaced laterally and inferiorly, an effort is made to reposition this medially and superiorly. Using 4-0 nylon suture and a small Keeth needle over Teflon bolsters, the lower lateral cartilage can be more appropriately positioned (Fig. 27).

Postoperative Care   Topical antibiotic ointment is placed on the suture line and arm restraints are applied. The wound is cleaned with half-strength hydrogen peroxide four or more times a day. Once there is no longer crusting, the use of antibiotic ointment is discouraged as occasionally allergic reactions occur. As alternatives, A&D ointment or cocoa butter with vitamin E can be continued to promote healing. Feedings are given with a syringe and attached flexible tubing. Breast feeding is acceptable. At 3 weeks, normal feeding is resumed and arm restraints discontinued. The use of a Logan's bow is not necessary.

PEARLS AND PERILS

1. Use a closure test to determine whether adequate lip length has been obtained.
2. When the advance flap is too short extend the advancement incision laterally along the vermilion cutaneous junction or use the c-flap to close the superior portion of the rotation defect.
3. Adequate muscle closure inferiorly will avoid a whistle deformity.
4. Align the vermilion cutaneous junction and close the skin and vermilion from this point.
5. A small nostril can be avoided by "active placement of the alar base."
6. Carefully compare lip and nasal symmetry at the completion of surgery and be prepared to redo the lip repair completely.

MANAGEMENT OF COMPLICATIONS

Bleeding and Infection

Significant bleeding with a cleft lip repair is an extremely rare complication and would be associated with a bleeding diatheses. Many surgeons do not routinely utilize antibiotics, yet the rate of infection remains remarkably low. If erythema of the surrounding skin develops, and this is not related to an allergic reaction to the antibiotic ointment, antibiotics are appropriate.

Dehiscence

On a rare occasion, a lip repair will dehisce. This is often associated with a history of trauma or a severe infection. Large bites of muscle with a PDS suture should limit this complication to only the most extreme circumstances.

Elevation of Cupid's Bow

Pseudo-elevation of the cupid's bow can occur due to widening of the scar, particularly at the vermilion cutaneous junction. This can give a false impression that the lip repair did not have adequate rotation release or that the advancement flap was inappropriately short. The use of a white roll flap has been felt to reduce this incidence; however, acceptance of this technique by surgeons is by no means universal.

Excessive Scar Contraction

Some patients have excessive amounts of scar contraction, which can take over a year to resolve. Massage and time are the patient's and surgeon's best ally.

Uneven Vermilion Fullness

This is a common complication that can be due to uneven vermilion fullness prior to the lip repair or to the surgeon's inattentiveness to the closure of the mucosa. It is relatively easily corrected through a mucosal lip reduction on the full side or a V-to-Y advancement on the nonfull side.

PEARLS AND PERILS

1. Massage wound with vitamin E ointment to diminish scarring.
2. Avoid lip revision until the scar is mature.

CONCLUSIONS

The treatment of an infant with unilateral cleft lip is complex and should be coordinated with a cleft team. At the initial evaluation, it is critical to establish rapport with the patient and family, as well as perform a feeding assessment and evaluate for other abnormalities. The surgery is technically demanding, but with proper diligence and effort, it yields excellent results.

✺ REFERENCES

1. McCarthy JG, May JW Jr, Littler JW. Cleft lip and cleft palate and craniofacial anomalies. In: McCarthy JG, ed. *Plastic surgery*, vol. 4. Philadelphia: WB Saunders, 1990:2581–2597, 2633.

2. Millard DR Jr. *Cleft craft: the evolution of its surgery. I. The unilateral deformity.* Boston: Little, Brown, 1976:79–88.

3. Pancoast JA. *A treatise on operative surgery.* Philadelphia: Carey and Hart, 1844:234.

4. Tennison CW. The repair of the unilateral cleft lip by the stencil method. *Plast Reconstr Surg* 1952;9:115–119.

5. Randall P. A triangular flap operation for the primary repair of unilateral clefts of the lip. *Plast Reconstr Surg* 1959;23:331–336.

6. Millard DR Jr. A primary camouflage of the unilateral hare-look. In: *Transactions of the First International Congress of Plastic Surgery, Stockholm, Sweden,* 1957:160–166.

7. *Recommended daily allowances,* 9th ed. Washington DC: National Academy of Sciences, 1980:76–78.

8. Stenstrom SJ. The alar cartilage and the nasal deformity in unilateral cleft lip. *Plast Reconstr Surg* 1966;38:223–231.

9. Sykes JM, Senders CW. Anatomy of cleft lip, palate, and nasal deformities. In: Myers AD, ed. *Biological basis of facial plastic surgery.* New York: Thieme, 1993:57–71.

10. Fara M, Dvork J. Abnormal anatomy of the muscles of palatopharyngeal closure in cleft palate. *Plast Reconstr Surg* 1970;46:488–497.

11. Gorlin RJ, Cohen MM Jr, Levin LS. *Syndromes of the head and neck.* New York: Oxford University Press, 1990:693–714.

12. Ness JA, Sykes JM. Basics of the Millard rotation-advancement technique for repair of the unilateral cleft lip deformity. In: *Facial plastic surgery.* New York: Thieme, 1993:167–176.

13. Sykes JM, Senders CW. Surgery of the cleft lip nasal deformity. *Op Tech Otolaryngol Head Neck Surg* 1990;1:219–224.

14. Senders CW, Sykes JM. Surgical treatment of the unilateral cleft nasal deformity at the time of lip repair. *Fac Plast Surg Clin North Am* 1995;3;1:69–77.

C.W. Senders and J. M. Sykes: Department of Otolaryngology—Head and Neck Surgery, University of California, Davis Medical Center, Sacramento, California 95817.

• *Practical Pediatric Otolaryngology*
• edited by Robin T. Cotton and Charles M. Myer, III
• Lippincott-Raven Publishers, Philadelphia © 1999

CHAPTER 49

Cleft Palate

Jonathan M. Sykes & Craig W. Senders

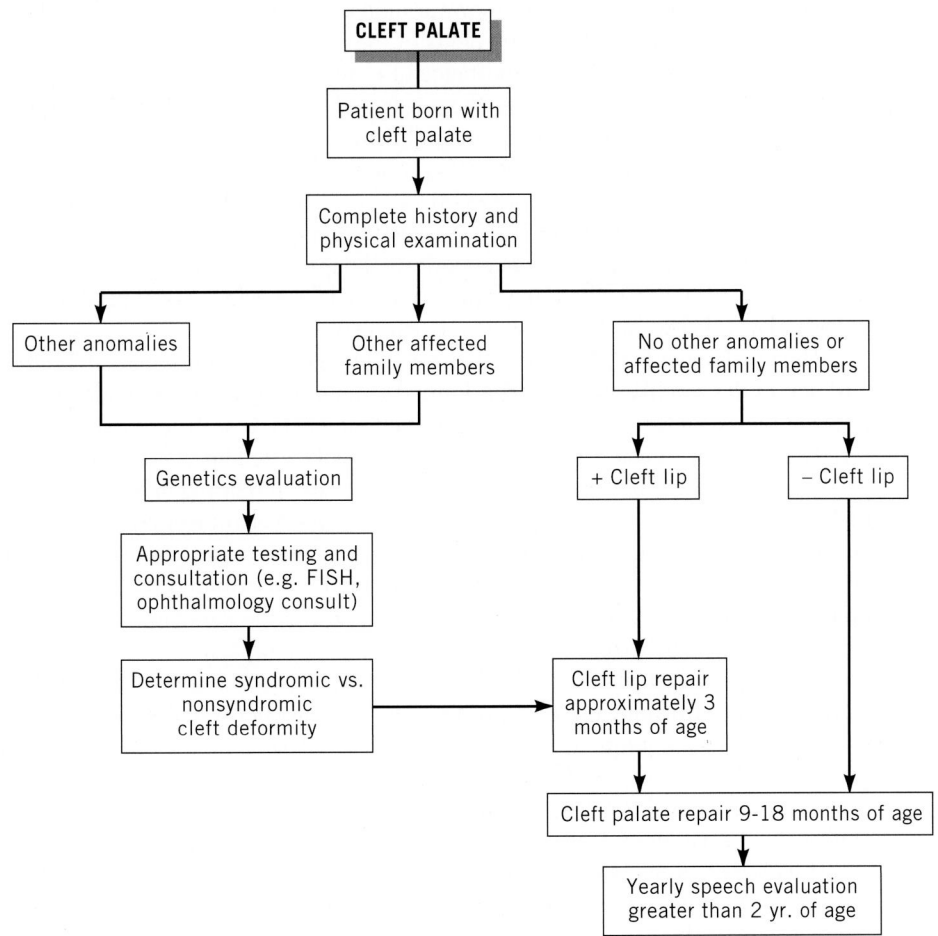

Evaluation and treatment of the patient with congenital cleft palate with or without cleft lip presents a challenge to the cleft surgeon. Appropriate treatment involves a coordinated effort by a multidisciplinary cleft team. Comprehensive care includes otologic, dental, and speech therapy, in addition to surgical treatment of the actual cleft deformity (1).

Initial evaluation of the patient with congenital cleft palate includes classification of the cleft type, identification of associated anomalies, and family teaching to ensure that the cleft patient receives adequate nutrition. Appropriate testing and genetics evaluation should be performed to identify whether the cleft is isolated or syndromic. After cleft palate repair, periodic speech evaluation should be accomplished to monitor normal speech development and identify velopharyngeal dysfunction. Ongoing evaluation by a pediatric dentist and orthodontist is performed to identify and treat malocclusion. This chapter will discuss the evaluation, classification, and comprehensive treatment of the patient with the cleft palate deformity.

🌀 HISTORICAL BACKGROUND

The first attempt at surgical closure of a cleft palate was performed by a French dentist named Le Monnier Rouen in 1764 (2). This technique involved cauterization of the cleft edges and one-layered palatal closure with heavy sutures. Following this initial surgical description, palatal obturation was the mainstay of treatment for the next 50 years.

During the early 19th century, several surgeons including von Graefe and Roux reported successful palatal closure on clefts of the soft palate only (3,4). In the mid-19th century, surgeons realized the importance of reducing tension across the suture line in cleft palate repair. Procedures were then designed to create flaps to reduce tension and minimize the risk of postoperative oronasal fistula. In 1828, Dieffenbach (5) described lateral relaxing incisions and osteotomies of the hard palate to facilitate closure of clefts involving the hard palate. Pancoast (1843), Warren (1828, 1843) (6,7), Fergusson (1845), and finally von Langenbeck (1861) (8) realized the importance of relaxing incisions and described elevation of bipedicle mucoperiosteal flaps to aid in hard palatal closure. This technique of raising and advancing bipedicle palatal flaps, which is still used by some surgeons today, is known as the von Langenbach repair.

The von Langenbach bipedicle flap technique has the disadvantage of limiting visualization of the vascular pedicle. This limited visualization can prevent adequate dissection and release of the soft tissues adjacent to the pedicle. If sufficient release is not performed, increased tension across the suture line will exist. This concept was recognized by Veau (1931) (9), who advocated connecting the lateral relaxing incisions with the medial cleft margin incisions. This posteriorly based unipedicle mucoperiosteal flap has the advantage of increased visualization of the pedicle, increased soft tissue release, and decreased tension across the cleft suture line. Veau also contributed the concept of a layered palatal closure by dissecting and separately closing the nasal layer.

In the 1930s, it became apparent that specific palatoplasty techniques could affect speech function. Wardill (10) and Kilner (11) independently modified Veau's three-flap technique by performing a V-to-Y pushback of the mucoperiosteal flaps to lengthen the soft palate. This technique has the disadvantage of leaving large areas of exposed hard palate laterally. This exposed bone may contribute to maxillary growth restriction in the transverse and anterior–posterior dimensions. Other advances in palatoplasty have included the formal dissection and reapproximation of the malaligned soft palatal musculature. This technique, known as intravelar veloplasty, was first advocated by Otto Kriens (12) in 1970. Although realignment of the tensor veli palatini and levator veli palatini muscles has the theoretical advantage of improving function of the soft palate, prospective, randomized studies have been unable to prove this (13).

In 1978, at the Southeastern Society of Plastic Surgeons, Leonard Furlow (14) described double opposing Z-plasties of the oral and nasal mucosa as a method of palatal repair. This technique has the theoretical advantage of realigning the soft palatal musculature and lengthening the palate. Although originally described for all types of palatal clefts, the double opposing Z-plasty (Furlow) technique is primarily used today for submucous clefts or clefts of the soft palate only (15).

Incidence and Genetics

The incidence of clefting of the lip and palate is approximately 1 in every 750 live births in the United States. Approximately three-fourths of all clefts involve the palate. Many

TABLE 1: Racial Incidence of Clefts

	Cleft lip and palate[a]	Cleft palate[a]
African American	0.2–0.7	0.2–0.5
White	1.0–1.4	0.3–0.5
Asian	1.2–2.1	0.2–0.6
Native American	1.0–4.3	0.5–0.6

[a]Per thousand.
(Modified from ref. 18, with permission.)

factors, such as race, gender, parental age, and exposure to a variety of drugs and medical conditions during pregnancy, affect the overall incidence of cleft palate. It is important to note that isolated cleft palate is genetically different from cleft palate occurring in association with cleft lip.

Cleft palate is seen more frequently in Native Americans, Latin Americans, and Asians; African Americans have the lowest incidence of both cleft palate and cleft lip (with or without cleft palate) (Table 1). Isolated cleft palate is twice as common in females as it is in males, and cleft lip (with or without cleft palate) is more frequent in males.

Parents often ask physicians to state the incidence of clefting of the palate, especially if a child or other family member has already been affected. Although many factors influence the incidence of clefting, a general rule of thumb is that 1 of 750 to 1,000 Americans will be born with some type of cleft, if no prior family history of clefting exists (Table 2). If one parent or one sibling has a history of a cleft, the incidence increases to about 3% to 5%. If one parent and one sibling is affected, the incidence increases to about 13%. Although exact percentages are easily obtained from tables, it is important that all high-risk children and families be referred for genetic consultation and counseling.

ANATOMIC CONSIDERATIONS AND CLASSIFICATION

The palate may be divided embryologically into the primary and secondary palate. The primary palate is located anterior to the incisive foramen and forms between the

TABLE 2: Percentage Recurrence Risk for Nonsyndromic Clefts

Affected relative	Cleft lip, palate (Average)		Cleft palate (Average)	
No parent				
No siblings	0.1		0.04	
One sibling	4–6	(5)	2–4	(3)
One sibling and 1st degree relative	10–20	(15)	10–20	(15)
Two siblings	9–14	(12)	10–17	(13)
One parent				
No siblings	2–4	(3)	3–7	(5)
One sibling	9–16	(13)	10–17	(13)
Two siblings	18–25	(22)	22–24	(23)
1st degree relative	10–20	(15)	10–20	(15)
Two parents				
No siblings	24–50	(37)	18–45	(32)
One sibling	31–54	(43)	30–52	(41)
Two sibling	37–57	(47)	45–55	(50)

(Modified from ref. 18, with permission.)

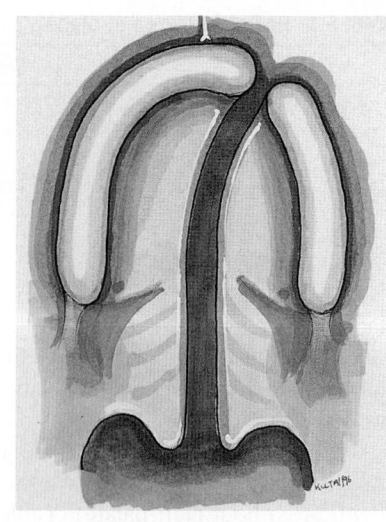

FIGURE 1 Complete unilateral cleft palate and alveolus.

fourth and sixth weeks of gestation. This gestational age coincides with the formation of the central aspect of the upper lip. The primary palate contains the developing tooth buds of the central and lateral incisors, and the remainder of the teeth are formed from the lateral palatal shelves.

The secondary palate is formed from the fusion of the paired palatal shelves, between the sixth and twelfth weeks of gestation. The palatal processes (or palatal shelves) of the secondary palate fuse in an anterior-to-posterior direction, beginning at the incisive foramen.

Interruption of the normal formation of the palate at any stage of development can result in a cleft palate. The process can be associated with clefting of the upper lip and alveolus or can occur in isolation. A cleft of the entire hard and soft palate is referred to as *complete*, and embryologically occurs in association with a cleft lip. A complete cleft palate may be associated with either a unilateral or a bilateral cleft lip (Figs. 1 and 2). A complete bilateral cleft lip and palate involves complete association of the two palatal shelves from the midline vomer and premaxilla.

An *incomplete*, or partial, cleft palate usually refers to a cleft that does not involve the primary palate. This clefting of the secondary palate is a malformation that inhibits fusion of the palatal shelves. An incomplete cleft palate may present as a submucous cleft (with bifid uvula), as a cleft of the soft palate only, or as a cleft of the entire secondary palate (Fig. 3 and 4).

FIGURE 2 Complete bilateral cleft palate and alveolus.

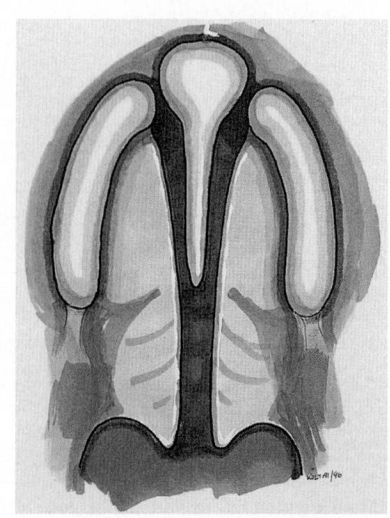

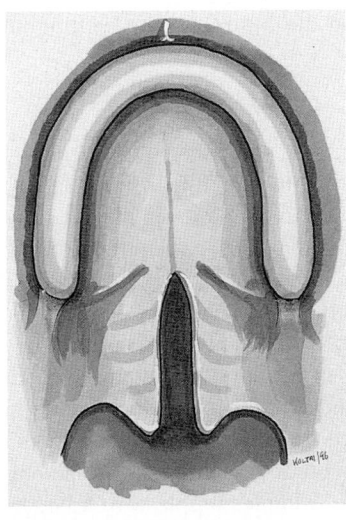

FIGURE 3 Cleft of the soft palate.

PATIENT ASSESSMENT

All patients with cleft palate should have a through history and physical examination, including a careful search for associated congenital abnormalities. Almost 300 syndromes have been associated with cleft lip and palate. Awareness of common syndromes is important as this will often suggest appropriate testing or consultation. For instance, a patient with Pierre Robin sequence (micrognathia, glossoptosis, and U-shaped cleft palate) is predisposed to having airway difficulties after cleft palate repair. This is important knowledge for any cleft surgeon. Additionally, the patient with Pierre Robin sequence should have an ophthalmology consultation as some of these patients will have early myopia or retinal problems. This syndrome (Pierre Robin sequence plus myopia or retinal problems) is known as Stickler's syndrome and warrants careful periodic ophthalmologic examinations. Other common syndromes associated with cleft palate include velocardiofacial, Treacher Collins, fetal alcohol, and orofaciadigital type 1 syndromes. Cleft palate syndromes with cleft lip, such as van der Woude's syndrome, also exist.

All patients with cleft palate and a significant family history of clefting, or with associated anomalies, should receive a genetic consultation. Appropriate testing (e.g., serum immunoassay in patients suspected of having velocardiofacial syndrome) or consultation (e.g., ophthalmology consultation in patients with Pierre Robin sequence) should be per-

FIGURE 4 Cleft of the secondary palate.

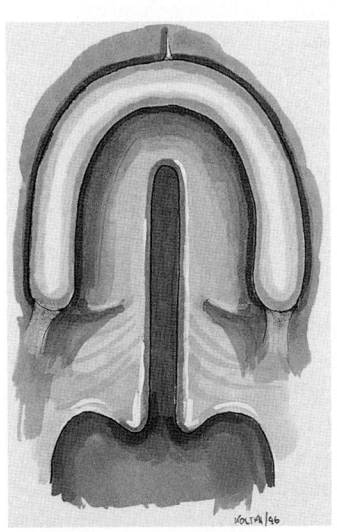

formed. Additionally, the family should be counseled on the future risks of clefting in subsequent births.

Feeding

All infants with a cleft palate will have some compromise in their ability to feed. In babies with isolated, nonsyndromic clefting of the palate (i.e., without other significant neuromuscular problems), family training by a nurse specialist is usually sufficient to enable the child to feed successfully.

The increased intraoral volume and lack of continuity of the palate result in an inability of the infant to suckle normally. The inefficient suckle mechanism can be overcome by (a) modifying the nipple and bottle used and (b) careful positioning of the child during feeding. Additionally, the parents should be warned that early feedings may require longer periods until both the parents and child have adjusted to the altered suckle mechanism. A Mead Johnson cleft palate nurser squeeze bottle is advised, as this allows coordinated squeezing with the infant's effort to suckle. A longer nipple with a larger opening may also be utilized. This will either occlude or bypass the opening in the palate. In almost all cases, infants and parents are able to adapt to the cleft, to achieve adequate oral intake.

The child with a cleft palate should be seen weekly until it is clear that adequate weight gain and nutrition are achieved. After a weight loss of about 10% (of birth weight) at 1 week, the infant should gain about 20 to 30 g per day. Weight gain of less than 15 g per day will usually require hospital admission and nasogastric feeding. The parents are advised to begin the child on a "cup" diet 3 weeks prior to the palatoplasty procedure. A cup diet refers to any food that can be spooned out of a cup. This diet is continued for approximately 3 weeks postoperatively. The change in diet is implemented well prior to the procedure to allow the child to adjust to the change. This hopefully will alleviate a difficult dietary change perioperatively, when oral pain may add to feeding difficulties.

PEARLS AND PERILS

Evaluation
1. All patients with clefts should undergo a careful examination for associated anomalies.
2. Awareness of common syndromes is important.
3. All high-risk families should be referred for genetic counseling.
Feeding
1. Children with unrepaired cleft palate have an altered suckle mechanism.
2. With proper training, most infants with cleft palate are able to achieve adequate oral intake.
3. Patients should be started on a "cup" diet 3 weeks prior to palatoplasty.

 TREATMENT RECOMMENDATIONS

Timing of Cleft Repair

The timing of repair of cleft deformities is outlined in Table 3. In all patients with cleft palate, tympanostomy tube placement is performed to aerate the middle ear and to minimize the chance of chronic ear disease. In patients with cleft lip and palate, cleft lip repair is performed at approximately 3 months of age. At the time of lip repair, tympanostomy tubes are also placed. Cleft palate repair occurs between 9 and 18 months of age, prior to the initial development of speech. Long-acting tympanostomy tubes are placed at the time of palatoplasty. After cleft palate repair, yearly speech evaluation, beginning

TABLE 3: Timing of Cleft Repairs

Procedure	Age
Cleft lip repair	3 months
Tip rhinoplasty	
Tympanostomy tubes	
Palatoplasty	9–18 months
T-tube placement	
Speech evaluation	3–4 years
Velopharyngeal insufficiency workup and surgery (if necessary)	4–6 years
Alveolar bone grafting	9–11 years
Nasal reconstruction	12–18 years
Orthognathic surgery (if necessary)	At completion of mandibular growth (>16 years)

at 2 years of age, is essential to identify velopharyngeal insufficiency (VPI). If VPI is identified, evaluation (including nasopharyngoscopy and videofluoroscopy) is performed to quantify the amount of velopharyngeal dysfunction.

Other interventions for the cleft patient (including orthodontic therapy, alveolar bone grafting, cleft nasal reconstruction, and orthognathic surgery) are related to the degree of the original deformity and the growth of the face. It can be noted that in cleft patients who do not undergo palatoplasty at a young age, midfacial growth is normal (16). Ross (17) has noted that midfacial growth disturbance is most related to the type of repair and timing of palatoplasty. The decision to perform palatoplasty at approximately 1 year of age is made to improve speech and with the knowledge that facial growth may be altered.

Goals and General Principles

The goals of palatoplasty are (a) to allow the patient to develop normal speech and (b) to prevent nasal regurgitation of food through the oronasal fistula. To prevent postoperative VPI, recreation of the velopharyngeal muscular sling should be performed. Successful repair of a cleft palate requires adherence to several surgical principles. (Table 4). These principles include (a) adequate flap mobilization to minimize wound tension, (b) atraumatic technique to minimize injury to vessels at the flap periphery, (c) two-layer closure of the oral and nasal mucosa to minimize postoperative fistula formation, and (d) recreation of the soft palate muscular sling to maximize velopharyngeal function and speech.

To maximize blood supply to the margins of the palatal flaps, meticulous atraumatic technique must be used when elevating and manipulating the palatal mucosa. A "no-touch" technique is advocated, in which the margins of the palatal flaps are never grasped with tissue forceps. Elevators, blunt-tipped suctions, and surgical hooks are used in careful atraumatic fashion.

Attempts are made to minimize use of monopolar cautery at the periphery of the palatal flaps. Vasoconstriction is achieved with careful injection of xylocaine 1% with 1:100,000 epinephrine into the entire palatal mucosa. Approximately 2 to 3 mL of solution are used in the 1-year-old patient prior to prepping and draping. A well-placed in-

TABLE 4: Principles of Palatoplasty

Minimize wound tension
Atraumatic technique
Two-layer closure of oral and nasal layers
Recreation of soft palate muscular sling

jection will markedly decrease intraoperative blood loss. If troublesome mucosal bleeding does occur, bipolar cautery should be carefully used for hemostasis.

Three-Flap Palatoplasty

The three-flap technique is used to repair clefts of the secondary palate (the entire soft palate and the hard palate posterior to the incisive foramen). This technique involves medial incisions along the cleft margin from the incisive foramen through the uvula bilaterally. Bilateral lateral incisions are made adjacent to the tooth crowns and carried around the maxillary tuberosity. The medial cleft margin and lateral relaxing incisions are joined anteriorly by oblique incisions extending from the cleft margin incisions laterally to the lateral alveolar incisions at the level of the canine teeth (Fig. 5A). These anterior communicating incisions convert the flaps into posteriorly based unipedicled mucoperiosteal flaps, which can be completely mobilized to minimize tension across the cleft wound.

After complete injection of the palate with a xylocaine–epinephrine solution, a Dingman mouth gag (with tongue and buccal mucosal retractors) is placed. All patients are placed in the reverse Trendelenberg position with a throat pack. Mucosal incisions are made with a #15 scalpel. The incisions are then recut to ensure complete and clean incision through the mucoperiosteum. Elevation of the posteriorly based palatal flaps is performed with a Woodsen elevator. The greater palatine neurovascular pedicle is identified, preserved, and carefully dissected from surrounding soft tissue.

Dissection is carried posterior to the neurovascular pedicle into the space of Ernst with a Woodsen elevator. The malinserted levator sling is bluntly dissected off the posterior free edge of the hard palate. The soft palate muscular sling is dissected with a curved blunt-tipped scissors, to facilitate reapproximation.

After dissection and elevation are completed, the mucosal margins of the oral flaps are advanced to determine mobility. If tension exists across the cleft margin, further dissection, usually around the neurovascular pedicle, must be performed. If necessary, the entire pedicle may be mobilized from its foramen by sharply skeletonizing the surrounding soft tissue, or by fracture of the bony plate at the foramen. It is essential that the closure be tension free, and this can be determined by advancing the flaps across the cleft gap.

The two posteriorly based mucoperiosteal flaps may be advanced posteriorly in a V-to-Y fashion to create increased length in the soft palate. This modification of the three-

FIGURE 5 A: Secondary palatal cleft. Dotted lines, incisions for three-flap palatoplasty. **B:** Oral closure of a secondary palatal cleft with three-flap palatoplasty. **C:** Closure of three-flap palatoplasty with V-to-Y pushback.

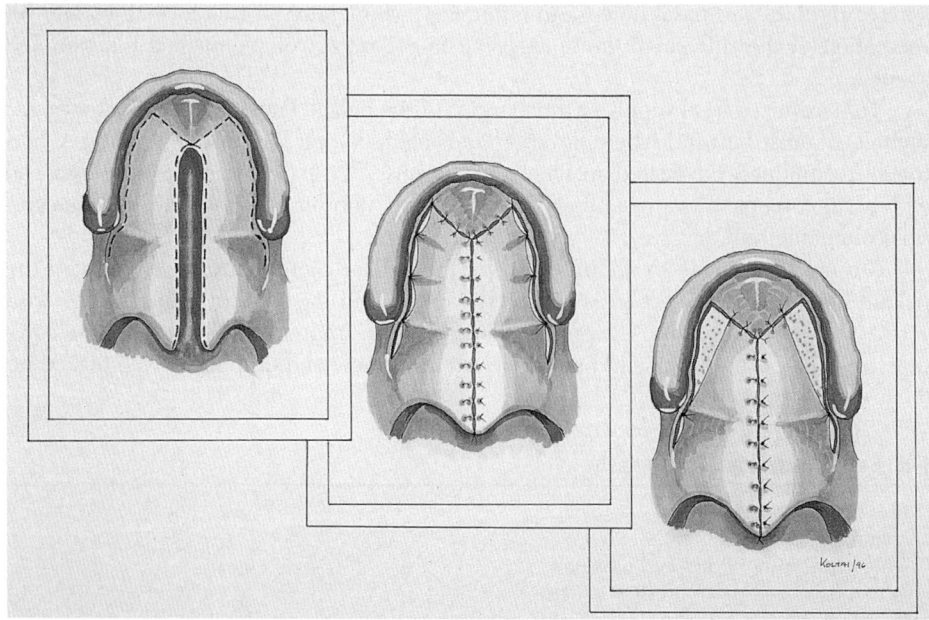

A-C

flap palatoplasty was described in 1937 by Wardill (10) and Kilner (11) and is referred to as the *pushback technique.* This technique has the advantage of adding palatal length, which theoretically can improve velopharyngeal function. However, the V-to-Y pushback does leave additional bone exposed laterally (Fig. 5C). This "raw" bone may cause transverse growth restriction of the maxilla and predispose to maxillary hypoplasia at full growth (17).

After mobilization of the posteriorly based mucoperiosteal flaps, dissection and release of the malaligned soft palatal musculature from the posterior edge of the hard palate is performed. This allows reorientation of the muscular sling from an oblique to a transverse (more physiologic) orientation. Closure of the velopharyngeal muscular sling allows a three-layered closure on the soft palate. Complete elevation and closure of nasal flaps is performed prior to any suturing, minimizing the chance of postoperative fistula. The nasal flaps are elevated in a *submucosal* plane, with a curved hockey-stick-shaped elevator to undermine behind the palatal shelves.

Closure of the palate is performed in layers, beginning with complete reapproximation of the nasal layer with a 4-0 chromic catgut suture on a J-shaped needle. A J-shaped needle is used when possible as this needle shape facilitates intraoral placement of sutures in difficult areas. In cases of very wide clefts of the secondary palate, separate vomerine nasal flaps may be elevated and used for closure of the nasal layer. After complete closure of the nasal layer, the soft palatal muscular sling is reapproximated with 4-0 synthetic braided absorbable suture. A J-shaped needle is again used. The muscular layer is the strength of the soft palatal repair and usually requires three to four carefully placed sutures. Closure of the oral layer is accomplished in a posterior-to-anterior direction with 4-0 braided absorbable suture (Fig. 5B). Alternating simple and vertical mattress sutures are placed to maximize eversion of the oral layer. At least one "tacking" simple suture is placed to coapt the oral and nasal layers at the midportion of the hard palate. This decreases the dead space and minimizes the risk of postoperative hematoma formation.

The technique of intravelar veloplasty involves a formal dissection of the levator veli palatini muscles from the cleft margin. This technique, first described by Kriens in 1970 (12), was originally thought to improve palatal function. A retrospective study by Dreyer and Trier (19) indicated a decrease in the need for a pharyngeal flap from 35% to 9% when using the intravelar veloplasty. However, a subsequent prospective, randomized study by Marsh et al. in 1989 (13) failed to confirm this hypothesis statistically. Debate continues as to whether dissection and closure of the levator veli palatini muscles provide long-term improved palatal function.

von Langenbeck Palatoplasty

In the early 19th century, elevation of bipedicle mucoperiosteal flaps to close clefts of the hard palate was first reported independently by Dieffenbach (5), Warren (6,7), and von Langenbeck (8). This method involves medial incisions (along the cleft margin) and lateral relaxing incisions (adjacent to the alveolar ridge). Undermining the bipedicled flaps in a mucoperiosteal plane allows flap release and advancement. The flaps can then be closed like a "drawbridge" in a tension-free fashion.

The medial (cleft margin) incisions are made with a #15 scalpel through the mucosa and the mucoperiosteum. The lateral incisions are made adjacent to the tooth roots and around the maxillary tuberosity (Fig. 6A). Atraumatic technique is then used to elevate the mucoperiosteal flaps with a Woodsen elevator. After complete elevation, the cleft margins are opposed manually to determine if a tension-free closure is possible. This step is crucial. If tension exists at the wound edge, further elevation and undermining is performed to ensure a tension-free closure. The cleft margin is then closed in layers with 4-0 braided absorbable suture. Two to three tacking sutures are used to close the lateral incision lines (Fig. 6B).

Several important principles of palatoplasty are used in the bipedicle flap palatoplasty (often called the von Langenbeck repair). These tenets include a two-layered clo-

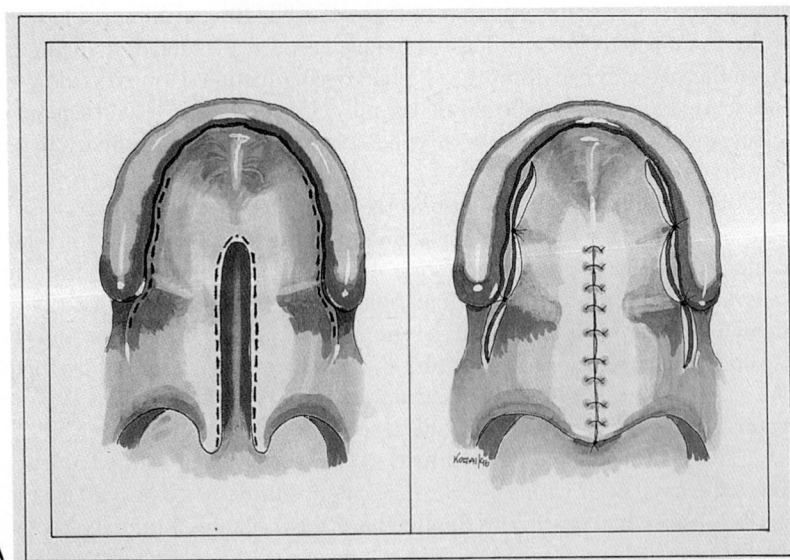

FIGURE 6 A: Bipedicle flap incisions for von Langenbeck palatoplasty in a secondary palatal cleft. **B:** Closure of the bipedicle flap palatoplasty.

sure (oral and nasal) of the hard palate and adequate flap mobilization to minimize tension across the wound. However, the bipedicle flap technique fails to visualize the vascular pedicle fully and may therefore be associated with increased wound tension when used in wide palatal clefts. For this reason, most surgeons connect the medial and lateral cleft incisions, thereby converting the bipedicle flaps (von Langenbeck) to posteriorly based unipedicled flaps. These three-flap (incomplete clefts) and two-flap (complete clefts) repairs allow increased pedicle visualization, increased flap mobilization, and decreased wound tension.

Two-Flap Palatoplasty

The two-flap technique is used to repair complete palatal clefts (of the entire primary and secondary palate). Two-flap palatoplasty may be used for both complete bilateral and unilateral clefts. In the complete unilateral cleft, the medial incisions are carried anteriorly almost to the alveolar ridge and joined to the curved lateral incisions (Fig. 7A). The incisions are again scored with a #15 scalpel and recut to ensure complete incision through the periosteal layer. Subperiosteal flap elevation with an atraumatic "no-touch" technique is performed to expose and isolate the neurovascular pedicle. Dissection posterior to the pedicle is accomplished to mobilize the oral palatal flap completely (Fig. 7B). The "pinch" technique is again used to ensure a tension-free closure. Nasal flaps are elevated with curved hockey-stick elevators.

After adequate flap elevation, two-layered closure over the hard palate is performed by closing both the nasal (4-0 chromic catgut) and oral layers (4-0 braided absorbable suture) (Fig. 8). In the region of the soft palate, the palatal muscles are dissected and separately reoriented and closed. This provides a three-layered closure in the soft palate. As in the three-flap palatoplasty, one or two coapting sutures are placed, tacking the oral layer to the nasal layer. This decreases the potential space between these layers.

If the palatal cleft is bilateral, a separate longitudinal incision is made in the mucosa over the vomer, creating two vomerian mucosal flaps (Fig. 9). The incisions are made with a #15 scalpel, and the flaps are elevated with Paget elevators. These two flaps are separately sutured to the nasal mucosa on each side with 4-0 chromic catgut suture. This creates two nasal closure layers anteriorly and one posteriorly. If the cleft is unilateral, only a single nasal suture line is created. In either the unilateral or bilateral complete cleft palate, a small area cannot be closed anteriorly at the alveolar ridge. This small residual alveolar cleft is usually closed when the patient is about 9 to 11 years of age, at the time of alveolar bone grafting.

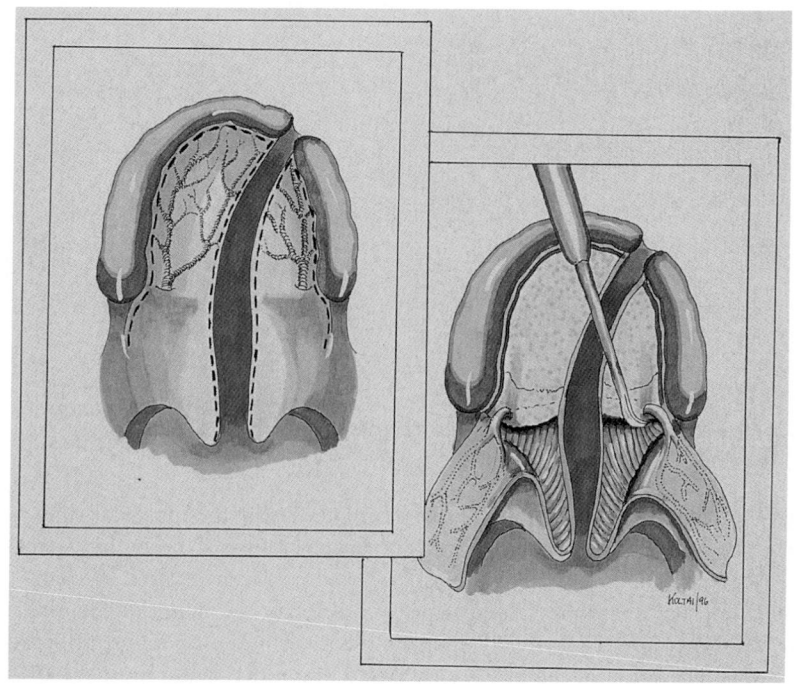

FIGURE 7 A: Complete unilateral cleft palate. Dotted lines, oral incisions for a two-flap palatoplasty. **B:** Elevation of mucoperiosteal flaps with skeletalization of the neurovascular pedicle. Note that skeletization is taking place posterior to the greater palatine neurovascular bundle in the space of Ernst.

Furlow Palatoplasty

The double reversing Z-plasty, or Furlow palatoplasty, is usually used to repair submucous cleft palate or clefts of the soft palate only. The technique, first introduced by Leonard Furlow (14,15) in 1978, involves opposing Z-plasties of the oral and nasal mucosa. The repair is designed to (a) lengthen the palate and (b) recreate the muscular sling of the soft palate. Theoretically, these two important features combine to improve function of the soft palate.

The central limbs of the double reversing Z-plasty technique are made at the cleft margin with a #15 scalpel (Fig. 10A). Incisions are then made extending from the cleft

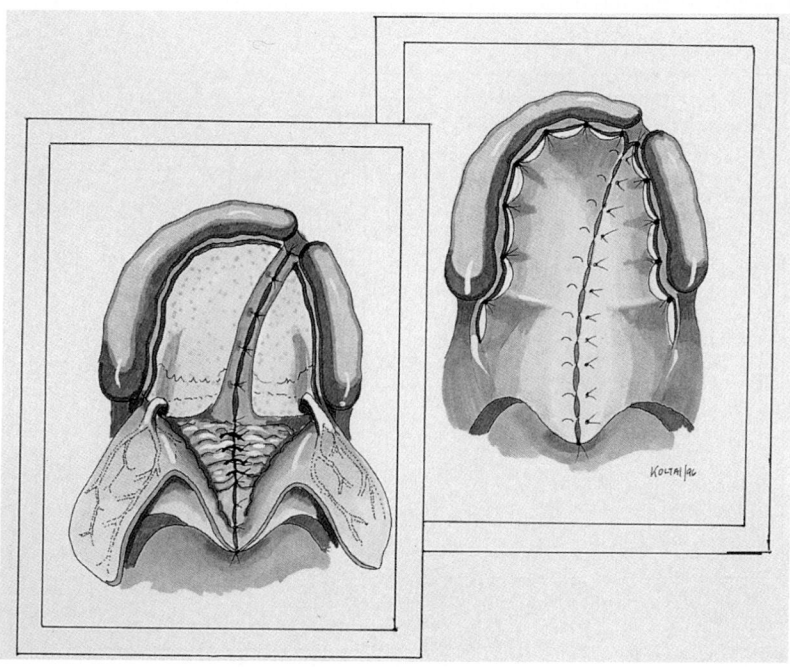

FIGURE 8 A: Two-flap palatoplasty after closure of the nasal flaps and soft palate musculature. **B:** Two-flap palatoplasty at completion after oral flap closure.

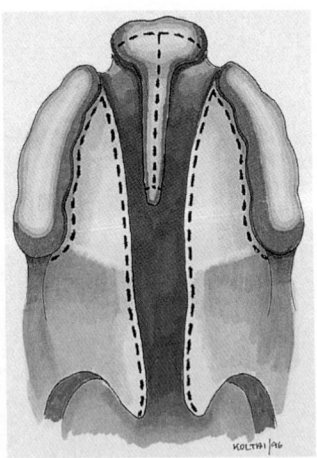

FIGURE 9 Designation of two-flap palatoplasty in a complete bilateral cleft. Dotted lines, oral mucosal incisions. Note the T-shaped incision on the vomer, indicating incisions for bilateral vomerian flaps.

margin obliquely toward the hamulus laterally. It is important that the muscular sling of the soft palate be reoriented to a horizontal direction during closure of the Z-plasty flaps. For this reason, the soft palate musculature must be based posteriorly within the flap.

The anterior oral incision parallels and is just posterior to the margin of the hard palate. The posterior incision extends medially from the uvula and is obliquely oriented toward the hamulus. Elevation of the posteriorly based oral mucosa and muscle flap is performed with a Woodsen elevator (Fig. 10B). The anteriorly based oral flap contains only oral mucosa and glands, and this dissection is easily accomplished with a long curved tenotomy scissors. After elevation of the oral flaps, a long right-angled scissors is used to create the nasal flaps by making opposite incisions on the nasal mucosa (Fig. 11).

The anatomy of the soft palate musculature is important in dissection and elevation of the oral and nasal flaps in this procedure. In that the levator veli palatini muscles are located immediately adjacent to the nasal (not the oral) mucosa, elevation of these muscles from the nasal mucosa is difficult (Fig. 12). Meticulous dissection of the flap containing the oral mucosa and muscle from the nasal mucosa is therefore required. Right-handed surgeons more easily perform this difficult dissection on the patient's left or contralateral side; left-handed surgeons should design the incisions in the mirror image.

After dissection of both oral and nasal flaps, transposition of all four flaps is accomplished. Closure of the nasal flaps is first performed with 4-0 chromic catgut su-

FIGURE 10 A: Schematic diagram of a Furlow palatoplasty indicating proposed incisions. **B:** Elevation of oral flaps in the Furlow palatoplasty. Note that the more difficult dissection of the palatomusculature from the nasal mucosa is performed on the patient's left side. The right side contains oral mucosa only, and the left side contains oral mucosa and muscle.

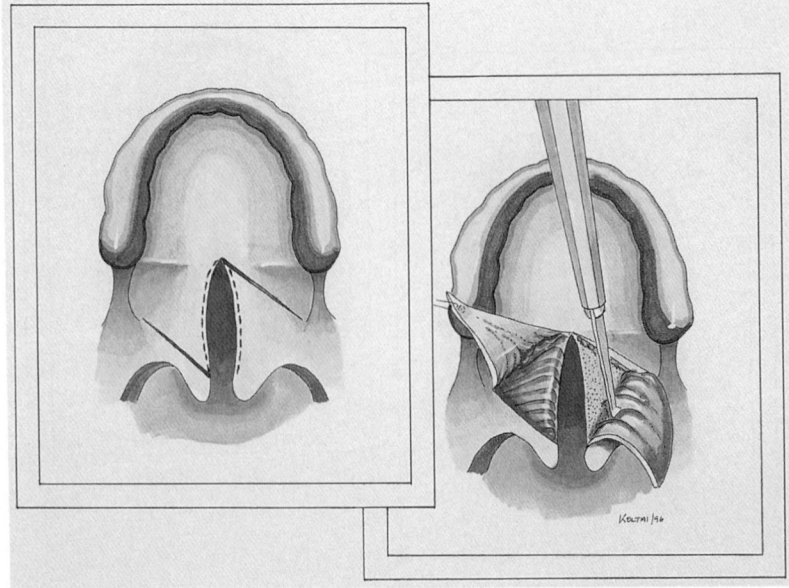

A

B

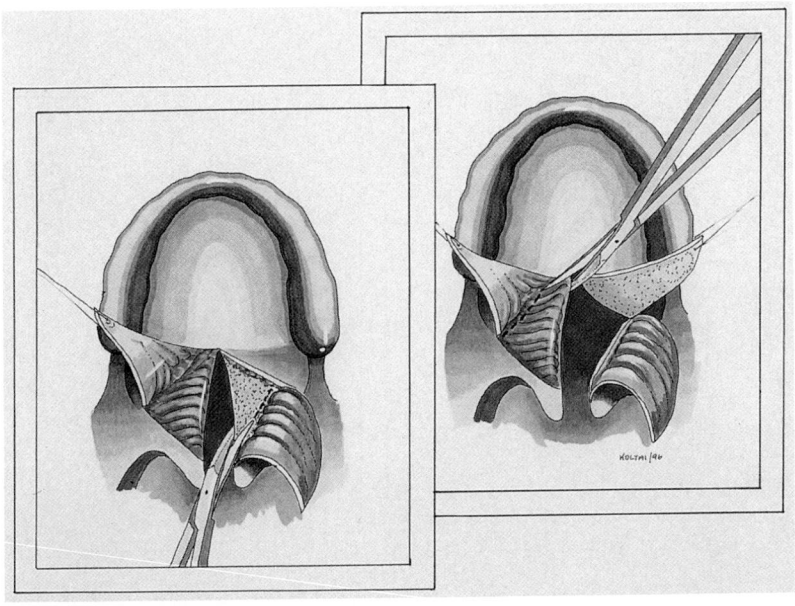

FIGURE 11 A, B: Incision of the nasal side flaps with a curved scissor.

ture (Fig. 13). The muscular sling is then reapproximated with 4-0 braided absorbable suture (Fig. 14A). The oral flaps and mucosa are also closed with 4-0 braided absorbable suture (Fig. 14B). In that the nasal and oral suture lines do not overlie one another, postoperative fistula are usually prevented and scarring is minimized. This technique can be combined with the two- or three-flap techniques anteriorly for complete or secondary palatal clefts.

Preferred Techniques

A summary of preferred surgical techniques for repair of cleft palate is listed in Table 5. They include two-flap palatoplasty for complete clefts, three-flap palatoplasty for incomplete clefts, and the double reversing **Z**-plasty for submucous clefts and clefts of the soft palate only.

PEARLS AND PERILS

1. Use atraumatic "no-touch" technique to maintain vascularity to flap periphery.
2. Ensure tension-free closure by testing flap mobility prior to closure.
3. Use two-layered closure over hard palate and three-layered closure on soft palate.
4. Recreate soft palate muscular sling.
5. Use "tacking" suture to coapt oral and nasal mucosa.

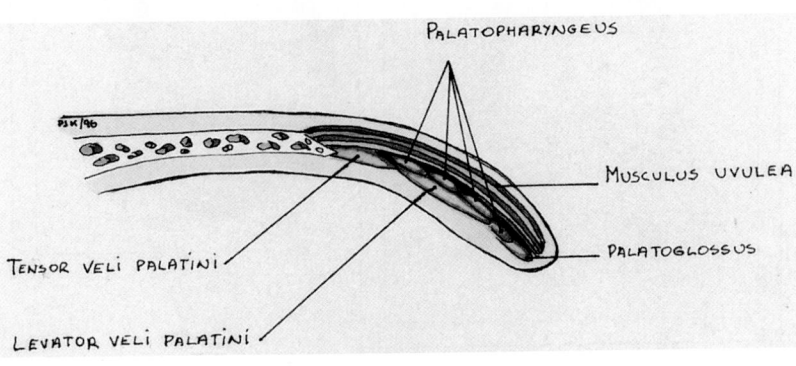

FIGURE 12 Schematic diagram of a sagittal section of the soft palate showing the relationship of the palatal muscles to the oral and nasal mucosa. Note that the levator veli palatini muscle is close to the nasal mucosa.

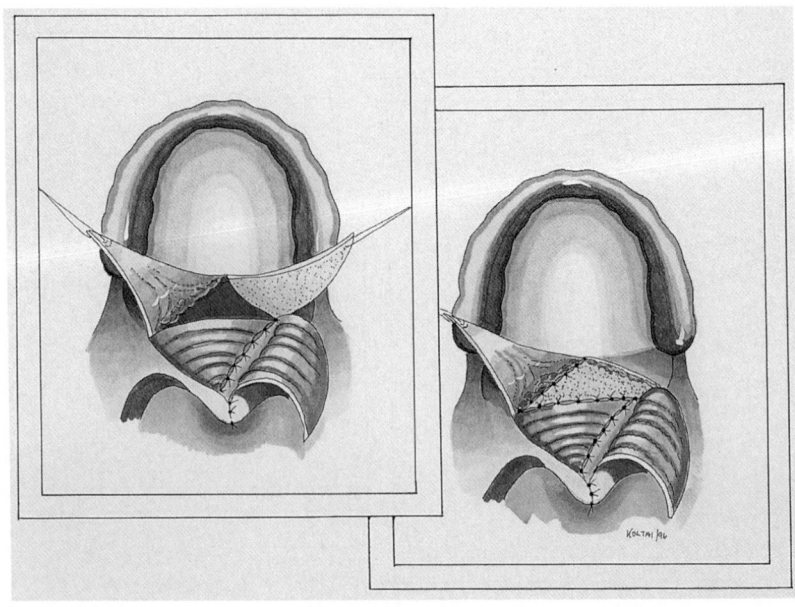

FIGURE 13 A, B: Closure of the nasal mucosa and the central limb of the double reversing Z-plasty flaps.

Postoperative Care

Cleft palate patients are placed on a pureed diet from a cup for 3 weeks. Arm restraints are also utilized for a 3-week interval. Care is taken to keep patients well hydrated postoperatively. A mist tent is used to prevent intraoral mucosal surfaces from excessive drying. Oral intake and oxygen saturation are carefully monitored. Patients are discharged from the hospital when they are taking 90% of their calculated daily oral fluid intake. Antibiotics are used for 3 days. Steroids are not routinely used.

MANAGEMENT OF COMPLICATIONS

Complications after palatoplasty are uncommon. Complications include bleeding, infection, airway obstruction, and oronasal fistula. Intraoperative bleeding can be minimized by judicious infiltration of a vasoconstrictive agent (1:100,000 epinephrine) and

FIGURE 14 A, B: Oral closure of the double reversing Z-plasty showing significant palatal lengthening after this closure.

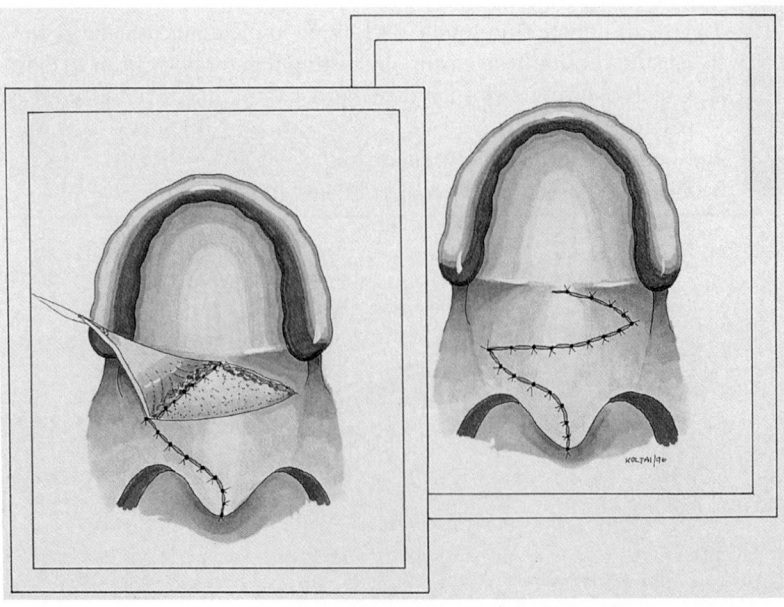

TABLE 5: Preferred Palatoplasty Techniques

Cleft type	Technique
Complete unilateral	Two-flap
Complete bilateral	Two-flap (with vomerian flaps)
Complete secondary palate	Three-flap
Soft palate	Double reversing Z-plasty
Submucous	Double reversing Z-plasty

meticulous intraoperative technique. The need for perioperative blood transfusion is rare. Although some airway compromise occurs in all postoperative cleft palate patients, significant airway obstruction is usually avoided. Periodic release of the mouth gag intraoperatively minimizes postoperative tongue edema. Careful postoperative care, including frequent suctioning of the pharyngeal secretions and use of a mist tent, will decrease obstructive symptoms. In patients at greater risk, a "tongue" suture may decrease the need for reintubation postoperatively.

With careful adherence to surgical principles, the incidence of oronasal fistula after cleft palate repair is rare. Care should be taken to minimize wound tension and maximize flap vascularity prior to closure of the palate. When a layered palatal closure is used, a minor early mucosal dehiscence often does not result in fistula formation.

SUMMARY

Cleft palate is a relatively uncommon congenital malformation often associated with clefting of the lip or other congenital anomalies. Repair is essential for the development of normal speech and eustachian tube function. Adherence to basic principles such as intraoperative hemostasis, adequate flap elevation to minimize wound tension, and meticulous layered surgical closure usually result in successful palatoplasty procedures. Complications such as bleeding, infection, and fistula formation are uncommon and usually can be avoided by following basic surgical principles.

 ## REFERENCES

1. Koepp-Baker H. The craniofacial team. In: Bzoch KR, ed. *Communicative disorders related to cleft lip and palate.* Boston: Little, Brown, 1979.
2. Rogers BO. History of cleft lip and palate treatment. In: Rosenstein SW, Bzoch KR, eds. *Cleft lip and palate.* Boston: Little, Brown, 1971:142.
3. Millard DR Jr. *Cleft craft, the evolution of its surgery.* Boston: Little Brown, 1980.
4. Randall P, LaRossa D. Cleft palate. In: McCarthy JG, ed. *Plastic surgery,* vol. 4. *Cleft lip and palate and craniofacial anomalies.* Philadelphia: WB Saunders, 1990.
5. Dieffenbach JF. Beitrage zur Gaumennath. *Lit Ann Heilk* 1828;10:322.
6. Warren JC. On an operation for the cure of natural fissures of the soft palate. *Am J Med Sci* 1828;3:1.
7. Warren JM. Operations for fissures of the soft and hard palate (palatoplastie). *N Engl Q J Med Surg* 1843;1:538.
8. von Langenbeck B. Operation der angebornen totalen Spaltung des harten Gaumens nach einer neuer Methode. *Dtsch Klin* 1861;3:321.
9. Veau V. *Division palatine, anatomie, chirurgie, phonetique.* Paris: Masson, 1931.
10. Wardill WEM. Techniques of operation for cleft palate. *Br J Surg* 1937;25:117.
11. Kilner TP. Cleft lip and palate repair technique. *St. Thomas Hosp Rep* 1937;2:127.
12. Kriens O. Fundamental anatomic findings for an intravelar veloplasty. *Cleft Palate J* 1970;7:27.
13. Marsh JL, Grames LM, Holtman B. Intravelar veloplasty: a prospective study. *Cleft Palate J* 1989;26:46.
14. Furlow LT Jr. Double reversing Z-plasty for cleft palate. In: Millard DR Jr, ed. *Cleft craft, alveolar and palatal deformities,* vol. 3. Boston: Little, Brown, 1980:519.

15. Furlow LT Jr. Cleft palate repair by double opposing Z-plasty. *Plast Reconstr Surg* 1986;78:724.
16. Innis CO. Some preliminary observations on unrepaired harelips and cleft palates in adult members of the Dusan tribes of North Borneo. *Br J Plast Surg* 1962;15:173.
17. Ross RB. Treatment variables affecting facial growth in complete unilateral cleft lip and palate. Part 7. An overview of treatment and facial growth. *Cleft Palate J* 1987;24:71.
18. Tatum S, Senders C. Perspectives on palatoplasty. Fac Plast Surg Int Q Monogr 1993;9:225.
19. Dreyer TM, Trier WL. A comparison of palatoplasty techniques. *Cleft Palate J* 1984;21:251.

J. M. Sykes and C.W. Senders: Department of Otolaryngology—Head and Neck Surgery, University of California, Davis Medical Center, Sacramento, California 95817.

• *Practical Pediatric Otolaryngology*
• edited by Robin T. Cotton
  and Charles M. Myer, III
• Lippincott-Raven Publishers,
  Philadelphia © 1999

Assessment and Management of Velopharyngeal Insufficiency

J. Paul Willging & Ann W. Kummer

The velopharyngeal valve is important for normal speech since it is responsible for regulating and directing the transmission of sound energy and air pressure in the cavities of the vocal tract. Incomplete closure of the velopharyngeal valve can affect the quality and clarity of speech and can also make speech production very difficult for the speaker.

NORMAL VELOPHARYNGEAL CLOSURE

Speech production requires the coordination of respiration, phonation, velopharyngeal valving for normal resonance, and articulation. As speech is initiated, air pressure from the lungs and sound energy from the vocal folds travel in a superior direction in the vocal tract. During the production of most speech sounds, the velopharyngeal valve closes, thus blocking off the nasal cavity from the oral cavity. This allows the sound energy and air pressure to be redirected anteriorly into the oral cavity.

The sound energy vibrates, or resonates, in the oral cavity prior to its release, thus resulting in oral resonance. The intraoral air pressure builds up in the oral cavity and provides the force for the production of oral consonants, particularly plosives, fricatives, and affricates. Plosive sounds (p, b, t, d, k, g) require a buildup of intraoral pressure prior to a sudden release. Fricative sounds (f, v, s, z, sh, th) require a release of air pressure through a small opening. Affricate sounds (ch, j) are a combination of a plosive and fricative since they require a buildup of intraoral air pressure and then slow release through a narrow opening. Nasal consonants (m, n, ng) are the only speech sounds that do not require velopharyngeal closure. In fact, they are produced with an open velopharyngeal valve. This allows sound energy to resonate in the nasal cavity for the production of these sounds.

Structures of the Velopharyngeal Mechanism

Normal velopharyngeal closure is accomplished by the coordinated action of the velum (soft palate), the lateral pharyngeal walls, and the posterior pharyngeal wall. During speech, the velum moves in a superior and posterior direction to contact the posterior pharyngeal wall. At the same time, the posterior pharyngeal wall often moves anteriorly to assist in achieving contact. The lateral pharyngeal walls move medially to close against the velum, or in some cases, to meet in midline behind the velum. Some normal and abnormal speakers will demonstrate a Passavant's ridge during velopharyngeal closure. Passavant's ridge consists of a muscle mass in the posterior pharyngeal wall that bulges forward during speech. Passavant's ridge has been thought to be a contributor to velopharyngeal closure. However, it is usually located well below the level of velar and lateral pharyngeal wall movement and therefore may not be a factor in velopharyngeal closure in most cases.

Patterns of Velopharyngeal Closure

In a population of normal speakers, there are several variations in the method of velopharyngeal closure, based on the relative contribution of the soft palate and pharyngeal walls (1). The coronal pattern of closure is the most common and is accomplished by the posterior movement of the soft palate against a broad area of the posterior pharyngeal wall. With this closure pattern, there is minimal contribution of the lateral pharyngeal walls to closure. The next most common pattern of closure is the circular pattern. This pattern occurs when the soft palate moves posteriorly, the posterior pharyngeal wall moves anteriorly, and the lateral pharyngeal walls move medially. In this case, all the velopharyngeal structures contribute equally, and the closure pattern resembles a true sphincter. The least common pattern of closure is the sagittal pattern. With this pattern, the lateral pharyngeal walls move medially to meet in the midline, and there is minimal posterior displacement of the soft palate to effect closure. These variations in normal closure are important to recognize in the evaluation process, since the type of velopharyngeal closure can impact on the type of surgical or prosthetic intervention that is planned.

Musculature

The velopharyngeal sphincter requires the coordinated action of six different muscles. The *levator veli palatini,* also known as the levator sling, originates from the petrous portion of the temporal bone and the inferior aspect of the eustachian tube (2). The levator inserts into the palatal aponeurosis and into the medial raphe of the palate. This muscle interdigitates with other muscle fibers composing the soft palate. The levator muscle is the main muscle mass of the soft palate and serves as the primary elevator of the soft palate. Contraction of the levator muscle forces the free edge of the soft palate to move in a superior and posterior direction to close against the posterior pharyngeal wall.

The *tensor veli palatini* muscle originates from the lateral hook of the eustachian tube cartilage. Additional slips arise from the lateral aspect of the medial pterygoid plate and the spine of the sphenoid. The tensor veli palatini courses vertically down from the skull base to pass around the pterygoid hamulous. This redirects the muscle tendon 90° medially, where it contributes to the palatine aponeurosis (3). The tensor veli palatini muscle is responsible for opening the eustachian tube to enhance middle ear aeration and drainage. Although it is the main contributor to the palatal aponeurosis, it contributes little to velopharyngeal closure.

The *musculus uvulae* is a paired muscle in the midline of the posterior soft palate and is the only intrinsic muscle of the velum. The bulk of this muscle is on the nasal surface of the soft palate (4). The musculus uvulae originates from the area of the palatal aponeurosis and extends to the free edge of the soft palate, superficial to the levator veli palatini. The palatoglossus and palatopharyngeus insert into the musculus uvulae to stabilize its position. Contraction of the musculus uvulae creates a budge on the posterior nasal surface of the soft palate that contributes significantly to velopharyngeal closure.

The *superior pharyngeal constrictor* muscle arises from the pterygoid hamulus, pterygomandibular raphe, posterior tongue, posterior mandible, and palatine aponeurosis. It inserts posteriorly in the midline pharyngeal raphe. This muscle is responsible for the medial displacement of the lateral pharyngeal walls to narrow effectively the velopharyngeal port. Passavant's ridge is the result of contraction of specific fibers of the superior pharyngeal constrictor muscle (5).

The *palatoglossus* muscle arises from the palatal aponeurosis of the anterior half of the soft palate and inserts into the posterior lateral aspect of the tongue. It is contained within the anterior tonsillar pillar and thus is subject to possible damage during tonsillectomy (6). The palatoglossus muscle acts antagonistically to the levator veli palatini to depress the velum or elevate the tongue.

The last muscle associated with the soft palate is the *palatopharyngeus.* It originates from the palatal aponeurosis and posterior border of the hard palate (7). This muscle is contained within the posterior tonsillar pillar. The function of this muscle is not well understood, although it is felt to be instrumental in lowering the soft palate. Horizontal fibers of this muscle may be associated with the superior pharyngeal constrictor and contribute to the formation of Passavant's ridge.

The tensor veli palatini receives neural innervation from the mandibular division of the trigeminal nerve. All other soft palate musculature contributing to velopharyngeal closure receives innervation from the pharyngeal plexus of the vagus nerve.

CAUSES OF VELOPHARYNGEAL INSUFFICIENCY

The velopharyngeal valve may be inadequate due to structural deficiencies resulting in a velum that is short relative to the posterior pharyngeal wall. The term *velopharyngeal insufficiency* is used to refer to a type of structural defect of the velopharyngeal valve. The velopharyngeal valve can also be affected by neuromotor dysfunction, which results in poor movement of the velopharyngeal structures. This type of disorder is correctly called *velopharyngeal incompetence.* Finally, inadequate velopharyngeal closure may occur during the production of some speech sounds due to mislearning of appropriate articulation patterns. This has been called *functional velopharyngeal insufficiency.* In practice, the term velopharyngeal insufficiency, or just VPI, is used most commonly as a generic term for all types of velopharyngeal dysfunction.

Structural Factors

VPI is found most commonly in patients with a history of cleft palate. Despite surgical repair of the cleft, approximately 20% of these patients will demonstrate VPI due to insufficient velar length or inadequate muscle structure and function.

Patients with submucous cleft palate often have characteristics of VPI, although the vast majority of these patients will have normal speech. Obvious characteristics of a submucous cleft may include a hypoplastic or bifid uvula, a bluish zona pellucida, visible diastasis of the soft palate musculature in the midline, or notching of the posterior border of the hard palate as noted through palpation (8) (Fig. 1). Some abnormalities, such as a hypoplastic musculus uvulae, can only be seen on the nasal surface of the velum and therefore must be detected through nasopharyngoscopy.

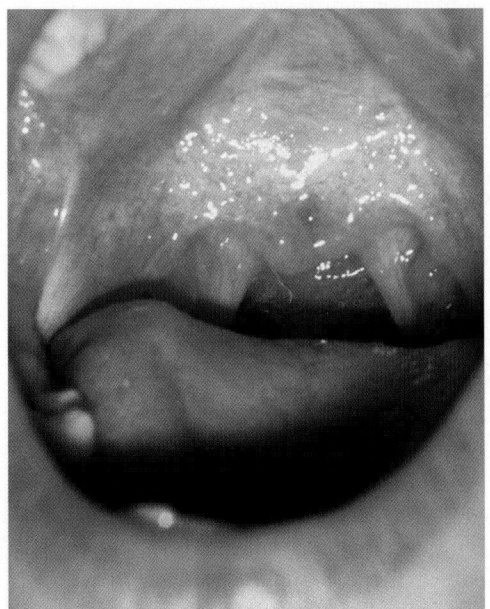

FIGURE 1 Submucous cleft palate demonstrating the zona pellucida, notch in the posterior hard palate, and bifid uvula.

Adenoidectomy can result in postoperative VPI, although the incidence is only approximately 1:1,500. Patients with a history of cleft palate or evidence of submucous cleft are at greatest risk for VPI following adenoidectomy due to the lack of reserve muscle mass or tenuous velar function. Patients with VPI following adenoidectomy, despite a lack of preoperative findings of velar abnormality, are often found to have subtle findings through nasopharyngoscopy postoperatively that would have been suggestive of velar abnormality in retrospect (9).

Patients with a history of cleft palate repair or with submucous cleft may begin to demonstrate evidence of VPI as they begin to reach adolescence. These patients may have had effective, although tenuous, velopharyngeal closure against the adenoid pad, but demonstrate inadequate closure as the adenoid tissue begins to atrophy.

Hypertrophic tonsils, on rare occasions, may cause velopharyngeal insufficiency. This can occur if the tonsil restricts the movement of the lateral pharyngeal wall or when the pole of the tonsil projects into the pharynx, between the velum and posterior pharyngeal wall, thus preventing an adequate velopharyngeal seal.

Neuromotor Disorders

Neuromotor disorders may lead to velopharyngeal insufficiency due to poor motor movement or coordination of velopharyngeal musculature. Patients with cranial nerve deficits may demonstrate VPI due to paralysis of the soft palate or pharyngeal musculature. Patients with a history of central neurologic injury may demonstrate dysarthric speech, which includes characteristics of VPI. *Dysarthria* is characterized by poor movement of all the speech articulators, including the velopharyngeal structures. Speech is often muffled due to weak consonants, and sentence length decreases because of the loss of air pressure nasally. Finally, patients with difficulty coordinating motor movements for speech due to *verbal apraxia* may demonstrate characteristics of VPI due to poor timing of velopharyngeal closure with the production of speech sounds (10).

Mislearning

Some patients develop articulation errors that include improper movement patterns of the velopharyngeal mechanism (11). Although the speech may sound similar to that of patients with VPI, these patients do not have a primary velopharyngeal valving disorder and therefore are not candidates for surgical or prosthetic intervention. Instead, speech therapy is very successful in correcting these functional problems.

EFFECTS OF VELOPHARYNGEAL INSUFFICIENCY ON SPEECH

Since velopharyngeal closure is important for the production of most speech sounds, any disruption in the function of this valve can result in an audible resonance and speech disorder. VPI causes inappropriate transmission of sound energy and air pressure into the nasal cavity during speech, resulting in one or more of the following perceptual characteristics:

Hypernasality and Other Forms of Abnormal Resonance

Hypernasality is the result of too much sound resonating in the nasal cavity during speech production, due to inadequate velopharyngeal closure. This can make speech sound muffled and unclear. Hypernasality is particularly evident on vowel sounds and is most noted during the production of connected speech. When hypernasality is severe, most oral phonemes sound as if they are substituted by the nasal sounds (m, n, ng). Hypernasality should not be confused with the opposite problem of *hyponasality*, which is due to obstruction of the nasopharynx or nasal cavity. When obstruction causes a reduction or elimination of nasal resonance, it is the nasal consonants that are adversely affected in that they sound as if they are substituted by their oral phoneme cognates (b, d, g). Common causes of hyponasality include hypertrophic adenoids, choanal atresia/stenosis, a markedly deviated nasal septum, midface deficiency, or transient factors such as the common cold or allergic rhinitis.

When a patient has velopharyngeal insufficiency and nasopharyngeal blockage, speech many be characterized by *mixed resonance,* with both hyper- and hyponasality. *Cul-de-sac resonance* can also occur when there is obstruction in the vocal tract, causing the transmission of sound energy to be trapped in a closed or blocked cavity. The resonance can become cul-de-sac in cases of severe adenotonsillar hypertrophy, resulting in sound energy trapped in the oropharynx. Velopharyngeal insufficiency, in combination with obstruction in the nasal cavity, can cause cul-de-sac resonance since the sound energy is forced to resonate within the closed nasopharynx.

Nasal Air Emission

Audible nasal air emission may occur during consonant production, particularly during production of pressure-sensitive sounds (plosives, fricatives, affricatives). As air pressure increases in the oral cavity, the air pressure leaks through the velopharyngeal valve and is emitted nasally. When this nasal air emission is turbulent, as often occurs when it is forced through a small opening, the distortion is appreciated audibly as a nasal rustle (12).

Weak or Omitted Consonants

Air pressure for production of consonants may be adversely affected if air pressure is leaked through the velopharyngeal valve. As a result, consonants may be very weak, both in intensity and pressure, or even completely omitted.

Short Utterance Length

Utterance length is determined, at least in part, by the supply of air pressure available for speech. When there is velopharyngeal insufficiency causing a leak of air pressure, this shortens the supply of oral air pressure for connected speech. As a result, utterance length is short, and connected speech is choppy due to a frequent need to replenish air pressure by taking more breaths.

Compensatory Articulation Productions

If intraoral air pressure is inadequate for the normal production of speech sounds, some patients learn to compensate by producing speech sounds in a different manner. These patients commonly learn to produce similar sounds in the area of the glottis or pharynx as a substitution for the oral sounds they cannot produce. Some common compensatory articulation productions include glottal stops, pharyngeal stops, and pharyngeal fricatives.

Dysphonia

In addition to the perceptual characteristics of VPI, some patients will demonstrate dysphonic characteristics, such as breathiness, hoarseness, and glottal fry. Breathiness may be compensatory, since it can mask hypernasality and nasal air emission. Vocal fold nodules can also be the cause of the dysphonia, however, particularly since nodules are common in children with VPI (13). Vocal fold nodules may develop secondary to the use of compensatory articulation productions, such as glottal stops, or they may result from strain in the entire vocal tract when velopharyngeal closure is attempted.

✪ PATIENT ASSESSMENT

Perceptual Evaluation

The perceptual evaluation of speech and resonance should be done by a qualified and experienced speech pathologist. This evaluation will begin with an assessment of resonance, which is best evaluated in connected speech. Since the production of longer utterances increases the demand on the velopharyngeal valving system, some deficiencies may not be apparent in single words or short utterances. Resonance is usually judged to be normal or hypernasal. If there is obstruction in the vocal tract, resonance may be determined to be hyponasal, cul-de-sac or characterized by a mixture of these types. For abnormal findings, the examiner will usually judge the severity to be mild, moderate, or severe in degree.

As part of the evaluation, the speech pathologist will assess for the presence of nasal air emission. If present, it is important to determine whether it occurs on all types of pressure-sensitive sounds, or only on specific phonemes. The speech pathologist will evaluate articulation and determine which articulation errors are compensatory errors due to VPI and which are merely placement errors. The adequacy of oral pressure will also be evaluated by noting the intensity of pressure-sensitive consonants.

An assessment of stimulability is a very important component of the examination. If a reduction or elimination of the nasal air emission or hypernasality can be accomplished by changes in articulatory placement, this suggests a good prognosis for correction with speech therapy. The articulation errors leading to hypernasality may be the result of faulty learning of oral–motor movements, rather than a primary velopharyngeal valving disorder.

Nasometric Assessment

The Nasometer (Kay Elemetrics, Pine Brook, NJ) is a computer-based instrument that measures acoustic energy emanating from both the nasal cavity and the oral cavity during speech. It computes a ratio of the nasal acoustic energy to the total acoustic energy produced and displays the score in real time. An average "nasalance" score is computed for a specific speech segment. When standardized passages are used, this score can be compared with normative data (14).

The Nasometer provides useful clinical information, but the results must be interpreted by the speech pathologist in the context of the perceptual assessment of nasal resonance and nasal air emission. A nasal rustle, which usually signifies a small velopharyngeal opening, can give a very high nasalance score, whereas a paretic palate with no velar movement may give a moderate nasalance score due to the lack of intensity of both oral and nasal acoustic energy.

Videofluoroscopic Speech Study

A videofluoroscopic speech study is a radiographic technique consisting of multiple views of the velopharyngeal sphincter. These views are obtained during speech production to evaluate the function of the velopharyngeal mechanism (15). The lateral view documents the length of the soft palate, depth of the pharynx, elevation and elongation of the soft palate with speech, and anterior motion of the posterior pharyngeal wall, which may contribute to closure. The frontal view allows assessment of the lateral pharyngeal wall motion and its contribution to velopharyngeal closure. The base view, taken at right angles to the plane of closure of the velopharyngeal sphincter, permits an *en face* view of closure. The contributions to closure of the entire sphincter, including the soft palate, lateral pharyngeal walls, and posterior pharyngeal wall, can be determined by the base view.

The lateral view is done without the use of barium. The other views require the use of a high-density barium instilled into the nasal passages through a catheter. The head of the patient is then rotated to encourage passage of the barium into the nasopharynx, where the soft palate and pharyngeal walls become coated with the contrast material. The barium can cause some discomfort and minor irritation, but most children tolerate the procedure without difficulty.

Videofluorosopy is a good technique for evaluation of the structure and function of the velopharyngeal mechanism. It is particularly helpful in assessing the extent and symmetry of lateral pharyngeal wall motion. The radiation exposure associated with videofluoroscopy is low, but it can be a concern when repeat examinations are required.

Nasopharyngoscopy

Nasopharyngoscopy is a minimally invasive endoscopic procedure that allows direct assessment of the velopharyngeal mechanism during speech (16). The endoscope is passed through the middle meatus and through the choana. It is then turned down to view the velopharyngeal port from above. With the endoscope in place in the nasopharynx, the adequacy of closure of the velopharyngeal sphincter can be directly assessed during connected speech. The degree and symmetry of soft palate and lateral wall motion is assessed. The nasal surface of the soft palate is also scrutinized for signs of a submucous cleft palate, or hypoplastic musculus uvula. Because of the high incidence of vocal fold nodules in patients with VPI, flexible laryngoscopy should also be performed as a matter of completeness.

Prior to the procedure, the nasal cavity is numbed for the patient's comfort. A 1:1 mixture of Afrin and 2% Pontocaine, introduced into the nasal cavity through a nasal spray, provides adequate anesthesia for the procedure and does not affect velopharyngeal closure. Nasopharyngosopy requires a moderate degree of cooperation from the patient to complete the study successfully, but with the topical anesthesia, it is usually well tolerated by children, even as young as 3 years of age. Nasopharyngoscopy results are complementary to radiographic studies and are superior in patients who have a small velopharyngeal gap or who have had a previously placed pharyngeal flap.

Team Approach to Evaluation

Children with velopharyngeal insufficiency offer complex diagnostic problems. A team approach to the management of these problems is therefore beneficial to the patient. Many of these patients are managed by a craniofacial anomaly team, which consists of a variety of professionals. Many patients are effectively managed by a subset of these professionals through a VPI clinic, particularly if there is no history of cleft palate or other obvious craniofacial anomalies. A VPI clinic should ideally include a speech pathologist, an otolaryngologist, and a geneticist.

The speech pathologist offers expertise in the assessment of speech and resonance. The gold standard for determining the need for intervention remains the perceptual quality of the speech. The speech pathologist can determine whether VPI exists, and if so, how it affects the quality and intelligibility of speech or whether the patient is stimulable, which may suggest correction with speech therapy. The speech pathologist is essential during the nasopharyngoscopy and videofluoroscopic examinations to determine the appropriate stimuli for the examination to emphasize the velopharyngeal closure defects, and also to evaluate the results of these studies and assist with recommendations for treatment.

The otolaryngologist assesses the structural aspects of the oral cavity, oropharynx, nasal cavity, and upper airway with respect to VPI. Associated problems are also identified, such as chronic ear problems, adenotonsillar hypertrophy, pharyngeal masses, or vocal fold nodules. Treatment recommendations are made in conjunction with the speech pathologist.

A geneticist offers expertise in the identification of syndromes associated with VPI. More than 200 recognized syndromes include palatal clefting as a manifestation. All patients with an obvious cleft of the palate, and those with VPI without signs of an overt cleft palate, need to be evaluated for other anomalies (telecanthus, maxillary or malar hypoplasia, retrognathia, malocclusion, craniosynostosis, microtia or aural atresia, facial nerve paralysis) that may be associated with a known syndrome.

Velocardiofacial (VCF) syndrome is a particularly common syndrome in patients with VPI but is thought to be an underdiagnosed condition. In addition to VPI, characteristics of VCF may include submucous cleft palate, various facial anomalies (malar flattening, maxillary excess, retrognathia, auricular anomalies), and minor cardiac anomalies. Other findings may include pharyngeal hypotonia, slender fingers, small stature, and learning disabilities (17). Nasopharyngoscopy may reveal tortuosity of the internal carotid arteries, with medial displacement against the posterior pharyngeal wall. These vessels can often be seen pulsating against the posterior pharyngeal wall. (They remain deep to the prevertebral fascia and should not be of concern when raising a conventional pharyngeal flap, but extra attention to the depth of the dissection is prudent.) The geneticist can do a physical examination and a DNA probe to determine whether the VPI is associated with VCF or another related genetic condition.

The VPI clinic team should be involved with comprehensive assessment of velopharyngeal function followed by the development of treatment recommendations for the patient. Early recognition of these patients and multidisciplinary management of corelated problems minimizes the impact of defective speech and other underlying congenital deformities by timely intervention. Follow-up examinations should also be performed by the team to assess the results of surgery or therapy objectively and to develop long-term treatment plans for the patient.

 ## TREATMENT RECOMMENDATIONS

Treatment for VPI falls into three general classifications: speech therapy, prosthetics, and surgical management. An accurate assessment of the degree of VPI, the etiology of the problem, and specific patient and family factors will lead to the proper treatment options for an individual patient.

Speech Therapy

Speech therapy cannot correct structural defects. Therefore, most patients with significant VPI will not benefit from speech therapy as the primary treatment approach. Speech therapy can be effective in patients who demonstrate a small velopharyngeal opening or inconsistent closure. It is also very effective in postoperative management. Despite surgical correction, the patient may need to be taught appropriate articulatory placement and oral airflow before normal speech can be obtained.

Speech therapy for patients with VPI is similar to the therapy used for articulation disorders. The emphasis of therapy is on reduction of compensatory articulation patterns and on improving oral resonance by changing the focus of articulation. Therapy should continue as long as the child is stimulable or shows progress (18). If hypernasality or nasal air emission persists, further evaluation of velopharyngeal function must be done to determine the need for further surgical intervention.

Prosthetic Management

Prosthetic devices, such as obturators or palatal lifts, are sometimes used in the treatment of VPI (Fig. 2). An obturator can be used when the velopharyngeal port cannot be adequately closed due to a short velum. The obturator extends into the velopharyngeal port to close the defect. A palatal lift can be effective when neurologic impairment results in poor velopharyngeal movement. The palatal lift holds the velum in a superior and posterior position, so that it can close against the posterior pharyngeal

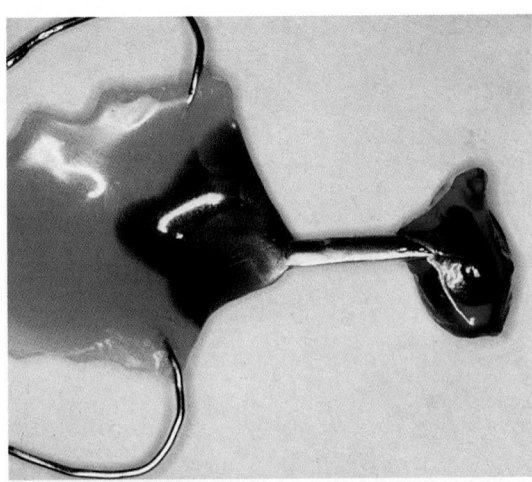
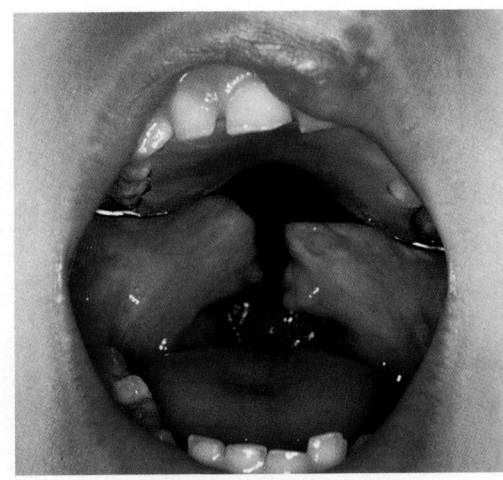

FIGURE 2 **A:** Obturator to fill void in velopharyngeal area. **B:** Device in place (prosthesis created by Dr. Gordon Huntress, D.D.S., University of Cincinnati Medical Center, Cincinnati, OH 45267).

wall. Both of these devices are usually made of acrylic and are anchored to the teeth with a palatal appliance (19).

Palatal appliances are often poorly tolerated by children. They can be uncomfortable, and they can be easily lost. They require frequent adjustments as the child grows. They are generally used when there are contraindications to surgical intervention. There has been renewed interest in utilizing obturators as a form of preoperative therapy, however. It is theorized that if an obturator can help to stimulate improved lateral pharyngeal wall motion prior to placement of a pharyngeal flap, a smaller flap may be required as a result.

Surgical Intervention

The surgical approach required to correct hypernasality depends on the size of the persistent velopharyngeal port and the closure pattern exhibited by the patient. A standard approach to all patients is inappropriate. A tailored surgical approach will yield the best final speech results with the lowest long-term morbidity.

Pushback Palatoplasty

A patient with a submucous cleft palate and good lateral pharyngeal wall motion may be a good candidate for a palatoplasty with pushback, prior to considering other surgical options for correction of VPI (Fig. 3). With the palatoplasty, the levator sling is reconstructed to improve soft palate motion, and additional length is obtained with a V-Y closure of the palatal incisions (20).

Posterior Pharyngeal Wall Augmentation

When velopharyngeal insufficiency results from a small gap, or an anterior–posterior defect of no more than 10 mm, posterior pharyngeal wall augmentation may be considered. The implant must be accurately placed at the place of the defect in the area of normal velopharyngeal closure. This is generally at the level of the atlas promontory. The implants are placed superficial to the prevertebral fascia, deep to the superior pharyngeal constrictors. Surgical approaches include an external lateral cervical approach, a transoral incision, or a transoral injection. Overcorrection is required for all injectable augmentation material, as the vehicle solution is absorbed.

Various materials have been used for posterior pharyngeal wall augmentation and include paraffin, otogenous cartilage, cadaver cartilage, fascia, fat, silicone, proplast, and polytetrafluoroethylene (Teflon). Teflon has been the main material used for posterior pharyngeal wall augmentation. The U.S. Food and Drug Administration has not ap-

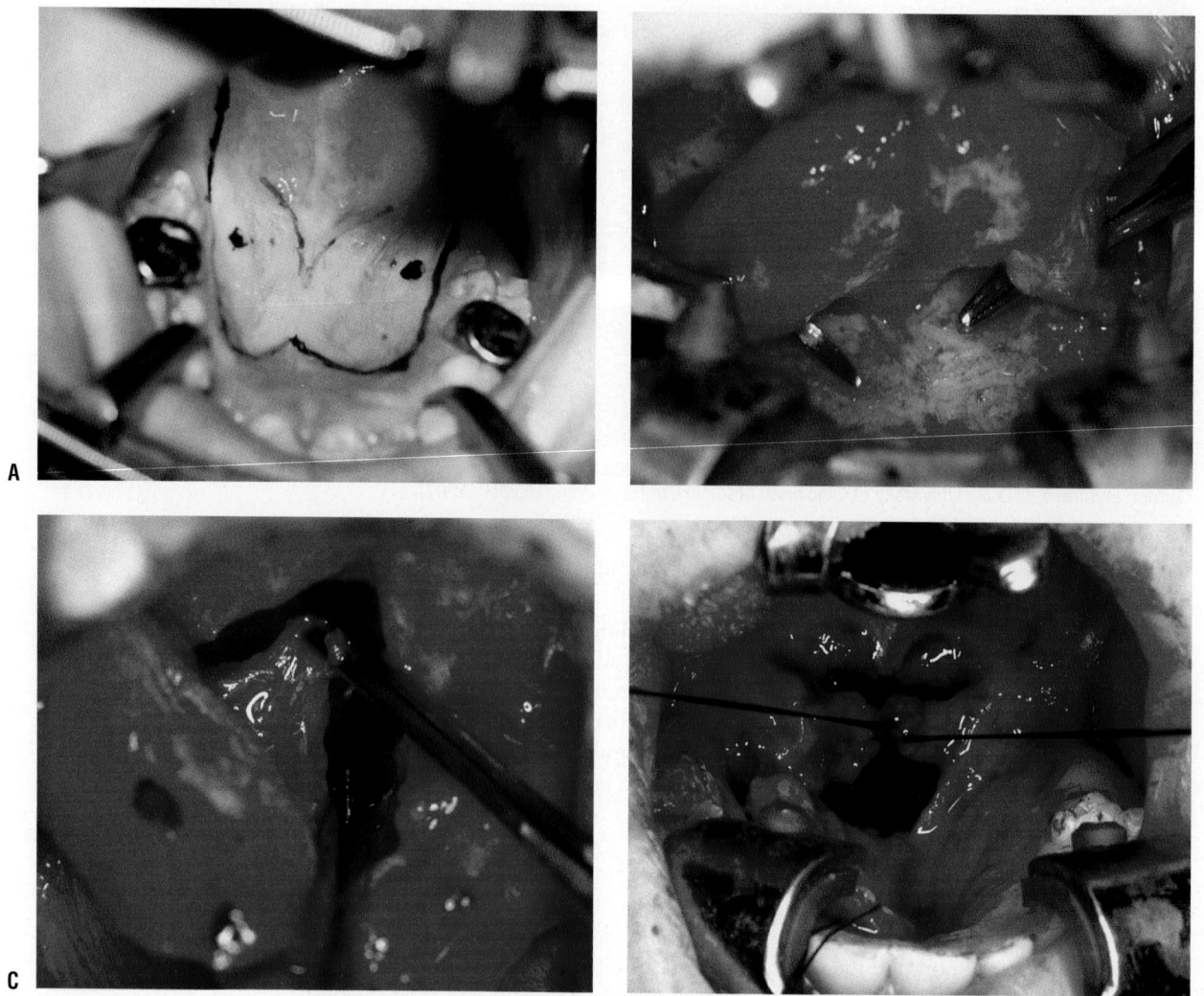

FIGURE 3 Pushback palatoplasty. **A:** Incision outlined on palate, with bony notch and greater palatine arteries identified. **B:** Circumferential isolation of greater palatine vessels. **C:** Isolation of levator palatini muscle from its attachments to the palatal shelf. **D:** Approximation of levator palatini muscle in the midline. Palatal flaps are closed in a V-Y fashion to maintain increased length of the palate.

proved the use of Teflon in the retropharynx, however, due to incidences of inadvertent injection of the material intravascularly. Recent articles in the urologic literature (Teflon is used around the ureters to correct reflux) suggest the possibility of brain and pulmonary embolization of the Teflon particles (21). Granuloma formation has also been associated with Teflon implantation. Other complications associated with posterior pharyngeal wall implantation include infection, extrusion, undercorrection, inappropriate positioning of the implant, and migration of the material after insertion.

Pharyngeal Flap

The superiorly based pharyngeal flap is a common procedure done to correct VPI (Fig. 4). The procedure involves raising a superiorly based flap from the posterior pharyngeal wall and then inserting the flap into the velum. Lining the muscular surface of the flap with mucosa obtained from the nasal surface of the soft palate reduces fibrosis and contracture narrowing of the flap over time. Lateral ports remain on each side of the flap for normal nasal breathing (22). In general, the lateral ports should be approximately 4 mm in diameter. During speech, the flap acts as an obturator against which the lateral pharyngeal walls can close. Good lateral pharyngeal wall motion is essential to close the

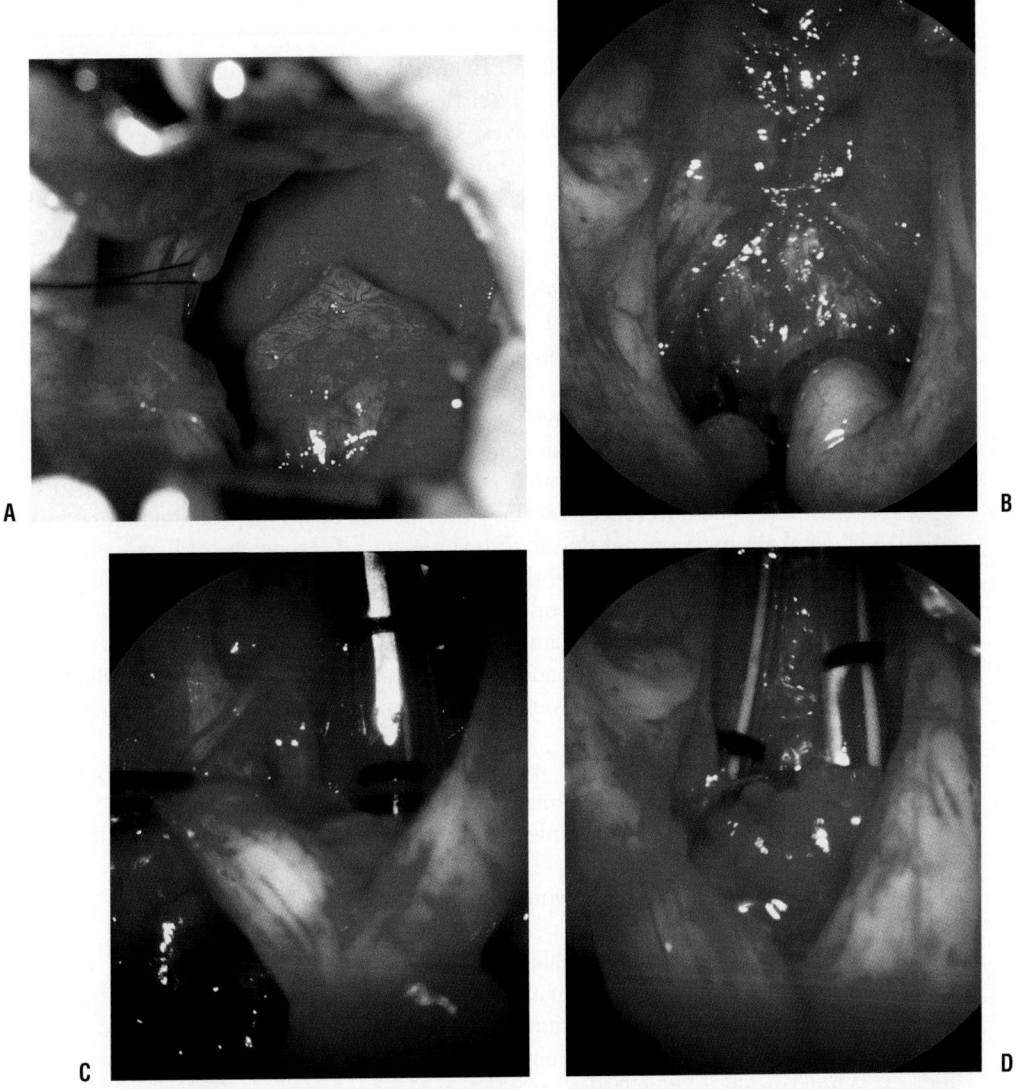

FIGURE 4 **A:** Creation of superiorly based pharyngeal flap. **B:** Closure of donor site. **C:** Incisions on posterior margin of the soft palate; an endotracheal tube acts as a stent. The flap is sewn around the stent, which creates the lateral velopharyngeal port. **D:** Bilateral stents with flap centrally. The soft palate is being retracted anteriorly and superiorly. The flap must be located at the level of velopharyngeal closure. An excessively long flap is at risk for draping inferiorly and residing below the level of velopharyngeal closure.

lateral ports created during the procedure. The preoperative nasopharyngoscopy examination may show poor lateral wall motion, but this should not exclude the patient from pharyngeal flap consideration. After the flap is in position and speech therapy sessions are begun, lateral wall motion is usually noted to improve.

The success of a pharyngeal flap often depends on its position in the nasopharynx. The flap must be positioned at the level of the hard palate and first cervical vertebrae, where velopharyngeal closure usually occurs. Flexible nasopharyngoscopy preoperatively allows identification of landmarks for accurate positioning of the flap with respect to the soft palate.

The width of the flap also affects the postoperative success. The width of the flap should be determined preoperatively based on a judgment of lateral pharyngeal wall movement. A patient demonstrating no lateral wall motion will require a wide flap, and a patient with a small central gap will be well managed with a narrow flap.

PEARLS AND PERILS

1. To evaluate speech for possible VPI, have the patient do the following:
   a. *Count from sixty to seventy:* The sixties contain a combination of sibilants, velar plosives, and alveolar plosives. These sounds require the generation and continuation of intraoral pressure that may overwhelm a tenuous velopharyngeal closure mechanism.
   b. *Sentence repetition:* Have the patient repeat sentences loaded with pressure-sensitive phonemes. This can accentuate nasal air emission and compensatory articulation. Examples are: Popeye plays baseball. Take Teddy to town. Give Kate the cake. Go get the wagon. Fred has five fish. Sally sees the sun in the sky. She went shopping. I eat cherries and cheese. John told a joke to Jim.
   c. *Prolong the vowel /ah/:* Have the patient prolong the vowel /a/ while opening and closing the nose by pinching the nares with the fingers. If there is a difference in quality, the resonance is hypernasal and there is evidence of VPI. If there is no difference, this does not rule out VPI. The problem may be just nasal air emission, cul-de-sac resonance, mixed resonance, or hyponasality.
   d. *Palpation of the nose:* Feel the sides of the nose during production of pressure-sensitive consonants or 60, 60, 60. If you feel a vibration during these repetitions, nasal air emission is suggested.
   e. *Air paddle:* Use a small, paper "paddle" under the nares during production of pressure-sensitive consonants. If the paper paddle moves, this suggests nasal air emission.
2. If nasal phonemes (m, n, ng) are distorted or sound like they are oral cognates (b, d, g), the problem is hyponasality, probably due to obstruction, not hypernasality due to VPI. An example of a nasal sentence is: My mama made lemonade.
3. Patients at risk for VPI following adenoidectomy:
   a. Preexisting VPI.
   b. Family history of VPI or palatal clefting.
   c. Obvious submucous cleft palate.
   d. History of nasal regurgitation or feeding difficulty as a child.
   e. Oral–motor or other neuromuscular problems.
4. When speech therapy is appropriate for velopharyngeal insufficiency:
   a. The patient demonstrates mild, inconsistent hypernasality.
   b. The patient is stimulable for a reduction of nasality with a change in articulation.
   c. Hypernasality is due to faulty articulation or associated with oral–motor dysfunction.
   d. The patient has had a surgery for correction of VPI and needs to learn how to use the new structure.
5. Evaluation and management of obstructive sleep apnea following pharyngeal flap:
   a. Sleep study to document severity of the problem.
   b. Trial of continuous positive airway pressure.
   c. Revision of the lateral ports to increase their diameter.
   d. Consider taking down the flap if severe obstructive apnea exists.

Prior to placement of a pharyngeal flap, the patient should be evaluated for adenotonsillar hypertrophy. It may be necessary to perform a tonsillectomy if the lateral ports will be obstructed postoperatively by this lymphoid tissue. The tonsillectomy must be separated from the pharyngeal flap operation by at least 6 weeks to minimize the risk of nasopharyngeal stenosis.

Most patients exhibit very loud snoring for some time following placement of the flap. Patients with retrognathia or neuromotor dysfunction are at a greater risk for postoperative airway obstruction causing sleep apnea following placement of the flap. This should be closely monitored postoperatively.

Sphincter Pharyngoplasty

A sphincteroplasty procedure involves the surgical creation of a dynamic sphincter to close lateral openings of the velopharyneal valve. This procedure is particularly appropriate when lateral pharyngeal wall motion is poor, or when the lateral pharyngeal recesses are deep, but central closure of the velopharyngeal port is present. With this procedure, bilateral superiorly based myocutaneous flaps are raised that include the palatopharyngeus muscle. The flaps are inset into a transverse incision in the nasopharynx, positioned at the level of velopharyngeal closure (23). The effect of the transposition is a narrowing of the lateral channel and a dynamic sphincter that closes with speech.

Complications associated with the sphincter pharyngoplasty are similar to those of the pharyngeal flap. The risk of postoperative obstructive sleep apnea, however, is much less with this procedure than with the pharyngeal flap.

CONCLUSIONS

VPI can have a significant effect on the quality and clarity of speech. This can affect the patient's social and emotional development and overall quality of life. The management of VPI is complex and requires the expertise of several professionals. Although most otolaryngologists and speech pathologists are technically qualified to evaluate and treat VPI, many do not have sufficient knowledge or experience to do this effectively. Referral to those professionals who specialize in this area should always be considered.

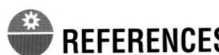 **REFERENCES**

1. Boorman JG, Sommerlad BC. Musculus uvulae and levator palati: their anatomical and functional relationship in velopharyngeal closure. *B J Plast Surg* 1985;38:333–338.
2. Ross MA. Functional anatomy of the tensor palati. Its relevance in cleft palate surgery. *Arch Otolaryngol* 1971;93:1–3.
3. Langdon HL, Klueber K. The longitudinal fibromuscular component of the soft palate in the fifteen-week human fetus: musculus uvulae and palatine raphe. *Cleft Palate* 1978;15:337–348.
4. Shprintzen RJ, McCall GN, Skolnick ML, Lencione RM. Selective movement of the lateral aspects of the pharyngeal walls during velopharyngeal closure for speech, blowing, and whistling in normals. *Cleft Palate J* 1975;12:51–58.
5. Kuehn DP, Azzam NA. Anatomical characteristics of palatoglossus and the anterior faucial pillar. *Cleft Palate J* 1978;15:349–359.
6. Dickson DR, Dickson WM. Velopharyngeal anatomy. *J Speech Hear Res* 1972;15:372–381.
7. Skolnick ML, Mc CG, Barnes M. The sphincteric mechanism of velopharyngeal closure. *Cleft Palate J* 1973;10:286–305.
8. Steward JM, Ott JE, Lagace R. Submucous cleft palate: prevalence in a school population. *Cleft Palate J* 1972;9:246–250.
9. Witzel MA, Rich RH, Margar-Bacal F, Cox C. Velopharyngeal insufficiency after adenoidectomy: an 8-year review. *Int J Pediatr Otorhinolaryngol* 1986;11:15–20.
10. Yorkston KM, Beukelman DR, Bell KR. *Clinical management of dysarthric speakers.* Boston: College Hill Press, 1988.
11. Trost JE. Articulatory additions to the classical description of the speech of persons with cleft palate. *Cleft Palate* 1981;18:193–203.
12. Kummer AW, Curtis C, Wiggs M, Lee L, Strife JL. Comparison of velopharyngeal gap size in patients with hypernasality, hypernasality and nasal emission, or nasal turbulence (rustle) as the primary speech characteristic. *Cleft Palate Craniofac J* 1992;29:152–156.

13. McWilliams BJ, Lavorato AS, Bluestone CD. Vocal cord abnormalities in children with velopharyngeal valving problems. *Laryngoscope* 1973;83:1745–1753.

14. Dalston RM, Warren DW, Dalston ET. Use of nasometry as a diagnostic tool for identifying patients with velopharyngeal impairment [published erratum appears in *Cleft Palate Craniofac J* 1991;28:446]. *Cleft Palate Craniofac J* 1991;28:184–188; discussion 188–189.

15. Skolnick ML. Videofluoroscopic examination of the velopharyngeal portal during phonation in lateral and base projections—a new technique for studying the mechanics of closure. *Cleft Palate J* 1970;7:803–816.

16. D'Antonio LL, Muntz HR, Marsh JL, Marty-Grames L, Backensto-Marsh R. Practical application of flexible fiberoptic nasopharyngoscopy for evaluating velopharyngeal function. *Plast Reconst Surg* 1988;82:611–618.

17. Shprintzen RJ, Goldberg RB, Lewin ML, et al. A new syndrome involving cleft palate, cardiac anomalies, typical facies, and learning disabilities: velo-cardio-facial syndrome. *Cleft Palate J* 1978;15:56–62.

18. D'Antonio LL, Crockett DM. Evaluation and management of velopharyngeal inadequacy. In: JD S, R B, eds. *Pediatric facial plastic and reconstructive surgery.* New York: Raven Press, 1993:173.

19. McGrath CO, Anderson MW. Prosthetic treatment of velopharyngeal incompetence. In: J B, HL M, eds. Multidisciplinary Management of Cleft Lip and Palate. Philadelphia: W B Sanders, 1990.

20. WE W. Technique of operation for cleft palate. *Br J Surg* 1937;25:117–125.

21. Aaronson IA, Rames RA, Greene WB, Walsh LG, Hasal UA, Garen PD. Endoscopic treatment of reflux: migration of Teflon to the lungs and brain. *Eur Urol* 1993;23:394–399.

22. Hogan VM. A clarification of the surgical goals in cleft palate speech and the introduction of the lateral port control (l.p.c.) pharyngeal flap. *Cleft Palate J* 1973;10:331–345.

23. Hynes W. Observations on pharyngoplasty. *Br J Plast Surg* 1967;20:224–256.

J. P. Willging: Department of Otolaryngology and Maxillofacial Surgery, University of Cincinnati, Children's Hospital Medical Center, Cincinnati, Ohio 45229-3039.   •   A. W. Kummer: Departments of Speech Pathology and Pediatrics, University of Cincinnati, Children's Hospital Medical Center, Cincinnati, Ohio 45229-3039.

• *Practical Pediatric Otolaryngology*
• edited by Robin T. Cotton
  and Charles M. Myer, III
• Lippincott-Raven Publishers,
  Philadelphia © 1999

CHAPTER
51

Otolaryngologic Manifestations of Down Syndrome

Sally R. Shott

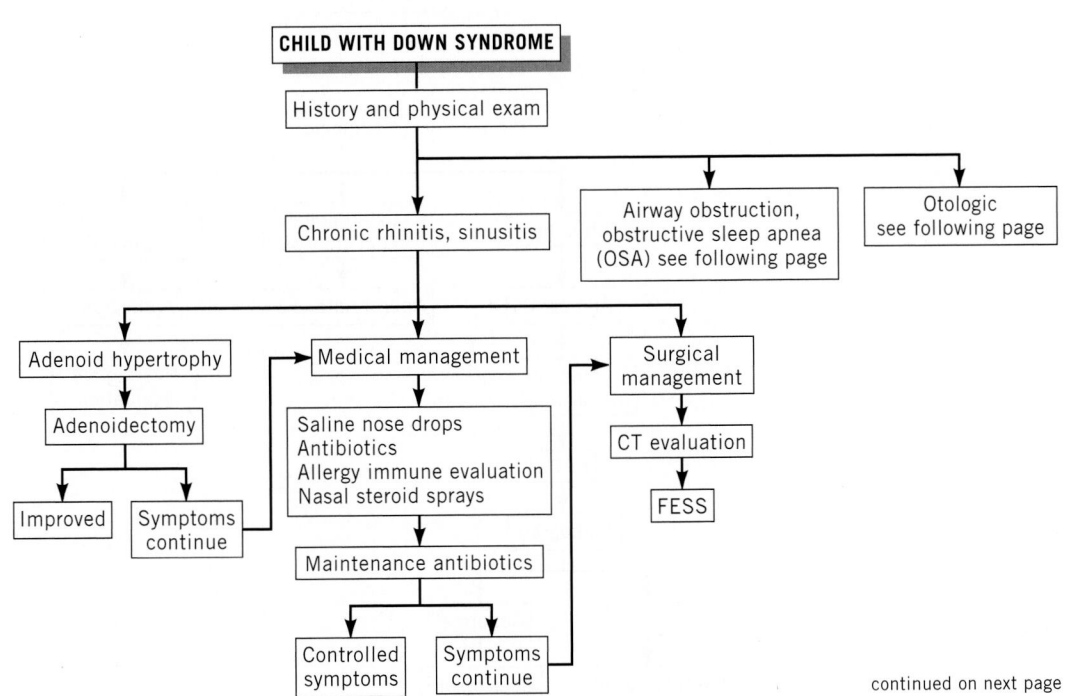

continued on next page

continued

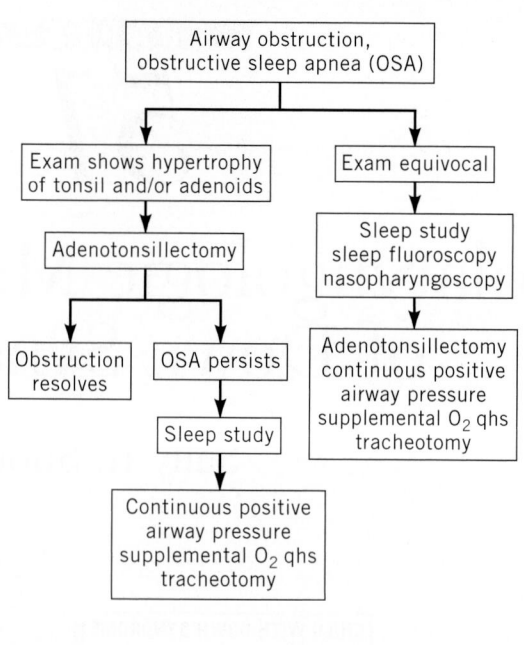

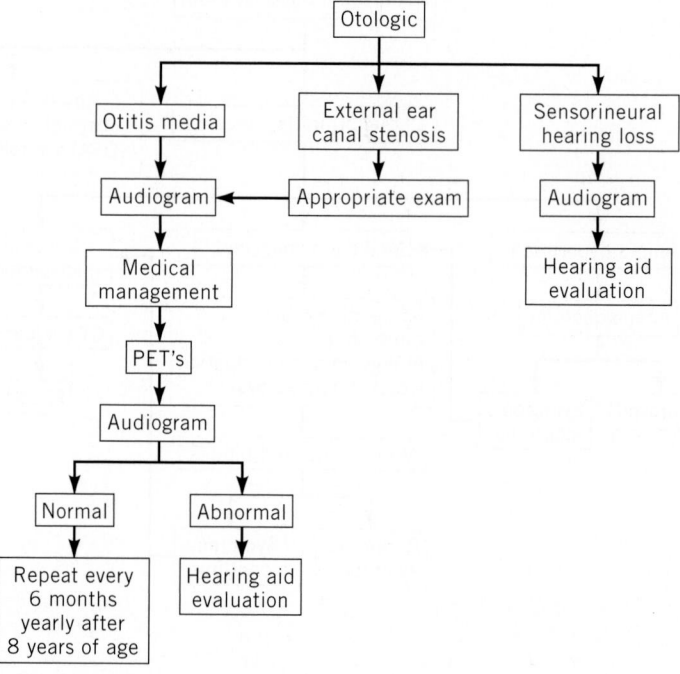

⊘ HISTORICAL BACKGROUND

John Langdon Down first described Down syndrome, caused by an aberrant chromosomal disorder, in 1865. Children with trisomy 21 constituted the largest population of institutionalized individuals in the United States in the early 1900s. These children are no longer "allowed to die"; life-saving cardiac surgery, once rarely done, is now commonplace, and more than 80% live past 30 years of age (1). In the United States, laws affirming the rights of these children to full medical care have been passed. Children with Down syndrome are no longer shuffled into institutions; now the emphasis is on integration into normal family life. The level of mental retardation associated with Down syndrome has been found to be quite variable, and positive effects are seen with early intervention programs, stimulation, and education.

As the care of children with Down syndrome has become more aggressive and proactive, multiple otolaryngologic problems common to children with Down syndrome have become apparent. These include an increased incidence of otologic infections and hearing loss, airway problems including obstructive sleep apnea and subglottic stenosis, problems with chronic rhinorrhea and sinusitis, and some very important anesthetic considerations.

With an incidence of approximately 1 in 1,000 live births, children with Down syndrome will commonly be a part of any busy pediatric otolaryngology practice (2). Appropriate treatment of the otolaryngologic manifestations of Down syndrome can be instrumental in allowing this patient population to achieve their full potential.

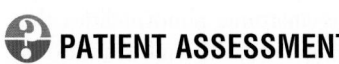

PATIENT ASSESSMENT

Specific questions should be oriented toward a potential history of chronic ear disease, possible airway obstruction, and possible history of chronic rhinorrhea and/or sinusitis.

Otologic Disease

External Ear Canal Stenosis

Stenotic ear canals are a common problem occurring in approximately 38% of newborns with Down syndrome (3). This makes detection of disease more difficult. The small ear canals are resultant cerumen impactions can obscure any type of middle-ear disease. Simple cleaning of the ear canals under the office microscope provides a big service to not only the patient but the patient's pediatrician. Stenotic ear canals are associated with an increased incidence of middle-ear effusion; approximately 80% of patients with stenotic ear canals are noted to have middle-ear effusion on examination (3). Strome (3) also reported a 100% incidence of middle-ear effusion in the presence of stenotic ear canals and chronic rhinorrhea.

Hearing Loss: Chronic Ear Disease

There is an increased incidence of chronic ear disease in children with Down syndrome, possibly due to the increased incidence of upper respiratory tract infections seen in these children, or possibly to the depressed immune system. Studies have shown a reduction of both T- and B-cell function in individuals with Down syndrome (4,5). In addition, there are some structural considerations. The anatomy of the midface, with an overall midface hypoplasia including the area of the nasopharynx, contributes to the increased incidence of ear disease. In addition to an abnormal insertion of the eustachian tube, the shape of the eustachian tube is more cylindrical than oval and smaller in width (6). The generalized hypotonia may also cause chronic middle-ear effusions secondary to decreased functioning of the tensor veli palatini muscle of the palate, resulting in poor eustachian tube function (3). On a histopathologic level, the decreased cartilage cell density within the eustachian tube in patients with Down syndrome may contribute further to the increased incidence of eustachian tube pathology (7).

As many as 78% of patients with Down syndrome have decreased hearing (8–10). Children with Down syndrome have a three times higher incidence of chronic ear disease and hearing loss than other children with mental retardation (9,11). Multiple studies have shown a relationship between even mild hearing loss and educational and emotional development (8,9,12). Hearing loss can also affect language development, and statistically significant IQ differences were demonstrated in some studies between children with mild hearing loss due to otitis media and matched controls (8). As pointed out by Balkany et al. (10), these studies were all done on otherwise normal children with hearing loss, and it should be assumed that the developmental problems from hearing loss may have a greater effect on children with the mental and physical handicaps associated with Down syndrome.

Balkany et al. (10) reported that 83% of the hearing loss in patients with Down syndrome was due to a conductive abnormality (10). Interestingly, of those with a conductive hearing loss, only 60% of the cases could be attributed to chronic ear disease such as middle-ear disease or tympanic membrane perforations. This observation led them to look for other sources of the conductive hearing loss; they conducted studies of temporal bones and also evaluated the middle-ear ossicles at surgery. Ossicular abnormalities included congenital fixation and suprastructure deformity of the stapes, as well as deformities of the malleus and incus including erosion and/or fixation. The latter were felt to be due to chronic inflammation. Twenty-five percent of the children evaluated through surgery for their conductive hearing loss had no obvious anatomic abnormalities that could explain the hearing loss. The reasons for this are still unclear, although Harado and Sando's (13) studies on temporal bone histopathology in Down syndrome postulate that remnants of mesenchyme tissue in the round window niche may contribute to this unexplained conductive hearing loss.

Although most hearing loss is conductive in nature, between 4% and 20% of patients with Down syndrome will have either a mixed hearing loss or a sensorineural hearing loss (9,10,14).

Initial evaluation should include a thorough examination, frequently under an office microscope. Otologic and audiologic assessment is sometimes hampered by the patient's underlying developmental delay and stenotic ear canals. Regardless, audiologic evaluation should start with a neonatal auditory brainstem response (ABR), followed by behavioral audiometry and pure tone testing every 6 months up to age 8 years, and then annual follow-up testing.

ABR testing can differentiate between sensorineural and moderate conductive hearing loss but may miss a mild conductive loss (15). Because of this limitation, appropriate examination and impedance testing is helpful for detection of middle-ear fluid or infection that may have a mild effect on hearing levels. In addition, even with a normal ABR, follow-up behavioral audiometry should be done to rule out a mild loss.

There is some controversy as to the presence or absence of abnormal ABR wave patterns in children with Down syndrome (9,15,16). Except for some delay in the waveforms, often due to middle-ear fluid, the audiology department at the author's institution does not feel that the mild variations in the waveforms affect diagnosis and treatment.

Airway Obstruction: Obstructive Sleep Apnea

Airway obstruction is common in children with Down syndrome. Predisposing factors include midface and mandibular hypoplasia. The abnormally small upper airway combined with superficially positioned tonsils lead to obstruction. Adenoids are relatively large in comparison with a contracted nasopharynx, contributing further to the obstruction. Macroglossia is another contributing factor. This can be true macroglossia but more commonly is a normal size tongue in an abnormally small pharynx, resulting in glossoptosis. Increased secretions, obesity, and the generalized hypotonia frequently seen in Down syndrome also contribute to the oropharyngeal collapse and obstruction during sleep. Sleep-related airway obstruction has been reported to occur in 50% to 100% of patients with Down syndrome (17,18). Marcus et al. (17) evaluated 53 patients with Down syndrome and found that 100% had abnormal sleep studies, 63% had obstructive sleep apnea, 81% had hypoventilation problems, and 56% had desaturations during their studies. Age, obesity, and the presence of congenital heart disease were not predictive for the presence or absence of these sleep disturbances. In almost 60% of these children, obstructive sleep apnea was totally unsuspected, with parents expressing no specific complaints or suspicions.

Obstructive sleep apnea (OSA) is frequently overlooked. Unfortunately, in some cases, the apnea is initially missed or not discussed, and many parents assume that their child's sleep disturbances are simply part of the Down syndrome spectrum. For a long time obstructive sleep apnea was not recognized as a potential health problem, as many of the sequelae of the obstructive sleep apnea disorders are conditions also associated with Down syndrome including failure to thrive, pulmonary hypertension, and behavior problems. The pulmonary hypertension was primarily believed to be due to congenital heart abnormalities, present in 50% of children with Down syndrome. However, pulmonary hypertension occurs at a much higher rate than would be expected if due only to cardiac abnormalities. Several studies have noted the association of not only pulmonary hypertension but also heart failure and cor pulmonale with chronic upper airway obstruction (17–20).

Even mild obstructive respiratory patterns during sleep may be associated with significant hypoxic sleep abnormalities (17). Evaluation for OSA includes a thorough history and examination. In the face of a positive history and enlarged tonsils and adenoids, appropriate surgical management may be indicated. Lateral neck x-rays and/or nasopharyngoscopy may further demonstrate the obstruction in the case of relatively minimally enlarged tonsils and adenoids in a contracted oropharynx and nasopharynx (see Fig. 1).

Sleep fluoroscopy is useful in demonstrating what level of the airway is causing the obstruction. For instance, in a child with a significant history of sleep obstruction but on examination small tonsils and adenoids, a sleep fluoroscopy may show more inferior hypopharyngeal collapse causing the obstruction. Sleep studies help to delineate the severity of obstruction and also better characterize the type of obstruction. Although true OSA may benefit from surgical intervention, central apnea also occurs in patients with Down syndrome and will not generally improve with surgical intervention.

Chronic Rhinorrhea/Sinusitis

Chronic rhinorrhea is a common clinical finding in children with Down syndrome. Anatomic considerations contribute to the increased incidence of nasal obstruction, rhinorrhea, and sinusitis. Because of growth retardation in the anterior–posterior dimension of the skull and the increase in the vertical growth in the parietal region, midface hypoplasia occurs. Orbital hypotelorism, an abnormal narrowing of the interorbital distance, further contributes to midface abnormalities (21). Palatal widths have been found to be narrower than normal with lengths shorter than normal (22,23). Posterior choanae are smaller in all dimensions, and the nasopharynx is significantly narrow in regards to both width and interior–posterior dimensions.

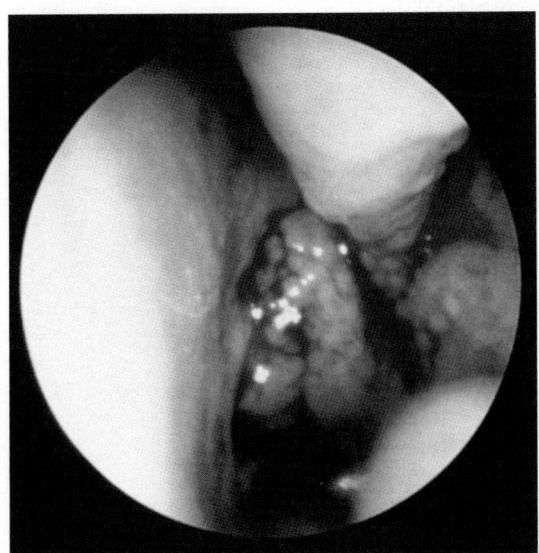

FIGURE 1 Adenoid tissue in a contracted nasopharynx can cause significant nasal obstruction, as seen in this transnasal view of the posterior choanae.

Because of immature immunologic development, children with Down syndrome tend to have more upper respiratory tract infections that are more chronic. Sinusitis is frequently seen. Radiologic studies have described abnormal development of the frontal, maxillary, and sphenoid sinuses including both hypoplasia and total nonpneumatization. The failure of the aeration of the sphenoid is believed to be due to a maturation defect of the basicranium (24).

Much of the rhinorrhea will improve with age and may be due to enlargement of the anatomic abnormalities with growth. With more emphasis on inclusion and mainstreaming however, the persistent runny nose can be a social problem. Despite the anatomic and immunologic factors that may predispose to chronic sinusitis, aggressive evaluation and management of chronic rhinorrhea and sinusitis can lead to clinical improvement. The chronic rhinorrhea should not be simply accepted as an inevitable characteristic of Down syndrome.

Assessment of chronic rhinorrhea and sinusitis should include evaluation of the upper airway to rule out obstruction. Nasopharyngoscopy is helpful to assess for relative enlargement of the adenoids in the case of a contracted nasopharynx. Immune workups are frequently helpful, as well as allergy evaluations to rule out any predisposing contributing factors. Risk factors, such as exposure to cigarette smoke, need to be identified and eliminated. Computed tomography (CT) scan evaluation and consideration of surgical intervention are also options if medical control is not possible.

Oral and Dental Abnormalities

A relative macroglossia is much more common than a true macroglossia and is present in approximately 60% of children with Down syndrome (1). A small oral cavity combined with decreased motor tone can exacerbate this problem. Tongue thrusting, a common neurologically based behavior in young children with Down syndrome, improves with age. In addition, better tongue control and an awareness of the tongue positioning also improve with age and surgical intervention is not usually necessary. However, in extreme cases, tongue reduction may be indicated.

Fissuring of the tongue and enlargement of the vallate papillae is common in children with Down syndrome. These are common, normal variants in the tongue architecture and no specific intervention or treatment is needed.

Fifty percent of children with Down syndrome have missing teeth (1). Malocclusion, particularly type III with mandibular protrusion, and posterior crossbite occur in most patients with Down syndrome (Fig. 2). It is possible that the upper airway obstruction and obstructive sleep apnea and resultant dental–facial changes may be contributing to these dental changes.

FIGURE 2 Type III malocclusion and a cross-bite in a 14-year-old boy with Down syndrome.

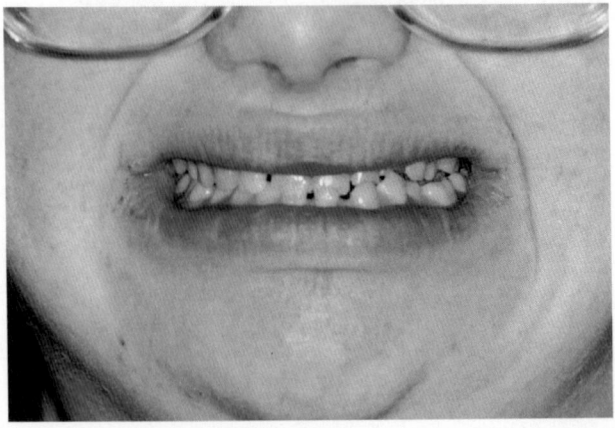

TREATMENT RECOMMENDATIONS

Otologic Problems

Because hearing loss effects intellectual, social, and psychological development, as well as language development, aggressive treatment of otologic infection and/or hearing loss is advocated. Otolaryngologists can first help by educating their referring physicians as to the need for appropriate diagnosis and treatment of all ear disease in this patient population. In this age of managed care, referrals should not be held back if examination is not possible because of stenotic ear canals. Treatment of stenotic ear canals is achieved by simple cleaning of the ears in the office with the assistance of a microscope and use of a small, 2-mm ear speculum. Repeated cleaning may be necessary. The author routinely sees children with stenotic ear canals every 3 months both to clean the canals and to diagnosis any type of ear infections better. Most ear canals enlarge with age, and canalplasty is rarely necessary.

Chronic suppurative otitis can be missed, particularly in children with stenotic ear canals, and can contribute to both conductive and sensorineural hearing loss. Atelectases, atrophic and adhesive disease, and ossicular damage can occur if left untreated. The need for repeated polyethylene tube placement is common and should be expected in most patients with Down syndrome.

Strome (3) found that less than 10% of the patients in his series were left with residual conductive pathology following treatment of their chronic otitis media. He stressed the importance of treating patients aggressively, initially with medical treatment and then with surgical placement of ventilation tubes if middle-ear fluid failed to resolve. He noted that treatment of the patient's purulent rhinorrhea seemed to improve their ear disease.

Balkany et al. (10) agreed with the need for aggressive medical and surgical management of middle-ear infections. However, some limitations were identified. They found little improvement in conductive hearing loss in patients with Down syndrome undergoing surgery for ossicular abnormalities and suggested a more conservative course such as amplification in patients who continue to have a conductive hearing loss following treatment for their chronic ear disease (10).

Amplification should be considered even if there is only a mild hearing loss, especially in view of the data linking even mild hearing loss with delays in educational, emotional, and language development (8,9,12).

Anesthetic Considerations

A high incidence of physical abnormalities associated with Down syndrome may require surgical intervention. With 50% of these children born with cardiac anomalies, it is quite likely that a general anesthesia will be needed at some point. Kobel et al. (25) reviewed 100 general anesthesia procedures on patients with Down syndrome, and although he found a very low rate of complications, he also stressed that the anesthesiologist must have a good understanding of the pathophysiology of patients with Down syndrome. For instance, not only is there a high rate of cardiac anomalies, the type of cardiac lesions in such children differs from those in the general population. Whereas 2% of all congenital heart disease is due to an atrioventricular cardiac defect, this accounts for 60% of the congenital heart anomalies in children with Down syndrome. There is an increased incidence of pulmonary hypertension, polycythemia in the neonatal population, thyroid function abnormalities, and a possible sensitivity to atropine. No differences were noted in regard to the response of patients to inhaled anesthesia agents (25).

Specific differences that may effect otolaryngologic surgery include the possibility of cervical spine abnormalities that may effect manipulation of the neck during surgery, a higher incidence of subglottic stenosis, and a potential for postoperative difficulties due to anatomic features of midface hypoplasia and macroglossia predisposing the patient to upper airway obstruction in the immediate postoperative period.

Subglottic Stenosis

An association between Down syndrome, stridor, and/or subglottic stenosis is frequently discussed in the anesthesia literature (24–26). It is common practice to use a smaller endotracheal tube when intubating children with Down syndrome. Kobel et al.'s (25) series of 100 patients undergoing intubation reported that 23% of the children with Down syndrome required endotracheal tubes one or two sizes smaller. Miller et al. (27) suggested that when intubation is performed in a child with Down syndrome, it would be wise to use a tube one-half size smaller in diameter than would be predicted by the patient's age. This is particularly important because this paper also reviewed a series of patients with Down syndrome who required laryngotracheal reconstruction for subglottic stenosis. They found that a successful repair was much more difficult to achieve in this population (27). The author's experience has led to the conclusion that a full one size smaller size tube be placed initially. In view of the variation in the airway size, it is also very important to test for an appropriate air leak around the endotracheal tube after it is placed.

Cervical Spine Abnormalities

Cervical spine abnormalities seen in Down syndrome include atlantoaxial instability (AAI), abnormal congenital fusion of the vertebral bodies, degenerative changes in the C-2 to C-3 and C-3 to C-4 cervical interspaces, and spinal cord compression.

Approximately 15% of patients with Down syndrome have AAI (28). This is caused by a combination of odontoid hypoplasia resulting in loss of the buttressing action of the dens during extension and laxity of the transverse ligament of the first and second vertebrae. With hyperextension, AAI can cause compression of the spinal cord. Lateral neck x-rays in the extension, flexion, and neutral position are currently used to document this condition (Fig. 3). Cervical spine films, however, are not particularly reliable and in asymptomatic children with AAI and abnormal cervical x-rays, up to 20% may have normal films if these are rechecked 3 to 6 years later (29). CT gives more detailed information about bony anomalies and spinal cord compression (30). No specific recommendations for its routine use are currently recommended. One of the difficulties surrounding AAI is that most individuals with AAI are asymptomatic. To date, there are no studies identifying which patients with Down syndrome and AAI are at risk for spinal cord injury (29).

In 1983, the Special Olympics began requiring that lateral neck x-rays be done on all individuals with Down syndrome before participating in the Special Olympics nationwide athletic competition. If any sign of AAI was present, these participants were restricted from certain activities and events associated with a risk to the cervical spine. In

FIGURE 3 Cervical spine film in the lateral flexion view of an 8-year-old boy with Down syndrome. The first cervical vertebra is hypoplastic. The space anterior to the dens is increased *(arrowheads)*, and the space posterior to the dens is markedly decreased *(arrows)*.

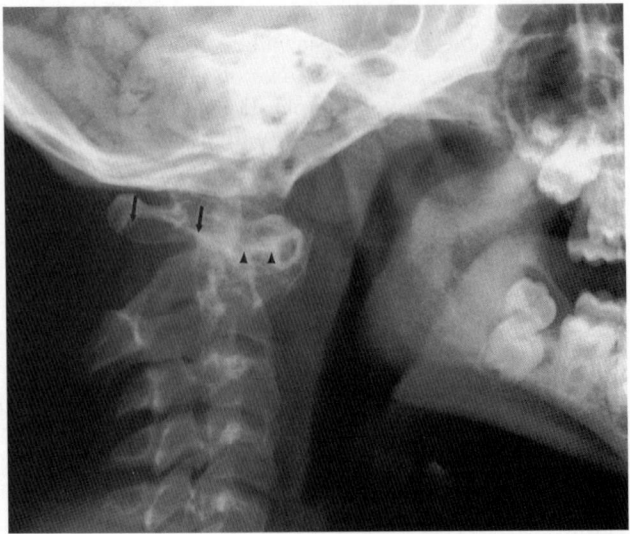

1984, the American Academy of Pediatrics published a statement agreeing with this decision. However, in July 1995, the American Academy of Pediatrics, Committee on Sports Medicine and Fitness published a subject review on AAI and Down syndrome stating that current evidence suggested that the presence of neurologic abnormalities may be more predictive of potential cervical spine injuries. Neurologic manifestations of symptomatic AAI include easy fatigability, difficulties in walking, abnormal gait, neck pain, limited neck mobility, torticollis or head tilt, incoordination and clumsiness, sensory deficits, spasticity, hyperreflexia, clonus, extensor–plantar reflex, and other upper motor neuron and posterior column signs and symptoms. In reviewing 41 cases of reported symptomatic AAI, this committee noted that nearly all the individuals who had experienced a catastrophic injury to the spinal cord had a history of less severe neurologic findings that had been present for weeks to years previously. Identification of patients who have complaints or physical findings consistent with AAI may be of more value than obtaining cervical spine films. The committee concluded that lateral plain x-rays of the cervical spine were "of potential but unproven value in detecting patients at risk for developing spinal cord injury during sports participation" (29).

Once identified, individuals with Down syndrome and AAI should be followed with serial neurologic exams. One to 2% may ultimately require cervical stabilization surgery (28).

Taking these issues as a whole, from an anesthetic standpoint, special attention should be placed to patient positioning on the operating table. Although it is small, there is a risk to the spinal column and because of the general anesthesia, subtle neurologic changes cannot be monitored. Harley and Collins (31), in their review of neurologic sequelae due to AAI in otolaryngologic surgery, recommend special precautions for adenotonsillectomy (because of the risk of hyperextension injury) and major otologic surgery (because of the risk of cord compression from rotary subluxation). For adenotonsillectomy, the patient should stay in as neutral a position as possible. Shoulder rolls should not be used.

It is recommended that prior to these surgical procedures, cervical spine films and neurologic assessment be done to rule out those at risk (28). There is minimal if any risk with a short ventilation tube placement procedure (31).

PEARLS AND PERILS

History and examination of children with Down syndrome should include evaluation of
1. Otologic disease—includes chronic otitis media and hearing loss.
2. Airway obstruction—ask about obstructive sleep apnea.
3. Chronic rhinorrhea, sinusitis—include allergy and immune workup.
4. Anesthetic considerations—check for air leak around the endotracheal tube and be aware of patient positioning during general anesthesia.

Airway Obstruction: Obstructive Sleep Apnea

Treatment of upper airway obstruction in children with Down syndrome is dependent on appropriate diagnosis of the source and level of the obstruction. In the face of a contracted oropharyngeal airway and relative enlargement of the tonsils and adenoids, adenotonsillectomy is indicated. Uvulopalatopharyngoplasty may be a more aggressive yet indicated approach in the adolescent or young adult with Down syndrome.

As pointed out by Marcus et al. (17), although most patients showed improvement after adenotonsillectomy, many of the children continue to have abnormal sleep studies. If there is any sign of obstruction postoperatively, children undergoing adenotonsillectomy should have a repeat polysomnogram. If the apnea persists, options in this situation include oxygen supplementation during sleep, continuous positive airway pressure (CPAP) ventilation during sleep, and/or tracheotomy. Weight reduction programs may also be helpful.

Borderline abnormal sleep studies should be followed with serial retesting, particularly in view of the relationship of chronic hypoxemia and chronic hypoventilation with pulmonary hypertension and congestive heart failure.

If the upper airway obstruction is due to hypopharyngeal collapse or glossoptosis, adenotonsillectomy would not significantly improve the upper airway obstruction. Supplemental oxygen during sleep and/or CPAP can be quite helpful in these situations. Tongue reduction surgery in the face of true macroglossia can also be considered. In severe cases, tracheotomy may be needed.

Because of the small nasal passage and midface hypoplasia, nasal obstruction from secretions and nasal crusting is quite common in children with Down syndrome. Simple use of normal saline spray can help keep the nasal passages clear, improving the upper airway. This very simple therapy can lead to dramatic improvement and should not be overlooked.

Chronic Rhinorrhea/Sinusitis

Although there are anatomic and physiologic reasons that predispose children with Down syndrome to chronic rhinorrhea and sinusitis, this should not affect one's treatment approach. Evaluation and treatment should include examination and surgical intervention if indicated for obstructing structures such as enlarged adenoids. Strome (3) did not find adenoidectomy to be significantly helpful in treatment of chronic rhinorrhea in children with Down syndrome. However, if near total posterior choanae obstruction is caused by the adenoids, this procedure should be considered.

Again, because of the decreased nasal airways, frequent nasal crusting is common and the use of normal saline spray to cleanse and moisturize nasal passages can be extremely helpful. The significant improvement achieved with this very simple form of therapy should not be underestimated. Rule out etiologic factors that may predispose to an increase in upper respiratory tract infections such as large day-care environment and exposure to cigarette smoke. A very strong admonishment against any exposure whatsoever to cigarette smoke is an absolute necessity.

Medical management of chronic rhinorrhea and sinusitis is similar to the treatment of these entities in general with the use of appropriate antibiotics and decongestants. Strome (3) noted a significant improvement in controlling his patients' chronic rhinorrhea with the use of maintenance antibiotics. This author's experience has been similar. A longer course of low-dose antibiotics, preferably one with a narrower spectrum such as amoxicillin, may be particularly helpful in view of the higher incidence of immunodeficiencies in children with Down syndrome.

Allergy evaluations should also be considered. Nasal steroids are quite helpful in controlling mild allergic-type rhinitis and its effect on chronic sinusitis. However, in patients who do not improve or respond to medical management, surgical intervention using functional endoscopic sinus surgery should be considered. Indications for surgical intervention are no different in treating children with Down syndrome. CT evaluation following maximization of medical management should be done to evaluate for the presence of chronic sinus mucosal disease and blockage of the osteomeatal complex. The CT scan will also delineate any type of sinus abnormalities and/or hypoplasia in preparation for surgery.

CONCLUSIONS

As otolaryngologists, we will play an active and important role in the medical and surgical care of children with Down syndrome. With an increased life expectancy and increased emphasis on inclusion and mainstreaming, the true potential of individuals with Down syndrome has yet to be established. With basic otolaryngologic problems such as ear disease and hearing loss, as well as upper airway obstruction and the potential for chronic hypoxemia so closely linked to physical, emotional, and educational development, it is important that we aggressively address and treat these very common otolaryngologic manifestations of Down syndrome.

REFERENCES

1. Cooley WC, Graham JM. Common syndromes and management issues for primary care physicians. Down syndrome—an update and review for the primary physician. *Clin Pediatr* 1991;30:233–253.
2. Down syndrome prevalence at birth—United States, 1983–1990. *MMWR* 1994;43:617–622.
3. Strome M. Down's syndrome—a modern otorhinolaryngological perspective. *Laryngoscope* 1981;41:1581–1594.
4. Spina CA, Smith D, Korn E, Fahey JL, Grossman HJ. Altered cellular immune functions in patients with Down's syndrome. *Am J Dis Child* 1981;135:251–255.
5. Gershwin ME, Crinella FM, Castles JJ, Trent JK. Immunologic characteristics of Down's Syndrome. *J Ment Defic Res* 1977;21:237–248.
6. Shibahara Y, Sando I. Congenital anomalies of the eustachian tube in children with Down syndrome. *Ann Otol Rhinol Laryngol* 1989;98:543–547.
7. Yamaguchi N, Sando I, Hashida Y, Takahashi H, Matsune S. Histologic study of eustachian tube cartilage with and without congenital anomalies: a preliminary study. *Ann Otol Rhinol Laryngol* 1990;99:984–987.
8. Balkany TJ, Downs MP, Jafek BW, Krajicek MJ. Hearing loss in Down's syndrome. *Clin Pediatr* 1979;18:116–118.
9. Brooks DN, Wooley H, Kanjhal GC. Hearing loss and middle ear disorders in patients with Down's syndrome (mongolism). *J Ment Defic Res* 1972;16:21–29.
10. Balkany TJ, Mischke RE, Downs MP, Jafek BW. Ossicular abnormalities in Down's syndrome. *Otolaryngol Head Neck Surg* 1979;87:372–384.
11. Dahle AJ, McCollister FP. Hearing and otologic disorders in children with Down syndrome. *Am J Ment Defic* 1986;90:636–642.
12. Holm V, Kunze L. Effect of chronic otitis media on language and speech development. *Pediatrics* 1969;43:833–839.
13. Harada T, Sando I. Temporal bone histopathologic findings in Down's syndrome. *Arch Otolaryngol* 1981;107:96–103.
14. Davies B. Auditory disorders in Down's syndrome. *Scand Audiol Suppl* 1988;30:65–68.
15. Maurizi M, Ottaviani F, Paludetti G, Lungarotti S. Audiologic findings in Down's children. *Int J Pediatr Otorhinolaryngol* 1985;9:227–232.
16. Folsom RC, Widen JE, Wilson WR. Auditory brain-stem response in infants with Down's syndrome. *Arch Otolaryngol* 1983;109:607–610.
17. Marcus CL, Keens TG, Bautista DB, von Pechmann WS, Davidson Ward SL. Obstructive sleep apnea in children with Down syndrome. *Pediatrics* 1991;88:132–139.
18. Southall DP, Stebbens VA, Mirza R, Lang MH, Croft CB, Shinebourne EA. Upper airway obstruction with hypoxaemia and sleep disruption in Down syndrome. *Dev Med Child Neuron* 1987;29:734–742.
19. Levine OR, Simpser M. Alveolar hypoventilation and cor pulmonale associated with chronic airway obstruction in infants with Down syndrome. *Clin Pediatr* 1982;21:25–29.
20. Rowland TW, Nordstrom LG, Bean MS, Burkhardt H. Chronic upper airway obstruction and pulmonary hypertension in Down's syndrome. *Am J Dis Child* 1981;135:1050–1052.
21. Gerald BE, Silverman FN. Normal and abnormal interorbital distances with special reference to Mongolism. *AJR* 1965;95:154–161.
22. Shapiro BL, Gorlin RJ, Redman RS, Bruhl HH. The palate and Down's syndrome. *N Engl J Med* 1967;2765:1460–1463.
23. Austin JH, Preger L, Siris E, Taybi H. Short hard palate in newborn: roentgen sign of mongolism. *Radiology* 1969;92:775–556.
24. Miller JDR, Capusten BM, Lampard R. Changes at the base of the skull and cervical spine in Down syndrome. *J Can Assoc Radiol* 1986;37:85–89.

25. Kobel M, Creighton RE, Steward DJ. Anaesthetic considerations in Down's syndrome: experience with 100 patients and a review of the literature. *Can Anaesth Soc J* 1982;29:593–598.

26. Sherry KM. Post-extubation stridor in Down's syndrome. *Br J Anaesth* 1983;55:53–55.

27. Miller R, Gray SD, Cotton RT, Myer CM III. Subglottic stenosis and Down syndrome. *Am J Otolaryngol* 1990;11:274–277.

28. Pueschel SM, Scola FH. Atlantoaxial instability in individuals with Down syndrome: epidemiologic, radiographic, and clinical studies. *Pediatrics* 1987;80:555–560.

29. American Academy of Pediatrics, Committee on Sports Medicine and Fitness. Atlantoaxial instability in Down syndrome: subject review. *Pediatrics* 1995;96:151–153.

30. Pueschel SM, Moon AC, Scola FH. Computerized tomography in persons with Down syndrome and atlantoaxial instability. *Spine* 1992;17:735–737.

31. Harley EH, Collins MD. Neurologic sequelae secondary to atlantoaxial instability in Down syndrome: implications in otolaryngologic surgery. *Arch Head Neck Surg* 1994;120:159–165.

S. R. Shott: Department of Otolaryngology and Maxillofacial Surgery, University of Cincinnati, Children's Hospital Medical Center, Cincinnati, Ohio 45229–3039.

• *Practical Pediatric Otolaryngology*
• edited by Robin T. Cotton
  and Charles M. Myer, III
• Lippincott-Raven Publishers,
  Philadelphia © 1999

52

Management of Craniosynostosis

Lawrence J. Marentette

 HISTORICAL BACKGROUND

Craniosynostosis is one of the most common congenital anomalies of the upper facial skeleton. The terms craniosynostosis and craniostenosis have been used interchangably to refer to the same condition, but a distinction exists between these two entities. *Craniosynostosis* refers to the premature fusion of sutures of the calvarium (Fig. 1). *Craniostenosis* is defined as lack of growth of the cranium as a result of premature sutural fusion. Craniosynostosis causes craniostenosis. Its existence was first recorded in the literature by Hippocrates, who described various abnormal cranial shapes that can be compared with coronal, lambdoid, or multiple sutural fusions. Cohen (1–3) has proposed the most useful classification of craniosynostosis: simple and compound. Under simple synostosis, the term brachycephaly refers to coronal synostosis, dolicocephaly to sagittal synostosis, trigonocephaly to metopic synostosis, and plagiocephaly to unilateral coronal or unilateral lambdoid synostosis. In the category of compound synostoses, acrocephaly refers to fusion of all sutures or fusion of various combinations, as seen in coronal and sagittal, cloverleaf skull malformation, and coronal and lambdoid. This then enables further classification of the patient's pathology into nonsyndromal or isolated craniosynostosis versus syndromal craniosynostosis.

Craniosynostosis is also classified as primary or secondary. Primary craniosynostosis refers to the pathologic basis directly resulting from premature fusion of a cranial suture. Secondary craniosynostosis, however, is a result of premature sutural fusion secondary to an established disorder. These disorders may be hematologic (polycythemia vera, sickle cell anemia, congenital hemolytic icterus, and thalassemia); metabolic (hyperthyroidism and ricketts; mucopolysaccharidosis associated (mucolipidosis III, Morquoi's syndrome, Hurler's syndrome, and beta-glucuronidase deficiency); congenital (encephalocele, holoprosencephaly, or microcephaly); or iatrogenic (decreased intracranial pressure as a result of ventricular peritoneal shunt for hydrocephalus).

It is important likewise to distinguish between isolated and syndromal craniosynostosis. Isolated craniosynostosis is typically corrected with one surgical procedure, and in the vast majority of cases, no further treatment is required. Syndromal craniosynostosis, however, requires multiple surgical corrections, as well as later midface corrections.

ETIOLOGY

Several etiologies have been proposed as causative factors of craniosynostosis. If possible, these etiologic factors should be elucidated as part of the assessment to allow the surgeon to individualize treatment planning, and also to advise the patient's family of the possible need for further surgical intervention. One theory holds that initial fusion occurs

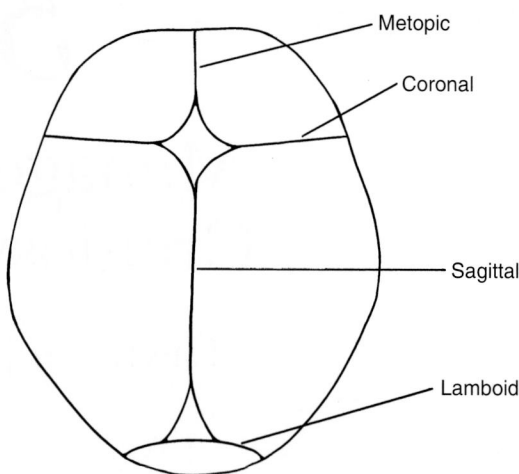

FIGURE 1 As viewed from above, the cranium is symmetric and all sutures are patent.

in the base of the skull resulting in dural tension, which then restricts further growth of the dura and brain, causing stimulus for suture separation to cease. The sutures fuse, resulting in synostosis.

It is important to note that identification of secondary craniosynostosis is significant because, although surgical treatment initially produced an excellent result, the failure to treat the underlying disorder will result in refusion of the sutures and the need for revision surgery. As has been previously mentioned, primary craniosynostosis is divided into isolated versus syndromal craniosynostosis. Syndromal craniosynostosis is further subdivided into three basic categories, which, again, can assist the surgeon in an overall treatment plan. The first category is referred to as monogenic syndromes. These are caused by a defect of one gene, transmitted as autosomal dominant, autosomal recessive, or X-linked. Classic examples of autosomal dominant inheritance would include Apert's syndrome, Crouzon's syndrome and Pfeiffer's syndrome. Examples of autosomal recessive inheritance include Carpenter's syndrome, Antley-Bixler syndrome, and Gorlin-Chaudhry-Moss syndrome. The second category, syndromal craniosynostoses, involves deletions or duplications of the long or short arms of chromosomes I, III, V, VI, VII, IX, XI, XII, XIII, and XV. The third category refer to environmentally induced syndromes which include retinoic acid syndrome and fetal hydantoin syndrome.

Craniosynostosis should not be thought of as merely a localized pathologic event resulting in premature fusion of a suture and resultant calvarial and facial deformity. The heterogeneous nature of this disorder's etiology has been well established by documentation of primary and secondary craniosynostosis.

Although most cases of simple craniosynostosis are sporadic, a small percentage of these cases, which may involve the coronal or the sagittal suture, are familial. In these families, the same suture or other sutures may be involved in successive generations. Syndromal craniosynostosis, for example Crouzon's syndrome, is known to occur as a sporadic mutation. However, once established, successive generations of the proband are susceptible to autosomal dominant expression of deformity. In some cases, offspring may exhibit the cloverleaf skull deformity, whereas a parent may only exhibit bilateral coronal craniosynostosis. Obviously, in the case of patients with Crouzon's syndrome, they will concomitantly manifest maxillary hypoplasia.

PATIENT ASSESSMENT

All patients with craniosynostosis should be evaluated by a craniofacial team, which typically consists of a craniofacial surgeon, geneticist, speech pathologist, oral maxillofacial surgeon, audiologist, orthodontist, and other specialists appropriate for evaluation of these types of patients. It is important to determine whether the patient can be classified into a specific syndrome category. If the patient manifests a syndrome, this would dictate the overall treatment protocol and sequence of treatment.

Syndromal Craniosynostosis

Crouzon's Syndrome

Patients with Crouzon's syndrome typically manifest bilateral coronal craniosynostosis, as well as maxillary hypoplasia and proptosis as a result of orbital deficiency. In some cases, in addition to the coronal suture synostosis, lambdoid suture synostosis and sagittal synostosis may occur, which can result in the cloverleaf skull deformity. In more severe cases of Crouzon's syndrome, the patients have significant ocular proptosis and exposure keratitis, eventually resulting in blindness. Likewise, as the patient grows, reduced orbital volume may lead to stretch of the optic nerve with resultant blindness.

Apert's Syndrome

In contrast to Crouzon's syndrome, in which the anterior fontanelle is typically fused, Apert's syndrome patients present with bilateral coronal craniosynostosis and an open, gaping anterior fontanelle. Midface hypoplasia is significant, and in most cases, more severe than in patients with Crouzon's syndrome. A hallmark of this syndrome is syndactlyly, which involves the second, third, and fourth fingers. Additionally, the maxilla is more severely affected, since there is a very high arched constricted palate that may be accompanied by a palatal cleft. Postmortem examination of patients with Apert's syndrome revealed malformation in the shape of the brain itself, and this may account for the more severe calvarial deformities seen in Apert's syndrome patients, compared with Crouzon's syndrome patients.

Pfeiffer's Syndrome

Patients with Pfeiffer's syndrome manifest bilateral coronal craniosynostosis with a very flat forehead and a more tower-shaped skull. Additionally, the thumb and great toe are broad and enlarged with respect to the other digits.

Antley-Bixler Syndrome

Patients with Antley-Bixler syndrome manifest bilateral coronal craniosynostosis with marked frontal bossing and significant retrusion of the upper portion of the midface, particularly at the nasal frontal suture. Additionally, they have radiohumeral synostosis, femoral bowing, and joint contractures. The midface is hypoplastic, ocular proptosis is quite apparent, and dysplastic ears are also part of this syndrome.

Jackson-Weiss Syndrome

These patients possess multiple sutural synostoses, including the lambdoid sutures and coronal sutures. The midface is hypoplastic but not as severely so as in patients with Apert's syndrome. A distinguishing feature of this syndrome is that the first metatarsals are wide, abnormally shaped and, in some cases, fused. Also, there may be other anomalies of the tarsal bones. Radiographs are important to distinguish Jackson-Weiss syndrome from Pfeiffer's syndrome.

Saethre-Chotzen Syndrome

Coronal synostosis is frequently seen in this syndrome, although not 100% of the time. These patients have a very flat forehead, eyelid ptosis, hypertelorism, and a low-set frontal hairline. The palpebral fissures are downslanting, and optic atrophy may be present. Syndactyly is common in this syndrome, with soft tissue webbing most frequently seen between the second and third digits but, in some cases, extending to include the fourth digit as well.

Nonsyndromal Craniosynostosis

Scaphocephaly

Scaphocephaly, or boat-shaped skull, describes a cranial shape resulting from sagittal synostosis (Fig. 2A). The cranial narrowing also causes a decrease in the upper transverse facial dimension. This is the most common form of craniosynostosis and is not associated with mental retardation. Although the correction of scaphocephaly produces excellent cosmetic results, the elimination of the psychosocial aspects of no correction should be considered a functional indication for correction.

Plagiocephaly

Plagiocephaly is a term referring to forehead asymmetry with one side of the forehead in a retruded position and the other side in a more forward position (Fig. 2B). It is important to distinguish plagiocephaly caused by coronal craniosynostosis as opposed to that caused by torticollis, i.e., fibrotic shortening of the sternocleidomastoid muscle. Facial analysis makes this distinction quite easy. In patients with unilateral coronal synostosis (CS), facial midlines deviate away from the affected side. Patients with torticollis have facial midline deviation toward the affected side. Frontal bossing is present on the affected side in patients with torticollis, whereas it is present on the contralateral side in patients with CS. This distinction is important to make as treatment modalities are very different for these two entities. Torticollis is best treated with helmet therapy and conservative neck brace treatment. If this fails to resolve the muscular shortening, then sternocleidomastoid muscle resection is indicated. However, unilateral coronal synostosis is treated with a frontal orbital advancement requiring an intracranial extracranial osteotomy of the upper craniofacial skeleton.

Brachycephaly

Bilateral coronal synostosis produces a widened skull with a decrease in the anterior–posterior dimension or brachycephaly (Fig. 2C). In nonsyndromal patients, retrusion is present in the nasoethmoid region. Midfacial hypoplasia is seen in syndromal patients, e.g., Crouzon's and Apert's syndromes. Mental retardation is not present in nonsyndromal patients but may be to varying degrees in syndromal. This may be caused by underlying brain anomalies or untreated hydrocephalus.

Trigonocephaly

Trigonocephaly, or triangle-shaped skull, is a result of metopic synostosis (Fig. 2D). The forehead has a prominent vertical midline ridge and there is recession of the lateral supraorbital rims. Varying degrees of bitemporal narrowing are also present. Interorbital distance is decreased, which results in orbital hypotelorism. Because of an association of trigonocephaly with corpus callosum agenesis or holoprosencephaly, a computed to-

FIGURE 2 Cranial shapes in craniosynostosis. **A:** Scaphocephaly, fused sagittal suture. **B:** Plagiocephaly, fused unilateral coronal suture. **C:** Brachycephaly, bilateral coronal fusion. **D:** Trigonocephaly, fused metopic suture. **E:** Posterior plagiocephaly, lambdoid suture fusion.

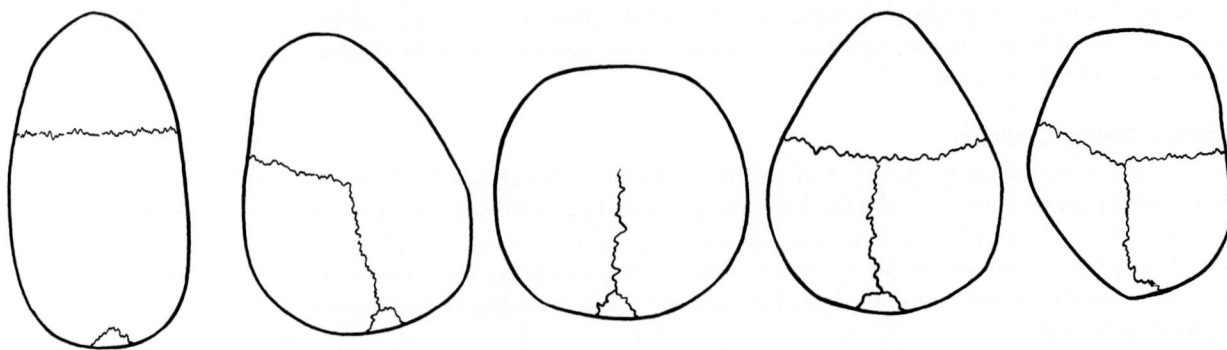

A-E

mography (CT) scan should be performed preoperatively to assess the potential of mental retardation.

Posterior Plagiocephaly

This deformity is caused by synostosis of a unilateral lambdoid suture (Fig. 2E). Synostosis of all other sutures can be clinically diagnosed by a palpable ridge at the fused suture. The ridge in lambdoid synostosis develops on the inner side of the skull. A CT scan will easily demonstrate this ridge and will distinguish between craniosynostosis and intrauterine molding, which will spontaneously correct occasionally. Contralateral coronal synostosis is present, which produces a twisted or slanted shape to the skull.

Radiographic Evaluation

Axial CT and three-dimensional CT scans are important initial tools in the evaluation of patients with craniosynostosis. The axial CT is quite accurate in delineating which sutures are fused, not only in the calvarium, but also in the skull base itself. The three-dimensional CT gives an overall picture of the patient's deformity and can be used as an aid in surgical planning. However, it is not a definitive tool when used in planning the appropriate surgery. When patients are old enough to be cooperative, lateral cephalogram evaluation is extremely helpful on an ongoing basis, as this can be used to determine patterns of facial growth and will provide the definitive planning tool for maxillary surgery. Panorex evaluation is likewise essential to determine dental eruption.

Genetic Counseling

It is important to offer genetic counseling to the patient's family as part of their overall treatment plan. If craniosynostosis is determined to be isolated rather than nonsyndromal, the family can be reassured that this has been a chance event and that further siblings are unlikely to be effected. It is important for the family to know whether a syndrome exists, so that they may counsel the patient in the future regarding chances for offspring to be affected. For example, Crouzon's syndrome is inherited through an autosomal dominant pattern, and it is important for the family to know that as the patient matures, there is a 50% chance of having offspring similarly affected.

TREATMENT RECOMMENDATIONS

Timing of Surgery

Proper timing is essential in the correction of patients with craniosynostosis. Early intervention, (at 3 to 6 months) is the general rule as the optimum time for correction of the cranial anomalies, which has a number of advantages as opposed to later correction at 2 to 4 or 5 years of age. Most importantly, brain growth is most rapid during the first year of life. Therefore, early correction allows the growing brain (the functional matrix) to guide the remodeled calvarium in a normal growth pattern. Second, early correction can avoid facial deformities, which would require further osteotomies in early teens. For example, unilateral coronal craniosynostosis producing plagiocephaly results in a facial deformity of the facial midlines being deviated away from the affected side. Early surgical correction allows normalization of facial growth. If later correction is contemplated, the facial asymmetry may require maxillomandibular orthognathic osteotomies in the teens to correct the residual facial deformity. Correction under 1 year of age has the advantage of calvarial regrowth. Most of the time, patients who undergo correction of craniosynostosis have resultant gaps in the calvarium where bone has been advanced or expanded. In the 3- to 6-month-old patient population, bone is rapidly deposited in these defects such that by 1 year of age the entire calvarium has been regenerated. This is due to the significant osteogenic potential possessed by the dura, the endosteum of the cranial bone. Although early intervention is ideal, this may not be possible in children with syndromal craniosynostosis, if there are multisystem anomalies, particularly in the case of cardiac deformities: Cardiac surgery may be necessary prior to the correction of the cranial anomaly. Therefore, surgery may have to be delayed until later in infancy, unless the child has concomitant hydrocephalus, common in patients with Apert's syndrome. In these patients, early ventricular peritoneal shunt is necessary to prevent neurologic injury. The incidence of hydrocephalus with craniosynostosis increases with the number of sutures that are involved, and in some patients with multiple craniosynostosis, early intervention and correction may be protective of cognitive skills as measured by IQ.

Surgical Procedures

As a general consideration, specific sutures that are fused will need to be opened and the affected area anatomically corrected. The deformity dictates the operation; a standard operation cannot applied to a specific deformity. In this way, each surgical procedure is tailored to the patient's specific problem.

Unilateral Coronal Synostosis

The correction of plagiocephaly as a result of unilateral coronal synostosis can be achieved with two specific osteotomies (Fig. 3), the first being a unilateral forehead advancement. This is performed by advancing the unilateral frontal bone, "green sticking" the frontal bone at the metopic suture in the midline of the forehead. A unilateral frontal craniotomy is performed with removal of the bone flap, after which a frontal orbital osteotomy is created with a tongue and groove cut made in the temporal fossa. This allows for adequate bone contact in this area following frontal orbital advancement. This procedure should be reserved for very specific cases in which the normal contralateral forehead abruptly deviates from the midline in a retruded fashion. If, on the other hand, a gentle sloping from the contralateral normal side to the affected side is found, unilateral forehead advancement will result in a midline groove in the forehead. This procedure is rarely done today as most patients manifest very gentle sloping asymmetry of the forehead in an anterior to posterior direction.

FIGURE 3 Plagiocephaly correction. **A:** The deformity is limited to the right forehead only. **B:** The forehead and upper orbit are advanced.

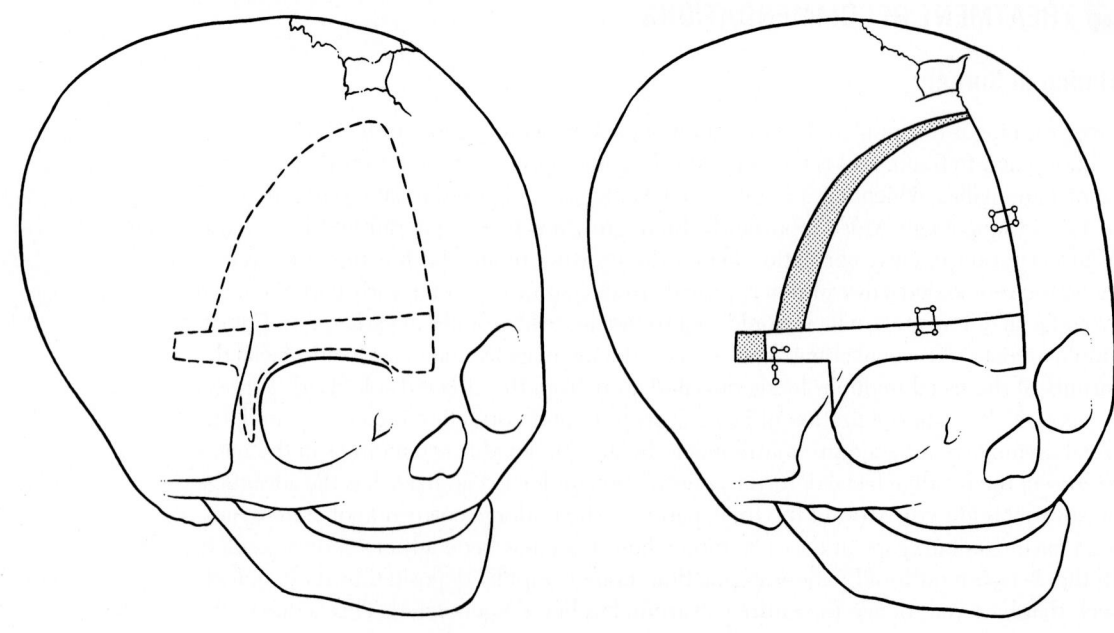

A   B

Bilateral Frontal Orbital Advancement

In bilateral frontal orbital advancement, a bilateral frontal craniotomy is performed, and bilateral frontal orbital osteotomies are created, with tongue and groove bone cuts made in the temporal fossa bilaterally (Fig. 4). This allows for total advancement of the frontal orbital bar, which contains the forehead and upper part of the orbits from the nasal frontal suture superiorly, and laterally encompassing the zygomaticofrontal suture and the upper portion of the lateral orbital rim. In this fashion, the forehead is advanced and the normal contour of the forehead is maintained. The frontal craniotomy bone flaps are then replaced, with a gap left on the side of the forehead that was advanced. If the surgery is performed at 3 to 6 months of age, the bone gap will fill in with calvarial bone such that by 1 year of age, the cranium will have reestablished its continuity, thereby avoiding any soft areas that may predispose the patient to brain injury secondary to trauma from a fall.

Frontal Orbital Correction of Metopic Synostosis

In patients with metopic synostosis who manifest trigonocephaly, the midline of the forehead is not advanced but rather maintained in this normal position (Fig. 5). A bifrontal craniotomy is performed, and the frontal bone flap is removed. Frontal orbital osteotomies are created, again in the same fashion as in a plagiocephaly correction, with a tongue and groove cut fashioned in the temporal fossa. However, the lateral aspects of the supraorbital rims and forehead are advanced, maintaining the midsection of the forehead in a central position. This involves a green stick fracturing of the sphenofrontal suture, which may require microplate fixation to stabilize this area following the lateral advancement. Then, the frontal craniotomy bone flap is sectioned in the midline and recontoured to fit the newly formed forehead profile.

Total Head Remodeling

Total head remodeling is performed in patients with moderate to severe scaphocephaly deformation as a result of sagittal suture synostosis (Fig. 6). In this procedure, the entirely of the calvarium is exposed with a coronal incision, and exposure of the calvarium is achieved extending from the supraorbital rims to the occiput. Anteriorly, a bifrontal craniotomy is created, as well as a frontal orbital osteotomy. These bones are removed and re-

FIGURE 4 Brachycephaly correction. **A:** The osteotomy is designed to advance the forehead and upper orbits, as is the case in Crouzon's syndrome. **B:** The frontoorbital complex is advanced into the correct position.

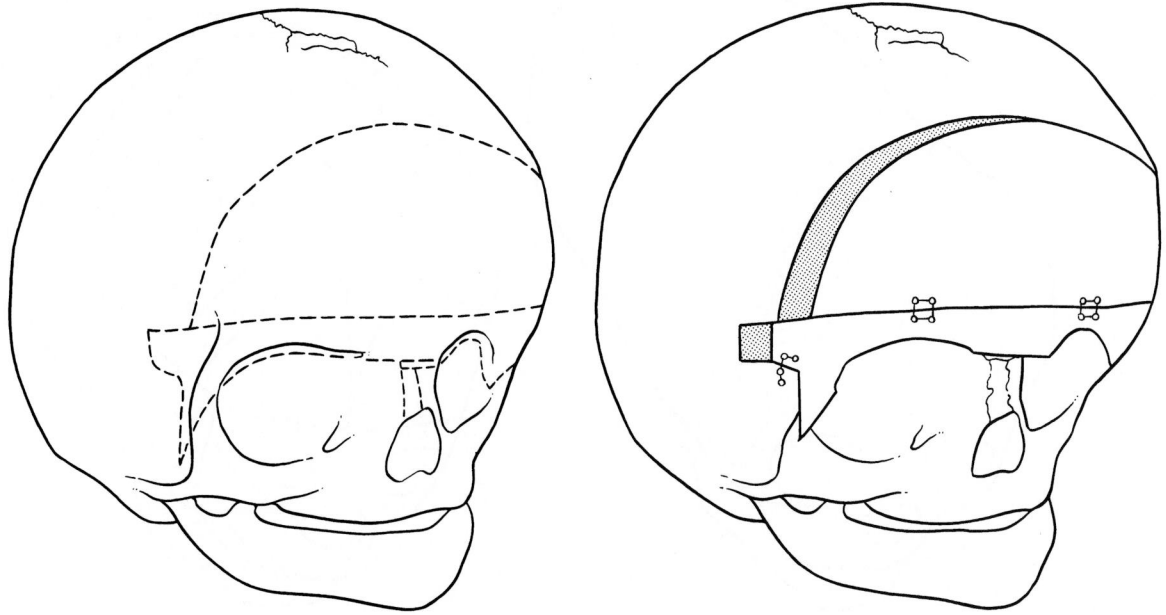

A   **B**

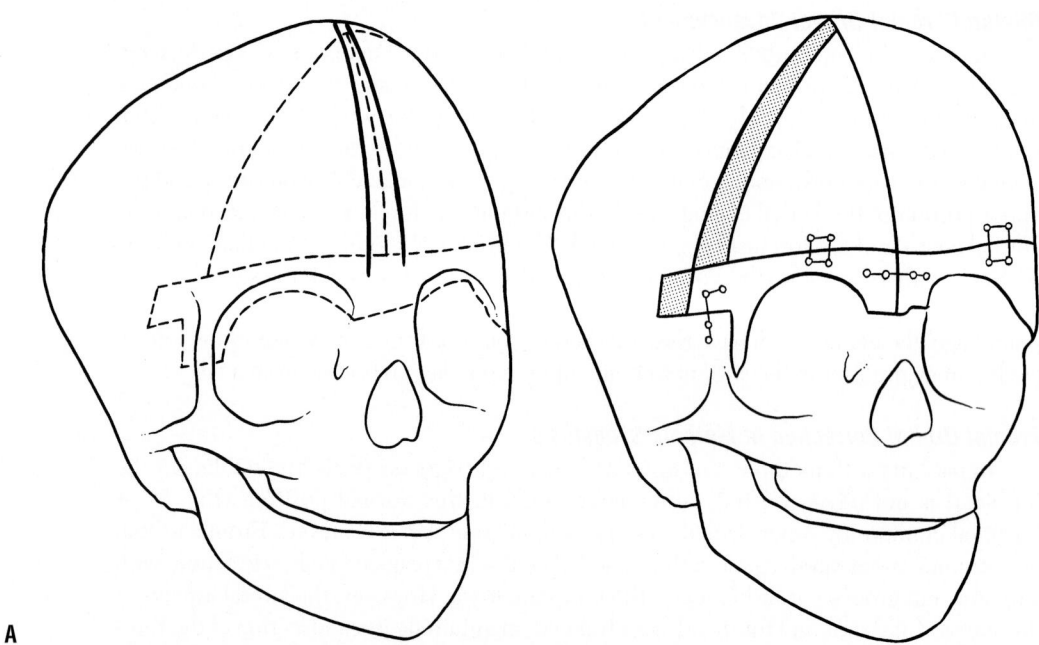

A

B

FIGURE 5 Trigonocephaly correction. **A:** Fused metopic suture resulting in midline vertical forehead ridge and bitemporal narrowing. **B:** The lateral frontoorbital complex is advanced, and the central portion is not. This increases bitemporal width and eliminates the vertical ridge.

modeled on the back table. Additionally, parietal and occipital osteotomies are created, and those bones are removed as well. At the discretion of the surgeon, the bones are replaced in the proper position to achieve normal head shape and then are fixed in position.

Lambdoid Synostosis

Lambdoid synostosis involves asymmetry of the occiput, which requires occipital re-modeling (Fig. 7). Correction of lambdoid synostosis involves a coronal incision with pos-

FIGURE 6 Scaphocephaly correction. **A:** Fusion of the sagittal suture has resulted in marked elonga-tion of the skull. **B:** Total remodeling includes decreasing the anterior–posterior dimension while in-creasing the transverse dimension.

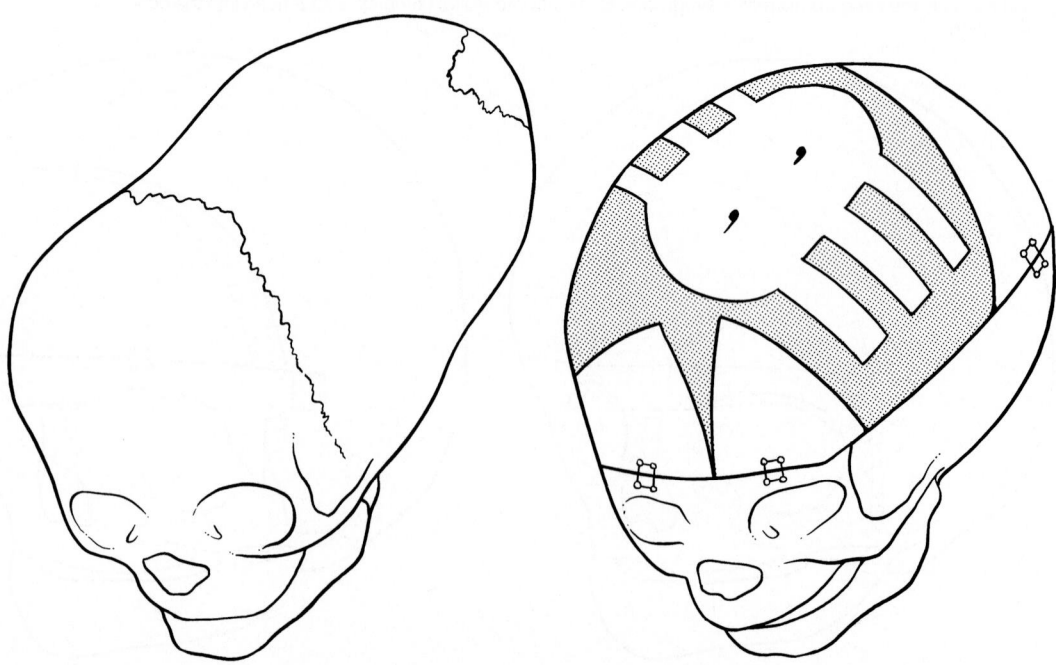

A

B

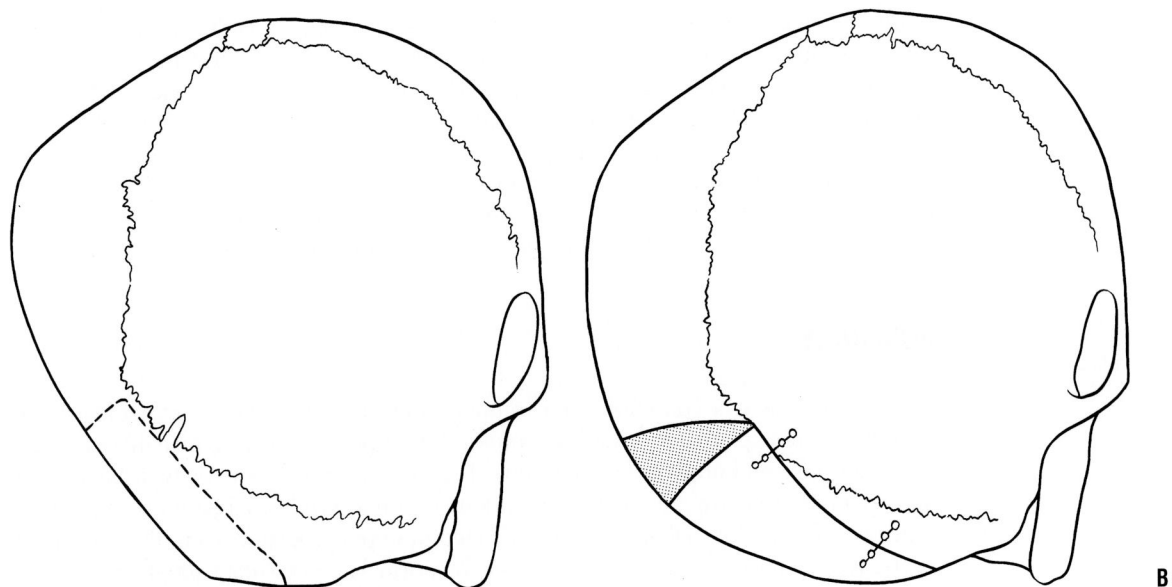

FIGURE 7 Lambdoid synostosis correction. **A:** Posterior flattening caused by unilateral lambdoid synostosis. **B:** The flattened occiput is removed and replaced in a normal position.

terior dissection extending from the vertex to the base of the skull posteriorly to the basiocciput. Osteotomies are then created along the fused lambdoid sutures, and the occipital bone is removed, including the portion extending down to the foramen magnum. The bone is then remodeled and replaced in a normal position. If the patient has a concomitant Chiari malformation, this may be corrected at the same time.

Rigid Fixation in Craniofacial Growth

Much debate has occurred over the use of microplate fixation in patients who undergo surgery for craniosynostosis. Evidence exists in the literature that plate fixation restricts growth of the cranial vault. When the material in Enlow (4) regarding cranial growth is reviewed, bone is seen to be deposited on the outside of the cranium and resorbed on the inside of the cranium as the underlying functional matrix brain grows. This would suggest that with time, plates would migrate from the extracranial to the intercranial side. Bone healing in these patients occurs very rapidly within 2 to 3 months; therefore, it is difficult to envision that plates would restrict growth. The diameter of the screws used in microplates, 1 mm, approximates that of wires used in past craniosynostosis repairs. Since repairs had not presented a problem in terms of restricting growth, it seems unlikely that plates would restrict plates as well. In the studies performed, patients with Crouzon's syndrome and Apert's syndrome were grouped together with patients who had isolated craniosynostosis. This is not appropriate, as patients with syndromal craniosynostosis often require multiple cranial remodeling surgeries, particularly patients with Apert's syndrome. It is more likely that in the animal experiments performed with plate and screw fixation, scar tissue of the surrounding functional matrix was responsible for growth retardation and not the actual rigid fixation systems used to stabilize the osteotomies.

Results of Treatment

Again, it is important to note that patients who have nonsyndromal craniosynostosis have a higher likelihood of not requiring reoperation. These patients typically undergo one surgical procedure for cranial vault correction, and the cranium continues to grow in a normal fashion. Similarly, any concomitant facial deformity normally self-corrects and does not require surgical intervention in the teenage years. In contrast to these patients, syndromal craniosynostosis patients require multiple cranial procedures, as well as mid-face procedures to achieve an ultimate point of treatment. The most frustrating of these patients are those with Apert's syndrome. They require multiple cranial vault corrections, and in spite of the best surgical efforts, cranial irregularities continue to occur. In spite of corrections of midface and orbital hypertelorism, they continue to manifest the stigmata of the Apert's syndrome in the best of surgical hands. More work needs to be done in the area of syndromal craniosynostosis correction to try to minimize the amount of surgical procedures needed to bring these patients to a relatively normal quality of life.

SUMMARY

Craniosynostosis is a condition seen frequently by the pediatric otolaryngologist; the overall treatment plan may be highly complex. It is important to categorize these patients into syndromal and nonsyndromal groups. The nonsyndromal patients typically require one operation to correct cranial deformations, whereas syndromal patients require the expertise of a craniofacial team; they may need multiple procedures and multiple interventions to achieve a result that at best may be normal and at worst suboptimal.

REFERENCES

1. Cohen MM Jr. History, terminology, and classification of craniosynostosis. In: Cohen MM Jr., ed. *Craniosynostosis: diagnosis, evaluation, and management.* New York: Raven Press, 1986:1–20.
2. Cohen MM Jr. The etiology of craniosynostosis. In: Cohen MM Jr., ed. *Craniosynostosis: diagnosis, evaluation, and management.* New York: Raven Press, 1986:59–80.
3. Cohen MM Jr. Syndromes with craniosynostosis. In: Cohen MM Jr., ed. *Craniosynostosis: diagnosis, evaluation, and management.* New York: Raven Press, 1986:413–590.
4. Enlow DH. *Facial growth.* 3rd ed. Philadelphia: WB Saunders, 1990:25–148.

RECOMMENDED READINGS

1. Garlin RJ, Cohen MM, Levin LS, eds. *Syndromes of the head and neck,* 3rd ed. New York: Oxford University Press, 1990.
2. Cohen MM Jr., ed. *Craniosynostosis: diagnosis, evaluation, and management.* New York: Raven Press, 1986.
3. Dufresne CR, Carson BS, Zinruich SJ, eds. *Complex craniofacial problems.* New York: Churchill Livingstone, 1992.

L.J. Marentette: Department of Otolaryngology, University of Michigan Medical Center, Ann Arbor, Michigan 48109–0312.

• *Practical Pediatric Otolaryngology*
• edited by Robin T. Cotton and Charles M. Myer, III
• Lippincott-Raven Publishers, Philadelphia © 1999

Auricular Reconstruction

Jonathan M. Sykes

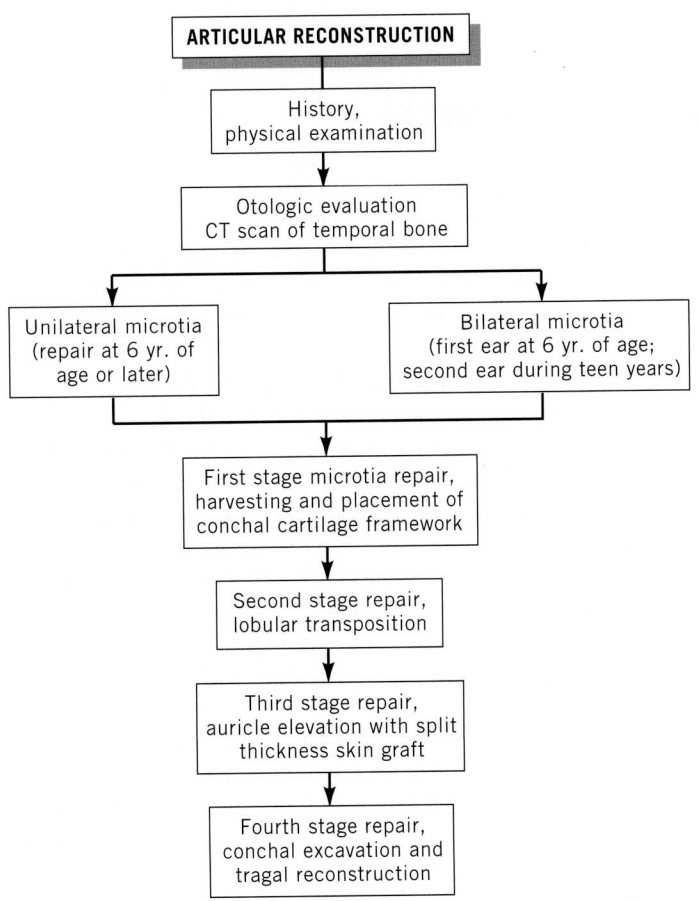

ARTICULAR RECONSTRUCTION

History,
physical examination

Otologic evaluation
CT scan of temporal bone

Unilateral microtia
(repair at 6 yr. of
age or later)

Bilateral microtia
(first ear at 6 yr. of age;
second ear during teen years)

First stage microtia repair,
harvesting and placement of
conchal cartilage framework

Second stage repair,
lobular transposition

Third stage repair,
auricle elevation with split
thickness skin graft

Fourth stage repair,
conchal excavation and
tragal reconstruction

HISTORICAL BACKGROUND

The creation of an external ear in the child with a congenital auricular deformity is both a challenging and rewarding experience. Over the years, many different methods and materials have been used in the repair of the microtic ear. These have included the fabrication and placement of external prostheses, the placement of auricular frameworks comprised of homograft cartilage (1) and various alloplasts (2,3), and staged reconstruction utilizing autologous cartilage grafts. The variation in approach and technique is indicative of the difficulty in achieving consistent, reproducible aesthetic results.

Historically, the search for the ideal material for an auricular framework has included use of irradiated homologous cartilage (1,4,5). This material tends to absorb over time, resulting in loss of size, shape, and definition of the created auricle. Various alloplastic materials, including solid silicone implants, have also been used for replacement of the auricle (6). Although these materials resist resorption, the potential for infection or extrusion is extremely high. The skin overlying any auricular framework is quite thin, and a firm alloplastic implant renders the reconstructed ear susceptible to even the slightest trauma.

Use of autogenous rib cartilage for creation of an auricular framework for microtia reconstruction was first described by Tanzer (7) in 1959. This staged technique has been refined and popularized by Brent (8–11). Auricular reconstruction results with this technique are reliable and relatively predictable, with minimal complications. Additionally, auricles reconstructed with autogenous cartilage can withstand the usual trauma of childhood (12,13). For these reasons, staged microtia repair with autogenous rib cartilage has become the gold standard against which other techniques should be compared.

🩺 PATIENT ASSESSMENT

The decision to perform microtia repair is a complex one. It requires consideration of developmental, medical, and psychological factors. Repair of this congenital deformity is best performed prior to the initiation of peer ridicule, but after sufficient growth of the thorax has occurred. Adequate rib growth is necessary to provide enough cartilage for the creation of an auricular framework. Additionally, the child must be generally aware of the problem and understand the surgical process to cooperate postoperatively. The exact timing of microtia repair should include (a) auricular growth, (b) size of the rib cage, (c) psychological needs of the patient, and (d) parental desires.

Growth of the external ear is usually 85% to 90% completed by age 6, and the rib cartilages are typically large enough to provide an adequate auricular framework by this age (14,15). If the normal ear is small and the child is large (rib cage), the first stage of the repair may be started by age 5. On the other hand, if the normal ear is large and the child small, auricular reconstruction is best delayed until after the age of 6. In any case, surgical construction of the microtic ear should not be started unless there is a strong communication between the family and surgeon, with attention to the psychological aspects by the surgeon, and an understanding of the staged nature of the surgery by the parents.

It is clear that the best results from microtia repair are usually from the first attempt, at a time when the native skin is previously unviolated. Thin skin drapes easily over the cartilaginous framework, allowing maximal visualization of auricular detail. If the skin of the ear has been violated by previous trauma or surgery, auricular detail is obscured, despite the creation of an anatomically correct cartilaginous framework. For these reasons, the family and child should be prepared to follow postoperative instructions carefully to avoid postoperative trauma.

Before initiating surgery, a detailed discussion should occur between the family and physician regarding the goals of surgery. Congenital microtia with external auditory canal atresia usually involves abnormality of the middle-ear space. Reconstruction of the external auditory canal, tympanic membrane, and ossicles is usually performed after all stages of auricular reconstruction are completed. Creation of an external canal usually requires soft tissue exposure and drilling of bone in the middle of the reconstructed auricle. If performed prior to, or during, auricular reconstruction, the canalplasty procedure usually compromises the appearance of the constructed auricle. The family should be made aware of the potential conflict between the functional canalplasty and ossicular reconstruction, and the staged auricular reconstruction procedures.

TABLE 1: **Stages of Auricular Reconstruction**

Stage	
1	Harvest, fabrication, and placement of auricular framework
2	Lobule transportation
3	Lateralization of the auricle (with split-thickness skin graft)
4	Tragal construction and conchal excavation

 TREATMENT RECOMMENDATIONS

Three to four stages are typically required for successful auricular reconstruction (16). (Table 1): (stage 1) harvest, fabrication, and placement of the auricular framework; (stage 2) lobule transposition; (stage 3) placement of a skin graft with creation of a postauricular sulcus; and (stage 4) tragal construction and conchal excavation. A minimum of 3 months between stages is required to allow swelling to subside and to increase vascularity to the overlying skin.

Preoperative Considerations

An individual's attractiveness is never defined by the beauty of their ears. However, a deformed or malpositioned auricle can detract from one's appearance. It is very important to keep these factors in mind when outlining surgical goals to the patient and family. Since most observers do not view both ears simultaneously, minor asymmetries of detail between the ears are often overlooked. However, gross differences in size or position of the two ears are easily noticed. It is therefore crucial to measure the size of the ear to be constructed carefully and to determine accurately the position and orientation of the auricular framework.

A detailed pattern of the opposite normal ear is traced on radiographic film. The pattern is then reversed to be used as an intraoperative template when harvesting and carving the auricular framework. The template is usually cut about 3 mm smaller than the outer dimensions of the normal ear to allow for the thickness of the skin overlying the ear. In cases of bilateral microtia, auricular size and template formation must be estimated from age-matched children. It is important in cases of bilateral microtia not to create too large a template, so as not to create too large an ear.

The position and orientation of the reconstructed ear is very important and should be determined preoperatively. This is accomplished in the surgeon's office by taping a reversed film pattern to the patient's head and tracing the outline of this pattern on the patient's head (Fig. 1).

The ear should be positioned approximately one full ear's length from the lateral canthus. A horizontal line (drawn parallel to the Frankfort horizontal) at the level of the lateral canthus should intersect the superior helical root. The anterior–posterior position of the newly constructed ear must often be modified in the patient with significant facial asymmetry (e.g., significant hemifacial microsomia) (17). If the microtic ear is associated with hemifacial microsomia, placement of the framework one ear's length from the lateral canthus will position the ear too far posteriorly. If the hairline only is used to position the new ear framework, the ear will be placed too anteriorly. In these cases, a compromise between these two positions should be used to determine the correct position for the auricular framework.

The orientation of the newly created ear is also very important. It is quite common for inexperienced surgeons to place the ear in too upright a position. The orientation of a normal ear is approximately 15° from vertical (Fig. 2). This can be approximated by halving the angle from vertical (0°) and that of the nasal dorsum (30° from upright).

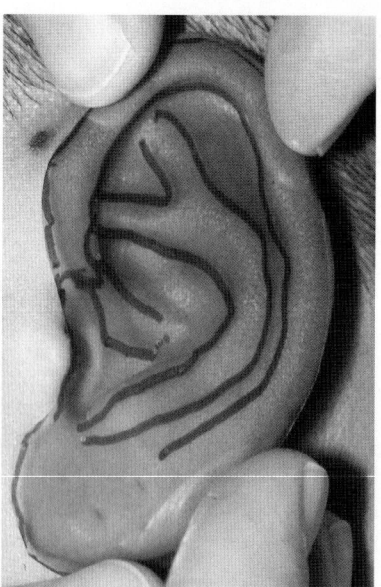

FIGURE 1 Establishment of the position and orientation of the reconstructed ear by tracing a pattern of the normal ear on radiographic film. Several of these templates are made to be used intraoperatively to determine the position and orientation of the ear and to determine the size of the costal cartilage to be harvested.

Proper position and orientation is crucial and should be determined and marked preoperatively.

Stage 1: Harvest, Sculpting, and Placement of the Auricular Framework

Preparation of the Skin Pocket

Prior to prepping and draping the patient, the position, size, and orientation of the auricle is checked and outlined over the microtic ear. It is important not to remove the outlined marking when prepping the patient, as the precise position and orientation of the auricular framework is a key factor in obtaining a good result. A sterile, clear plastic drape is used over the face to allow visualization of both sides of the head simultaneously.

Removal of the cartilaginous portion of the microtic remnant and dissection of the pocket is usually performed after harvest of the rib cartilage and sculpting of the auricular framework. This waiting period is used for vasoconstriction, as rib harvest and sculpting of the framework usually requires more than 2 hours. Prior to preparing the auricular pocket, a small amount of xylocaine 1% with epinephrine 1:100,000 is used for

FIGURE 2 Schematic diagram of the position and orientation of a normal ear, showing it approximately one full ear's length from the lateral canthus of the eye and 15° from a vertical orientation.

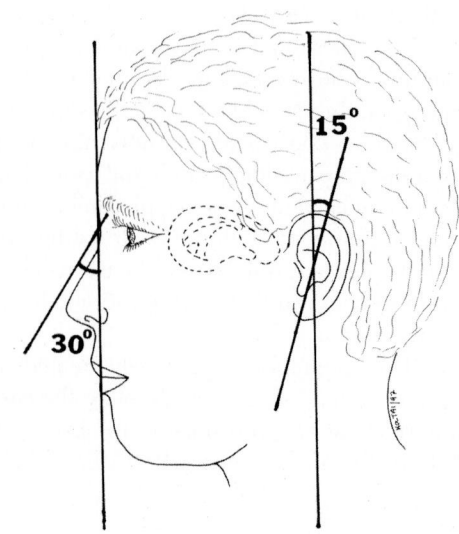

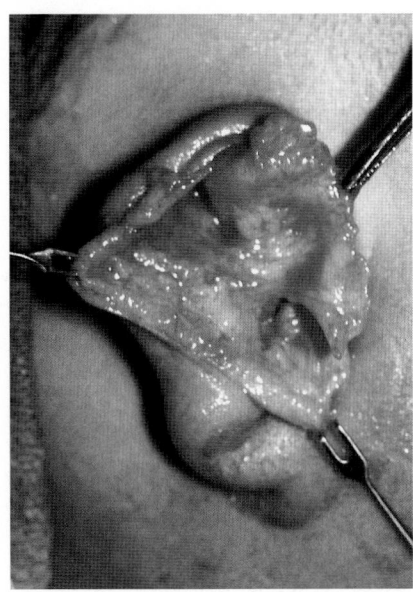

FIGURE 3 Intraoperative view of a microtic ear using an anterior incision to remove the auricular cartilage remnant completely.

vasoconstriction. An incision is made just anterior to the microtic remnant. This incision should be just large enough to allow placement of the carved auricular framework and removal of the existing cartilage remnant. The entire auricular cartilage is then removed (Fig. 3). However, the soft tissue of the microtic remnant is preserved for later reconstruction of the auricular lobule. Complete cartilage removal will enhance coaptation of the skin to the newly created auricular framework. Careful dissection of the pocket in the subdermal plane is then performed. The area dissected should extend slightly beyond the premarked outline to create sufficient skin laxity for skin redraping over the auricular framework (Fig. 4). The skin should then be thinned to allow maximal re-

FIGURE 4 Schematic diagram of the premarked dissection pocket for the auricular framework.

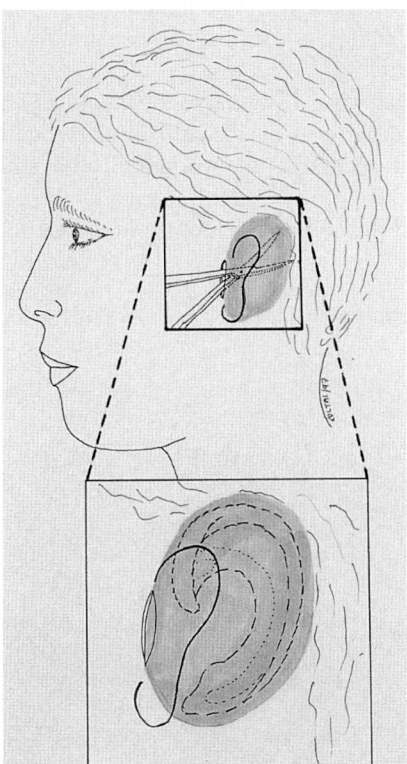

draping. In ears that have had prior surgery, increased skin thickness may prevent fine auricular definition.

Harvesting the Rib Cartilage

The configuration of the contralateral rib cage forms the most favorable material for auricular grafting (Fig. 5). The three-dimensional nature of the naturally shaped ear requires a multilevel framework. The floating, or mobile, rib is well suited to form the helix and helical root, while the synchondrosis of ribs 6 and 7 will form the framework body (superior and inferior crura, antihelix, and conchal bowl).

The floating rib is palpated, and an oblique incision is marked just superior to the costal margin. Vasoconstriction is obtained with infiltration of epinephrine 1:100,000. An oblique incision (measuring three-fourths the length of the costal margin) is made parallel and just inferior to the costal margin. The upper fibers of the rectus abdominus muscles are divided to expose the thorax, and a large self-retaining retractor is used for exposure. A precut separate sterilized film template (of the normal ear) is placed directly in the chest wound to determine the size and orientation of the cartilage to be harvested. Meticulous subperichondrial dissection is performed to separate the rib cartilages from the parietal pleura. Special care must be taken in the lateral intercostal spaces, where dense adherence of the pleura to the ribs may occur. If a small hole is made in the pleura, closure of the hole is performed with a purse string suture (4-0 braided synthetic suture) around a soft catheter. After the purse string suture is placed, the catheter is removed on forced mechanical (bagged) ventilation during expiration. Watertight closure may be checked by filling the wound with saline and looking for bubbles during deep inspiration. If these methods are used, postoperative pneumothorax is rare.

After subperiosteal dissection of the rib cartilages is completed, the floating rib (or ribs) and the synchondrotic portion of the graft are removed separately (Fig. 6). Care must be taken to remove the entire floating rib, as this portion is often deficient in length.

The chest wound is closed in layers with a 3-0 braided synthetic absorbable suture used for muscle and a 4-0 absorbable suture for dermal closure. A running intracuticular 5-0 monofilament suture is used for skin closure. A small soft passive drain is used in the subcutaneous tissues, and a tight pressure dressing is used for 48 hours.

Sculpting the Auricular Framework

A thorough knowledge of normal auricular anatomy is essential to the creation of a precise framework. Formation of the well-known patterns of normal convexities and concavities of the external ear are dependent on (a) accurate framework fabrication and (b) coaptation of the overlying skin. Precise creation of the auricular framework is based on a detailed knowledge of auricular anatomy and the ability to sculpt these shapes accurately.

FIGURE 5 Schematic diagram of the rib cage showing the area of synchondrosis for harvesting of the auricular framework body. Note the contralateral rib cage forms the most favorable configuration for the auricular framework.

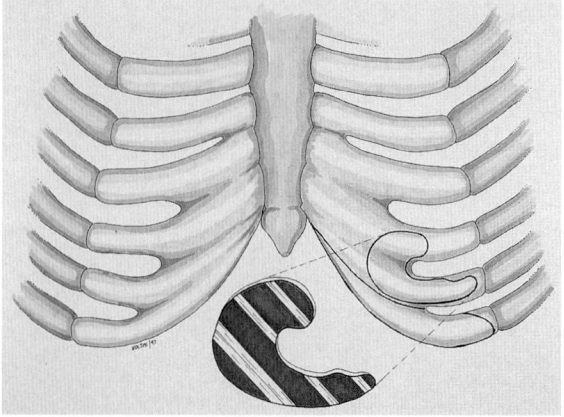

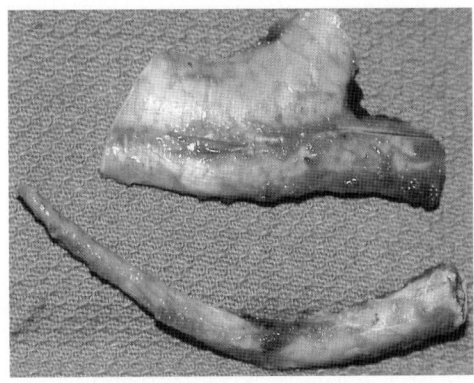

FIGURE 6 Typical appearance of the floating rib and synchondrotic portion of the sixth and seventh ribs prior to sculpting into an auricular framework.

Carving the auricular framework requires several #10 and #15 scalpel blades and sharp wood-carving tools. A set of wood-carving gouges can be purchased at any arts and crafts store and facilitates deepening of small areas, such as the triangular fossa, the scaphoid fossa, and the conchal bowl. The surgeon should hone his or her skills by practicing on a potato or an apple. In addition, observing an experienced microtia surgeon aids in developing a carving method.

The auricular framework body is first carved from the synchondrotic portion of the rib graft (Fig. 7A). The general size of the framework is first achieved by using a #10 scalpel blade (Fig. 7B). Further "gross" carving of the framework is accomplished with a #15 scalpel. The fine detail of the framework body is achieved by using curved and beveled gouges from the wood-carving set (Fig. 7C). Creation of maximal differential in heights between the framework and the carved areas will allow maximal definition of the constructed ear postoperatively. The original template (cut from radiographic film) is used as a guide to ensure that the contours are located in the proper position. Occasionally, a small piece of cartilage is sutured to the framework to augment a desired area.

After the framework body is sculpted, the helix is carved from the floating rib (Fig. 8). To create adequate flexion of the floating rib, this cartilage is carefully "thinned" using a #15 scalpel. Thinning of the floating rib is performed on the outer surface to facilitate bending in the opposite (inner) direction. The helix is then affixed to the framework

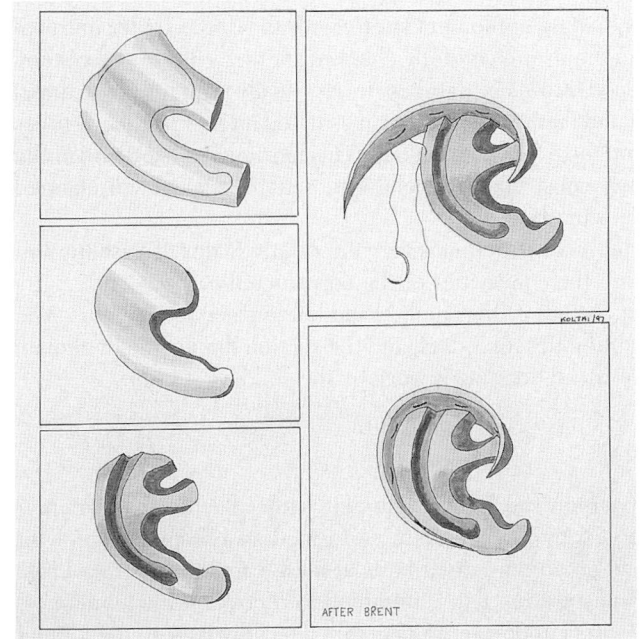

A
B
C
D
E

AFTER BRENT

FIGURE 7 A–C: Sculpting of the auricular framework body. **D, E:** After sculpting and thinning of the auricular helix from the floating rib, this is affixed to the framework body with 4-0 monofilament permanent sutures.

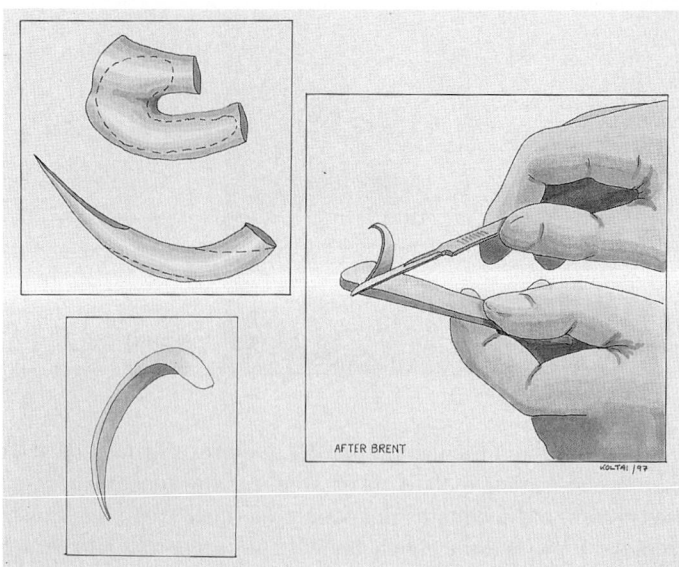

FIGURE 8 Thinning of the floating rib to create a curved appearance for the auricular helix.

body with 4–0 clear monofilament permanent suture (Fig. 7D and E). Several horizontal mattress sutures are used for stability, with the knots being buried on the undersurface of the cartilage framework. Projection of the helix (lateral to the framework body) should be maximized. Augmentation of the helix (to increase lateral projection) is sometimes necessary and requires an additional cartilage graft sutured onto the undersurface of the affixed floating rib.

Placement of the Framework

After the auricular framework is sculpted and stabilized with sutures, placement of the framework into the skin pocket is performed. Additional thinning of the skin is achieved just prior to framework placement. Two self-contained petite vacuum drains are placed to prevent hematoma formation and to facilitate coaptation of the skin pocket. The drains are placed prior to placement of the framework and sutured into position. The framework is then positioned into the skin pocket and digitally manipulated. If the skin pocket is too small, the graft is removed and the pocket dissection increased. The skin wound is then closed with 5–0 monofilament suture with the drains under maximal suction. After skin closure, the drains are carefully checked for any leaks in the system. The two suction drains are placed into vacuum tubes (tubes usually used for blood drawing) (Fig. 9). The nursing staff and family are carefully instructed on how to change tubes to maintain adequate suction on the overlying skin flap. This maximizes coaptation of the flap and definition of the newly constructed auricle. The patient is usually discharged from the hospital with the drains in place.

The dressing after auricular reconstruction is very important. Strips of Vaseline-impregnated gauze are placed into the concavities of the constructed ear (Fig. 10). A dry pressure dressing with fluff gauze pads is then applied and left in place for 48 hours. The patient is maintained on oral antibiotics for 7 days, and the suction drains usually remain in place for 5 days. A protective head dressing is worn by the child for 4 weeks.

Stage 2: Lobule Transposition

Although some surgeons reposition the lobule remnant while placing the auricular framework, lobule transposition is more accurately performed as a second stage. This procedure is usually performed on an outpatient basis at least 3 months after cartilage graft placement. A modified transposition flap is designed to reposition the lobule posteriorly and inferiorly (Fig. 11). It is important to maintain a healthy base to the lobular

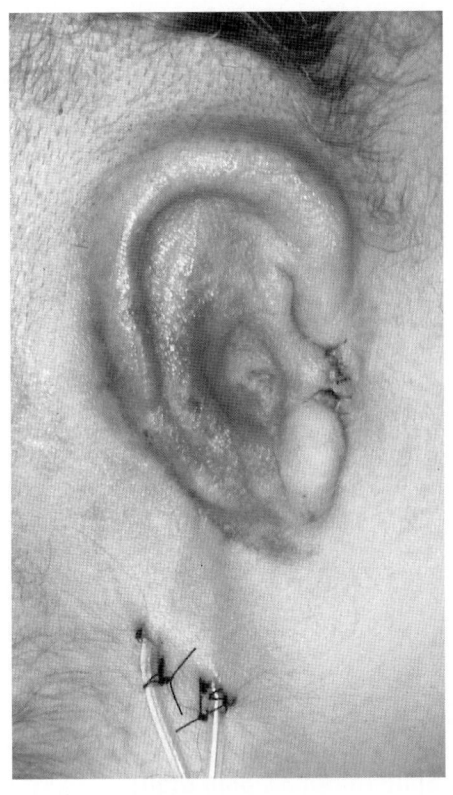

FIGURE 9 Intraoperative appearance after placement of two suction drains and the auricular framework. Note that the lobule is malpositioned at this time.

transposition flap to ensure adequate vascularity of the flap. Dissection under the inferior aspect of the cartilage graft is accomplished with slight elevation of the graft. The lobule remnant is then fileted with a portion of this soft tissue being placed deep to the cartilage graft (Figs. 12 and 13). This creates bulk and support in this area of transition and prevents depression of the scar. If soft tissue support of this transition zone (between the framework and the native lobule) is not adequate, an unsightly depression is formed (Fig. 14). The subcutaneous soft tissues are sutured into position with 4–0 braided synthetic absorbable suture. Skin closure is accomplished with interrupted 5–0 monofilament sutures.

FIGURE 10 Placement of a conforming dressing into the crevices of the newly created auricular framework.

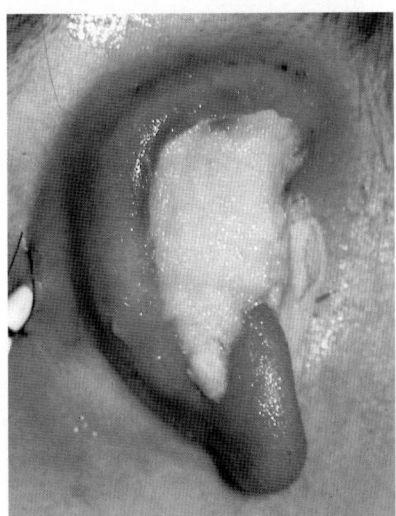

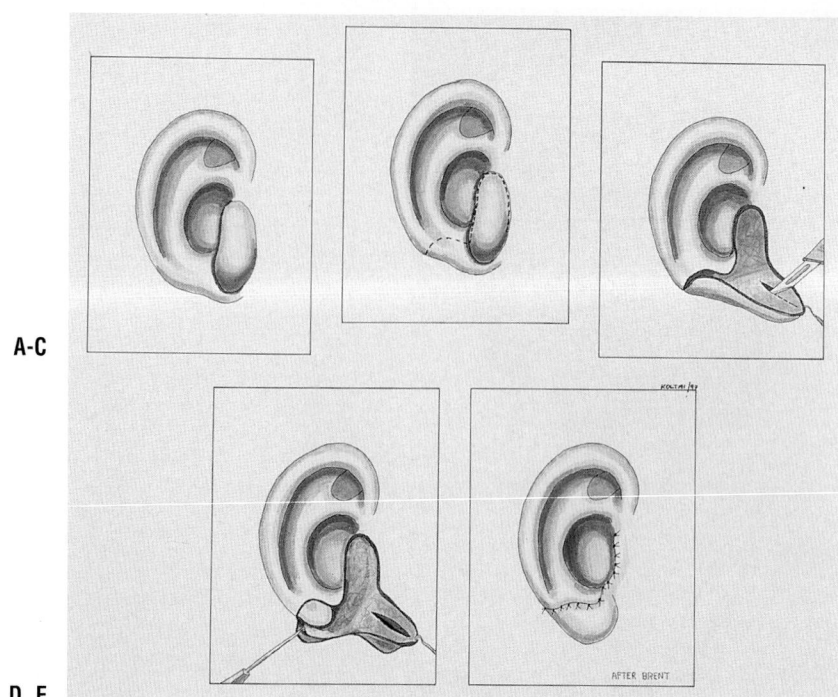

A-C

D, E

FIGURE 11 A–E: Schematic diagram of transposition of the lobule with fileting of the lobule.

Stage 3: Lateralization of the Auricle (with Split-Thickness Skin Graft)

Although the overall size, shape, and configuration of the constructed ear is determined after the first two reconstructive stages, the ear usually lacks sufficient lateral projection at this point. This lack of projection occurs because the three-dimensional cartilage framework is placed into a two-dimensional skin-soft tissue pocket. To increase the auriculocephalic angle and create a postauricular sulcus, significant mobilization of the graft and placement of a postaruicular skin graft is performed. Again, this procedure is performed at least 3 months after lobule transposition (or 6 months after placement of the original auricular framework).

A generous incision is made at the posterior margin of the graft from the superior helix to the lobule inferiorly (Fig. 15A). The graft is then dissected entirely from the head, leaving a layer of soft tissue on the posterior surface of the graft (Fig. 15B). The

FIGURE 12 Intraoperative view with fileting of the lobule and creation of a transposition flap.

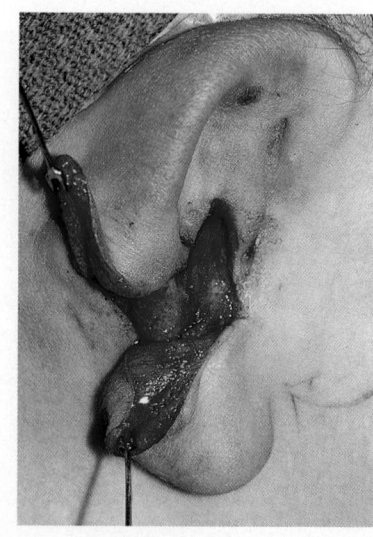

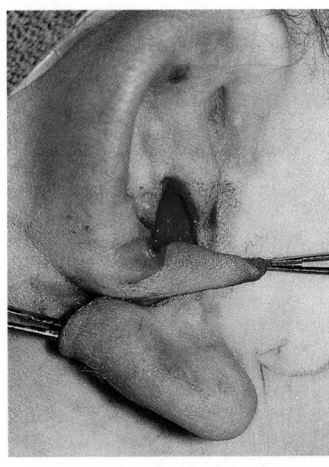

FIGURE 13 Intraoperative photograph of transposition of the lobular remnant.

skin overlying the mastoid is then undermined and advanced anteriorly (Fig. 15C). At this point, a split-thickness skin graft (approximately 15/1,000 inch thick) is harvested from the upper, outer thigh. The skin graft is then sutured onto the posterior aspect of the auricular framework (Fig. 15D). It is important to resurface the postauricular (mastoid) bone with skin advanced from the retroauricular scalp, rather than with harvested skin graft. The postauricular skin is undermined, advanced, and sutured into position with 3–0 braided synthetic absorbable suture. This will deepen the sulcus, project the ear, and prevent tethering of the reconstructed ear. A retroauricular bolster is placed (to define the sulcus) for 7 days (Fig. 15E).

Stage 4: Conchal Excavation and Tragal Reconstruction

After completion of the first three stages of microtia repair, the correct size, shape, orientation, and projection of the ear are obtained. At this point, many patients are satisfied and request no further surgical procedures. In motivated patients, however, a fourth stage can be performed that improves the definition and contour of the anterior ear.

A composite chondrocutaneous graft is harvested from the symba concha of the opposite ear using a curved incision on the anterior surface of the ear. A J-shaped incision is made in the conchal bowl of the reconstructed ear, and the bowl is deepened by defatting the soft tissue from the conchal floor. The same curved J-shaped incision is used to both deepen the conchal bowl and to insert the composite graft for tragal reconstruction. The excavated concha is resurfaced with a small full-thickness skin graft from the

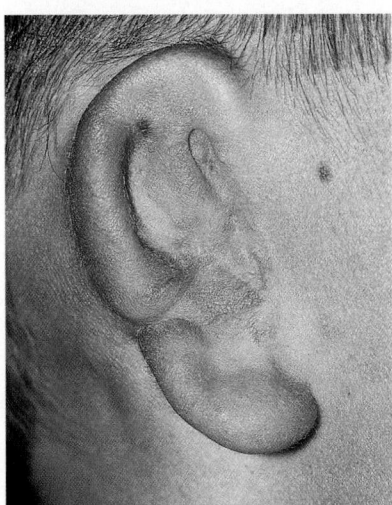

FIGURE 14 Postoperative view after lobular transposition showing good position of the lobule but lack of soft tissue fullness in the area of the suture line. This creates an unsightly depression in the region of transposition.

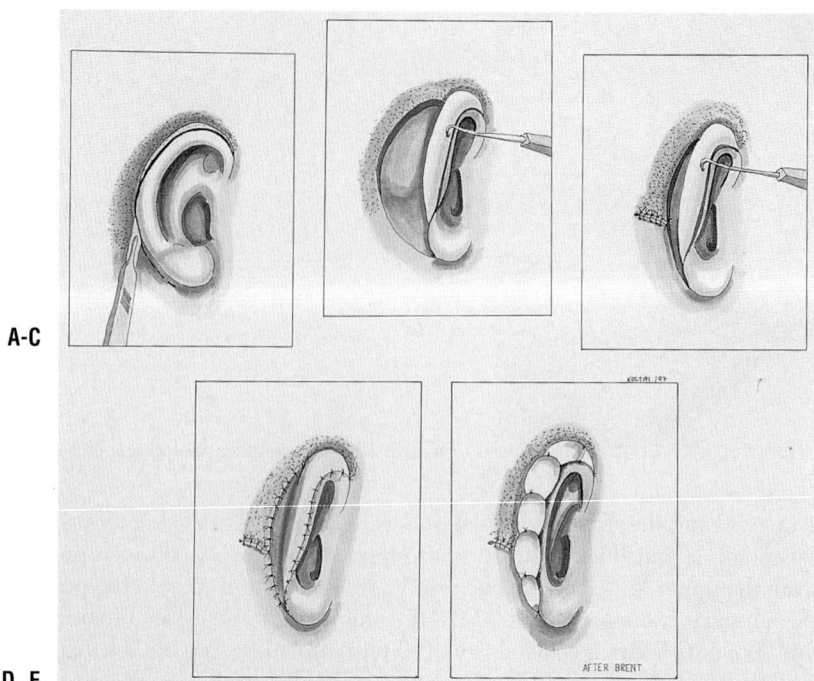

FIGURE 15 A–E: Schematic diagrams showing lateralization of the auricle with advancement of postauricular skin and placement of a split-thickness skin graft on the posterior aspect of the auricle. A bolster is then placed to ensure immobility of the graft.

opposite lobule, and the tragus is reconstructed with the composite graft from the opposite symba concha. Vaseline-impregnated gauze is placed in the canal and on the conchal floor, and a pressure dressing is placed for 5 days.

Secondary Auricular Reconstruction

In many instances, the native skin envelope will not be of sufficient amount or quality to support a successful microtia repair. Lack of sufficient skin may result from prior trauma to the auricular skin, or from a prior failed attempt at microtia repair. Failed auricular reconstruction is usually caused by infection, hematoma, or extrusion of an alloplast or auricular autograft. In any case, the overlying skin covering is crucial to the final reconstruction, and poor vascularity of the skin significantly compromises the result (Fig. 16).

FIGURE 16 Example of a poor result from an auricular reconstruction. Poor vascularity and thickness of the overlying skin prevented sufficient auricular detail.

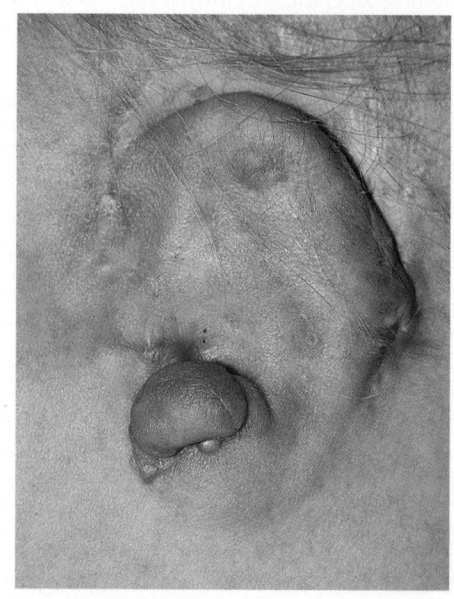

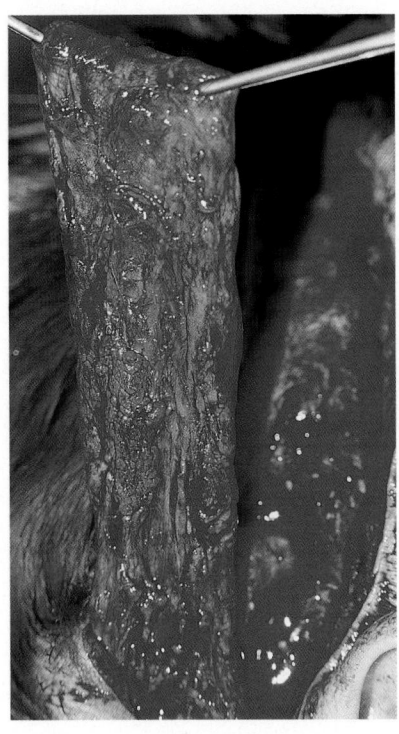

FIGURE 17 Intraoperative photograph of an elevated temporoparietal fascia flap prior to transposition.

In cases with insufficient skin covering, elevation of a pedicled temporoparietal fascia flap (TPFF) can be used to cover the auricular framework graft (18). The TPFF is a thin, well-vascularized transposition flap proximate to the operative field (19) (Fig. 17). It has a hearty blood supply that serves as a rich bed to support a split-thickness skin graft.

The temporoparietal fascia (TPF) is located in the temporal region deep to the subcutaneous tissue and superficial to the deep temporal fascia. It is supplied by the superficial temporal artery (one of the two terminal branches of the external carotid artery) and vein. Other important structures that travel within the TPF include the auriculotemporal nerve and the frontal branch of the facial nerve. The TPF is an extension of the superficial musculoaponeurotic system fascia of the lower face and is continuous with the galea aponeurosis of the forehead and scalp. The TPF is densely adherent to the overlying skin but loosely connected to the underlying deep temporal fascia by loose areolar tissue between the fascial layers. This areolar tissue allows the TPF to slide on the deeper fascial layers.

Elevation of the Temporoparietal Fascia Flap

When performing secondary auricular reconstruction, a TPFF is outlined large enough to drape over the entire auricular framework. After removal of the poorly vascularized skin and auricular remnant, a hemicoronal scalp incision is made superficially into the subcutaneous tissue of the scalp. It is important that the surgeon not violate the TPFF, which is located superficially. Sharp elevation of the skin and subcutaneous tissue is accomplished using a #10 scalpel in a meticulous fashion. This densely adherent plane is unnatural, and the dissection is time consuming.

After skin elevation, the vascular TPF layer can be visualized. A rectangular TPFF is then outlined and marked. Care must be taken not to transect the frontal branch of the facial nerve with the anterior limb of the TPFF. The location of this nerve should be marked on the patient to avoid transection. The course of the frontal branch can be outlined by drawing a line between the external auditory canal and a point 2 cm above the lateral eyebrow. If the anterior limb of the outlined TPFF is posterior to the course of the frontal branch of the facial nerve, injury to the nerve will be avoided.

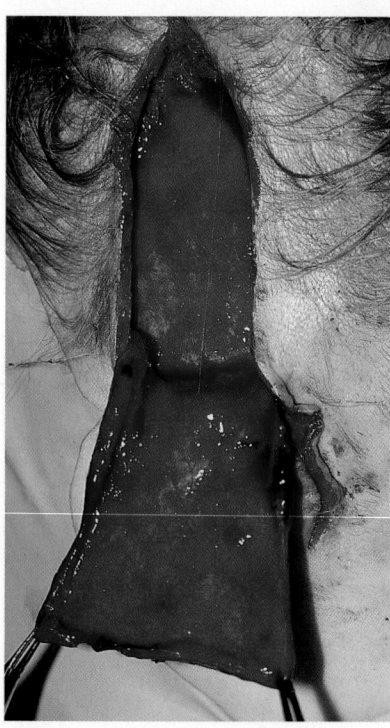

FIGURE 18 Transposition of a temporoparietal fascia flap in a secondary auricular reconstruction.

Dissection of the flap off the deep temporal fascia is easily accomplished in a blunt fashion. Transposition of this flap is performed by turning the flap 180° inferiorly, after the new auricular framework graft is secured in position with periosteal fixation sutures (4–0 monofilament absorbable sutures) (Fig. 18). The TPFF/auricular framework sandwich is then covered with a split-thickness skin graft (Fig. 19). Dressings and drains are performed as with primary microtia repair. Dressings are kept in place for 48 hours, and drains are usually left in for 4 to 5 days.

MANAGEMENT OF COMPLICATIONS

Complications after auricular reconstruction include hematoma, infection, graft exposure and extrusion, and skin breakdown (Table 2). In each of these situations, compli-

FIGURE 19 Intraoperative view of a secondary auricular reconstruction after transposition and attachment of a temporoparietal fascia flap (TPFF). The new auricular framework has been positioned underneath the TPFF and is awaiting placement of a split-thickness skin graft.

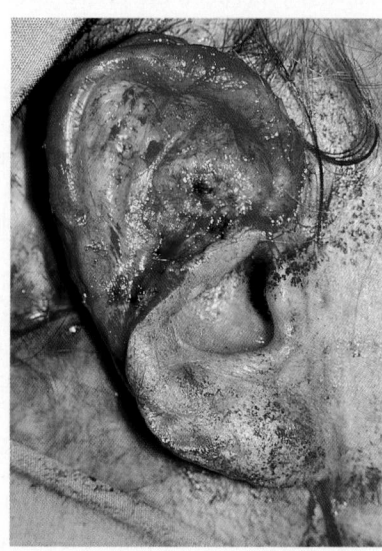

TABLE 2: Complications of Microtia Repair

Site of constructed auricle
   Infection
   Hematoma
   Graft exposure
   Graft extrusion

Rib harvest
   Infection
   Hematoma
   Pneumothorax

Temporoparietal fascia flap
   Injury to frontal branch cranial nerve VII

cations usually contribute to poor vascularity of the overlying skin and compromise detail of the constructed auricle. Loss of definition usually requires revision surgery and recruitment of vascularized tissue for coverage of a new auricular framework.

Other complications from harvest of the rib cartilage include hematoma, infection, and pneumothorax. Although small tears in the pleura are common during rib harvest, pneumothorax is uncommon if these are repaired in the manner outlined. Complications from elevation and transposition of TPFFs include injury to the frontal branch of the facial nerve.

SUMMARY

Reconstruction of congenital auricular deformities is a challenging task. Experience has shown that microtia reconstruction is best accomplished with staged procedures utilizing a carved autologous rib framework. The size, position, and orientation of the sculpted autologous graft and the vascularity and pliability of the overlying skin determine the appearance of the constructed auricle. Alloplasts are generally not used due to an increased rate of infection, extrusion, and susceptibility to trauma. In cases of failed microtia repair, revision surgery is performed with pedicled temporoparietal fascial transposition flaps and split-thickness skin grafts. With strict adherence to learned principles of microtia reconstruction, complications are rare and results very acceptable.

⚙ REFERENCES

1. Musgrave RH. The impracticality of preserved cartilage homografts in reconstructing the microtic ear. In: *Transactions of the Third International Congress on Plastic Surgery*, 1963:454.
2. Cronin TD. Use of a Silastic frame for total and subtotal reconstruction of the external ear: preliminary report. *Plast Reconstr Surg* 1966;37:399.
3. Cronin TD. Use of a Silastic frame for construction of the auricle. In: Tanzer RC, Edgerton, MT, eds. *Symposium on reconstruction of the auricle*. St. Louis: CV Mosby, 1974.
4. Limberg AA Jr. Late results of homotransplantation with chopped cartilage. *Acta Chir Plast (Prague)* 1962;4:59.
5. Steffenson WH. Comments on reconstruction of the external ear. *Plast Reconstr Surg* 1955;16:194.
6. Tanzer RC. Discussion of Silastic framework complications. In Tanzer RC, Edgerton MT, eds. *Symposium on reconstruction of the auricle*. St. Louis: CV Mosby, 1974:87–88.
7. Tanzer RC. Total reconstruction of the external ear. *Plast Reconstr Surg* 1959;23:1.
8. Brent B. Ear reconstruction with an expansile framework of autogenous rib cartilage. *Plast Reconstr Surg* 1974;53:619.
9. Brent B. The correction of microtia with autogenous cartilage grafts. I. The classic deformity. *Plast Reconstr Surg* 1980;66:1.

10. Brent B. The correction of microtia with autogenous cartilage grafts. II. Atypical and complex deformities. *Plast Reconstr Surg* 1980;66:13.
11. Brent B. Reconstruction of the microtic ear with autogenous rib cartilage. In: Jackson IT, ed. *Recent advances in plastic surgery,* 2nd ed. New York: Churchill Livingstone, 1981.
12. Tanzer RC. An analysis of ear reconstruction. *Plast Reconstr Surg* 1963;31:16.
13. Brent B. Auricular repair with autogenous rib cartilage grafts: two decades of experience with 600 cases. *Plast Reconstr Surg* 1992;90:355.
14. Farkas LG. Growth of normal and reconstructed auricles. In: Tanzer RC, Edgerton MT, eds. *Symposium on reconstruction of the auricle.* St. Louis: CV Mosby, 1974.
15. Farkas LG. *Anthropometry of the head and face,* 2nd ed. New York: Raven Press, 1994.
16. Bardach J. Reconstruction of the microtic auricle in a fourstage operation. *Otorhinolaryngology* 1974;78:349.
17. Lauritzen C, Munro IR, Ross RB. Classification and treatment of hemifacial micorsomia. *Scand J Plast Reconstr Surg* 1985;19:33.
18. Edgerton MT, Bacchetta CA. Principles in the use and salvage of implants in ear reconstruction. In: Tanzer RC, Edgerton MT, eds. *Symposium on reconstruction of the auricle.* St. Louis: CV Mosby, 1974.
19. Cheney ML. Free flaps; fascial and fasciocutaneous flaps. Temporoparietal fascia. In: *Atlas of regional and free flaps for head and neck reconstruction,* vol. 14. New York: Raven Press, 1995:197–211.

J. M. Sykes: Department of Otolaryngology—Head and Neck Surgery, University of California, Davis Medical Center, Sacramento, California 95817.

- *Practical Pediatric Otolaryngology*
- edited by Robin T. Cotton
  and Charles M. Myer, III
- Lippincott-Raven Publishers,
  Philadelphia © 1999

54

Otoplasty

Vito C. Quatela & Mark A. Clymer

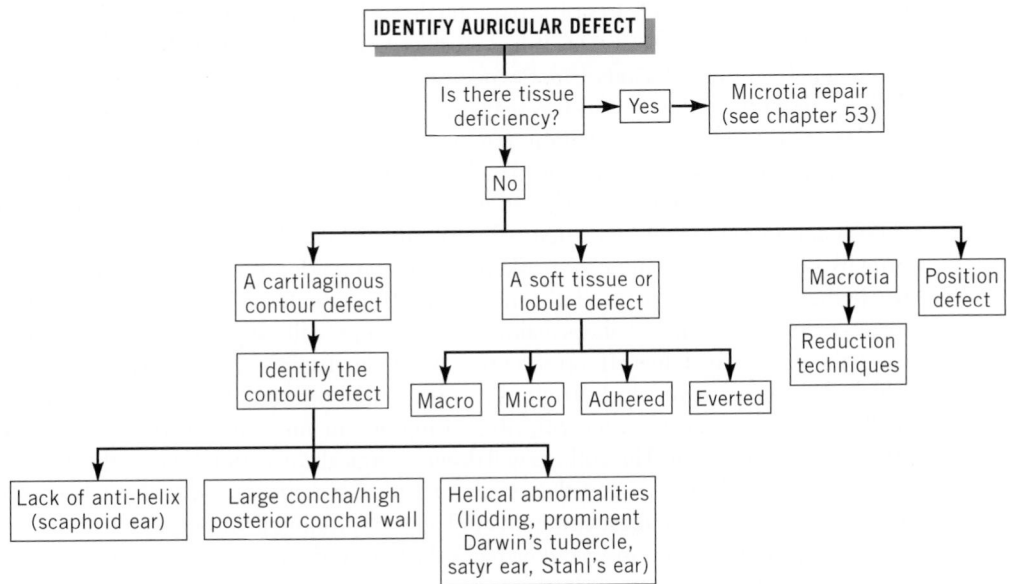

The human auricle is one of the most architecturally intricate facial features. Many variations in size, shape, and configuration exist, and each may fall within the realm of "normal." However, obvious malformations exist that fall outside these bounds. One may assess an ear subjectively, noting the shape, configuration, size, and relationship to other facial features to determine if it appears "normal." Anthropomorphic measurements, as described by Farkas (1), help to identify those aspects of an auricle that make it appear malformed and thereby guide surgical correction. Attempts to define appropriate surgical approaches further have led to the development of a variety of classification schemes. These are summarized well by Aguilar (2). Among the different systems Aguilar cites, Weerda's classification (3) divides auricular deformities into first-, second-, and third-degree dysplasia. First-degree dysplasia is defined as an ear with mostly normal architecture, whose reconstruction does not require the use of additional skin or cartilage. These abnormalities include macrotia, protruding ears, cryptotia, absence of the upper helix, small deformities such as absent tragus, satyr ear, Stahl's ear, prominent Darwin's tubercle, colobomata, lobule abnormalities, and cup ear deformities. Second- and third-degree dysplasia are more severe deformities that require reconstruction by addition of cartilage, skin, or both. Reconstructions of second- and third-degree deformities are better addressed in a discussion of microtia repair (which is covered in Chapter 53). The focus will be on otoplasty on those ears that are misshapen or malpositioned, or have contour irregularities, and would be classified by Weerda as first-degree dysplasia. These deformities primarily consist of outstanding or protuberant ears.

Auricular form varies considerably between individuals, with mild degrees of deformity found relatively frequently. Gender differences for prominent ears vary according to the reference. Adamson et al. (4) noted an equal male to female ratio, whereas Goode and Profitt (5) reported a 4:1 male to female ratio. This finding supports a presumed autosomal dominant mode of inheritance for protuberant ears (5).

Correction of this deformity can be gratifying for the surgeon, patient, and family members. It is indicated to avoid adverse psychosocial effects on the child's development. Prior to age 7 to 9, criticism and ridicule do not impact the child significantly. Thereafter, the effects of peer ridicule may adversely affect the child's self-confidence, self-image, and sense of self-worth. Consultation is often sought by parents when the child complains of teasing and name calling at school. It is important to assess both the child's and parents' motivation for improvement in the appearance of the auricular abnormality. Surgical alteration of the auricle in a child who is neither concerned nor criticized by playmates merely to satisfy parental desires for improvement are not in the best interest of the patient. However, it is a mistake to assume that the child who does not complain about the deformity is not concerned. The child may fear expressing negative feelings about the deformity, as this may expose an uncomfortable vulnerability (6).

We will discuss the evaluation and treatment of auricular deformities involving shape, size, contour, and protrusion. To plan surgical correction of prominent ears, a decision tree is useful. This allows the surgeon to identify the abnormality correctly and to choose appropriate techniques that will give an aesthetically pleasing final result. The primary distinction that must be made prior to intervention for auricular abnormalities is whether an absolute tissue deficiency exists. If adequate tissue is present, but lacks form or possesses contour abnormalities, the surgeon will employ techniques that address the particular defect. If, on the other hand, an absolute tissue deficiency exists in which there is a greater than 20-mm size differential between the normal ear and the malformed ear, reconstruction with rib grafting in a manner similar to microtia reconstruction is undertaken. The authors will discuss surgical correction for ears that have adequate tissue present. As noted above, microtia reconstruction is covered in Chapter 53. The focus will be on the most common etiologies of prominent auricles, lack of the antihelical fold, and a high posterior conchal wall. Before discussion of techniques, a brief historical overview and a more in-depth discussion of patient evaluation are warranted.

HISTORICAL BACKGROUND

Surgical alteration of the auricle dates back to the 10th century writings of Sushruta and the 16th century writings of Tagliacozzi (7). However, the first to receive credit for treatment of the protruding ear was Ely in 1881 (8). He made an incision through the anterior skin, cartilage, and posterior skin and excised a crescent-shaped piece of cartilage "measuring 1⅛ in. by ⅓ in." and a piece of skin that was "considerably larger than this" to correct a prominent ear (8). In 1896, Jacques Joseph, considered by many the father of rhinoplasty, performed his first plastic surgical procedure, a reduction otoplasty. He excised skin from the postauricular sulcus for setback and a wedge excision for size reduction on a 10-year-old boy (9). In 1903, Gersuny (10) published an article on correction of an outstanding ear using conchal mastoid sutures. This technique was again proposed and used by Furnas in 1968 (11). Luckett (12) in 1910 is credited for identification of the primary defect in a prominent ear, the lack of the antihelical fold. He used cartilage excision techniques to correct this. He excised a strip of cartilage along the antihelix and fixed the new antihelical fold with mattress sutures. This gave correction of the antihelical fold but left an operated look, with a sharp edge of cartilage along the new antihelical fold. Subsequent attempts to correct this operated look gave rise to incisional and suture techniques (12). Becker (13) and Converse et al. (14) were among the first to address the sharp, operated look of the prior excisional techniques. They combined incisional techniques, both anterior and posterior, with suture fixation to give a more smooth and natural look to the antihelical fold.

The evolution of otoplasty from excisional techniques to incisional was carried further to purely suture fixation by Mustardé in 1963 (15). This is one of the most commonly employed techniques today. Further attempts at even less invasive techniques have been proposed by Fritsch (16), who reported a series of otoplasty cases corrected with mattress sutures placed transcutaneously, without a skin incision, that he refers to as "incisionless otoplasty."

Overall, the trend has been from excision of skin and cartilage to incision and shaping to suture fixation. Surgeons today continue to use a variety of these techniques to achieve an aesthetically pleasing result in otoplasty. The authors' preferred techniques are reshaping with Mustardé type mattress sutures combined with concha–mastoid setback, avoiding cartilage resection or skin removal, except in highly select cases. These techniques will be outlined below.

To individualize a treatment plan and choose an otoplastic technique, one must first assess the patient and identify and analyze the deformity. This requires knowledge of the embryology and anatomic landmarks of the auricle. With this fundamental understanding, one can determine the goals of correction and the timing of repair and then implement techniques to achieve these goals.

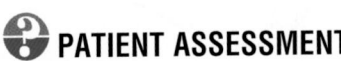

PATIENT ASSESSMENT

Embryology

To understand the final auricular architecture, one needs to understand the embryologic events that lead up to the final appearance of the ear. His first described the embryologic development of the auricle in 1885. Six hillocks of His, or tuberosities, may be seen on the lateral aspect of the 39-day-old embryo; these arise along the margins of the first branchial groove and are produced by proliferation of mesenchyme from the first and second branchial arches. The first branchial arch gives rise to hillocks 1, 2, and 3. The second branchial arch gives rise to hillocks 4, 5, and 6. The auricle develops in the upper part of the future neck region, and as the mandible develops, the auricles move to the side of the head. With subsequent growth, they ascend to the level of the eyes. As growth occurs, the contribution of the first branchial arch, i.e., hillocks 1, 2, and 3, becomes relatively reduced. The last part of the auricle to develop is the lobule. Figure 1 shows the hillocks in the embryo and their corresponding locations in the fully formed ear (17).

Abnormalities in development may occur with each of the hillocks and with varying degrees. This gives rise to a myriad of potential auricular deformities. Davis (18) has correlated some of the more common abnormal hillock development patterns with clinical appearance. Davis organizes his discussion of hillock abnormalities based on the timing of maturation of the auricular structures. Therefore, he begins with hillock 3, as this is where the first branchial groove begins closing at the upper cephalic end of the embryo. Abnormal closure here will lead to malformed superior–anterior helices. This may range from a mild form with absent anterior helix to the classical "lop" ear with its lack of superior crus of the antihelix and the shortened scapha. Irregular fusion of hillocks 3 and 4 may lead to an irregular border of the superior aspect of the helix with a cleft, much the same as in formation of a cleft lip. Davis refers to this as a "3-4 ear cleft." Malformations of hillock 4 alone give rise to abnormally shaped helical domes and adjacent scapha. Mild degrees of malformation lead to absence of the upper helix, a flattened scapha or scaphoid ear, or absence of the scapha, as shown in Fig. 2A. More severe malformations result in loss of scapha and sharp angulation of the superior helix, giving rise to a satyr ear, as shown in Fig. 2B. Abnormal fusion of hillocks 4 and 5 leads to a prominent Darwin's tubercle. This results from poor fusion of hillocks 4 and 5, giving rise to an angu-

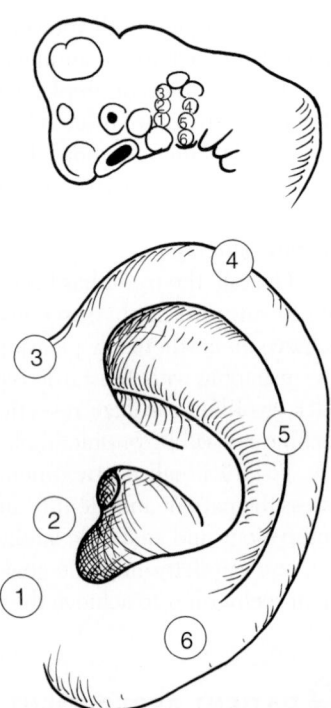

FIGURE 1 The hillocks of His in the embryo. These arise from the first and second branchial arches. Their corresponding locations in the fully developed auricle are shown.

lated posterior–superior helical rim (Fig. 3). A more severe malformation than Darwin's tubercle is the "4-5 ear cleft," in which there is discontinuity of the helical rim with severe angulation of the posterior aspect of the rim, similar to that seen with the "3-4 cleft." Radial folds may be seen coursing across the scapha from the antihelix to the helical rim at the location of Darwin's tubercle, which is referred to as "Stahl's ear." Hillock 5 forms the descending helix, antitragus, and part of the concha. Malformations range from lack of the inferior scapha to absence of the posterior middle third of the ear and concha, leading to the "mini ear." Abnormalities of fusion of hillocks 5 and 6 result in abnormal fusion in the region of the inferior helix, antitragus, and lobule. This may lead to a cleft appearance, the "5-6 ear cleft." Hillock 6 is responsible for lobule development, and subsequently, lack of this hillock leads to congenital absence of the lobule. Abnormal fusion of hillocks 6 and 1 leads to congenital bifid lobule, as shown in Fig. 4. Tragal and inferior helical root abnormalities are the result of fusion abnormalities of hillocks 6 and 1, as well

FIGURE 2 A: Mild degrees of hillock 4 maldevelopment result in absence of the scapha, as shown here. **B:** Abnormal development of the posterior hillock 4 can give rise to flattening of the scapha or, when more severe, will result in development of a satyr ear, as shown here.

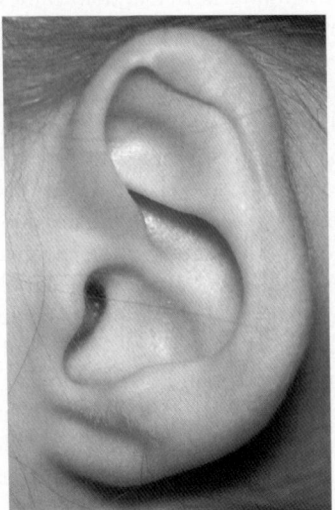

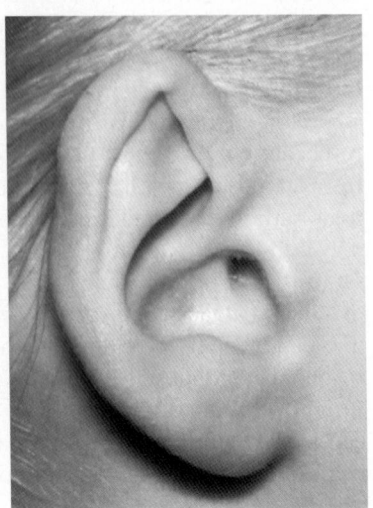

A   B

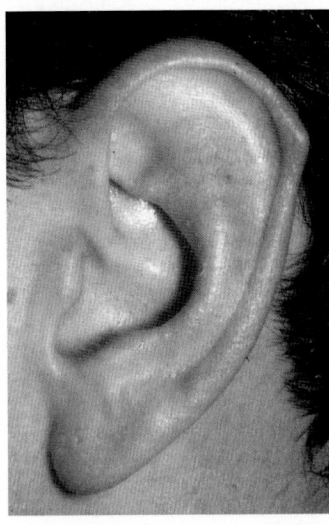

FIGURE 3 A prominent Darwin's tubercle, resulting from incomplete fusion of hillocks 4 and 5.

as hillocks 1 and 2. Hypergenesis of hillock 2 leads to preauricular tags and polyotia (cartilage containing supranumary ear appendages) anterior to the helical root and tragal area.

Maldevelopment of hillocks 2, 3, 4, and 5 leads to classic microtia. There may also be combinations of other abnormalities that lead to varying degrees of agenesis. Various nomenclatures have been assigned to these deformities, such as canoe ear, snail shell ear, peanut ear, and others. These are more severe types of auricular maldevelopment and should be considered degrees of microtia. They should be reconstructed with techniques used for microtia reconstruction as these add tissue to the auricle.

In addition to understanding the embryologic events involved in development of the auricle, the otoplastic surgeon must understand the maturation and development of the auricle after birth. At birth, ear size is the same in boys and girls, but growth rates differ as the children age (19). Adamson et al. state (20) that 85% of the auricular growth occurs in both sexes by age 3. According to Maniglia and Maniglia (21), cartilaginous growth of the ear is nearly complete by age 5 or 6. Farkas (22) quantifies this by stating that the ear reaches 85% of its adult size by age 6, 90% by age 9, and 95% by age 14. The width of the ear and its distance from the scalp also change only minimally after age 10 (23). Therefore, timing of surgery is usually between ages 5 and 10. This allows the ear to reach nearly its adult size, and correction may be performed before the stigmata of peer ridicule negatively impact the child.

FIGURE 4 Abnormal development of hillock 6 gives rise to the congenital bifid lobule. Incidentally, this patient also has a port wine stain involving the auricle.

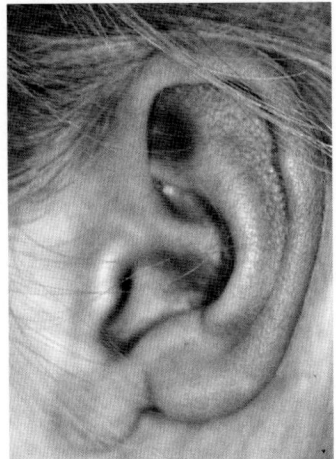

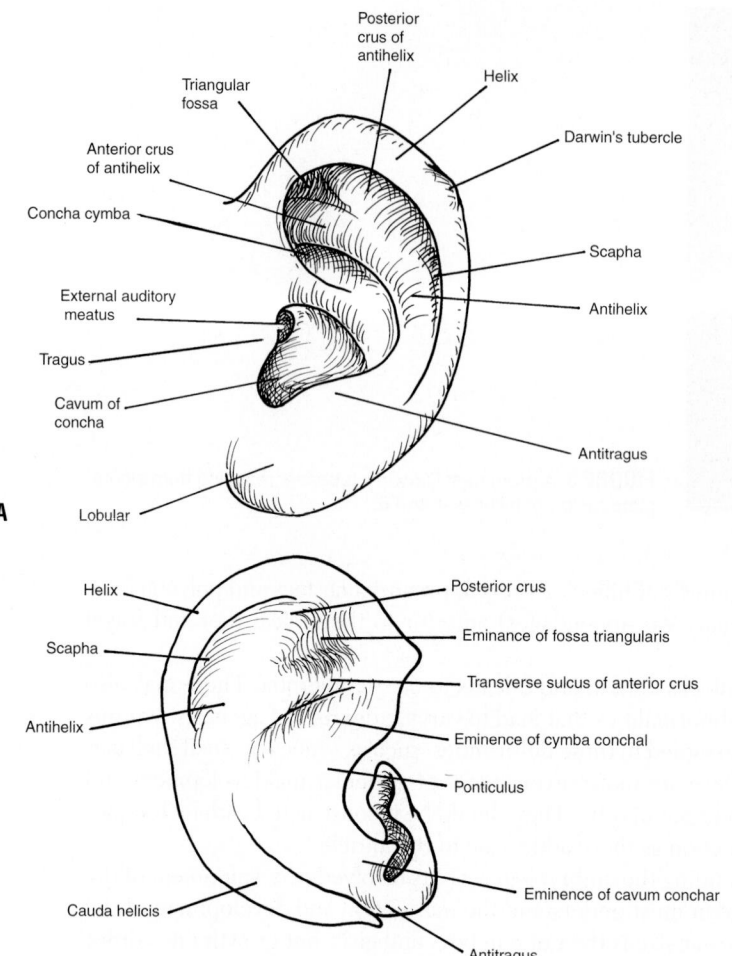

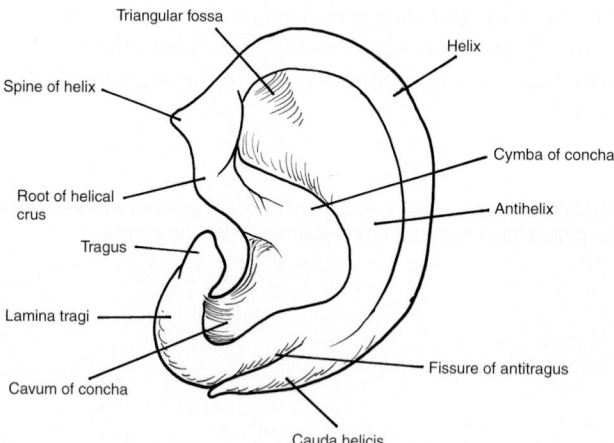

FIGURE 5 **A:** The surface anatomic landmarks of the auricle. **B:** Cartilaginous framework of the auricle.

Anatomy

Understanding normal anatomy and architecture of the auricle is paramount if one is to restore a malformed ear to a more visually pleasing state. External landmarks of importance include the helical crus, the helical rim, the scaphoid fossa, the antihelix, the triangular fossa, Darwin's tubercle, the tragus, antitragus, and the lobule. These are shown in Fig. 5A. The corresponding anatomic structures of the underlying cartilaginous framework that gives the ear its unique shape are shown in Fig. 5B.

The relationship of size, position, and prominence of these landmarks compared with one another gives the ear its characteristic shape. Farkas (24) has described reference points that may be used to measure these relationships (Fig. 5C). These are useful landmarks to standardize pre- and postoperative measurements and to analyze the differing sizes, shapes, and positions of various auricles. These are the landmarks by which a normal range may be defined. Farkas has studied facial relationships in an attempt to characterize average measurements in certain control populations (25–27). He defines as normal those measurements that are greater than two standard deviations above or below the mean for a particular ethnic control group. These measurements help guide the surgeon in both assessment of the degree of malformation and surgical correction. The width of the ear (preaurale to postaurale) for boys 6 years of age is reported to be 34 mm, and at 18 years of age 36 mm. Girls at age 6 have an ear width of 34 mm, which remains the same on average at age 18 (34 mm). The auricular length (supraaurale to subaurale) for boys age 6 is 55 mm, and at age 18 increases to 62 mm. Girls also show ear elongation from an average of 54 mm at age 6 to 58 mm at age 18. The ear index may be used to compare patient populations or pre- and postoperative measurements for an individual patient. The ear index is equal to the ear width multiplied by 100, divided by the ear length (ear index = ear width × 100/ear length).

The relationship of the auricle to the head, eyes, mandible, and nose is also of utmost importance. The angle between the posterior skin of the ear and the mastoid is generally less than 30° or an absolute distance of less than 20 to 25 mm (28). The incline of the ear is the angle between the medial longitudinal axis of the ear and the vertical plane. The artistic rule of thumb is that this incline is parallel to the incline of the dorsum of the nose. However, Farkas et al. (26) have shown the ear incline to be slightly more vertical

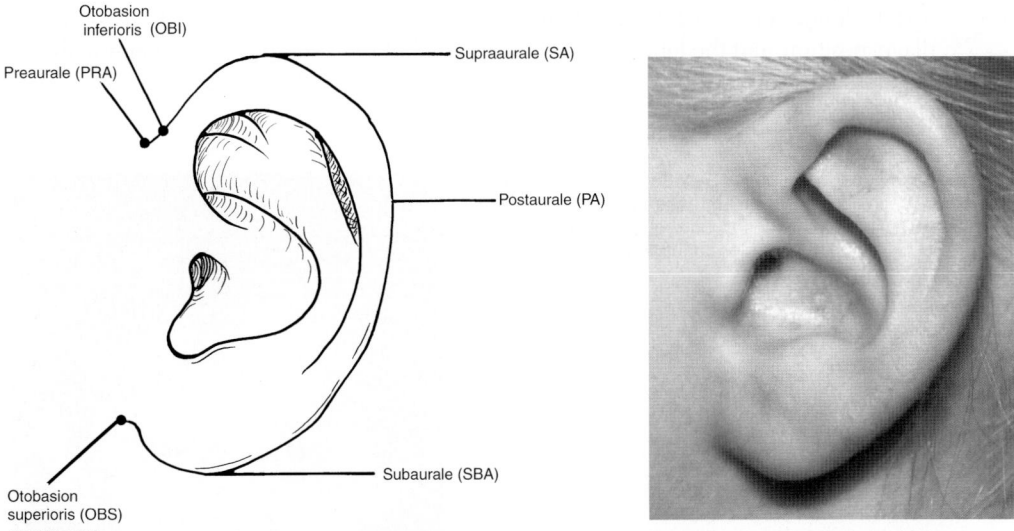

FIGURE 5 *Continued.* **C,D:** Reference points used in measuring auricular size, shape, and location with respect to other facial features: supraaurale (SA), the highest point of the free helical periphery; subaurale (SBA), the lowest point of the free lobular border; length of the auricle, SA to SBA distance; preaurale (PRA), the most anterior point of the ear, located just in front of the helical rim attachment to the head; postaurale (PA), the most posterior point of the free helical periphery; otobasion superius (OBS), the attachment point of the helix in the temporal area; otobasion inferius (OBI), the attachment point of the lobe to the cheek.

than the axis of the nose in 91% of the population. In boys, the mean angle of inclination is 21° from the vertical, with girls having a mean inclination of 20° (1). The distance from the lateral canthus to the helical crus determines the anterior–posterior position of the auricle. This should be approximately equal to the length of the ear (supraaurale to subaurale distance), or roughly 69 mm.

These measurements serve as a guideline for the surgeon in determining the degree of surgical correction needed for each patient. Understanding these anatomic relationships arms the otoplastic surgeon with the knowledge necessary to identify individual auricular deformities correctly, which will, in turn, help plan appropriate surgical correction.

Deformity Identification

Understanding the embryologic development and anatomy of the mature auricle gives the otoplastic surgeon the ability to identify correctly the various auricular anomalies encountered and therefore plan treatment. The decision tree outlines this process. The first question one must ask is, "Is there an absolute tissue deficiency?" If the ear has classic microtia the answer to this question is relatively straightforward. Milder degrees of microtia are more difficult to assess. If the contralateral ear is of normal size, the affected ear must be smaller by 20 mm or more for the difference to be perceptible. If there is greater than a 20 mm difference in size between the two ears, the affected ear suffers from an absolute tissue deficiency that is great enough to require reconstruction in a manner similar to that of classic microtia. If both ears are malformed, the absolute size of each must be considered, guided by the proportions reported by Farkas (25–27). Each ear must be addressed individually, as one ear may require techniques similar to those required for microtia, and the contralateral ear may require otoplastic techniques for protrusion, excessive height of the conchal bowl, or other contour irregularities. The boy in Fig. 6 demonstrates this situation. His left ear lacks a sufficient antihelical fold, and the posterior conchal bowl is excessive. The right ear is significantly smaller and shows not only prominence of the conchal bowl, but superior lidding. This ear will require tissue addition to correct this deformity; the left ear will be addressed with Mustardé sutures and concha–mastoid setback (Fig. 6).

Ears that do not suffer from an absolute tissue deficiency have defects in contour, position, lobule size, and/or shape or an excess amount of cartilage and are addressed with techniques that differ from those used in microtia repair. Defects of excessive cartilage, position, and the lobule will be addressed, but the focus will be on contour abnormalities, as these are the most common defects encountered.

FIGURE 6 Patient with a greater than 20% size discrepancy between the two ears. The smaller ear will require tissue addition techniques, similar to those used in classic microtia; the larger ear is best addressed using techniques to correct protrusion that results from the lack of an antihelical fold and a high posterior conchal bowl.

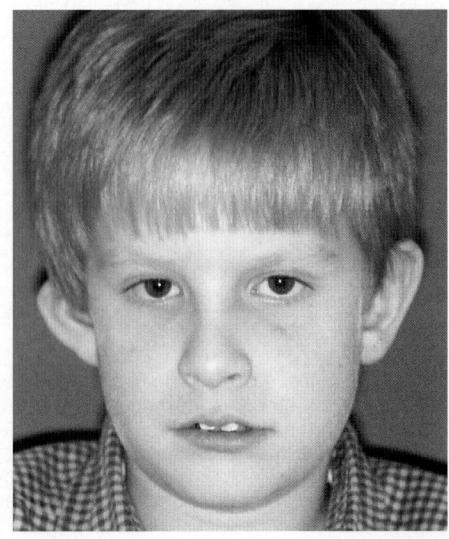

Excessively large ears may be reduced in a variety of ways, ranging from full-thickness wedge excisions to resection of portions of the scapha. A more difficult situation to correct is that of a malpositioned ear. The location of the external ear canal and the size and shape of the mandible, maxilla, and cranium play roles in this problem. The mandible and maxilla may be altered, but the position of the external ear canal and the size and shape of the cranium are variables the surgeon has little ability to change. Therefore, the best alternative in these cases is often to reconstruct the most aesthetically pleasing ear located in its present position. Lobule defects include excessive tissue (macrolobule), insufficient tissue (microlobule), bifid lobules, everted or adhered lobules, or absent lobules. Davis (29) gives an excellent discussion of surgical correction of these deformities, and his work is recommended for review.

Contour defects include the two most common auricular defects, lack of the antihelical fold and a high posterior wall of the conchal bowl, as well as less common abnormalities described earlier. Surgical correction of these defects has evolved from primarily an excisional approach, to an incisional approach, to suture techniques combined when indicated with alteration of the conchal bowl. The authors' preferred technique for correction of prominent ears is the suture technique described by Mustardé (15) combined with conchal bowl setback in selected cases. This technique will be discussed and illustrated with a case representative of the most commonly encountered defect: the lack of an antihelical fold and a prominent posterior conchal wall.

PEARLS AND PERILS

1. Note the size discrepancy between ears.
2. Keep in mind the anatomic relationships to other facial structures (e.g., brow, nasal dorsum, mandible).
3. Identify the defect as one of size, contour, position, protrusion, or a combination thereof.
4. Individualize the treatment approach based on the anatomic defect.

TREATMENT RECOMMENDATIONS

Photo Documentation

After the initial consultation with the child and parents, a treatment plan is formulated based on the decision tree described above. Prior to implementing this plan, photo documentation of the child's auricles is obtained. Full facial views are obtained with a magnification of 1:10 for all patients. These include frontal, right and left oblique, and right and left lateral views, as well as a posterior view with the child facing away from the camera. It is important to place the hair in an elastic band to keep it from obscuring the view of the relationship of the auricle to the side of the head. Closeup views of each auricle are obtained to show contour and shape irregularities better. A frontal view at a magnification of 1:4 is obtained to include the eyes and ears. All photographs are taken with attention to keeping the Frankfort horizontal plane parallel with the floor.

Anesthesia

Otoplasty may be performed under local anesthetic with sedation or a general anesthetic. In adult patients, the authors' method of choice is local, with sedation. However, in the pediatric population commonly undergoing these procedures, a general anesthetic is often preferred. Communication and collaboration with anesthesia colleagues in determining which method is preferable for a particular patient allow individualization of the anesthetic.

Surgical Technique

This discussion will focus on the more commonly encountered deformities, the lack of an antihelix and a prominent conchal bowl. Lobule techniques will also be addressed.

Following induction of either a general or sedation anesthetic, the patient's ears are prepped with Betadine solution. Both ears are left exposed in all cases, even those undergoing unilateral otoplasty. A clear drape with a central circular opening is placed over the ear on each side. These two drapes are then rolled together in the midline and a hemostat used to secure them to one another. This technique is modified when sedation is used, so as to leave the airway exposed. Draping in this fashion allows visualization of the child's face during the procedure, as well as intraoperative comparison between each side. Preoperative measurements are taken at three points along the auricle: the supraaurale (upper pole), the postaurale (middle third), and the subaurale (lobule). A ruler is held gently against the scalp and the lateral aspect of the auricle at the positions described above, and measurements are recorded for intraoperative reference and inclusion in the operative note. Accuracy is imperative to achieving an excellent result, which may be ensured by obtaining measurements at a preoperative appointment or at the beginning of the procedure and *prior* to injection of local anesthetic.

Once measurements are complete, local anesthetic is injected into the postauricular incision site and over the mastoid cortex. Care is taken to avoid instilling excessive local anesthetic as this may distort the auriculocephalic angle or scaphal architecture. The next step is to determine the proper suture placement. One technique to determine placement of the Mustardé sutures is to place 30-gauge needles transcutaneously through the auricle. The authors prefer to substitute 5-0 silk suture for the 30-gauge needles. A 5-0 silk suture is passed through the skin on the lateral aspect of the ear, through the underlying cartilage, continuing subcutaneously deep to the skin of the medial side of the ear, and returning through the cartilage and skin of the lateral aspect of the ear. The entrance point and exit points through the skin and underlying cartilage correspond to the position in the cartilage where the subcutaneous nylon (Mustardé) sutures will be placed. Four to five silk sutures are usually placed, each approximately 1 cm apart. One silk suture is placed for each nylon suture necessary to correct the protuberant ear and reestablish the antihelical fold (Fig. 7).

The postauricular incision is then made in a curvilinear fashion on the posterior aspect of the auricle. Care is taken to incise only the skin; then, using small tenotomy scissors, the subcutaneous tissue is dissected with a spreading motion. This allows identification of the underlying silk suture without cutting it (Fig. 8). Once the silk suture is identified, careful scissor dissection is then performed to the level of the helical rim and posteriorly over the soft tissue covering the mastoid (Fig. 9). Elevation of the postauricular skin in this fashion allows the surgeon to visualize the cartilaginous framework both

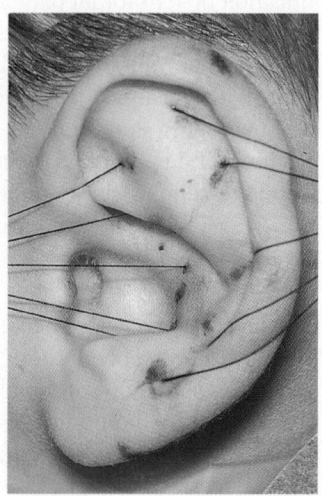

FIGURE 7 Placement of silk marking sutures. These travel in the subcutaneous plane on the posterior side of the auricle. Each silk suture corresponds to the location of a nylon (Mustardé) suture that will be placed via the postauricular approach.

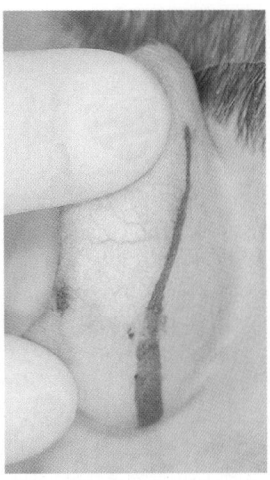
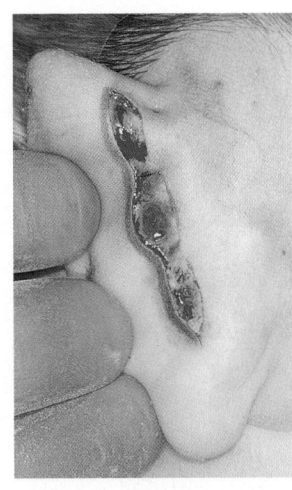
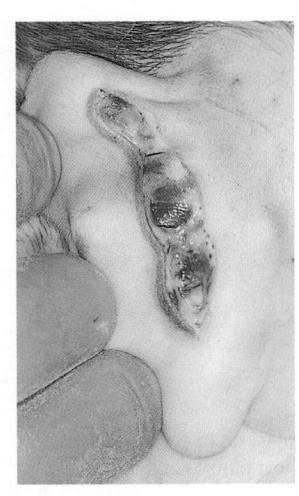

A-C

FIGURE 8 **A:** Planned incision. **B:** Incision made through skin but not through the silk sutures. **C:** After spreading technique with scissors to expose silk marking sutures.

medial and lateral to the scapha. This will facilitate accurate placement of the Mustardé sutures. It also allows visualization of the soft tissue between the conchal bowl and the mastoid cortex.

With exposure of the 5-0 silk marking sutures accomplished, 4-0 clear nylon Mustardé sutures are placed. The nylon suture is passed from the posterior aspect of the auricle, through the cartilage at the entrance point of the silk marking suture. The needle is directed in a subcutaneous plane underneath the lateral skin of the auricle and exits the cartilage on the posterior surface of the auricle. Prior to delivering the needle from the substance of the cartilage, the lateral aspect of the ear is inspected to ensure subcutaneous placement of the nylon suture. The needle is then delivered from the cartilage. The nylon suture is then placed at the exit point of the same silk suture in the fashion described above. This horizontal mattress suture is tightened to inspect the degree of bending of the antihelix. If it is satisfactory, a hemostat is placed and the identical sequence of steps is repeated for each silk suture. When all nylon sutures have been placed, the silk sutures are removed, and the nylon sutures are tied down, beginning superiorly and proceeding inferiorly. The antihelical fold is recreated and contoured precisely by controlling the tension placed on each of the Mustardé sutures (Fig. 10B).

In highly selected cases in which the cartilage resists remolding with Mustardé sutures alone, the authors will perform cartilage scoring. A #15 blade is used to incise the cartilage from the postauricular incision. Two parallel incisions are made, essentially creating a bipedicled cartilage strut. The incision is not carried through the lateral auricular

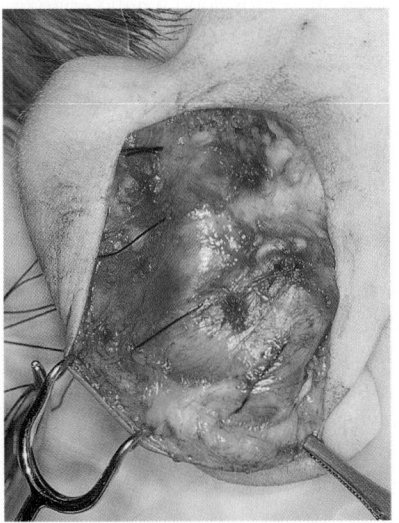

FIGURE 9 Scissor dissection is performed to the helical rim and over the mastoid soft tissue. This allows visualization of the antihelix for placement of Mustardé sutures, as well as exposure of the soft tissue overlying the mastoid for removal in the concha–mastoid setback procedure.

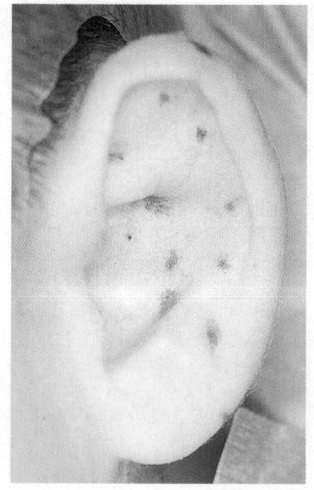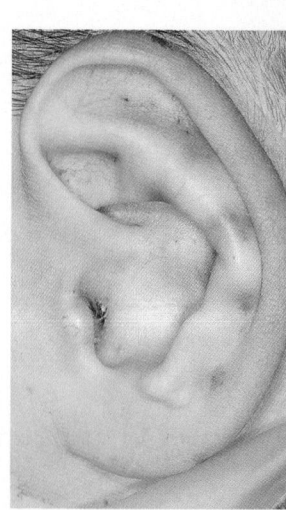

A   B

FIGURE 10 **A:** Auricular shape prior to tightening the Mustardé sutures. **B:** Recreation of the antihelical fold after Mustardé sutures are tied down.

skin. The cartilage strut between the incision lines is then weakened by grasping with Adson-Brown forceps and partially morselizing the cartilage to release the inherent spring. The Mustardé sutures are then tightened as described above.

Having recreated the antihelical fold, concha–mastoid setback is now performed (if indicated by preoperative analysis). Working through the same postauricular incision, the subcutaneous soft tissue and muscle that overlie the mastoid periosteum are removed with scissors. This resection is taken anteriorly to the spine of Henle, but no further. Resection of tissue more anteriorly would weaken the junction of the external auditory canal with the mastoid and result in forward displacement of the posterior cartilaginous canal. This leads to a buckling of the cartilage and a decrease in the cross-sectional diameter of the opening of the external auditory canal.

After resection of the concha–mastoid soft tissue, 4–0 clear nylon is used to set back the conchal bowl. The suture is passed through the conchal bowl cartilage (again taking care to ensure the subcutaneous placement by inspecting the lateral aspect of the conchal bowl) and then through the mastoid periosteum. Two sutures are generally placed, and the more lateral on the bowl these are placed, the greater the setback. However, care must be taken not to place them too far laterally, as this can lead to forward displacement of the conchal bowl and narrowing of the external auditory canal.

Hemostasis is achieved throughout the case with bipolar cautery, and at the conclusion of the case the wound is irrigated with Lincocin antibiotic solution prior to closure. The incision is closed with a running 5–0 nylon suture. Rarely do the authors find a need for skin excision. There is often skin redundancy, which allows for good wound edge eversion; this slightly raised incision line resolves spontaneously during the postoperative period. Measurements are repeated at the end of the procedure and are included with the preoperative measurements in the operative note. Antibiotic ointment is placed over the incision, and a light mastoid pressure dressing is applied. The authors do not use any transauricular bolster sutures.

Postoperative Care

The mastoid dressing is removed the following morning. The ear is inspected for any hematoma formation. Attention must be paid to the newly created antihelical fold, as the skin here is generally tight, and skin perfusion is inspected for any areas of decreased viability. The patient and parents are instructed in the use of a soft headband that is worn continuously for the first 7 postoperative days. Following this, the headband is worn only at night for the next 6 weeks. Sutures are removed on postoperative day 5, and Steri-strips are applied for another 4 to 5 days. The results of this technique are shown in Fig. 11.

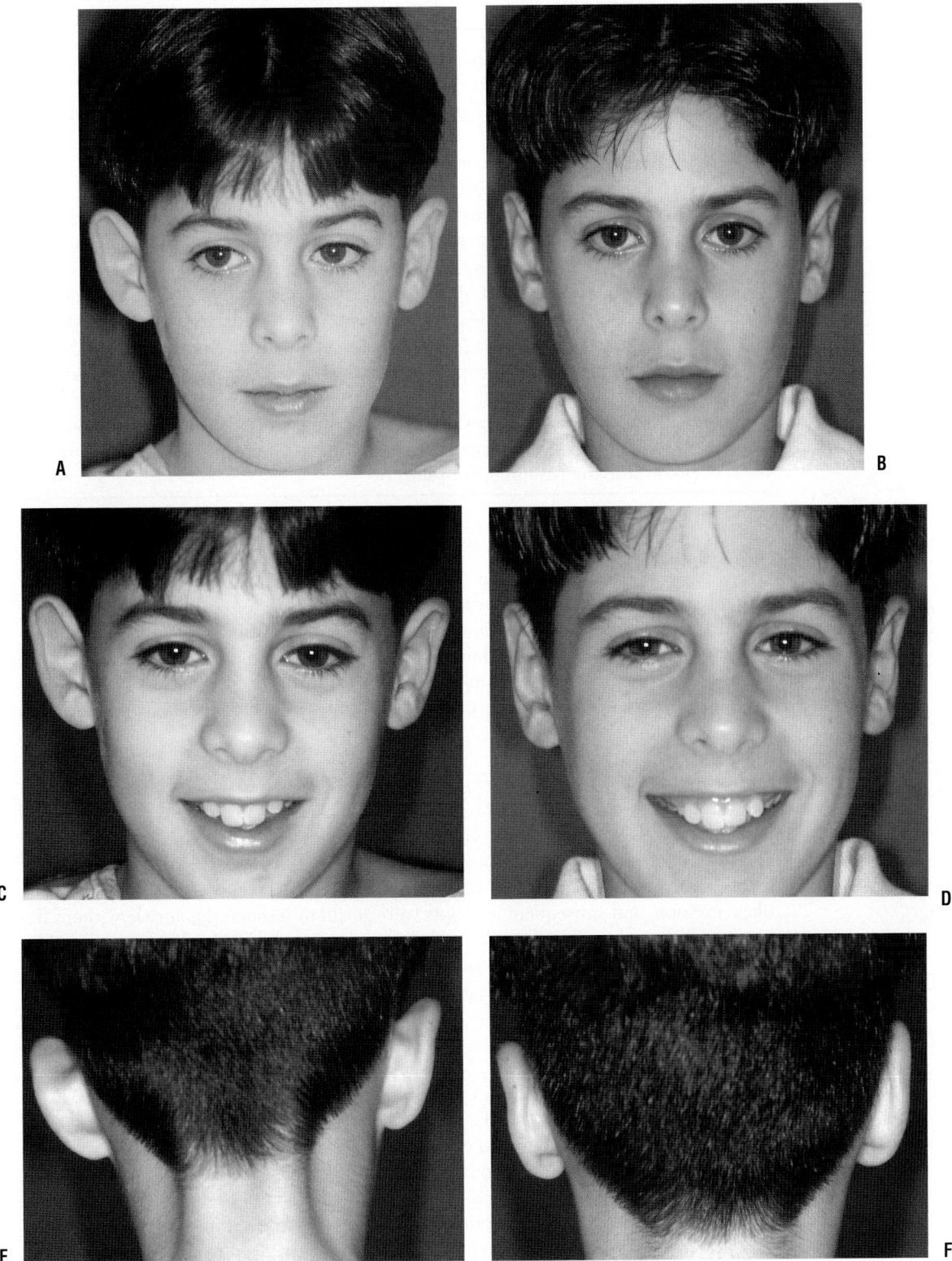

FIGURE 11 Pre- and postoperative views of a youngster with protruberant ears. The postoperative result showing correction of the absent antihelical fold and reduction in conchal bowl prominence. **A:** Preoperative frontal view. **B:** Postoperative frontal view. **C:** Preoperative close-up. **D:** Postoperative close-up. **E:** Preoperative posterior view. **F:** Postoperative posterior view.

> **PEARLS AND PERILS**
>
> 1. Take measurements at the superior pole, middle pole, and lobule *prior* to injection of local anesthetic.
> 2. The use of silk marking sutures facilitates accuracy and ease of placement of the Mustardé sutures.
> 3. Cartilage sparing techniques are used—no cartilage incision or excision or skin excision is routinely performed.
> 4. Do not remove concha–mastoid soft tissue anterior to the junction of the external auditory canal and the conchal bowl, as this leads to narrowing of the meatus of the external auditory canal.
> 5. Inspect the lateral aspect of the ear after placement of the 4–0 clear nylon needle to ensure its subcutaneous placement. Once confirmed, the needle may be delivered from the cartilage. If it is transcutaneous, the needle may be backed out and replaced. This helps prevent cartilage weakening and tearing with repeated suture placement.
> 6. Care must be taken in performing these procedures during winter months in cold climates, as the postoperative numbness associated with the procedure may predispose the patient to frostbite.

Other Methods

A number of methods have been reported in the literature for correction of the various auricular deformities. The evolution of otoplasty has been from cartilage excision, to incisional techniques, to suture techniques. Combinations of these techniques have been employed as well. Some of the many techniques for cartilage excision and cartilage incision and scoring will be discussed briefly, and the authors will note the recently reported "incisionless" otoplasty technique.

Cartilage Excision

Cartilage excision techniques were among the first used in otoplasty. Davis and Kitlowski (30) used excision, incision, and shaving techniques to create the antihelix. Farrior (31) described a method of excising wedges of cartilage to break the spring and thereby recontour the auricle. These techniques often left irregular contours at the edges of cartilage excision, and subsequent attempts were made to reshape the auricle without the resultant sharp edges that gave an unnatural "operated" look. This led to the development of incisional and sculpting techniques. This did not, as will be discussed below, solve the problem of sharp cartilage contours and an unnatural postoperative appearance.

Cartilage Incision/Scoring

Cartilage incisional techniques were reported by Converse et al. (14) in 1955. He used parallel incisions along the planned antihelical fold combined with wire brush thinning and sutures in an attempt to create a rounded antihelical contour and avoid the sharp edge associated with excisional techniques. The concept of cartilage scoring was based on work by Gibson and Davis (32), who showed that removal of perichondrium in rib cartilage released the tension provided by the elastic fibers immediately beneath the perichondrium. By removal of the perichondrium, the cartilage would bend toward the side that still had a perichondrial layer (32). This principle was utilized by Stenstrom (33), Chongchet (34), and others (35). Stenstrom (33) used a postauricular approach and created an anterior tunnel along the planned antihelix. He then scored the perichondrium and cartilage to release the antihelical region and allow it to bend posteriorly, recreating the antihelical fold. Chongchet (34) used a transcartilaginous incision to approach the anterior antihelical region and then scored the cartilage and perichondrium with parallel incisions. This technique was modified by Nolst Trenite (36). He performed more shallow anterior incisions and placed posterior mattress sutures to allow more controlled bending of the antihelix.

Incisionless Otoplasty

"Incisionless otoplasty" is a term used by Fritsch (16) in his description of a suture technique for otoplasty. This is similar to the Mustardé otoplasty, but the sutures are placed transcutaneously. As the suture is passed back through the cartilage to form the figure-of-eight stitch, the needle is passed beside the exit of the suture so as not to bury epithelium. He advocates this approach and cites histologic analysis supporting the lack of epithelial inclusion that could result if proper stitch placement were not performed (16).

⊕ MANAGEMENT OF COMPLICATIONS

Otoplasty is a well-tolerated procedure with fortunately relatively few complications. When they do occur, they may divided into early and late complications.

Early Complications

Hematoma

The incidence of postoperative hematoma is estimated to be between 0.08% and 3.0% (5,37,38). Meticulous intraoperative hemostasis and a postoperative pressure dressing reduces this likelihood. The cardinal sign of a hematoma is unilateral pain. If the patient complains of this, the dressing should be removed and the ear examined. Once identified, the hematoma must be evacuated and the bleeding site identified. This should be performed under sterile technique, and for children is best done by returning them to the operating room. The wound is cleaned (as hematoma may act as a nidus for infection) and the bleeding site identified and cauterized. The wound is irrigated with antibiotic solution and then closed. A small closed suction drain or rubber band drain may be utilized. The pressure dressing is reapplied.

Infection

Postoperative infection may be a serious sequela of otoplasty, and therefore many surgeons advocate the use of prophylactic antibiotics (39,40). We routinely administer antistaphylococcal antibiotics such as a first-generation cephalosporin intravenously at the beginning of the case and continue this postoperatively in an oral form for 3 days. Should a postoperative infection develop, prompt identification and aggressive management is warranted. This most commonly develops in the second to fourth postoperative day. If a collection of purulent material is identified, it should be drained and the contents sent for culture and sensitivity testing. A small drain may be left in place to facilitate irrigation with antibiotic solution. Chondritis is fortunately rare in otoplasty, occurring in fewer than 1% of patients (5,37). Pain, erythema, and edema of the auricle are the hallmark signs of chondritis. Once the diagnosis of chondritis is made, aggressive management should ensue with intravenous antibiotics that cover staphylococcus and *Pseudomonas* organisms. Once cultures have been obtained and results of identification of the organism and its sensitivity to different antibiotics are available, the treatment regimen may be tailored accordingly. Local wound care including warm compresses, elevation of the head of the bed, drainage of any purulent material, and removal of any infected foreign bodies is also useful. This aggressive approach is mandatory, because if cartilage necrosis develops from the infection, it will lead to a permanent deformity. Conservative debridement of obviously necrotic cartilage is warranted in the management of postoperative chondritis.

Skin Necrosis

This is a rare problem due to the excellent vascularity of the auricle. The region to be attentive to is the newly created antihelical fold, which has the greatest amount of tension as the result of the correction. Mild bruising is not uncommon in this area, but overt skin loss is. The development of skin necrosis should be managed conservatively with local wound care including cleaning and antibiotic ointment. Oral antibiotics are also warranted to prevent secondary soft tissue infection or chondritis. Conservative debridement of the eschar may be performed, but aggressive debridement is only warranted if overt infection is present. If there is loss of only skin, and viable perichondrium is present, early application of a skin graft should be considered. This is performed when the wound is clean and granulation has begun, but prior to significant wound contraction. This is best performed in the first 1 to 2 weeks after the development of necrosis, depending on the degree of loss and the rate of secondary healing. If skin loss is accompanied by perichondrial loss as well, small perforations may be made in the cartilage with a 1.0- or 1.3-mm punch to allow granulation tissue formation from the posterior perichondrium. Once formed, this may act as the nutrient bed for a skin graft.

Late Complications

Recurrence of Deformity

Estimates of recurrence of deformity range from 6% (41) to 33% (42). This recurrence is often likely due to the execution of a particular technique, and not the technique itself. Adults have thicker and more noncompliant cartilage, so recurrence rates may be higher in this population. Children have more pliable cartilage that responds well to the suture and setback techniques described above. Correct execution of these suture techniques is mandatory as the placement and number of sutures used will determine success or failure. Late failure may also be the result of rupture of one of these sutures. Depending on how long after surgery this occurs, the suture may or may not need to be replaced. The authors' experience is that suture rupture more than 1 year after operation rarely requires replacement of the suture.

Another cause of loss of correction is patient compliance. Wearing a protective headband continuously during the first week and then nightly not only holds the auricle in the fixed position, but also protects it from inadvertent bending that may break a suture or pull the suture through the soft cartilage. Should the deformity recur, early intervention is discouraged to allow time for scar maturation to occur prior to a revision procedure.

Telephone Ear

A distinct type of postoperative deformity is the telephone ear. This is more likely to occur in patients with wide scaphas and a protruding cauda helicis. It occurs from overcorrection of the middle third, leaving the superior and inferior thirds more prominent. This leads to the shape resembling a telephone. The "reverse telephone deformity" occurs as the result of overcorrection of the superior and inferior poles, or inadequate correction of the middle third, including inadequate tissue removal in a conchal setback procedure. Careful attention to suture placement and tightening with postoperative measurements helps to avoid these complications.

Hypertrophic Scars and Keloids

The incidence of hypertrophic scars has been estimated to be 0.7%, and the incidence of keloid formation in blacks was found to be 11% (37). For this reason, anterior incisional techniques in dark-skinned individuals (skin types V and VI) should be avoided (43). Careful preoperative counseling with individuals with a prior history of hypertrophic scars or keloid formation is mandatory. If keloid formation should occur, management includes intralesional steroid administration and massage.

Hypoesthesia

Sensory deficits immediately after operation are common. These resolve in most patients within the first weeks to months after surgery.

Surface Irregularity

With cartilage incision and excision techniques, the edges may be visible or palpable. These contour irregularities are one of the driving forces behind the evolution of otoplasty toward suture and repositioning techniques, and away from techniques that disrupt the cartilage framework. Suture techniques may result in surface irregularities especially in thin-skinned individuals if the sutures are visible or palpable across the postauricular sulcus. This may occur years after the original surgery but need not be treated unless it is bothersome to the patient, becomes infected, or extrudes. Should removal become necessary, removal years after the surgery usually does not necessitate replacement of the suture. The cartilage and the soft tissue scarring hold the auricle in the desired position.

CONCLUSIONS

Otoplasty is a procedure performed on both adults and children. Intervention to prevent the psychological sequelae suffered from peer ridicule is an important factor when considering pediatric otoplasty. These effects do not permanently impact the child before age 7 to 9. Therefore, intervention is best performed shortly before this age, since the auricle has reached near adult proportions and the child is not yet permanently adversely affected by peer ridicule. The otoplastic surgeon must counsel both the child and the parents preoperatively to assess the child's and the parents' motivation. If the child is not bothered by the protuberant ears and feels none of the adverse sequelae from his or her peers, then intervening to satisfy parental desires is not in the best interest of the child.

The evolution of otoplastic techniques has been from cartilage excision to cartilage incision to suture techniques. We have presented our preferred technique for treatment of the most common deformity, the lack of the antihelical fold and a prominent conchal bowl. This technique has met with a high degree of success, patient satisfaction, and parental satisfaction.

REFERENCES

1. Farkas LG. Anthropometry of the normal and defective ear. *Clin Plast Surg* 1990;17:213–221.
2. Aguilar EA. Classification of auricular congenital deformities. In: Papel ID, Nachlas NE, eds. *Facial plastic and reconstructive surgery.* St. Louis, MO: Mosby-Year Book, 1992:532–534.
3. Weerda H. Classification of congenital deformities of the auricle. *Fac Plast Surg* 1988; 5:385–388.
4. Adamson PA, McGraw BL, Tropper GJ. Otoplasty: critical review of clinical results. *Laryngoscope* 1991;101:883–888.
5. Goode RL, Profitt SD. Complications of otoplasty. *Arch Otolaryngol* 1970;91:352–355.
6. Knorr NJ, Edgerton MT, Barberie M. Psychologic factors in reconstruction of the ear. In: Tanzer RC, Edgerton MT, eds. *Symposium on reconstruction of the auricle.* St. Louis, MO: CV Mosby, 1974:183–186.
7. Adamson PA, Morrow, TA. Otoplasty. In: Lucente FE, Lawson WE, Novick WL, eds. *The external ear.* Philadelphia: WB Saunders, 1995:220–242.
8. Ely ET. An operation for prominence of the auricles. *Arch Otol* 1881;10:97.
9. Natvig P. *Jacques Joseph, surgical sculptor.* Philadelphia: WB Saunders, 1982.
10. Gersuny R. Uber einige kosmetische Operationen. *Wien Med Wochenschr* 1903;53:2253.
11. Furnas DW. Correction of prominent ears by conchamastoid sutures. *Plast Reconstr Surg* 1968;42:189–193.

12. Luckett WH. A new operation for prominent ears based on the anatomical deformity. *Surg Gynecol Obstet* 1910;10:635.

13. Becker OJ. Correction of the protruding deformed ear. *Br J Plast Surg* 1952;5:187.

14. Converse JM, Nigro A, Wilson FA, Johnson N. A technique for surgical correction of lop ears. *Plast Reconstrut Surg* 1955;15:411.

15. Mustardé JC. The correction of prominent ears by using simple mattress sutures. *Br J Plast Surg* 1963;16:170.

16. Fritsch MH. Incisionless otoplasty. *Laryngoscope* 1995;105(No. 5, Part 3)[Suppl 70]:1–11.

17. Moore KL. The eye and the ear. In: *The developing human: clinically oriented embryology.* Philadelphia: WB Saunders 413–431.

18. Davis J. Surgical embryology. In: *Aesthetic and reconstructive otoplasty.* New York: Springer-Verlag, 1987:93–185.

19. Farkas LG. Anthropometry of normal and anomalous ears. *Clin Plast Surg* 1978;5:401–412.

20. Adamson JF, Horton CE, Crawford HH. The growth pattern of the external ear. *Plast Reconstruct Surg* 1965;36:466–470.

21. Maniglia AJ, Maniglia JV. Congenital lop ear deformity. *Otolaryngol Clin North Am* 1981;14:83–93.

22. Farkas LG. Growth of normal and reconstructed auricles. In: Tanzer RC, Edgerton MT, eds. *Symposium on reconstruction of the auricle.* St. Louis: CV Mosby, 1974:24–31.

23. Tardy ME Jr, Dennis D. Otoplasty: a contemporary survey. *Am J Otolaryngol* 1981;2:43–47.

24. Farkas LG. Otoplastic architecture. In: Davis J, ed. *Aesthetic and reconstructive otoplasty.* New York: Springer-Verlag, 1987:13–52.

25. Farkas LG, Hreczko TA, Kolar JC, Munro IR. Vertical and horizontal proportions of the face in young adult North American Caucasians: revision of neoclassical canons. *Plast Reconstruct Surg* 1985;75:328–337.

26. Farkas LG, Sohn P, Kolar JC, Katic MJ, Munro IR. Inclinations of the facial profile: art versus reality. *Plast Reconstruct Surg* 1985;75:509–519.

27. Farkas LG. *Anthropometry of the head and face in medicine.* New York: Elsevier, 1981.

28. Nachlas NE, Smith HW, Keen MS. Otoplasty. In: Papel ID, Nachlas NE, eds. *Facial plastic and reconstructive surgery.* St. Louis, MO: Mosby-Year Book, 1992:256–269.

29. Davis J. Earlobe and tragus. In: Davis J, ed. *Aesthetic and reconstructive otoplasty.* New York: Springer-Verlag, 1987:119–212.

30. Davis JS, Kitlowski EA: Abnormal prominence of the ears: a method of readjustment surgery. *Surgery* 1937;2:835.

31. Farrior RT. Modified cartilage incisions in otoplasty. *Facial Plast Surg* 1985;2:109.

32. Gibson T, Davis WB. The distortion of autogenous cartilage grafts: its cause and prevention. *Br J Plast Surg* 1958;10:257.

33. Stenstrom SJ. A natural technique for correction of congenitally prominent ears. *Plast Reconstr Surg* 1963;32:283.

34. Chongchet V. A method of antihelix reconstruction. *Br J Plast Surg* 1963;16:268.

35. Courtiss EH, Webster, White MF. Otoplasty: direct surgical approach. In: Masters FW, Lewis JR, eds. *Symposium on aesthetic surgery of the nose, ears, and chin.* St. Louis, MO: CV Mosby, 1973.

36. Nolst Trenite GJ. A modified anterior scoring technique. *Facial Plast Surg* 1994;10:255–266.

37. Baker DC, Converse JM: Otoplasty: a twenty year retrospective. *Aesthetic Plast Surg* 1979;2:36.

38. Maniglia AJ, Maniglia JJ, Witten BR. Otoplasty—an eclectic technique. *Laryngoscope* 1977;87:1359–1368.

39. Adamson PA. Complications of otoplasty. *Ear Nose Throat J* 1985;64:568–574.

40. Furnas DW. Complications of surgery of the external ear. *Clin Plast Surg* 1990;17:305–318.

41. Spira M. Reduction otoplasty. In: Goldwyn RM, ed. *The unfavorable results in plastic surgery; avoidance and treatment.* Boston: Little, Brown, 1984:307.

42. Messner AH, Crysdale WS. Otoplasty. Clinical protocol and long term results. *Arch Otolaryngol Head Neck Surg* 1996;122:773–777.

43. Quatela VC, Ries WR. Aesthetic facial surgery. In: Krespi YP, Ossoff RH, eds. *Complications in head and neck surgery.* Philadelphia: WB Saunders, 1993:385–436.

• *Practical Pediatric Otolaryngology*
• edited by Robin T. Cotton and Charles M. Myer, III
• Lippincott-Raven Publishers, Philadelphia © 1999

V. C. Quatela: Facial Plastic and Reconstructive Surgery, Strong Memorial Hospital, University of Rochester, Rochester, New York 14607. • M. A. Clymer: Facial Plastic and Reconstructive Surgery, Indiana West, PC, Terre Haute, Indiana 47802.

55

Congenital Vascular Lesions of the Head and Neck

Milton Waner & C. M. Bower

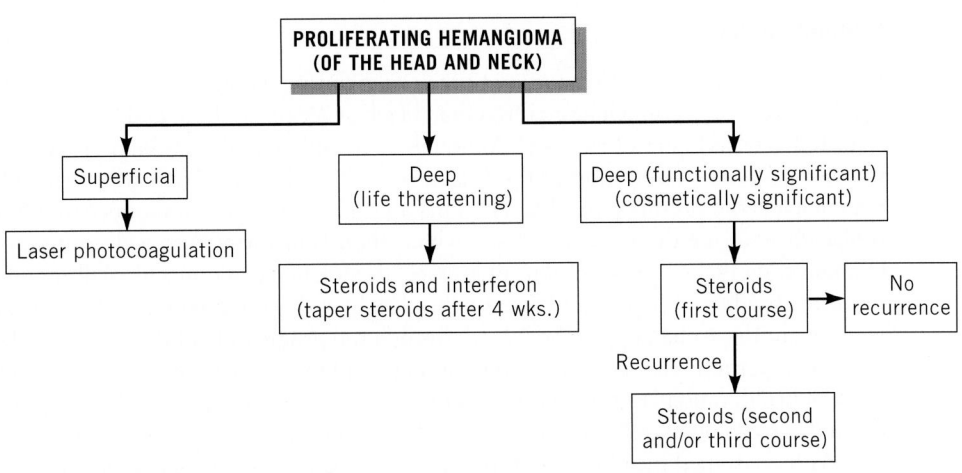

Laser photocoagulation
- Flashlamp pumped dye laser
- 4 – 6 weekly treatments
- 6.5 – 8 J/cm^2 face and head
- 6.0 J/cm^2 – neck

Steroid (first course)
- Prednisone or Prednisalone
- 3 – 5 mg/kg/day in divided doses
- 6 wks. course, then taper

Steroids (second or third course)
- Prednisone or Prednisalone
- 3 – 5 mg/kg/day
- Attempt taper every 6 wks.
- If recurrence noted, back into full dosage

Interferon
- INH α ZA
- 3×10^6 units/m^2
- Daily S.C. injections
- 6 – 10 months (no taper necessary)

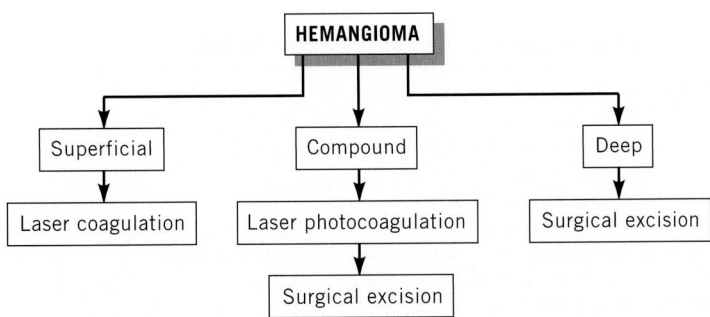

THE CLASSIFICATION OF CONGENITAL VASCULAR LESIONS

Until recently, the term *hemangioma* was used in a generic sense to describe all congenital vascular lesions. This was confusing since some "hemangiomas" involuted, while others clearly did not. Furthermore, some were present at birth whereas others were not. Recognizing these differences, Mulliken and Glowacki (1) reclassified congenital vascular lesions. In what was called the "biological" classification, they recognized two distinct entities, *hemangiomas* and *vascular malformations* (1) (Tables 1,2). Hemangiomas were usually *not* present at birth, *proliferated* during the first year of life, and then proceeded to *involute*. On the other hand, vascular malformations were *always* present at birth, *never proliferated,* and *never involuted*. As its name implies, there was a biologic basis to this classification. Hemangiomas are made up of plump, proliferating endothelial cells during their proliferative phase, whereas vascular malformations are made up of flat, inactive endothelial cells.

Hemangiomas

Hemangiomas are the most common tumors seen during infancy. By all accounts, white children are affected much more often than black or Asian children, and the incidence is reported to be as high as 12% (1–6). Although up to 30% may already be present at birth, the vast majority present during the first few weeks of life (7). The earliest sign of hemangioma is the presence of a blanched macule. This often goes unnoticed and is soon replaced by an erythematous macule, which then transforms into a discrete area of telangiectasia (4). As proliferation progresses, the telangiectatic macule will proliferate to form a bright-red papule and eventually a bright-red bosselated mass. The histologic correlate of these changes can be traced through the progression of the endothelial cells from an apparently flat, normal configuration to a plump, proliferating variety, the hallmark of proliferation (Fig. 1). As the endothelial cells become more active, they plump up, and in so doing, they "squeeze" the blood out of the vessels, hence the blanched macule. With continued proliferation, the number of vessels greatly increases as does their diameter, hence the erythematous, the telangiectatic macule and eventually the papular mass.

The exact cause and origin of these lesions are not known. Whether or not they originate from a single stem cell or a "sick field" has yet to be determined. However, in a review of several hundred cases, Waner et al. (*unpublished data*) determined that there were definite sites of predilection and that these appeared to correlate with the lines of embryologic fusion. What is obvious is the fact that hemangiomas may be superficial, deep, or compound (1,8). Superficial lesions present as red papular masses, and deep lesions, because of their depth, as bluish masses (Fig. 2–4). Therefore, compound lesions have both superficial, red components and deep, bluish components. The previous nomenclature for these was confusing and included names such as capillary or strawberry nevus, and cavernous and capillary cavernous hemangiomas. Although the rate and the extent of proliferation may vary, proliferation usually slows by the age of 6 months usually ceases by the end of the first year of life. The first 4 to 12 weeks of life and the fourth

TABLE 1: The Classification of Congenital Vascular Lesions

Hemangiomas
Vascular malformations
    Venular malformations (frequently, port-wine stains).
    Venous malformations
    Arteriovenous malformations
    Lymphatic malformations
    Mixed malformations (made up of one or more of the above)
    Mixed venous lymphatic malformations
    Mixed venous venular malformations

TABLE 2: The Clinical Differences between Hemangiomas and Venous Malformations

Hemangiomas	Vascular Malformations
Usually not present at birth (30% may be present at birth)	Always present at birth (may not always be apparent)
Proliferate during first year of life (hyperplasia)	Never involute. Increase in size throughout life (hyperplasia hypertrophy)
Involution	
More common in females—3:1	Male-female ratio—1:1

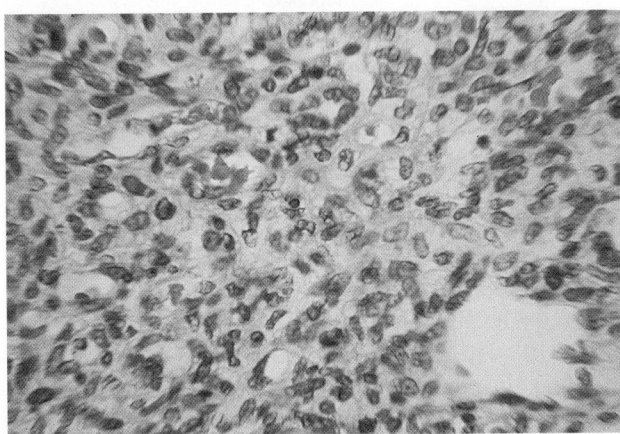

FIGURE 1 Hematoxylin-eosin staining of a section of a proliferating hemangioma. Most of the plump proliferating endothelial cells with frequent mytoses.

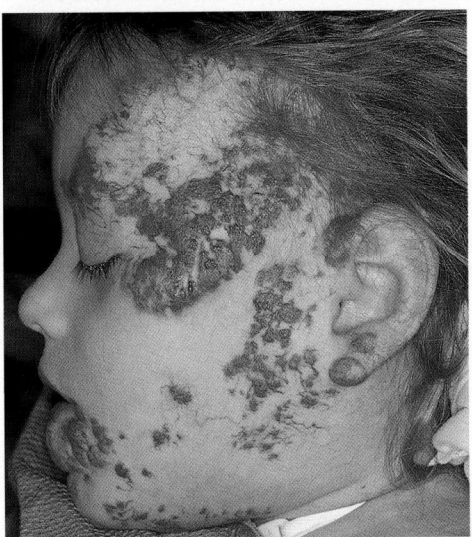

FIGURE 2 A 2-year-old with a superficial hemangioma.

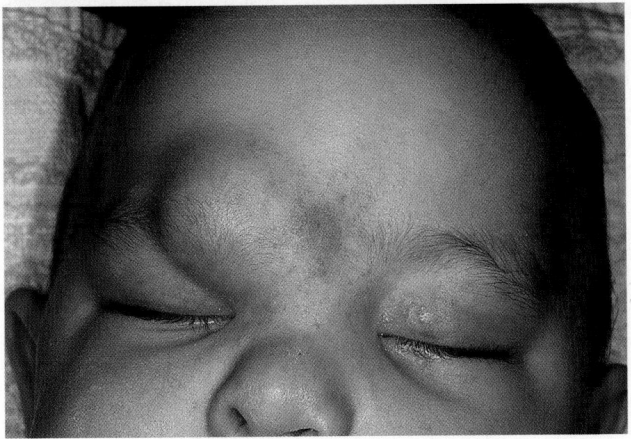

FIGURE 3 A 6-month-old with a deep hemangioma.

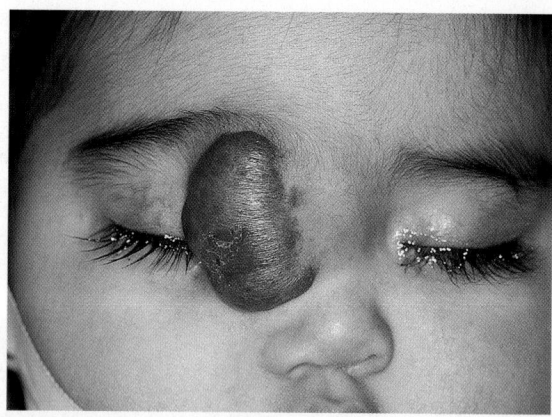

FIGURE 4 A 9-month-old with a compound hemangioma.

to the sixth months of life appear to be periods of rapid growth. The clinical features of proliferation depend on the depth of the lesion. Superficial lesions are tense and appear as bright-red bosselated masses. Deep lesions present as a tense, bluish soft tissue mass that does not empty easily with compression, and expands when the child cries.

The transition from proliferation to involution is gradual and usually commences by the end of the first year of life (5,9,10). The parents of the child will notice a definite diminution in the growth rate. In time, the hemangioma becomes less tense to palpation and no longer expands as much when the child cries. The lesion empties with compression, and eventually, a diminution in size will be obvious. Superficial lesions assume a more dusky, maroonish color but, as can be expected, no color change is obvious in deep lesions. The cause of involution is unknown and has left much room for speculation. That all hemangiomas involute is an absolute. However, we must define what is meant by *involution*. It appears that in the context of hemangiomas, involution merely means shrink. The speed and the extent of involution will vary (5,9,10). The misconception that all hemangiomas will involute and disappear completely within a short period is widespread and led to the policy of benign neglect. Therefore, all but the most complicated hemangiomas were left untreated. Recent evidence suggests that, broadly speaking, hemangiomas that involute rapidly are more likely to do so completely (7). This means that rapidly involuting lesions are less likely to require corrective surgery than those that involute more slowly. The cutoff seems to be at the age of approximately 5 years. Only 40% of lesions that involute completely by the age of 5 to 6 years require corrective surgery, whereas 80% or more of those that take longer than 5 years to involute require corrective surgery (7) (Fig. 5). In addition to this, hemangiomas in certain anatomic sites are

FIGURE 5 A digrammatic representation of the life cycle of the hemangioma. More hemangiomas grow during the first year of life and then involute during the remainder of childhood. Group I lesions involute rapidly and 60% of these will have a complete response. Group II lesions involute slowly, taking longer than 6 years, and only 20% will have a complete response.

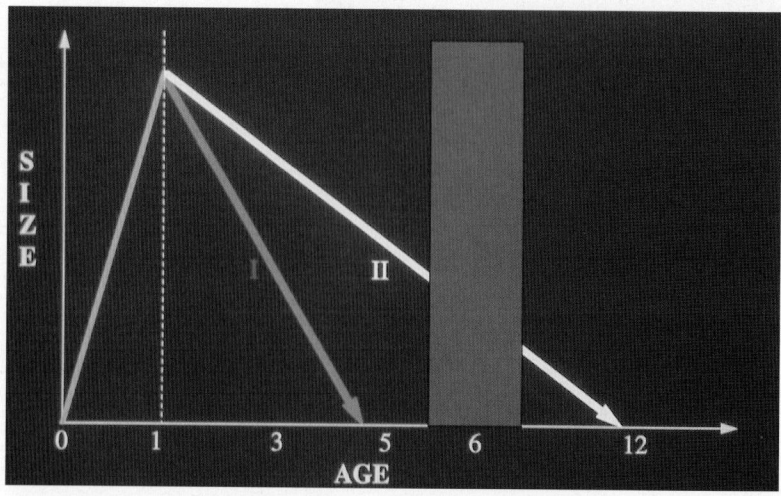

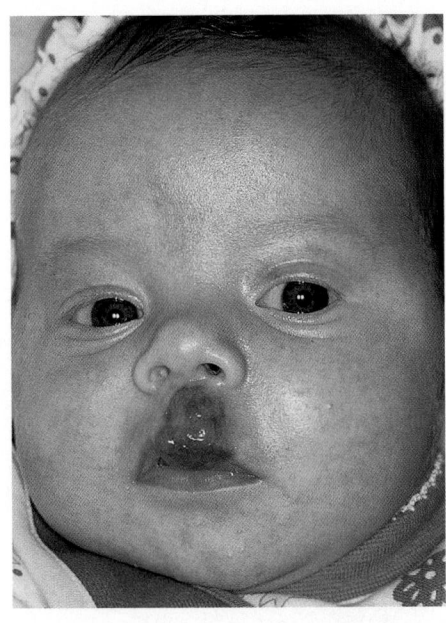

FIGURE 6 A child with an upper-lip hemangioma showing ulceration of the lesion.

less inclined to involute completely. These sites (5,11) include the nasal tip; the lower lip, especially where there has been lengthening of the lip; and the anterior chest wall. Analysis of these data suggests that the likely outcome of involution is complete resolution in only 40% of patients. The rest will have some residuum, the nature of which depends on the depth of the lesion. Superficial lesions are likely to leave epidermal atrophy and residual telangiectasia, whereas deep lesions are likely to leave a residuum of excess fibrofatty tissue.

While most hemangiomas progress through the various stages of their life cycle in an orderly manner, some develop complications:

1. **Ulceration.** This is the most common complication and is usually seen during the stage of rapid proliferation (10). During this stage, the hemangioma will stretch the overlying skin, which may then split with minor trauma and result in an ulcer. As long as the hemangioma continues to proliferate at a greater rate than the basal layer of the epidermis, the ulcer will not heal (Fig. 6).
2. **Airway obstruction.** Laryngeal involvement, either supraglottic, paraglottic, or subglottic, may embarrass the airway. Occasionally, a large parapharyngeal or cervical lesion will obstruct the airway.
3. **High-output cardiac failure.** Hemangiomas are high-flow vascular lesions and act as arteriovenous shunts. The larger the lesion, the higher the shunt fraction. Thus, left ventricular hypertrophy is not an uncommon finding but frank failure is much less common and is usually seen only with giant lesions. High-output failure may be insipient and usually persists through the earliest phases of involution. The mortality rate is high (55%) and death is usually the result of congestive cardiac failure (12).
4. **Ophthalmic complications.** Deprivation amblyopia may result from a relatively short period of visual obstruction. Even a small lesion that does not obstruct the visual axis may bring about astigmatism, which, if severe, may also lead to deprivation amblyopia (13).
5. **Kasabach-Merritt syndrome.** Platelet sequestration and destruction within the hemangioma and the spleen gives rise to this thrombocytopenic coagulopathy (14). Kasabach-Merritt syndrome carries a 60% mortality rate. Clinical features include pitting edema around the lesion and ecchymoses (Fig. 7). The platelet count will be low and the serum level of fibrin degradation products will be elevated.
6. **Psychosocial consequences.** The effect of a child with a hemangioma on the dynamics of the entire family can be profound. Parental guilt coupled with overindul-

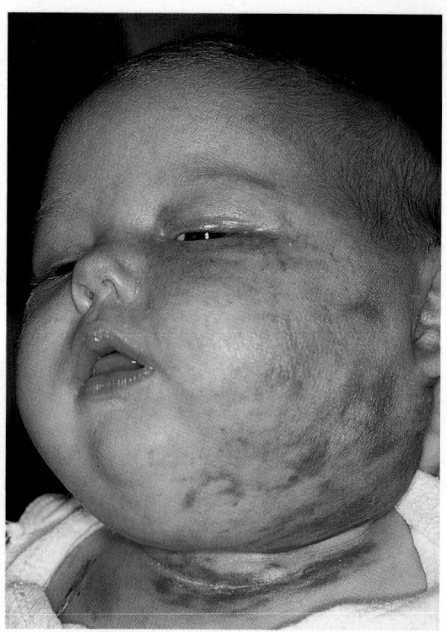

FIGURE 7 A 6-month-old with Kasabach-Merritt syndrome. Note the diffuse edema and the ecchymoses. These are hallmarks of Kasabach-Merritt syndrome.

gence is common. Older siblings are often neglected and may harbor deep-seated resentment to the newcomer with the hemangioma.

Vascular Malformations

Vascular malformations behave quite differently. Unlike hemangiomas, they are always present at birth, never proliferate, and never involute. Instead, slow, steady, relentless enlargement throughout the life of the patient is the norm. Periods of rapid enlargement may punctuate this normal progression. These occur in association with hormonal changes, trauma, or infection.

Vascular malformations can be subdivided in accordance with their vascular content (see Table 1).

Vascular malformations are true developmental abnormalities, and although they may occasionally not be apparent at birth, by definition, they are always present at birth. Furthermore, unlike hemangiomas, the lesion expands by a process of hypertrophy and not proliferation. This distinction is important and forms the basis of the biologic classification. Hypertrophy is a process whereby the lesion expands by enlargement of existing structures, in this instance, progressive ectasia of the preexisting component vessels. No increase in the number of vessels is seen. Hyperplasia, on the other hand, results in expansion through an increase in the number of cells and in this way an increase in the number of vessels. This is the mechanism whereby hemangiomas expand.

Venous Malformations

These lesions are made up of anomalous, disorganized, dilated veins and may be localized or diffuse, superficial or deep. Commonly involved sites include the buccal fat space, buccal mucosa, tongue, floor of the mouth, lips, nasal tip, and the neck (15). Superficial lesions are readily visible as bosselated maroon masses whereas deeper lesions will be more bluish (Fig. 8). Therefore, the diagnosis is usually obvious with regard to superficial lesions, but deeper lesions may be mistaken for hemangiomas or arteriovenous malformations and should be distinguished from these by the history. Venous malformations are usually soft and compress easily. They readily expand in a dependent position and with raised venous pressure. A rather unique feature is their tendency to form phleboliths. These can sometimes be felt with deep palpation but are readily visible on computed tomography (CT) scans and magnetic resonance images (MRIs).

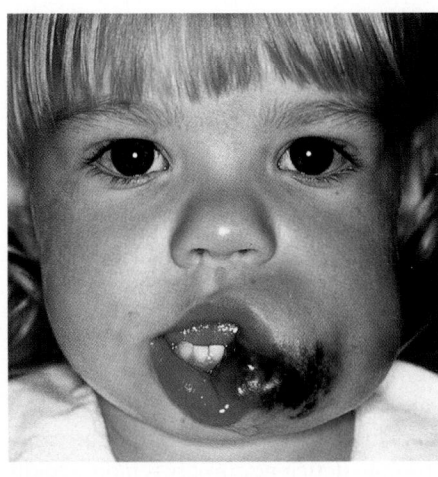

FIGURE 8 An 18-month-old with a buccal fat space venous malformation extending forward to involve the oral commissure.

Venular Malformations

As was the case with vascular lesions in general, some confusion existed. The term *nevus flammeus* has been used collectively to describe all cutaneous vascular stains. Classic port-wine stains, referred to by Mulliken and Glowacki (1) and others as *capillary malformations*, are in fact made up of postcapillary venules. Therefore, a more appropriate name for them would be *venular malformations* (Fig. 9). Midline lesions, commonly referred to as "stork bites" or "angel kisses," are a separate entity and although they look like port-wine stains, they behave quite differently. Sixty percent of these disappear by the age of 6 years and those that do persist never hypertrophy. The term *midline venular malformation* is probably best; the reason will become obvious later.

Venular malformations occur in 0.3% of the population and are equally as common in the male and female population (16). They are always present at birth as light-pink macules but may not be noticed for the first few days of life. Their distribution seems to correspond with one or more sensory dermatomes, and they may be confluent or nonconfluent (geographic) in their involvement of that dermatome (17). At least 80% are found in the head and neck, and their distribution usually corresponds with one or more

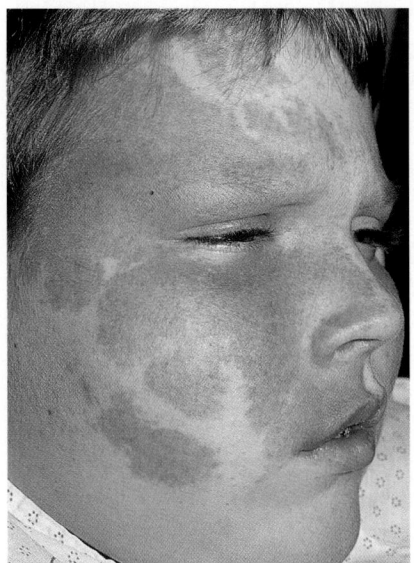

FIGURE 9 A child with a VI and a VII venular malformation (port-wine stain).

of the trigeminal dermatomes. Mucosal or gingival involvement in continuity with a cutaneous lesion is common, especially in the presence of a midfacial lesion. In contradistinction with midline venular malformations, venular malformations persist throughout life and progressively darken and thicken with advancing age. Eventually, cobblestones will form in most. These changes are due to progressive ectasia of the venules.

Midline venular malformations, on the other hand, never progress and up to 60% disappear the by the age of 6 years (18). They are most commonly seen on the central part of the forehead (angel kisses) or on the nape of the neck (stork bites) (Fig. 10). Forehead lesions are usually stippled light-pink macules and form a V on the central part of the forehead, extending up from the glabellum. The upper eyelids, nasal alae, and philtrum may also be involved (19).

Smoller and Rosen (20) postulated that an altered or absent neural innervation of the cutaneous vascular plexus is responsible for the ectasia. Orten et al. (17) suggested that a relative or absolute deficiency in autonomic innervation of the plexus led to the variation in the rate of progression. Lesions with an absolute deficiency progress more rapidly whereas those with a relative deficiency do so more slowly. The only possible explanation for midline lesions is that autonomic innervation of the venular plexus has not fully developed by birth in these patients and does so soon thereafter in most. In those in whom the lesion persists, there is only a very slight deficiency in innervation and so progression is slow if at all.

Arteriovenous Malformations

Arteriovenous malformations are congenital developmental anomalies whereas arteriovenous fistulas are acquired, usually posttraumatically (21). Furthermore, an arteriovenous fistula is usually made up of a single fistulous tract whereas there are multiple fistulous tracts in a congenital arteriovenous malformation. As is the case with all other congenital vascular malformations, arteriovenous malformations are always present at birth, although they may not become apparent until much later. Occasionally, they may present for the first time in the second, third, or even fourth decade of life (22). An arteriovenous malformation is made of a nidus and afferent blood supply and a venous drainage. The nidus is the root of the abnormality and is made up of an ectatic capillary bed (23). Recent work showed that the fundamental defect is in the regulation of flow from the arterioles into the capillary bed. Under normal circumstances, this flow is controlled by precapillary sphincters. An absence of these sphincters, or alternatively a deficient autonomic nerve supply, is the probable underlying cause (23). Without this control, blood shunts into the capillary bed and out again unhindered. This continuous flow

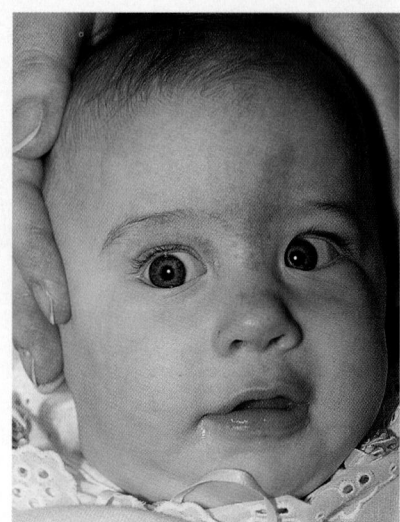

FIGURE 10 An infant with a midline venular malformation involving the distribution of the supraorbital and supratrochlear nerves. The lesion is V-shaped, extending from the nasion cephalad.

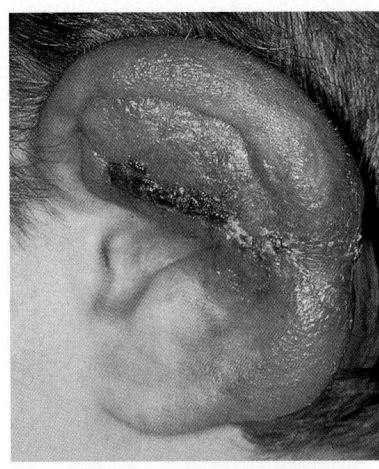

FIGURE 11 An arteriovenous malformation involving the pinna. Note the ulceration of the skin.

through the capillary bed will cause progressive ectasia of the bed, which in turn forms the nidus of the arteriovenous malformation. Prolonged flow through the arterioles will, in turn, result in arteriolar hypertrophy and, continuous shunting of a considerable volume of blood into the venous system will cause venous dilation (23).

An arteriovenous malformation usually presents as a soft tissue mass. Unlike venous malformations, the lesion is of a hard-soft consistency. The lesion will empty with compression, but only after considerable compression. Occasionally, a pulsation or a fluid thrill can be felt. Long-standing arteriovenous malformation will usually have evidence of arterial hypertrophy and venous dilatation. As is often the case, scars from previous surgical attempts at extirpation will be obvious. The overlying skin may also be involved, in which case a vascular blush will be evident (Fig. 11). A severe arterial venous malformation with significant shunting may cause flow reversal and subsequent skin necrosis. In these cases, ulceration with a history of profuse, spontaneous bleeding will be noted. The bleeds are spectacular with regard to their projection. The patient may bleed a considerable volume in a very short time, and spontaneous cessation of bleeding often happens with the same degree of rapidity as did the start of hemorrhage.

Lymphatic Malformations

This term is used to describe all congenital malformations of the lymphatic system. Terms such as *lymphangioma* and *cystic hygroma* are misleading and their use is inappropriate. Furthermore, the suffix (*-oma*) implies proliferation (1). Since all lymphatic malformations are characterized by a normal rate of endothelial turnover, usage of this suffix is inaccurate.

As with all other vascular lesions, lymphatic malformations may be superficial or deep, localized, or diffuse. Deep lesions are usually clinically obvious as hard doughly masses. They are much more difficult to compress than are arteriovenous or venous malformations, but they will readily pit on digital compression, indicating the presence of lymphedema. In general, lesions involving the neck tend to be more localized whereas extensive cervicofacial or facial lesions are much more diffuse. Superficial involvement, either mucosal or cutaneous, is characterized by the appearance of small, 1- to 2-mm fluid-filled vesicles (commonly referred to as *frog eggs*) (Fig. 12).

Mixed Malformations

Lesions made up of more than one vascular component are not uncommon. These lesions will have features of the constituent vascular components and the dominant appearance will depend on the vascular content. Examples include mixed venous lymphatic malformations, mixed venous venular malformations, and mixed arterial venous capillary malformation.

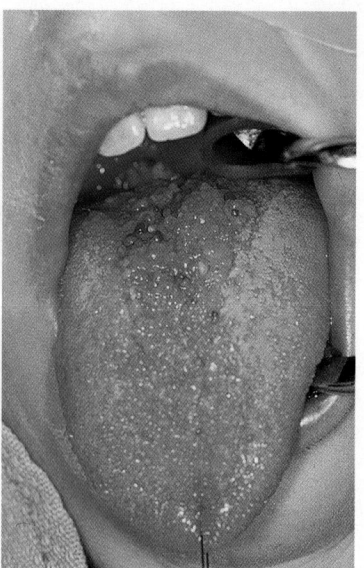

FIGURE 12 An extensive lymphatic malformation involving the dorsum of the tongue. Note the small fluid-filled vesicles (frog eggs) involving the midline, all the way down to the tip of the tongue.

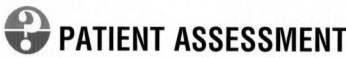

PATIENT ASSESSMENT

An accurate history and physical examination are usually sufficient to render a diagnosis. Only rarely is it necessary to resort to special investigations.

History

An accurate history is of paramount importance in distinguishing between a hemangioma and a vascular malformation. To do this, three questions must be answered.

First, was the lesion present at birth? Although this question is important, the answer may confuse the issue. Remember, by definition, all vascular malformations are present at birth. Unfortunately, they may not be noticed and may therefore only present in the first few weeks of life. Furthermore, arteriovenous malformations may present for the first time in the second, third, or even fourth decade of life. Hemangiomas, on the other hand, are usually not present at birth, although up to 30% may already be present at birth. Consideration of the answer to this question, in conjunction with the answer to the next question, will be more indicative.

Second, has it grown? A history of proliferation during the first year of life, or more specifically during the first 6 months of life, is a clear indication of hemangioma. On the other hand, slow steady expansion of the lesion, more or less commensurate with the growth of the child, is likely to indicate a vascular malformation. This process is much slower and is less impressive than the growth seen with hemangiomas.

Third, has it gotten any smaller? After the first year of life, only hemangiomas involute. Therefore, any history of involution is indicative of hemangioma. A pure lymphatic malformations has a tendency to swell with a concurrent upper respiratory tract infection, and then shrink back to its original size. This, however, will be obvious on further questioning.

Examination

While an accurate history will distinguish between a hemangioma and a vascular malformation, the examination will very often clinch the diagnosis. In general, superficial hemangiomas are bright red during proliferation and a dusky red during involution. Deep hemangiomas, on the other hand, are firm and bluish during proliferation, but are softer and less bluish during involution. Superficial venous malformations are a maroonish color and deep venous malformations are, like involuting hemangiomas, bluish. Arteriovenous malformations are usually deeper, colorless lesions. Therefore, they may be mistaken for a deep venous malformation or a deep lymphatic malformation. Occasionally, cutaneous involvement will be evident. In this instance, a pink to light-red vascular blush will be present. Lymphatic malformations are colorless.

With regard to consistency, venous malformations are very soft and compressible whereas lymphatic malformations are much harder and much more difficult to compress. They do exhibit a degree of pitting with digital compression. The consistency of an arteriovenous malformation is somewhere between these two extremes. Hemangiomas are firm to palpation during proliferation, but during involution, they are not dissimilar in consistency from a venous malformation.

PEARLS AND PERILS

1. A deep hemangioma: a history of proliferation and involution will be given.
2. A deep venous malformation: soft, compressible; empties on compression.
3. An arteriovenous malformation: harder, compressible, does not empty.
4. Lymphatic malformation: doughy feel, pitting, edema, does not empty with compression.

Special Investigations

Special investigations are only necessary if the diagnosis is in doubt, or alternatively, the result of the investigation is likely to influence the course of management. From a diagnostic perspective, MRI is by far the most informative investigation. If the diagnosis remains in doubt, MRI will determine the nature of the lesion with a high degree of accuracy.

Hemangiomas are high-flow, parenchymatous lesions of intermediate intensity on T_1-weighted images and of high intensity on T_2-weighted images. Flow voids are usually seen on both T_1- and T_2-weighted images.

Arteriovenous malformations are also high-flow lesions, but lack the parenchymatous structure and therefore do not enhance as readily on T_2-weighted images. Once again, since they are high-flow lesions, flow voids are characteristically seen on both T_1- and T_2-weighted images.

Venous malformations are low-flow lesions and appear only slightly more intense than muscle (intermediate intensity on T_1-weighted images). The signal from a venous malformation will be very intense on T_1-weighted presaturation images. Phleboliths will appear as low-intensity punctate areas on T_2-weighted images.

Lymphatic malformations are also slow-flow lesions not dissimilar in their characteristics from those seen with venous malformations. The main difference between these two is that lymphatic malformations do not enhance with gadopentetate dimeglumine (gadolinium). Cystic lymphatic malformations will be obvious whereas diffuse noncystic lesions will show a significant solid tissue mass with a high-intensity signal on T_2-weighted images.

Angiograms are occasionally helpful in distinguishing between hemangiomas and arteriovenous malformations in a very young patient. Since both appear to be high-flow lesions, the distinction between the two can usually be made with an angiogram. In addition to this, an angiogram is often helpful in preoperative planning. Digital subtraction angiography will establish the primary as well as the collateral blood supply to a lesion. It will also delineate the extent of the nidus, and since treatment is aimed at complete removal of the nidus, this is extremely important. Both MRI and digital subtraction angiography should be used to evaluate the extent of this nidus.

TREATMENT RECOMMENDATIONS

Hemangiomas

In 1938, Lister (9) first reported that a group of vascular lesions he called *strawberry nevi* involuted spontaneously. This led to the status quo of nonintervention, and since then, all vascular lesions were called *hemangiomas* and left untreated. This policy, now known as *benign neglect,* has only recently been seriously challenged. The fact that a cosmetically unacceptable result is often left at the end of involution, together with the severe psychosocial trauma of a readily visible hemangioma during the formative years of a child's life and the recent technologic advances with regard to both chemotherapeutic agents and surgical lasers, all necessitated a reevaluation of this policy.

Since hemangiomas pass through several stages, each with its own distinct clinical and histologic features, a logical approach to the management of hemangiomas would be to consider each stage in the life cycle as a distinct entity. In addition to this, several treatment modalities can be used, each with its indications and contraindications. These modalities should all be incorporated into the management of hemangiomas and used where they are best suited. The treatment plan that follows considers each phase in the life cycle separately and recommends the modalities best suited to that phase.

Early Proliferation

Destruction of the proliferating endothelial cells results in complete eradication of the hemangioma. Unfortunately, given the limited depth of penetration of the currently available lasers, it is only possible to accomplish this with very superficial lesions (Fig. 13). Treatment with a flash lamp pumped dye laser has been found to be effective in these circumstances (24). Using a 5-mm spot size and overlapping the spots by 10%, one can treat the entire lesion between 6.5 and 8 J per square centimeter to an end point of uniform purplish-gray discoloration. This may require several pulses of the same area during the same treatment. Treatment should commence at the earliest sign of the lesion and be repeated every 4 to 6 weeks until the lesion has been completely destroyed. It must be stressed that only the most superficial of lesions will respond to this form of treatment. A deeper lesion or a deeper portion of the hemangioma will continue to proliferate unabated because it is beyond the reach of this laser system. This will present as a bluish discoloration or mass. Previous claims that treatment of the surface of a deep lesion will slow proliferation or induce a more rapid rate of involution are anecdotal and remain unsubstantiated.

FIGURE 13 A superficial hemangioma before **(A)** and after **(B)** six treatments with a flash lamp pumped dye laser. All treatments were performed with general anesthesia.

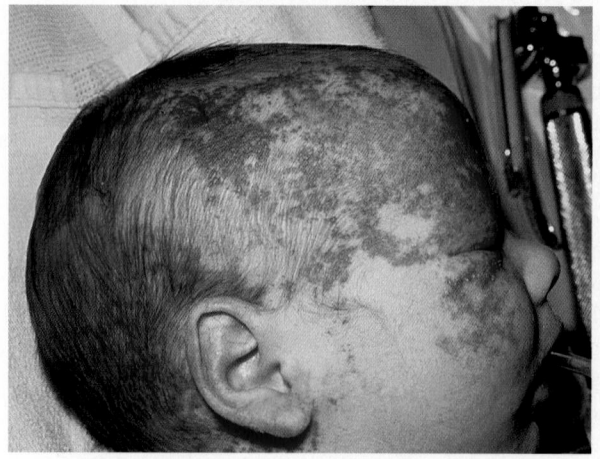
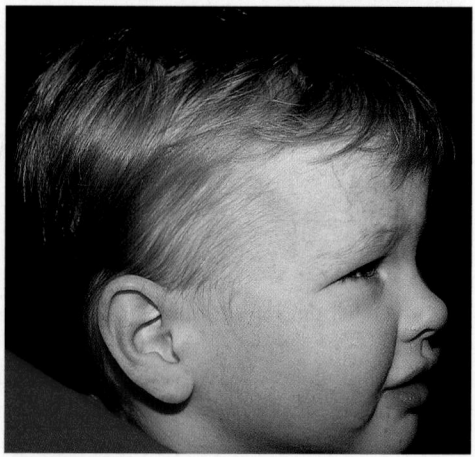

A   B

Late Proliferation

During late proliferation, the lesion has acquired a thickness or depth beyond which a flash lamp pumped dye laser will penetrate. Treatment with a laser is therefore no longer effective. At this point, a decision should be made whether or not a treatment is warranted. It is the authors' policy to recommend treatment if the lesion is life-threatening or functionally or cosmetically significant. *Life-threatening* lesions are those that result in Kasabach-Merritt syndrome or high-output cardiac failure. A *functionally significant* lesion is one that affects a vital function, such as breathing, swallowing, or vision. Airway obstruction is also obviously life-threatening. A *cosmetically significant* lesion is one that involves the face or neck and is thus clearly visible and cannot easily be hidden. The authors' first line of treatment is oral prednisone or prednisolone. A 4-week course of oral prednisone or prednisolone at a dose of 3 to 4 mg per kilogram of body weight and tapered over a additional 2 weeks is usually effective during active proliferation. A significant response is usually seen in about 75% of patients. However, growth will resume during the taper or within a few days of completion of this course in 40% of patients. If this happens, steroids should be started again at the same dose as before and continued for another 6 weeks. After this, one should again attempt to taper the dose, using hemangioma growth as the indicator. A resumption of growth should be countered with continuation of the steroids for another month or until involution is underway. The child should be followed closely by a pediatrician and monitored for any significant side effects. The immunization schedule should be appropriately modified until after cessation of prednisone. Surprisingly, few side effects have been encountered with this regimen. Moon facies appears to be the most common and is seen in about half the patients. Fortunately, it is only temporary and disappears soon after completion of treatment. In a large study, only 2 of 60 patients experienced growth retardation (11). Both of these infants received unusually prolonged treatment but reached their expected weight within a few months after cessation of therapy.

Intralesional injections of steroids were first described in 1970. It was thought that this would eliminate the systemic side effects sometimes seen with oral prednisone. Although this advantage is not conclusive, intralesional steroids should be reserved for small well-localized lesions. The recommended dose should not exceed 14 mg of triamcinolone and 6 mg of betamethasone. An initial response rate of up to 80% has been reported, but a second or even third injection may be necessary at 6-week intervals (25). One should bear in mind that triamcinolone is a colloid suspension. Retinal artery occlusion with ipsilateral and even contralateral blindness has occurred with periorbital injections. In addition to this, cutaneous necrosis and epidermal atrophy are also not uncommon. The authors therefore do not recommend intralesional steroids for periocular lesions.

The role of interferon alfa-2a is uncertain. In the past, interferon was only used to treat life-threatening complications. However, it may be advantageous to treat functionally significant lesions as well. A dose of 3 million per square meter given as a daily subcutaneous injection is effective. Furthermore, it may be necessary to administer interferon for an average of 6 to 10 months to obtain a sustained effect. Side effects, such as low-grade fevers (up to 39°C) for the first 2 weeks of therapy, are common. An oral dose of acetaminophen prior to the injection of interferon may prevent this. Other side effects include an increase in liver transaminases, transient neutropenia, and anemia. These effects subside once the infant is off interferon. An alarming side effect is the appearance of spastic diplegia. Careful neurologic assessment every month during the regimen is thus essential.

Surgical resection should be reserved for lesions that have either not responded to steroids or interferon, or both, or have regrown after adequate therapy and still warrant further treatment. A preoperative MRI will delineate the full extent of the lesion and is advisable. Although surgical excision is usually reserved for the phase of involution, resecting a rapidly expanding lesion does have advantages:

1. During proliferation, the lesion will develop a soft tissue plane or false capsule around it. This is an extremely useful plane for dissection as it is relatively bloodless and will facilitate hemostasis.
2. The lesion will often act as a skin expander, which will often enable a surgeon to obtain primary closure after resection. This advantage may be lost if one waits until the lesion has involuted.

During surgery, meticulous attention must be paid to hemostasis. The authors have found both the contact neodymium:yttrium-aluminum-garnet (Nd:YAG) laser and the Shaw thermoscalpel to be useful in this regard. With these instruments and good surgical technique, it should rarely be necessary to perform a transfusion. While the surgeon should always aim at complete removal of the lesion, bearing in mind that all hemangiomas eventually involute, a small pocket of hemangioma in an inaccessible, cosmetically important or difficult area may well be left alone unless the lesion is rapidly proliferating. The surgeon should exercise clinical judgment in these decisions.

Complications

Treatment of *ulceration* with a flash lamp pumped dye laser has been shown to beneficial. The laser probably temporarily retards a rim of superficial proliferated hemangioma, which then enables the epidermis to finally close. Usually, only one or two treatments, spaced at 4- to 6-week intervals, are necessary to accomplish this.

High-output cardiac failure should be treated medically in the first instance. In resilient cases, both prednisone and interferon alfa-2a may be tried. It may also be necessary to resect the lesion, especially where a large, solitary hemangioma has been incriminated.

The management of *airway obstruction* has traditionally been conservative. An attempt at establishment of an airway with a carbon dioxide (CO_2) laser may be made. However, failing this, a tracheotomy should be fashioned until the lesion has involuted sufficiently. Wiatrak et al. suggested resecting these lesions where appropriate. However, it may be possible to prevent tracheotomy by treating the patients in the first instance with prednisone and then interferon. Since the effect of interferon is usually delayed by 1 to 2 weeks, commencing the two drugs simultaneously and then tapering the steroid dose may prove beneficial.

Ophthalmologic complications should be treated in conjunction with an ophthalmologist. In the presence of amblyopia, taping the good eye periodically may be necessary to preserve vision. Once again, a large hemangioma obstructing the visual axis and having failed to respond to conservative measures may require resection. Also, given that the presence of a hemangioma on the upper eyelid may result in astigmatism, surgical excision is once again beneficial, as one is able to rapidly relieve the abnormal pressure on the globe.

Patients with *Kasabach-Merritt syndrome* must be treated aggressively. The patient should be started on both prednisone and interferon alfa-2a simultaneously. The response can be monitored through the level of fibrinogen and fibrin degradation products. Once a response has been achieved, it may be possible to taper and discontinue the steroid dose. However, interferon should be continued until the child is somewhere between the ages of 10 and 12 months. Unfortunately, early withdrawal has been known to result in a recurrence. Use of platelets and blood products should be avoided if at all possible, as these may be trapped within the lesion and further accentuate growth. This may not be practical in the setting of a dangerously low platelet count; under these circumstances, platelets should be given judiciously, knowing that aggressive replacement may be counterproductive. Heparin, the mainstay for treatment of disseminated intravascular coagulation, is specifically contraindicated in Kasabach-Merritt syndrome, as it has been known to cause accelerated growth of the hemangioma.

Involution

Once the process of involution has begun, the patient can be treated expectantly. Periodic follow-up visits are essential to keep in touch with the patient. The frequency of these visits will depend on the parents. Statistics have shown that broadly speaking, hemangiomas can be divided into two groups with respect to involution: those that involute slowly and those that involute rapidly (see Fig. 5). A given hemangioma has a 50% chance of involuting rapidly. The cutoff age between rapid and slow involution appears to be between 5 and 6 years. This means that 50% of all hemangiomas will involute before the age of 5 years. Further research has shown that rapidly involuting hemangiomas are more likely to leave an adequate cosmetic result at the end of involution. Hemangiomas that involute slowly are less likely to leave an adequate cosmetic result and will require corrective surgery in 80 to 90% of patients. Overall, therefore, 60% of all patients with hemangiomas will require some form of intervention. A logical approach to management would be to wait until the ages of 3 to 4 years. By this stage, the physician will know whether the lesion is likely to involute rapidly or not. In the face of rapid involution, the parents can be informed of the likely outcomes, and a decision can be made on this basis. However, in the face of slow involution, the parents should be informed that a favorable outcome is highly unlikely, and to spare the child any further psychosocial trauma, treatment should be commenced as soon as possible. In this way, those that are likely to involute completely are left to do so, whereas those that are less likely to do so are treated in a proactive manner.

Intervention should follow the same principles discussed previously. Superficial lesions should be treated with laser photocoagulation and deep lesions should be surgically excised (Figs. 14 to 16). Compound hemangiomas may need to be treated with both modalities. Both flash lamp pumped dye lasers and copper vapor lasers have been shown to be useful. The flash lamp pumped dye laser is safe and easy to use with a very low risk of complications. With a 5-mm spot size, any cutaneous telangiectasia should be photocoagulated to an end point of purpura. Individual impaction points should be overlapped by about 10% until this is achieved. Several treatments, spaced at 6- to 8-week intervals, will eventually resolve any cutaneous telangiectasia. Residual epidermal atrophy has been shown to respond well to skin recontouring with a CO_2 laser. The technique used is not dissimilar from that used to recontour the face of a patient with rhytidosis. The technique involves the use of a 9-mm silk touch scanner (Sharplan Lasers, Allendale, NJ) and 16 W of power. The scan duration is 0.45 second. A pass using 9-mm scans is undertaken, and these scans are overlapped just sufficiently to remove all of the epidermis. Following this, the proteinaceous debris should be meticulously removed with wet saline-soaked sponges. The surface should then be dried and treated again with the same parameters. Heating the collagen of the papillary dermis in this way will result in shrink-

FIGURE 14 A full-thickness hemangioma involving the lower lip before **(A)** and after **(B)** surgical resection. The lip was stretched by 2 cm as a result of the hemangioma.

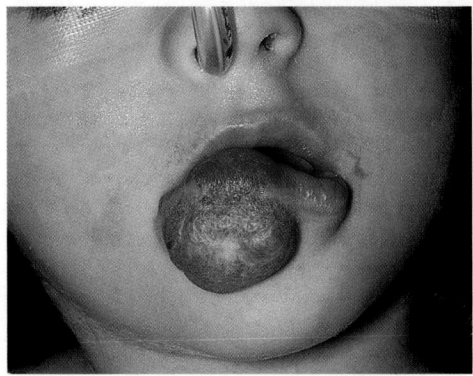
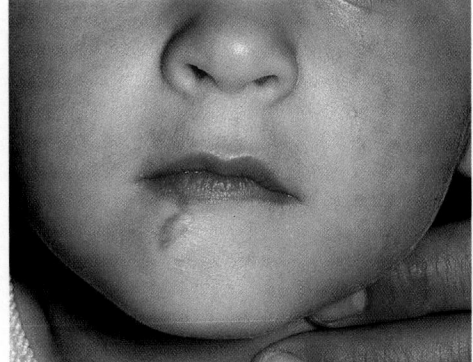

A B

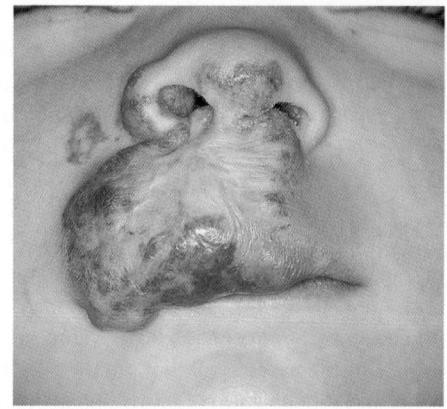 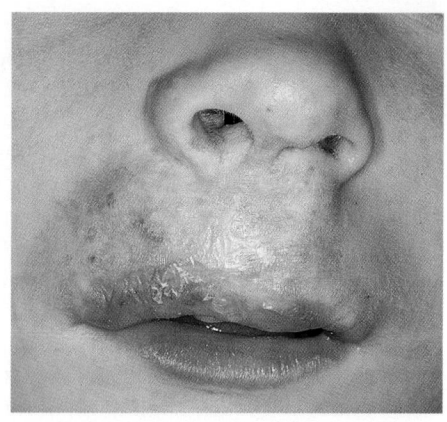

FIGURE 15 An upper-lip hemangioma before **(A)** and after **(B)** resection, flash lamp pumped dye laser treatment, and skin resurfacing. An 18-month interval separates these pictures.

ing of the collagen and smoothing of the surface irregularities. Rarely, a high spot should be treated with a third pass. In this way, the entire surface can be smoothed and reepithelialization will take place within 10 to 12 days. Postoperative wound care consists of twice-daily cleansing with a gentle soap and the application of a hydrogel or a hydrocolloid type dressing. Although the technique described uses a Silktouch system, similar results can be expected with any of the skin-resurfacing lasers.

Residual fibrofatty tissue or any contour abnormality should be treated with surgical resection. Once again, during resection, meticulous attention should be paid to hemostasis and either a Shaw scalpel or contact Nd:YAG laser surgical techniques are helpful. The resection should be individualized for each patient and should follow the principles of cosmetic surgery. It should be noted that it is often not necessary to completely resect a residual hemangioma. Debulking or partial resection may be all that is necessary as the objective is to obtain adequate cosmesis. Any residual hemangioma will continue along its process of involution and eventually become fibrofatty tissue. If this is known and taken into consideration, the patient may be spared an unnecessary resection.

In an approach to a compound hemangioma, the principles described above should be followed. When one is planning treatment, the cutaneous component should always be dealt with first. In this way, the surgeon will be able to incise through treated skin and raise a flap in a relatively bloodless plane. The skin is thus available for reconstruction.

FIGURE 16 An extensive parotid hemangioma with early ulceration in a child before **(A)** and after **(B)** resection. This child was left with weakness in the marginal mandibular branch. All other branches were intact.

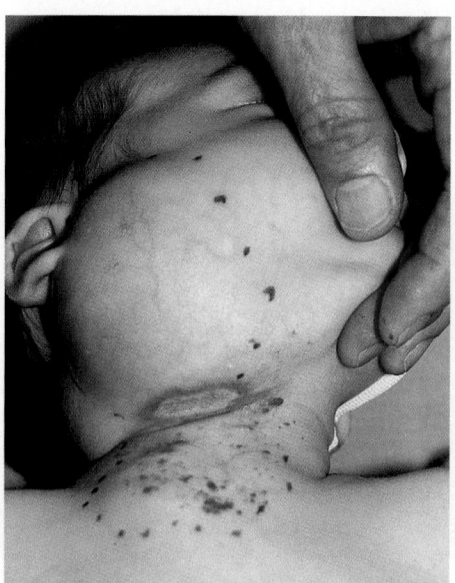 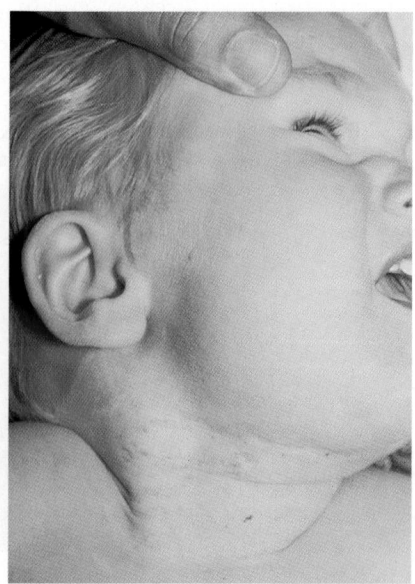

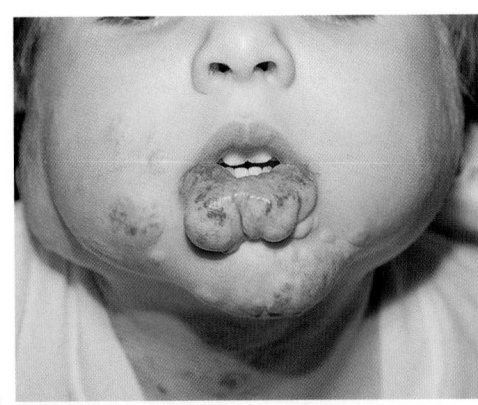
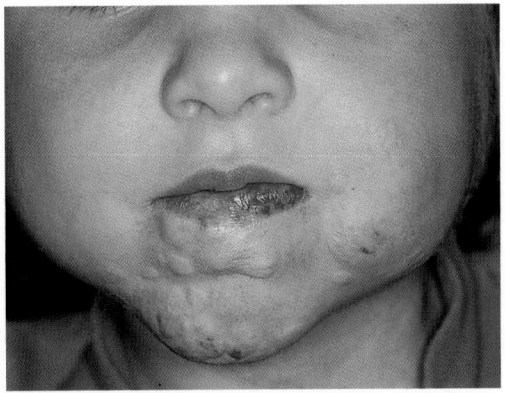

A   B

FIGURE 17 An extensive lower-lip hemangioma before **(A)** and after **(B)** resection.

Late Involution

During this phase, most of the vascular channels have disappeared. However, a few persist as dilated vessels. These will be visible as cutaneous telangiectasia in a superficial hemangioma. Unfortunately, the hemangioma will have replaced the papillary dermis with fibrofatty tissue and an atrophic scar is common. Excessive subcutaneous fibrofatty tissue may also be left at the end of involution. In general, the telangiectasia can be treated with a copper vapor laser or a flash lamp pumped dye laser. The atrophic scarring responds well to skin resurfacing with a silk touch or an ultrapulse CO_2 laser system and the residual fibrofatty tissue should be resected where appropriate (Fig. 17).

Vascular Malformations

Given that vascular malformations never involute, the rationale for their treatment requires no justification. However, the choice of treatment will depend on several factors; these include the vascular content of the lesion, its anatomic location, and its depth.

One should also bear in mind the natural history of the lesion and choose the most appropriate time for treatment. In general, superficial lesions are best treated with laser photocoagulation, deeper lesions should be surgically excised, and compound lesions treated with a combination of laser photocoagulation and then surgical resection.

Arteriovenous Malformations

Arteriovenous malformations are among the most difficult of the vascular malformations to manage. The object of treatment should be complete irradiation of the nidus of the arteriovenous malformation, and surgical resection is the only way to accomplish this (Fig. 18) (23). Since the margins of the nidus are often unclear, it is very difficult to know just how much to resects. Any residium left behind at the end of surgery will invariably result in a recurrence. Embolization is not curative but can be used as a temporizing measure. Ligation of a feeding vessel should be discouraged, since these lesions have such a rich collateral circulation and will invariably revascularize. Furthermore, if a branch of the external carotid artery is tied off, and a collateral develops from a branch of the internal carotid system, preoperative immobilization will become impossible.

Preoperative planning is essential. The full extent of the nidus should be determined and both digital subtraction angiography and MRI are useful. The surgeon may elect to embolize the lesion 24 to 48 hours preoperatively. This is sometimes helpful in reducing intraoperative hemorrhage. At operation, it is imperative to identify and remove the entire nidus. The dilated venous drainage and hypertrophied afferent blood supply need not be removed together with the nidus, as they have developed in response to the increased shunting across the nidus. Removal of the nidus will usually reverse these processes. The presence of a vascular blush involving the overlying skin is indicative of the

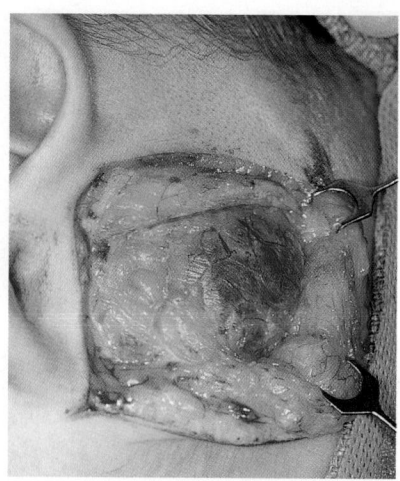

FIGURE 18 A nidus of an arteriovenous malformation.

fact that the overlying skin is involved in the disease process and therefore should be resected en bloc with the nidus. Intraoperative frozen section control is difficult to interpret, since many of the changes are dynamic and are more related to the increased shunting than the underlying abnormality itself. If possible, the margins of resection should be well beyond the anatomic confines of the nidus (as determined by MRI and angiography).

Venous Malformations

The advent of lasers has enhanced the ability to treat these lesions. The choice of treatment will once again depend on several factors. These include the depth of the lesion, its anatomic location, and its extent. In general, a Nd:YAG laser or a copper vapor laser should be used to treat the superficial component of the lesion, whereas surgical resection should be reserved for a deeper component. A lesion involving a cutaneous or mucosal surface, as well as deeper structures, should be treated in the first instance with laser photocoagulation and then followed with surgical resection. The role of sclerosing agents is still not yet settled. Sclerotherapy has evolved into a viable alternative and can be used alone or in conjunction with laser photocoagulation or surgical resection. The choice of sclerosing agent is largely up to the surgeon or interventional radiologist. Hypertonic saline (23.4%), sodium tetradecyl sulfate (Sotradecol), and Ethiblock have all been used with some degree of success. It is currently believed that sclerosing agents should be used more as an adjuvant rather than as a sole modality of treatment.

Laser Photocoagulation   The impressive vasoconstriction seen with laser photocoagulation is often sufficient to completely eradicate a superficial lesion. Although the precise mechanism of this vasoconstriction is still unknown, it is believed to be due to thermal coagulation of the wall of the blood vessel and its surrounding tissue. Copper vapor lasers are appropriate for very superficial lesions and are used in the following way: With a 150-μm spot size and 300 mW of power, the laser light is chopped or gated at 0.2-second intervals. The focused spot should be moved slowly over the entire lesion, looking for an end point of vasoconstriction. This technique works best for mucosal lesions, especially those involving the lips and buccal mucosa. Deeper components, often found in areas such as the tongue, lips, and buccal mucosa, are beyond the depth of penetration of light emitted by a copper vapor laser and are best treated with a Nd:YAG laser. The near infrared wavelength emitted by this laser will penetrate up to 3 mm of tissue and will cause nonspecific thermal heating, which, in turn, results in vasoconstriction. The tissue will then heal with scar formation, and fibrous tissue will replace the ectatic vascular malformation. The technique by which this laser is used has been well described. A 600-mm fiber is held perpendicular to and about 2 mm off the surface of the tissue. Using be-

TABLE 3: Treatment with a Neadymium Yttrium-Aluminum-Garnet Laser

Flat cut fiber held perpendicular and 1–2mm off surface
Series of impactions 1–2mm apart
30-W 0.2–0.3-sec exposures (mucosal)
30-W 0.1-sec exposures (skin)

tween 30 and 40 W of power and an exposure time of between 0.2 and 0.3 second, a grid of treatment spots is placed, 2 mm apart (Table 3). Since the epicenter of the thermal effect is just below the surface of the mucosa, a small blanched spot less than 1 mm in diameter, seen on the surface of the mucosa, is an appropriate end point (Fig. 19). Any more than this is excessive and will result in confluent necrosis. If deeper penetration is required, the surface can be compressed with a glass slide and treated through the slide. This technique is most useful for full-thickness tongue lesions, as well as deep mucosal lesions.

Although the Nd:YAG laser has been used to treat through skin, the risk of scarring is far greater, and this laser should be used with caution in this circumstance. To avoid extensive skin damage, the exposure time should never be greater than one-tenth of a second and the points of treatment should be at least 2 mm apart. If necessary, two or even three treatments, using these parameters and spaced at 6-week intervals, will be appropriate. The most obvious immediate effect is a reduction in the volume of the lesion caused by the combined effect of vasoconstriction and coagulative necrosis of the interstitium. However, swelling soon sets in and may last up to 5 or 6 days. This can be prevented or diminished by a short 3-day course of oral prednisone. An exudative slough will appear around day 3 and will finally separate once the area has been fully reepithelialized (around 14 to 21 days). Secondary hemorrhage seen between 7 and 10 days after treatment is possible but is usually self-limiting and can be controlled with gentle, but firm pressure. Occasionally, a bleeder needs to be oversewn.

Postoperatively, frequent application of an antibiotic ointment or simple petrolatum, or if the oral cavity has been treated, frequent mouthwashes are all that is necessary. Pain is not usually severe and can be easily remedied with a nonnarcotic analgesic. Nonsteroidal antibiotics should be avoided owing to effect on platelets.

Surgery   Dissection of massive thin-walled ectatic veins that frequently cross tissue planes can be challenging. Since these lesions expand much more slowly, they are nonen-

FIGURE 19 A venous malformation involving the buccal mucosa before **(A)** and immediately after **(B)** neodymium:yttrium-aluminum-garnet laser treatments. Each of the blanched dots represents an area of treatment. Note the 2 to 3 mm separation of the treatment spots. Note the considerable shrinkage of the venous malformation immediately following treatment.

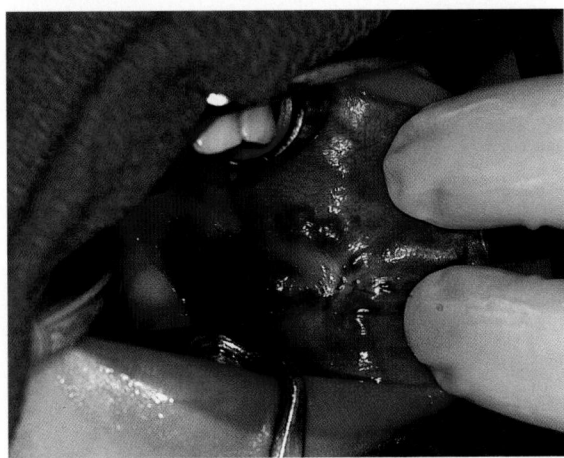
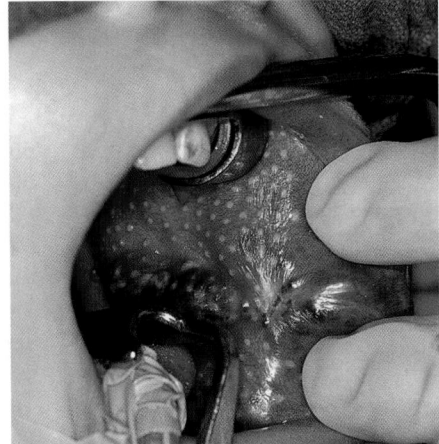

A   B

capsulated and are more inclined to infiltrate soft tissue structures, especially muscle. It is therefore imperative that the surgeon be fully appraised of the full anatomic extent of the lesion. Once again, a Shaw scalpel or contact Nd:YAG laser is helpful and particular attention should be paid to hemostasis. The surgeon should attempt to dissect completely outside the malformation since the thin-walled vessels are very difficult to coagulate once they have been transected. In the face of uncontrolled intraoperative bleeding, the surgeon may have to resort to the use of hemoclips to control the hemorrhage. Bipolar electrocautery is essential when dissecting around the facial nerve (Fig. 20).

Sclerotherapy   Sclerosing agents should be used more as an adjuvant to surgery or laser photocoagulation. Since there are no valves within the facial veins, the middle third of the face should be avoided, as cavernous sinus thrombosis may complicate sclerotherapy. Several sclerosing agents have been used. These include hypertonic saline (23%), Ethoxysclerol, Ethiblock, and sodium tetradecyl sulfate (Sotradecol). It is best to administer the sclerosing agent with the help of screening. An indwelling catheter should be inserted transcutaneously into the venous malformation. A test dose of dye should then be given to ascertain the direction of flow. Flow away from the central nervous system, toward the internal jugular vein, is favorable and will enable one to proceed with the administration of the sclerosing agent. If, on the other hand, the test dose of dye proceeds through the cavernous sinus, no sclerosing agent should be given and the procedure should be aborted.

Lymphatic Malformations

Lymphatic malformations may be localized or diffuse, superficial or deep. Localized cystic lesions are more inclined to occur in the neck, whereas diffuse involvement of the lower third of the face is much more common. Superficial, mucosal, or cutaneous involvement is manifested by the presence of small, fluid-filled vesicles. These are commonly referred to as *lymphangioma circumscriptum*. The treatment of the superficial mucosal lesions depends on whether or not a deeper component is present. In the presence of a deeper component, an attempt should be made to excise the entire lymphatic malformation as completely as possible. If this is not possible, a CO_2 laser can be used to vaporize the mucosal vesicles. Since each vesicle is connected to a deeper reservoir of lymphatic fluid, the CO_2 laser vaporization technique should be aggressive. In the presence of vesicles on the tongue, vaporization should be continued into the muscle of the tongue in an attempt to vaporize the deeper component of the lymphatic vesicle. It may be advisable to treat individual strips of tongue, since reepithelialization will take place from the sides of the untreated areas.

Surgical resection is extremely difficult since the lymphatic malformation will usually cross tissue planes. Muscular involvement is common, so complete resection of the

FIGURE 20 The extensive venous malformation shown in Figure 8 was treated surgically. All the branches of the facial nerve were preserved and functioning.

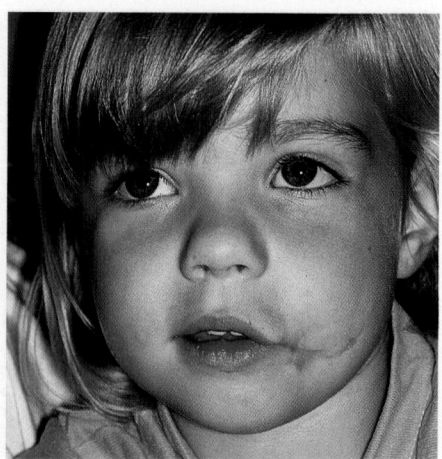

lesion is extremely difficult. Recurrence is frequent, and several procedures may need to be undertaken to eradicate the lesion. During resection of extensive cervicofacial lesions, one must expect to have to return to the same anatomic area at some later stage. It is therefore prudent to place some sort of marker in close proximity to important structures, such as the facial nerve. This will facilitate subsequent procedures.

Venular Malformations

Midline venular malformations respond well to treatment with a flash lamp pumped dye laser. Usually only one or two treatments are necessary to obtain a complete response (17). With a 5-mm spot size and a power setting of between 6 and 6.65 J per square centimeter, the lesion is treated in the usual manner with a 10% overlap of the spots, so that the entire surface of lesion has been covered. An end point of purpura is appropriate.

For the most part, *venular malformations* are also treated with a flash lamp pumped dye laser. The technique is the same as that described previously. For facial lesions, up to 7.5 to 8.0 J-per square centimeter may be necessary. Neck lesions should be treated with caution, since the neck is an underprivileged area and is thus more apt to scar. A fluence of up to 6 J per square centimeter is appropriate. Postoperatively, the patient is instructed to avoid excessive trauma to the area. The skin should be washed two to three times a day in a normal fashion and blotted dry rather than rubbed dry. Any scabbing should be covered with frequent applications of a thin film of bacitracin or bacitracin zinc–polymyxin B sulfate (Polysporin) ointment. The purpura, as well as any scabs, can be expected to resolve within a 10- to 12-day, period. Postinflammatory hyperpigmentation is a fairly frequent complication but will resolve spontaneously within 6 to 8 weeks of treatment. Multiple treatments spaced at 12- to 24-week intervals may be necessary. Up to 10 to 12 treatments may need to be administered, until a satisfactory response has been obtained.

Thick, hypertrophic, or cobblestoned port-wine stains may first need to be treated with a copper vapor laser using the same technique as that described for venous malformations; the entire lesion can be treated in stages. Using an end point of blanching or graying of the lesion, one can expect some epidermal destruction. Therefore, crusting will develop and a moist wound dressing, such as hydrogel or hydrocolloid, is preferable. Complete healing can be expected within 10 to 12 days, and subsequent treatments can usually be carried out with a flash lamp pumped dye laser (Fig. 21). The object of using the copper vapor laser in the first instance is to destroy the thick, hypertrophied, or cobblestoned areas of the port-wine stain. Once this has been accomplished, treatment with a flash lamp pumped dye laser will be sufficient to destroy the ectatic vascular tissue.

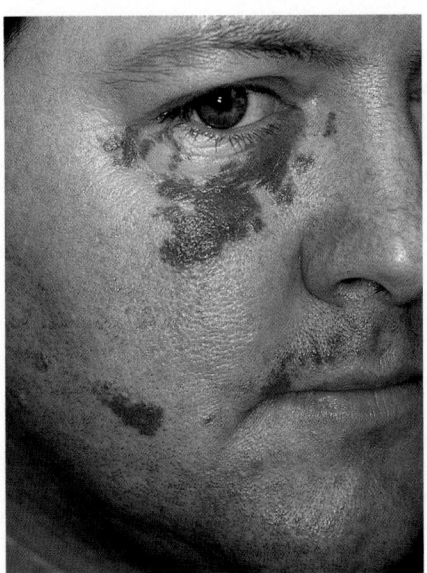 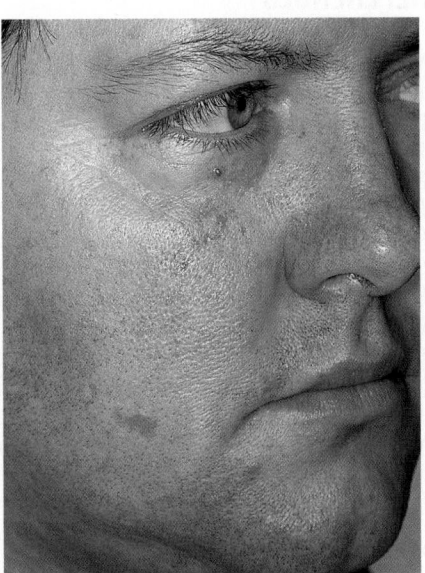

A   **B**

FIGURE 21 A venular malformation before **(A)** and after **(B)** treatment with a copper vapor laser followed by a flash lamp pumped dye laser.

Recently, several investigators began using skin-resurfacing techniques with a CO_2 laser to treat thick, cobblestoned, or hypertrophied areas of a port-wine stain. With these techniques and three or four passes with an appropriate CO_2 laser, it is possible to ablate the hypertrophied areas of a port-wine stain. The mechanism of skin resurfacing appears to be thermal-related collagen denaturation, which, in turn, results in a shrinking of the papillary dermis. Since the ectatic vessels that make up the port-wine stain are situated within the papillary dermis, shrinking of this layer will tend to ablate the vessels. At the same time, treatment with a flash lamp pumped dye laser in the usual fashion will result in a synergistic effect. It is believed that this technique is probably safer than using a copper vapor laser and will become the treatment of choice for thick hypertrophied port-wine stains.

With the above techniques, only between 15% and 20% of port-wine stains will clear completely. However, the vast majority will lighten significantly and between 10 and 12 treatments may be necessary to accomplish this. It is therefore important the patient be made aware of this at the commencement of treatment. Complications include epidermal atrophy, hypertrophic scarring, and postinflammatory hyperpigmentation. Hypopigmentation is also seen, especially after repeated treatments. The complication rate is low and remains at around 1% to 2%. A rather disturbing finding was recently reported by Waner and Orten (26). In a long-term follow-up of over 100 patients, they found that port-wine stains which had not completely disappeared appeared to return after a variable period. The recurrence rate is not known and the time to recurrence appears to be variable. The longer the interval between the last treatment and the follow-up, the higher the recurrence rate. Since a port-wine stain is considered to be a "sick dermatome" in which the cutaneous plexus is devoid of autonomic innervation, any remaining vessels will simply undergo progressive ectasia and therefore the port-wine stain will recur. To prevent this, it may be necessary to administer maintenance treatments at 3- to 4-year intervals. This possibility is currently being investigated.

Mixed Malformations

The treatment of a mixed malformation should be determined by the vascular components present. In keeping with the principles prescribed throughout this chapter, a superficial lesion should be treated with a laser, whereas a deep lesion should be excised. Compound lesions should be treated first with laser photocoagulation and then with excision.

 REFERENCES

1. Mulliken JB, Glowacki J. Hemangiomas and vascular malformations in infants and children: a classification based on endothelial characteristics. *Plast Reconstr Surg* 1982;69:412–422.
2. Holmdahl K. Cutaneous hemangiomas in premature and mature infants. *Acta Paediatr* 1955;44:370.
3. Jacobs AH. Strawberry hemangiomas: the natural history of the untreated lesion. *Cal Med* 1957;86:8.
4. Hidano A, Nakajima S. Earliest features of the strawberry birthmark in the newborn. *Br J Dermatol* 1972;87:138.
5. Pratt AG. Birthmarks in infants. *Arch Dermatol* 1967;67:302.
6. Waner M, Suen JY. Treatment of hemangiomas of the head and neck. *Laryngoscope* 1992;102:1123–1132.
7. Finn MD, Glowacki J, Mulliken JB. Congenital vascular lesions: clinical application of a new classification. *J Pediatr Surg* 1983;18:894.
8. Margileth AM, Museles M. Cutaneous hemangiomas in children: diagnosis and conservative management. *JAMA* 1965;194:135.
9. Lister WA. The natural history of strawberry naevai. *Lancet* 1938;1:1429–1434.
10. Bowers RE, Graham EA, Tomlinson KM. The natural history of the strawberry nevus. *Arch Dermatol* 1960;82:667.

11. Sadan N, Wolach B. Treatment of hemangiomas of infants with big doses of prednisone. *J Pediatr* 1996;128:141–146.
12. Berman B, Lim HWP. Concurrent cutaneous and hepatic hemangiomata in infancy: report of a case and a review of the literature. *J Dermatol Surg Oncol* 1978;4:869.
13. Robb RM. Refractive errors associated with hemangiomas of the eyelids and orbit in infancy. *Am J Ophthalmol* 1977;83:52.
14. Kasabach HH, Merritt KK. Capillary hemangioma with extensive purpura. *Am J Dis Child* 1940;59:1063.
15. Waner M, Kincannon J. Vascular malformations of the lips. *Arch Otolaryngol Head Neck Surg (in press)*.
16. Barsky SH, Rosen S, Geer DE, Noe J. The nature and evolution of port wine stains: a computer assisted study. *J Invest Dermatol* 1980;74:154.
17. Orton S, Waner M, Flock S. A longterm follow-up of the treatment of port wine stains. *Arch Otolaryngol Head Neck Surg (in press)*.
18. Oster J, Nielson A. Nudra naevi and intercapular telangiectasis. *Acta Paediatr Scand* 1970;59:416.
19. Pratt AG. Birthmarks in infants. *Arch Dermatol* 1967;67:302.
20. Smoller BR, Rosen S. Port wine stains: a disease of altered neural modulation of blood vessels. *Arch Dermatol* 1986;122:177.
21. Young AE. Arteriovenous malformations. In: Mulliken JB, Young AE, eds. *Vascular birthmarks, hemangiomas and malformations.* Philadelphia: WB Saunders, 1988.
22. Sako Y, Varco R. Arteriovenous fistula: results of management of congenital and acquired forms, blood flow measurements, and observations on proximal arterial degeneration. *Surgery* 1970;67:40.
23. Baker L, Waner M, Suen JY. Arteriovenous malformations. *Arch Otolaryngol Head Neck Surg (in press)*.
24. Waner M, Suen JY, Dinehart S, Mallory SB. Laser photocoagulation of superficial proliferating hemangiomas. *J Dermatol Surg Oncol* 1994;20:1–4.
25. Mulliken JB, Lawrence MB, Kozbe T, Oblnis L, Folkmar J, Eyekowitz AB. Pharmacologic therapy for endangering hemangiomas. *Curr Opin Dermatol* 1995 :109–113.
26. Waner M, Orten S. A recurrence of port wine stains after treatment. *Dermatol Surg (in press)*.

M. Waner and C. M. Bower: Department of Otolaryngology, University of Arkansas for Medical Sciences, and Arkansas Children's Hospital, Little Rock, Arkansas 72205.

• *Practical Pediatric Otolaryngology*
• edited by Robin T. Cotton and Charles M. Myer, III
• Lippincott-Raven Publishers, Philadelphia © 1999

Difficult Cases in Pediatric Otolaryngology

Section Editors

Brian J. Wiatrak & George H. Zalzal

Management of Frontal Sinusitis

Thomas M. Andrews

❓ INITIAL PRESENTATION

A 12-year-old girl presented to the office with symptoms of chronic sinusitis for the last 5 to 7 months. Her major symptoms included frontal headache and maxillary facial pain. She had complaints of postnasal drip, occasional periorbital swelling, and irritability, as well as losing interest in sports. She had been treated in the past with multiple antibiotics including beta-lactamase-stable antimicrobials with some minimal relief, although symptoms returned when therapy was discontinued. The patient had had a complete allergy/immunology workup, which was negative. She had been treated with antihistamines and decongestants without relief. She continued to see an allergist and use nasal steroids intermittently. The family history was positive for inhalant allergies. There was no history of gastroesophageal reflux or related symptoms. There was no family history of headaches. Past radiographic examinations included plain films demonstrating maxillary and right frontal sinus opacification. The child did not have reactive airway disease, cystic fibrosis, any immune deficiency by testing, or diabetes, nor did she complain of frequent ear infections. She had no previous sinus surgery.

❓ PHYSICAL EXAMINATION

On physical examination, the patient was a healthy, well-developed, well-nourished white girl. She had no facial swelling. The only positive findings were the nasal mucosa, which appeared slightly erythematous but not atopic, bilateral posterior cervical adenopathy and point tenderness over the right frontal sinus, and tenderness over both temporomandibular joints with tenderness of the temporalis muscle bilaterally. A recent evaluation by an orthodontist showed no dental or occlusal problems.

❓ DIFFERENTIAL DIAGNOSES

The patient exhibited signs and symptoms suggestive of sinusitis, temporomandibular joint (TMJ) syndrome, or migraine headaches. Most obvious were signs and symptoms of sinusitis, such as postnasal drip, periorbital swelling, maxillary facial pain, and frontal headaches. The differential diagnosis included TMJ syndrome. She exhibited classic physical examination signs of this syndrome demonstrated by TMJ tenderness and temporalis muscle pain. Other cranial neuralgias were less likely given the patient's signs and symptoms. The differential diagnosis should also include migraine headache; however, she did not have classic migraine symptoms, such as prodrome, visual changes, or nausea with headache pain. There was no family history of migraine headaches.

At this point history and physical examination were most consistent with frontal sinusitis and TMJ syndrome.

💬 INITIAL MANAGEMENT

The patient was treated with soft diet, warm compresses, and ibuprofen, as well as systemic and topical decongestants and beta-lactamase-stable oral antimicrobials. TMJ pain resolved after approximately 4 days of treatment. The patient continued to have significant headaches and frontal sinus tenderness. Medical therapy continued for 30 days, including intranasal steroids, systemic decongestants, and alternating 10-day courses of second- and third-generation oral cephalosporins. Coronal and axial computed tomography (CT) scans of the paranasal sinuses were obtained (Fig. 1).

💬 SURGICAL MANAGEMENT

The patient underwent an endoscopic approach to both ethmoid and maxillary sinuses to alleviate obstruction of the osteomeatal complex. The right nasofrontal duct was approached endoscopically. The patient did well after surgery and had immediate relief of her symptoms. She remained symptom free for several months, after which she returned with complaints of recurrent frontal headaches. She was treated with topical and systemic decongestants and Augmentin. After 3 weeks of therapy with no diminution in symptoms, the patient had a repeat coronal (limited) CT scan demonstrating bilateral frontal sinus disease. The patient underwent a revision endoscopic approach to both maxillary and frontal sinuses. This revealed purulent material draining from both frontal sinuses that demonstrated no bacterial growth.

Minor relief occurred after this procedure, but she continued to have frontal headaches. External frontal sinusotomies were performed revealing a copious amount of

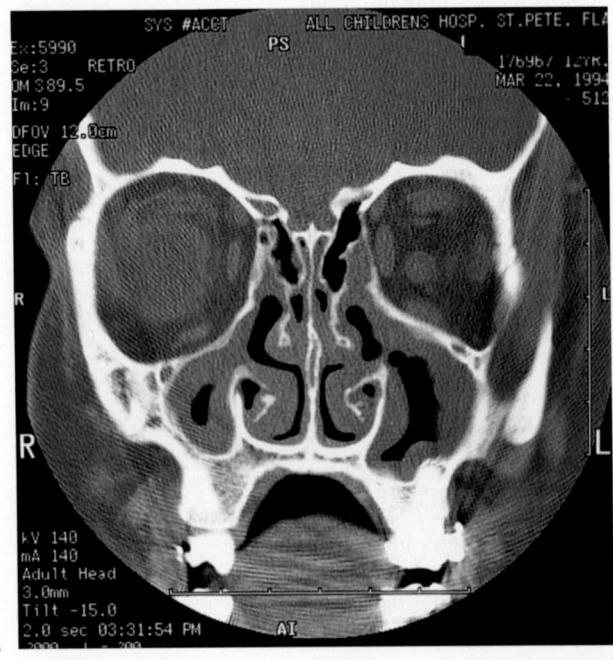
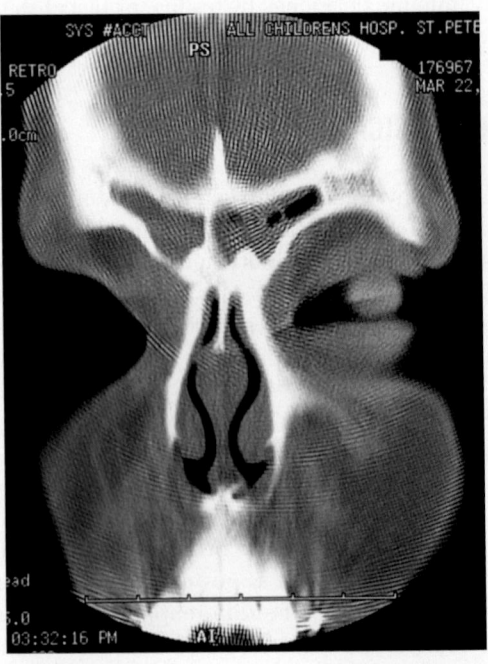

FIGURE 1 Initial coronal computed tomography scan with evidence of bilateral maxillary **(A)** and frontal **(B)** sinus disease.

polyploid tissue and purulent discharge. Microbiologic cultures did not demonstrate growth (including fungal and anaerobic). Pathologic cultures revealed chronic inflammatory infiltrates. The patient was symptom free after this procedure for several months.

Six months later the patient presented complaining of frontal headaches and was initially treated with oral antimicrobials. This time, oral steroids (Pediapred 20 mg per day) were added. Her headaches continued to worsen and the patient was admitted for intravenous antibiotics (Timentin). A CT scan of the head was performed to rule out any intracranial extension of her previously known frontal sinus disease; the scan was negative. Steroids were discontinued, the patient was placed on cefuroxime i.v. (150 mg per kilogram per day), and topical and systemic decongestants were used. After 72 hours, she had some minor relief, and after 5 days, she had much milder headaches. Treatment was continued for 10 days, and then a coronal CT scan revealed persistent bilateral frontal sinus disease. At this time, a combination intranasal and external approach to the frontal sinuses was performed. Surgical findings included polypoid tissue obstructing both nasofrontal ducts and a thick, mucoid fluid in both frontal sinuses. A culture revealed *Hemophilus influenzae*, (not beta-lactamase positive) and *Moraxella catarrhalis*. The patient received intravenous Cefuroxime postoperatively for an additional 10 days.

She remained symptom free on prolonged therapy with an oral antimicrobial (Cefprozil 15 mg per kilogram per day) for approximately 2 months when, once again, she developed severe headaches. A coronal CT scan revealed frontal sinus disease.

Decision Point 1

The options at this time included additional intravenous antibiotics, a repeat frontal sinus trephination, and/or placement of a nasofrontal stent. The decision is based on the degree of symptoms, amount of outflow tract obstruction, and the possibility of further scarring.

Two stents made from size 1 Shiley pediatric tracheotomy tube shafts were placed from the frontal sinus to the middle meatus using a widened trephine combined with an endoscopic intranasal approach (Fig. 2). Ciliary biopsies were taken and found to be normal. Pathology revealed chronic inflammatory infiltrates, and cultures grew rare *Staphylococcus aureus* and rare *H. influenzae* type III.

The stents were pulled after 4 months, and endoscopic evaluation revealed well-mucosalized nasofrontal ducts. The patient did well for 6 weeks, when she returned with a frontal headache. A CT scan found the frontal sinuses clear and the nasofrontal duct patent.

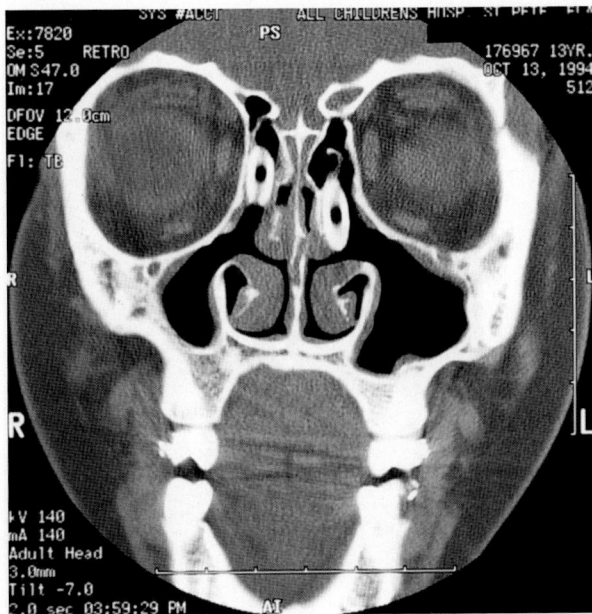

FIGURE 2 Coronal CT after placement of nasofrontal stents.

Decision Point 2

With continued symptoms and a negative CT scan, other etiologies considered were osteomyelitis, migraine headaches, or intermittent nasofrontal duct obstruction. Technetium bone scan revealed no evidence of osteomyelitis (1). A neurology consult was obtained, and migraine headache treatment was initiated without significant resolution of her symptoms after several medical trials.

She presented once again with disabling headaches while using Toradol for headache pain. CT scan showed evidence of mucosal thickening within both frontal sinuses and opacification consistent with continued mucosal changes and a nonpatent nasofrontal duct. It was clear the patient suffered from nonpatent nasofrontal ducts. A frontal sinus obliteration was performed through a bicoronal flap utilizing autologous cancellous bone from the right hip. The nasofrontal ducts were sealed with temporalis muscle and fascia. The patient had complete resolution of headaches. A recent CT scan demonstrates ossification of her frontal sinuses (Fig. 3).

FINAL OUTCOME

The patient has now resumed her normal lifestyle and activities, has had no cosmetic complaints from the bicoronal flap, and has had no discomfort, chronic pain, or ambulation difficulties from the right hip cancellous bone graft.

PROBLEM-FOCUSED DISCUSSION

The patient with chronic frontal sinusitis can be an extremely difficult management problem. Aggressive medical therapy is the treatment of choice in most cases of frontal sinusitis. Surgical instrumentation of the nasofrontal duct or ostia may lead to stenosis and subsequent long-term difficulties.

In 50% of frontal sinusitis cases, aggressive medical management consisting of intravenous antibiotics is successful (2). This was previously the treatment of choice for frontal sinus disease. Mild cases of frontal sinusitis are treated with beta-lactamase-stable antimicrobials, intranasal steroids, and/or decongestants, as well as systemic decon-

FIGURE 3 Coronal CT demonstrating ossification of frontal sinus 2 years after autologous cancellous bone graft.

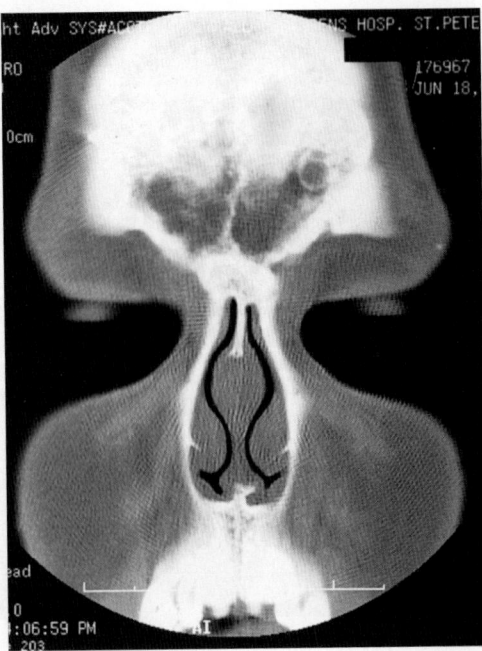

gestants on an outpatient basis. Appropriate testing should be obtained to assess allergies, systemic illnesses such as ciliary dysfunction, or cystic fibrosis in appropriate cases.

Indications for surgery include failure to resolve symptoms with medical therapy, progression of disease, or impending complications. Surgical management includes endoscopic and open techniques. The endoscopic approach should be considered initially, with a goal of opening the nasofrontal duct, thereby allowing decompression of the frontal sinuses (3,4). External frontal sinusotomies (or trephines) can be utilized for placement of irrigation catheters to flush the sinus, allowing visualization intranasally of the nasofrontal duct. With recently developed instrumentation, the nasofrontal duct may be decompressed without injuring the mucosa, thus averting stenosis. Avoidance of trauma to the nasofrontal duct will help lead to long-term patency.

More aggressive external approaches may be used combining wide frontal sinus trephination with nasal endoscopy. Endoscopic sinus instruments can be used through the trephination (5,6). Flaps may be used to reconstruct the nasofrontal duct once it has become occluded (7). Stents have also been used to ensure patency of the nasofrontal duct (8). The optimal length of time for stent placement has not been determined, but the author uses a minimum of 12 weeks.

Once the nasofrontal duct has been traumatized, either surgically or by placement of a stent, there is a certain irreversibility of that action, for if that maneuver fails there are only a few options left to the surgeon if disease recurs. Endoscopic enlargement of the nasofrontal duct may be attempted (3,4). Another method is the modified Lothrop procedure, which has recently become more popular (9). This procedure allows endoscopic decompression by removal of the floor of the frontal sinus and widening the nasofrontal duct, thus making it less likely to stenose.

A more aggressive procedure is obliteration of the frontal sinus cavity itself. This can be done with either autologous tissue (fat or cancellous bone) or synthetic materials. The use of fat for obliteration, although it has led to several problems, has been very successful in the past (10,11). The most challenging problem is diagnosis of a patient with recurrent frontal sinus headaches or pain with an autologous fat graft in place in which saponification has occurred. Current imaging studies are able to distinguish between infection and fat necrosis and/or saponification when both CT and magnetic resonance imaging are obtained (12).

Autologous cancellous bone graft was successful in this patient. It removes the diagnostic dilemma of recurrent infection versus fat saponification if the patient returns with recurrent symptoms (13). It should only be considered when normal medical and surgical management techniques have been exhausted.

PEARLS AND PERILS

1. Frontal sinusitis should initially be treated with aggressive medical management including antimicrobials, decongestants, and nasal steroids.
2. In the face of recurrent frontal sinusitis, consider underlying conditions that may lead to treatment failure (i.e., allergies, ciliary dysfunction, cystic fibrosis) and obtain appropriate testing.
3. In surgical therapy of the frontal sinus, care should be taken not to traumatize the nasofrontal duct.
4. With improved instrumentation and visualization, an endoscopic approach to the frontal sinus has improved the surgical outcome in this disease without extensive obliterative procedures.
5. Procedures involving extensive endoscopic resection, such as the modified Lothrop procedure, should first be attempted on cadaveric specimens prior to clinical use.
6. Frontal sinus obliteration is an extreme but successful surgical option for patients who have failed more traditional endoscopic open techniques.

⚙REFERENCES

1. Goshen E, Zwas ST, Sadan M, Kronenberg J. The combined use of classified bone and gallium scans in the management of frontal sinusitis. *Nucl Med Commun* 1994;15:331–336.
2. Middleton WG, Briant TDR, Fenton RS. Frontal sinusitis—a 10 year experience. *J Otolaryngol* 1985;14:197–200.
3. Har-El G, Lucente FE. Endoscopic intra-nasofrontal sinusotomy. *Laryngoscope* 1995;105:440–443.
4. Perko D. Endoscopic surgery of the frontal sinus without external approach. *Rhinology* 1989;27:119–123.
5. Rawest L, Jannert M, Malm L. Resection of the interfrontal sinus septum in chronic or recurrent frontal sinusitis. Pre- and post-operative evaluation of the naso-frontal duct. *Clin Otolaryngol* 1985;10:151–155.
6. Gerber ME, Myer CM III, Prenger EC. Transcutaneous frontal sinus trephination with endoscopic visualization of the nasofrontal communication. *Am J Otolaryngol* 1993;14:55–59.
7. Boyden GL. Surgical treatment of chronic frontal sinusitis. *Ann Otol Rhinol Laryngol* 1952;61:558–566.
8. Metson R. Endoscopic treatment of frontal sinusitis. *Laryngoscope* 1992;102:712–716.
9. Becker DG, Moore D, Lindsey WH, Gross WE, Gross CW. Modified transnasal endoscopic Lothrop procedure: further considerations. *Laryngoscope* 1995;105:1161–1166.
10. Montgomery WW. *Surgery of the upper respiratory system.* Philadelphia: Lea & Febiger, 1979:117–165.
11. Schenck NL. Frontal sinus disease: III. Experimental and clinical factors in the failure of the frontal osteopathic operation. *Laryngoscope* 1975;85:76–92.
12. Catalano PJ, Lawson W, Som P, Biller HF. Radiographic evaluation and diagnosis of the failed frontal osteoplastic flap with fat obliteration. *Otolaryngol Head Neck Surg* 1991;104:225–234.
13. Shumrick KA, Smith CP. The use of cancellous bone for frontal sinus obliteration and reconstruction of frontal body defects. *Arch Otolaryngol Head Neck Surg* 1994;120:1003–1009.

T.M. Andrews: Departments of Otolaryngology and Pediatrics, University of South Florida, St. Petersburg, Florida 33701.

Laryngeal Trauma

Thomas M. Andrews

❓ INITIAL PRESENTATION

A 4-year-old girl suffered a dog bite injury to the larynx from a Rottweiler. Initially, she underwent emergency examination and workup at an outlying community hospital. The cervical spine was cleared, and head and neck examination revealed dog bite puncture wounds near the anterior thyroid cartilage, including the cricothyroid membrane. An emergency cricothyroidotomy was performed through the existing dog bite injury. Two days later the patient was transferred to a children's hospital.

❓ PHYSICAL EXAMINATION

Examination revealed that the cricothyroidotomy was still in place. The patient was aphonic, and abrasions around the anterior neck were noted. The tracheotomy site was revised in the operating room. Microlaryngoscopy and bronchoscopy revealed that the patient had a right true cord avulsion injury (Fig. 1).

❓ DIFFERENTIAL DIAGNOSES

In cases of penetrating laryngeal trauma, other cervical structures such as the carotid sheath, cranial nerves, pharynx, or esophagus may be injured and should be assessed. Angiography will be necessary in cases of expanding hematomas or suspicious vascular trauma and zone I or zone III injuries (Fig. 2). Angiography is necessary in zone I injury due to the high likelihood of great vessel involvement in the upper chest and medi-

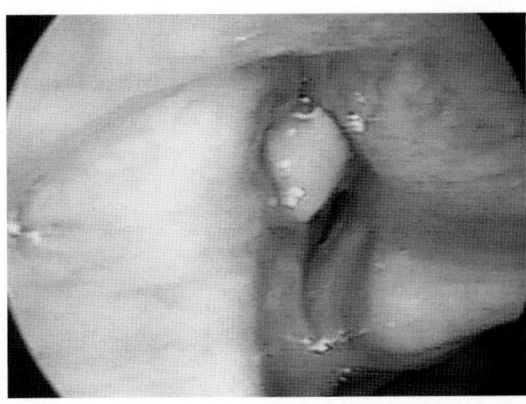

FIGURE 1 Endoscopic view of the traumatized larynx demonstrating an avulsed right true vocal cord.

FIGURE 2 Regions of the neck.

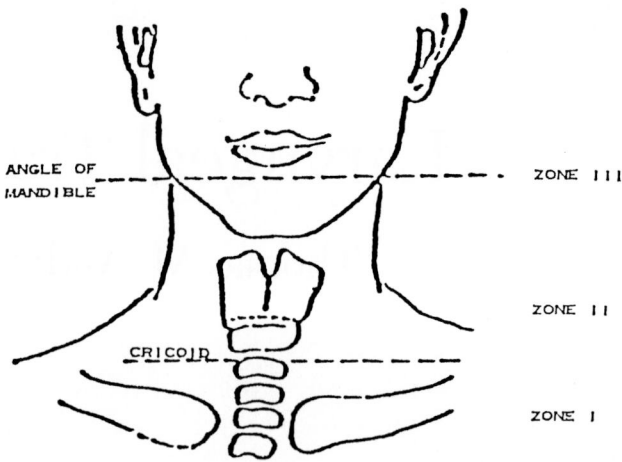

astinum. In zone III injuries, angiography is necessary to diagnose vascular injury at the skull base, where exposure may be difficult. Endoscopy should include microlaryngoscopy, bronchoscopy, and esophagoscopy. Vertebral fractures and subluxations can occur as the result of penetrating or blunt laryngeal trauma, and radiographic evaluation should be obtained on initial presentation to rule out any cervical spine injury.

 INITIAL MANAGEMENT

The patient was initially observed and found to be stable with a tracheotomy tube through a cricothyroidotomy (original dog bite). Radiographic evaluation showed no vertebral or facial skeleton fracture. Microlaryngoscopy, bronchoscopy, and esophagoscopy showed an avulsed right true vocal cord, subglottic mucosal tears, and high (cricothyroid) tracheotomy. No other soft tissue cervical injuries were seen.

 SURGICAL MANAGEMENT

Delay in transfer to our institution allowed edema and inflammation to resolve. The avulsed right cord could easily be identified and separated from the left true cord (Fig. 3).

The patient underwent reattachment of the right true vocal cord through a laryngofissure. The posterior aspect of the cord was sutured to the vocal process using a 6-0 prolene with a mattress stitch. Exact placement during suturing was accomplished with simultaneous endoscopic evaluation by a second surgeon. Subglottic granulation tissue

FIGURE 3 Endoscopic view of the larynx after separation of the avulsed cord.

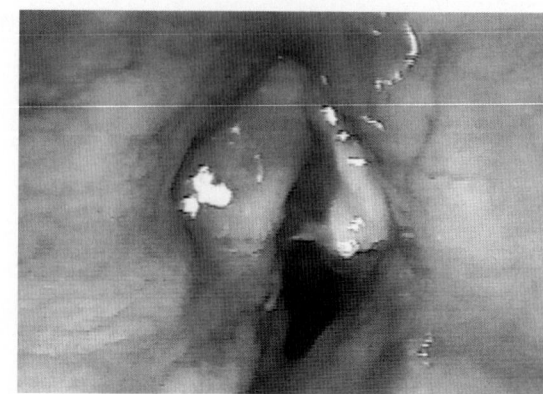

was removed and a 7.0 Cotton-Lorenz (Walter Lorenz Surgical Instruments, Jacksonville, FL) stent was placed above and separate from the tracheotomy. The stent was removed on postoperative day 9, revealing a widely patent airway. Two weeks later, endoscopic evaluation showed granulation tissue at the anterior commissure. The right true cord appeared to be healing satisfactorily. Over the next 2 months, the patient developed recurring anterior glottic granulation tissue, which was treated with CO_2 laser vaporization. Nevertheless, anterior commissure blunting developed, and a laryngeal keel was placed through an open procedure. The keel was left in place for 2 months and then removed. The patient was then decannulated without incident.

Since that time, the patient has undergone flexible endoscopy to evaluate her vocal cord function. The right true cord is mobile and appears normal. She does not show any sign of right arytenoid joint trauma or inflammation. Her voice continues to improve.

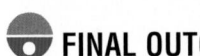 **FINAL OUTCOME**

The patient is now 2 years post injury, has been decannulated for 18 months, and has shown steady improvement in her voice with twice-weekly therapy sessions (Fig. 4).

PROBLEM-FOCUSED DISCUSSION

Laryngeal trauma in children is rare. Although laryngeal trauma in adults may be as frequent as 1 in 15,000 emergency room visits annually, pediatric laryngeal trauma is much more unusual, because fewer children are involved in altercations and as unrestrained passengers in motor vehicle accidents.

Their anatomy also allows better protection of their laryngotracheal complex (1). The thyroid cartilage rides high up under the hyoid bone until late in childhood and is well protected by the mandible. The laryngeal framework, including the thyroid and cricoid cartilages, are not ossified in childhood and therefore are more elastic and malleable.

This case represents penetrating laryngeal trauma. This is even more unusual in children as most penetrating neck trauma is due to stabbing injuries or gunshot wounds. However, it should be noted that use of deadly force among teenagers is rising, especially in urban areas, and this statistic may change in the future. Blunt and penetrating laryngeal trauma will be discussed.

FIGURE 4 Postoperative endoscopic view of the larynx.

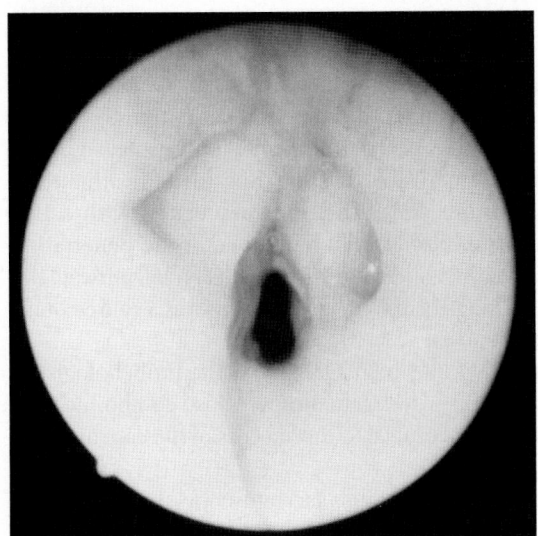

TABLE 1: Laryngotracheal Injury Classification

Group	Findings	Management
I	Minor endolaryngeal hematoma without detectable fracture	Close observation Monitoring Serial laryngoscopy Humidified air CT scan selectively used
II	Edema, hematoma, minor mucosal disruption without exposed cartilage, nondisplaced fracture	Tracheotomy Laryngoscopy Bronchoscopy Esophagoscopy CT scan selectively used
III	Massive edema, mucosal tears, exposed cartilage, cord immobility	Tracheotomy Endoscopy Open repair
IV	Group III findings plus more than 2 fracture lines or massive trauma to larynx	Tracheotomy Endoscopy Open repair
V	Complete laryngotracheal separation	Bronchoscopy Tracheotomy Open repair

(From ref. 4, with permission.)

Initial evaluation in laryngeal trauma is crucial. Patients may be classified by a scale first described by Schaefer (2,3) and modified by Fuhrman et al. (4). This classification groups the traumatic injury prognostically (Table 1).

In children, because the framework of the larynx is cartilaginous, it will stretch or bend, causing avulsion injuries of the cords, arytenoids, and mucosa. There are two disadvantages to a pediatric patient with laryngeal trauma. First, more swelling takes place because of loose connective tissue, and second, this swelling and the relatively small size of the airway quickly leads to encroachment of the lumen of the airway by edema and/or hematoma, resulting in rapid airway compromise.

Tracheotomy can be done in the face of laryngeal trauma once general mask anesthesia has been induced. It is important to continue spontaneous ventilation, as this will allow easier maintenance of an airway even when it is fractured or disrupted (5). Once a patient is placed under neuromuscular blockade, the airway may collapse, and ventilation through a mask may become increasingly difficult, leading to a hurried and traumatic intubation.

Patients with significant respiratory distress should have the airway secured by tracheotomy first. Emergency tracheotomy can be performed while the patient is maintaining spontaneous ventilation. Diagnostic endoscopic evaluation is next. Specifically, the endoscopist should evaluate for vocal cord paralysis, hematoma, arytenoid dislocation, anterior/posterior collapse, telescoping injuries, and mucosal disruptions.

When hematoma or internal derangement is noted, the tracheotomy is placed below the trauma site. Any group 2 and higher injury (Table 1) should be treated with a temporary tracheotomy (3). This case illustrates the difficulties associated with a tracheotomy tube placed through a cricothyroidotomy, which was one of the penetrating wounds. Initially performed in time to save the child's life and establish a safe airway, the otolaryngologist must recognize it is not a long-term solution and serves as a source of infection, granulation tissue, and possible stenosis.

In selected cases of tracheal disruption, it may be necessary for the bronchologist to use the bronchoscope to secure the airway prior to tracheotomy. Close communication between the endoscopist and anesthesiologist is crucial to the success of the case and survival of the patient.

If the patient is not in respiratory distress, flexible laryngoscopy should be performed to assess the function of the larynx. The endoscopist should record the presence or absence of trauma, as noted above. If any esophageal injury is suspected but not delineated by esophagoscopy, follow-up radiographic swallowing studies may be necessary.

Radiographic evaluation of the neck should be undertaken in either blunt or penetrating laryngeal trauma. Cervical spine films should be taken to rule out any injury prior to attempting intubation if possible. Radiographic evaluation of the airway may become important later in delineating the extent of the injury. Computed tomography (CT) scanning is useful when findings will have a direct impact on management. Patients with true vocal cord hematomas, slight arytenoid dislocation, and poor vocal cord mobility may have radiographic explanations for these findings delineated by CT scan that may allow for conservative therapy (6). In an unstable airway, CT scanning should not be attempted until tracheotomy is performed. In cases of significant laryngeal injury in which open reduction is mandatory, CT scanning is not warranted.

Schaefer group I (Table 1) patients may be watched closely. Many advocate serial flexible laryngoscopy to evaluate the lesion (1). The patient can be followed symptomatically, but should be placed in a monitored setting due to the risk of airway deterioration.

In group II to group V patients, in whom mucosal lacerations, hematoma, and fractures are present in the most minimal cases, immediate examination at the time of tracheotomy should be performed. The examination should include the larynx, subglottis, trachea, main stem bronchi, and esophagus. Care should be taken to delineate whether the arytenoids are mobile and whether there is vocal cord function. Bilateral vocal cord paralysis has long been known to portend a poor prognosis for recovery of nerve function and extubation failure (5).

In cases of laryngotracheal separation, immediate reanastomosis should be performed. The anterior trachea may be sutured to the end of the tracheotomy incision to facilitate reanastomosis. In these cases, loss of recurrent nerve function is likely due to the injury. There is little evidence to suggest that nerve function will return satisfactorily, despite reanastomosis.

In cases of laryngeal trauma, it is crucial to repair immediately any mucosal lacerations or denuded cartilage that may lead to further damage. Stenting is necessary when internal structures or the laryngeal skeleton needs support. When endolaryngeal damage has occurred and mucosal flaps are being supported, and when the cartilaginous framework is intact, stents can be removed as early as 3 to 5 days depending on circumstances. In cases of laryngeal fracture with an unstable skeletal framework, stents should be left in place for 4 to 6 weeks. Soft stents, such as packed finger cots, are ideal for short-term support of mucosal tears. Formed, rigid stents, such as Montgomery (Boston Medical Products, Boston, MA) and Cotton-Lorenz stents, should be used when longer support of the laryngeal framework is necessary.

The use of steroids in the first 24 hours after trauma, in a patient with a stable larynx and no open fracture, may help to reduce edema. It is important that all patients with any endolaryngeal mucosal violation, especially open fractures, be covered with broad-spectrum antimicrobials given intravenously (e.g., cefuroxime, ticarcillin/clavulanate).

If supraglottic structures have been affected (i.e., loss of petiole support, prolapse of preepiglottic fat into the glottis), then postoperative management may be especially challenging. The best advice for supraglottic lesions is to repair the wound immediately. Repair is best performed in one stage. Minor mucosal tears without exposed cartilage can be observed without repair. However, exposed cartilage usually leads to formation of granulation tissue, scarring, and/or adhesions.

Once the traumatized larynx has healed, the patient is ready for decannulation. Adequate vocal cord function should be noted by flexible laryngoscopy. Bilateral vocal cord paralysis is the most frequent reason for failure to decannulate (5). Patients with normal arytenoid joint mobility and vocal cord paralysis should be observed for return of function at least 12 months prior to surgical intervention. Vocal cord lateralization, a reversible procedure, may be one option in these patients.

Rehabilitation of the paralyzed larynx prior to decannulation may include arytenoid lateralization or arytenoidectomy. The first priority is an adequate airway, and the secondary consideration is voice, although most patients will view these priorities as reversed. In cases of lateralization of one cord due to scarring, Gelfoam or fat injections may be used to demonstrate whether medialization techniques, such as thyroplasty, will be successful. Teflon injections are also used, although they do not have the reversibility of thyroplasty. Arytenoid joint fixation, if unilateral, may not require intervention. Bilateral arytenoid joint fixation may require arytenoidectomy prior to decannulation. This condition must be distinguished from vocal cord paralysis.

Repair of posttraumatic laryngeal stenosis is covered more completely elsewhere. The best treatment is prevention of stenosis, scarring, and adhesion formation by timely repair and support of the acutely injured larynx. Open laryngotracheal reconstruction may be necessary for decannulation.

One of the most important aspects of recovery from laryngeal injury is the support of a speech/language pathologist in helping to assess vocal cord function and response to therapy.

PEARLS AND PERILS

---

1. Blunt and penetrating laryngeal trauma in the pediatric population is unusual. Pediatric patients are more likely to present in respiratory distress due to bleeding or edema within loose subcutaneous tissues and relatively smaller airways.
2. Initial evaluation should include function and anatomy of the larynx, as well as cervical spine evaluation.
3. Initial management of the laryngotracheal trauma patient consists of securing the airway. In Schaefer group II to IV injuries, the airway should be secured by a temporary tracheotomy. Intubation in laryngotracheal injury should be avoided, but when absolutely necessary should be done by the most experienced endoscopist present.
4. A high index of suspicion is necessary when examining a child with blunt or penetrating laryngeal trauma. The child with significant laryngotracheal disruption may present with minimal respiratory distress.
5. Surgical repair of laryngotracheal injuries should be performed as soon as the patient is stable. Immediate repair should include mucosal tears, denuded cartilage, and dislocated arythenoids.
6. Computed tomography may be helpful in the selected patient to demonstrate laryngeal framework abnormalities and may explain voice changes and slight internal derangements when no mucosal interruptions are present.
7. Immediate assessment, repair, and careful follow-up are necessary to avoid infection, scarring, adhesions, and stenosis.

⚙ REFERENCES

1. Willging JP, Myer CM III. Blunt pediatric laryngeal trauma. In: Myer CM, Cotton RT, Shott, eds. *The pediatric airway.* Philadelphia: JB Lippincott, 1995:181–194.
2. Schaefer SD. Primary management of laryngeal trauma. *Ann Otol Rhinol Laryngol* 1982;91:399–402.
3. Schaefer SD, Close LG. Acute management of laryngeal trauma. *Ann Otol Rhinol Laryngol* 1989;98:98–104.
4. Fuhrman GM, Stieg III FH, Buerk CA. Blunt laryngeal trauma: classification and management protocol. *J Trauma* 1990;30:87–92.
5. Myer CM III, Orobello P, Cotton RT, Bratcher GO. Blunt laryngeal trauma in children. *Laryngoscope* 1987;97:1043–1048.
6. Schaefer SD, Brown OE. Selective application of CT in the management of laryngeal trauma. *Laryngoscope* 1983;93:1473–1475.

T.M. Andrews: Departments of Otolaryngology and Pediatrics, University of South Florida, St. Petersburg, Florida 33701.

Laryngeal Cleft

George H. Zalzal

INITIAL PRESENTATION

A 7-year-old South American girl with mild myotonic muscular dystrophy presented with a history of stridor, limited exercise tolerance, and occasional circumoral cyanosis. She had a history of three episodes of croup within a period of 6 months around 1 year previously. Her voice was normal. There was no history of endotracheal intubation or aspiration. However, when the child was younger, there were many episodes of choking and poor voice that improved with time. Accompanying films indicated presence of subglottic stenosis (Fig. 1).

On physical examination, the ears, nose, mouth, and throat were normal. There was no stridor or respiratory difficulties. Fiberoptic endoscopy showed no significant abnormality, and the vocal cords were mobile.

DIFFERENTIAL DIAGNOSIS

This child had a history of intermittent stridor and recurrent croup with radiologic evidence of subglottic stenosis and normal vocal cord mobility. The differential diagnosis in such a case is limited to subglottic stenosis, cysts, or hemangioma. Several radiologic evaluations in Ecuador had included laryngeal tomography, which showed subglottic stenosis, and a barium swallow, which showed no aspiration.

INITIAL MANAGEMENT

The child was scheduled for a diagnostic laryngoscopy and bronchoscopy with the intention of assessing the severity of the subglottic stenosis. The procedure was performed with the patient under general anesthesia and spontaneous respiration. The larynx was initially visualized with the Miller blade laryngoscope. There seemed to be some posterior glottic redundancy, and the vocal cords were mobile. Reexamination of the larynx using a 4-mm telescope showed a redundancy in the posterior glottic area (Fig. 2) with mucosal collapse into the laryngeal lumen on inspiration that was reducing the lumen size. Further manipulation with the telescope revealed a posterior laryngeal cleft that was extending down through the upper portion of the cricoid cartilage posteriorly. The inferior part of the cricoid cartilage was present and was rigid, with minimal narrowing in the subglottic area. The rest of the trachea and main stem bronchi were normal.

SURGICAL MANAGEMENT

At this point, treatment options were discussed with the family in light of the severity of her symptoms. They consisted of open surgical repair of the cleft through an anterior laryngofissure or the possibility of endoscopic repair because of the mild nature of the cleft.

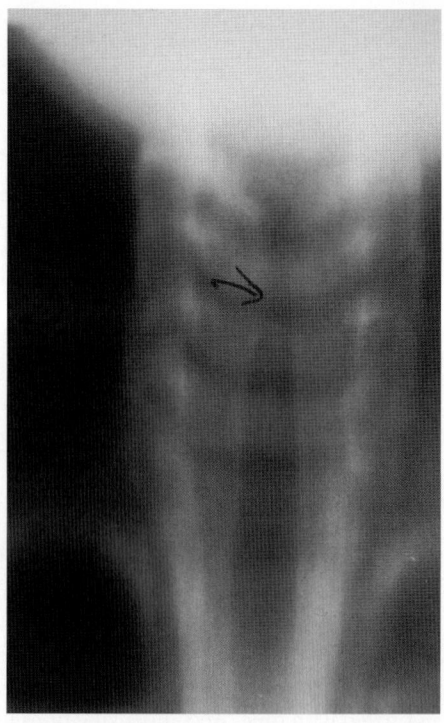

FIGURE 1 Tomogram of the larynx showing subglottic narrowing.

An endoscopic approach was chosen. With the patient under general anesthesia, using 5.0 endotracheal tube, the larynx was suspended using a specially designed laryngoscope that exposes the posterior larynx and allows bimanual manipulation of the posterior larynx. An operating microscope was used to visualize the larynx using a 400-mm lens. Vicryl, 4-0, was passed through the superior part of the mucosa over the arytenoids on each side and used as retraction sutures (Fig. 3). One percent lidocaine with epinephrine (1:100,000) was injected in the edges of the cleft, and the edges were freshened by removing the mucosa. Care was taken not to remove excessive mucosa. With laryngeal needle holders, 5-0 Vicryl sutures on P2 needles were used to approximate the freshened edges of the cleft using two layers of closure to the arytenoid level but not at the arytenoid level. Examination after endotracheal tube removal showed a repaired cleft

FIGURE 2 Endoscopic view of the larynx. Note the mucosal redundancy in the posterior glottis.

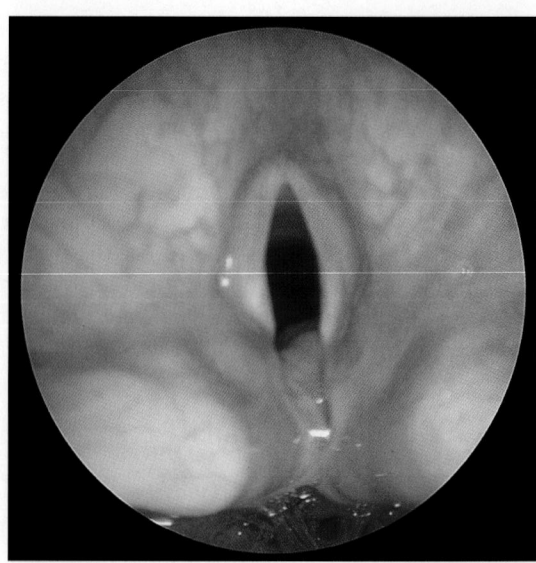

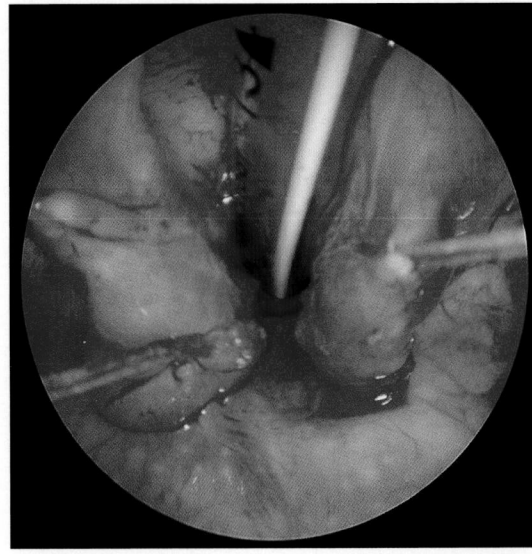

FIGURE 3 Endoscopic exposure of the cleft during repair.

with no redundant mucosa prolapsing into the laryngeal lumen (Fig. 4). The vocal cords were mobile, with no fixation of the arytenoids. The patient was extubated and tolerated the procedure well. Amoxicillin and clavulanic acid 250 mg by mouth three times daily for 10 days was given. A soft diet was started 24 hours after surgery, and the patient was discharged on the fifth postoperative day.

FINAL OUTCOME

The patient continued to do well, and endoscopic assessment 3 weeks after surgery showed the vocal cords to be mobile (Fig. 5). The cleft has healed up to the level of the arytenoids, and the redundant mucosa of the cleft has been placed posteriorly into the esophageal inlet. Minimal protrusion of mucosa-covered scar into the laryngeal and subglottic lumen posteriorly could be seen. The patient continues to do well 4 years postoperatively.

FIGURE 4 Repaired cleft. Note mucosal swelling immediately after surgery.

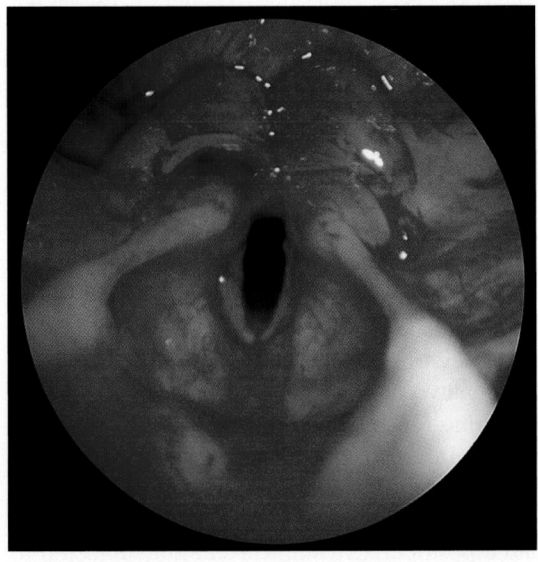

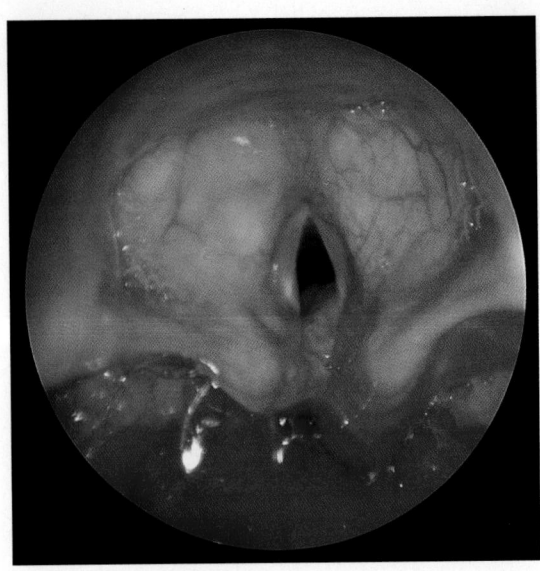

FIGURE 5 Larynx after healing.

🔖 PROBLEM-FOCUSED DISCUSSION

The presentation of this child was atypical in that she was older, with only intermittent symptoms. The stridor would occur erratically, and aspiration, if present, was clinically insignificant. This clinical presentation is consistent with what Evans (1) termed type I cleft in his clinically oriented classification of laryngeal clefts: type I—stridor; type II—aspiration on feeding, recurrent pneumonias, and abnormalities of cry; and type III—severe aspiration, cyanosis, and cardiorespiratory failure. This classification is very helpful clinically.

It is essential that other congenital anomalies be ruled out, specifically the G syndrome (Opitz oculo-genital-laryngeal syndrome/Opitz BBB/G syndrome/Opitz-Frias syndrome). These patients have hypertelorism with other midline abnormalities, including hypospadias in the male; the inheritance is autosomal dominant (2).

Evaluation workup of stridor initially includes fiberoptic laryngoscopy, which may not be adequate to detect a posterior laryngeal cleft (3). High kilovoltage airway films may or may not show subglottic narrowing depending on the severity and type of cleft and the amount of redundant mucosa prolapsing into the airway lumen. A modified barium swallow is extremely helpful in cases with aspiration. However, if the cleft is mild, as in this case, barium may not penetrate the larynx. A normal barium swallow may give the impression that the airway is normal. The method of choice for diagnosis is direct laryngoscopy and bronchoscopy. The posterior larynx should be palpated with blunt instruments to assess the presence and severity of the cleft. In this case, initial inspection on direct laryngoscopy was normal. However, under spontaneous inspiration, there was posterior laryngeal mucosal prolapse into the lumen indicating the presence of cleft.

Surgical repair will depend on the severity of the cleft. Dubois et al. (4) suggested endoscopic repair for type I clefts using microsurgical instruments. However, with types II to IV, an open approach must be used and a tracheotomy is a universal requirement, sometimes for an extended period. The anterior laryngofissure approach may be the preferred choice over the lateral one because of the advantage of excellent and easy exposure of the anomaly without jeopardizing the laryngeal nerves. Although there may be a theoretical disadvantage of postoperative laryngeal instability, clinically this is not significant (5,6).

Intraoperative airway management during repair of severe clefts is difficult, especially if the cleft reaches the carina or beyond. Bifurcated long endotracheal tubes to cannulate the main stem bronchi have been described. However, extracorporeal membrane oxygenation begun intraoperatively and continued for several days after surgery offers adequate intraoperative oxygenation and a postoperative surgical site not subjected to contact with foreign bodies (endotracheal tubes) (7). For clefts that do not extend through the inferior border of the posterior cricoid, endoscopic repair is technically difficult but feasible with good results. Evans et al. (8) reported on 44 patients of whom 25 (56%) had associated congenital anomalies. Fourteen (32%) were treated conservatively, 16 (36%) underwent primary endoscopic surgical repair, 8 (18%) underwent primary repair via anterior laryngofissure, and 6 (14%) underwent primary repair via lateral pharyngotomy. Morbidity and mortality were reduced by securing the airway, controlling gastroesophageal reflux, and using a multidisciplinary pediatric team. They recommended the anterior laryngofissure approach because of the ease of surgical access.

PEARLS AND PERILS

1. A high index of suspicion is necessary to diagnose a laryngeal cleft, especially if aspiration is not pronounced.
2. Fiberoptic laryngoscopy may not be adequate to determine the presence of a laryngeal cleft.
3. A modified barium swallow may not be sufficient to diagnose a laryngeal cleft.
4. Palpation of the posterior larynx using blunt instruments, during direct laryngoscopy is essential for diagnosis.
5. In type I clefts that are severe enough to cause symptoms and that cannot be managed with observation alone, the endoscopic approach is recommended.
6. Posterior laryngeal exposure can be difficult for bimanual manipulation, and a specially designed laryngoscope may be needed.
7. Long instruments, especially a laryngeal needle holder, are very important for successful repair.
8. A two-layer repair using 4-0 Vicryl sutures is important.
9. Endoscopic repair can be accomplished without the performance of a tracheotomy. It reduces postoperative morbidity and accelerates discharge of the patient.

Endoscopic exposure of the posterior larynx can be difficult, especially for bimanual work. In certain instances, using a Dingman retractor can expose the larynx adequately. In most cases, a laryngoscope should be used and a specially designed laryngoscope in which most of its posterior border is open to allow bimanual work has been used successfully (Fig. 6). The advantage of endoscopic repair is avoidance of a tracheotomy with

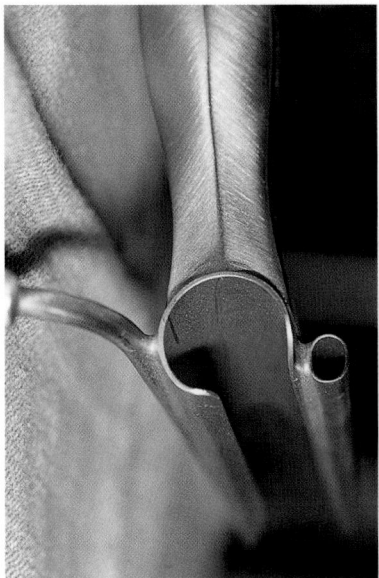

FIGURE 6 Specially designed laryngoscope with a large posterior opening that allows bimanual work on the posterior larynx.

discharge of the patient soon after the procedure. For more extensive clefts, a laryngofissure is recommended along with a tracheotomy and, in appropriate cases, gastrostomy and fundoplication when gastroesophageal reflux is present.

✴ REFERENCES

1. Evans JN. Management of the cleft larynx and tracheoesophageal clefts. *Ann Otol Rhinol Laryngol* 1985;94:627–630.
2. Conlon BJ, O'Dwyer T Jr. The G syndrome/Opitz oculo-genital-laryngeal syndrome/Opitz BBB/G syndrome/Opitz-Frias syndrome. *J Laryngol Otol* 1995;109:244–246.
3. Zalzal GH. Stridor and airway compromise. *Pediatr Clin North Am* 1989;36:1389–1402.
4. Dubois JJ, Pokorny WJ, Harberg FJ, Smith RJ. Current management of laryngeal and laryngotracheosoephageal clefts. *J Pediatr Surg* 1990;25:855–860.
5. Berkovits RN, Bax NM, Van der Schans EJ. Surgical treatment of congenital laryntracheoesophageal cleft. *Prog Pediatr Surg* 1987;21:36–46.
6. Myer CM III, Cotton RT, Holmes DK, Jackson RK. Laryngeal and laryngotracheoesophageal clefts: role of early surgical repair. *Ann Otol Rhinol Laryngol* 1990;99:98–104.
7. Geiduschek JM, Inglis AF Jr, O'Rourke PP, Kozak FK, Mayock DE, Sawin RS. Repair of a laryngotracheoesophageal cleft in an infant by means of extracorporeal membrane oxygenation. *Ann Otol Rhinol Laryngol* 1993;102:827–833.
8. Evans KL, Courteney-Harris R, Bailey CM, Evans JM, Parsons DS. Management of posterior laryngeal and laryngotracheosophageal clefts. *Arch Otolaryngol Head Neck Surg* 1995;121:1380–1385.

G.H. Zalzal: Departments of Otolaryngology and Pediatrics, George Washington University, Children's National Medical Center, Washington, DC 20010.

Laryngomalacia

George H. Zalzal

INITIAL PRESENTATION

An 8-week-old healthy boy born at the 75th percentile for weight presented with stridor since birth that had been increasing in severity and was associated with severe feeding difficulties. Apnea was reported by the mother to last for a few seconds. The child's weight was failing to increase and was 8 pounds, 1½ ounces (10th percentile). He was a slow feeder, and barium swallow to assess his feeding difficulties showed no aspiration; however, there was a transit delay. His pediatrician had placed him on ranitidine (Zantac) and metoclopramide (Reglan) for a presumed diagnosis of gastroesophageal reflux. He had a good cry.

Physical examination showed normal ears and nose. Mouth and throat examination was normal except for a *Candida* thrush of the lips, palate, and tongue, which was being treated by Mycostatin suspension. He had supraclavicular, infraclavicular, suprasternal, and substernal retraction and nasal flaring. Fiberoptic laryngoscopy showed very severe laryngomalacia; the vocal cords could not be visualized. Anteroposterior and lateral neck airway films showed no airway abnormality.

SURGICAL MANAGEMENT

His condition was discussed with the parents, the pulmonary physician, the gastroenterologist, and the pediatrician. He was admitted overnight, during which oxygen desaturation fell to the low 80s. Epiglottoplasty was performed the following day with immediate improvement in breathing and feeding.

With the patient in the supine position and following induction of general anesthesia with a ventilating mask, the supraglottic region was sprayed with lidocaine. The supraglottic area was examined with a 7200A Hopkins telescope, and marked prolapse of the posterior half of the supraglottis into the glottis was evident. Most of the redundant tissue was seen over the aryepiglottic folds and the arytenoids (Fig. 1). The epiglottis itself was quite short and did not collapse posteriorly. The subglottis and trachea were normal, with the exception of very mild narrowing of the subglottis. A 3.5 endotracheal tube was used to size the subglottic narrowing, which would not allow air leak up to a pressure of 50 cm H_2O. A 3.0 endotracheal tube was used to intubate the patient with air leak at 19 cm H_2O. The larynx was suspended using a small Dedo laryngoscope, and the supraglottic area was exposed. A CO_2 laser with settings of 4 W power, 0.1 pulse width, and 0.1 pulse rate was used to obliterate the redundant tissue over the posterior aryepiglottic folds (Fig. 2). The interarytenoid mucosa was kept intact. This procedure was done under apneic technique. Once the child was fully awakened, he was extubated and sent to the intensive care unit. Cefpodoxime (Vantin) and beclomethasone (Vanceril) inhalers were used for 2 weeks along with ranitidine and metoclopramide for gastroesophageal

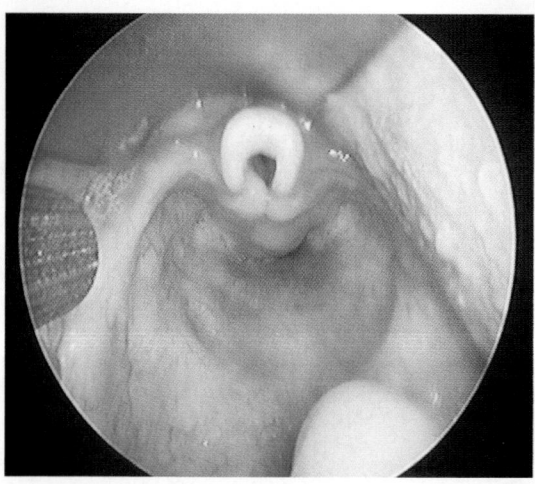

FIGURE 1 Preoperative view of larynx showing laryngomalacia.

reflux and nystatin p.r.n. for thrush. He was discharged home 5 days later on an apnea monitor to rule out any further occurrences of apnea. The monitor disk recorder was downloaded two times at 1-month intervals. Good parental compliance and absence of apnea were documented. The monitor was discontinued.

⬤ FINAL OUTCOME

On follow-up 2 weeks postoperatively, the child was adding weight with good voice and normal breathing. Fiberoptic laryngoscopy showed a healed supraglottis with an open inlet and normal vocal cord mobility. Reexamination 2 months later showed the child was continuing to add weight with good feeding and breathing and no decompensation during severe upper respiratory infection. Fiberoptic laryngoscopy continues to show an open laryngeal inlet.

& PROBLEM-FOCUSED DISCUSSION

Laryngomalacia (congenital laryngeal stridor) is a relatively benign self-limiting condition. The first report describing this condition was by Barthez and Rilliet (1) in 1843. Among the congenital laryngeal anomalies, it is the most common, and comprised 59.8% of Holinger's (2) series. Narcy et al. (3) found an incidence of 50% among a series of 687

FIGURE 2 Postoperative view of larynx after laser ablation of redundant tissue; note good view of vocal cords.

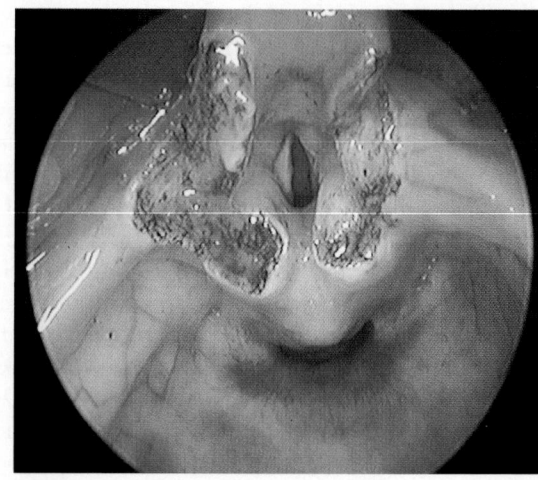

patients with laryngeal anomalies. The anatomic abnormalities that cause laryngomalacia are long and curled epiglottis that prolapses posteriorly on inspiration, bulky arytenoids that prolapse forward on inspiration, and short aryepiglottic folds. Children with laryngomalacia present with inspiratory stridor that is intermittent with variable intensity augmented by agitation and reduced with neck extension. There is a normal cry and (rarely) dyspnea, cyanosis, or feeding disorder. Presentation is usually during the first 10 days of life, and the symptoms are exacerbated by upper respiratory infections.

This child presented with severe symptoms at a very young age, which is not typical of laryngomalacia; thus, other conditions must be ruled out. The differential diagnosis includes other congenital anomalies, such as bilateral vocal cord paralysis in which the cry is weak and there is severe stridor. Children who have unilateral vocal cord paralysis present with cough and choking on feeding, with positional stridor that may improve during sleep. However, the louder stridor appears when the patient is awake, compared with laryngomalacia, which is noisier when the patient is asleep, and vascular sling problems in which feeding problems are often present with reflex apnea. Subglottic hemangioma usually appears late, and around half the patients have skin hemangiomata. Stridor in laryngomalacia and innominate artery tracheal compression decreases with the patient in a prone position with the neck extended.

Airway films were taken to help in assessing the lower airway, which is not adequately done with a fiberoptic laryngoscope, especially in this child, in whom severe collapse prevented adequate vocal cord examination and the subglottis could not be visualized. High kilovoltage neck airway films are usually requested. Barium swallow, fluoroscopy, or computed tomography are rarely needed. Diagnosis is by fiberoptic laryngoscopy during which the assessment of severity is made, and a correlation between the symptoms and the anatomic abnormality is made. If the symptoms are more pronounced than the severity of the laryngomalacia, then the possibility of a significant second airway lesion becomes greater (4).

PEARLS AND PERILS

1. Laryngomalacia is the most common congenital laryngeal anomaly but may be confused with vocal cord paralysis. Fiberoptic laryngoscopy is essential for diagnosis.
2. History taking should focus on clinical severity by assessing severity of airway obstruction, presence of apnea and oxygen desaturation, and associated feeding difficulties with failure to thrive.
3. If the physical examination shows that severity is not commensurate with clinical presentation, a second airway lesion should be suspected, and a bronchoscopy is indicated.
4. Surgical intervention is indicated only in very severe cases with feeding difficulties, failure to thrive, and apnea in whom flexible laryngoscopy shows collapse of the laryngeal inlet with inability to see the vocal cords. Careful clinical judgment is needed when only part of the anterior vocal cords can be seen.
5. Both laryngeal instruments and laser can be used to trim excess supraglottic tissue, the advantages of the laser being a bloodless field and better precision. In both techniques, excessive resection of tissue is contraindicated to avoid supraglottic stenosis. Excision of tissue from the interarytenoid area is contraindicated to avoid arytenoid fixation.

In mild cases, watchful waiting is the treatment of choice, and improvement usually occurs within 18 months. However, around 10% to 15% of children do poorly and do not resolve on their own (5). Severe cases, such as this patient, will need treatment to avoid continued airway obstruction with development of cor pulmonale. Inability to feed well leads to failure to thrive. Although tracheotomy is 100% effective in relieving airway obstruction from laryngomalacia, it carries considerable risk of mortality and requires continuous monitoring. Epiglottoplasty can replace tracheotomy in most cases and consists of supraglottic tissue excision. It was initially described using laryngeal instruments (6). The CO_2 laser is an alternative; when used carefully, it is more accurate and bloodless but may be more time consuming. The anesthetic technique can be either apneic or by insufflation with spontaneous respiration. It is extremely important that full evaluation of the airway by bronchoscopy be performed to avoid missing any significant second airway lesion that could be contributing to airway obstruction. Epiglottoplasty is indicated in patients with severe stridor not resolving with time that may be associated with feeding difficulties and failure to thrive, cor pulmonale, and apnea. The decision to proceed with surgical intervention (supraglottoplasty) is guided by symptom severity. However, the inability to view the true vocal cords with flexible nasopharyngoscopy because of laryngeal inlet collapse, is an indicator of severe laryngomalacia and surgical success is likely. Overzealous removal of supraglottic tissue or mucosa in the interarytenoid area can lead to supraglottic stenosis.

The case described displayed clear indications for surgery: apnea, oxygen desaturation, and feeding difficulty with failure to thrive. Spontaneous improvement occurred, and concomitant problems, such as gastroesophageal reflux, were attended to. The patient added weight significantly and continues to do well 1 year postoperatively.

✱ REFERENCES

1. Barthez E, Rilliet F. *Traite clinique et pratique des maladies des enfants.* Paris: G. Baillière, 1843:484–488.
2. Holinger LD. Etiology of stridor in the neonate, infant and child. *Ann Otol Rhinol Laryngol* 1980;89:397–400.
3. Narcy P, Bobin S, Contencin P, Le Pajolec C, Manach Y. Laryngeal anomolies in newborn infants. Apropos of 687 cases. *Ann Otolaryngol Chir Cervicofac* 1984;101:363–373.
4. Mancuso R, Choi S, Zalzal GH, Grundfast KM. Laryngomalacia. The search for the second lesion. *Arch Otolaryngol Head Neck Surg* 1996;122:302–306.
5. Fearon B, Ellis D. The management of long term airway problems in infants and children. *Ann Otol Rhinol Laryngol* 1971;80:669–677.
6. Zalzal GH, Anon JB, Cotton RT. Epiglottoplasty for the treatment of laryngomalacia. *Ann Otol Rhinol Laryngol* 1987;96:72–76.

G.H. Zalzal: Departments of Otolaryngology and Pediatrics, George Washington University, Children's National Medical Center, Washington, DC 20010.

Congenital Tracheal Rings

George H. Zalzal

☺ INITIAL PRESENTATION

A 19-month-old child with Down syndrome born at 28 weeks presented with a long-standing history of stridor necessitating eight hospitalizations. Endotracheal intubation for about 2 hours after birth was needed, after which the child did well. Most of the admissions to the hospital were related to croup, occasionally associated with pneumonia, but not requiring respiratory assistance. The child had normal feeding habits with no history of cyanosis or apnea. His voice was occasionally high pitched.

Physical examination showed cerumen impaction in both ear canals, which were narrowed. The cerumen was removed, and the eardrums were normal. Mouth and throat were also normal. This was a Down syndrome child with developmental delay and stridor and no respiratory distress.

❞ INITIAL MANAGEMENT

Magnetic resonance imaging (MRI) films (Fig. 1) accompanying the family showed lower tracheal stenosis consistent with congenital complete tracheal rings extending over a length of 2.5 cm and ending around 1 cm above the carina.

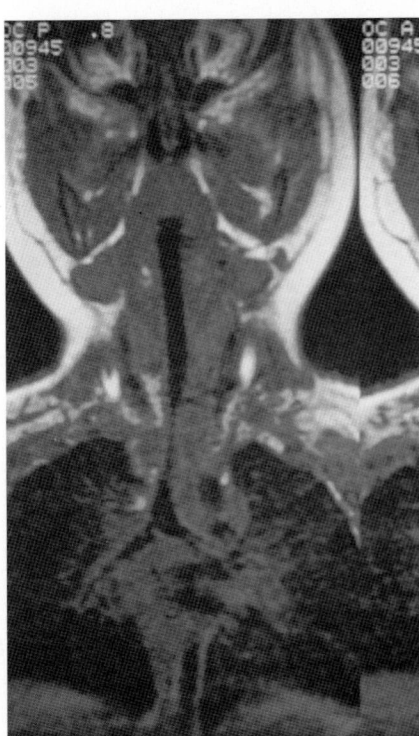

FIGURE 1 Magnetic resonance imaging (MRI) showing tracheal narrowing.

Direct laryngoscopy and bronchoscopy were performed under general anesthesia with spontaneous respiration. The larynx was normal except for anterior subglottic narrowing (Fig. 2A). The upper trachea had an adequate lumen, but the lower trachea was extremely narrowed (Fig. 2B) to the extent that a 27018A Hopkins telescope (2.7-mm diameter) could not be passed through. The procedure was terminated at this stage.

🌐 SURGICAL MANAGEMENT

The patient underwent direct laryngoscopy and bronchoscopy with tracheal reconstruction using a pericardial patch under partial cardiopulmonary bypass. A median sternotomy was performed. The pericardium was split to the right of the midline to allow for harvesting of a large pericardial patch. The right atrium was cannulated with number 28 single venous canula, and a 5.2 highflow SARNS cannula was placed in the ascending aorta after heparinization. The innominate vein was absent.

The trachea was exposed from high in the neck to the level of the bifurcation; obvious narrowing extended to just above the carina. Cardiopulmonary bypass was instituted maintaining normothermia and a beating heart. Bronchoscopy was performed, and a needle was passed through the trachea to identify the upper end of the stenosis. An endotracheal tube was inserted. An anterior tracheal wall incision was made involving all of the tracheal rings that were complete and narrow. There were eleven tracheal rings with a total length of 3.6 cm. Bleeding was moderate and was controlled by neurosurgical pledgets soaked with epinephrine 1:10,000. A piece of pericardium measuring about 3.8 cm in length and 1 cm in width was sutured to the edges of the open trachea, which were distracted. A 3.5 endotracheal tube was passed through the trachea so as to be just above the carina. Suturing of the pericardial patch to the edges of the trachea was performed using 5-0 Dexon. Care was taken not to enter the tracheal lumen. After the suturing, the lungs were hyperinflated, and three areas of air leak were sealed with additional sutures. The sternum was wired closed. Previously placed proline sutures were used to suspend the innominate artery anteriorly, thus alleviating anterior pressure on the pericardial patch. Skin and subcutaneous layers were closed. The patient tolerated the procedure well and was transferred to the intensive care unit.

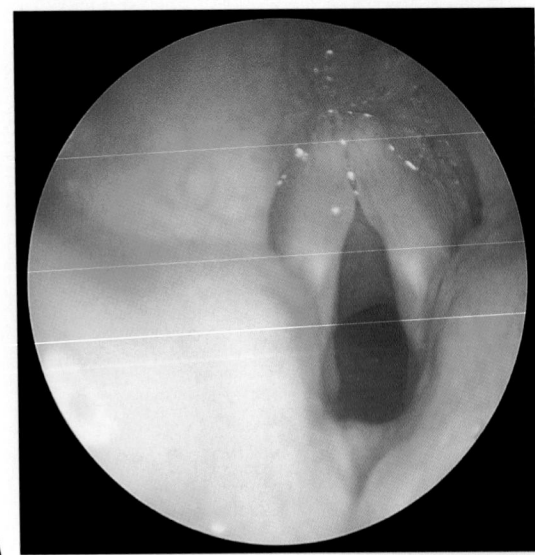 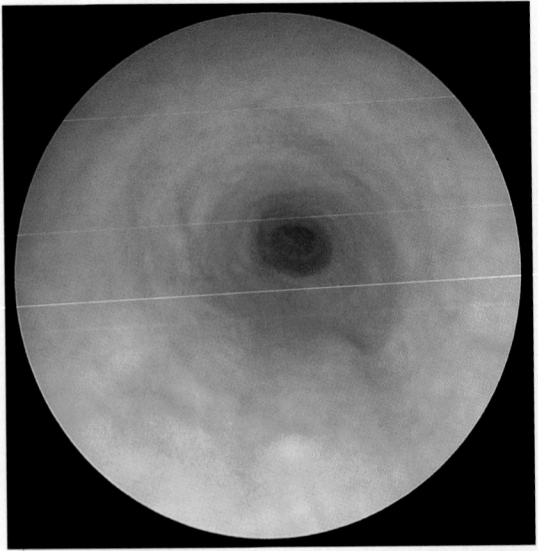

A   B

FIGURE 2 **A:** Endoscopic view showing anterior subglottic stenosis. **B:** Endoscopic view showing complete rings narrowing the tracheal lumen.

Twenty-four hours later the endotracheal tube was blocked with a blood clot and was changed. The patient was examined in the operating room; both main stem bronchi were filled with serosanguinous secretions that were suctioned out. The site of repair was patent, with the pericardial patch adequately in place anteriorly. There was no evidence of any tears in the graft or loose sutures. A number 4.0 endotracheal tube was used instead of 3.5 to provide better ventilation and avoid any further endotracheal tube blockage.

Because of the presence of anterior subglottic stenosis and the need for further endotracheal intubation with a larger endotracheal tube, a cricoid split was done 6 days later. The cricoid split was not done during the tracheoplasty for fear of creating a pneumomediastinum with air going out of the cricoid and back into the mediastinum. The procedure was uneventful.

FINAL OUTCOME

The patient was intubated for a total of 3 weeks during which heavy sedation and intermittent muscle paralysis were used. On extubation, he did very well, and endoscopy showed a patent airway (Fig. 3) with no granulation tissue and complete mucosalization of the pericardial graft. Methadone had to be used for 2 weeks because of drug withdrawal. His recovery was prolonged because of drug-induced hypotonia superimposed on his basic hypotonia and developmental delay. Physical and rehabilitative treatment were instituted. He continues to do well 3 years after the surgery with adequate exercise tolerance.

PROBLEM-FOCUSED DISCUSSION

This patient, like most with congenital tracheal rings, presented with airway difficulties early in life. Watchful waiting was not successful, and the narrow tracheal segment did not increase in size. Several hospital admissions were needed during upper respiratory infections. Diagnosis of this lesion involves plain airway films for initial assessment followed by bronchoscopy. If the child tolerates sedation, then more involved radiologic procedures can be performed, such as MRI and computed tomography (CT). These modalities will add more information about the vasculature in the mediastinum since

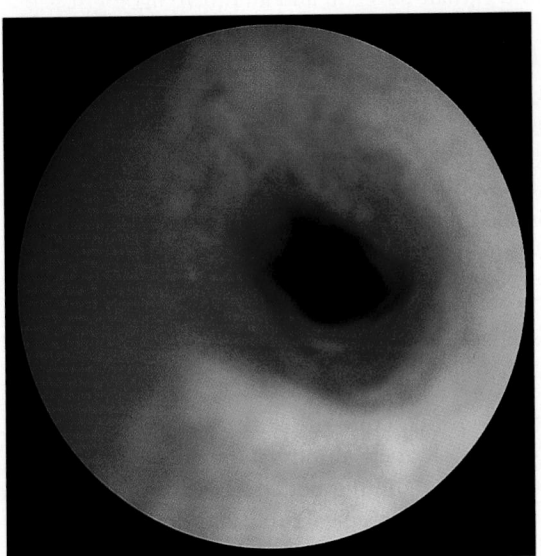

FIGURE 3 Endoscopic view showing a larger tracheal lumen after repair.

many of these patients have vascular anomalies, which can impact on the technical aspects of repair. The commonly accepted diagnostic procedure involves history, physical examination, and plain radiograph studies, followed by bronchoscopy and CT scan or MRI if possible (1,2).

It is essential to assess the length of the stenotic segment and whether it involves the carina or the main stem bronchi. Involvement of the carina will lead to poor results with high mortality (3). If this information can be obtained through radiologic evaluation or endoscopy, then a clear picture can be presented to the parents preoperatively regarding successful repair and associated morbidity and mortality.

Surgical repair requires a team consisting of a cardiothoracic surgeon and an otolaryngologist. The approach involves a median sternotomy with partial normothermic cardiopulmonary bypass. Not infrequently, vascular anomalies are encountered. A key part of the otolaryngologist's task includes endoscopic location of the superior edge of the stenosis, anterior tracheal split, and suturing of the pericardial patch obtained by the cardiac surgeon. Airtight closure is mandatory to avoid postoperative pneumediastinum, pneumothorax, and mediastinitis. The pericardial patch has given the best results, as described initially by Idriss (4). However, resection of up to eight tracheal rings can be possible, and other methods, such as anterior and posterior tracheal split, anterior castellated tracheal incision, and cartilage grafts, have been tried (2). Once an anterior tracheal split is performed for congenital tracheal rings, the rings spring open and the lumen is significantly increased. Using a pericardial patch will create a membranous trachea anteriorly. A theoretical disadvantage of cartilage grafts is poor nutrient supply, which may lead to cartilage resorption. The stenotic segment can extend from the cricoid all the way to the carina. Involvement of the carina or the main stem bronchi leads to significant intraoperative and postoperative complications with a high mortality rate. In general, lesions that do not involve the carina do well; the overall mortality rate is around 47% (2) and has been reported to range from 0 to 70%.

PEARLS AND PERILS

1. Presentation of congenital tracheal rings is early in life.
2. Vascular anomalies are associated with this anomaly.
3. When the symptoms are severe, surgical repair is needed; a wait and see policy is very dangerous.
4. Adequate preoperative diagnosis, specifically as to the involvement of the carina, is mandatory.
5. A team approach consisting of a cardiac surgeon and an otolaryngologist is essential.
6. Postoperative management should be in an intensive care unit, and the procedure should be performed in a tertiary center.
7. Concomitant presence of subglottic stenosis with a skip lesion of normal trachea followed by lower tracheal stenosis presents a peculiar setup, since a pericardial patch can not be extended all the way to the subglottis to perform an airtight seal closure. A cricoid split is advisable to improve the subglottic airway, which may necessitate two separate procedures.
8. Postoperative paralysis and heavy sedation may cause neuromuscular complications.

Subglottic narrowing and Down syndrome added to the difficult course of this patient. After repair of the pericardial patch, endotracheal intubation is needed for anywhere from 7 to 21 days; the shorter the intubation, the better. However, on the first postoperative day, a blood clot blocked his 3.5 endotracheal tube, and the endotracheal tube had to be changed to a larger 4.0. Because of the congenital subglottic narrowing and fear of causing acquired subglottic stenosis, a cricoid split was considered but not performed at the same time as the pericardial patch because of fear of inducing subcutaneous emphysema and pneumomediastinum from air leak around the cricoid split. A trial of endotracheal intubation with a small tube (3.5) proved dangerous, and a cricoid split was performed on the seventh postoperative day. This necessitated another 12 days of intubation to give the child an adequate subglottic and tracheal airway.

Sedation was sufficient early on to control the child's movement; eventually it became necessary to paralyze him intermittently, which led to prolonged lower extremity paresis superimposed on hypotonia secondary to trisomy 21. Prolonged muscular weakness after reversal of vecuronium has been reported (5). Atelectasis has been reported in 48% of the patients; however, the author's patient managed not to develop atelectasis. After extubation, physical therapy helped significantly, and the patient continues to do well.

 REFERENCES

1. Cosentino CM, Backer CL, Idriss FS, Holinger LD, Gerson CR, Mavroudis C. Pericardial patch tracheoplasty for severe tracheal stenosis in children: indeterminate results. *J Pediatr Surg* 1991;26:879–884; discussion 885.
2. Andrews TM, Cotton RT, Bailey WW, Myer CM III, Vester SR. Tracheoplasty for congenital complete tracheal rings. *Arch Otolaryngol Head Neck Surg* 1994;120:1363–1369.
3. Dunham ME, Holinger LD, Backer CL, Mavroudis C. Management of severe congenital tracheal stenosis. *Ann Otol Rhinol Laryngol* 1994;103:351–356.
4. Idriss FS. Tracheoplasty with pericardial patch for extensive tracheal stenosis in infants and children. *Thorac Cardiovasc Surg* 1984;88:527–536.
5. Palasti S, Respler DS, Fieldman RJ, Levitt J. Anterior cricoid split for subglottic stenosis: experience at the Children's Hospital of New Jersey. *Laryngoscope* 1992;102:997–1000.

G.H. Zalzal: Departments of Otolaryngology and Pediatrics, George Washington University, Children's National Medical Center, Washington, DC 20010.

Vocal Cord Paralysis

Sukgi S. Choi

 INITIAL PRESENTATION

A 5-year-old boy was referred by a speech/language pathologist for persistent hoarseness. The patient had been delivered vaginally without significant birth trauma. There were no pre- or postnatal difficulties. The patient's past medical history was significant for adenotonsillectomy and bilateral myringotomy and tube insertion at age 2. Following this procedure, the patient experienced transient stridor, which resolved spontaneously. There were no other past surgeries. The patient had a history of mild difficulty with his balance and with fine and gross motor activities, for which he received a short-term physical therapy. In addition, he had delay in his speech and language development with poor articulation, and speech therapy had been started at age 4.

On examination, patient had a mild inspiratory stridor and hoarseness. A flexible laryngoscopy showed paralysis of the left true vocal cord in paramedian position. A chest x-ray was normal. Magnetic resonance imaging (MRI) of the brain and upper cervical spine showed (a) three abnormal nodular foci of signal lining the superior aspect of the left ventricle (Fig. 1), (b) Chiari I malformation with 13-mm downward herniation of the cerebellar tonsils (Fig. 2), (c) patulous spinal canal at the C-1 to C-2 level, and (d) no cervical syrinx.

The patient was referred for neurologic evaluation, which revealed mild dysfunction of cranial nerves IX to XII and a mild cerebellar deficit. The patient has been followed with serial neurologic examination over the ensuing 18 months with no changes in his clinical examination. No surgical intervention has been necessary to date.

 DIFFERENTIAL DIAGNOSIS

Hoarseness in children is most commonly secondary to vocal cord nodules, recurrent respiratory papillomatosis, and vocal cord paralysis. With the use of a flexible laryngoscope, these diagnoses can easily be made in the clinic setting.

 PROBLEM-FOCUSED DISCUSSION

The etiology of vocal cord paralysis in children is different from that in adults. In adults, vocal cord paralysis is often the result of surgical procedures, trauma, and neoplasms of the head and neck. In children, vocal cord paralysis is more often secondary to birth trauma, central nervous system (CNS) abnormalities, Arnold-Chiari malformation, and heart and great vessel abnormalities.

Thirty percent to 62% of cases of pediatric vocal cord paralysis are reported to be bilateral (1). Bilateral vocal cord paralysis often requires either intubation or tracheotomy

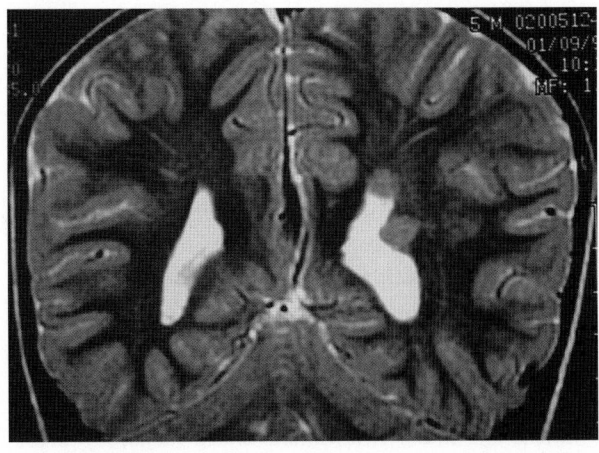

FIGURE 1 Three heterotopic foci in the vicinity of the left ventricle due to migrational defect.

for establishment of an airway. Unilateral vocal cord paralysis rarely requires any airway intervention and thus may not be diagnosed until a child is older.

Evaluation of any child with suspected vocal cord paralysis consists of a thorough history including birth and trauma history. This is followed by physical examination, which is geared toward detecting any underlying etiology and other associated congenital anomalies. A flexible fiberoptic examination of the larynx is an integral part of this evaluation.

Because of the previously mentioned differences in the etiology of vocal cord paralysis in children and adults, further evaluation depends on the age of the patient. In adults, evaluation of vocal cord paralysis includes chest x-ray followed by MRI or computed tomography (CT) of the chest. The area scanned depends on the side of involvement: if the left side is involved, imaging should include the neck and chest to the level of the aorta; if the right side is involved, then only the neck is imaged (2). In children, CNS involvement should be suspected, and evaluation of any child with vocal cord paralysis must include a CT or MRI of the brain (3,4).

The Chiari malformations are a group of cranial–cervical junction abnormalities that involve the cerebellum, medulla, and skeletal anatomy of the posterior cranial fossa (5).

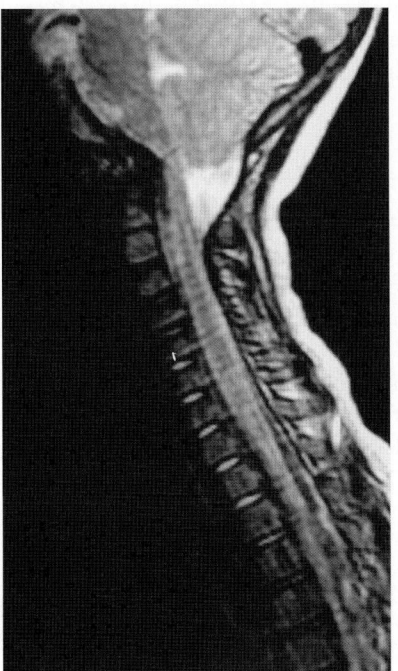

FIGURE 2 Sagittal magnetic resonance imaging (MRI) showing a Chiari I malformation with patulous upper cervical spinal canal.

These malformations can be subdivided into four categories. Chiari type I malformation consists of elongation of the cerebellar tonsils and medial portions of the inferior lobes of the cerebellum, which is displaced into the upper cervical vertebral canal. In Chiari type 2 malformation, often referred to as Arnold-Chiari malformation, there is a greater degree of elongation and caudal displacement of the brainstem. There is also caudal displacement of the fourth ventricle and cerebellar vermis into the upper cervical canal. This malformation is often associated with meningomyelocele and hydrocephalus. In Chiari type 3 malformation, there is herniation of the cerebellum, which then forms a high cervical meningocele, and in Chiari type 4 malformation, a generalized hypoplasia of the cerebellum is seen. Types 3 and 4 are uncommon.

The association of Chiari type 2 malformation (Arnold-Chiari malformation) and vocal cord paralysis has been well established (6–11). Bilateral vocal cord paralysis is more commonly seen than unilateral paralysis. Four mechanisms for etiology of vocal cord paralysis have been proposed (6): (a) traction on cervical rootlets of the vagus, (b) direct compression of the medulla and cranial nerves in the foramen magnum, (c) increased intracranial pressure causing injury to the brainstem, and (d) dysgenesis of the brainstem. Whatever the mechanism, the vocal cord paralysis is often reversible if the intracranial pressure is relieved promptly (7). Although less commonly seen, other CNS abnormalities and mass lesions, such as a brain tumor, may present with isolated vocal cord paralysis (3,4).

The child in this case had soft, nonlocalizing neurologic signs and symptoms. Since his vocal cord paralysis was unilateral, no significant airway obstruction was seen, and his hoarseness was assumed to be a part of his speech and language problems. He was eventually referred to the otolaryngologist for persistent hoarseness. This case demonstrates that any child with hoarseness should be evaluated using the flexible fiberoptic laryngoscope to determine the underlying cause.

Once the diagnosis of vocal cord paralysis was established, MRI of his brain was obtained; it showed Chiari type 1 malformation, as well as several heterotopic foci near the left ventricle. It is possible that this patient's signs and symptoms of Chiari malformation were minimized by the presence of patulous spinal canal, which prevented compression of the brainstem. Whether the migration defect of the gray matter, resulting in heterotopic foci, or Chiari malformation is the etiology primarily responsible for the vocal cord paralysis and dysfunction of cranial nerves IX to XII cannot be determined.

Although this child has not required surgical intervention, MRI of his brain detected an underlying condition that needs close monitoring and may eventually require surgery. This case illustrates the importance of imaging the CNS in any child with vocal cord paralysis.

PEARLS AND PERILS

1. Flexible fiberoptic laryngoscopy must be a part of the evaluation of any child with a history of hoarseness and/or stridor.
2. Imaging of the CNS by MRI or CT scan must be part of evaluation of vocal cord paralysis in any child even if the diagnosis is first made in later childhood.
3. Since bilateral vocal cord paralysis seen in Arnold-Chiari malformation is often reversible if prompt attention is given to the underlying etiology, early diagnosis and management are essential to avoid a permanent tracheostomy.

✳ REFERENCES

1. Bower CM, Choi SS, Cotton RT. Arytenoidectomy in children. *Ann Otol Rhinol Laryngol* 1994;103:271–278.
2. Terris DJ, Arnstein DP, Nguyen HH. Contemporary evaluation of unilateral vocal cord paralysis. *Otolaryngol Head Neck Surg* 1992;107:84–90.

3. Boey HP, Cunningham MJ, Weber AL. Central nervous system imaging in the evaluation of children with true vocal cord paralysis. *Ann Otol Rhinol Laryngol* 1995;104:76–77.

4. Ross DA, Ward PH. Central vocal cord paralysis and paresis presenting as laryngeal stridor in children. *Laryngoscope* 1990;100:10–13.

5. Weber PC, Cass SP. Neurotologic manifestations of Chiari I malformation. *Otolaryngol Head Neck Surg* 1993;109:853–860.

6. Hesz N, Wolraich M. Vocal cord paralysis and brainstem dysfunction in children with spina bifida. *Dev Med Child Neurol* 1985;27:528–531.

7. Bluestone CD, Delerme AN, Samuelson GH. Airway obstuction due to vocal cord paralysis in infants with hydrocephalus and meningomyelocele. *Ann Otol* 1972;81:778–783.

8. Cohen SR, Geller KA, Birns JW, Thompson JW. Laryngeal paralysis in children. *Ann Otol Rhinol Laryngol* 1982;91:417–424.

9. Holinger LD, Holinger PC, Holinger PH. Etiology of bilateral abductor vocal cord paralysis. a review of 389 cases. *Ann Otol* 1976;85:428–436.

10. Holinger PC, Holinger LD, Reichert TJ, Holinger PH. Respiratory obstruction and apnea in infants with bilateral abductor vocal cord paralysis, meningomyelocele, hydrocephalus, and Arnold-Chiari malformation. *J Pediatr* 1978;92:368–373.

11. Snow JB, Rogers KA. Bilateral abductor paralysis of the vocal cords secondary to the Arnold-Chiari malformation and its management. *Laryngoscope 1965;75:316–321.*

S.S. Choi: Department of Otolaryngology, George Washington University, Children's National Medical Center, Washington, DC 20010.

Thyroglossal Duct Cyst

Sukgi S. Choi

INITIAL PRESENTATION

A 10-year-old boy presented to the clinic with a 6-year history of a mass overlying the hyoid bone. There had been several episodes of infection of this mass, which were successfully treated with antibiotic therapy. The mass had gradually enlarged over time. There was no significant past medical history. On examination, the patient had a soft, partially mobile mass in the submental triangle. The mass appeared to be attached to the hyoid bone and moved on deglutition. A thyroid scan was obtained, which showed the thyroid gland in its normal position (Fig. 1).

DIFFERENTIAL DIAGNOSIS

The likely diagnosis in this case is a thyroglossal duct cyst. Such cysts are the most commonly seen midline neck mass in children. Other possible diagnoses are ectopic thyroid, dermoid cyst, and lymphadenopathy. In general, for a pediatric midline neck mass, a thyroid scan is obtained preoperatively. This verifies the presence of a normally located and functioning thyroid, thus excluding the possibility of an ectopic thyroid. Computed tomography (CT) scan or sonography of the thyroid gland can be used in place of a thyroid scan; however, these two imaging modalities only provide anatomic information about the thyroid gland and not its functional status (1). CT scan can be valuable in defining the precise location and extent of the thyroglossal duct anomalies, particularly when there is an unusual presentation (2).

FIGURE 1 Thyroid scan showing the thyroid gland in its normal position.

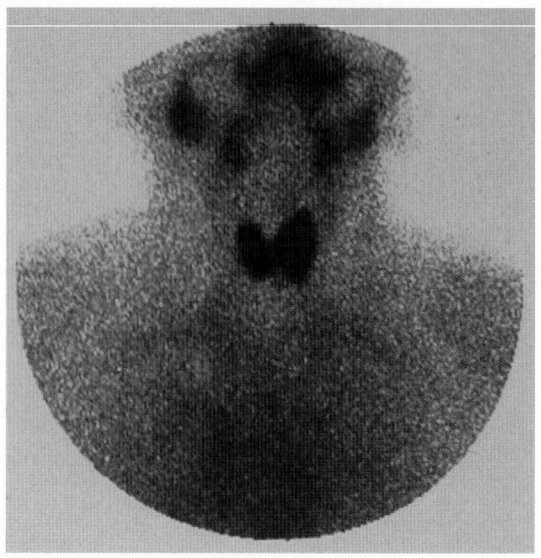

The traditional view that preoperative thyroid scan should be obtained has recently been challenged. Radkowski et al. (3), in their review of 229 pediatric patients with midline neck masses, found that with careful preoperative history and physical examination directed toward detecting mild hypothroidism, as well as thyroid function tests (specifically thyroid-stimulating hormone), thyroid scan is needed only in a select patient population. Stevens and Gray (4) have expressed a similar opinion. However, in some cases, the final diagnosis may only be possible at the time of surgery and with pathologic evaluation of the specimen.

SURGICAL MANAGEMENT

The patient was taken to the operating room for excision of the mass. The mass was approached through a horizontal incision over its midportion. It was deep to the mylohyoid muscle and was dissected out from the surrounding muscle. A tract was found in the inferior portion of the mass, and this was followed to the midportion of the hyoid bone (Fig. 2). There was no superior tract. The mass was removed in continuity with the midportion of the hyoid bone. The patient had an uneventful recovery.

Surgical pathology showed a 2.7 × 2.2 × 1.8-cm cystic mass attached to the hyoid bone by a fibromembranous tissue. The cyst was lined by keratinizing, stratified squamous epithelium with few attached skin appendages. The lumen was filled with keratinous debris. This was consistent with a diagnosis of dermoid cyst.

PROBLEM-FOCUSED DISCUSSION

Thyroglossal duct anomalies (TGDA) are the most common congenital neck masses in children (5). They usually present as an asymptomatic anterior midline neck mass. However, they can become repeatedly infected with upper respiratory infections and can also (rarely) undergo malignant degeneration (6). Thus, TGDA requires surgical excision.

Embryologically, the thyroid gland develops during the third week of gestation as an invagination of the endodermal cells on the pharyngeal floor at the eventual site of the foramen cecum. The thyroid anlage then migrates caudally as an epithelium-lined tube known as the thyroglossal duct (TGD). In its descent, TGD becomes intimately related to the central portion of the hyoid bone (7). By the seventh week, the thyroid gland reaches its final pretracheal position, and the TGD atrophies. Persistence of TGD results in TGDAs, including cysts, sinuses, and fistulae.

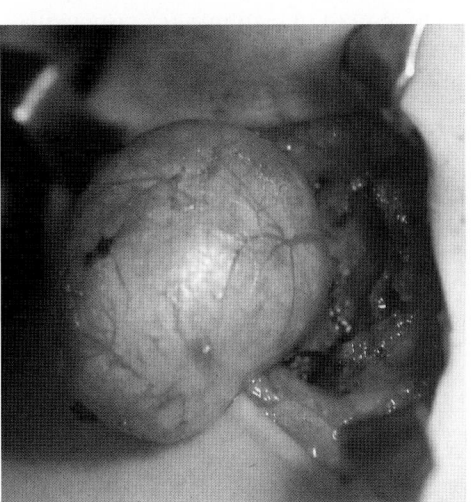

FIGURE 2 A large midline mass with attachment to the hyoid bone.

Historically, TGDAs were incised and drained. However, this approach resulted in an unacceptably high rate of recurrence of over 50% (8). In 1893, Schlange (9) proposed the removal of the central portion of the hyoid bone with TGDA; this reduced the recurrence rate of TGDA to 20%. Subsequently, in 1920, Sistrunk (10) recommended the removal of a tissue core 5 mm in diameter from the hyoid bone center up to and including the foramen cecum in addition to the midportion of the hyoid bone and TGDA. The Sistrunk procedure has reduced the recurrence rate of TGDA to 3% to 5%. This low recurrence rate associated with the Sistrunk procedure can be explained by the embryology of TGDA.

The differential diagnosis of TGDA includes ectopic thyroid gland, dermoid cyst, branchial anomalies, sebaceous cyst, lymphadenopathy, cystic hygroma, and laryngocele (11). These other cervical masses do not require a Sistrunk procedure but rather a simple excision with shorter operating time and lower morbidity.

Although it is generally thought that TGDA is an easy diagnosis to make, misdiagnosis is a persistent problem, even in tertiary referral centers (12). The differentiation of TGDA from other midline cervical masses pre- and intraoperatively is also not always reliable. In addition, a number of midline cervical cysts show features of both TGDA and dermoid. Therefore, deMello et al. (13) have recommended treating all midline cervical masses with the Sistrunk procedure. Generally, the morbidity of the Sistrunk procedure can be considered acceptable, and the additional time required to do this procedure may be reasonable in all midline cervical cysts if the recurrence rate for TGDA can be further reduced.

In this patient, although intraoperatively the mass was felt to represent a TGDA, pathologic examination made a diagnosis of a dermoid cyst. This case illustrates that the Sistrunk procedure is the surgical procedure of choice for midline neck masses suspected of being TGDA.

PEARLS AND PERILS

1. A preoperative thyroid scan should be considered in any child suspected to have a midline neck mass to rule out the possible diagnosis of ectopic thyroid.
2. A midline neck mass in the vicinity of the hyoid bone is a TGDA until proved otherwise, and a Sistrunk procedure should be performed to excise these lesions, to decrease the rate of recurrence.
3. In performing a Sistrunk procedure, dissection should be carried out superiorly, as well as inferiorly, to ensure excision of the entire lesion.

 REFERENCES

1. Lim-Dunham JE, Feinstein KA, Yousefzadeh DK, Ben-Ami T. *AJR* 1995;164:1489–1491.
2. Ward RE, Selfe RW, St. Louis L, Bowling D. *Otolaryngol Head Neck Surg* 1986;95:93–98.
3. Radkowski D, Aronald JA, Healy GB, McGill T, et al. *Arch Otolaryngol Head Neck Surg* 1991;117:1378–1381.
4. Stevens MH, Gray S. *Arch Otolaryngol Head Neck Surg* 1994;120:113.
5. Santiago W, Rybak LP, Bass RM. *J Otolaryngol* 1985;14:261–264.
6. Weiss SD, Orlich CC. *Br J Surg* 1992;79:1248–1249.
7. Ellis D, Van Nostrand P. *Laryngoscope* 1977;87:765–770.
8. Noyek AM, Friedberg J. *Otolaryngol Clin North Am* 1983;14:187–201.
9. Schlange H. *Arch Klin Chir* 1893;46:390–392.
10. Sistrunk WE. *Ann Surg* 1920;7:121–123.
11. Ward PH, Strahan RW, Acquarelli M, Harris PF. *Trans Am Acad Ophthalmol Otolaryngol* 1970;74:310–318.
12. Pelausa EO, Forte V. *J Otolaryngol* 1989;18:325–333.
13. deMello DE, Lima JA, Liapis H. *Arch Otolaryngol Head Neck Surg* 1987;113:418–420.

S.S. Choi: Department of Otolaryngology, George Washington University, Children's National Medical Center, Washington, DC 20010.

Sialorrhea and Aspiration

Brian J. Wiatrak

🔆 INITIAL PRESENTATION

An 8-year-old boy with a history of severe cerebral palsy presented with a history of significant drooling, which had worsened over recent years. There were occasional episodes of aspiration. He had been hospitalized 2 years previously for aspiration pneumonia, which resolved with medical therapy, and had not had a recurrent episode since that time. The family stated that he had to have his bibs changed six to ten times a day and that at times the skin on his chin and upper neck became very raw and macerated. He had had a gastrostomy tube placed 4 years previously, and most of his alimentation was obtained through this route. Occasionally, however, he could tolerate thickened feedings. He had excessive stertorous breathing at night but no obvious stridor. He was a chronic mouth breather.

The patient was a well-nourished boy with obvious severe neurologic impairment and spastic changes in his extremities. He did have adequate head control and responded when asked questions, although he was unable to speak. He had significant sialorrhea with maceration of the skin of his chin and anterior neck. Oral examination showed satisfactory dentition. His tonsils were mildly enlarged and noninflamed. He was mouth breathing and had evidence of bilateral purulent rhinorrhea. His lungs sounded clear to auscultation.

Initial Diagnostic Tests

A chest radiograph revealed no evidence of chronic pulmonary changes. A modified barium swallow revealed poor control of the oral phase of swallowing with a minimal amount of aspiration. Flexible nasopharyngoscopy performed with topical nasal decongestant and local anesthesia revealed significant hypertrophy of the adenoidal pad, obstructing the right and left choanae. A large amount of salivary secretions was noted in the hypopharynx and pooling in both pyriform sinuses. Vocal cord mobility appeared to be normal, and there was adequate glottic closure with protection of the larynx when the larynx was touched with the tip of the fiberoptic endoscope.

🔆 DIFFERENTIAL DIAGNOSIS

The patient had severe neurologic impairment with pronounced sialorrhea. He had poor control of the oral phase of swallowing and may have had chronic subclinical aspiration. Although there was one episode of aspiration pneumonia 2 years ago, this had not been a recurrent problem, and the chest x-ray did not reveal chronic pulmonary changes. The patient's primary problem at this time was most likely related to sialorrhea, and aspiration appeared to be a minimal concern at this time.

🕨 INITIAL MANAGEMENT

A speech therapy consultation was obtained to evaluate further the patient's swallowing function. The speech pathologist felt that there was poor neuromuscular control of the oral phase of swallowing and recommended only thickened feedings if the patient was to be fed orally. The possibility of utilizing anticholinergic medication to control the excessive sialorrhea was discussed with the family. They stated that this had been attempted in the past and the patient had not tolerated the side effects, leading to discontinuation of the medication.

🕨 SURGICAL MANAGEMENT

Because the excessive sialorrhea caused a significant quality-of-life problem for the patient and his family, and the patient had low-grade intermittent aspiration, it was felt that surgical intervention was warranted to control the sialorrhea. This included adenoidectomy to relieve the nasal obstruction and bilateral submandibular gland excision with bilateral parotid duct ligation. This was performed, and the patient tolerated the procedure well.

🕧 FINAL OUTCOME

Three months postoperatively, the patient is doing very well, with a significant decrease in sialorrhea and a major improvement in his quality of life. His nasal obstruction is much improved. Although he does intermittently mouth breathe and has occasional stertorous breathing at night, this is improved over his preoperative condition. The family reported a transient episode of bilateral swelling of the cheek region in the first postoperative week that subsequently subsided over a period of 1 week.

A repeat modified barium swallow was obtained showing a marked decrease in pooling of hypopharyngeal secretions with no evidence of aspiration.

🙵 PROBLEM-FOCUSED DISCUSSION

The management of sialorrhea and associated aspiration can constitute a significant problem in a neurologically impaired child. Medical therapy is often inadequate and may have secondary side effects. Surgical therapy may also have associated postsurgical complications, and at this time, there is no consensus of the best surgical treatment for sialorrhea. Poor neurologic control of swallowing may result in sialorrhea and aspiration. Surgical management of chronic aspiration is often quite radical and may lead to permanent loss of vocal function. In certain patients, aggressive management of sialorrhea in itself may control aspiration, as was the situation in this case.

Sialorrhea in neurologically impaired patients is generally the result of an impaired oral phase of deglutition, not the result of excessive salivary production. Deglutition is divided into three phases: I, oral; II, pharyngeal; and III, esophageal. Whereas pharyngeal and esophageal swallowing are primarily under autonomic control, the oral phase of swallowing is primarily a voluntary act. Cineradiographic studies have shown that patients with cerebral palsy have disruption of the voluntary or oral phase of swallowing (1). Other associated factors that may lead to sialorrhea include the patient's head position and posture, malocclusion, tongue control and size, perioral sensation, and nasal obstruction. In this case, sialorrhea was probably the result of nasal obstruction secondary to adenoid hypertrophy causing chronic mouth breathing in addition to the incoordination of swallowing.

Salivary production is regulated by automonic control of the major and minor salivary glands, primarily through parasympathetic innervation (2). Preganglionic parasympathetic fibers reach the submandibular and sublingual glands from the superior salivary nuculeus in the medulla, synapsing with postganglionic fibers of the submandibular ganglion. They travel primarily with the chorda tympani nerve. Parasympathetic preganglionic fibers reach the parotid gland from the inferior salivary nuculeus in the medulla, traveling with the glossopharyngeal nerve and synapsing with postganglionic fibers in the otic ganglion in the pterygopalatine fossa.

In some neurologically impaired children, the combination of poor oral motor control and poor motor and sensory function of the hypopharynx and larynx can lead to chronic aspiration. Controlling the problem of sialorrhea in selected patients may secondarily decrease aspiration, obviating the need for more radical surgical intervention. Surgical intervention for sialorrhea in certain neurologically impaired children has been shown to control chronic aspiration in these patients (2).

The diagnostic evaluation of a child with sialorrhea and aspiration should include a thorough head and neck examination. Causes of nasal obstruction and chronic mouth breathing should be evaluated, i.e., the nasal septum and evidence of adenotonsilar hypertrophy. Correction of these problems may lead to better oral motor control of salivary secretions and secondarily help control aspiration. Flexible fiberoptic nasopharyngoscopy should also be utilized in these patients to help assess laryngeal function, vocal cord mobility, pooling of secretions, and sensation of the hypopharynx and larynx.

The management of sialorrhea in neurologically impaired children may be medical or surgical. In general, medical management utilizing drugs, such as anticholinergic agents, may lead to significant side effects and, in general, are not tolerated well by patients (1,2).

PEARLS AND PERILS

1. Chronic aspiration in neurologically impaired children may be the result of poor oral motor control of salivary secretions.
2. Medical or surgical control of sialorrhea may improve chronic aspiration secondarily in selected neurologically impaired patients.
3. The diagnostic evaluation of patients with sialorrhea should include assessment of underlying causes of nasal obstruction and chronic mouth breathing, i.e., nasal septal deviation and adenotonsillar hypertrophy.
4. Radical surgical intervention, i.e., tracheal diversion procedures, may be required in neurogically devastated patients with chronic aspiration. Although the ideal surgical procedure for sialorrhea is still debatable, excellent results have been obtained utilizing bilateral submandibular gland excision and bilateral parotid duct ligation.

The surgical management of sialorrhea in neurologically impaired children remains controversial; multiple surgical modalities have been described in the literature. Crysdale (4) reported excellent results for surgical rerouting of the submandibular ducts (Wharton's ducts). Theoretically, rerouting Wharton's ducts will result in redirected salivary flow to a more posterior location in the oral cavity. However, the actual amount of salivary production is not changed. Complications from this surgical modality include stenosis of Wharton's duct (5,6) and ranulas (7,8). Satisfactory results have resulted from the Wilkie procedure, which includes bilateral submandibular gland excision and rerouting of Stensen's duct (9). Again, in this situation, rerouting of the parotid ducts transfers flow more posteriorly into the oral cavity; however, parotid salivary flow is not actually decreased. Utilization of bilateral submandibular gland excision and bilateral parotid duct ligation leads to excellent results with very few cases of xerostomia (8). Although recanalization of the parotid ducts is possible, the actual incidence of this has never been documented. Complications include transient parotid swelling, which is usually short-lived. Finally, disrupting the autonomic innervation of the salivary glands through an exploratory tympanotomy approach has been described. This involves sectioning of the chorda tympani nerve and disruption of the tympanic plexus (10,11). Unfortunately, high failure rates have been described, and the obvious loss of taste may be debilitating to the patient.

An alternative to surgical intervention may be physical therapy initiated in neurologically impaired children to help control sialorrhea. Although the results have been relatively disappointing (1), physical therapy may play a significant adjunctive role to other treatment modalities (4,5).

In patients with devastating neurologic injuries, control of salivary secretions alone will not help control chronic aspiration, which at times may become life threatening. In these situations, radical surgical intervention may be required, such as laryngeal closure procedures or tracheal diversion procedures, i.e., the Lindeman procedure (12–14).

REFERENCES

1. Myer CM III. Sialorrhea. *Pediatr Clin North Am* 1989;36:1495–1500.
2. Lew KM, Younis RT, Lazar RH. The current management of sialorrhea. *Ear Nose Throat* 1991;70:99–105.
3. Gerber ME, Gaugler M, Myer CM III, Cotton RT. Chronic aspiration in children. When are bilateral submandibular gland excision and parotid duct ligation indicated? *Arch Otolaryngol Head Neck Surg* 1996;122:1368–1371.
4. Crysdale WS. The drooling patient: evaluation and current surgical options. *Laryngoscope* 1980;90:775–783.
5. Cotton RT, Richardson MA. The effect of submandibular duct rerouting in the treatment of sialorrhea in children. *Otolaryngol Head Neck Surg* 1981;89:535–541.
6. Ray SA, Bundy AC, Nelson DL. Decreasing drooling through techniques to facilitate mouth closure. *Am J Occup Ther* 1983;37:749–753.
7. Crysdale WS, Mendelsohn JD, Conley S. Ranulas-Mucoceles of the oral cavity: experience in 26 children. *Laryngoscope* 1988;98:296–298.
8. Shott SR, Myer CM III, Cotton RT. Surgical management of sialorrhea. *Otolaryngol Head Neck Surg* 1989;101:47–50.
9. Wilkie TF. The problem of drooling in cerebral palsy: a surgical approach. *Can J Surg* 1967;10:60–67.
10. Michel RG, Johnson KA, Patterson CN. Parasympathetic nerve section for control of sialorrhea. *Arch Otolaryngol* 1977;103:94–97.
11. Frederick FJ, Stewart IF. Effectiveness of transtympanic neurectomy in management of sialorrhea occuring in mentally retarded patients. *J Otolaryngol* 1982;11:289–292.
12. Eavey RD. Airway interruption in encephalopathic children: a clinical and histological analysis. *Laryngoscope* 1985;95:1455–1460.
13. Kirsch JP, Solomon JW. Evaluation and mangement of chronic aspiration. *J L State Med Soc* 1993;145:75–80.
14. De Vito MA, Wetmore RF, Pransky SM. Laryngeal diversion in the treatment of chronic aspiration in children. *Int J Pediatr Otorhinolaryngol* 1989;18:139–145.

B.J. Wiatrak: Department of Surgery, Division of Otolaryngology—Head and Neck Surgery, The University of Alabama at Birmingham, Children's Hospital of Alabama, Birmingham, Alabama 35233–1711.

Sigmoid Sinus Thrombosis

Brian J. Wiatrak

🔮 INITIAL PRESENTATION

A 6-year old girl presented with a 1-day history of progressive right otalgia, mild right temporal headache, and a protruding right auricle. She had had fevers as high as 101.5°F but had not been treated with antimicrobials. She had no significant otologic history and was otherwise healthy. She had no significant history of prior ear disease.

🔮 PHYSICAL EXAMINATION

The patient was alert, awake, and cooperative for examination. The right ear was prominent, with loss of the postauricular crease. She was tender over the mastoid area. Although postauricular edema was present, there was no obvious fluctuance. Facial movement was intact and bilaterally symmetric. Her tympanic membrane on the left was normal and on the right was erythematous and bulging, with evidence of acute otitis media and purulent material in the middle-ear space. Her ear canal was tender on examination, especially in the posterior superior quadrant. However, the bone was intact, and there was no fluctuance on palpation. The remainder of her head and neck examination was unremarkable. The last time she had had anything to eat or drink was 6 hours previously. Fundoscopic examination was normal with no evidence of papilledema.

Initial Diagnostic Tests

A complete blood count with differential was obtained; she had a white blood cell count of 19,000 cells/mm^3 with a shift to the left. Computed tomographic (CT) scan with contrast revealed opacification of the right mastoid air cells with no obvious bony erosion or coalescence of the mastoid air cells.

🔮 DIFFERENTIAL DIAGNOSIS

The most likely diagnosis at this time was acute mastoiditis. The diagnosis of coalescent mastoiditis could not be made, based on the CT scan and the fact that the patient did not appear toxic at this time. Other causes of periauricular edema that may cause a prominent ear include periauricular cellulitis from acute otitis externa and possibly auricular chondritis. However, the evidence of acute otitis media on otologic examination made these entities much less likely. Intracranial complications of otitis media should always be considered when managing a patient with mastoiditis. However, the absence of papilledema, severe headache, or lethargy made this possibility unlikely.

🗨 INITIAL MANAGEMENT

The patient was taken to the operating room for myringotomy and ventilating tube placement in the right ear. On incision of the tympanic membrane, purulent debris was encountered and sent for culture and sensitivity. A great deal of bleeding from the tympanic membrane occurred, and polypoid mucosa was noted behind the tympanic membrane in the middle-ear space. The patient was admitted to the hospital and begun on intravenous antimicrobial therapy and topical otic antibiotic drops. In addition, she was scheduled to have her myringotomy tube examined and, if necessary, suctioned under the microscope on a daily basis. Antimicrobial coverage utilizing a third-generation cephalosporin (Ceftriaxone) and clindamycin was initiated to cover beta-lactamase producing strains of *Hemophilus influenzae, Streptococcus pneumoniae, Staphylococcus aureus,* and anaerobic bacteria. More specific antimicrobial therapy was planned after the culture and sensitivity results were obtained.

Interval Management

For 24 hours following myringotomy tube placement, the right ear continued to be prominent, with slightly increased tenderness and edema over the mastoid region. There was no nuchal rigidity. The white blood cell count had risen to 21,000 cells/mm^3 with a shift to the left. Fevers were now spiking to 103°F. The patient complained of a persistent right temporal headache. On fundoscopic examination, mild papilledema was present. In addition, the patient's clinical appearance had deteriorated and she appeared toxic. Blood cultures were sent for evaluation.

⅜ DIFFERENTIAL DIAGNOSIS

The patient's condition had clearly deteriorated despite drainage of the middle-ear space and placement of a ventilation tube and continuation of aggressive antibiotic therapy. The increased headache, worsening fever spikes, increased white blood cell count, increased periauricular edema, and the appearance of papilledema suggested an intracranial

FIGURE 1 Computed tomography scan with contrast demonstrating a superior lateral orbital subperiosteal abscess associated with sinusitis.

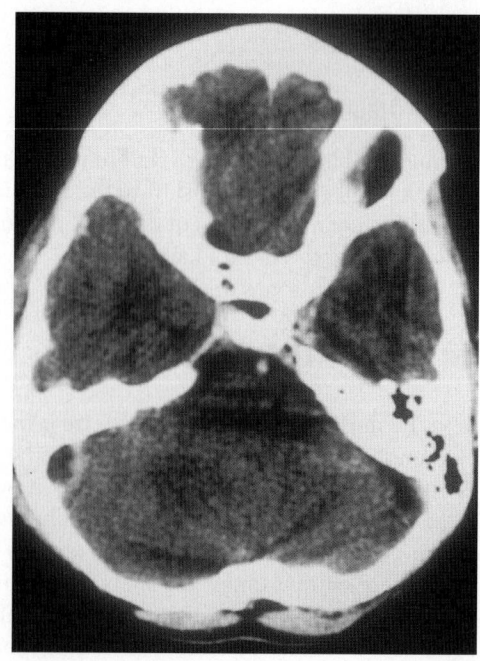

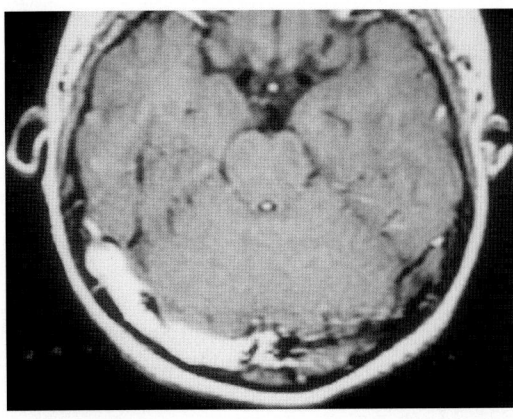

FIGURE 2 Magnetic resonance imaging scan demonstrating obstructive blood flow through the right lateral sinus.

complication. This would include the possibilities of lateral sinus thrombosis, brain abscess, or possibly an epidural abscess. A repeat CT scan with contrast was obtained and showed evidence of right sigmoid sinus thrombosis (Fig. 1). Subsequently, a magnetic residence imaging scan was obtained confirming the presence of lateral sinus thrombosis (Fig. 2).

SURGICAL MANAGEMENT

The patient was taken to the operating room immediately for tympanomastoidectomy. During the cortical mastoidectomy, polypoid edematous mucosa was encountered with no obvious purulence. The lateral cortical bone of the mastoid was intact, and there was no obvious dehiscence in the region of the mastoid tegmen. Granulation tissue was noted overlying the region of the sigmoid sinus, and the overlying bone was dehiscent (Fig. 3). An 18-gauge needle was placed into the lumen of the sigmoid sinus, and no blood flow was obtained. The sinus was incised and the granulation tissue debrided. Some purulence was encountered. The entire cavity was thoroughly irrigated. The middle-ear space was explored, revealing polypoid mucosa, some purulence, and no evidence of cholesteatoma. The incision was closed over a rubber band drain.

FINAL OUTCOME

The patient's clinical status improved dramatically over the next 48 hours, with complete defervescence and return of her white blood cell count to normal in 72 hours. The

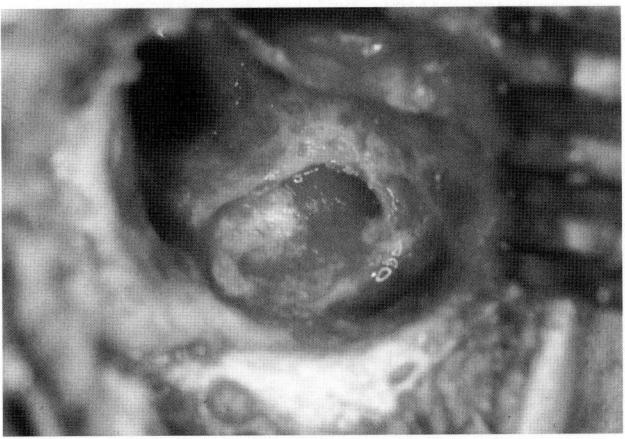

FIGURE 3 Granulation tissue overlying exposed, thrombosed right sigmoid sinus.

patient continued on a 1-week course of intravenous antimicrobial therapy and was discharged on a three-week course of amoxicillin/clavulanic acid. The final culture results of the ear revealed *S. pneumoniae*, penicillin-sensitive. There was no growth in the blood cultures.

PROBLEM-FOCUSED DISCUSSION

Fortunately, lateral sinus thrombosis is a rare complication of acute suppurative mastoiditis. However, when present; it may lead to more extensive intracranial complications and possibly death. The mortality from lateral sinus thrombosis has been reported to be as high as 36% (1). However, mortality rates as low as 5% have also been reported 2–4). It is important to note that as the incidence of pneumococcal-penicillin resistance increases, current antimicrobial treatment regimens may be less successful, thus leading to increasing mortality rates (5).

Typically, acute mastoiditis is a complication of acute supurative middle-ear disease. As inflammation creates obstruction at the aditus ad antrum, purulent debris may accumulate in the mastoid cavity, leading to subsequent demineralization of bone and the formation of osteitis. This process of coalescence within the mastoid cavity subsequently may lead to further intratemporal complications such as labyrinthitis and petrositis or, more worrisome, intracranial complications such as meningitis, epidural or subdural empyema, brain abscess, or lateral sinus thrombosis.

Prompt treatment of acute mastoiditis may prevent development of these complications. High-dose intravenous antimicrobials (with adequate coverage of *S. aureus*, aerobic and anarobic streptococcus, beta-lactamase-producing *H. influenzae*, upper respiratory tract anaerobes, and *Proteus* species) will provide excellent initial empiric therapy until more specific therapy can be guided by cultures (2). It is also important to provide middle-ear and mastoid drainage by wide myringotomy or placement of a myringotomy tube. A CT scan of the temporal bone is an important initial diagnostic test that may show evidence of mastoid coalescence. If this is demonstrated, then urgent cortical mastoidectomy is required.

An intracranial complication should be suspected when initial treatment for acute mastoiditis has not resulted in significant resolution of symptomatology or reduced the white blood cell count. In cases of acute mastoiditis in which fever spikes continue with associated malaise and headache despite aggressive medical therapy, lateral sinus thrombosis should be considered. Signs of increased intracranial pressure such as papilledema, altered consciousness, and seizures may be present. The diagnosis is best made utilizing CT scans with contrast in combination with magnetic residence imaging with contrast. A lumbar puncture should be performed only after a cranial CT scan has ruled out a space-occupying lesion, which may predispose the patient to brain herniation. Typically, in lateral sinus thrombosis, the lumbar puncture is sterile, with very few white cells present, unless a patient has coexistent meningitis; the intracranial pressure is usually normal unless the disease process has progressed to otitic hydrocephalus. More invasive tests may be utilized, such as digital subtraction angiography, retrograde jugulography, and carotid arteriography. However, complications may results from theses test (1).

The treatment for lateral sinus thrombosis includes high-dose intravenous antimicrobial therapy and cortical mastoidectomy with unroofing of the sigmoid sinus. A needle should be placed into the sigmoid sinus; if free blood flow is obtained, no further intervention is warranted. If no blood flow is detected, the sinus should be opened, and any infected clot should be evacuated. Typically, exuberant amounts of granulation tissue will be encountered overlying the sigmoid sinus, often with dehiscent bone at the time of cortical mastoidectomy.

REFERENCES

1. Teichgraeber JF, Per-lee JH, Turner JS. Lateral sinus thrombosis: a modern day perspective. *Laryngoscope* 1982;92:744–751.
2. Garcia RDJ, Baker AS, Cunningham MJ, Weber AL. Lateral sinus thrombosis associated with otitis media and mastoiditis in children. *Pediatr Infect Dis J* 1995;14:617–623.
3. Samuel J, Fernandes CMC. Lateral sinus thrombosis: a review of 45 cases. *J Laryngol Otol* 1987;101:1227–1229.
4. Mathews TJ. Lateral sinus pathology (22 cases managed at Groote Schuur Hospital). *J Laryngol Otol* 1988;102:118–120.
5. Poole MD. Otitis media complications and treatment failures: implications of pneumococcal resistance. *Pediatr Infect Dis J* 1995;14:23–26.

B.J. Wiatrak: Department of Surgery, Division of Otolaryngology—Head and Neck Surgery, The University of Alabama at Birmingham, Children's Hospital of Alabama, Birmingham, Alabama 35233–1711.

Membranous Tracheitis

Brian J. Wiatrak

INITIAL PRESENTATION

A 5-year-old white boy presented to the emergency room with significant respiratory distress preceded by a 1-week history of an upper respiratory tract infection and a 1-day history of fever and increasing productive cough. Over the previous 24 hours, the patient's temperature had reached 103.5°F at one point. The patient had received albuterol aerosol treatment in his pediatrician's office without improvement.

PHYSICAL EXAMINATION

On physical examination, the patient was having obvious respiratory distress with evidence of inspiratory and expiratory stridor. He was sitting upright and drooling, and he had a temperature of 101.5°F. He was having supraclavicular and intercostal retractions. There was evidence of subcutaneous emphysema in his neck and supraclavicular regions. On auscultation, there was evidence of bilateral wheezing. However, breath sounds were equal on both sides.

Before the otolaryngology service was consulted, the emergency room staff obtained cervical airway radiographs and anterior–posterior and lateral chest radiographs. These revealed a small right-sided pneumothorax, pneumomediastinum, and subcutaneous emphysema (Fig. 1). The cervical radiographs were of poor quality, and the epiglottis could not be accurately assessed, nor could the subglottic and tracheal airway be seen clearly on the radiograph, although there was evidence of subglottic narrowing. A complete blood count with differential revealed a white blood cell count of 26,100 cells/mm³, hematocrit of 41.9%, with 81% segmented neutrophils, 12% bands, and 4% lymphocytes. At this point, the otolaryngologist was consulted.

DIFFERENTIAL DIAGNOSIS

The differential diagnosis in this age group should include (a) epiglottitis, (b) bacterial tracheitis, (c) foreign body aspiration, and possibly (d) peritonsillar abscess with deep neck infection. A patient of this age with stridor and obvious respiratory distress with evidence of systemic infection should be considered to have epiglottitis until proved otherwise. Patients with epiglottitis typically are in significant respiratory distress, and no effort should be made to manipulate the patient in any way that may provoke anxiety, thus worsening the fragile respiratory condition. Attempts at flexible laryngoscopy, oral examination with a tongue blade, drawing blood, or obtaining radiographs should be discouraged. In this particular situation, the emergency room staff elected to obtain radiographic examinations before the otolaryngology consultation. Children with bacterial

964

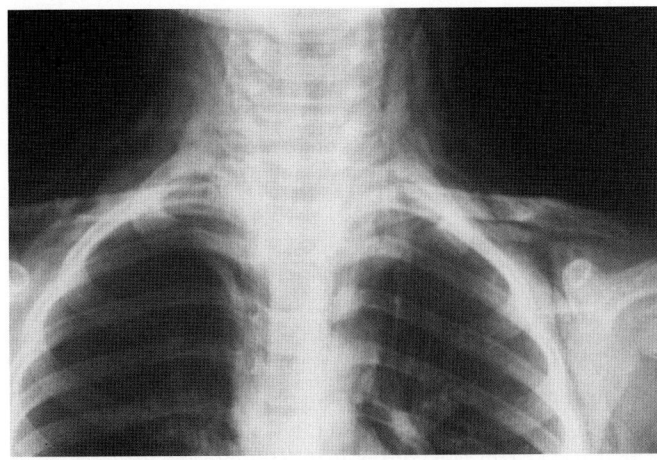

FIGURE 1 Posterior–anterior chest radiograph revealing cervical subcutaneous emphysema, a small right apical pneumothorax, and evidence of pneumomedia stinum.

tracheitis may also present with similar symptomatology, systemically ill and toxic appearing. When epiglottitis is being seriously considered, endoscopic intervention in the operating room should be considered early. If a radiographic evaluation is performed, the patient should be accompanied to the radiology suite by a physician. The parents should also be present to allay the child's anxiety. In this particular situation, the cervical airway radiographs were noncontributory in the assessment of the airway due to poor-quality films. Therefore, these two entities could not be differentiated. Foreign body aspiration should also be considered in this patient. The presence of subcutaneous emphysema and a small pneumothorax indicated the possibility of severe air trapping, which may have caused a rupture into the pleural space. The presence of systemic symptomatology, high fever, and elevated white blood count with a shift to the left argues against foreign body aspiration. However, when a foreign body has been present for a long period (more than a few days) secondary infection, pneumonia, and systemic symptomatology as well as mediastinitis may be present. Although the chest radiograph showed evidence of a pneumothorax and massive subcutaneous emphysema, there was no obvious hyperinflation of the lung and no evidence of pneumonia. A severe broncospastic episode may also present with severe respiratory difficulty and similar radiologic findings, but the high fever and systemic toxicity argued against it.

SURGICAL MANAGEMENT

Preparations were made to take the patient to the operating room immediately for laryngoscopy and bronchoscopy. The patient was given supplemental oxygen through a nasal cannula and kept with his parents to allay as much anxiety as possible. An intravenous line was not started at this point due to the patient's significant distress and anxiety; this would be started once general anesthesia had been initiated.

Preparations in the operating room need to be complete before general anesthesia is actually initiated. It is important that the nurses staffing the operating room be comfortable with the endoscopy equipment and familiar with assisting on this type of procedure. It is crucial that all personnel be prepared for the possibility that the patient's airway may deteriorate rapidly. All endoscopy equipment needs to be tested to make sure the appropriate-sized telescopes, bronchoscopes, and foreign body forceps are present and fit together correctly, that all light sources are functioning properly, and that appropriate flexible and rigid suction catheter devices are present. It is extremely important to have a tracheotomy tray present in the room and open, ready for immediate use if the need should arise. General anesthesia is initiated utilizing halothane through a face mask. It is important that this step of the procedure not be rushed, that the patient be allowed to be affected by the halothane gradually, and not be agitated in any way. Once the patient becomes anesthetized, the endoscopy may be performed. It is important not to use neuromuscular paralysis at this point since this may abruptly cause loss of the airway and have potentially catastrophic results. Halothane and oxygen may be insufflated while the patient is breathing spontaneously through a suction port of the laryngoscope or simply by having the open anesthesia circuit presented to the corner of the mouth during the procedure. The important diagnostic maneuver at this point is to examine the supraglottic larynx carefully. In this particular situation, the patient's supraglottic airway, particularly the epiglottis, appeared completely normal with no evidence of edema or other abnormalities. The vocal cords appeared erythematous and edematous. At this time, an appropriately sized bronchoscope was passed through the true vocal cords and the anesthesia circuit then connected to the bronchoscope for ventilation.

First, the entire trachea appeared significantly inflamed and edematous (Fig. 2). There was obvious exudate within the trachea down to the level of the carina. Second, the anesthesiologist related that it was still very difficult to ventilate the patient, even through the bronchoscope was placed at the level of the midtrachea. Both lung fields failed to ventilate appropriately, and the patient was having significant difficulty maintaining his blood oxygen saturation.

A more distal examination of the tracheobronchial tree revealed thick, inspissated mucus in the right and left main stem bronchi, which had formed obvious casts or plugs obstructing both the right and left main stem bronchi. This required urgent removal to provide ventilation and maintain oxygen saturation. Optical foreign body forceps were present in the room, and the casts were removed with straight grasping alligator forceps (Fig. 3). Immediately, there was significant improvement of ventilation. Oxygen saturation reached 100%, and full expansion of the lungs was obtained.

At this point, cultures were sent from the trachea for culture and sensitivity. The patient was then intubated with an appropriately sized endotracheal tube, and ventilation continued to be easy. A repeat chest x-ray was obtained in the operating room, which revealed a small residual right apical pneumothorax. To evaluate the pneumothorax, a pediatric surgeon was consulted who felt that the lesion was small enough to avoid placement of a chest tube. The patient was empirically begun on antibiotics (nafcillin and cefotaxime) to cover *Staphylococcus aureus* and respiratory pathogens, such as *Hemophilus influenzae*. The final culture and sensitivity results revealed negative growth for blood cultures and tracheal cultures. However, the patient had been on antimicrobial therapy for his upper respiratory tract infection beginning 1 week prior to admission to the hospital.

Postsurgical Management

The patient was admitted for observation to the pediatric intensive care unit (PICU) postoperatively and was successfully extubated on the third day of hospital admission. By

FIGURE 2 Endoscopic appearance of lower trachea.

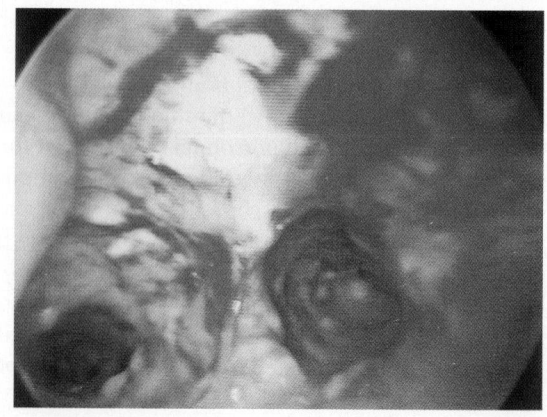

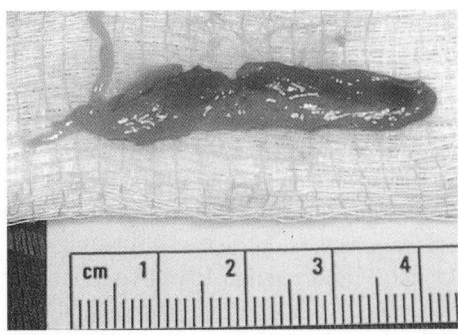

FIGURE 3 One of two casts removed from the proximal right and left main stem bronchi.

the second day of his admission to the PICU, the patient's white blood count had returned to normal and evidence of the pneumothorax had completely resolved on chest radiographs.

🔴 FINAL OUTCOME

The patient was discharged from the hospital 6 days after admission, at which time he was having no respiratory difficulty and had been afebrile for 48 hours. He was discharged on a 10-day course of amoxicillin with clavulanic acid.

& PROBLEM-FOCUSED DISCUSSION

Bacterial tracheitis is a potentially life-threatening respiratory illness that occurs most commonly during the winter months (1). This illness often presents with features common to viral croup (laryngotracheobronchitis) and epiglottitis. The initial presentation of bacterial tracheitis is not uncommonly confused with epiglottitis, as was the situation in this case. However, over recent years, due to the advent of the *H. influenzae* type B (HIB) vaccine, there has been a dramatic reduction in the incidence of epiglottitis (2–5). Gallagher and Myer (6) reported 18 cases of bacterial tracheitis between 1986 and 1988. During that same time, there were 34 cases of epiglottitis within their institution.

Bacterial tracheitis may be preceded by a prodrome of a viral upper respiratory tract illness for a period of 1 to 2 weeks. This is usually mild in severity with subsequent rapid deterioration in the patient's status. Epiglottitis, on the other hand, is not associated with a viral prodrome, and acute respiratory distress typically develops rapidly. Patients with bacterial tracheitis usually present with respiratory distress consisting of cough, inspiratory and expiratory stridor, and retractions. Patients prefer to be in the prone position as opposed to sitting up and leaning forward. In addition, drooling is a very common finding in patients with epiglottis and not in patients with bacterial tracheitis. The diagnosis is usually made on the basis of clinical presentation, radiographic findings, and flexible endoscopy. In Friedman et al.'s (1) series of ten cases of bacterial tracheitis, seven cases were diagnosed by direct laryngoscopy and bronchoscopy. Gallagher and Myer (6) reported that laryngoscopy and bronchoscopy was diagnostic in all eight cases in which it was utilized and that, in addition, flexible bronchoscopy was diagnostic of tracheitis in the eight cases in which it was performed. Eckel et al. (7) reported 11 patients with bacterial tracheitis. It was their feeling that no reliable predictive factors existed for the diagnosis of bacterial tracheitis and that no single clinical radiologic or laboratory test was a reliable diagnostic predictor for bacterial tracheitis. The only definitive diagnostic procedure to distinguish bacterial tracheitis accurately from other entities was direct laryngoscopy and bronchoscopy in the operating room. In addition to being a diagnostic modality, there was therapeutic value in all cases, with the ability to suction all tracheal secretions aggressively, aiding in pulmonary toilet.

Blood cultures typically reveal no growth, and tracheal aspirates usually grow *S. aureus* in addition to other aerobic pathogens, including *Streptococcus pyogenes, Streptococcus viridans, H. influenzae,* and *Moraxella catarrhalis* (1,6).

Patients respond well to aggressive medical therapy following endoscopy. This therapy should include appropriate antimicrobial therapy and possibly corticosteroids and/or racemic epinephrine. When ventilatory support is required, endotracheal intubation may be utilized for periods of time. Gallagher and Myer (6) reported that 10 of 18 patients required endotracheal intubation for a mean of 5.9 days, whereas Friedman et al. (1) reported that 3 of 10 patients required endotracheal intubation; these authors felt that younger patients were more likely to require endotracheal intubation for ventilatory support. The duration of endotracheal intubation should be minimized to avoid the sequela of prolonged intubation.

PEARLS AND PERILS

1. The presentation of bacterial tracheitis may be confused with that of acute epiglottitis.
2. Do not provoke anxiety in a patient suspected of having acute epiglottitis by performing overly invasive examinations and diagnostic procedures.
3. In any patient, when the diagnosis of acute epiglottitis is entertained, endoscopic evaluation should be performed in the operating room.
4. It is important to have a tracheotomy set immediately available in patients being evaluated in the operating room for acute respiratory distress in case the airway should deteriorate suddenly. Laryngoscopy and bronchoscopy are both diagnostic and therapeutic in cases of bacterial tracheitis. They provide the ability to suction tracheal secretions, remove crusts, and obtain tracheal cultures.
5. Until definitive cultures have been obtained, broad-spectrum antimicrobial agents that cover *S. aureus* and common respiratory pathogens are mandatory.
6. Patients who do not respond well to aggressive medical therapy or who require ventilatory support will require endotracheal intubation. It is possible that younger patients may be more likely to require endotracheal intubation in the management of bacterial tracheitis.

 ## REFERENCES

1. Friedman EM, Jorgensen K, Healy GB, McGill TJI. Bacterial tracheitis—two-year experience. *Laryngoscope* 1985;95:9–11.
2. Ryan M, Snowberger T. A changing pattern of epiglottitis. *Clin Pediatr* 1992;31:532–535.
3. Frantz TD, Rasgon BM. Acute epiglottitis: changing epidemiologic patterns. *Otolaryngol Head Neck Surg* 1993;109:457–460.
4. Gorelick MH, Baker MD. Epiglottitis in children. *Arch Pediatr Adolesc Med* 1994;148:47–50.
5. Gonzales Valdepena H, Wald ER, Rose E, Ungkanont K, Casselbrant ML. Epiglottitis and *Haemophilus influenzae* immunization: the Pittsburgh experience—a five-year review. *Pediatrics* 1995;96:424–427.
6. Gallagher PG, Myer CM III. An approach to the diagnosis and treatment of membranous laryngotracheobronchitis in infants and children. *Pediatr Emerg Care* 1991;7:337–342.
7. Eckel HE, Widemann B, Damm M, Roth B. Airway endoscopy in the diagnosis and treatment of bacterial tracheitis in children. *Int J Pediatr Otorhinolaryngol* 1993;27:147–157.

B.J. Wiatrak: Department of Surgery, Division of Otolaryngology—Head and Neck Surgery, The University of Alabama at Birmingham, Children's Hospital of Alabama, Birmingham, Alabama 35233–1711.

Laryngeal Saccular Cyst

Brian J. Wiatrak

INITIAL PRESENTATION

An infant was born after a normal term pregnancy and immediately experienced severe airway obstruction and respiratory distress. Endotracheal intubation was performed, described as difficult, with poor visualization of the vocal cords. No audible cry was noted at birth. Initial laryngoscopy at a community hospital by a general otolaryngologist revealed distorted laryngeal anatomy and a laryngeal mass completely obstructing the airway. Therefore, a tracheotomy was performed. Upon transfer for a second opinion, flexible laryngoscopy confirmed the presence of a right-sided laryngeal mass. Subsequently, direct laryngoscopy and bronchoscopy were performed in the operating room and an obvious right-sided cystic laryngeal mass was noted (Fig. 1). The tracheotomy site looked good, with no evidence of suprastomal granuloma formation or collapse. The remainder of the trachea and the proximal bronchi were normal.

Initial Tests

A magnetic resonance imaging (MRI) scan was obtained after the laryngoscopy and bronchoscopy (Fig. 2).

DIFFERENTIAL DIAGNOSIS

At this point, the differential diagnosis should include (a) laryngeal saccular cyst, (b) laryngocele, and (c) lymphangioma. The lesion involves the right side of the larynx, primarily at the level of the supraglottis. This eliminates the possibility of subglottic hemangioma and other congenital subglottic and tracheal lesions. This particular location also explains the absence of any audible cry after birth. The lesion appears to be covered by mucosa, which is typical for a laryngeal saccular cyst or laryngocele. However, lymphangioma will have a more irregular and infiltrating appearance. The MRI scan, which was performed with contrast, revealed no significant enhancement, which is consistent with a cystic mass and argues against a vascular lesion. This is most likely a laryngeal saccular cyst and not a laryngocele, which is typically filled with air. Laryngeal lymphangiomas typically have multiple septae within them and often have a component external to the larynx within the soft tissue of the neck. This was not the case on this scan. Based on the clinical, endoscopic and MRI findings, a laryngeal saccular cyst was considered the most likely diagnosis.

SURGICAL MANAGEMENT

At this point, surgical options were discussed with the family. One option is endoscopic drainage and marsupialization of the cyst utilizing the CO_2 laser. This may require

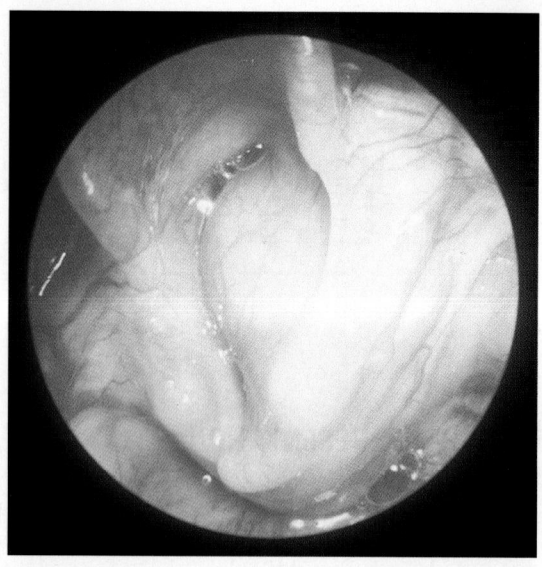

FIGURE 1 Endoscopic view of right-sided supraglottic laryngeal mass.

multiple procedures due to the recurrent nature of a laryngeal saccular cyst. Complete resection of the mass utilizing an external cervical approach to the thyrohyoid membrane is another option, which was chosen in this case.

The surgical procedure involved an incision overlying the upper aspect of the right thyroid cartilage to expose the thyrohyoid membrane. This was divided with care to prevent damage to the superior laryngeal nerve and its branches. The cyst was encountered almost immediately on the inner aspect of the thyroid ala and was completed dissected down to a pedicle in the region of the saccular orifice leading to the region of the ventricle. This was ligated with a suture; the saccular cyst was excised completely and noted to be filled with thick, viscous mucus. At this point, the wound was closed over a Penrose drain. The tracheotomy was removed and the patient intubated. Extubation was performed successfully on the third postoperative day and there have been no further problems. Voice quality has improved significantly since surgery and is normal now.

FIGURE 2 Magnetic resonance imaging scan with contrast of the laryngeal mass.

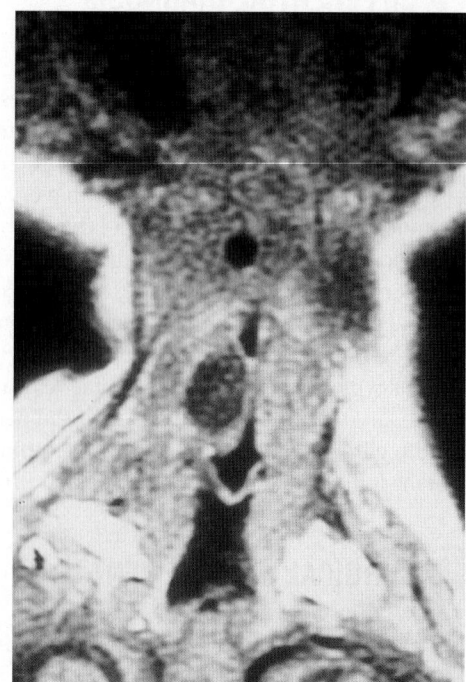

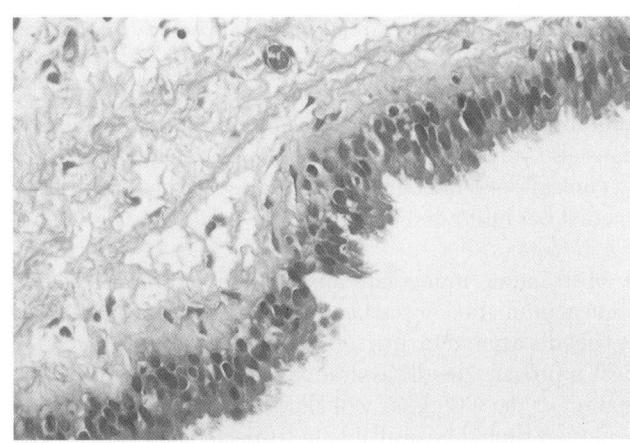

FIGURE 3 Histologic section of the laryngeal cyst demonstrating respiratory epithelium.

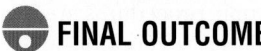 ## FINAL OUTCOME

Eight weeks postoperatively, an interval direct laryngoscopy and bronchoscopy was performed in the operating room revealing a well-healed larynx with a very adequate supraglottic and glottic airway. The final histologic diagnosis was laryngeal cyst lined with respiratory epithelium (Fig. 3).

PROBLEM-FOCUSED DISCUSSION

Saccular cysts are unusual congenital laryngeal anomalies. They are very similar in their embryologic development and presentation to laryngoceles. Both lesions arise from a vestigial laryngeal structure known as the saccule, which was first described by Galen in 300 AD (1). Typically, the saccule communicates with the internal laryngeal lumen through an orifice located in the anterior portion of the ventricle. Saccular cysts have no communication with the internal laryngeal lumen and are filled with thick, viscous fluid. By contrast, laryngoceles do communicate with the lumen and are intermittently filled with air, causing them to dilate and protrude into the laryngeal lumen (internal laryngocele) or the neck (external laryngocele). Both lesions tend to be very unusual. In a review of 200 cases of laryngeal stridor in children, Birch (2) reported 4 cases of laryngeal cyst, and Holinger et al. (3) reported 20 cases of congenital laryngeal cysts and laryngoceles over a 30-year experience with congenital laryngeal anomalies. DeSanto (4) clarified the

FIGURE 4 Laryngeal lymphangioma.

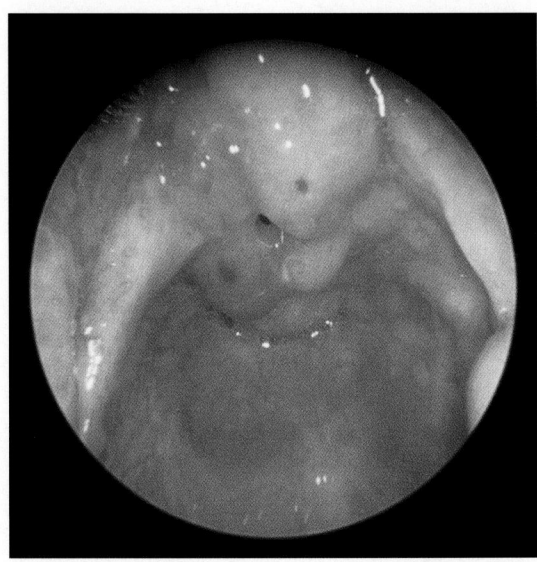

terminology of laryngeal cysts, describing those that extend posterosuperiorly into the region of the false vocal cord and aryepiglottic fold, and an anterior saccular cyst that extends medially and posteriorly, protruding into the laryngeal lumen between the true and false vocal cords. Saccular cysts are submucosal lesions and are covered with normal mucosa.

A laryngeal lymphangioma is also very unusual and has an appearance quite different from that of a saccular cyst, clinically and radiographically. These lesions usually represent a cervical lymphangioma that has infiltrated the larynx. An isolated laryngeal lymphangioma is very unusual (Fig. 4) (5).

In cases of severe airway obstruction, immediate airway intervention will be required, utilizing either endotracheal intubation or tracheotomy. Surgical management of laryngeal saccular cysts includes needle aspiration, marsupialization, or surgical resection through an external transcervical approach. Needle aspiration or marsupialization of the cyst utilizing sharp instrumentation or the CO_2 laser will allow acute decompression of the cyst. Appropriate instrumentation should be available in suspected cases. However, recurrence of the cyst is not unusual, and often multiple endoscopic procedures are required to attain a satisfactory result. Donegan et al. (1) reported on a case requiring eight separate endoscopic needle aspirations and marsupialization procedures to attain decannulation. Holinger et al. (3) reported on ten children with laryngeal saccular cysts who required an average of 7.5 endoscopic procedures for each infant. One patient eventually required external transcervical excision after 11 endoscopic procedures. Ward et al. (6) described four patients who underwent external resection of congenital laryngeal saccular cysts for recurrent problems that did not respond to repeat aspiration and marsupialization. Surgical resection of these lesions appears to be warranted in cases of recurrent saccular cysts and for very large obstructive lesions that would otherwise require long-term endotracheal intubation and possibly tracheotomy for an extended period.

PEARLS AND PERILS

1. The differential diagnosis for infants presenting with dysphonia and airway obstruction should include congenital laryngeal web and laryngeal saccular cyst. If a supraglottic mass is noted endoscopically, then a laryngeal saccular cyst is the most likely diagnosis.
2. Computed tomography or MRI may be beneficial to delineate the laryngeal mass better. This may help differentiate a saccular cyst from a laryngocele or lymphangioma.
3. Surgical options include needle aspiration, CO_2 laser marsupialization, and transcervical surgical excision.
4. Surgical resection is beneficial in recurrent saccular cysts and may be of benefit for large obstructive lesions.

REFERENCES

1. Donegan JO, Strife JL, Seid AB, Cotton RT, Dunbar JS. Internal laryngocele and saccular cysts in children. *Ann Otol Rhinol Layngol* 1980;89:409–413.
2. Birch DA. Laryngeal stridor in infants and children. *J Laryngol Otol* 1961;75:833–840.
3. Holinger LD, Barnes DR, Smid LJ. Laryngocele and saccular cysts. *Ann Otolaryngol* 1978;87:675–685.
4. DeSanto LW. Laryngocele, laryngeal mucocele, large saccules, and laryngeal saccular cysts: a developmental spectrum. *Laryngoscope* 1974;84:1291–1296.
5. Myer CM III, Bratcher GO. Laryngeal cystic hygroma. *Head Neck Surg* 1983;6:706–709.
6. Ward RF, Jones J, Arnold JA. Surgical management of congenital saccular cysts of the larynx. *Ann Otol Rhinol Laryngol* 1995;104:707–710.

B.J. Wiatrak: Department of Surgery, Division of Otolaryngology—Head and Neck Surgery, The University of Alabama at Birmingham, Children's Hospital of Alabama, Birmingham, Alabama 35233–1711.

Allergic Fungal Sinusitis

Brian J. Wiatrak

🌓 INITIAL PRESENTATION

A 14-year-old boy had progressive right-sided nasal obstruction, right frontal headaches, increasing right facial pressure sensation, and intermittent epistaxis, primarily from the right side. His history was significant for previous recurrent sinusitis (not requiring surgery), a history of inhalant allergies (which had required desensitization therapy), and mild reactive airway disease controlled with bronchodilators alone. The symptoms had worsened gradually over the previous 3 months.

🌓 PHYSICAL EXAMINATION

The patient was well nourished and in no acute distress. He was obviously mouth breathing and demonstrated evidence of very mild proptosis of the right eye. The remainder of his ophthalmologic evaluation was normal. His nasal examination revealed a large, fleshy polyp filling a significant amount of the right nasal cavity arising from the region above the inferior turbinate (Fig. 1). It had a very friable appearance. The left nasal cavity revealed no evidence of polyps or masses, although the turbinates were boggy and hypertrophied. There was mild right maxillary and right frontal tenderness. There was no erythema or evidence of acute infection. The remainder of the head and neck examination was unremarkable.

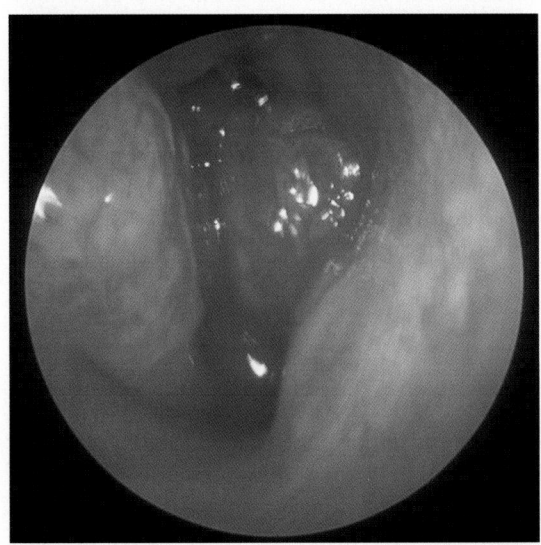

FIGURE 1 Endoscopic view of right nasal polyp.

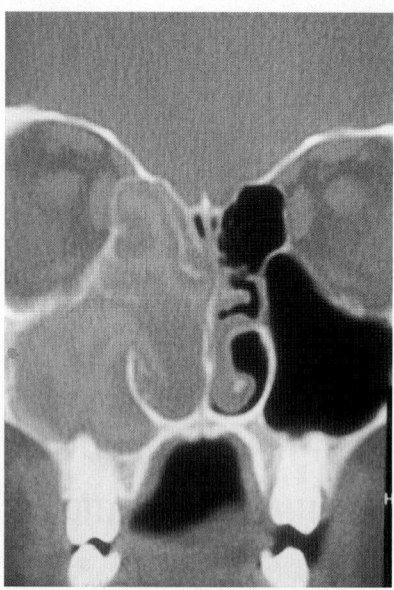

FIGURE 2 Computed tomography scan with contrast demonstrating a rim-enhancing lesion suggestive of right-sided sigmoid sinus thrombosis.

Diagnostic Texts

A computed tomographic (CT) scan of the paranasal sinuses with contrast (Fig. 2) revealed right-sided pansinus opacification involving the ethmoid and maxillary sinuses; a distinct heterogeneous appearance was noted with evidence of bone destruction in the medial wall of the maxillary sinus. No obvious orbital or intracranial invasion was noted. The axial portion of the scan did not reveal any involvement of the nasopharynx. Since this was a child with a nasal polyp, a sweat chloride test was performed. There was a history of reactive airway disease, and the CT scan confirmed expansile sinusitis. The sweat chloride test was within normal limits.

DIFFERENTIAL DIAGNOSIS

A juvenile nasopharyngeal angiofibroma should be considered a possibility in any case of a progressively enlarging nasal mass with nasal obstruction and epistasis in an adolescent boy. This particular lesion did not enhance with contrast on the CT scan, and there was no evidence of nasopharyngeal involvement. Therefore, this diagnosis was less likely. Expansile sinusitis in a child associated with nasal polyposis may also be a manifestation of cystic fibrosis. Although it is unusual, cystic fibrosis may present later in life and may initially present to the otolaryngologist as sinusitis (1). The fact that the patient was obviously well nourished, had no significant nutritional problems, and had strictly unilateral paranasal sinus disease with a normal sweat chloride test made cystic fibrosis highly unlikely. Allergic fungal sinusitis frequently presents with unilateral expansile sinusitis with a typical heterogeneous appearance on CT scan in older children and young adults. This patient had a significant atopic history with reactive airway disease, making allergic fungal sinusitis very probable at this point.

INITIAL MANAGEMENT

Surgical intervention was considered at this time. In patients with suspected allergic fungal sinusitis or other conditions causing extensive polypoid disease, it is often beneficial to administer a course of oral corticosteroids to decrease the vascularity and size of the nasal polyps before surgery is performed. Allergic fungal disease responds significantly to corticosteroid therapy. The patient was started on prednisone (60 mg per day) and 4 weeks later underwent surgery for extirpation of disease. Due to the extensive nature of this patient's paranasal sinus disease, the lesion was approached endoscopically and through a Caldwell-Luc procedure. An extensive amount of the intranasal polyp was removed and sent for culture and histology. The remainder of the polypoid tissue was removed utilizing powered instrumentation. Upon opening the maxillary sinus through an anterior maxillary antrostomy, viscous greenish brown fluid was encountered. Diseased tissue was completely removed from the maxillary sinus. The histologic specimens stained with hematoxylin and eosin from the initial surgical procedure revealed amorphous layers of mucus mixed with eosinophils, which, under high magnification, demonstrated Charcot-Leyden crystals. KOH stain revealed extramusocal hyphae, which appeared scarce and fragmented.

Postoperative Management

Based on the surgical, CT, and histologic findings, as well as the patient's history, a diagnosis of allergic fungal sinusitis was made. The patient was maintained on oral prednisone, eventually tapering off completely over a period of 2 months. Since there was no evidence at this time to support systemic antifungal agents, none were utilized. Frequent nasal endoscopic examinations will be required since the recurrence rate for allergic fungal sinusitis is extremely high. In the case of recurrent disease, a repeat CT scan would be required, as well as corticosteroid therapy. If the recurrence does not resolve with these measures, then revision surgery would be required, and longer term therapy with corticosteroids should be considered.

FINAL OUTCOME

The fungal culture, 8 weeks postoperatively, eventually grew *Curvularia* species. One year postoperatively, a nasal polyp recurred on the right side, arising within the middle meatus. A CT scan revealed recurrent disease, primarily in the ethmoid sinuses. The patient was started on oral corticosteroid therapy and subsequently underwent revision endoscopic sinus surgery with elimination of the disease.

PROBLEM-FOCUSED DISCUSSION

Fungal sinusitis is currently divided into four categories: 1, acute (invasive); 2, chronic-indolent (invasive); 3, mycetoma (fungus ball); and 4, allergic fungal sinusitis (2). Fungal sinus disease was first described in 1791 (3). Allergic fungal sinusitis was first described by Katzenstein et al. (4) in 1983, and pediatric allergic fungal sinusitis was first described by Manning et al. in 1989 (5). Invasive fungal sinusitis typically involves immunosuppressed individuals, most commonly those with diabetic ketoacidosis; however, it may be associated with immunosuppressed patients after bone marrow or organ transplantation. The fungus is usually *Rhizopus* species, typically *Mucor*. Radical surgical resection is often required in adults. Less radical surgical debridement utilizing nasal endoscopes has been shown to be beneficial in children (6). Chronic invasive sinusitis usually involves immunocompetent patients, with disease eventually extending beyond the confines of the sinus cavity, requiring extensive surgical debridement and intravenous antifungal therapy. Mycetomas, or fungus balls, typically are limited to the maxillary sinus and involve *Aspergillus* species. Patients with allergic fungal sinusitis typically have unilateral sinus disease, expansile sinusitis demonstrated on CT scan, and a significant history of atopy. Pediatric patients may have significant facial abnormalities resulting from long-standing, progressive expansile sinusitis (5). Bent and Kuhn (2) described five diagnostic criteria for allergic fungal sinusitis, including (a) hypersensitivity, (b) nasal polyposis, (c) characteristic CT findings, (d) eosinophilic mucus with no fungal invasion into sinus tissue and (e) positive fungus stain of sinus contents. Although *Aspergillus* was initially described as the etiologic agent, other fungal species have been identified, i.e., *Curvularia* species, *Bipolaris, Alternaria,* and *Exserohilum.*

Radiologically, the CT scan typically demonstrates unilateral disease with a significant expansile component often associated with demineralization or overt bone destruction with a classic heterogenous appearance. This may be caused by ferromagnetic elements produced by the fungi. Magnetic resonance imaging may also be of benefit in cases of allergic fungal sinusitis, demonstrating hypointense regions in the paranasal sinus cavity surrounded by regions of inflammation that are hyperintense. This is in contrast to neoplasms, which are moderately hyperintense throughout and typically do not have this classic heterogenous appearance (2).

Management involves surgical and medical therapy. Most authors agree that high-dose oral corticosteroids are of benefit pre- and postoperatively (2,5,7–9). Although utilization of systemic antifungal agents is controversial, most authors feel that for allergic sinusitis, systemic antifungal therapy is not of benefit. Long-term nasal steroid sprays and possibly nebulized cortocosteroids may be of benefit.

Surgical therapy requires an endoscopic approach. Powered instrumentation allows relatively bloodless dissection. However, the endoscopic approach may not be adequate to extirpate disease completely from the maxillary sinus, and a Caldwell-Luc procedure may also be required in patients over 10 years of age.

Fungal cultures obtained at surgery may not show fungal growth until approximately 6 to 8 weeks postoperatively. However, frequently there is no growth of the culture. Histologic findings have been described previously and are fairly classic for allergic fungal sinusitis. Typically, there are scant fungal hyphae noted with KOH stain and no obvious tissue invasion.

Despite aggressive medical and surgical therapy, recurrence rates are high, ranging from 32% to 100% (10,11). Frequent follow-up utilizing nasal endoscopy and CT scans will be necessary for long-term follow-up of these patients.

PEARLS AND PERILS

1. Children with nasal polyposis and expansile sinusitis on CT scan should have a sweat chloride test to rule out cystic fibrosis.
2. Allergic fungal sinusitis demonstrates a classic heterogenous appearance of expansile sinusitis on computed tomographic scan. Magnetic resonance imaging may also be beneficial.
3. Although endoscopic sinus surgery should be utilized first, a Caldwell-Luc procedure may be necessary in particularly extensive and aggressive cases.
4. High-dose corticosteroids for long periods may be helpful and may decrease recurrence rates. In children, long-term steroid use should be used cautiously due to the metabolic effects.
5. There is no demonstrated benefit at this time for the use of systemic antifungal agents.
6. Tissue at surgery should be stained for fungal hyphae and cultured for fungus in addition to routine histologic staining.
7. Recurrence rates are very high, and close long-term follow-up is necessary in these patients.

REFERENCES

1. Wiatrak BJ, Myer CM III, Cotton RT. Cystic fibrosis presenting with sinus disease in children. *Am J Dis Child* 1993;147:258–260.
2. Bent JP, Kuhn FA. Diagnosis of allergic fungal sinusitis. *Otolaryngol Head Neck Surg* 1994;111:580–588.

3. Waxmann JE, Spector JG, Sale SR, Katzenstein ALA. Allergic Aspergillus sinusitis: concepts in diagnosis and treatment of a clinical entity. *Laryngoscope* 1987;97:261–266.

4. Katzenstein ALA, Sale SR, Greenberger PA. Allergic Aspergillus sinusitis: a newly recognized form of sinusitis. *J Allergy Clin Immunol* 1983;72:89–93.

5. Manning SC, Vuitch F, Weinberg AG, Brown OE. Allergic aspergillosis: a newly recognized form of sinusitis in the pediatric patient. *Laryngoscope* 1989;99:681–685.

6. Wiatrak BJ, Willging JP, Myer CM III, Cotton RT. Functional endoscopic sinus surgery in the immunocompromised child. *Otolaryngol Head Neck Surg* 1991;105:818–825.

7. Corey JP. Allergic fungal sinusitis. *Otolaryngol Clin North Am* 1992;25:225–230.

8. Cody DTI, Neel HB, Ferreiro JA, Roberts GD. Allergic fungal sinusitis: the Mayo Clinic experience. *Laryngoscope* 1994;104:1074–178.

9. Roth M. Should oral steroids be the primary treatment for allergic fungal sinusitis? *Ear Nose Throat J* 1994;73:928–930.

10. Sher TH, Schwartz HJ. Allergic Aspergillus sinusitis with concurrent allergic bronchopulmonary aspergillus: a report of a case. *J Allergy Clin Immunol* 1988;81:844–846.

11. Schweitz LA, Gourly DS. Allergic fungal sinusitis. *Allergy Proc* 1992;13:3–6.

B.J. Wiatrak: Department of Surgery, Division of Otolaryngology—Head and Neck Surgery, The University of Alabama at Birmingham, Children's Hospital of Alabama, Birmingham, Alabama 35233–1711.

Orbital Subperiostal Abscess

Brian J. Wiatrak

INITIAL PRESENTATION

An 8-year-old boy presented to the emergency room with right periorbital edema and right eye pain that had progressed rapidly over the previous 24 hours. This was preceded for 1 week by a presumed viral upper respiratory tract infection. Over the previous 24 hours, the patient had spiked temperatures up to 102.5°F. He also complained of mild right frontal headaches and right facial pain. He had no significant history for prior sinus disease and no recent history of facial or periorbital trauma.

PHYSICAL EXAMINATION

His physical examination was significant for right periorbital edema. There was no evidence of visual acuity problems or proptosis. The eye was tender to palpation but not tense. He had a normal light reflex and no evidence of chemosis. There was limited right lateral gaze in the right eye. His nasal examination revealed boggy, inflamed nasal mucosa bilaterally and purulent drainage in the right nasal cavity. There was shotty lymphadenopathy, primarily on the right side, and evidence of right-sided ethmoid and maxillary tenderness.

Initial Diagnostic Tests

A computed tomography (CT) scan was not performed at this time, since the patient's clinical examination was consistent with preseptal cellulitis secondary to sinusitis and not consistent with orbital subperiosteal abscess (SPA). A complete blood count was obtained, which revealed a white blood cell count of 19,000 cells/mm^3, with a significant shift to the left.

DIFFERENTIAL DIAGNOSIS

Based on clinical presentation, the patient most likely had preseptal cellulitis secondary to right-sided pansinusitis. The presence of chemosis, visual acuity changes, and proptosis would suggest a postseptal process such as orbital SPA. Neoplastic causes of mass lesions in the orbit were unlikely due to the obvious presence of acute sinusitis and the presence of a high white blood cell count and fever, implying active infection.

INITIAL MANAGEMENT

The patient was begun on aggressive medical therapy consisting of an intravenous antibiotic (Cefuroxime) and nasal decongestants (oxymetazoline and phenyl-

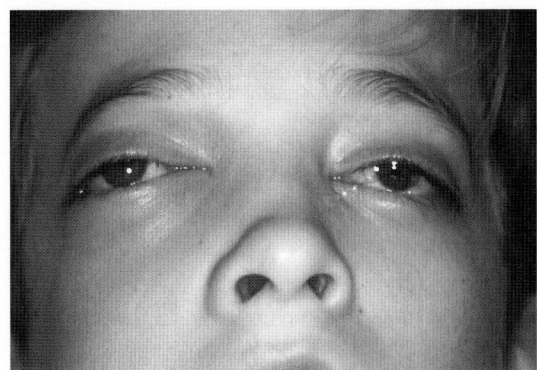

FIGURE 1 Patient with right-sided periorbital cellulitis.

propanolamine). The ophthalmology service was consulted and agreed with the assessment of normal vision and no proptosis at that time.

The following day, the patient's condition deteriorated. Moderate proptosis developed, along with mild chemosis, increased orbital tenderness, and decreased ocular motility on lateral and downward gaze. Fever persisted, up to 102.5°F, and the white blood cell count rose to 22,000 cells/mm³ with a shift to the left.

Interval Test

At this point, a thin-section axial and coronal CT scan with contrast was obtained of the paranasal sinuses (Fig. 1). This was highly suggestive of a right medial orbital SPA.

🗫 SURGICAL MANAGEMENT

The patient was taken to the operating room for surgical drainage of a presumptive right SPA and pansinusitis. This can be performed via an open external ethmoidectomy approach with an intranasal antral puncture or an antrostomy. Alternatively, an endoscopic approach to the ethmoid/maxillary sinuses can be employed, as was done in this case. The nasal cavity on the right side was decongested with oxymetazoline. Utilizing endoscopic sinus instrumentation, the uncinate process was removed and the maxillary sinus ostium identified and opened to allow drainage of purulent material. The ethmoid bulla was identified and the anterior and (subsequently) posterior ethmoid cells opened. A minimal amount of purulence was encountered along with edematous, inflamed mucosa. The lamina papyracea was carefully identified and palpated using a J-curette. The eggshell bone was opened carefully into the region of the suspected orbital SPA. Purulence was immediately encountered, which was sent for culture and sensitivity. The lamina papyracea was only opened as far as purulent material was encountered.

🖝 FINAL OUTCOME

Postoperatively, the patient becames afebrile within 24 hours, and the white blood cell count returned to normal within 48 hours. By postoperative day 3, the proptosis and periorbital edema had resolved completely. The final culture results for the SPA revealed *Streptococcus pneumoniae.* The patient was discharged on the fourth postoperative day on oral amoxicillin with clavulanic acid. The patient returned for a follow-up visit in 3 weeks with no orbital or sinus symptomatology. A well-healed sinus cavity was visualized on nasal endoscopy.

& PROBLEM-FOCUSED DISCUSSION

Periorbital cellulitis is a very common problem in the pediatric population; orbital SPA is uncommon. Page and Wiatrak (1) reported on 158 patients admitted with the diagnosis of periorbital cellulitis. Nineteen of these patients were diagnosed with postseptal orbital inflammation by CT scan, of whom 14 underwent surgical drainage for suspected orbital SPA. The most common etiology of acute orbital SPA in children is paranasal sinus disease (2,3). However, many other potential causes do exist. Due to the close anatomic proximity of the orbits and paranasal sinuses, primarily the ethmoid sinus, inflammatory processes in the sinus may spread quickly to involve the orbital contents. The orbital septum is the primary barrier for spread of infection from the preseptal to the postseptal region. However, bony dehiscences of the lamina papyracea or the valveless venous drainage system of the face and orbit may provide quick routes of spread for sinus disease to involve the orbit. Chandler et al. (2) divided orbital complications of sinusitis into five groups: group 1, periorbital or preseptal cellulitis; group 2, orbital cellulitis; group 3, orbital subperiosteal abscess; group 4, orbital abscess; and group 5, cavernous sinus thrombosis, although this is actually an intracranial process. Orbital SPA typically presents with proptosis, chemosis, and decreased extraocular motility. When orbital abscess exists, complete ophthalmoplegia usually results, along with marked proptosis and significant visual loss. A CT scan of the paranasal sinuses is the diagnostic modality of choice in cases of suspected orbital SPA. A rim-enhancing mass in the medial orbital region immediately adjacent to the ethmoids and medial rectus muscle may be apparent, possibly displacing the medial rectus muscle (Fig. 2). It should be stressed that orbital SPA cannot be diagnosed with CT scan alone, and the entire clinical picture must be taken into account (4).

It is important to differentiate between preseptal and postseptal inflammatory processes since this will affect the management of these patients. Patients with normal visual acuity, no chemosis, and no proptosis may have a process limited to the preseptal region, although significant periorbital edema exists. In this situation, it is appropriate to pursue aggressive medical therapy before obtaining a CT scan. If the patient's clinical appearance deteriorates or if there is no improvement in 48 hours, a CT scan is warranted. If the clinical examination is not consistent with an orbital SPA and a CT scan has been obtained revealing sinusitis and a possible medial orbital subperiosteal abscess, aggressive medical therapy is warranted. If the patient's examination deteriorates or if there is no improvement in 48 hours, surgical intervention is warranted. Permanent loss of visual

FIGURE 2 Computed tomographic scan with contrast demonstrating a rim-enhancing lesion in the medial orbit associated with right pansinus opacification.

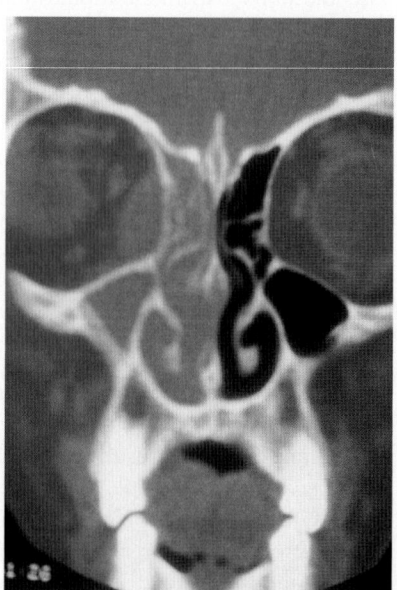

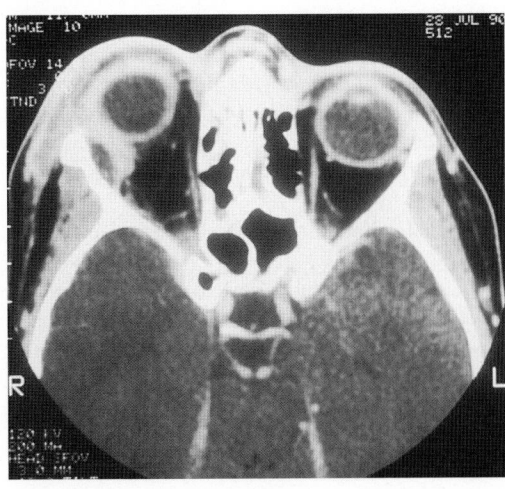

FIGURE 3 Computed tomographic scan with contrast demonstrating rim-enhancing lesion in right lateral–superior orbit.

acuity may result from orbital SPA (5). Surgical management may be performed through an external ethmoidectomy approach, exposing and carefully opening the lamina papyracea, elevating the periorbita, and opening the ethmoids to provide continued drainage. An intranasal maxillary antrostomy is recommended to drain the maxillary sinus if this is noted to be involved on CT scan. More recently, endoscopic sinus surgery has been advocated for the surgical management of orbital SPA in children (1,6,7). Page and Wiatrak (1) demonstrated that postsurgical hospitalization is significantly reduced when an endoscopic surgical approach is utilized. It also saves the patient an external ethmoidectomy incision. However, when there is significant mucosal edema, inflammation, and intraoperative bleeding, an external ethmoidectomy approach may be necessary.

Although orbital SPA is limited to the medial orbital region, it is possible to have a simultaneous abscess in the superior lateral aspect of the orbit (Fig. 3). In this situation, a separate incision in the lateral brow region may be necessary to drain the second abscess. This possibility should always be considered in cases of orbital SPA; it is more commonly found in patients with simultaneous frontal sinus disease (8).

PEARLS AND PERILS

1. Sinus disease is the most common etiology of periorbital inflammatory disease in children.
2. It is important to determine the presence of a preseptal or postseptal inflammatory process to guide management. A CT scan is the diagnostic modality of choice for evaluation of suspected orbital SPA.
3. An ophthalmology consultation should be obtained in all patients with suspected orbital SPA.
4. In cases of suspected preseptal cellulitis with no associated proptosis, visual acuity changes, or chemosis, aggressive medical therapy is warranted before obtaining a computed tomographic scan.
5. Endoscopic drainage of orbital SPA may decrease postsurgical hospital stay. However, an external ethmoidectomy approach may be warranted when endoscopic visualization is poor, or the operator does not feel comfortable with such an approach.

REFERENCES

1. Page E, Wiatrak BJ. Endoscopic vs. external drainage of orbital subperiosteal abscess. *Arch Otolaryngol* 1996;122:737–740.

2. Chandler JR, Langenbrunner DJ, Stevens ER. The pathogenesis of orbital complications in acute sinusitis. *Laryngoscope* 1907;80:1414–1428.
3. Moloney JR, Badham NJ, McRae A. The acute orbit. *J Laryngol Otol* 1987;12:1–18.
4. Andrews TM, Myer CM III. The role of computed tomography in the diagnosis of subperiosteal abscess of the orbit. *Clin Pediatr* 192;31:37–43.
5. Schramm VLJ, Curtin HD, Kennerdell JS. Evaluation of orbital cellulitis and results of treatment. *Laryngoscope* 1982;92:732–738.
6. Manning SC. Endoscopic management of medial subperiosteal orbital abscess. *Arch Otolaryngol* 1993;119:789–791.
7. Arjmand EM, Lusk RP, Muntz HR. Pediatric sinusitis and subperiosteal orbital abscess formation: diagnosis and treatment. *Otolaryngol Head Neck Surg* 1993;109:886–894.
8. Garcia CE, Cunningham MJ, Clary RA, Joseph MP. The etiologic role of frontal sinusitis in pediatric orbital abscesses. *Am J Otolaryngol* 1993;14:449–452.

B.J. Wiatrak: Department of Surgery, Division of Otolaryngology—Head and Neck Surgery, The University of Alabama at Birmingham, Children's Hospital of Alabama, Birmingham, Alabama 35233–1711.

Penetrating Injury of the Carotid Artery

Kenneth M. Grundfast

INITIAL PRESENTATION

A 14-year-old girl presented with severe sore throat, ipsilateral sore neck, and fever to 102° F. The sore throat had developed over the preceding 2 days and had begun to localize to the right side on the day the patient presented to the emergency room of a local hospital.

PHYSICAL EXAMINATION

The patient was uncomfortable because of sore throat and fever but otherwise appeared healthy. She had difficulty opening her mouth. When the tongue was gently depressed, the pharynx could be partially visualized. There was erythema and fullness on the right side of the soft palate, and the right tonsil appeared medially displaced. There were enlarged and tender upper cervical nodes on the right side of the neck.

DIFFERENTIAL DIAGNOSIS

Findings are consistent with a diagnosis of peritonsillar abscess, but the possibility of peritonsillar cellulitis also needs to be considered. Customarily, in this situation, needle aspiration of the area of fullness is undertaken both for the purpose of differentiating cellulitis from abscess and also to drain the abscess if one is encountered (1–5).

INITIAL MANAGEMENT

An otolaryngologist at the local hospital inserted an 18-gauge needle into the area of fullness superior and lateral to the right tonsil. When attempting to aspirate pus by pulling back the plunger on the 10-ml syringe to which the needle was attached, no pus could be aspirated into the barrel of the syringe, and no blood entered the barrel.

FINAL OUTCOME

Eight hours after the attempt to aspirate pus from the area of peritonsillar fullness, the patient became restless; on further examination, a left hemiparesis was noted. A com-

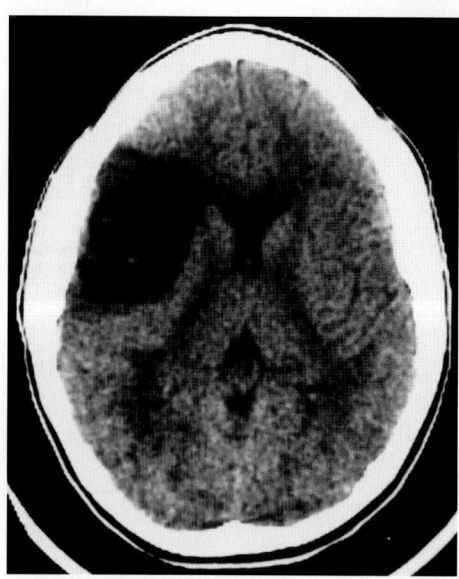

FIGURE 1 Computed tomography scan of the cerebral hemispheres demonstrates massive infarct of the right frontoparietal region in distribution of the middle cerebral artery.

puted tomography (CT) scan of the head revealed a nonenhancing radiolucency in the distribution of the right middle cerebral artery with mild surrounding edema and slight compression of the right cerebral ventricle (Fig. 1).

The patient was transferred to the Children's National Medical Center in Washington, DC. Doppler flow studies of the right carotid artery revealed diminished flow. A carotid artery angiogram revealed a pseudoaneurysm of the right internal carotid artery at the level of the C-1 to C-2 interspace with narrowing of the lumen superior to the aneurysm (Fig. 2 and 3). There was markedly diminished flow in the distribution of the right middle cerebral artery. The patient was placed on bed rest, and aspirin was administered.

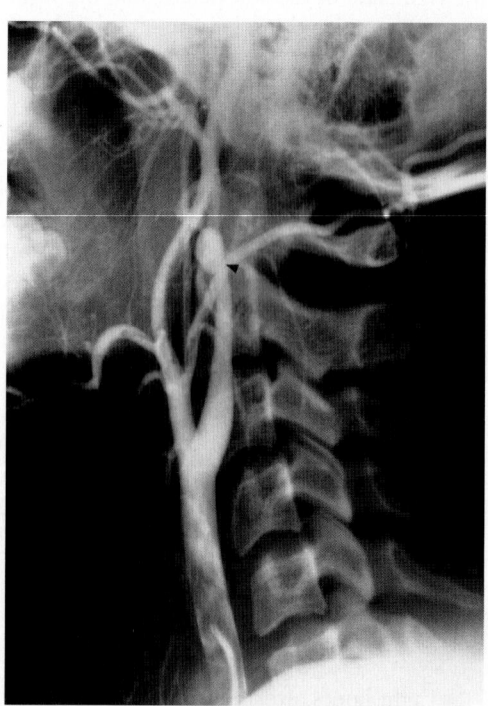

FIGURE 2 Arteriogram of right carotid artery shows pseudoaneurysm of internal carotid artery with distal narrow arterial lumen.

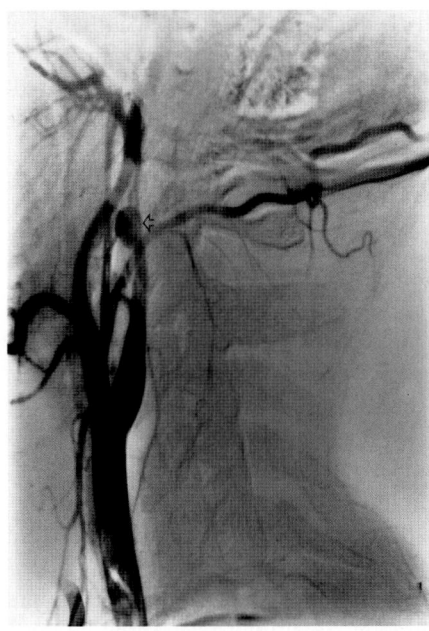

FIGURE 3 Subtraction arteriogram. Arrow points to pseudoaneurysm.

On the third day after admission to the Children's Hospital, the patient developed right-sided myoclonic seizure activity; a repeat CT scan demonstrated extension of the infarcted area. The patient was treated with Dilantin, and the seizure activity diminished.

On the eleventh hospital day, the patient suddenly became comatose; an emergency CT scan demonstrated a large intracerebral hemorrhage with evidence of herniation (Fig. 4). Subsequently, the patient's condition continued to deteriorate until she died on the thirteenth day after admission.

Postmortem Examination

Postmortem examination revealed a large area of liquefactive necrosis in the right frontoparietal area of the brain. In addition, there was evidence of meningitis, inflammation

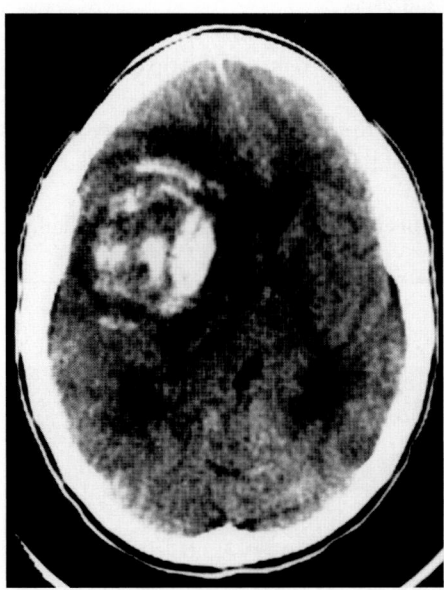

FIGURE 4 Computed tomography scan showing progression of infarct compared with infarct seen in Figure 1. Now there is compression of the lateral ventricle and evidence of intracerebral hemorrhage.

of the mucous membranes of the sphenoid and ethmoid sinuses, and pus in the right parapharyngeal space although no abscess cavity could be identified. There was a false aneurysm of the right internal carotid artery without evidence of a needle track in or adjacent to the vessel.

& PROBLEM-FOCUSED DISCUSSION

Although needle aspiration in children is reportedly safe and efficacious (6), complications can occur. Presumably, the etiology of the false aneurysm was the attempted needle aspiration done 8 hours prior to the onset of neurologic symptoms. The fact that no pus or blood was aspirated suggests that the tip of the needle may have punctured the arterial wall without entering the lumen. Indirect injury to the internal carotid artery with serious neurologic sequelae has previously been reported. Furthermore, it seems apparent that the pseudoaneurysm did not develop as a result of direct extension of cellulitis or abscess, because no pus was recovered at the time of the initial attempted needle aspiration, and the findings at the time of initial presentation were more consistent with cellulitis than with abscess. Since needle aspiration of a fluctuant appearing peritonsillar mass can result in complications, needle aspiration must be done cautiously and properly (7–9). Indeed, in children, needle aspiration should not necessarily be done early for diagnosis or management. Children under the age of 8 years are usually frightened by the sight of a syringe and needle being inserted into the mouth. Even teenagers have difficulty cooperating for an office needle aspiration of a peritonsillar abscess. Although in adults needle aspiration helps to differentiate peritonsillar abscess from cellulitis, in children, simply treating with parenteral antibiotics for 24 to 48 hours usually helps to differentiate abscess from cellulitis. Children with peritonsillar cellulitis usually show rapid signs of improvement when treated with parenteral antibiotics. The area of redness diminishes rapidly, and the area of fullness becomes smaller if the child has cellulitis, whereas the area of fullness remains erythematous and full if the child has an abscess. If the child continues to show signs of peritonsillar abscess, then a quinsy tonsillectomy, also known as tonsillectomy aux chad, can be done (10).

PEARLS AND PERILS

1. Use caution in aspirating the peritonsillar area.
2. When attempting to aspirate pus from the peritonsillar area, wrap adhesive tape around the needle used for aspiration leaving only 6 mm of the tip exposed (Fig. 5).
3. When aspirating, do *not* insert the needle tip lateral to an imaginary line extending superiorly from the medial edge of the anterior faucal tonsil pillar (Fig. 6).
4. Consider quinsy tonsillectomy; that is, tonsillectomy at the time peritonsillar abscess has been diagnosed.

FIGURE 5 Wrapping adhesive tape around an 18-gauge syringe needle leaving only 6 mm of the tip exposed helps to prevent penetration of the needle deep into the pharyngeal musculature.

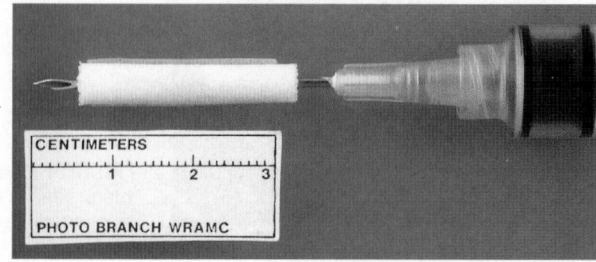

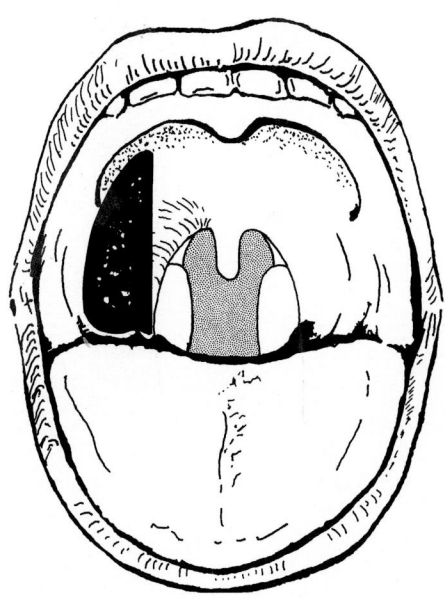

FIGURE 6 When aspirating a presumed peritonsillar abscess, the needle should not be inserted lateral to an imaginary line extending superiorly from the plane of the medial edge of the anterior faucal tonsil pillar.

REFERENCES

1. Bonding P. Routine abscess tonsillectomy: late results. *Laryngoscope* 1976;86:286–290.
2. Nielsen VM, Greisen O. Peritonsillar abscess II. Cases treated with tonsillectomy a chaud. *J Laryngol Otol* 1981;95:801–807.
3. Richardson KA, Birck H. Peritonsillar abscess in the pediatric population. *Otolaryngol Head Neck Surg* 1981;89:907–909.
4. Yung AK, Cantrell RW. Quinsy tonsillectomy. *Laryngoscope* 1976;86:1714–1717.
5. Spires JR, Owens JJ, Woodson GE, Miller RH. Treatment of peritonsillar abscess. A prospective study of aspiration vs incision drainage. *Arch Otolaryngol Head Neck Surg* 1987;113:984–986.
6. Weinberg E, Brodsky L, Stanievich J, Volk M. Needle aspiration of peritonsillar abscess in children. *Arch Otolaryngol Head Neck Surg* 1993;119:169–72.
7. Salinger S, Pearlman SJ. *Arch Otolaryngol* 1933;18:464–509.
8. Blum DJ, McCaffrey TV. Septic necrosis of the internal carotid artery: a compilation of peritonsillar abscess. *Otolaryngol Head Neck Surg* 1983;91:114–118.
9. Shanon E, Cohn D, Streifler M, Rapoport Y. Penetrating injuries of the parapharyngeal space. *Arch Otolaryngol* 1972;96:256–259.
10. Lockhart A, et al. *Ann Otol Rhinol Laryngol* 1991;100:569–571.

K.M. Grundfast: Department of Otolaryngology—Head and Neck Surgery, Georgetown University Medical Center, Children's National Medical Center, Washington, DC 20007.

• *Practical Pediatric Otolaryngology*
• edited by Robin T. Cotton and Charles M. Myer, III
• Lippincott-Raven Publishers, Philadelphia © 1999

Subject Index

Page numbers in *italic* indicate figures and tables.